Volume 1

BRAIN SURGERY

COMPLICATION AVOIDANCE AND MANAGEMENT

Volume 1

BRAIN SURGERY

COMPLICATION AVOIDANCE AND MANAGEMENT

Edited by

Michael L.J. Apuzzo, M.D.

Edwin M. Todd/Trent H. Wells Jr. Professor
Department of Neurological Surgery
University of Southern California School of Medicine
Los Angeles, California

With illustrations by Diane Abeloff, M.A., A.M.I.

Churchill Livingstone
New York, Edinburgh, London, Melbourne, Tokyo

Library of Congress Cataloging-in-Publication Data
Brain surgery : complication avoidance and management / edited by
   Michael L.J. Apuzzo ; with illustrations by Diane Abeloff.
         p.   cm.
      Includes bibliographical references and index.
      ISBN 0-443-08709-1
      1. Brain—Surgery—Complications.   I. Apuzzo, Michael L. J.
      [DNLM: 1. Brain Diseases—surgery. 2. Intraoperative
Complications—prevention & control.   3. Intraoperative
Complications—therapy. 4. Postoperative Complications—prevention
& control. 5. Postoperative Complications—therapy.   WL 368 B814]
   RD594.B76 1993
   617.4'8101—dc20
   DNLM/DLC   92-49409
   for Library of Congress   CIP

Distributed in the United Kingdom by Churchill Livingstone, Robert Stevenson House,
1-3 Baxter's Place, Leith Walk, Edinburgh EH1 3AF, and by associated companies,
branches, and representatives throughout the world.

Accurate indications, adverse reactions, and dosage schedules for drugs are provided in
this book , but it is possible that they may change. The reader is urged to review the
package information data of the manufacturers of the medications mentioned.

The Publishers have made every effort to trace the copyright holders for borrowed
material. If they have inadvertently overlooked any, they will be pleased to make the
necessary arrangements at the first opportunity.

Acquisitions Editor: *Toni M. Tracy*
Assistant Editor: *Ann Ruzycka*
Copy Editor: *Donna C.Balopole*
Production Designer: *Patricia McFadden*
Production Supervisor: *Sharon Tuder*
Indexer: *Irving Conde Tullar*
Cover design: *Jeannette Jacobs*

Printed in the United States of America

First published in 1993   7 6 5 4 3 2 1

To my parents,
Dominic John and Ann Lawrence Apuzzo

Contributors

E. Francois Aldrich, M.D., M.Med., FCS.
Associate Professor, Division of Neurosurgery,
University of Texas Medical Branch at Galveston,
Galveston, Texas

Eben Alexander, Jr., M.D.
Professor Emeritus, Department of Neurosurgery,
Bowman Gray School of Medicine of Wake Forest
University, Winston-Salem, North Carolina

Ossama Al-Mefty, M.D.
Professor, Division of Neurological Surgery,
Department of Surgery, Loyola University of Chicago
Stritch School of Medicine, Maywood, Illinois

Lee V. Ansell, M.D.
Assistant Professor, Division of Neurosurgery,
Department of Surgery, University of Texas Health
Science Center, San Antonio, Texas

Jason A. Apuzzo, B.A.
Yale College, New Haven, Connecticut

Michael L.J. Apuzzo, M.D.
Edwin M. Todd/Trent H. Wells Jr. Professor,
Department of Neurological Surgery, University of
Southern California School of Medicine,
Los Angeles, California

James I. Ausman, M.D., Ph.D.
Professor and Head, Department of Neurosurgery,
University of Illinois College of Medicine at Chicago,
Chicago, Illinois

Stanley L. Barnwell, M.D., Ph.D.
Associate Professor, Division of Neurosurgery,
Department of Surgery and the Charles Dotter Institute
of Interventional Therapy, Oregon Health Sciences
University School of Medicine, Portland, Oregon

Daniel L. Barrow, M.D.
Associate Professor, Department of Neurosurgery,
Emory University School of Medicine, Atlanta, Georgia

H. Hunt Batjer, M.D.
Associate Professor, Department of Neurological
Surgery, University of Texas Southwestern Medical
Center, Dallas, Texas

Ulrich Batzdorf, M.D.
Professor, Division of Neurosurgery, Department
of Surgery, University of California, Los Angeles,
UCLA School of Medicine; UCLA Medical
Center and Wadsworth Veterans Administration
Hospital, Los Angeles, California

Abdolmajid Bayat, M.D.
Assistant Professor of Clinical Anesthesiology,
University of Southern California School of Medicine,
Los Angeles, California

Robert J. Bernardi, M.D.
Division of Neurosurgery, Department of Surgery,
Saint Louis University School of Medicine,
Saint Louis, Missouri

Peter McL. Black, M.D., Ph.D.
Franc D. Ingraham Professor of Neurosurgery,
Department of Surgery, Harvard Medical School;
Neurosurgeon-in-Chief, Brigham and Women's
Hospital and Children's Hospital, Boston,
Massachusetts

Susan Black, M.D.
Assistant Professor, Department of Anesthesia and
Critical Care, University of Chicago Division of the
Biological Sciences Pritzker School of Medicine,
Chicago Illinois

Linda I. Bland, M.D.
Instructor of Surgery, Division of Neurological
Surgery, University of Rochester Medical Center;
Department of Neurological Surgery, University of
Rochester School of Medicine and Dentistry,
Rochester, New York

Derald E. Brackmann, M.D.
Clinical Professor, Department of Otolaryngology,
University of Southern California School of Medicine,
Los Angeles, California

Robert E. Breeze, M.D.
Assistant Professor, Department of Surgery
(Neurosurgery), University of Colorado Health
Sciences Center; Head, Section of Cerebrovascular
Surgery, and Section Chief (Neurosurgery),
Veterans Affairs Medical Center, Denver,
Colorado

Douglas Brockmeyer, M.D.
Department of Neurosurgery, University of Utah School
of Medicine, Salt Lake City, Utah

Willis E. Brown, Jr., M.D.
Professor, Division of Neurosurgery, Department of
Surgery, University of Texas Health Science Center,
San Antonio, Texas

Jeffrey N. Bruce, M.D.
Assistant Professor, Departments of Neurosurgery
and Pathology, Columbia University College of
Physicians and Surgeons; Assistant Attending
Neurosurgeon, Department of Neurological Surgery,
Presbyterian Hospital in the City of New York,
New York, New York

James Brunberg, M.D.
Associate Professor, Department of Radiology,
and Director, Division of Neuroradiology,
University of Michigan Medical School, Ann Arbor,
Michigan

William A. Buchheit, M.D.
Professor and Chairman, Department of Neurosurgery,
Temple University School of Medicine, Philadelphia,
Pennsylvania

Peter W. Carmel, M.D.
Professor of Clinical Neurosurgery, The Neurological
Institute, Columbia University College of Physicians
and Surgeons; Director, Division of Pediatric
Neurosurgery, Columbia-Presbyterian Medical Center,
New York, New York

Howard N. Chandler, M.D.
Department of Neurosurgery, University of Florida
College of Medicine, Gainesville, Florida

Parakrama T. Chandrasoma, M.D.
Associate Professor, Department of Pathology,
University of Southern California School of Medicine;
Chief, Department of Anatomic Pathology,
Los Angeles County–University of Southern California
Medical Center, Los Angeles, California

Thomas C. Chen, M.D.
Clinical Instructor, Department of Neurological
Surgery, University of Southern California School of
Medicine, Los Angeles, California

Lawrence S. Chin, M.D.
Clinical Instructor, Department of Neurological
Surgery, University of Southern California School of
Medicine, Los Angeles, California

Shelley N. Chou, M.D., Ph.D.
Professor, Department of Neurosurgery, University of
Minnesota Medical School—Minneapolis, Minneapolis,
Minnesota

Ivan S. Ciric, M.D.
Clinical Professor, Division of Neurosurgery,
Northwestern University Medical School, Chicago,
Illinois; Bennett-Tarkington Chair and Head, Division
of Neurosurgery, Evanston Hospital, Evanston, Illinois

H. Bushnell Clarke, M.D.
Section of Neurosurgery, Department of Surgery,
University of Michigan Medical School, Ann Arbor,
Michigan

William F. Collins, M.D.
Professor and Chairman, Department of Surgery, and
Harvey and Kate Cushing Professor of Neurological
Surgery, Yale University School of Medicine, New
Haven, Connecticut

Paul R. Cooper, M.D.
Professor, Department of Neurosurgery, New York
University School of Medicine, New York, New York

Peter D. Costantino, M.D., Major USAF MC
Clinical Assistant Professor, Department of
Otolaryngology–Head and Neck Surgery,
Loyola University of Chicago Stritch School of
Medicine, Maywood, Illinois; Director of Departmental
Education and Research, Department of
Otolaryngology–Head and Neck Surgery,
Wilford Hall USAF Medical Center,
Lackland AFB, Texas

William T. Couldwell, M.D., Ph.D.
Assistant Professor, Department of Neurological
Surgery, University of Southern California School of
Medicine, Los Angeles, California

Robert M. Crowell, M.D.
Associate Professor, Department of Surgery, Harvard
Medical School; Director of Cerebrovascular Surgery,
Neurosurgical Service, Massachusetts General Hospital,
Boston, Massachusetts

Roy F. Cucchiara, M.D.
Professor, Department of Anesthesiology, University of
Florida College of Medicine, Gainesville, Florida

Manuel Cunha e Sa, M.D.
Consultant, Department of Neurological Surgery,
Hospital Egaz Moniz, Lisbon, Portugal

Arthur L. Day, M.D.
Professor, Department of Neurosurgery, and James
Newton Eblen Eminent Scholar of Cerebrovascular
Surgery, University of Florida College of Medicine,
Gainesville, Florida

John Day, M.D.
Clinical Instructor, Department of Neurological
Surgery, University of Southern California School of
Medicine, Los Angeles, California

Christopher M. DeGiorgio, M.D.
Assistant Professor, Department of Neurology, and
Director, Adult Epilepsy Program, University of
Southern California School of Medicine, Los Angeles,
California

Johnny B. Delashaw, M.D.
Adjunct Associate Professor, Division of Neurosurgery,
Oregon Health Sciences University School of Medicine,
Portland, Oregon

Lew Disney, M.D., Ph.D.
Division of Neurosurgery, Department of Surgery,
University of Alberta Faculty of Medicine;
University of Alberta Hospital, Edmonton,
Alberta, Canada

Vinko V. Dolenc, M.D., Ph.D.
Professor and Chairman, Department of Neurosurgery,
University Medical Center Ljubljana, Ljubljana, Slovenia

Christopher F. Dowd, M.D.
Assistant Professor, Departments of Radiology and
Neurological Surgery, University of California,
San Francisco, School of Medicine, San Francisco,
California

Charles G. Drake, M.D., F.R.C.S.(C.)
Professor, Department of Clinical Neurological
Sciences, University of Western Ontario Faculty of
Medicine, London, Ontario, Canada

Howard M. Eisenberg, M.D.
Professor and Chief, Division of Neurosurgery,
University of Texas Medical Branch at Galveston,
Galveston, Texas

Fred J. Epstein, M.D.
Professor and Director, Division of Pediatric
Neurosurgery, Department of Neurosurgery,
New York University School of Medicine, New York,
New York

Jean-Pierre Farmer, M.D., F.R.C.S.(C.)
Postgraduate Fellow, Division of Pediatric
Neurosurgery, Department of Neurosurgery,
New York University School of Medicine,
New York, New York

Donald I. Feinstein, M.D.
Professor, Department of Medicine, University of
Southern California School of Medicine; Chief,
Department of Medicine, University Hospital
and Kenneth Norris Jr. Cancer Hospital and Research
Institute, Los Angeles, California

J. Max Findlay, M.D., Ph.D.
Associate Professor, Division of Neurosurgery,
Department of Surgery, University of Alberta Faculty of
Medicine; University of Alberta Hospital, Edmonton,
Alberta, Canada

Eugene S. Flamm, M.D.
Charles Harrison Frazier Professor and Chairman,
Division of Neurosurgery, University of Pennsylvania
School of Medicine, Philadelphia, Pennsylvania

Ana Flisser, Ph.D.
Biologist, Doctor in Science, and Senior Research
Scientist (Professorial), Instituto de Investigaciones
Biomedicas of the National Autonomous University of
Mexico, Mexico City, Mexico

John L. Fox, M.D.
Clinical Professor, Division of Neurosurgery, University
of Nebraska Medical Center, Omaha, Nebraska

Takanori Fukushima, M.D., D.M.Sc.
Professor, Department of Neurological Surgery,
University of Southern California School of Medicine,
Los Angeles, California

Eugene D. George, M.D.
Professor and Chairman, Division of Neurosurgery,
Department of Surgery, University of Rochester School
of Medicine and Dentistry; Strong Memorial Hospital,
Rochester, New York

Timothy M. George, M.D.
Clinical Instructor, Section of Neurosurgery,
Department of Surgery, Yale University School of
Medicine, New Haven, Connecticut

Steven L. Giannotta, M.D.
Professor, Department of Neurological Surgery,
University of Southern California School of Medicine;
Chief of Service, University of Southern California
University Hospital, Los Angeles, California

Atul Goel, M.D.
Fellow, Department of Neurosurgery, University of
Pittsburgh School of Medicine, Pittsburgh,
Pennsylvania

David J. Gower, M.D.
Assistant Professor, Neurosurgical Section, Department
of Surgery, University of Oklahoma College of
Medicine, Oklahoma City, Oklahoma

Robert G. Grossman, M.D.
Professor and Chairman, Department of Neurosurgery,
Baylor College of Medicine; Professor and Chairman,
Department of Neurological Surgery, The Methodist
Hospital, Houston, Texas

Robert L. Grubb, Jr., M.D.
Professor, Department of Neurology and Neurological
Surgery, Washington University School of Medicine;
Director, Department of Neurological Surgery, Jewish
Hospital; Neurosurgeon, Barnes Hospital and
Children's Hospital, Saint Louis, Missouri

Peter Gruen, M.D.
Clinical Instructor, Department of Neurological
Surgery, University of Southern California School of
Medicine, Los Angeles, California

Van V. Halbach, M.D.
Associate Professor, Departments of Radiology and
Neurological Surgery, University of California, San
Francisco, School of Medicine, San Francisco,
California

Jules Hardy, O.C., M.D., F.R.C.S.(C.)
Professor, Division of Neurosurgery, Department of
Surgery, University of Montreal Faculty of Medicine;
Adjunct Professor, McGill University; Service of
Neurosurgery, Notre-Dame Hospital and Montreal
General Hospital, Montreal, Quebec, Canada

Milton D. Heifetz, M.D.
Clinical Professor, Department of Neurological Surgery,
University of Southern California School of Medicine,
Los Angeles, California; Visiting Professor, Department
of Surgery–Neurological Surgery, Brigham and
Women's Hospital, Harvard Medical School, Boston,
Massachusetts

M. Peter Heilbrun, M.D.
Professor and Chair, Department of Neurosurgery,
University of Utah School of Medicine, Salt Lake City,
Utah

Roberto C. Heros, M.D.
Lyle A. French Professor and Department Head,
Department of Neurosurgery, University of Minnesota
Medical School—Minneapolis, Minneapolis, Minnesota

Grant B. Hieshima, M.D.
Professor, Departments of Radiology and Neurosurgery,
University of California, San Francisco, School of
Medicine, San Francisco, California

Randall T. Higashida, M.D.
Associate Professor, Departments of Radiology and
Neurological Surgery, University of California,
San Francisco, School of Medicine, San Francisco,
California

Charles J. Hodge, M.D.
Professor and Chairman, Department of Neurosurgery,
State University of New York Health Science
Center at Syracuse College of Medicine,
Syracuse, New York

Julian T. Hoff, M.D.
Professor of Surgery and Head, Section of
Neurosurgery, Department of Surgery, University of
Michigan Medical School, Ann Arbor, Michigan

**Harold J. Hoffman, M.D., B.Sc.(Med),
F.R.C.S.(C.)**
Professor, Division of Neurosurgery, Department of
Surgery, University of Toronto Faculty of Medicine;
Neurosurgeon-in-Chief, Service of Neurosurgery,
Hospital for Sick Children, Toronto, Ontario,
Canada

Paul D. Holtom, M.D.
Assistant Professor of Clinical Medicine, Department
of Medicine, University of Southern California
School of Medicine; Chief, Division of Infectious
Diseases, University of Southern California University
Hospital, Los Angeles, California

Robin P. Humphreys, M.D., F.R.C.S.(C.)
Professor, Department of Surgery, University of
Toronto Faculty of Medicine; Senior Neurosurgeon and
Associate Neurosurgeon-in-Chief, Hospital for Sick
Children, Toronto, Ontario, Canada

John A. Jane, M.D., Ph.D.
David D. Weaver Professor of Neurosurgery and
Chairman, Department of Neurosurgery, University
of Virginia School of Medicine, Charlottesville, Virginia

Peter J. Jannetta, M.D.
Professor and Chairman, Department of Neurological
Surgery, University of Pittsburgh School of Medicine,
Pittsburgh, Pennsylvania

Patrick Juneau, M.D.
Department of Surgery, Harvard Medical School;
Department of Neurosurgery, Brigham and Women's
Hospital and Children's Hospital, Boston,
Massachusetts

Neal F. Kassell, M.D.
Professor, Department of Neurosurgery, University of
Virginia School of Medicine; Professor, Department of
Neurosurgery, University of Virginia Hospital,
Charlottesville, Virginia

David T. Kawanishi, M.D.
Associate Professor, Division of Cardiology,
Department of Medicine, and Director,
Cardiac Catheterization Laboratory,
George C. Griffith Laboratory, and Pacemaker
Center, University of Southern California School of
Medicine, Los Angeles, California

Michael Kazim, M.D.
Assistant in Clinical Ophthalmology, Columbia
University College of Physicians and Surgeons and
Edward S. Harkness Eye Institute, New York,
New York

David L. Kelly, Jr., M.D.
Professor and Chairman, Department of Neurosurgery,
Bowman Gray School of Medicine of Wake Forest
University, Winston-Salem, North Carolina

John S. Kennerdell, M.D.
Adjunct Professor of Surgery (Ophthalmology),
Medical College of Pennsylvania; Chairman,
Department of Ophthalmology, Allegheny General
Hospital, Pittsburgh, Pennsylvania

E. Leon Kier, M.D.
Professor, Section of Neuroradiology, Department of
Diagnostic Radiology, Yale University School of
Medicine, New Haven, Connecticut

Glenn W. Kindt, M.D.
Professor, Department of Surgery (Neurosurgery),
University of Colorado Health Sciences Center,
Denver, Colorado

Shigeaki Kobayashi, M.D.
Professor and Chairman, Department of Neurosurgery,
Shinshu University School of Medicine, Asahi,
Matsumoto, Japan

Douglas Kondziolka, M.D., M.Sc., F.R.C.S.(C.)
Assistant Professor, Department of Neurological
Surgery, University of Pittsburgh School of Medicine;
Associate Director, Specialized Neurosurgical Center,
Pittsburgh, Pennsylvania

Alexander N. Konovalov, M.D.
Director, Burdenko Neurological Institute, Moscow,
Russia

Kazuyoshi Korosue, M.D.
Assistant Professor, Department of Neurosurgery,
University of Minnesota Medical School—Minneapolis,
Minneapolis, Minnesota

Theodore Kurze, M.D.
Visiting Professor, Department of Neurological Surgery,
University of Pittsburgh School of Medicine,
Pittsburgh, Pennsylvania

Edward R. Laws, Jr., M.D.
Professor, Department of Neurosurgery, University of
Virginia School of Medicine, Charlottesville, Virginia

John M. Leedom, M.D.
Hastings Professor of Medicine, Department of
Medicine, University of Southern California
School of Medicine; Chief, Division of Infectious
Diseases, Los Angeles County–University of
Southern California Medical Center, Los Angeles,
California

Michael L. Levy, M.D.
Clinical Instructor, Department of Neurological
Surgery, University of Southern California School of
Medicine, Los Angeles, California

N. Scott Litofsky, M.D.
Clinical Instructor, Department of Neurological
Surgery, University of Southern California School of
Medicine, Los Angeles, California

John R. Little, M.D.
Spine and Neurologic Surgery Center, Naples, Florida

Don M. Long, M.D., Ph.D.
Harvey Cushing Professor of Neurosurgery, and
Director, Department of Neurological Surgery,
Johns Hopkins University School of Medicine;
Neurosurgeon-in-Chief, The Johns Hopkins Hospital,
Baltimore, Maryland

L. Dade Lunsford, M.D.
Professor of Neurological Surgery, Radiology, and
Radiation Oncology, Department of Neurological
Surgery, University of Pittsburgh School of Medicine;
Director, Specialized Neurosurgical Center,
Pittsburgh, Pennsylvania

Mark A. Lyerly, M.D.
Department of Neurosurgery, Bowman Gray School of
Medicine of Wake Forest University, Winston-Salem,
North Carolina

Ignacio Madrazo, M.D., D.Sc.
Professor of Neurosurgery and Head,
Department of Experimental Neurology and
Neurosurgery, Instituto Mexicano del Seguro
Social Universidad Nacional Autónoma de México;
Director of the Hospital, Centro Médico Nacional
"Siglo XXI," Departments of Neurosurgery and
Experimental Neurology and Neurosurgery,
Instituto Mexicano del Seguro Social Universidad
Nacional Autónoma de México,
Mexico City, Mexico

William W. Maggio, M.D.
Assistant Professor, Division of Neurosurgery,
Department of Surgery, University of Texas Medical
Branch at Galveston, Galveston, Texas

Leonard I. Malis, M.D.
Professor, Department of Neurosurgery, Mount Sinai
School of Medicine of the City University of New York;
Attending Neurosurgeon, The Mount Sinai Hospital,
New York, New York

Joseph C. Maroon, M.D.
Professor of Neurosurgery, Medical College of
Pennsylvania; Chairman, Department of Neurosurgery,
Allegheny General Hospital, Pittsburgh, Pennsylvania

David Masel, M.D.
Department of Neurosurgery, Henry Ford Hospital,
Detroit, Michigan

Masao Matsutani, M.D.
Associate Professor, Department of Neurosurgery,
University of Tokyo Hospital, Hongo, Bunkyo-ku,
Tokyo, Japan

Robert E. Maxwell, M.D., Ph.D.
Professor, Department of Neurosurgery, University
of Minnesota Medical School—Minneapolis;
Professor, Department of Neurosurgery, University
of Minnesota Hospitals and Clinic, Minneapolis,
Minnesota

Peter L. Mayer, M.D.
Section of Neurosurgery, Department of Surgery, Yale
University School of Medicine, New Haven,
Connecticut

J. Gordon McComb, M.D.
Professor, Department of Neurological Surgery,
University of Southern California School of Medicine;
Head, Division of Neurosurgery, Children's Hospital of
Los Angeles, Los Angeles, California

Ian E. McCutcheon, M.D.
Montreal Neurological Institute, Division of
Neurosurgery, McGill University Faculty of Medicine,
Montreal, Quebec, Canada

George McDonald, J.D.
Member of the California and U.S. Supreme Court,
and all federal bars in California; Diplomate,
American Board of Trial Advocates; affiliated with
George McDonald and Associates, South Pasadena,
California

David G. McLone, M.D., Ph.D.
Professor, Division of Neurosurgery, Department of
Surgery, Northwestern University Medical School;
Professor and Head, Department of Pediatric
Neurosurgery, Children's Memorial Hospital, Chicago,
Illinois

Arnold H. Menezes, M.D.
Professor and Vice Chairman, Division of Neurosurgery,
Department of Surgery, University of Iowa College of
Medicine; University of Iowa Hospitals and Clinics,
Iowa City, Iowa

Sean Mullan, M.D.
John Harper Seeley Professor of Neurological Surgery,
Division of Neurosurgery, Department of Surgery,
University of Chicago Division of the Biological
Sciences Pritzker School of Medicine; University of
Chicago Medical Center, Chicago, Illinois

Paul J. Muller, M.D., F.R.C.S.(C.)
Associate Professor, Department of Surgery, University
of Toronto Faculty of Medicine; Chief, Division of
Neurosurgery, Department of Surgery, St. Michael's
Hospital, Toronto, Ontario, Canada

Raj Murali, M.D.
Associate Professor of Clinical Neurosurgery,
Department of Neurosurgery, New York University
School of Medicine; Vice-Chairman, Department
of Neurological Surgery, St. Vincent's Hospital and
Medical Center of New York, New York, New York

Russ P. Nockels, M.D.
Assistant Professor, Department of Neurological
Surgery, University of California, San Francisco,
School of Medicine; Assistant Chief, Department of
Neurosurgery, San Francisco General Hospital,
San Francisco, California

Christopher S. Ogilvy, M.D.
Assistant Professor, Department of Surgery, Harvard
Medical School; Assistant and Visiting Neurosurgeon,
Neurosurgical Service, Massachusetts General Hospital,
Boston, Massachusetts

George A. Ojemann, M.D.
Professor, Department of Neurological Surgery,
University of Washington School of Medicine, Seattle,
Washington

Robert G. Ojemann, M.D.
Professor, Department of Surgery, Harvard Medical
School; Professor of Surgery and Visiting Neurosurgeon,
Neurosurgical Service, Massachusetts General Hospital,
Boston, Massachusetts

Russel H. Patterson, Jr., M.D.
Professor of Surgery (Neurosurgery), Division of
Neurological Surgery, Cornell University Medical
College; Attending in Charge, Division of
Neurosurgery, The New York Hospital, New York,
New York

John A. Persing, M.D.
Professor of Plastic Surgery and Neurosurgery, and
Chief, Section of Plastic Surgery, Yale University
School of Medicine; Chief, Department of Plastic
Surgery, Yale-New Haven Hospital, New Haven,
Connecticut

David G. Piepgras, M.D.
Professor and Chairman, Department of Neurologic
Surgery, Mayo Medical School and Mayo Clinic,
Rochester, Minnesota

Joseph M. Piepmeier, M.D.
Associate Professor, Section of Neurosurgery,
Department of Surgery, Yale University School of
Medicine, New Haven, Connecticut

Webster H. Pilcher, M.D., Ph.D.
Assistant Professor, Division of Neurosurgery,
Department of Surgery, University of Rochester School
of Medicine and Dentistry; Strong Memorial Hospital,
Rochester, New York

Dennis S. Poe, M.D.
Senior Otolaryngologist, Departments of Neurosurgery
and Otolaryngology, Lahey Clinic, Burlington,
Massachusetts

Michael Pollay, M.D.
Professor and Chief, Neurosurgical Section, University
of Oklahoma College of Medicine; Oklahoma City,
Oklahoma

Jeffrey M. Preuss, M.D.
Department of Emergency Medicine, Louisiana State
University School of Medicine in New Orleans, New
Orleans, Louisiana

David Primrose, M.D.
Assistant Professor, Department of Neurosurgery,
State University of New York Health Science Center
at Syracuse College of Medicine, Syracuse, New York

Donald O. Quest, M.D.
Professor of Clinical Neurological Surgery,
Department of Neurological Surgery, Columbia
University College of Physicians and Surgeons;
Attending Neurological Surgeon, Department of
Neurosurgery, Columbia-Presbyterian Medical Center,
New York, New York

Craig Rabb, M.D.
Clinical Instructor, Department of Neurological
Surgery, University of Southern California School of
Medicine, Los Angeles, California

Adrian L. Rabinowicz, M.D.
Epilepsy Fellow, Department of Neurology,
University of Southern California School of Medicine,
Los Angeles, California

Corey Raffel, M.D., Ph.D.
Associate Professor, Department of Neurological
Surgery, University of Southern California School of
Medicine; Staff Neurosurgeon, Division of
Neurosurgery, Children's Hospital of Los Angeles,
Los Angeles, California

Joseph Ransohoff, M.D.
Professor, Department of Neurosurgery, University
of South Florida College of Medicine, Tampa,
Florida

Mark U. Rarick, M.D.
Assistant Professor, Department of Medicine,
University of Southern California School of Medicine,
Los Angeles, California

Setti S. Rengachary, M.D.
Professor and Chief, Section of Neurological Surgery,
University of Missouri–Kansas City School of Medicine;
Chief, Neurosurgery Service, Truman Medical Center,
Kansas City, Missouri

Albert L. Rhoton, Jr., M.D.
R.D. Keene Professor and Chairman, Department of
Neurological Surgery, University of Florida College of
Medicine, Gainesville, Florida

James T. Robertson, M.D.
Professor and Chairman, Department of Neurological Surgery,University of Tennessee, Memphis, College of Medicine, Memphis, Tennessee

Jon H. Robertson, M.D.
Associate Professor, Department of Neurosurgery, University of Tennessee, Memphis, College of Medicine; Semmes-Murphey Clinic, Memphis, Tennessee

Jack P. Rock, M.D.
Neurosurgical and Senior Staff, Department of Neurosurgery, Henry Ford Hospital, Detroit, Michigan

Szymon Rosenblatt, M.D.
Instructor, Division of Neurosurgery, Northwestern University Medical School, Chicago, Illinois; Evanston Hospital, Evanston, Illinois

Robert H. Rosenwasser, M.D.
Associate Professor and Chief, Section of Cerebrovascular Surgery, Department of Neurosurgery, and Associate Professor, Department of Physiology, Temple University School of Medicine, Philadelphia, Pennsylvania

Richard L. Rovit, M.D.
Professor of Clinical Neurosurgery, Department of Neurosurgery, New York University School of Medicine; Chairman, Department of Neurological Surgery, St. Vincent's Hospital and Medical Center of New York, New York, New York

John R. Ruge, M.D.
Clinical Assistant Professor, Department of Surgery, University of Chicago Division of the Biological Sciences Pritzker School of Medicine; Attending Neurosurgeon, Department of Neurosurgery, Lutheran General Children's Medical Center, Chicago, Illinois

W. George Rusyniak, M.D.
Assistant in Surgery, Division of Neurosurgery, Department of Surgery, University of Rochester School of Medicine and Dentistry; Strong Memorial Hospital, Rochester, New York

Balaji Sadasivan, M.B., B.S., F.R.C.S.
Consultant, Department of Neurosurgery, Tan Tock Sang Hospital, Singapore

Michael Salcman, M.D.
Clinical Professor, Department of Neurosurgery, George Washington University School of Medicine, Washington, D.C.; Attending Physician, Union Memorial and Sinai Hospitals, Baltimore, Maryland

Duke S. Samson, M.D.
Professor and Chairman, Department of Neurological Surgery, University of Texas Southwestern Medical Center, Dallas, Texas

Keiji Sano, M.D., D.M.Sc.
Emeritus Professor of Neurosurgery, University of Tokyo Faculty of Medicine, Tokyo, Japan; Professor, Department of Neurosurgery, Teikyo University School of Medicine, Tokyo, Japan; Director, Fuji Brain Institute and Hospital, Fujinomiya, Japan

Kimberlee J. Sass, Ph.D.
Assistant Professor, Section of Neurosurgery, Department of Surgery, Yale University School of Medicine, New Haven, Connecticut

Richard L. Saunders, M.D.
Professor and Chairman, Section of Neurosurgery, Department of Surgery, Dartmouth Medical School; Dartmouth-Hitchcock Medical Center, Hanover, New Hampshire

Henry H. Schmidek, M.D.
Neurosurgeon, Department of Neurosurgery, St. Luke's Hospital, New Bedford, Massachusetts

Daniel J. Scodary, M.D.
University of Cincinnati College of Medicine, Cincinnati, Ohio; Attending Neurosurgeon, De Paul Medical Center and Christian Northeast Medical Center, Saint Louis, Missouri

Laligam N. Sekhar, M.D.
Co-Director and Professor, Department of Neurosurgery, University of Pittsburgh School of Medicine; Presbyterian-University Hospital, Pittsburgh, Pennsylvania

Chandra N. Sen, M.D.
Associate Professor, Department of Neurosurgery, The Mount Sinai Hospital, New York, New York

R.P. Sengupta, F.R.C.S.
Consultant Neurosurgeon, Newcastle General Hospital, Newcastle-Upon-Tyne, Great Britain

Christopher I. Shaffrey, M.D.
Departments of Neurosurgery and Orthopaedics, University of Virginia School of Medicine, Charlottesville, Virginia

Mark E. Shaffrey, M.D.
Department of Neurosurgery, University of Virginia School of Medicine, Charlottesville, Virginia

William Shucart, M.D.
Professor and Chairman, Department of Neurosurgery, Tufts University School of Medicine; Chief, Department of Neurosurgery, New England Medical Center, Boston, Massachusetts

Kenneth R. Smith, Jr., M.D.
Professor and Chairman, Division of Neurosurgery, Department of Surgery, Saint Louis University School of Medicine, Saint Louis, Missouri

Maurice M. Smith, M.D.
Clinical Instructor, Division of Neurosurgery, Virginia Commonwealth University Medical College of Virginia School of Medicine, Richmond, Virginia

Robert R. Smith, M.D.
Professor and Chairman, Department of Neurosurgery, University of Mississippi School of Medicine, Jackson, Mississippi

Carl H. Snyderman, M.D.
Assistant Professor, Department of Otolaryngology, University of Pittsburgh School of Medicine, Pittsburgh, Pennsylvania

Robert A. Solomon, M.D.
Associate Professor, Department of Neurological Surgery, Columbia University College of Physicians and Surgeons; Associate Attending, Presbyterian Hospital in the City of New York, New York, New York

Dennis D. Spencer, M.D.
Professor and Chairman of Neurosurgery, Section of Neurosurgery, Department of Surgery, Yale University School of Medicine, New Haven, Connecticut

Stephen N. Steen, Sc.D., M.D.
Professor of Clinical Anesthesiology and Director of Research, University of Southern California School of Medicine, Los Angeles, California

Bennett M. Stein, M.D.
Byron Stookey Professor and Chairman, Department of Neurological Surgery, Columbia University College of Physicians and Surgeons; Director of Service, Department of Neurological Surgery, The Neurological Institute, Presbyterian Hospital in the City of New York, New York, New York

Jim L. Story, M.D.
Professor and Head, Division of Neurosurgery, Department of Surgery, University of Texas Health Science Center, San Antonio, Texas

Kenichiro Sugita, M.D.
Professor and Chairman, Department of Neurosurgery, Nagoya University School of Medicine, Nagoya, Japan

Peter Sunderland, Ph.D., R.N.
Assistant Professor, Department of Neurosurgery, University of Utah School of Medicine, Salt Lake City, Utah

Thoralf M. Sundt, Jr., M.D.
Professor, Department of Neurologic Surgery, Mayo Medical School and Mayo Clinic, Rochester, Minnesota

Dana L. Suskind, M.D.
Department of Surgery, University of Pennsylvania School of Medicine, Philadelphia, Pennsylvania

William H. Sweet, M.D., D.Sc.
Emeritus Professor of Surgery, Harvard Medical School; Senior Neurosurgeon, Neurosurgical Service, Massachusetts General Hospital, Boston, Massachusetts

Kintomo Takakura, M.D.
Professor and Chairman, Department of Neurosurgery, University of Tokyo Hospital, Hongo, Bunkyo-ku, Tokyo, Japan

Masakazu Takayasu, M.D.
Assistant Professor, Department of Neurosurgery,
Nagoya University School of Medicine,
Nagoya, Japan

Yuichiro Tanaka, M.D.
Assistant Professor, Department of Neurosurgery,
Shinshu University School of Medicine, Asahi,
Matsumoto, Japan

Edward C. Tarlov, M.D.
Senior Neurosurgeon, Departments of Neurosurgery
and Otolaryngology, Lahey Clinic, Burlington,
Massachusetts

Ronald R. Tasker, M.D.
Professor, Department of Surgery, Division of
Neurosurgery, University of Toronto Faculty of
Medicine; Toronto Hospital, Toronto, Ontario,
Canada

Charles H. Tator, M.D., Ph.D., F.R.C.S.(C.)
Professor and Chairman, Division of Neurosurgery,
Department of Surgery, University of Toronto Faculty
of Medicine; Head, Division of Neurosurgery,
Toronto Hospital, Toronto, Ontario, Canada

John M. Tew, Jr., M.D.
Professor and Chairman, Department of Neurosurgery,
University of Cincinnati College of Medicine; Mayfield
Neurological Institute, Cincinnati, Ohio

George T. Tindall, M.D.
Professor and Chairman, Department of Neurosurgery,
Emory University School of Medicine, Atlanta,
Georgia

William Tucker, M.D., F.R.C.S.(C.)
Associate Professor, Division of Neurosurgery,
Department of Surgery, University of Toronto
Faculty of Medicine; Head, Trauma Service,
Department of Surgery, Saint Michael's Hospital,
Toronto, Ontario, Canada

Howard Tung, M.D.
Clinical Instructor, Department of Neurological
Surgery, University of Southern California School of
Medicine, Los Angeles, California

John C. VanGilder, M.D.
Professor and Chairman, Division of Neurosurgery,
Department of Surgery, University of Iowa College of
Medicine; University of Iowa Hospitals and Clinics,
Iowa City, Iowa

Joan Venes, M.D.
Professor of Surgery (Neurosurgery), Department of
Surgery, University of Michigan Medical School,
Ann Arbor, Michigan

Franklin C. Wagner, Jr., M.D.
Professor and Chairman, Department of Neurological
Surgery, University of California, Davis, School of
Medicine, Davis, California; Chief, Department of
Neurological Surgery, University of California, Davis,
Medical Center, Sacramento, California

John D. Ward, M.D.
Professor of Neurosurgery, Chief of Pediatric
Neurosurgery, and Director of Neuroscience Intensive
Care Unit, Division of Neurosurgery, Department of
Surgery, Virginia Commonwealth University Medical
College of Virginia School of Medicine, Richmond,
Virginia

John P. Weaver, M.D.
Clinical Instructor, Division of Neurosurgery,
Department of Surgery, Virginia Commonwealth
University Medical College of Virginia School of
Medicine, Richmond, Virginia

David Weinsweig, M.D.
Instructor, Division of Neurosurgery, Northwestern
University Medical School, Chicago, Illinois; Division
of Neurosurgery, Evanston Hospital, Evanston, Illinois

Bryce K. Weir, M.D.
Professor and Chief, Division of Neurosurgery,
Department of Surgery, University of Chicago Division
of the Biological Sciences Pritzker School of Medicine,
Chicago, Illinois

Martin H. Weiss, M.D.
Professor and Chairman, Department of Neurological
Surgery, University of Southern California School of
Medicine; Chairman, Department of Neurosurgery,
Los Angeles County–University of Southern California
Medical Center, Los Angeles, California

Robert H. Wilkins, M.D.
Professor and Chief, Division of Neurosurgery,
Department of Surgery, Duke University Medical
Center, Durham, North Carolina

Charles B. Wilson, M.D.
Tong-Po Kan Professor and Chairman,
Department of Neurological Surgery, University of
California, San Francisco, School of Medicine,
San Francisco, California

Eric J. Woodard, M.D.
Assistant Professor, Department of Neurosurgery,
Emory University School of Medicine; Emory Clinic
Spine Center, Atlanta, Georgia

Harold F. Young, M.D.
Professor and Chairman, Division of Neurological
Surgery, Department of Surgery, Virginia
Commonwealth University Medical College of Virginia
School of Medicine, Richmond, Virginia

Ronald F. Young, M.D.
Professor and Chief, Division of Neurological
Surgery, Department of Surgery, University of
California, Irvine, College of Medicine, Irvine,
California; Chief, Department of Neurosurgery,
University of California, Irvine, Medical Center,
Orange, California

Chi-Shing Zee, M.D.
Associate Professor, Department of Radiology,
University of Southern California School of Medicine,
Los Angeles, California

Vladimir Zelman, M.D., Ph.D.
Professor of Clinical Anesthesiology, Neurological
Surgery, and Neurology, and Director of
Neuroanesthesiology, University of Southern California
School of Medicine, Los Angeles, California

Foreword

With the publication of Sir William Macewen's *Pyogenic Infective Diseases of the Brain and Spinal Cord* in 1883, neurological surgery as a recognized discipline within the field of surgery was born, at least in the English-speaking countries. Cushing's speech in November, 1904, to the Cleveland Academy of Medicine, titled "The Special Field of Neurological Surgery" gave impetus to the development of this specialty. Early on in this century it became apparent that no one individual could write authoritatively about all aspects of the operative experience. An outgrowth of this perception was the multivolume approach edited by an eminent practitioner who assembled the views of his peers. The benchmark by which all subsequent efforts were to be measured was established by two encyclopedic compendia. W.W. Keen's five-volume 1908 work, *Surgery*, was graced by a splendid treatise from Harvey Cushing; and in 1932, Walter Dandy's classic contribution, *The Brain*, appeared in Dean Lewis's *Practice of Surgery*. It appeared as the first chapter (682 pages) of Volume XII. In 1944, it was revised and was subsequently published separately.

In 1931, Cushing, in a presentation to the International Neurological Congress in Berne, Switzerland, reported on the surgical mortality in his series of 2,000 verified brain tumors. The following year, he published a monograph on these data, in which he carefully recorded his "score" or operative mortality. In the Preface, he stated "The laying bare of one's mere mortality percentages, however, is only a start toward what will ultimately be called for: namely, figures relating to the expectancy of life of those who have survived tumour extirpations. And still more important would be figures for each kind of tumour which would show the percentage of surviving patients whose wage-earning capacity has been restored by operation and for how long a time." In this monograph, he foresaw the logical next step, the advent of subspecialization within our field when he wrote "Neurological surgery is a large subject and the surgery of brain tumours is a special field within it. Indeed, the day may well enough come when certain surgeons will find enough to keep themselves fully occupied by attending exclusively to tumours of a single type."

I firmly believe that *Brain Surgery: Complication Avoidance and Management* represents a crucial event in that it brings together a most stellar array of world-class neurosurgeons. The wisdom, pictorial displays, and background reference materials contained in these volumes are incomparable, and with its publication, a new standard has been set. I congratulate Michael Apuzzo and his collaborators for their handiwork, which will be the Bible for neurosurgeons everywhere, young and old.

Hugo V. Rizzoli, M.D.
Professor Emeritus
Department of Neurosurgery
George Washington University
School of Medicine and Health Sciences
Washington, D.C.

Preface

In the most rudimentary sense, optimization of surgery of the brain and perineural intracranial space may be viewed as accomplishing a task or corrective endpoint while creating no harm or undue cost in attaining the goal.

Each particular surgical enterprise has inherent risks and pitfalls—certain key or hazardous steps or maneuvers in its methodology. Rather than proceeding in a surgical undertaking by "cookbook" fashion, the refined and truly intellectual surgeon holds a firm comprehension of the scope of these pitfalls and the problems that are attendant to each stage of a given surgical enterprise. Mastering the art of avoidance of both intraoperative and postoperative problems is a key factor in operative excellence and optimization of outcome.

Competence in management of problems should they occur during the intraoperative or postoperative period is a hallmark of completeness in the development of the neurological surgeon. Levels of skill in complication avoidance and management in a given situation represent the true essence of surgical competence.

Development of precision of thought and action in relation to complication avoidance and management requires absolute comprehension of individual steps in a surgical enterprise, potentially hazardous maneuvers, the spectrum of potential immediate and late problems, and individual refinement of those issues of thought to the case presented.

Philosophically these elements of thought and skill represent the true essence of any surgical enterprise in the most sophisticated fashion and separate the experienced and thoughtful surgeon from the neophyte or journeyman.

Brain Surgery: Complication Avoidance and Management attempts to approach this essential feature of intracranial surgery by presenting in detail elements of surgical preparation, concepts of strategy, steps of operative enterprise, and a compendium of complication potential, avoidance methodology, and management modes for problems should they occur intraoperatively or postoperatively.

The information is presented within three major topics, the first dealing with the supratentorial space, the second with the infratentorial compartment, and the third with the cranial base. Each section begins by describing in broad and general terms the spectrum of strategies, problems, and techniques attendant to the pathology and surgeries for their amelioration or correction. This general overview is followed by chapters dealing with the major groups of surgical pathology and their subgroups, with an effort to present specific strategies and techniques with the focus on the major theme of complications, their avoidance and management.

This concept of problem avoidance provided the seed for a massive project with seven years of undertaking and preparation. All senior authors were selected because of their recognized expertise and unusual experiences associated with an individual topic. Most had not approached their topic formally from this perspective at any time in the past. The reappraisal and analysis at times was difficult in spite of its essential character and supportive fiber within their own established fabric of expertise and unusual competence.

Although the individual chapters in certain situations would seem to stand alone, it is more appropriate to view these volumes as a whole with multiple components giving integration and support to the individual statements in the development of the concept of maximal intellectual and technical neurosurgical competence in surgery in and around the brain.

Michael L.J. Apuzzo, M.D.

Acknowledgments

This project required a seven-year evolution and necessitated a number of key resolved, dedicated, and loyal people to bring it to fruition.

Toni Tracy, President of Churchill Livingstone Inc., believed in and underwrote the effort sustaining it in appropriate balance between the editor's need for perfection and the contemporary realities of publishing.

Carolyn Soter helped in launching the organization of the initial conception at the University of Southern California–Los Angeles County Medical Center. This effort was sustained with major commitment and furious energy by *Gabriela Saavedra* over the long period of the publication's genesis. *Reynalda Guzman* dedicated herself to critical support in the important stages of the book's completion.

At Churchill Livingstone, remarkable patience, intelligence, and professionalism were consistently evident in *Ann Ruzycka* and *Donna Balopole* as polish and order were conferred on rough manuscripts. *Patricia McFadden* professionally handled the design process.

Finally, special praise is in order for illustrator *Diane Abeloff,* who worked with incredible dedication, patience, and resolve bringing her own special stamp of excellence to the fabric of this atlas text.

What Is A Complication In Neurological Surgery?
A Practical Approach

There is considerable diversity in what neurosurgeons consider a complication. This commentary presents the results of a questionnaire sent to a sample of neurosurgeons about what is listed as a complication at their institution, discusses the concept of a neurosurgical complication, and closes with some suggestions about the general problem of assessing complications in neurological surgery.

A Neurosurgical Questionnaire about Complications

We sent a questionnaire to 18 leading neurosurgical academic centers asking about the ways they define complications, who decides what goes on the list, and whether certain specific problems would be considered a complication. Table 1 is a reprint of the questionnaire. Some of the definitions of complications provided by the respondents are as follows:

- Unexpected event that delays discharge
- Results that are less than optimal that we discuss among ourselves as neurosurgeons
- Any unexpected harmful outcome
- Adverse happening that alters treatment and/or affects the patient
- Any ill effect associated with surgery in a cause-effect manner
- Any unsatisfactory outcome related to a surgical procedure
- Any occurrence or event that has not been discussed (preoperatively)
- A deterioration of the patient's neurological or physical state, usually considered to be an *unexpected* deterioration
- Any events that extend hospitalization, cause readmission, require additional medications, cause a neurological deficit, etc.

Table 1. Questionnaire about Complications

1. Does your service have an explicit written definition of what should be considered a neurosurgical complication? (If so, could you append it here? If not, would you briefly describe your own concept of a complication?)
2. How do you decide what will be presented at an M&M conference?
   Residents decide _____ Staff decide _____ Other_____
3. Do you count complications as:
   a. Any adverse event within 48 hours of surgery _____
   b. Any adverse event within a week of surgery _____
   c. Any adverse event within a month of surgery _____
   d. Any adverse event that happened while the patient was in the hospital? _____
   e. Any adverse event happening with reasonable assurance as a result of the neurosurgical manipulation _____
   f. Other _____
4. Are the following problems surgical complications? Why or why not?
   a. Complete hearing loss in a patient with an acoustic neuroma who had 50% hearing loss before surgery.
   b. Deep vein thrombosis three weeks after surgery, diagnosed two weeks after discharge from the hospital.
   c. Acute myocardial infarction occurring 10 days after surgery while the patient is still in the hospital.
   d. Myocardial infarction occurring 10 days after surgery at home.
5. Do you have any general comments about what kind of events should be considered complications in neurosurgery?

◆ Any event that compounds the patient's course

◆ An unintended and nonbeneficial event following an operative procedure and caused by it

◆ Anything related to the procedure at any time

◆ Any untoward or adverse event within a month of surgery or while the patient is still in the hospital

◆ Any untoward event that delays the patient's discharge beyond the anticipated date or leaves the patient with a minor or major temporary or permanent disability

◆ Anything occurring in hospital or anything in the first two postoperative months related to surgery

◆ Any event that deviates at all from a direct recovery

One respondent gave very specific categories: wound infection, "delayed" wound hematoma, or cerebrospinal fluid leak; all system infections; all new neurological deficits; all deaths; all symptomatic variation in all electrolytes; seizure or other unexpected event. One respondent said their institution divided complications by cause: patient's disease, delay in diagnosis, error in diagnosis, delay in treatment, error in treatment, error in technique, or other.

In 4 institutions the residents decided what counted as a complication, in 2 the staff did so, and in 10 both groups were involved. Several respondents drew a distinction between listing an adverse event as such and calling it a complication.

Overall, the respondents suggested three general groups of complications: adverse events while the patient was in the hospital, adverse events within a month of surgery, and any adverse events resulting from surgery no matter when they happened. Six of the 18 respondents said that complications were any adverse event occurring while in the hospital; 4, anything occurring within one month of surgery; 4, anything related to surgery; and 4, all of the above.

In the questionnaire, four situations were described and the respondents were asked to identify whether or not they would be counted as a complication.

1. *Complete hearing loss in a patient with an acoustic neuroma who had 50 percent loss before surgery.* 7 respondents answered yes; 9 said no. Among those who said yes, some said it depended on what the patient expected or the size of the tumor. Those who said no argued it was an expected outcome to lose hearing in this situation.

2. *Deep venous thrombosis 3 weeks after surgery diagnosed 2 weeks after discharge.* 15 said yes; 2 said no.

3. *Acute myocardial infarction 10 days after surgery while the patient is still in the hospital.* 14 said yes; 3 said no, 2 because it was a medical complication.

4. *Myocardial infarction occuring within 10 days after surgery at home.* 10 said yes; 5 said no, presumably because it occurred at home.

The Components of a Complication

Most of the descriptions of complications just presented emphasize that complications are adverse outcomes and many introduced the concept of being unexpected. From them it is possible to derive a general statement about complications. A complication is an unexpected and undesirable event associated with management of a particular condition. Each of these events has elements worthy of discussion.

Unexpected

For quality assurance screening criteria, the unexpected nature of a complication seems most important. Table 2 presents the screening criteria at one institution—in all cases "unplanned" is a critical element.

This component of a complication arises in part from the doctor-patient relationship. There is a certain range of outcomes anticipated and complications lie outside these. This should not hide the fact that some adverse effects may be anticipated but are still "bad"—for example, a third nerve palsy after basilar aneurysm clipping or facial paralysis after acoustic neuroma resection. Present thinking suggests that these, because they are an accepted result of the procedure, are not as noteworthy as those problems that are unanticipated; presumably this is because the patient has an opportunity to anticipate them and takes them into account in agreeing to have any surgery done.

Undesirable

Undesirability may be defined by doctor, by patient, or by a third party. Surgeons may not have as rigorous a view of what is undesirable in patients as patients do—

Table 2. Screening Criteria, Department of Surgery, Brigham and Women's Hospital, Boston

---

1. Unplanned readmissions within 30 days of hospital discharge or day surgical procedure due to a postoperative complication or misdiagnosis.
2. Unplanned return to the operating room within the same admission of the primary surgery, for the same condition, or to correct an operative occurrence or postoperative complication.
3. Unplanned removal, injury, or repair of an organ or structure.
4. Unplanned transfer to the intensive care unit.
5. Death—review all cases.

---

every neurosurgeon, for example, has probably had one or two patients who say that their memory and concentration are not as good after a craniotomy as they were before. Insurance carriers may complain that an outcome that seems acceptable to both physician and patient is undesirable because of its cost.

Associated with Management

Patients may not understand that the natural history of a particular disease is worse than surgical intervention even with a bad outcome. Neurosurgeons may forget that not acting in some cases may lead to worse complications than proceeding with surgery. The complex issues of acting versus not acting to get a certain result has not been addressed carefully.

Duration

A problem that will steadily improve is much better tolerated than one which is stable.

Severity

A mild problem after surgery (urinary tract infection, superficial abrasion from poor turning) is much better tolerated than a major one. There are some complications (e.g. persistent vegetative state as a result of surgery) that must be reported in some states.

Degree of Control by the Surgeon

"Medical" complications, such as increased diabetes mellitus with steroid use, are often minimized in neurosurgical discussion.

General Comments

Although this book is about complication avoidance and management and although there is little question that most of the problems described here qualify as complications, there are several important questions left to answer about complications.

1. Can and should a uniform definition be adopted by neurosurgeons?
2. Who should decide to call something a complication—doctor, patient, insurance carrier, quality review board, or other?
3. How important is the degree of the defect in an anticipated result?
4. If an imperfect result was anticipated, does this relieve the physician of the responsibility for its imperfection?
5. Should complications be managed, as they now are, by insurance carriers and occasional law suits, which may or may not be justified, or should there be some kind of no-fault system as part of general tort reform?

These questions will have increased relevance as hospitals are mandated to maintain physician provider profiles that will record, among other things, how many complications each participating physician has. Recognizing, recording, and avoiding complications is an important part of neurosurgical practice. In the future it may be a matter of professional survival.

Peter McL. Black, M.D., Ph.D.

Neurosurgical Complications
A Philosophical Commentary

Complicate [*L. complicatus*, pp. of *complicare* to fold together, fr. *com-* + *plicare* to fold—more at PLY)

Complication 1 a: COMPLEXITY, INTRICACY; *esp*: a situation or a detail of character complicating the main thread of a plot **b:** a making difficult, involved, or intricate **c:** a complex or intricate feature or element **d:** a difficult factor or issue often appearing unexpectedly and changing existing plans, methods, or attitudes **2:** a secondary disease or condition developing in the course of a primary disease or condition

Webster's Ninth New Collegiate Dictionary

Although hard, logical definitions of complications may be offered and in fact are presented as the practical reality of these volumes, thoughtful individuals must ponder beyond what to most in one way or another is obvious. All practical definitions of complications have substance and relevance to neurosurgical practice. Certain philosophical and perhaps moral issues are attendant to the matter of *complicare.*

The patient is more than a collection of anatomical parts and physiological functions. The surgical experience must function in cognizance of the impact on the *balance of the integrity of the person.* Without a truly positive impact on the disease process, actions in themselves complicate with or without negative impact on functional soundness. Questions of the equilibrium between action and cost are the ethical issue.

As neurosurgeons we are entering a difficult era. Being blessed with a spectrum of unique technical adjuvants, we are at the same time burdened with a true dilemma of application. Currently the area of cranial base surgery presents a practical example of this dilemma. Patients present frequently with minimal complaints or deficits but harbor lesions that will devour them functionally with time. The cost of "possibility" of cure or palliation is frequently considerable. What is the balance of true benefit versus detriment in these cases? How should the term "complication" be defined in these cases where potential risks are high and the possibility for negative impact through "therapeutic" effort is broad in scope? What negative impact on function is to be expected in the individual case? What is the expected deficit in the individual case?

What should be the limit of application of surgical skills of an individual whether master, journeyman, or neophyte? Viewed morally, an approach that places the individual patient at unnecessary risk regardless of outcome is complicated by added threat. Practical manifestation of a complication may signal an error in judgment that may be manifest by various actions. Proper strategy of surgical undertaking reduces risks and amplifies logic of the management. Lack of the same philosophically complicates the management. One must ponder what is correct: (1) a complete tumor excision with functional impairment or (2) an incomplete excision in a fully functional patient? These questions are reductionistic but hopefully present moral dilemmas and raise questions of the complete definition of complication.

A complication may be viewed as an unsatisfactory result. A token surgical enterprise with risk of exposure even though a patient may be returned to physiological baseline can be viewed as an amateurish and morally repugnant action.

Each individual in applying procedures described in these volumes must look beyond the practical definition of complication and apply a moral and philosophical yardstick to himself and his endeavors as the balance of benefit versus risks is evaluated and outcome, both satisfactory or unsatisfactory, is truly perceived.

Michael L.J. Apuzzo, M.D.
William T. Couldwell, M.D., Ph.D.
Jason A. Apuzzo, B.A.

Contents

Volume 2

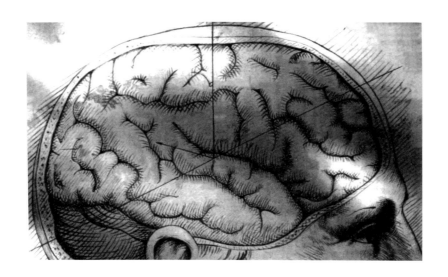

Supratentorial Procedures

Part 1: General Topics

1 Preoperative and Surgical Planning for Avoiding Complications

Robert G. Grossman

The goal of this chapter is to provide a systematic approach to preventing the complications of neurosurgical operations. The importance of preoperative planning is emphasized, and strategies for avoiding the common complications of neurological surgery are described.

The neurosurgeon who in the early stages of training assists in a major neurosurgical operation may be only partially aware of the complex series of steps that are taken by an experienced surgeon to bring the patient safely to and through the operation. Attempts to emulate the surgery itself without carrying out all of the preoperative steps may result in an unsuccessful outcome. The thought processes of planning for neurosurgery and the behavior of the neurosurgeon in carrying out successful surgery are made manifest in this chapter.

To avoid the complications of neurosurgery it is first necessary to consider the types of occurrences that constitute a complication and then to identify the causes of such occurrences. A complication of surgery can be defined as an occurrence that meets the following three criteria: it is *unwanted;* it is *unplanned;* and it *does not commonly occur.* An occurrence that fulfills only one or two of these criteria may not necessarily be a complication. For example, an unwanted occurrence is damage to the facial nerve during the excision of an acoustic neuroma. However, injury to the facial nerve during the excision of a large acoustic tumor is a common and even expected occurrence. Most neurosurgeons would not

therefore consider facial nerve injury in such an instance to be a complication of the surgery. An example of an unwanted occurrence, which nevertheless is planned, is the sectioning of a nerve to allow resection of a tumor or the clipping of an aneurysm. In this instance, the unwanted occurrence is deliberately produced to achieve a surgical goal. In both of these examples the loss of function is expected or unavoidable and is inextricably tied to an appreciation of the overall risks and benefits of the procedure for the patient. To classify these unwanted postoperative deficits under the pejorative term *complication* is neither reasonable nor appropriate.

Some authors have defined a complication as an occurrence that is avoidable. In the present discussion the ideas of avoidable or unavoidable have been subsumed under the concepts of expected or unexpected, based on knowledge of the statistical outcome of specific procedures. The exact frequency of occurrence at which an unwanted surgical outcome is no longer an expected outcome of surgery but instead is a complication cannot, of course, be given. Similarly, there is no exact definition of the temporal relationship of an unwanted occurrence to the time of surgery in classifying the occurrence as a complication. However, various guidelines have evolved over time, such as assigning deaths that occur within the first month after surgery to the operative mortality rate.

It is also necessary to have an understanding of the common causes of complications in order to devise methods that will prevent their occurrence. The causes of surgical complications can be divided into three major classes:

1. Lack of information, incorrect information, or confusion regarding data in planning surgery, during surgery, or in the postoperative period
2. Incorrect judgment in planning, during surgery, or in the postoperative period
3. Incorrect execution during surgery or in the postoperative period

Examples of the types of complications caused by each of these sources of error are given in Table 1-1. There can, of course, be considerable overlap between these categories, as is indicated in the table.

THE PREVENTION OF COMPLICATIONS

The intellectual and emotional attitudes that the surgeon brings to each phase of treatment are paramount in preventing complications and in achieving consistently good results. A commitment to meticulous attention to detail and to expending the time necessary to prepare and to execute flawlessly all aspects of the surgery is essential. As an example, the outcome of a perfectly performed microsurgical procedure can be compromised during the closure of the incision by the hasty and improper placement of a single suture, resulting in cerebrospinal fluid (CSF) leakage and infection.

Table 1-1.   Causes and Examples of Neurosurgical Complications

I. Lack of information, incorrect information, or confusion regarding data
  A. Incorrect or confused data
    1. Wrong patient undergoing surgery
    2. Wrong side operated on
    3. Wrong spinal level operated on
    4. Administration of wrong medication, blood, or fluids
  B. Complications due to failure to recognize and treat medical conditions
    1. Bleeding disturbances
    2. Diabetes mellitus
    3. Endocrinopathies
    4. Electrolyte imbalance
    5. Cardiovascular disturbances
    6. Pulmonary disturbances
    7. Allergic reactions
II. Incorrect judgment
  A. Wrong operation (failure to recognize the pathology)
  B. Inadequate operation (failure to remove adequate amount of pathology)
  C. Wrong side operated on
  D. Wrong spinal level operated on
  E. Inadequate access to pathology (incorrect approach)
III. Incorrect execution
  A. Incorrect or inadequate patient positioning
    1. Compromised venous drainage
    2. Compromised chest expansion
    3. Spinal cord injury due to neck flexion or extension
    4. Pressure-induced skin damage
    5. Pressure-induced nerve injuries
    6. Scalp and skull injuries due to pin fixation
  B. Intraoperative technical and physical complications
    1. Inability to cannulate the lateral ventricle
    2. Tearing of the dura
    3. Brain retractor-induced trauma
    4. Laceration or occlusion of major arteries
    5. Compromise of perforating arteries
    6. Disturbance of major venous drainage
    7. Damage to sensory, motor, or eloquent areas of the cortex
    8. Damage to the spinal cord or cauda equina
    9. Damage to cranial or spinal nerve roots

  C. Intraoperative physiological complications (often related to technical complications as well as to lack of information and to errors of judgment)
    1. Brain swelling
    2. Air embolus
    3. Hypertension
    4. Arrhythmias
    5. Hemorrhage
    6. Upward or downward herniation of the brain
  D. Postoperative complications (often related to the intraoperative complications as well as to lack of information and to errors of judgment)
    1. Physical complications
      a. CSF leakage
      b. Subgaleal fluid collections
      c. Poor wound healing or wound dehiscence
      d. Wound infection
      e. Systemic infection
      f. Poor cosmetic result of incision, including muscle weakness due to injury to the facial nerve or temporalis muscle by scalp incision
      g. Intracranial hematomas
      h. Pneumocephalus
    2. Physiological complications
      a. Arrhythmias
      b. Hypotension, hypertension
      c. Hypoxia
      d. Seizures
      e. Bacterial meningitis
      f. Aseptic meningitis
      g. Sepsis
      h. Fluid and electrolyte disturbances, especially hyponatremia
      i. Metabolic disturbances, especially hyperglycemia
      j. Pulmonary embolism
      k. Myocardial infarction

A consideration of the causes and types of operative complications indicates that many of the most serious complications are due to insufficient factual information about the patient or to an inadequate understanding of the patient's problem. Since surgery is a manual skill, improving one's surgical skills will reduce the incidence of specific technical complications. However, improving the interaction between the physician and the patient during all stages of treatment will result in prevention of the greatest number of complications.

The key to avoiding operative complications lies in aggressive and comprehensive preparation for the surgery. Neurosurgeons are fond of the term "aggressive," as in "aggressive management" and "aggressive surgery." However, "aggressive preparation" is more important than either. Meticulous planning of each of the steps required to perform the best possible operation for each patient should be carried out as aggressively as the surgery itself.

The process of surgical treatment can be divided into five phases:

1. Preoperative interaction with and evaluation of the patient
2. Formulation of the correct diagnosis
3. Choice of and planning of the operation
4. Execution of the operation
5. Postoperative and long-term care of the patient

Mental rehearsal of each of the steps in the five phases will identify the actions that need to be taken to decrease the possibility of complications during and after surgery.

Preoperative Interaction With and Evaluation of the Patient

Patients should be involved in the process of decision making concerning their surgery. The patient and the family should understand the entire sequence of studies necessary to make a diagnosis and the alternative medical therapies and surgical procedures that are available. Patients should have an understanding of the goals of surgery and of the technical and medical problems that must be dealt with in their care. An appreciation of the anatomy and physiology and of the healing processes relevant to their condition will help the patients deal with the prolonged period of pain, immobility, and disruption of work and home life that surgery entails. Explaining the anatomy of the skull, brain, and spine with models is very useful to helping patients to understand the techniques, goals, and limitations of the surgery they will undergo. It will also help the surgeon to understand the expectations of the patient concerning the surgery and will thereby aid in planning an operation that will come as close as possible to fulfilling those goals. Preoperative discussions also function to make manifest the events that can occur in each phase of investigation and treatment and can help the patient to understand that an unwanted, but expected result of the surgery is not a complication.

In addition to the surgeon's intellectual and emotional interaction with the patient concerning the neurosurgical illness, the general medical condition of the patient must be carefully evaluated. Hematological, cardiovascular, pulmonary, and endocrine functions should be analyzed. Any medications that the patient is taking should be reviewed, with special attention given to any that interfere with platelet function or blood coagulation or that interact with anesthetics or anticonvulsants. Any allergies to medications should also be identified.

Formulation of the Correct Diagnosis

One pitfall for the surgeon that can lead to complications is forming a preconception of the diagnosis. This danger increases as neurosurgeons assume more of the role of tertiary referral specialists and do less primary investigation of patients with neurological illness. Patients are now frequently referred to neurosurgeons with a specific diagnosis after having undergone extensive diagnostic studies, including magnetic resonance imaging (MRI) scans. The diagnosis that the patient bears at the time of referral can bias the surgeon's perception of the pathology and thus obscure the true diagnosis or mask secondary conditions. For example, a patient referred with the diagnosis of cervical spondylosis and myelopathy may have those conditions but may also have amyotrophic lateral sclerosis. Therefore it is important to start with a fresh view of each patient and to search for alternative explanations for the signs and symptoms. The significance of radiological abnormalities, particularly on myelography, must be carefully evaluated in terms of the patient's symptoms and signs.

Present governmental and insurance company regulations make it increasingly difficult to schedule patients for preoperative evaluations and surgery in a manner that allows adequate time to evaluate their neurological and medical status. The advent of "same-day admissions" for major surgery has, in practice, made it no longer possible for neurosurgeons, neurologists, neuroradiologists, and other involved specialists to see patients and evaluate their diagnostic studies and to meet together on the day before surgery in the hospital in order to discuss diagnosis and treatment in detail. Instead, the care of the patient has become fragmented. Therefore today, even more so than in the past, it is essential that the surgeon develop systematic methods to gain a thorough understanding of all aspects of the patient's history, neurological examination, laboratory studies, and radiological findings prior to performing surgery.

Choice of and Planning of the Operation

Each operation should be individualized, taking into consideration the patient's age and physiological status, job requirements, and factors such as the patient's willingness to accept a neurological deficit to accomplish a cure. These factors can only be understood by thorough preoperative interaction between patient and surgeon.

A surgeon should master a variety of surgical approaches and not be rigidly bound to doing a particular operation to treat a class of illnesses. For example, only using anterior or posterior approaches to the cervical spine may result in some patients not receiving optimal operative care. There are functional and anatomical situations in which one approach or another will better serve the individual patient.

A knowledge of topographic neuroanatomy and its variations will help to prevent complications. The anatomies of the different "corridors" leading to the base of the brain and to the ventricles should be well understood. When planning an approach to an intracranial lesion, it is important to have a three-dimensional mental image of the ventricular system, the anatomy of the cerebral hemispheres, the location of the sensory, motor, and eloquent areas, and the arterial supply and venous drainage of the brain. The visualization of these structures is particularly important for surgery for vascular malformations. Making drawings of the positions of the ventricular outlines and of the locations of arteries and veins by superimposing tracings of the different phases of the arteriograms will assist the surgeon in conceptualizing where the vessels will be found in the surgical approach that is chosen. Stereoscopic angiography can be particularly helpful when planning the surgery of arteriovenous malformations. MRI angiography to display vessels in three dimensions can also be useful.

The surgeon should be able to "run through" each step of the operation in his or her mind, visualizing each step. This will often alert the surgeon to particular technical patterns that must be solved, such as methods of controlling bleeding from major venous sinuses if they must be resected.

Execution of the Operation

The physical and mental states of the surgeon are important in obtaining good surgical results. It is important to obtain sufficient sleep and not to be fatigued. It is also important not to enter the operating room with a sense of irritation or frustration, which can be brought on by the tight schedules that are part of today's practice, as well as by the delays and frustrations that occur in obtaining operating room time.

Communication between all members of the operating team is a major factor in the prevention of complications. The team includes the anesthesiologist, the neuropathologist, often the infectious disease specialist, the operating room nurses, and the recovery room and intensive care nursing staffs. It is helpful to the nursing staff if the operation is properly posted on the operating room schedule, indicating the side of surgery and the position and any special equipment that will be needed, such as the ultrasonic aspirator or laser.

Communication with the anesthesiologist prior to induction of anesthesia is of the greatest importance. The extent to which the patient's neck can be extended during intubation should be discussed, as should the possible need for awake, fiberoptic intubation. The surgeon should be present during intubation and should personally support and guide the patient's head during positioning. The blood pressure levels that should be maintained, the amount of blood volume that can be lost without replacement, whether the patient will be likely to have air embolism, how much fluid should be administered, and whether adjuncts—such as osmotic or renal diuretics, antibiotics, anticonvulsants, and corticosteroids—will be used should all be discussed. Even with good preoperative communication with the anesthesiologist, however, it is still wise for the surgeon during the operation to check frequently the patient's blood pressure, volume of blood loss, urinary output, and amounts and types of fluids infused. Toward the end of the procedure, the surgeon should discuss with the anesthesiologist preparations to block postoperative hypertension, particularly in cases of posterior fossa surgery. Whether the patient will be kept intubated in the postoperative period should also be discussed.

If a large amount of blood loss is expected during surgery, preoperative arrangements should be made with the blood bank and the hematology service for possible treatment of coagulopathy after major transfusion. The use of the cell saver may be very helpful in some cases.

If neuropathological examination of tumorous biopsy material will be critical in determining the course of surgery, particularly when only a small piece of tissue will be available (as in the biopsy of an intramedullary spinal cord tumor or in stereotactic biopsy), preoperative discussion should be held with the neuropathologist.

Neurophysiological monitoring is gaining greater importance in neurosurgery, particularly during surgical removal of acoustic neuromas, tumors of the cavernous sinus, and intramedullary spinal tumors and vascular malformations. Preoperative discussion with the neurophysiologist should define the scope and goals of surgery and the parameters of the electrophysiological potentials that will be monitored.

The equipment that will be needed for the operative procedure should be discussed with the operating room nurses and should be laid out in a logical fashion prior to surgery. Instruments should be tested for proper functioning prior to the operation. Stylets should be removed from cannulas to be certain they can be removed after insertion, and they should be flushed to be certain that their lumens and apertures are open.

The relative positions of the patient, surgeon, operating microscope, nurses, and anesthesiologist should be envisioned prior to setting up the operating room. There are two goals in positioning a patient for surgery: (1) to provide the best physiological state for the patient and (2) to place the patient so that the surgeon can operate without becoming fatigued, and without experiencing undue bending of the body or prolonged elevation of the arms. The obese patient undergoing spinal surgery requires special consideration, with positioning on frames that prevent abdominal and thoracic compression. Patients should also be positioned to allow roentgenographs of the head or spine to be taken if they are needed for localization.

A prerequisite for performing successful surgery is that the surgeon be comfortable during surgery. I believe that most intracranial microsurgical operations should be done with the surgeon sitting. Individuals who work with their hands in situations demanding a high degree of control and precision, such as diamond cutters and engravers, generally sit while working to achieve greater steadiness of their hands and to reduce fatigue. Fatigue usually becomes a factor late in most major operations, just when particular technical problems must be faced, such as preserving the seventh nerve by dissecting it from the capsule of an acoustic tumor or avoiding damage to perforating arteries around basilar and anterior communicating artery aneurysms. Operating while sitting and using arm and wrist supports will reduce fatigue and can thereby reduce the incidence of complications. Fatigue can also be prevented by having another surgeon relieve the primary surgeon after a number of hours. While surgeons may pride themselves in their stamina and in being able to operate for long periods of time, fatigue impairs efficiency and judgment, particularly at critical points late in the course of an operation.

Another fundamental principle is always to have good lighting and good exposure. The use of headlight and loupe magnification and of the operating microscope for procedures requiring true microsurgical technique will improve outcome.

When positioning the operating microscope for use during surgery, the surgeon should take into consideration where it would also best help the assistants. For example, when operating on the right cerebellopontine angle (CPA) with the patient in the sitting position, the assistant can work better standing on the right side of the surgeon. However, when operating on the right CPA with the patient in the lateral prone position, the assistant is able to reach the operative field more easily if on the left side of the surgeon. The surgeon must also place the microscope in the position that will best visualize the pathology. For example, when performing a cervical foraminotomy with the patient in the prone position, the surgeon will have a better view of the pathology when standing on the side opposite to the foraminotomy so that the microscope can be used to look directly out into the foramen. Some additional points that are useful in avoiding intraoperative complications are as follows:

1. Always keep in mind the position of the patient's head in space when operating on the brain. To accomplish this, it is helpful to mark the orbitomeatal line (Reid's baseline) on the patient's scalp and to remember its orientation with respect to the floor of the operating room. To visualize its orientation, the sagittal MRI, computed tomography (CT) lateral scout view, or lateral angiogram or skull films should be taped on the view box with the orbitomeatal line drawn on the films and placed in the same spatial orientation as the line on the patient's scalp. This practice is especially helpful in avoiding going too posteriorly when operating in the interhemispheric fissure for a transcallosal approach to the third ventricle and in cannulating the frontal or occipital horn of the lateral ventricle.

2. The surgeon's goal is the restoration of normal anatomy and function. To accomplish this, it is essential to understand the normal anatomical planes. This is particularly important in suboccipital and cervical dissections. The muscles should be opened and identified layer by layer, and the muscles should be carefully closed in layers. An anatomical closure will almost always prevent CSF leakage. If hydrocephalus is present and has not been relieved by the surgery,

shunting or CSF diversion procedures should be carried out prior to closure.

3. An operating room policy should exist for double-checking the identity of the patient and the side and level of surgery. The surgeon, the assistant, the nurse, and the anesthesiologist all should verify the identity of the patient, the side of surgery, and the site of the surgery. Roentgenograms should be placed on the operating room view-boxes in such a way as to make identification of the side of pathology obvious. Many surgeons orient the films so that the anatomy is displayed in the same orientation as will be used in the operating field. For posterior approaches to the spine the surgeon will initially view the patient caudorostrally so that the right side of the patient is seen on the surgeon's right side. The films are therefore placed on the view-box in the same orientation.

4. The phenomenon of the surgeon becoming spatially disoriented during surgery, specifically with right-left and rostrocaudal disorientation, is a subject about which very little has been written. I believe that it is not an uncommon experience for surgeons, who clearly know which side of the brain or spinal cord they are operating on, nevertheless to have at some time during an operation a mental image of the expected anatomy that is disoriented with respect to the field. For example, when operating on the right internal acoustic meatus, the surgeon can be thinking of the arrangement of the divisions of the vestibulocochlear nerve as they lie in the left meatus. Rostrocaudal disorientation can also occur particularly when operating on the spinal cord. Disorientation is more likely to occur when using loupes or the operating microscope, which, despite the visual advantages that they confer, do limit the diameter of the visual field and reduce depth-of-field perception. The awareness of the possibility of spatial disorientation is the best form of defense against its occurrence. When using the microscope, it is helpful to look at the field directly at intervals to maintain proper orientation.

5. All containers, glasses, and vessels on the instrument table holding fluids, medication, or contrast material should be clearly labeled.

6. All surgeons encounter technical difficulties at times, and the surgeon's reactions at these times play a major part in overcoming the problem. A calm and measured approach will produce a more successful outcome than an approach characterized by extreme or hasty measures. Even major bleeding, particularly venous bleeding, can almost always be controlled by tamponade, providing time to organize for blood transfusion and to obtain equipment needed to control the bleeding if it is not present in the operating room.

7. Sponge, needle, and cottonoid counts should not be slighted. Any small object used in large numbers, such as Michel clips, should be counted. When tedious counts are made at the end of a long operation, the surgeon's patience may be tried, but this part of the procedure should not be hurried. If a count is not correct, a roentgenogram or CT scan should be obtained, the precise technique to be used being chosen on the basis of its technical capacity to identify the presumed retained object.

8. If a bone flap falls on the floor, a reasonable approach to this complication is to scrub it with an iodine-containing surgical scrub solution. The bone flap can then be wired into position in the usual manner.

9. The incidence of complications, particularly of infection, can be reduced by having a neat and clean operative field and by using irrigation liberally, but carefully, so as not to saturate the drapes.

10. The incidence of complications can be reduced by attention to detail and by concentration on all phases of the operation. Conversation should be confined to asking for instruments, discussing the patient's condition, and teaching. Playing and listening to music during surgery is probably not conducive to concentration by the entire operating team. Video display of the surgical field of the operating microscope is helpful in maintaining the concentration of the entire team on the operation.

11. Operative notes should be dictated immediately after a procedure is completed even if the procedure is completed late in the evening. Only then are the details of the procedure fully in the surgeon's mind. This is particularly important if a complication has occurred. The nature of the occurrence and the steps taken to treat it should be described clearly and dispassionately both in the dictated note and in the handwritten note in the chart. The transcribed operative notes should be read carefully and completely. Transcription errors, which occur frequently when technical procedures are described, should be corrected. Corrections should be initialled and dated. Incorrect statements in radiological, neuropathological, or laboratory reports should be noted and discussed with the physicians generating the reports. If the incorrectness of the report is verified, the report should be corrected or reissued.

Postoperative Care

The decision to extubate or to leave the patient intubated, particularly after postoperative fossa surgery, will generally be made during the latter stages of the operation based on the stability of the patient's physiological signs and the scope of the surgical removal. Postoperative physiological monitoring of intracranial and intra-arterial pressures and pulse oximeter measurement of arterial oxygen saturation are important continuous guides to the patient's physiological status. If increased intracranial pressure is likely during the postoperative period, cannulation of the lateral ventricle and postoperative monitoring of the intracranial pressure can be a lifesaving procedure.

The intensive care unit and recovery room staffs should receive a briefing about the surgery and about any problems that might occur in the postoperative period. The surgeon should frequently review the medication cardex, as this will at times reveal the omissions of a medication the surgeon thought was being administered or the continuation of a medication thought to have been discontinued. Postoperative notes detailing the patient's neurological status should be made frequently so that any change of status can be recognized.

PHYSICIAN-PATIENT INTERACTION AFTER COMPLICATIONS

When a complication has occurred there should be a complete discussion of the facts with the patient and the family as soon as the complication is identified. The reasons for the occurrence of the complication, the steps taken to treat the complication, and the prognosis should be fully discussed. When a complication occurs, the most important thing that the surgeon can do for the patient is to be supportive in all aspects of the patient's care while the patient is in the hospital and during long-term care.

EVALUATING AND IMPROVING OUTCOME

One of the most efficient methods of preventing complications is to know the frequency of their occurrence and then to modify practice and techniques in order to reduce their occurrence. The monthly mortality and morbidity conference is an important mechanism for improving the outcome of surgery.

MAXIMS CONCERNING COMPLICATIONS

Some aphorisms that are useful in guiding one's practice to avoid complications are as follows:

1. There is no such thing as a *simple* neurosurgical operation.
2. It is easier to stay out of trouble than to get out of trouble.
3. The time expended in avoiding complications will be more than recompensed by the time saved in not having to treat them.
4. The patient's well-being is paramount. A neurosurgeon should never hesitate to request consultation, or assistance, during surgery.
5. There is no situation in which the application of the Golden Rule is more apposite than in surgery. Surgeons should always operate with the meticulousness that they would wish for if they were the patient. It is salutary exercise for surgeons to think of their own feelings and reactions if they had to undergo the procedures being carried out.

2 Anesthetic Considerations

Susan Black
Roy F. Cucchiara

PREOPERATIVE ASSESSMENT

Principles

The preoperative assessment of a patient scheduled to undergo a supratentorial craniotomy is designed to determine if the patient is in optimal condition to undergo the stress of anesthesia and surgery (and, if not, to determine what further steps need to be taken to minimize risk), to evaluate risk to the patient related to the anesthetic and operative procedures, and to guide the choice of anesthetic techniques and appropriate perioperative monitoring. The evaluation of anesthetic risk, which is most predictive of postoperative morbidity and mortality, is the determination of the American Society of Anesthesiologists (ASA) physical status. Patients are classified as ASA physical status I through V based on condition for which they are coming to surgery, associated conditions, and other underlying but unassociated medical problems (Table 2-1).[36] Also included in the ASA classification is whether the operative procedure is elective or emergency, with emergency procedure designated by an "E" after the physical status. Perioperative morbidity and mortality rates are higher with higher physical status and in emergency versus elective procedures.

Routine preoperative work-up for any patient coming to the operating room for a surgical procedure should be performed whether local anesthesia with sedation, regional anesthesia, or general anesthesia is planned. Accepting lower standards for patients scheduled for local or regional anesthesia can lead to serious problems. Significant complications can occur with all types of anesthetics. One should not assume that local or regional anesthesia is safer and therefore requires less preoperative testing or intraoperative monitoring than does general anesthesia. Also the possibility that the local or regional anesthesia may become inadequate and thus that general anesthesia becomes necessary, due either to problems related to the anesthetic or to the operative procedure, must be considered. Clearly it is not feasible to stop at that point and complete the work-up that should have been done preoperatively.

The preoperative anesthetic evaluation should begin with a complete history and physical examination. There are several areas of particular concern to the anesthesiologist. Prior history of exposure to anesthesia, any problems associated with prior anesthetics, and family history of problems related to anesthesia are important. These problems include allergic reactions to anesthetic agents such as the local anesthetics (most commonly the esters and only rarely the amide local anesthetics) or thiopental (rare but potentially lethal) and unusual reactions to drugs such as prolonged muscle paralysis following use of succinylcholine (due to a genetic deficiency in the enzyme responsible for its breakdown). The nature of any supposed allergic reaction should be described. Frequently what the patient describes as an allergic reaction may be only a common side effect of the drug that does not necessarily preclude its use. A rare but potentially fatal complication of anesthesia is malignant hyperthermia (MH), and a personal or family history of MH must be sought. MH is a genetic disorder that results in an abnormal response of the skeletal muscle to certain anesthetic agents, the muscle relaxant succinylcholine and the volatile anesthetic agents. This response is characterized by a

Table 2-1. American Society of Anesthesiologists Physical Status Classification for Surgical Patients

Category	Description
I	Healthy patient
II	Mild systemic disease, no functional limitation
III	Severe systemic disease, definite limitations
IV	Severe systemic disease that is a constant threat to life
V	Moribund patient not expected to survive 24 hours

severe increase in temperature, acidosis, cardiac arrhythmias, seizures, myoglobinuria, renal failure, and death if not promptly diagnosed and correctly treated.[11] Most often patients who have survived a prior episode of MH or have an MH-susceptible relative will be well informed and volunteer that information. Occasionally, however, the only clue is a history of an unexpected and unexplained death under anesthesia in a relative, and this should be investigated by an anesthesiologist prior to proceeding with an elective procedure. It is possible to administer a safe anesthetic to an MH-susceptible patient as long as certain anesthetic drugs ("triggering agents") are avoided and appropriate precautions taken.

Other areas in the history of particular interest to the anesthesiologist are allergies to other drugs, current medications, symptoms of esophageal reflux, and history of cardiorespiratory, renal, or liver diseases. Medications the patient is taking may alter response to the anesthetic, and a few medications, such as the monoamine oxidase inhibitors, probably should be discontinued prior to an elective procedure. Most drugs should be continued up to the time the patient is brought to the operating room. Complications related to their withdrawal are frequently more common and more severe than are those associated with their use in the perioperative period. Symptoms of esophageal reflux indicate that the patient is at increased risk of aspiration of gastric contents with induction of general anesthesia, as are patients who have eaten prior to the procedure. Changes in the technique of induction of anesthesia in these patients are necessary. Significant cardiac or respiratory disease may alter the induction technique used and the necessary monitoring. Renal and hepatic disease alter the metabolism and elimination of many of the anesthetic agents, and alterations in dosing are indicated.

The preoperative physical examination should be thorough, with special attention paid to certain areas. The anatomy of the airway should be examined for indications of possible difficulty with intubation. Cervical range of motion should be determined to aid in positioning the patient intraoperatively. Once the patient is anesthetized and paralyzed, the head can be positioned in such a way as to cause injury to the cervical spinal cord or brachial plexus. Knowledge of the patient's range of motion when awake and not exceeding that after induction of anesthesia will greatly reduce the risk. Physical examination for signs of cardiac or respiratory disease is, of course, important.

The routine ordering of a large battery of preoperative tests is not necessary, cost effective, or indicated. Rather it is more appropriate to chose tests based on the patient's age, history, and physical examination. Only laboratory tests that are likely to give additional information that will aid in the perioperative management of the patient need be utilized.

Cardiology

Patients with cardiac disease present a special challenge in the perioperative period. Patients with coronary artery disease are at risk for perioperative myocardial ischemia with or without long-term complications. Preoperative assessment of these patients begins with a thorough cardiac history, including congestive heart failure (CHF), arrhythmias, and anginal pattern. The timing of any prior myocardial infarctions (MIs) should be reviewed, as well as current cardiac medications. Appropriate preoperative evaluation of a patient with suspected coronary artery disease depends on the likelihood of significant disease. Electrocardiogram (ECG) is routine. Further work-up (which may include exercise treadmill, dypridamole-thallium scans, and cardiac catheterization) to evaluate risk for perioperative myocardial ischemic events depends on the severity and stability of the patient's symptoms. If the patient is known to have suffered a prior MI or to have symptoms suggestive of CHF, some evaluation of cardiac function should be performed. Noninvasive precordial echocardiogram will detect ischemic wall motion patterns and major valvular defects and give a quantitative measure of ejection fraction (EF). A low EF value (<25 percent) is an important finding that indicates increased risk, specific anesthetic considerations, and likely need for increased cardiovascular monitoring intra- and postoperatively. Prior to any elective surgical procedure the patient's medical status should be optimized and stabilized. This may require further work-up or medication, a change in medical management, or coronary revascularization.

Those who have suffered a recent (within 6 months) MI are at significantly increased risk for perioperative infarction and death compared with those with more distant prior MI.[39] When possible, surgery should be postponed until 6 months or more following an MI. When this is not possible, intensive intraoperative and postoperative (up to 48 hours) monitoring and treatment has been shown to decrease the risk for perioperative cardiac morbidity and mortality.[34]

Patients with a history of cardiac failure have an increased risk for perioperative morbidity, and evaluation of their current myocardial function should guide in the choice of anesthetic technique and perioperative monitoring. This can be accomplished with a history and physical examination. However, obtaining preoperative echocardiography is often very useful and is noninvasive, presenting little if any risk to the patient. This test should be considered in any patient with a history of myocardial dysfunction. Likewise, a history of valvular heart disease requires further evaluation of current cardiac status. This often can be accomplished with the combination of a history and physical examination combined with echocardiography.

Uncontrolled or poorly controlled hypertension should be treated prior to any elective procedure. Uncontrolled hypertension can increase the hemodynamic lability intraoperatively and will alter the cerebral autoregulatory response, shifting the cerebral autoregulatory curve to the right (see below). These patients may experience a decrease in cerebral blood flow at a higher blood pressure than a patient with a normal autoregulatory response. Controlling the blood pressure will, with time, return the autoregulatory curve to normal.[27] The optimal duration of treatment of hypertension prior to surgery is not known, but is a matter of weeks rather than days.

Respiration

Patients with significant preoperative pulmonary dysfunction are at greater risk for pulmonary complications in the postoperative period. This risk can be evaluated by history and physical examination complimented by pulmonary function testing when indicated by the severity of the symptoms. Any reversible or improvable component of the pulmonary dysfunction should be treated preoperatively. It is important to ensure that patients with significant pulmonary disease have their medical status optimized prior to any elective procedure. In spite of this, there are a few patients who will have significant pulmo-nary complications postoperatively that may result in the need for long-term ventilatory support.

Neurology

It is important for the anesthesiologist to have a thorough understanding of the patient's neurological disease. In patients with mass lesions, the degree and potential for increase in intracranial pressure (ICP) are important considerations. During the perioperative period, there are numerous interventions that the anesthesiologist can make to alter the ICP. The need for this can only be anticipated if the preoperative status is known. Any preoperative neurological deficits, especially cranial nerve deficits, give important clues to possible postoperative problems. For example, patients with deficits of the ninth and tenth cranial nerves preoperatively may well have difficulty protecting their airway postoperatively and should only be extubated after very careful consideration and evaluation. In patients with vascular lesions, the timing of any prior hemorrhage will indicate potential perioperative problems with either re-bleeding or vasospasm. Information from computed tomography (CT) scans, magnetic resonance imaging (MRI), or angiography concerning the size, location, and vascularity of the lesion will indicate risk for significant blood loss intraoperatively and therefore the need for intravenous access, monitoring, and blood products. The more information available to predict potential intraoperative and postoperative problems, the better able the anesthesiologist will be to avoid or to lessen the risk for those events.

PREPARATION IN THE OPERATING ROOM

Monitoring Principles

Neurosurgical procedures are generally considered major surgery, and anesthetic monitoring is influenced by that assessment as well as by concomitant disease from which the patient may suffer. Whenever special techniques are to be employed to offer the surgeon an advantage in the operative field, more specialized patient monitoring may become necessary to manage the physiological changes induced. The use of those noninvasive monitors that have extremely low complication rates is desirable whenever such monitors can meet the requirements of the situation in response time, accuracy, and reproducibility. Many neurosurgical cases require on-line real-time monitoring systems because the situation can change quickly, and rapid response to the change is necessary before large swings in vital signs occur. Rapid assessment of the treatment is also necessary to avoid inducing impairment of physiological function by overtreatment. A concept that is frequently poorly understood is that of redundancy in monitoring. Back-up systems for all parameters are clearly important should the primary system of monitoring fail at a crucial part of the procedure. But they are equally important as a check system to be sure that the values reported by redundant systems agree. Because of the crucial nature of the data in decision making, it is vital that the data be correct and verified. Thus what can appear to the untrained as "too many gadgets" is a complex functioning system of primary and secondary monitors that provides the necessary redundancy to manage patients undergoing significant physiological trespass.

The ASA has recommended minimal monitoring standards for surgical cases. In short, these standards require an oxygen monitor of the anesthesia circuit, pulse oximetry, end-tidal CO_2 analysis, a ventilator alarm, ECG, and blood pressure and temperature measurements. Nearly all supratentorial cases require somewhat more complex intraoperative monitoring than the minimum standards suggest.

Vascular Access

Direct arterial pressure monitoring via an indwelling arterial catheter provides beat to beat information about blood pressure and the character of the pulse wave; it permits the sampling of arterial blood for gas tensions (arterial blood gases), glucose, electrolytes, and drug blood levels. We find it best to try to place the arterial catheter in the radial artery of the arm that is in sight of the anesthesiologist. This permits early detection of dislodgement of the line and of hematoma formation. It has been demonstrated that an Allen's test for collateral circulation is not too helpful in preventing ischemic injury to the extremity. If there are identification armbands on the arm where the radial cannula is placed we usually cut them, especially when it is necessary to place the arterial line in an extremity that we cannot observe during the case. This prevents the occasional case of hematoma formation with tight constriction of the arm by the band. Careful attention must be paid to securing the arterial line so that accidental dislodgement is unlikely. Some physicians use sutures for this task. We use a tape technique that seems to be just as effective without running the risk of impaling or trap-

ping the radial nerve or its superficial branches with a suture. We flush the catheter with a few milliliters of saline and observe the site for blanching. If blanching occurs it suggests that the saline has perfused a superficial branch of the artery and deprived the skin of its blood flow. When that happens we are careful to keep future flush efforts to a minimum so as to decrease the likelihood of late formation of a skin ulcer at that site. The decision as to whether to place the arterial catheter while the patient is awake or immediately after induction depends on the presence of concomitant disease and on the patient's general condition. When other risks are small we place the arterial catheter soon after anesthesia is induced, using the blood pressure cuff until then. Accurate placement of the transducer is necessary to obtain a pressure reading that can be referred to the organ at greatest risk (the brain). In general we visualize a line connecting the external auditory meati and place the transducer at a level crossing the center of that line. This technique ensures that the transducer is always related to cerebral perfusion pressure no matter the body or head position, thus preventing confusion among the paramedical personnel who assist us in this task. When radial artery cannulation is difficult or unsuccessful, we do not hesitate to use the arteries of the feet, the dorsalis pedis being technically easier to cannulate than the posterior tibial artery. The use of arterial catheters in neurosurgical patients seems to be quite safe, especially regarding ischemic problems. The catheters can generally be removed within 24 hours, and there is seldom a low output state that predisposes to extremity ischemia.

We find the use of a single intravenous (IV) line for induction of anesthesia to be quite acceptable. There is little reason to subject the routine patient to the unpleasantness of having more than one intravenous (IV) line started prior to induction. The sequence of line placement deserves comment. Generally we work to obtain arterial cannulation before proceeding to obtaining multiple venous access routes. The reason for this is to monitor the patient's pressure optimally during the period when we are concentrating on perhaps difficult IV access or placement of a central line. It is very easy for all personnel to get so involved in the immediate task at hand that the overall status of the patient may be unobserved for a short time. The arterial waveform helps to prevent that distraction. The decision as to the number of IVs necessary in a given case is a clinical decision. We usually have two IVs or the ready access to visible veins, which ensures that we can quickly get a second IV if things go poorly. Additional IVs may be needed as separate lines for the infusion of vasoactive agents. Trying to piggyback these agents into existing IV lines can lead to problems as the drugs accumulate in the line and are suddenly flushed in by changing the infusion rate. Thus it is safest and most controllable to have these types of drugs on infusion pumps running directly to a dedicated IV. When the surgical plan includes the intraoperative use of mannitol we try to place a single IV just for this purpose, to be removed as soon as surgery is completed to try to avoid the inflammation of the vein associated with that agent. The location of IV placement is not critical. When we need multiple IVs for a large patient we do not hesitate to use the veins of the feet. However, we are careful not to give irritating drugs through these catheters, and we try to remove them as soon as possible after surgery is completed to reduce the likelihood of thromboembolic complications.

Decisions on placement of central venous lines are based on several considerations. We have concerns about central line placement from the internal jugular route (although we often use it) for fear of puncturing the carotid artery and reducing arterial flow to the brain or somehow obstructing the venous outflow from the brain when the head is turned with a catheter in place, but we have found no clinical evidence that this occurs. The advantages of the technique in the perioperative setting are that there is a much lower risk of pneumothorax than with cannulation of the subclavian vein, and most anesthesiologists have more experience with this approach. The subclavian approach is effective, carries different risks, and is useful in our hands. We avoid administering mannitol or other irritating agents through an atrial central line, because we think this has caused thrombus formation and serious embolization in one of our patients. Meningiomas and metastatic tumors to the brain have a tendency to bleed, increasing the likelihood that the ability to monitor hemodynamic parameters will be useful. Procedures that have a likelihood of exposing a cerebral venous sinus to the atmosphere (e.g., a tumor invading the sinus) suggest special monitoring for early detection of venous air embolism. A right heart catheter may be lifesaving in these patients in the event of massive air embolism through an open dural sinus.

Airway Control

The basic principles of airway control for any situation apply in neurosurgical cases as well. However, the margin for error may be considerably smaller in dealing with patients with elevated ICP since both hypoxia and hypercarbia are potent stimuli to cerebrovasodilatation, increased cerebral blood volume, and thus further increase in ICP to dangerous levels. In addition, it is likely that compromised areas of brain tissue do not have the reserve capacity to tolerate episodes of hypoxia as well as normal brain tissue.

We have found that simply placing the mask on the patient's face frequently causes the ICP to increase slightly, even before we have administered any agents. Some suggest that patients should be asked to hyperventilate themselves while awake to decrease carbon dioxide, cerebral blood flow (CBF), and ICP prior to induction. We have not felt this to be necessary, since our primary induction agent is thiopental, which dramatically reduces CBF and ICP at the moment of induction of anesthesia. We feel that the small increase in anxiety and ICP that occurs with the placement of the mask is outweighed by the opportunity to complete a preoxygenation scheme that fills the lungs with a high concentration of oxygen. This is especially true of the functional residual capacity of the lung, that volume that is not quickly exchanged during ventilation but that is, in effect, a pulmonary reservoir of oxygen should the airway become obstructed.

For one of us (R.F.C.) a rapid sequence induction with thiopental is routinely utilized with succinylcholine whenever possible for facilitation of tracheal intubation. The thiopental reduces ICP, and the slight increase with succinylcholine does not usually bring the ICP back up to baseline. While this technique carries the risk of inadequate paralysis, it helps to protect against regurgitation and aspiration. Many anesthesiologists (including S.B.) prefer a more controlled induction with an intravenous agent and use of a nondepolarizing muscle relaxant with slower onset but more predictable effect when the patient is not at increased risk for aspiration. This requires a period of ventilation before the endotracheal tube can be placed, but paralysis can be assured by neuromuscular monitoring and the blood pressure response can be titrated by using smaller quantities of drugs over a longer period of time. Either method is effective when properly utilized.

As stereotactic neurosurgery becomes increasingly popular, additional airway problems are imposed on the anesthesiologist. Those patients having neurodiagnostic studies performed the same day as their surgery come to the operating room with the head frame in place. All of our frames have a removable piece over the mouth. Limitation of extension of the neck by the frame against the back of the shoulders may prevent adequate laryngoscopy for smooth tracheal intubation. There are basically three techniques available for such patients. Standard laryngoscopy can often be used, especially if supplemented by first passing an intubating stylet into the larynx and sliding the tube in over it. It is difficult to predict which patients are good candidates for this approach. Mask fit is difficult, and ventilation may be difficult as well. Use of the fiberoptic bronchoscope or some variant of it is extremely helpful in securing the airways in these patients. This can be performed in the asleep or awake patient but in any case requires careful attention to topical anesthesia of the laryngeal innervation to prevent coughing and straining. Lastly, when these techniques do not succeed readily, one can use a retrograde wire-modified Seldinger technique (Fig. 2-1). A steel 18-gauge needle is introduced at the tracheal rings, and a long wire is passed up through the larynx into the mouth. A tube is placed on the wire and slid down into the larynx and the wire removed. In our experience placement of the wire entry at the cricothyroid membrane, as is usually described, results in too short a distance between the cords and the wire exit point such that the tube does not seat well into the larynx and tends to deflect when the wire is pulled. If the tube is pushed, the wire may kink into an S pattern and be very difficult or impossible to remove. Use of a standard teflon needle over steel entry into the trachea sometimes fails because of kinking of the catheter when the steel is removed. The wire should not be passed through the Murphy eye of the tube as is frequently suggested, because it tends to get caught at

the glottis as it is passed. This technique can be performed with the patient awake or asleep, but when awake, the patient suffers discomfort and coughs, which is undesirable.

The use of a pulse oximeter is very helpful in performing these more difficult intubations because of the warning of hypoxia before clinical signs become visible to the naked eye. We always use such a device in these patients because of the manipulations involved and the significantly added risk to the airways.

Cardiac Monitoring

The use of the ECG is a "standard" in anesthesia practice. Further levels of monitoring are dictated by the patient's condition and by the risks of the surgical procedure. The use of invasive monitors follows these principles as well. The pulmonary artery catheter is useful to evaluate left ventricular function and cardiac filling pressures as well as for detection of myocardial ischemia. Except in cases of known or likely left ventricular dysfunction, significant coronary artery disease, or anticipated massive vascular volume shifts, the pulmonary artery catheter offers no advantage. The right atrial catheter is a less sensitive but reasonably effective intravascular volume monitor in patients with good cardiac function. In the usual cases of venous air embolism it offers a possible pathway for aspiration of the bubbles if properly

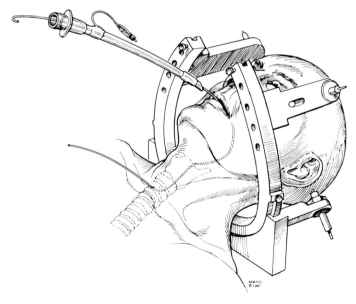

Figure 2-1. Use of the Seldinger retrograde wire/intubation technique for difficult airway management in a head frame patient. (By permission of Mayo Foundation.)

placed and is much more effective for air aspiration than a pulmonary artery catheter. Echocardiography has emerged as a reasonably sensitive, noninvasive measure of left ventricular dysfunction and a very sensitive detection device for venous air embolism. It is not widely used for supratentorial cases.

Intracranial Pressure

The measurement of ICP has received considerable attention in both clinical practice and research. Neither preoperative placement of a ventricular catheter nor the preoperative/intraoperative use of the Ladd monitor or the Richmond bolt is widely practiced. Drainage of cerebrospinal fluid (CSF) from the lumbar space is an effective technique to decrease ventricular volume size and thus the need for marked retraction, and it can be used to measure lumbar CSF pressure. There are several methods by which this can be accomplished. Our feeling is that the person placing the CSF drain must be the person responsible for maintaining it if it should need an alteration in position. This is because of the subtleties of placement that only the operator knows about in a given patient. We use a malleable spinal needle made of a nickel-silver alloy so that it will not break when changes in patient position put lateral stresses on the shaft. It is more difficult to place than a standard nonreusable needle because of its metallurgic properties. The tip does not have the same sharpness of point that the single-use needle has, perhaps making nerve impalement less likely. This needle can be redirected should the flow of fluid cease at a critical point in the operation. Another popular method is the use of an indwelling catheter threaded into the lumbar subarachnoid space. We have not been as happy with this system because the catheters seem to kink as they warm and the removal of CSF can be very slow. However, many feel this system is adequate for their needs and utilize it with unreported success rates.

Neurological Monitoring

For intraoperative neurological monitoring to be of value it is necessary that the structure monitored be at risk for intraoperative injury, that the monitor is sensitive to any intraoperative insult, and that if a change is detected some intervention is possible to reduce the risk for permanent damage. The modalities available for intraoperative neurological monitoring include neurological assessment of the awake patient, electroencephalogram (EEG), sensory evoked potentials (SEPs), motor evoked potentials (MEPs),

and electromyography (EMG). The need for and feasibility of utilizing any monitoring modality intraoperatively must be determined preoperatively. This will not only ensure that the equipment will be available but also will encourage communication between the neurosurgeon, neurologist, and neuroanesthesiologist, which is essential for successful use of the monitoring modality.

Monitoring the neurological status of the awake patient has been utilized during thalamotomy, carotid endarterectomy, and seizure surgery. It clearly provides an accurate prediction of postoperative neurological function. However, it presents the obvious difficulty of performing a major operative procedure on an awake patient. Should any untoward intraoperative event necessitate the institution of general anesthesia, the risk of this may be greatly increased by the limited access the anesthesiologist will likely have to the patient and his airways. Successful use of this technique requires the cooperation of a skilled surgical and anesthetic team as well as a cooperative and motivated patient.

The EEG is generated by spontaneous electrical activity of the brain. It has been used intraoperatively during neurosurgical procedures to detect cerebral ischemia such as might occur during carotid endarterectomy or aneurysm clipping and to guide surgical resection during epilepsy surgery. The "gold standard" for EEG monitoring is the unprocessed 16-channel EEG. This technique requires the expertise of an experienced electroencephalographer, which may not be readily available in many operating rooms. With the advent of computer-processed EEG, intraoperative EEG monitoring has become more readily available. However, there are several limitations of processed EEG that must be kept in mind. There must be some representation of both frequency and amplitude, or some intraoperative changes may be missed. As the signal becomes more and more processed and remote from the raw data, it will become more difficult to apply what we know about unprocessed EEG to the processed signal. In general, fewer channels will be analyzed by a processed EEG machine than by the standard 16-channel EEG. This is usually adequate for intraoperative use. Finally, some changes that can occur intraoperatively are unilateral and others bilateral. It is important that both hemispheres be monitored and displayed so that bilateral and unilateral changes can be diagnosed, as very different intraoperative events will lead to the two types of changes.[4]

SEP include somatosensory evoked potentials (SSEPs), brainstem auditory evoked potentials

(BAEPs), and visual evoked potentials (VEPs). All have been used intraoperatively during a wide variety of procedures with varying degrees of success. All types of SEPs consist of recorded electrical potentials generated by repetitive stimulation of a sensory nerve. In monitoring SEPs the generated waveform is analyzed, and the latency preceding the generated waveforms and their amplitudes are measured.

SSEPs are generated by repetitive stimulation of a peripheral sensory nerve and recording the resulting electrical potential at several points along its course, including the peripheral nerve itself, the plexus, lumbar, or cervical spinal cord, and over the sensory cortex. SSEP monitoring has been used extensively in operative procedures, placing either the sensory pathway or adjacent structures at risk. Common indications include spine surgery such as scoliosis correction or decompressive laminectomy, brainstem procedures, and cerebrovascular procedures such as aneurysm clipping, arteriovenous malformation (AVM) resection, and carotid endarterectomy. A major limitation of this technique is that it does not directly monitor motor function, and it is possible during some procedures for isolated motor deficits to occur that SSEP monitoring would not detect.[4,13]

BAEPs are generated by repetitive auditory stimulation and recording of the resulting electrical potential as it passes from the auditory nerve and to the brainstem with recording electrodes placed on the scalp. Intraoperatively these have been utilized most commonly during posterior fossa procedures such as cranial nerve decompressions and acoustic neuroma resection.[4,13]

VEPs are generated with repetitive delivery of flashes of light to the eye and recording of generated potentials over the occipital cortex. These have been utilized during procedures that place the optic pathways at risk, such as ophthalmic artery aneurysm clipping and pituitary tumor resection. However, they are the least reliable of the SEP and as a result are infrequently utilized.[4,13,35]

MEPs involve a modality that is still in the experimental stages of intraoperative use. MEPs are generated by delivering a magnetic stimulation over the motor cortex and monitoring over the path of the motor tracts at the level of the spinal cord, peripheral nerve, or muscle. Although they have great potential especially during spine surgery, they appear to be difficult to record reliably in the operating room environment.[4,17]

EMG recordings are generated by stimulation of a peripheral motor nerve and recording the resulting action potential in the muscle innervated by that nerve. They are of use only when the peripheral nerve is at risk, such as the facial nerve during acoustic neuroma resection. In that procedure, EMG monitoring has been shown to be effective in presenting facial nerve function.[14]

INTRAOPERATIVE MANAGEMENT

Principles

The goal of neuroanesthesia for supratentorial brain lesions is to facilitate surgical exposure consistent with maintenance of organ system function. ICP control is a key element in achievement of this goal. Because ICP is not strictly related to symptoms, one can never be sure where on the intracranial elastance ($\Delta p/\Delta v$) curve a given patient is situated preoperatively. We know that various anesthetic agents have quite profound effects on ICP, primarily by their effects on CBF and cerebral blood volume (Fig. 2-2). In the practical control of ICP during induction of anesthesia, agents that lower ICP markedly are preferred.

Maintenance of blood pressure to prevent cerebral ischemia requires a balance between the ICP, myocardial oxygen consumption, and cardiac perfusion. Sophisticated intraoperative monitoring is occasionally being used and requires modification of the anesthetic techniques of which the surgeon should be aware. The ergonomics of the anesthetist's work station is receiving increasing attention, as studies reveal its importance in prevention of anesthesia mishaps.

Anesthetic Management

ICP Control During Induction

Many things occur sequentially during induction (Table 2-2). Timing is important. Approaches that seem generally similar may produce very different patient responses because of timing and duration of pharmacologic intervention to balance stimulation.

One popular technique is preinduction voluntary hyperventilation. While hyperventilation decreases ICP, the application of a face mask to some awake brain tumor patients has been shown to transiently elevate ICP, perhaps because of anxiety. The ability to adequately preoxygenate the patient outweighs this concern in most situations. We do not know whether we can predict which response will occur in a given patient. On the other hand, that may not be critical because thiopental dramatically decreases ICP in doses commonly used for induction. It is this

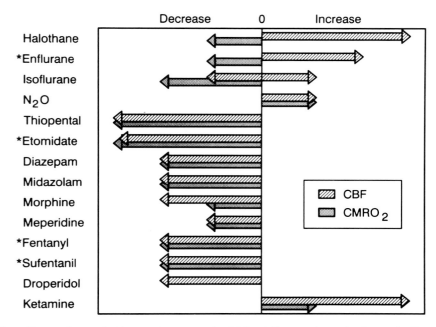

Figure 2-2. The effects of anesthetic agents on cerebral blood flow and cerebral metabolism. (From Cucchiara et al.,[7] with permission.)

effect on ICP that makes thiopental such a valuable induction agent in tumor patients. In addition, it very rapidly produces unconsciousness, it is well tolerated by most patients, and it is a drug that most anesthesiologists feel comfortable using. However, it is short acting.

One of the most common mismatches in timing relative to ICP control is the use of thiopental and nondepolarizing muscle relaxants. Techniques that use the approach are valuable and are to be recommended. However, total paralysis is sought to avoid an elevation of ICP during intubation. Depending on dose, this level of relaxation may take 3 minutes to achieve, during which time the central nervous system (CNS) effects of the thiopental are decreasing, the patient's anesthetic level is lightening, CBF is coming up toward control, and the reduction in ICP is being reversed. Intubation at this point will likely

result in elevation of blood pressure and a probable increase in ICP. Thus the proper selection of drugs may not give the anticipated results. Additional thiopental just before intubation will blunt those responses. It may also be helpful to supplement the induction drugs with fentanyl or a β-blocker. Fentanyl is a cerebral vasoconstrictor and will reduce ICP, and β-blockade will prevent hypertension with high perfusion pressures that allow breakthrough in autoregulation.

Some are concerned with the use of nitrous oxide because of studies suggesting that it causes an increase in cerebral metabolic rate for oxygen ($CMRO_2$), CBF, and thus ICP. It is true that nitrous oxide studies show these effects. These studies are not clinically very worrisome because the effect of nitrous oxide on CBF is easily blunted by the concomitant use of thiopental or hyperventilation during induction. Although we most frequently utilize intravenous inductions, it may be necessary in some uncooperative patients (especially young children) to perform an inhalation induction, usually with nitrous oxide and a volatile agent. When using an inhalation induction, it is prudent to start an IV line as soon as possible for administration of drugs such as thiopental to control ICP or hemodynamics.

Succinylcholine (SCh) can cause an elevation in ICP by contraction of the abdominal muscles or by a complex mechanism affecting muscle spindles. Again, these effects can be clinically eliminated by

Table 2-2. Control of ICP on Induction

Thiopental
Narcotic
Nondepolarizing muscle relaxant
Hyperventilation, ensure high SaO_2
Blunt stress of intubation
   Deepen anesthetic
      Narcotic, thiopental
      Lidocaine
      β-blockade (short acting)
Prompt intubation

induction doses of thiopental. Nondepolarizing muscle relaxants are generally preferred because they do not increase ICP either directly or indirectly.

Blood pressure control during induction may be important when there is loss of autoregulation in areas of pathology. Since flow is pressure dependent in areas without autoregulation and ICP is related to CBF via cerebral blood volume, and since we do not know which, if any, areas have lost autoregulation, it seems clinically prudent to control blood pressure to levels that the patient sustained awake. Blunting the hemodynamic response to intubation can be achieved by increasing the depth of anesthesia or by blocking the cardiovascular response with vasoactive agents.

Choice of Anesthetic

Most, but not all, anesthetics can be used safely in patients with cerebral lesions. There are specific effects of the agents that may require certain ancillary techniques in their administration to ensure appropriate pharmacological and physiological responses. The effects of the agent on ICP, cerebral perfusion pressure (CPP), CBF, cerebral metabolic rate (CMR), promptness of return of consciousness, drug-related protection from cerebral ischemia or edema, blood pressure control, and compatibility with neurophysiological monitoring techniques are important considerations.

Most craniotomy surgery in the United States is probably performed following a thiopental induction of anesthesia with intubation of the trachea after a nondepolarizing relaxant and maintenance with nitrous oxide–isoflurane–fentanyl in various combinations during hypocarbia to $PaCO_2$ levels of 28 to 33 mmHg. This is our preferred technique as well.

If the volatile agents are used to produce deeper levels of anesthesia with normocarbia an increase in ICP is an expected pharmacological result. However, this is rarely done in neurosurgery. Most commonly, minimum alveolar concentration (MAC) less than 1.0 of a volatile agent is combined with moderate hyperventilation to provide an adequate level of anesthesia and to avoid increases in ICP. The greatest reduction in cerebral vascular resistance and the greatest increase in ICP is produced by halothane. In humans, this can be blunted or even eliminated by establishing hypocarbia before administration of the agent.[2] Isoflurane also reduces cerebral vascular resistance and increases ICP at normocarbia, but this response can be blocked by simultaneous introduction of hyperventilation in tumor patients.[1] It has been suggested that patients with a midline shift on CT scan

are more likely to show an elevation in ICP during isoflurane anesthesia, but the clinical applicability of the data is not striking.[12] On balance, human studies suggest that isoflurane is a safe anesthetic drug when used with hyperventilation for intracranial surgery.[20]

Intravenous anesthetics (e.g., thiopental, fentanyl) decrease $CMRO_2$ and CBF together. This allows a reduction in ICP to be accomplished by modification of the vascular compartment. Thiopental safely produces a profound linked reduction in $CMRO_2$ and CBF to near one-half of the awake values.[8] The dramatic reduction in ICP that can be achieved with this drug clinically is secondary to these cerebral effects. Over the decades there has been a waxing and waning of enthusiasm for thiopental as an induction and maintenance agent in neurosurgical anesthesia. It is still our preferred induction agent in cerebral tumor patients. The effectiveness of thiopental as a cerebral protective drug should probably be viewed as applicable to the experimental conditions for which protection is most solidly demonstrated, that is, cerebral ischemia by vascular occlusion techniques. Cerebral protection produced by lowering ICP in cerebral tumor patients is a distinctly different, although useful, concept. Etomidate decreases $CMRO_2$ with a lesser reduction in CBF and is a useful induction agent for special situations of hemodynamic instability. It is known to produce myoclonus and possible seizure activity.

Of the short-acting narcotics, fentanyl has been the most completely studied. It decreases CBF slightly more than it decreases $CMRO_2$.[20] This imbalance could theoretically predispose to cerebral ischemia, but such a consideration does not seem to be clinically important. Fentanyl is useful in neurosurgical anesthesia because it lowers ICP through a decreased CBF and affords maintenance of stable heart rate and blood pressure during surgical stimulus. Although it has not been studied as thoroughly yet, sufentanil seems to have a different effect on CBF. Acutely, it produces a dramatic increase in CBF and ICP in animals and in humans.[22,29] Alfentanil does not increase ICP if the blood pressure is allowed to fall, but it does increase ICP if blood pressure is maintained (Michenfelder, JD, unpublished data).

Choice of Muscle Relaxants

Muscle relaxants can probably affect the conduct of a neuroanesthetic as much as can the primary agent. SCh as yet appears unequaled in achieving total rapid paralysis for the rapid sequence intubation of the trachea. There is still controversy regarding SCh-induced increases in ICP.[21,30] However, such increases are probably clinically insignificant, except, perhaps, in the most extreme cases of intracranial hypertension. Since complete flaccidity is required to avoid coughing and straining during intubation of the trachea and thus avoid ICP increases, it is reasonable to use a nerve stimulator during induction and intubation in these cases. The shorter acting, nondepolarizing muscle relaxants (vecuronium, atracurium) are well suited for intubation paralysis in cases of elevated ICP. They do not increase ICP and have little or no effect on heart rate and blood pressure.[31,40]

Hemiplegia from cerebral ischemia or from cerebral tumor is associated with differences in response to nondepolarizing muscle relaxants on the two sides of the body. The affected extremities are resistant to neuromuscular blockade by nondepolarizing muscle relaxants.[5,10] In most operating room arrangements, the face and endotracheal tube are turned toward the anesthetist so that the operative field is uppermost. This places the extremities contralateral to the tumor in a position that allows easy monitoring of neuromuscular transmission. However, that arm is likely to be more resistant to nondepolarizing muscle relaxants than is the rest of the body, thus leading us to use a relative overdose of drug, making timely reversal difficult or impossible. However, it ensures that the patient will not move intraoperatively, because we are providing neuromuscular blockade of the most resistant muscles. SCh is associated with a significant complication in the hemiplegic patient, that of hyperkalemia.[6] The time of sensitivity is not well defined, but cases are reported from 1 week to 6 months after onset of hemiplegia.

Intraoperative Management of "Tight Brain"

Intracranial hypertension can result in the extrusion of brain tissue when craniotomy is performed. The first sign of difficulty is usually noted by the neurosurgeon as the craniotomy flap is removed and the dura is bulging and tense. The term *tight brain* gives no clue as to etiology or course of treatment. Some characteristics can help to assess the severity and intractability of the situation. If the dura is tense and bulging only at the lower portion of the craniectomy, palpation may reveal that the brain tissue is easily displaced upward and that the superior dura is tense only from being pushed out at the lower level. Surgical exposure may be slightly compromised in this situation, and some maneuvers may improve the situation. If the dura is tense at all edges of the craniectomy and palpation reveals fairly immobile brain beneath, surgical exposure may be severely compro-

mised. Maneuvers may help the situation but are unlikely to bring the brain profile to the bone edge. A large dural incision will result in brain extrusion, with trapping at the edges and little room to achieve exposure. A small dural incision allows the surgeon some control of the brain while seeking to obtain exposure. While the usual cause of such extreme tenseness of the dura is not amenable to anesthetic maneuvers, it is important to rule out correctable problems (Table 2-3). The usual cause is intracranial hypertension because of the tumor mass itself. As resection is performed, the dural opening can be enlarged and the offending mass will be removed, eventually leaving a cavity where, previously, there was bulging brain. An ominous cause of such swelling is occult acute bleeding into the tumor. Vital signs give a clue to this. Hypertension may develop without apparent cause and appears unusually resistant to increasing anesthetic depth. Heart rate may initially rise, but then slows. This response is somewhat masked by the complexity of pharmacologic and surgical interventions superimposed during anesthesia. Timing is also important. If the brain begins to bulge vigorously where it was slack before, intracerebral hemorrhage must be strongly suspected. It is helpful to the surgeon to be informed of the subtle vital sign changes suggesting this etiology, because the surgeon will need to proceed more rapidly and boldly with decompression. Because of the relationship of CPP to ICP and blood pressure, it may be unwise to try to reduce blood pressure before decompression, despite the probability of bleeding.

With the use of the operating microscope, the surgeon may adjust the position of the table for best exposure without realizing that the patient is slowly being placed horizontal or head down. Readjusting the operating table to allow the head to be slightly elevated can dramatically improve the situation. Venous drainage may be compromised by extreme head positions and go unnoticed until the dura is exposed. Repositioning the alignment of head and chin to the body may be necessary.

Table 2-3. Therapeutic Maneuvers to Improve Tight Brain

Position, venous return
PCO_2, PO_2
Volatile anesthetic agent, nitrous oxide
Thiopental
Muscle relaxants
Diuretics
Spinal fluid drainage
Steroids
Pneumocephalus

Because it is a powerful cerebral vasodilator, an increase in $PaCO_2$ may cause a dramatic increase in ICP. Hypoxic cerebral vasodilation may produce the same effect. Reassurance that hypocarbia is achieved and that hypoxia is absent can be obtained by arterial blood gas determinations supported by pulse oximetry and capnography.

Despite the overall evidence of safety of volatile anesthetics, it seems prudent to discontinue such drugs and to utilize an opioid in the presence of tight brain. There may be no causal connection between volatile drugs and brain size, but changing to an opioid anesthetic eliminates any such possibility. Nitrous oxide may increase CBF, but its effect is likely to be less pronounced and easily altered by thiopental or opioids. Nonetheless, discontinuance of nitrous oxide eliminates any concern of its being a causative agent for the problem. Acute administration of a sleep dose of thiopental can be expected to reduce ICP. Lack of any visible response of the brain to thiopental suggests a serious situation. In theory, sequential changes in anesthetics can help to identify the agent responsible, although rarely is this helpful clinically. It is usually more practical to make several changes at once to effect a reduction in intracranial mass as quickly as possible.

Patients receiving antiseizure medications may have a shortened response to nondepolarizing muscle relaxants.[25] Return of abdominal and thoracic muscle tone during light anesthesia can raise central venous pressure and thus cerebral venous pressure (the presumed origin of the saying that "curare relaxes the brain"). Evaluation of the level of neuromuscular blockade is an important subtle step in seeking a cause for tight brain.

Osmotic diuretics have long been shown to be effective in reducing brain size in normal brain tissue by drawing water from the interstitial tissue. In patients with intact autoregulation, mannitol results in no change in CBF and in a decrease in ICP by 27 percent at 25 minutes. However, in patients with impaired autoregulation, the CBF increases by 5 percent and there is less decrease in ICP (18 percent) at 25 minutes.[32] Furosemide in fairly large doses (e.g., 80 mg) reduced ICP, but its mechanism of action is not entirely clear.[37]

Drainage of CSF is a rapid and effective method of reducing intracranial bulk directly. Generally effective methods include subarachnoid needle and catheter techniques. Rarely, pneumocephalus may be present from some previous diagnostic test and can increase with the use of nitrous oxide.

Ergonomics

We believe that major advances will be made in the design of the anesthesia workstation in the next two decades. This is made necessary by the increased complexity of monitoring modalities to reduce unknown physiological trespass and is made possible by the vast computer power now available in reduced size and cost. Until now, each additional monitor has been hung or stacked onto the anesthesia machine or placed on a stand of its own in the operating room. The practical concept of ergonomics in this generation consists more of helpful practices to avoid mishaps. In the future it is more likely to involve "heads up" displays, computer-driven infusion pumps and vaporizers, integrated neurological, cardiovascular, and neuromuscular monitoring, and computer alarms when certain sets of circumstances approach a pattern that is preprogrammed to be worthy of immediate attention. The utility of these workstations remains for future generations to evaluate. At present we have more mundane methods of preventing anesthesia mishaps. Our monitoring systems have gone a long way to provide early detection of vital sign changes, alterations in tissue oxygenation, carbon dioxide elimination, adequacy of ventilation, and neurological dysfunction. Mechanical or electronic device failure is an infrequent cause of anesthetic "critical events." More likely is the erroneous interpretation of data, drug errors in type or dose, or technical errors in performance. We do simple things to reduce the chance for errors. Reducing the numbers of IV bags that are hanging when they contain various vasoactive drugs so that they will not be plugged in by accident when other IVs run out and removing from the room drugs that are packaged in concentrated form, which might lead the user to administer a gross overdose thinking he was administering the more dilute form (e.g., esmolol), and checking the patient's blood carefully long before bleeding starts and the tempo of the situation picks up substantially are examples. Careful drug labeling and removing SCh from the countertop when a patient has a CNS lesion likely to result in hyperkalemia with its administration are examples of workstation care. Having anesthetists crawling under the drapes to adjust the operating table or whatever puts their backs to all the sophisticated equipment distracts from the real task to which they should be directed. It has been found that relief of the anesthetist is the point at which some impending "critical events" are discovered, showing the error of the old adage that one person should stay and do the entire anesthetic without relief like our surgical colleagues often do. There is still much to learn about the human factors that go into the tasks and decision making that this role requires.

Cerebral Ischemia

Cerebral ischemia will develop if the delivery of oxygen and nutrients to a region of the brain is inadequate to meet metabolic needs. The outcome following cerebral ischemia will depend on the severity and duration of the ischemic episode. Although inadequate cerebral oxygen supply can develop intraoperatively as a result of systemic hypoxia, the most common etiology during neurosurgical procedures is inadequate CBF. Normal CBF is 50 ml/100 g/min. Decreases in CBF will first lead to loss of neuronal function, with maintenance of cellular integrity. Restoration of CBF to normal levels will result in a return of neuronal function. Further decreases in CBF will cause not only a loss of neuronal function but also a loss of cellular integrity. This can cause irreversible cell damage and cell death, leading to permanent neurological deficits. The critical CBF at which these changes occur depends on the metabolic requirements of the cell. Conditions such as general anesthesia or hypothermia, which decrease CMR, will lower the critical CBF. In patients undergoing carotid endarterectomy the critical CBF for loss of neuronal function (as determined by EEG) is 18 to 20 ml/100 g/min under halothane/nitrous oxide anesthesia, 15 to 18 ml/100 g/min[38] during enflurane/nitrous oxide or Innovar/nitrous oxide anesthesia,[23] and 8 to 10 ml/100 g/min under isoflurane/nitrous oxide anesthesia.[24] In awake primates the critical CBF for loss of neuronal function is 23 ml/100 g/min and the lower critical CBF at which cellular damage occurs is 8 to 9 ml/100 g/min.[15] Therefore, when accessing critical CBF, it is important to keep in mind not only the CBF but also the CMR at the time of the ischemic episode.

Decreases in CBF may be due to either occlusion of the artery supplying the region or decreased CPP. Occlusion of a major vessel may be transient, as during temporary occlusion of the parent vessel during aneurysm clipping, or permanent, as during AVM resection or trapping of an aneurysm. Neurological outcome during temporary occlusion depends on the duration of the occlusion, CMR during the occlusion, and adequacy of collateral flow. Factors that can be altered by the anesthesiologist intraoperatively include decreasing CMR of the potentially ischemic area prior to temporary occlusion or attempting to improve the collateral flow by increasing CPP following placement of the clips. Maneuvers to decrease CMR prior to placement of the temporary clips include hypothermia and the administration of drugs such as thiopental or isoflurane, which are known to have cerebral protective effects. Neurological outcome following permanent occlusion of an extracranial or intracranial cerebral artery depends on the adequacy of collateral flow. This should be assessed when the patient is awake, as general anesthesia will alter the critical CBF at which ischemia will occur.

Cerebral ischemia can also occur as a result of global decreases in CPP, which may occur because of decreases in systemic mean arterial pressure (MAP) or increases in ICP. In a normotensive patient CBF is autoregulated over a range of CPP from 50 to 150 mmHg (Fig. 2-3), meaning that, within this range of CPP, CBF is constant. At CPP below 50 mmHg CBF will begin to fall, and at CPP above 150 mmHg CBF will increase. In patients with hypertension, this autoregulatory curve is shifted to the right so that CBF begins to fall at a CPP greater than 50 mmHg and increases in CBF do not occur until a CPP greater than 150 mmHg is exceeded. This change in the cerebral autoregulatory curve can be reversed toward normal with chronic treatment of the hypertension.[27]

Deliberately inducing hypotension is a technique that is sometimes helpful during intracranial procedures, especially vascular procedures. During resection of an AVM it may be possible to reduce intraoperative blood loss by decreasing CPP. Induced hypotension during aneurysm clipping may reduce the risk for intraoperative rupture and facilitate clip placement by decreasing the pressure within the aneurysm sac, "softening" the aneurysm.

Although there are few absolute contraindications to induced hypotension, the list of relative contraindications is long and varies greatly from author to author. Most consider significant ischemic cerebrovascular disease, coronary artery disease, significant anemia or hypovolemia, severe hypertension, or extremes of age to increase the risk for induced hypotension.[16,19] However, with intensive monitoring and careful control of the lower level to which the pressure is reduced, induced hypotension can be utilized in these patients.[3]

The commonly accepted lower limit for induced hypotension is the lower limit of cerebral autoregulation, an MAP of 50 mmHg. As long as CPP is main-

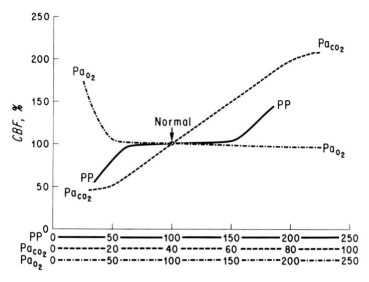

Figure 2-3. The relationship of cerebral blood flow to perfusion pressure (PP), $PaCO_2$, and PaO_2. Units on the abscissa are in millimeters of mercury. (From Michenfelder,[26] with permission.)

tained above this level CBF should remain within the normal range. As discussed above, in the chronic hypertensive patient the lower limit of cerebral autoregulation is shifted to a higher pressure. As a result the lower limit for safe induced hypotension will be at a higher MAP. Most would consider a decrease of MAP by 30 percent from the patient's normal MAP to be a safe lower limit for induced hypotension in these patients.[3]

Complications following induced hypotension are primarily the result of hypoperfusion. Ischemic cerebrovascular accidents, MI, retinal artery thrombosis, and renal failure have all been reported following induced hypotension. Fortunately the incidence of cerebral, coronary, or retinal artery thrombosis, renal failure, or hepatic failure following induced hypotension are each less than 1 percent.[18,19] When properly administered, induced hypotension can be a valuable and safe technique.

There are many agents that have been utilized to induce hypotension, including the volatile anesthetic agents (most commonly isoflurane), direct vasodilators (nitroprusside, nitroglycerin, hydralazine), ganglionic blocking agents (trimethaphan), and sympathetic blocking agents (esmolol, labetalol). Each of these agents has advantages and disadvantages. The safe conduct of induced hypotension can be accomplished with all of these agents. Choice of a specific agent or combination of drugs for a given patient depends on the level of induced hypotension needed, other potential intraoperative needs (such as the need

for cerebral protection, which might make isoflurane a good choice), and any underlying medical problem the patient may have.

It is important to remember that these patients must be intensively monitored. Direct arterial pressure must be continuously monitored, as should the adequacy of perfusion of vital organs. ECG evidence of myocardial ischemia should be sought and adequacy of renal perfusion assessed by measuring urine output. Adequacy of ventilation and oxygenation must be ensured. Levels of induced hypotension that might otherwise be safe could lead to major complications if combined with undetected hypoxia. Vigilance, intensive monitoring, and careful control of the lower limit of blood pressure reduction are the keys to safe use of deliberate hypotension.

Facilitation of CNS Monitoring

The purpose of intraoperative neurological monitoring is to improve the neurological outcome of the operative procedure. As discussed above, to accomplish this goal the structure monitored must be at risk during the operative procedure, the monitor must be sensitive to damage, and if a change is detected there must be some intervention possible. Changes detected by the monitors may be due to surgical compromise of the monitored structure, changes in the depth of anesthesia, or other systemic changes such as changes in systemic pressure or temperature.

One important goal of the anesthetic management during procedures in which intraoperative neurological monitoring is used is to minimize any systemic changes that can affect the monitor. This is especially important during crucial periods in the operative procedure when neurological structures are likely to be at risk. EEG changes suggestive of cerebral ischemia are first a decrease in fast activity with more prominent high amplitude slow activity, followed by a decrease or loss of all activity as the ischemic insult becomes more severe. The same changes can be caused by increasing depth of anesthesia with most of the commonly utilized agents. During SEP monitoring the changes suggestive of damage are an increased latency of the waveform and a decrease in its amplitude. SEP changes caused by many of the commonly used agents are listed in Table 2-4. In general BAEPs are the most resistant to the effects of anesthetic agents and VEPs the most sensitive.[4] Many of the anesthetic agents cause changes in the SEPs that are similar to those changes indicative of intraoperative damage.

Although many of the anesthetic agents cause changes in both the EEG and SEP that mimic those caused by neurological injury, the use of these agents is not contraindicated by the need to use the monitor. The anesthetic-induced changes are dose dependent, and it is possible to design an anesthetic plan that leaves the ability to monitor intact. A level of anesthesia must be selected that does not obliterate the monitored waveforms. During critical periods in the operative procedure the depth of anesthesia must re-

main stable, so that any change in the monitored modality can be accurately attributed to a change in the operative field. However, as more and more neurological monitors are coming into use in the operating room, the difficulty of selecting an anesthetic plan that preserves the ability to utilize all the monitors and still to keep the patient safely and adequately anesthetized increases. In some patients, this may not be possible, and the anesthetic risk to the patient may be increased by use of the neurological monitors. In this situation, any proven benefits of the monitor must be balanced against the increased risk of the anesthetic occurring as a result of the use of the monitor.

When intraoperative changes are detected in either the EEG or SEP, it is important to quickly identify the likely etiology of the change. If it is thought that it is due to systemic changes such as a decrease in systemic arterial pressure, these systemic changes must be promptly reversed. The response of the monitor to correction of the systemic variable should be assessed to see if the monitored waveforms have returned to baseline. If it is felt that the detected change is not due to systemic changes but rather due to some change in the operative field that is causing injury to the monitored neurological structure, this too must be quickly identified. The surgical maneuver thought to have resulted in the change must be reversed or altered. The neurological monitor must then be carefully observed for signs of recovery.

Control of Blood Pressure and Heart Rate

At various points in the intraoperative period, hypertension and tachycardia may develop. This is most commonly due to a change in the level of stimulation such that the depth of anesthesia is not adequate to block the sympathetic response to the increased stimulation. Common points in the operative course for hypertension and/or tachycardia to develop include during laryngoscopy and intubation, surgical incision, surgical stimulation of cranial nerves or their nuclei, and surgical closure and emergence from anesthesia. Common to these events are a sudden and intense increase in the level of stimulation or an increase in the degree of stimulation at a time when the anesthetic depth is being decreased (closure and emergence).

It is appropriate to attempt to control or prevent these increases in blood pressure and heart rate. Increases in blood pressure to levels that exceed cere-

Table 2-4. Drug Effects on Sensory Evoked Potentials

Drug	SSEPs		BAEPs		VEPs	
	LAT	AMP	LAT	AMP	LAT	AMP
Isoflurane	↑	↓	↑	0	↑	↓
Enflurane	↑	↓	↑	0	↑	↓
Halothane	↑	↓	↑	0	↑	0
Nitrous oxide	0	↓	0	0	↑	↓
Barbiturates	↑	↓	↑	0	↑	↓
Etomidate	↑	↑	↑	↓		
Droperidol	↑	↓				
Diazepam	↑	↓	0	0		
Midazolam	0	↓				
Fentanyl	↑	↓	0	0		
Morphine	↑	↓				
Meperidine	↑	↑ / ↓				

Abbreviations: SSEPs, somatosensory evoked potentials; BAEPs, brainstem auditory evoked potentials; VEPs, visual evoked potentials; LAT, latency; AMP, amplitude.
(From Black and Cucchiara,[4] with permission.)

bral autoregulation can lead to dangerous increases in CBF and ICP in patients with mass lesions, while any increase in blood pressure can increase the risk for bleeding in cerebrovascular procedures. In addition, increases in blood pressure and especially heart rate will lead to increases in myocardial oxygen demand and decreases in myocardial oxygen supply (tachycardia). In patients with coronary artery disease these adverse changes may result in myocardial ischemia and should be prevented or promptly treated.

Hypertension and tachycardia occurring as a result of the sympathetic response to stimulation can be prevented or treated either by increasing the depth of anesthesia or by blocking the systemic response to the sympathetic stimulation. While most anesthetic agents can be utilized to increase the depth of anesthesia, high doses of the newer synthetic narcotics such as fentanyl and sufentanil are more effective at completely blunting the sympathetic response to stimulation.[9] However, a high-dose narcotic technique will often result in delayed awakening following the operative procedure. Decisions regarding the choice of anesthetic agent or combination of agents must balance the importance of completely blocking the sympathetic response against the importance of prompt postoperative awakening in an individual patient. In patients with severe coronary artery disease, the need to prevent untoward hemodynamic changes may outweigh the desire for prompt postoperative neurological assessment, and a high-dose narcotic anesthetic may be chosen. In other patients, a different combination of agents may be utilized that might provide less complete blocking of the sympathetic response but be compatible with prompt postoperative awakening.

At some points, such as during surgical closure and emergence from anesthesia when hypertension develops in up to 90 percent of craniotomy patients, increasing the depth of anesthesia is not appropriate.[33] In these situations drugs to block the systemic response to the stimulation can be utilized. Many agents have been successfully utilized, including the direct vasodilators and sympathetic blocking agents. Sympathetic blocking agents such as labetalol and esmolol have been shown to be particularly effective in this situation decreasing both blood pressure and heart rate.[33] The vasodilators might be expected to be more effective in the treatment of hypertension in the presence of a slow heart rate. As in all points of the perioperative period, careful monitoring and rational choice of a therapeutic agent are more important than which specific agent is utilized.

IMMEDIATE POSTOPERATIVE MANAGEMENT

Principles

As anesthetic agents are being developed, manufacturers are aware of the usefulness of agents that have two specific features: they permit rapid emergence from anesthesia and their concentration or effect can be measured so that titration of the agent, especially near the end of the surgery, is possible (Table 2-5). This is an attempt to put more science into the anesthetic art of having a patient awaken quietly within minutes of the completion of the surgery. In general, the need to have the patient awake at the end is historical. There were no easy diagnostic tests to determine the effect of the surgery on the patient's mental state or if the patient had suffered a hemorrhagic (or ischemic) complication after the dura was closed. Despite the increased availability of CT and MRI scanning, these are still somewhat cumbersome, time-consuming, and probably impractical for every patient immediately postoperatively. Some neurosurgeons prefer to have the patients remain asleep and intubated overnight and to follow them with intermittent scans. The price of this approach is inability to assess neurological function continuously to obtain early warning if there is an intracranial complication. Our surgeons feel that their best neurological function monitor is the patient's own mental state, and the sooner after surgery that can be determined the more accurate will be their subsequent judgments in the handling of complications. Our goal then is to have the patient responding to commands when the head dressing is completed or immediately when the last stitch is placed. We do not always wait until the pins are removed from the head holder to have the patient awake and responding, and we have had no patients remember discomfort from the pins. The artists of emergence realize that deeper anesthesia is needed to blunt the stimulus from the endotracheal tube during movement of the head for the head dressing than is needed to place the last skin sutures. If one chooses to plan for emergence following the

Table 2-5. Anesthesia Goals in Immediate Postoperative Management of the Supratentorial Tumor Patient

Rapid early emergence
Progressive neurological improvement
Extubation as early as safely possible
Pain relief without obtundation
Immediate response to complications

head dressing, it is likely to take extra minutes for that reason. But these minutes are not critical to the patient's well being in terms of diagnosis of complications. There is benefit to the anesthesia team as well to have unimpeded access to the patient's head after the surgeon has completed the dressing. It is important that the surgeon and anesthesiologist discuss an emergence pattern that they find mutually acceptable. Light anesthesia during closing may result in patient movement, which some surgeons find completely intolerable, whereas other surgeons find that inconvenience acceptable in exchange for very early emergence and evaluation. There are not data to suggest that either position is better, but agreement on a singular pattern makes the crucial time of emergence more smoothly manageable. If the patient does not awaken at the end of the operation the surgeon has the right to expect the anesthesiologist to state accurately whether this is an anesthesia effect or not. Of course, there is some variation in emergence times based on a myriad of factors that are not measurable. But certainly within 15 to 30 minutes we should be able to give a fairly accurate assessment as to the contribution of anesthesia to the situation of slow arousal.

Our judgment on the likelihood of complications is heavily linked to progressive neurological improvement. If the patient emerges slowly but continues to improve fairly quickly we usually do not perform an immediate scan. However, if the patient is emerging more slowly than the anesthesiologist thinks wise in this anesthetic situation or if the patient fails to progress steadily to the neurological level the surgeon feels should be obtained based on the surgery, we do proceed with a CT scan to rule out an acute intracranial complication. This area is where the experience of the anesthesiologist and recovery room nurses can add the extra edge against time to help the surgeon identify these problems early and to act early to correct them.

The stimulus of the endotracheal tube in the throat, larynx, and trachea is quite considerable. The patient response is usually "bucking" (cough reflex without the ability to close the glottis) on the tube and hypertension with tachycardia. Some feel that this pattern does not really affect the likelihood of intracerebral complications. There are no data on this issue. We feel it is important to extubate the patient as early as possible to minimize these responses. Caution is important because patients who are likely at risk for aspiration or who require mechanical ventilation must not be treated the same as the otherwise healthy patient with a cerebral lesion. If one chooses to leave the endotracheal tube in place, one must be prepared to treat the cardiovascular stimulation with β-blockers and vasodilators, the cough reflex with narcotics and perhaps even muscle relaxants, and the cerebral stimulation with sedatives even to the point of making it difficult to evaluate the patient neurologically.

Fortunately, the pain is not usually a major problem following craniotomy, but pain relief is often necessary immediately postoperatively. We try to prevent obtundation and use shorter acting narcotics so that the effects will dissipate quickly if there is any question about progressive neurological improvement.

Management of Complications

Prophylactic management of seizures is always utilized when the risk is high. Motor seizures are the easiest to identify, and the end point of treatment is fairly clear. We manage these aggressively with intravenous agents. If they are resistant we are prepared, at our surgical colleagues' request, to place the patient in a barbiturate coma in the intensive care unit. The risks of this therapy are considerable, and it is not undertaken lightly. In many medical centers, the manpower and technical resources that this requires are simply not available.

The problem of slow arousal following surgery can be a difficult one, but the real question is whether it is due to the anesthetic, to the surgical intervention, or to an intracranial complication. The CT scan is very helpful in the differential diagnosis and usually provides the data necessary to direct therapeutic intervention.

Intracranial hematoma is a complication that requires emergent responses. At the first signs of neurological deterioration a CT scan is sought, and there is usually time to do this. However, it is still very appropriate to make this diagnosis clinically and go directly to the operating room. The anesthesia team must recognize the importance of time in this therapy, and compromises may have to be made in usual anesthetic techniques to allow for a very rapid surgical approach. Irreversible damage occurs within a very few hours and may occur sooner in compromised brain tissue.

Cerebral ischemia due to the circulatory system following supratentorial tumor surgery is uncommon. When ICP is high, perfusion pressure must also be allowed to rise, but it is difficult to know when to control blood pressure immediately postoperatively. The balance between cerebral ischemia and increasing the risk of bleeding from a tumor bed is difficult to assess. Consultation between neurosurgeon and anesthesiologist is useful to arrive at a judgment as to how to intervene in these cases.

REFERENCES

1. Adams RW, Cucchiara RF, Gronert GA et al: Isoflurane and cerebrospinal fluid pressure in neurosurgical patients. Anesthesiology 54:97, 1981
2. Adams RS, Gronert GA, Sundt TM, Michenfelder JD: Halothane, hypocapnia, and cerebrospinal fluid pressure in neurosurgery. Anesthesiology 37:510, 1972
3. Black S: Cerebral aneurysm and arteriovenous malformation. p. 223. In Cucchiara RF, Michenfelder JD (eds): Clinical Neuroanesthesia. Churchill Livingstone, New York, 1990
4. Black S, Cucchiara RF: Neurologic monitoring. p. 1185. In Miller RD (ed): Anesthesia. 3rd Ed. Churchill Livingstone, New York, 1990
5. Brown JC, Charlton JE: Study of sensitivity to curare in certain neurological disorders using a regional technique. J Neurol Neurosurg Psychiatry 38:34, 1975
6. Cooperman LH, Strobel GE, Kennell EM: Massive hyperkalemia after administration of succinylcholine. Anesthesiology 32:161, 1970
7. Cucchiara RF, Black S, Steinkeler JA: Anesthesia for intracranial procedures. p. 849. In Barash PG, Cullen BF, Stoelting RK (eds): Clinical Anesthesia. JB Lippincott, Philadelphia, 1989
8. Cucchiara RF, Michenfelder JD: The effect of interruption of the recticular activating system on metabolism in canine cerebral hemispheres before and after thiopental. Anesthesiology 39:3, 1973
9. de Lange S, Boscoe MJ, Stanley TH, Pace N: Comparison of sufentanil-O_2 and fentanyl-O_2 for coronary artery surgery. Anesthesiology 56:112, 1982
10. Graham D: Monitoring neuromuscular block may be unreliable in patients with upper motor neuron lesions. Anesthesiology 52:74, 1980
11. Gronert GA, Schulman SR, Mott J: Malignant hyperthermia. p. 935. In Miller RD (ed): Anesthesia. 3rd Ed. Churchill Livingstone, New York, 1990
12. Grosslight K, Foster R, Colohan AR, Bedford RF: Isoflurane for neuroanesthesia: risk factors for increases in intracranial pressure. Anesthesiology 63:533, 1985
13. Grundy BL: Intraoperative monitoring of sensory evoked potentials. p. 624. In Nodar RH, Barber E (eds): Evoked Potentials II. Butterworth, Boston, 1984
14. Harner SG, Daube JR, Ebersold MJ: Electrophysiologic monitoring of facial nerve during temporal bone surgery. Laryngoscope 96:65, 1986
15. Jones TH, Morawetz RB, Crowell RM et al: Thresholds of focal cerebral ischemia in awake monkeys. J Neurosurg 54:773, 1981
16. Lam AM: Induced hypotension. Can Anaesth Soc J 31:556, 1988
17. Levy WJ, York DH, McCaffrey M, Tanzer F: Motor evoked potentials from transcranial stimulation to the motor cortex in humans. Neurosurgery 15:287, 1984
18. Lindop MJ: Copmlications and morbidity of controlled hypotension. Br J Anaesth 47:799, 1975
19. Little DM: Induced hypotension during anesthesia and surgery. Anesthesiology 16:320, 1955
20. Madsen JB, Cold GE, Hansen ES, Bardrum B: The effect of isoflurane on cerebral blood flow and metabolism in humans during craniotomy for small supratentorial cerebral tumors. Anesthesiology 66:332, 1987
21. Marsh ML, Dunlop BJ, Shapiro HM et al: Succinylcholine-intracranial pressure effects in neurosurgical patients. Anesth Analg 59:550, 1980
22. Marx W, Shah N, Long C et al: Sufentanil, alfentanil, and fentanyl: impact on cerebrospinal fluid pressure in patients with brain tumors. J Neurosurg Anesth 1:3, 1989
23. McKay RD, Sundt TM, Michenfelder JD et al: Internal carotid artery stump pressure and cerebral blood flow during carotid endarterectomy. Modification of halothane, enflurane, and Innovar. Anesthesiology 45:390, 1976
24. Messick JM Jr, Casement B, Sharbrough FW et al: Correlation of regional cerebral blood flow (rCBF), with EEG changes during isoflurane anesthesia for carotid endarterectomy: critical rCBF. Anesthesiology 63:344. 1987
25. Messick JM, Maass L, Faust RJ, Cucchiara RF: Duration of pancuronium neuromuscular blockade in patients taking anticonvulsant medication, abstracted. Anesth Analg 61:203, 1982
26. Michenfelder JD: Anesthesia and the Brain. Churchill Livingstone, New York, 1988
27. Michenfelder JD: Cerebral blood flow and metabolism. p. 1. In Cucchiara RF, Michenfelder JD (eds): Clinical Neuroanesthesia. Churchill Livingstone, New York, 1990
28. Michenfelder JD, Theye RA: Effects of fentanyl, droperidol, and Innovar on canine cerebral metabolism and blood flow. Br J Anaesth 43:630, 1971
29. Milde LN, Milde JH, Gallagher WJ: Effects of sufentanil on cerebral circulation and metabolism in dogs. Anesth Analg 70:138, 1990
30. Minton MD, Stirt JA, Bedford RF: Increased intracranial pressure from succinylcholine: modification by prior nondepolarizing blockade. Anesthesiology 65: 165, 1986
31. Minton MD, Stirt JA, Bedford RF, Haworth C: Intracranial pressure after atracurium in neurosurgical patients. Anesth Analg 64:1113, 1985
32. Muizelaar JP, Lutz HA, Becker DP: Effect of mannitol on ICP and CBF and correlation with pressure autoregulation in severely head-injured patients. J Neurosurg 61:700, 1984
33. Muzzi DA, Losasso TJ, Black S, Cucchiara RF: Labe-

talol and esmolol in the control of hypertension following intracranial surgery. Anesth Analg 70:103, 1990

34. Rao TLK, Jacobs KH, El-Etra AA: Reinfarction following anesthesia in patients with myocardial infarction. Anesthesiology 59:499,1983

35. Raudzens PA: Intraoperative monitoring of evoked potentials. Ann NY Acad Sci 388:308, 1982

36. Ross AF, Tinker JH: Anesthesia risk. p. 715. In Miller RD (ed): Anesthesia. 3rd Ed. Churchill Livingstone, New York, 1990

37. Samson D, Beyer CW: Furosemide in the intraoperative reduction of intracranial pressure in the patient with subarachnoid hemorrhage. Neurosurgery 10:167, 1982

38. Sharbrough FW, Messick JM Jr, Sundt TM Jr: Correlation of continuous electroencephalograms with cerebral blood flow measurements during carotid endarterectomy. Stroke 4:674, 1973

39. Steen PA, Tinker JH, Tarhan S: Myocardial reinfarction after anesthesia and surgery. JAMA 239:2566, 1978

40. Unni VK, Gray WJ, Young MB: Effects of atracurium on intracranial pressure in man. Anaesthesia 41:1047, 1986

3 Basic Techniques and Surgical Positioning

John M. Tew, Jr.
Daniel J. Scodary

PATIENT POSITION

Surgical positioning of the patient is an integral part of the operative procedure.[2,5] Restrictions of movement in the operating theater are caused by the addition of many technical advances that require space and accurate positioning. Small surgical exposures and approaches to deep surgical targets require precise localization so as to ensure the creation of the most direct corridor to the lesion. Moreover, prolonged neurosurgical procedures create the need for a comfortable position for the surgeon and the patient. The operating table is an important adjunct in the positioning process. The table must be stable, well padded, and provide adequate access for the surgeon and the radiographic units. Remote control of table positions is essential for the sequential changes in patient position (Fig. 3-1A).

Adequate access to the patient for the anesthesiologist to maintain lines, airways, and monitors is mandatory. Many patients require additional access for physiological monitoring, electroencephalography (EEG), evoked potentials, electromyography (EMG), and auditory responses. Intraoperative radiological procedures, angiography, fluoroscopic imaging, and intravascular interventional techniques place additional requirements on space and access. As a result of the need for staged access to the head of the patient, we prefer to orient the anesthesiologist and his equipment at the left side or the feet of the patient (Fig. 3-1B; see also Fig. 3-4A). Once all preparations are made and lines and airways are secured, members of the team take their places in their assigned positions. We have found this tactic very effective for all members of the team.

All anatomical pressure areas and traction points require attention. If a position can be uncomfortable or cause hemodynamic compromise in the awake patient, its effects under anesthesia are exaggerated.

The nurse and assistants must have adequate visual access to the video monitors, assistant microscope, and surgical field. The final position of the patient should be acceptable to the surgeon when making the skin incision and visualizing the relationship of the surgical target to the table, body, and topography of the room and microscope. Access to a skull and the brain images enable the surgeon to plan the approach as a three-dimensional road map for a complex journey. The surgeon must pay careful attention to each of these details for each position and procedure. Attentive study of the images, planning of the position, and flap placement will ensure the selection of proper exposure and execution of the corridor to the lesion.

A thermal blanket should be placed over the patient, as a significant fall in temperature may be anticipated in most procedures. Warm humidified inspired gases and fluids should be used.

We recommend only two basic positions for all operative procedures on the nervous system. These positions are either supine or lateral oblique. The supine position is used for procedures to gain exposure from the anterior cervical spine through the occiput. The lateral oblique position is used for exposure of the occipital region through the lumbar spine. Once the head and body are fixed, needed variations in positions are obtained by changing the position of the operating table.

No position in neurosurgery is more versatile than the supine position. It can be used for most craniot-

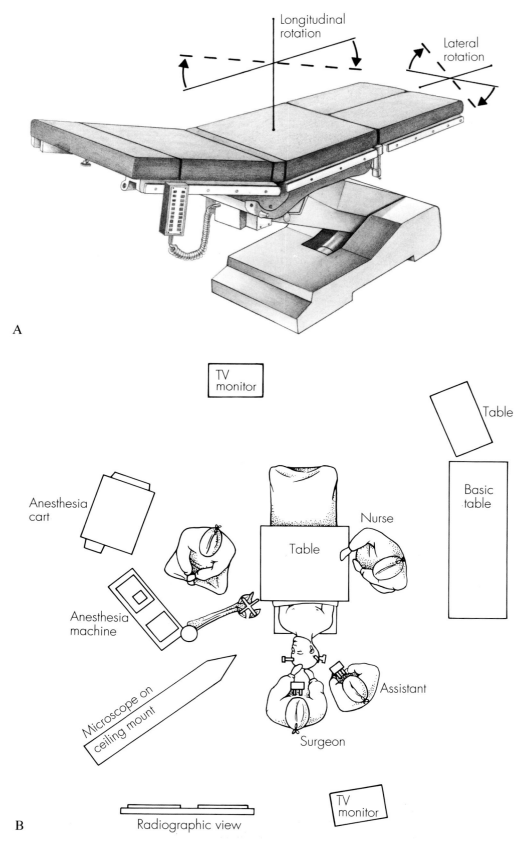

Figure 3-1. **(A)** Remote control surgical table. **(B)** Position for right pteronial approach. (*Figure continues.*)

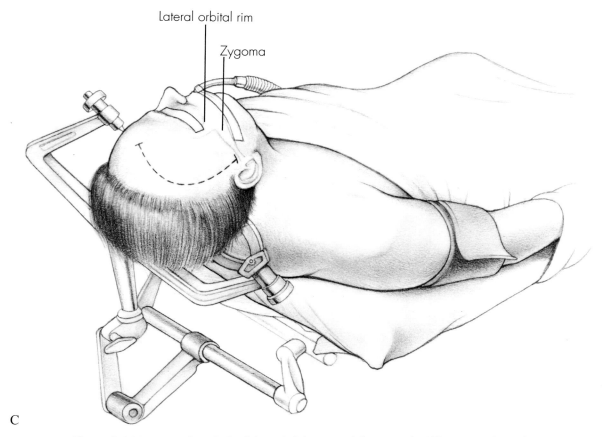

Lateral orbital rim

Zygoma

C

Figure 3-1 (*Continued*). **(C)** Incision of right pteronial approach. (*Figure continues.*)

omy approaches; frontal, temporal, and skull base approaches; and transsphenoidal, transoral, and petrosal approaches, which provide exposure of the supra- and infratentorial spaces. Some surgeons also prefer the supine position for lateral suboccipital approaches. We recommend the lateral oblique position in order to avoid excessive rotation of the neck.

The patient is placed supine on the operating table (Fig. 3-1C). A reinforced (armored) endotracheal tube will prevent kinking of the airway in positions that require rotation of the head (temporal and petrosal positions). Particular attention should be directed to maintenance of adequate venous return in patients when the head is rotated. The endotracheal tube must be securely affixed to the skin and to the skull clamp to avoid migration or dislodgement. The surgeon and the anesthesiologist must be responsible for protecting the airways. The corneas are lubricated, and the lids are taped closed to avoid desiccation and abrasions. The globes are protected from sources of pressure in all positions.[4] We use a rigid Mayfield skull fixation device (Ohio Medical Instrument Co.,

Cincinnati) for all craniotomies. The sterile pins are inserted in a manner so as not to interfere with the cranial incision and to facilitate attachment of the halo self-retaining retractor. The hair and scalp have been shampooed with Phisohex soap preoperatively. It is not necessary to shave the pin sites. Air embolism has been associated with the pin head holder used for the sitting position.[3] We have never encountered this problem in supine and oblique positions. The cranium is positioned in a posture that rotates the pterion to 12 o'clock and tilts the vertex toward the floor in order to bring the skull base into maximal line of view. The zygoma is the highest point in the surgical field. A radiolucent skull frame is used if imaging or angiographic procedures are anticipated. The arms are placed at the patient's side and secured to avoid ulnar nerve pressure points. A soft gelatin roll is placed under the shoulder to reduce neck rotation and to improve venous drainage. The thorax and head are elevated 10 degrees to improve venous return. Both knees are slightly flexed, and pressure wraps are placed on the legs to reduce venous stasis.

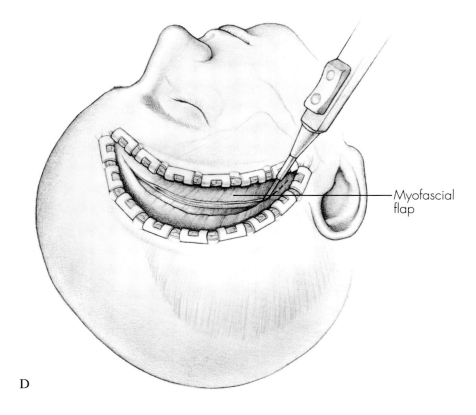

D

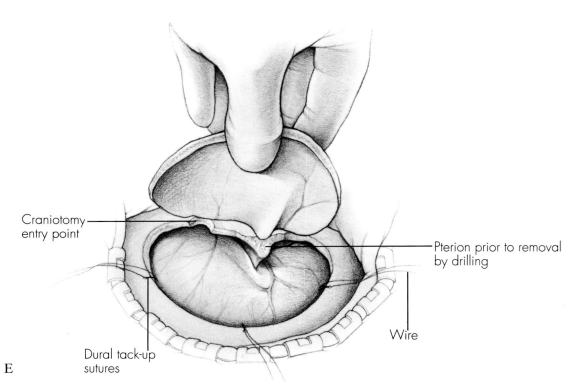

E

Figure 3-1 (*Continued*). **(D)** Opening of temporal fascia. **(E)** Removal of pteronial bone flap. (*Figure continues*.)

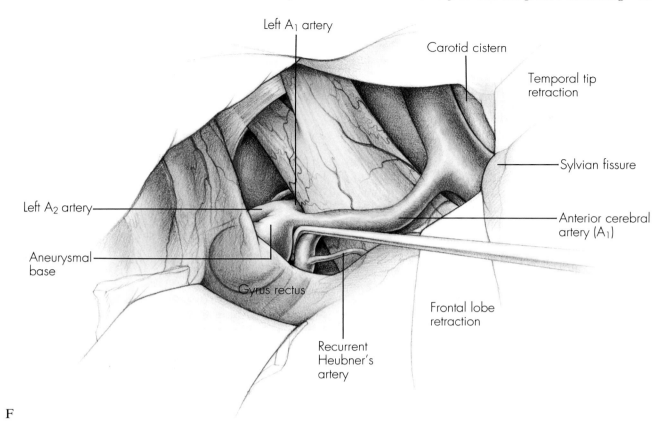

Left A$_1$ artery

Carotid cistern

Temporal tip retraction

Sylvian fissure

Left A$_2$ artery

Anterior cerebral artery (A$_1$)

Aneurysmal base

Gyrus rectus

Frontal lobe retraction

Recurrent Heubner's artery

F

Figure 3-1 (*Continued*). **(F)** Supraoptic dissection for an anterior communicating aneurysm lesion.

PTERIONAL APPROACH

The operating table is moved to a location in the room that achieves maximal access for the team and provides access to the operating microscope and other devices that may be required during the procedure. Careful placement of the table is required if a ceiling microscope is used. If the surgical team depends on overhead lights for illumination, the ceiling illumination fixtures deserve consideration in positioning of the patient's head. The anesthesiologist and gas columns are positioned to the left side of the patient, so the nurse and the surgical assistant can be positioned on the right side of the field for all cases. We prefer to stand during the cranial exposure and use a comfortable chair for the microsurgical portion of the procedure (Fig. 3-1A).

The anesthesiologist retains a control panel for the surgical table to adjust height, lateral tilt, and elevation or depression of the head at any time during the course of the procedure. Accordingly, the patient should be firmly secured to the table because the po-sition may be changed drastically during a procedure. The cranium is fixed to the table for vascular surgery with a radiolucent headholder (angiographic unit) on a metal device for standard procedures. The scalp incision should be marked prior to draping the cranium. The surgeon should keep the target in mind in order to allocate appropriate exposure of the frontal and temporal fossa. The exposure is centered on the pterion and directed to the frontal or temporal orientation, depending on the need to expose the anterior communicating area or the basilar cisterns.

The incision in the skin should begin at the zygoma, 1 cm anterior to the auricle, and extend cephalad across the superior temporal line and course posterior to the hairline. The base of the skin flap should be equal to the height in order to avoid necrosis of the skin margin. Circumstances determine the need to expand the size of the cranial opening. The temporal fascia and muscle are incised and reflected with the skin flap to avoid frontalis paralysis and atrophy of the temporalis muscle. A superior cuff of fascia should be retained on the bone in order to permit reattachment of the muscle to the bone flap. Otherwise, the bone is completely free of the muscle flap (Fig. 3-1D).

A single-entry burr hole is made at the anterior aspect of the superior temporal line. The Midax Rex Craniotome (Midas Rex, Ft. Worth, TX) is used to turn a bone flap that is broken across the base after the pterion has been grooved with a drill (Fig. 3-1E). The remainder of the pterion is removed with a high-speed drill until the periorbitum is visualized. Complete removal of the bony ridge facilitates access to the lateral carotid cistern and to the base of the sylvian fissure. This point is the site for the beginning of access to all of the basal approaches.

The dura is opened with a triangular flap that is sutured to the base of the reflected temporal muscle, which has been secured with multiple hooks. Multiple narrow retractors are placed on the frontal and temporal lobe, which has been covered with a protective coating of sponge or cottonoid material. Gentle retractor pressure is exerted to gain exposure of the basal cisterns in order to release cerebrospinal fluid (CSF) and gain further brain relaxation. Arachnoid pathways are opened widely as CSF is removed, and further exposure of the structures is achieved. The veins of the temporal lobe entering the sphenoid sinus may be sectioned as needed to open the sylvian fissure or to gain infratemporal exposure. Temporal veins should be spared if possible. The anatomic vein of Labbé should always be preserved. Self-retaining retractors are attached to the Budde halo ring (Ohio Medical Instrument Co., Cincinnati). Multiple narrow retractors are used to retain the dissection planes. Retractor pressure is always minimal. Exposure is facilitated by use of CSF drainage by opening the CSF pathways or by use of lumbar spinal drainage. Use of osmotic diuretics and placement of the cranium in a dependent position also facilitates brain relaxation. Brain damage due to laceration, venous stasis, and arterial compression can be avoided by adherence to these techniques.[1]

Figure 3-1F demonstrates the approach to the anterior communicating aneurysm lesions. The position of the patient and the orientation of the head is identical for approaches to all aneurysms that are exposed by the pterional approach. The position of the patient's skull is altered by adjustments of the mechanical table as needed. The adjustments in the skin incision, bone removal, and dissection planes are changes for variations in location of anterior circulation and basilar terminus aneurysms. The retractors are placed on the gyrus rectus as the sylvian fissure is opened medial to the carotid terminus. Dissection of the right and left A_1 segments of the artery is attained

prior to retraction of the aneurysmal dome. Dissection of the aneurysm neck, dome, and anterior communicating artery is achieved prior to placement of a clip. Hypotension is induced immediately prior to dissection of the lesion. Retraction is minimized until sharp dissection frees the adhesions about the chiasmal cistern. After clipping the aneurysm, the sac is aspirated and rotated to visualize perforators at the base of the sac and contralateral A_2 segment of the artery. The angle of approach should ensure that the clip placement is proper and that the aneurysm has been completely clipped and no perforating vessels lie within the blades of the clip. Intraoperative angiography may be advisable if there is any concern as to the adequacy of clipping and the exclusion of critical vessels.

Clot removal is pursued by dissection of the cisterns and vigorous irrigation. Subarachnoid clot removal may reduce vasospasm. Postoperatively, hemodilution and elevation of blood pressure will increase cerebral perfusion.

Closure

Closure of the craniotomy is thusly performed: a CSF tight dural closure is obtained with continuous suture and pericranial graft as needed. Dural tenting sutures were placed when the skull was opened. These sutures are spaced such that the dura is securely tented against the bone edge. An additional suture is placed in the center of the bone flap. Wire sutures are also placed through the same bone openings to secure the bone flap. The skull flap is rigidly secured with wire sutures. The stainless steel wire sutures are tucked into the bony openings to avoid irritation of the overlying skin. Cranioplastic closure of any bone defects is performed to eliminate any potential cosmetic defects. The muscle and fascia are reattached. A subgaleal drain is placed and attached to continuous aspiration. The drain is removed after 24 hours when the flap is adherent to the cranium. The galea is closed with absorbable sutures, and the skin is closed with metallic clips. A light pressure dressing and turban are applied.

SUBTEMPORAL APPROACH

The subtemporal approach is the approach of choice to large basilar terminus aneurysms (illustrated in this chapter), midbasilar aneurysms, trigeminal neuromas limited to the middle fossa, extradural petrous tumors, and certain petroclival meningiomas. For basilar terminus aneurysms that lie low in the posterior fossa (at or below the posterior clinoid) the subtemporal approach is ideal. Exposure is facilitated by placement of a lumbar catheter for CSF drainage.

The patient is positioned in a supine position. A right-sided approach is preferred if anatomical considerations permit. The right shoulder is raised with a gelatin pad, and the sagittal suture is placed parallel to the floor (Fig. 3-2A). The skull is fixed with a radiolucent headholder angiographic unit. The cranium is tilted so that the zygoma is the highest point in the field. This positioning facilitates exposure of the skull base and the tentorial edge. A skin flap is initiated posterior to the midpoint of the mastoid process and is carried upward to the superior temporal line before descending to inscribe a flap that is practically square, based on the ear, and terminates at the mid zygoma. The temporalis muscle is reflected after a myofascial cuff is retained at the superior temporal line to facilitate closure (Fig. 3-2B). The muscle flap is reflected downward on the zygoma unless a zygomatic or orbitozygomatic osteotomy is needed to gain a lower approach to the infratemporal fossa. For

the standard approach, the temporal squama is removed to the floor of the temporal fossa. A single-entry hole is made at the anterior-inferior margin of the flap. The craniotome inscribes the flap, and the drill removes the inferior bone to the floor of the middle fossa. The dura is tented at multiple sites, and wires are placed for subsequent stabilization of the flap. The dural flap is opened near the base of the skull, and cuts are extended vertically while the flap falls to cover the temporal lobe. The remainder of the cortex is protected with cottonoids or telfa sheets. The halo retractor system is attached to the skull fixation (Fig. 3-2C). The self-retaining retractor blades are placed and gentle retraction is induced as CSF is removed and brain relaxation follows the effect of osmotic diuretics. The anterior temporal veins and anastomotic vein of Labbé are preserved as we approach the medial edge of the tentorium. Resection of the anterior temporal lobe (4 cm) may be required for some complex cases. The arachnoid is incised medial to the oculomotor nerve, and CSF is removed further. Precise retraction of the medial edge of the tentorium and oculomotor and trochlear nerves later-

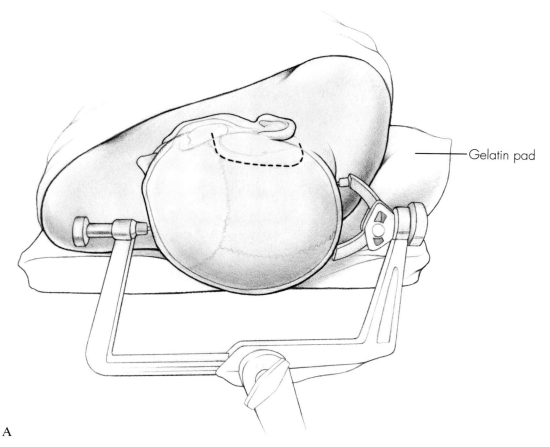

Gelatin pad

A

Figure 3-2. (A) Right subtemporal position and incision. (*Figure continues.*)

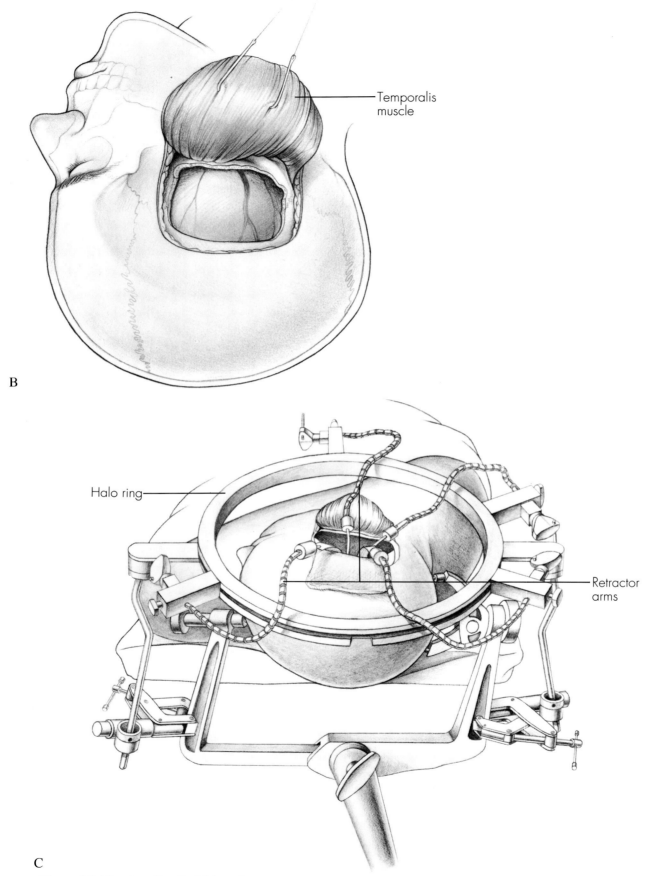

Temporalis
muscle

B

Halo ring

Retractor
arms

C

Figure 3-2 (*Continued*). **(B)** Right subtemporal myocutaneous flap and craniotomy. **(C)** Halo retractor system in place for subtemporal approach. (*Figure continues.*)

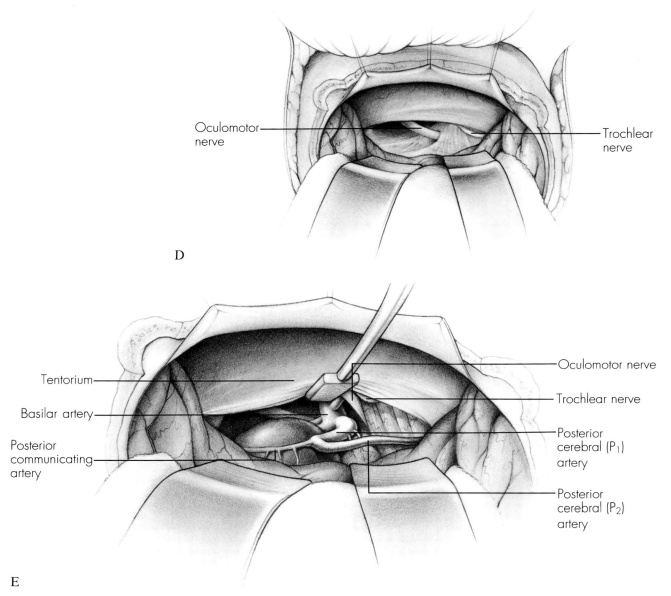

Figure 3-2 (*Continued*). **(D)** Initial right subtemporal exposure. **(E)** Right subtemporal excision of a basilar artery aneurysm.

ally may achieve adequate exposure of the membrane of Liliequist and the basilar caput (Fig. 3-2D). Sharp dissection of the arachnoid planes and subsequent retractor placement provides definition of the basilar anatomy (Fig. 3-2E).

Identification of the proximal basilar artery is a first priority that will enable the placement of a proximal clip if needed. Dissection of the posterior cerebral (P_1, P_2, and posterior communicating) and superior cerebellar branches are needed to prepare the site for clip application. Section of the posterior communicating at its junction with the posterior cerebral or the use of a fenestrated clip may facilitate clip placement, which will avoid occlusion of the posterior cerebral artery. A final microsurgical retractor may be placed on the peduncle to gain additional exposure of the perforators on the reverse side of the aneurysm and basilar artery. Section of the tentorium posterior to the insertion of the trochlear nerve and drill removal of the posterior clinoid facilitates better exposure of the proximal basilar artery. This tactic is best applied when the terminus lies low on the clivus.

An approach through the lateral wall of the cavernous after orbitozygomatic osteotomy facilitates exposure of the high-riding basilar terminus. This approach eliminates the need to retract the temporal lobe excessively, resect the anterior temporal lobe, or perform a pterional approach with wide opening of the sylvian fissure. The direct lateral approach provided by the subtemporal and infratemporal approaches allows the surgeon to visualize the base of the aneurysm and to separate the perforating vessels from the occluding clip. Failure to spare perforators will invariably lead to a poor operative result due to mesencephalic infarction. The subtemporal approach is also preferred for giant aneurysms (>2.5 cm), particularly for those that have some thrombus in the fundus of the lesion. Adequate exposure must be achieved by infratemporal approach or temporal lobe resection to isolate the aneurysm.

The use of temporary clips or the placement of an intraluminal balloon may be necessary to collapse the aneurysm. Aspiration of blood with a large-bore needle and removal of thrombus by ultrasonic aspiration is essential to collapse the aneurysm and gain precise clip placement. The advantage provided by a direct lateral trajectory and long fenestrated and reinforcing clips cannot be overemphasized in executing the approach to complex distal basilar aneurysms. Final evaluation of the results is provided by intraoperative digital subtraction angiography.

Closure

Removal of subarachnoid clot is performed by arachnoid dissection and copious irrigation with warm saline. The aspirated CSF is replaced with buffered saline, and the dura is tightly closed and secured to the bone edges to obliterate the extradural space. A tack-up suture is placed through the center of the bone flap. The flap is rigidly secured to the skull with wire. Bone defects are repaired with methylmethacrylate. The myofascial flap is reattached to the skull. A self-contained drain is placed beneath the galea. The galea and skin are closed in layers with absorbable suture and skin clips.

INTERHEMISPHERIC APPROACH

The interhemispheric approach is used to expose certain anterior cerebral aneurysms, lesions of the third and lateral ventricles, and lesions of the basal ganglia and thalamus. In this chapter, we direct our attention to an example approach to an arteriovenous malformation of the anterior horn of the lateral ventricle, caudate, and thalamus.

The patient's body remains supine; a gelatin roll under the shoulder allows the cranial axis (sagittal suture) to be placed parallel to the floor (Fig. 3-3A).

Some prefer to orient the vertex toward the ceiling. However, we recommend the lateral direction. This inclination permits maximal visibility along the axis of the falx. The lesion side is placed in a dependent position so as to allow maximal dependent retraction of the hemisphere. The skull is fixed with a radiolucent headholder (angiographic unit). An armored tube is used to avoid obstruction of the airways. Attention to the head rotation is indicated for the purpose of avoiding venous obstruction.

Preoperative evaluation of venous drainage of the hemisphere allows selection of a corridor along the midline that will avoid injury to critical bridging veins. The cranial opening is sited on the coronal suture and parallel to the sagittal sinus. Two entry holes are made adjacent to the sinus. The sinus is dissected free of the bone prior to using the Midas Rex Craniotome. Care is taken in raising the flap to avoid injury to the cortex, venous drainage, and sagittal sinus. The dural flap is placed on the border of the sagittal sinus and reflected medially (Fig. 3-3B). As the hemisphere is dependent, minimal retraction is needed as the adhesions of the frontal lobe are freed from the falx. The Budde halo retractor device is secured to the skull clamp, and the self-retaining retractor blades are prepared to overlie the padded aspect of the medial hemisphere. As dissection approaches the cingulate gyrus, the callosal marginal artery is identified. Further dissection with bipolar forceps and scissors frees the cingulate gyrus to fall dependently. One must be aware that the cingulate gyrus can be confused with the corpus callosum. The pericallosal arteries come into view and must be separated, right to right and left to left by incising the arachnoid and carefully evaluating the location of the arteries. Frequently, the pericallosal arteries may wander across the midline, may cross each other, and may be adherent. Proper identification is needed to ensure that the right pericallosal artery is taken to the right. The pearly white surface of the corpus callosum is identified deep to the cingulate gyrus and pericallosal arteries. The corpus callosum is opened in the midline with a carbon dioxide laser (Fig. 3-3C). A ruler is used to measure the opening and to ensure that the corpus split is limited to 2 cm. Limited opening of the corpus reduces the likelihood of postoperative disconnection syndrome. As the corpus is opened, the ependyma appears superficial to the CSF. Drainage of CSF exposes the anterior horn of the lateral ventricle. The choroid plexus is traced to the foramen of Monroe (Fig. 3-3D). Doing so, the correct ventricle is identified. Absence of the septum allows visualization of both the lateral ventricles simultaneously.

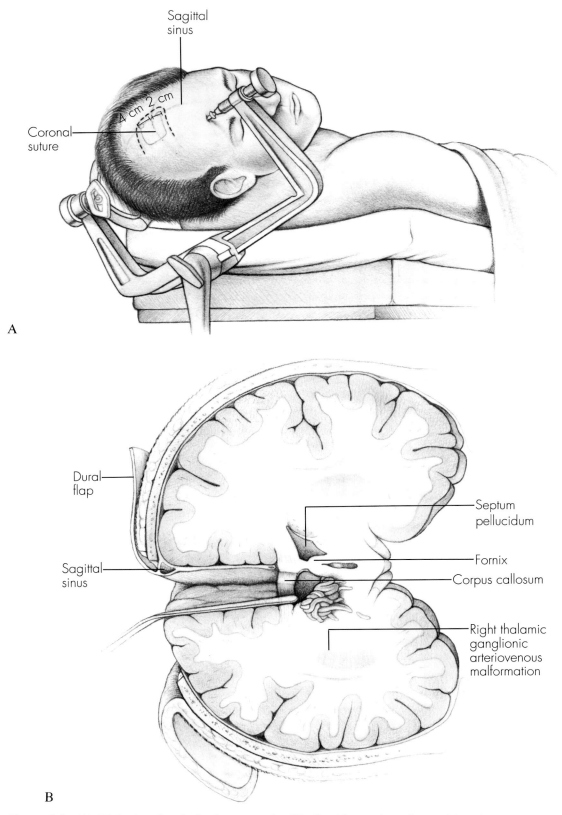

Figure 3-3. (A) Right interhemispheric approach. **(B)** Corridor to lateral ventricle of right hemispheric approach. (*Figure continues.*)

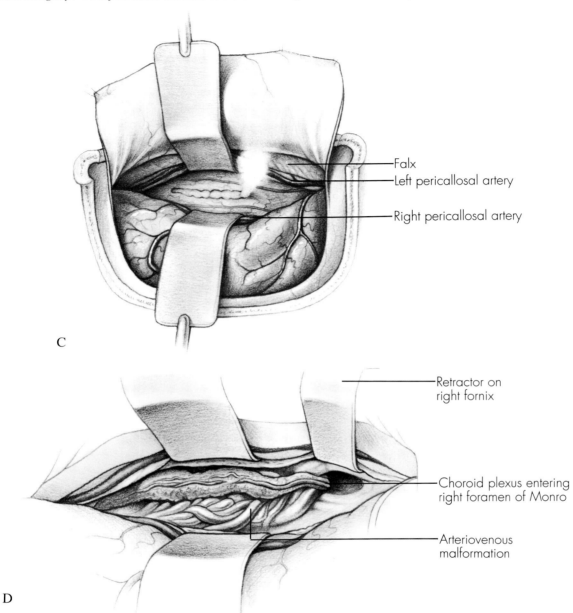

Falx
Left pericallosal artery
Right pericallosal artery

C

Retractor on
right fornix

Choroid plexus entering
right foramen of Monro

Arteriovenous
malformation

D

Figure 3-3 (*Continued*). **(C)** Colostomy of right interhemispheric approach. **(D)** Identification of choroid plexus and tract of foramen of Monroe.

Identification of the choroid plexus of the dependent ventricle enables us to localize the subchoroidal fissure inferior to the third ventricle and pinpoint the fornix, foramen of Monroe, and internal cerebral vein. Avoidance of damage to the fornices is essential to prevention of recent memory deficit. Damage to the internal cerebral vein may lead to internal hemorrhage into the third ventricle. The choroid plexus must be eliminated in order to obliterate posterior choroidal arterial supply to the vascular nidus. Staining of the basal ganglia or thalamus from hematoma and the venous drainage into the internal cerebral

vein establish the site of the vascular nidus, which must be dissected from the parenchyma of the thalamus and caudate. The hematoma cavity associated with the arteriovenous malformation assists with localization and dissection of the vascular nidus. Intraoperative angiography is essential to document total removal of the malformation. Retention of residual malformation is likely to be associated with the high risk of delayed postoperative hemorrhage.

Great care must be given to localizing the internal capsule and motor sensory thalamus to avoid major complications. Intraoperative evoked potentials and capsular stimulation may be needed to localize the critical pathways and nuclei.

Closure

The dura is closed tight with continuous suture. The bone flap is secured with multiple wire sutures. Galea and skin are closed in layers over a closed drainage system.

SUBLABIAL TRANSSPHENOIDAL APPROACH TO THE PITUITARY

The sublabial transsphenoidal approach is used to gain access to the sphenoid sinus and sella turcica for removal of pituitary tumors, cystic craniopharyn-

giomas, and other intrasellar lesions. This approach may be used to gain access to some lesions that extend into the medial cavernous sinus and upper one-third of the clivus.

The patient is placed in a supine position, with the cranium cradled in a modified cerebellar headrest, Hardy attachment, Mayfield headrest (Ohio Medical Instrument Co., Cincinnati) in order to permit the head to be angled and rotated during various aspects of the deep-narrow approach to the sella turcica. Figure 3-4A illustrates the room arrangement that is utilized for transsphenoidal and transoral approaches. Oral intubation is performed with an armored tube, and the tube is secured to the face prior to the anesthesiologist's movement to the end of the table. The endotracheal tube is securely packed away with moist sponge to avoid contact with the carbon diox-

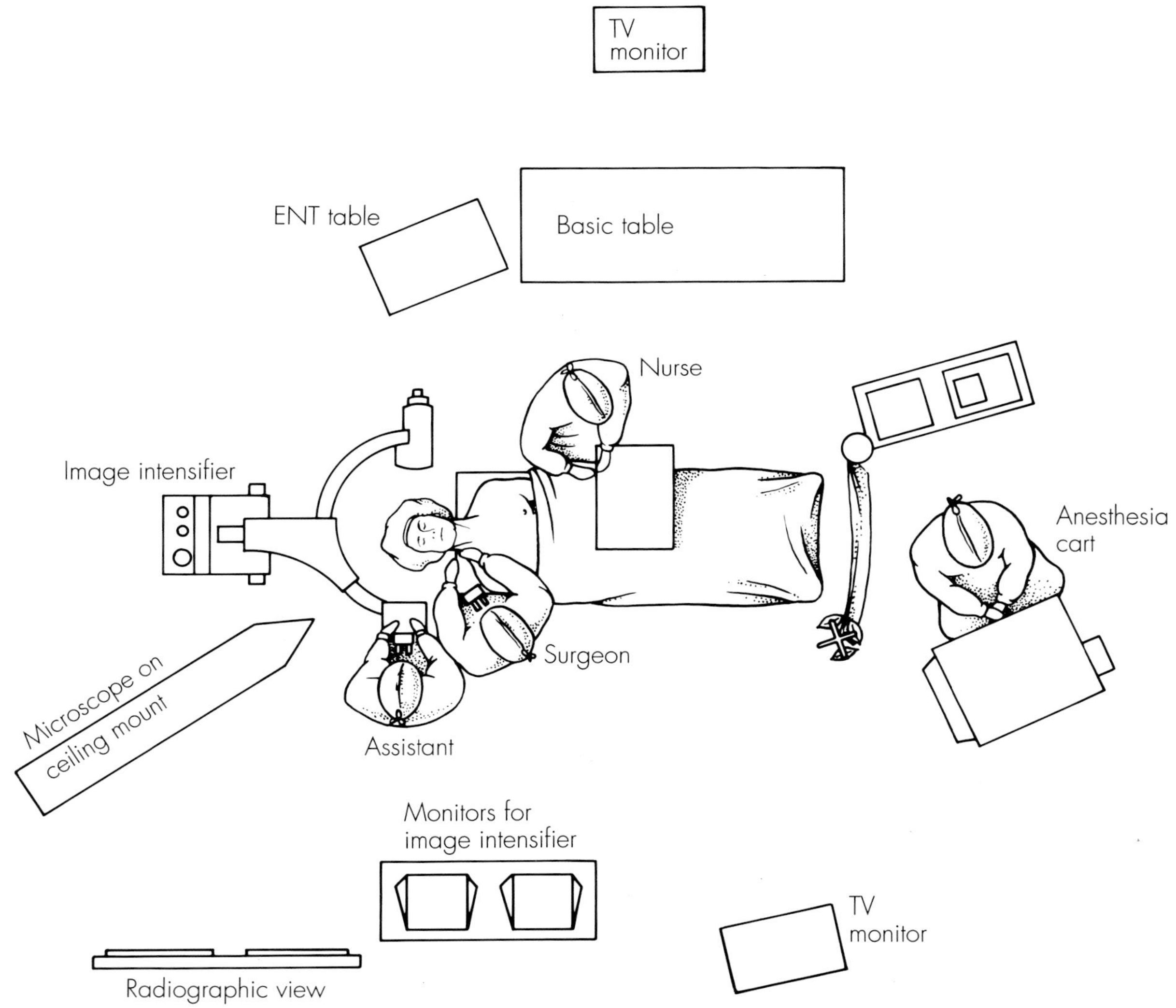

Figure 3-4. (A) Patient position for midfacial transsphenoidal approach. (*Figure continues.*)

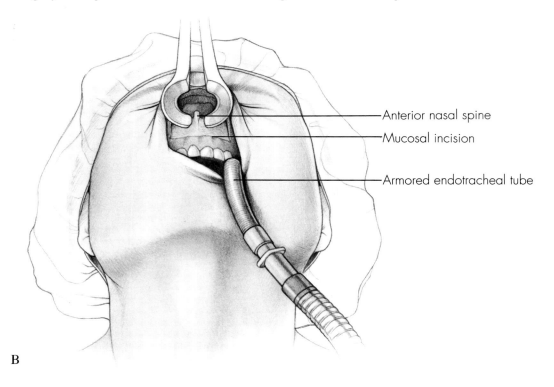

B

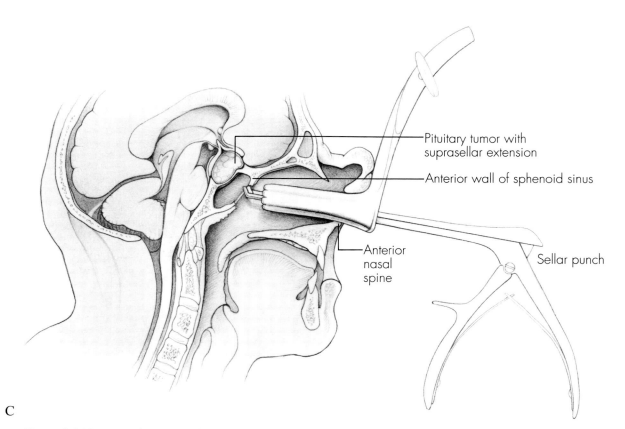

C

Figure 3-4 (*Continued*). **(B)** Position of transsphenoidal nasal speculum. **(C)** Lateral view of opening of the sphenoid sinus. (*Figure continues*.)

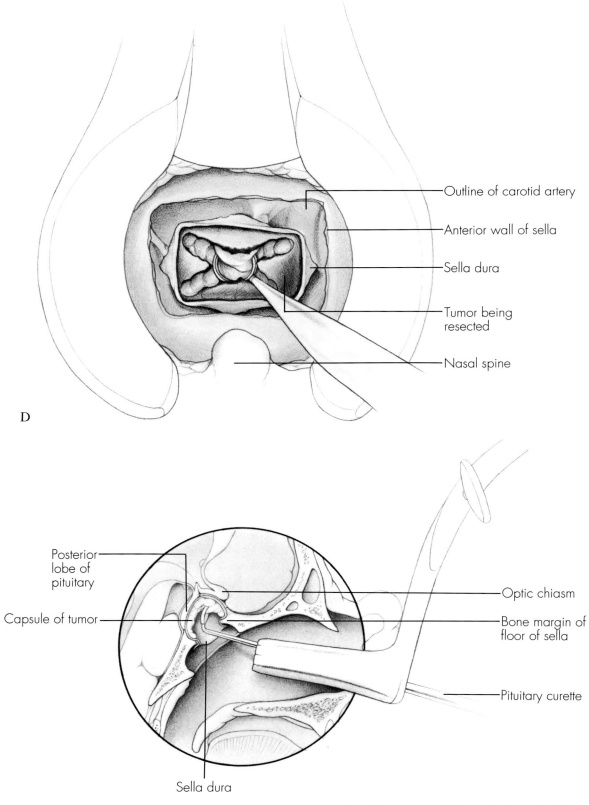

D

Outline of carotid artery

Anterior wall of sella

Sella dura

Tumor being resected

Nasal spine

Posterior lobe of pituitary

Capsule of tumor

Optic chiasm

Bone margin of floor of sella

Pituitary curette

Sella dura

E

Figure 3-4 (*Continued*). **(D)** Intraoperative view of curettage of a sellar tumor. **(E)** Lateral view of sellar tumor curettage. (*Figure continues.*)

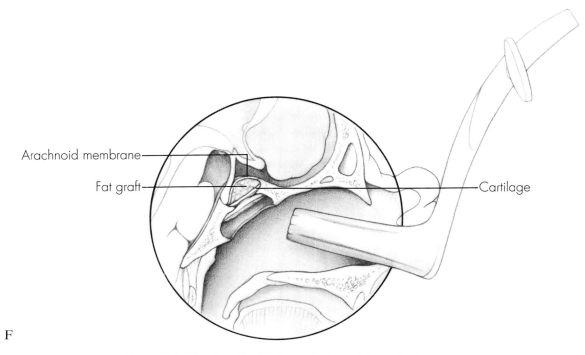

Arachnoid membrane

Fat graft

Cartilage

F

Figure 3-4 (*Continued*). **(F)** Lateral view of fat graft closure.

ide or Yag laser sources during the performance of the operation. Penetration of the endotracheal tube with the laser energy may result in an endobronchial explosion, which is a catastrophe.

All parenteral lines and monitoring devices are transferred to the foot of the table. This positioning of the room frees the top of the table for access by surgeons and for placement of the image intensifier, which is used throughout most of the procedure.

The corridor to the sella is made after injection of the septal, nasal, and paranasal mucosa with vasoconstrictor agents. The sublabial mucosa is incised and elevated to gain entry into the base of the nasal cavity (Fig. 3-4B). The nasal spine is spared and the mucosa is dissected from either side of the septum. The cartilaginous septum is excised, to be utilized in subsequent closure of the floor of the sella. As the mucosa is reflected off the floor of the nasal cavity, the turbanates are fractured laterally with a nasal speculum. The anterior nasal spine is spared to avoid subsequent depression of the nose and denervation of the teeth. The mucosa is reflected off the anterior wall of the sphenoid sinus, and the image intensifier is used to ensure that the trajectory is proper for entering the sphenoid sinus.

A chisel entry of the sphenoid sinus is followed by removal of the anterior wall of the sinus and extraction of the sinus mucosa (Fig. 3-4C). A wide removal of the anterior wall of the sinus is needed to gain a broad view of the anterior sella anatomy. The image intensifier is used to ensure that entry into the floor of the sella is gained at the junction of the sella with the clivus. Entry near the roof of the sella must be avoided in order to guard against injury to the optic nerve, chiasm, and arachnoid diverticulum over the pituitary gland.

The sella must be entered in the midline; the midline is located by identifying the nasal spine and aligning the perpendicular plate of the ethmoid and the nasal spine. Alignment of these two points will direct the entry into the midline of the sella. The anterior sellar wall is penetrated under radiographic control with a chisel. The remainder of the sella wall is removed with a small punch. Exposure is continued until both cavernous sinuses and the connecting sinuses above and below are visualized. The dura is opened in the midline, near the floor of the sella, and extended in a cruciate fashion toward each of the exposed sinuses. The entire sella can be explored through this wide exposure.

The pituitary capsule can be dissected free of the medial wall of the cavernous sinus unless the tumor invades this barrier and lies free in the cavernous sinus. Most tumors can be extracted from the cavernous sinus providing they do not encircle the carotid artery. Bleeding is controlled by application of Gelfoam or oxidized cellulose soaked with thrombin. Complete dissection of the tumor in the cavernous sinus is planned according to the preoperative magnetic resonance images (Figs. 3-4D & E). If the tumor extends through the diaphragma sella into the supra sella space, the mass will then fall into the empty sella from whence the tumor has been evacuated.

This maneuver is aided by injection of buffered saline into the CSF via a lumbar catheter. Injected air will aid in determining when the mass has been satisfactorily dislocated into the sella. The appearance of the chiasmal cistern and the infundibular recess is examined by the image intensifier. Further, the arachnoid will herniate into the sella when the tumor mass has been extracted. The intact arachnoid should be maintained to limit CSF leakage. The arachnoid should be displaced into the suprasellar space during closure to avoid chiasmal herniation into the sella. Arachnoid herniation may lead to delayed CSF leak. Chiasmal herniation will lead to a progressive altitudinal field defect.

Closure

Closure of the sella is very important to avoidance of complications (visual field cuts, CSF leak, and infection; see Table 3-1). The closure technique consists of aspiration of CSF to permit the arachnoid to recede into the suprasellar area. The sella is then covered with a layer of thrombin-soaked Surgicel. The sella is then filled with autologous fat. The floor of the sella is closed with a flexible piece of cartilage taken from the nasal septum (Fig. 3-4F). The cartilage is placed deep to the dura and the bony wall of the sella. It is secured by injecting tissue glue or medical adhesive into a layer of Surgicel. The adhesive creates a firm layer between the dura, bone, and cartilage implant to establish a strong reconstruction of the sella floor. A fat-fascial implant is placed into the sphenoid sinus and attached to the sella with adhesive. The nasal mucosa is returned to the septum. Residual cartilage and bone is returned to the septal pouch, and the septal mucosa is approximated with absorbable sutures that include both mucosal layers and the septum. The septum is reattached to the anterior nasal spine with a suture. Retention of the septal mucosa and closure of any septal perforations is essential to preventing crusting and air escape through the nostrils. Retention of the nasal spine and septum is necessary to avoid flattening of the nasal bridge. Excessive removal of the nasal spine may lead to denervation and discoloration of the canine teeth. Both nasal cavities are packed with antibiotic-impregnated dressing. The sublabial incision is closed with absorbable suture.

Table 3-1.   Possible Complications

Complication	Prevention
Position	
Skin pressure	Position and padding
Nerve pressure	Avoid pressure points
Venous obstruction	Avoid excessive neck rotation
Intubation	
Obstruction	Armored tube
Dislocation airway	Secured tube
Laser fire	Protect tube
Homeostasis	
Hypothermia	Warming blanket, warm fluids, monitor temperature
Hypotension	Supine position, avoid air embolism
Hypoxia	Control airway, adjust ventilation
Eye injury	
Eye abrasion (cornea)	Closure of lids
Blindness	Avoid pressure
Skeletal fixation	
Air embolism, infection at pin sites	Antibiotic paste at pin sites
Laceration at scalp	Secure pin placement
Exposure	
Scalp necrosis	Adequate base, proper storage of skin flap
Frontalis paralysis	Avoid fascial frontal branch
Temporalis atrophy	Reflect muscle with skin
Cosmetic bone defects	Single-entry hole closure all defects with methylmethacrylate
Cerebral edema	Proper exposure, gentle retraction, brain relaxation, osmotic diuretics, CSF drainage, position of skull
Neurological deficit	Good exposure, maintain gentle traction, sharp dissection
Cerebral ischemia	Proper clip placement, spare perforators, prevent vasospasm
Closure	
CSF leak	Complete dural closure, wax bone, close bony sinuses with grafts and adhesives
Pneumocephalus	Replace air with CSF, close sinus opening
Subdural hematoma	Hemostasis
Epidural hematoma	Hemostasis, dural testing sutures
Poor cosmetic closure	Secure bone flap with wire or plates, inbed wire, close all bone defects, approximate muscle fascia, close skin and galea
Infection	Subgaleal drain, intraoperative antibiotics, obliteration of all spaces, aseptic technique

Postoperative antibiotics and lumbar CSF drainage are maintained for 24 hours. If a large opening was produced in the arachnoid, or closure was less than perfect, the lumbar drain is converted to a percutaneous lumboperitoneal shunt. Antibiotics are not continued beyond 24 hours to avoid superinfection. Nasal packing is removed after 48 hours.

TRANSORAL APPROACH

The transoral approach is utilized to gain access to the extradural lesions of the lower one-third of the clivus and craniocervical junction such as chordoma and atlantoaxial instability. Intradural lesions, meningioma, and vertebrobasilar aneurysms may be accessed through the lower clivus. The palate obscures the approach to the midclival region, and the corridor provided by the transoral approach is narrow and limited laterally. The midpalatal approach afforded by a Le Fort I osteotomy or unilateral extended maxillary osteotomy provides the lateral and vertical exposures needed for more extensive lesions of the clivus. These approaches essentially give a broader approach to the clivus and upper cervical spine. The exposure and closure are substantially the same with all of the anterior approaches to the skull base region.

The transoral approach is achieved by placing the patient in the supine position with arrangements identical to those demonstrated for the transsphenoidal approach. An armored endotracheal tube is placed by oral intubation. The tube is protected from laser contact by wet packing. Nasal intubation, or tracheostomy, is rarely needed for these approaches. The Crockard retractor (Codman, Randolph, MA) is placed over the tongue, and counterforce is placed against the incisor teeth (Fig. 3-5A). Maximal opening of the mouth is needed to widen the corridor to the skull base. The corridor may be increased by placing a suture in the tip of the uvula and pulling the suture into the nostril with a flexible catheter. Further vertical exposure is gained by incising the soft palate and osteotomy of the hard palate. However, palatal split and bony removal may lead to dysphonia and short-term nasal regurgitation of fluids. Closure of the soft palate in two layers and avoidance of shortening of the uvula limits these complications. A midpalatal approach may be needed if these tactics are not feasible.

The palate is opened in the midline if an extradural approach is planned. A pharyngeal flap based on the upper clivus is structured in order to elevate the longus colli muscles and create a two-layer closure. The muscles and fascia are dissected from the anterior surface of the clivus. The image intensifier is used to identify the anterior arch of the atlas. Subperiosteal dissection is followed by drilling of the arch of the atlas and the inferior margin of the clivus. Precise determination of the midline is necessary in order to determine the width of the clival osteotomy and the vertical limitations of the bone dissection. The odontoid is removed only as low as necessary. Removal of the complete odontoid results in destruction of the transverse atlantal ligament and causes instability of the atlantoaxial articulation. Upward retraction of the soft palate, removal of the clivus and odontoid, followed by exposure of the tectorial membrane and ligaments of the odontoid (alar and transverse atlantal ligaments) provide ample midline exposure of the retroclival dura and brainstem (Fig. 3-5B). The tissues are greatly thickened when involved with chronic instability of the atlantoaxial joint and infiltrated by clival meningiomas. Removal of this tough and richly vascular tissue is greatly facilitated by carbon dioxide laser dissection. The basal dura should be preserved in all extradural lesions. In cases of intradural pathology, such as meningioma (Fig. 3-5C), the dura must be widely vaporized with the laser in order to eliminate the blood supply of the tumor. Wide excision of the dura eliminates the origin of the tumor and allows the mass to be liberated from its cavity in the brainstem. The remainder of the lesion is sharply separated from the brainstem, vessels, and cranial nerves.

Closure

The closure is initiated by procurement of hemostasis and a dry field by aspiration of CSF with the lumbar catheter. A fat graft is placed in the tumor bed (Fig. 3-5D). A fascial graft obtained from the fascia lata is approximated to the residual dural edge with fibrin glue or medical adhesive. Another layer of Surgicel adhesive is applied. The closure is buttressed with a thin bone graft secured from the iliac crest or bone bank. The bone implant is wedged into the clivus and odontoid. It is secured mechanically and sealed with another layer of adhesive. The mucosa-muscle flap is restored and sutured in two layers. Any defects in the pharyngeal wall are closed with pharyngeal rotation flaps or a myofascial flap transplanted from the temporalis muscle. This tactic is rarely needed except in previously irradiated patients. The CSF drainage via a lumbar catheter is converged into a lumboperitoneal shunt on postoperative day three. Antibiotics are discontinued after 24 hours to avoid superinfection by fungus. Postoperatively, stability is determined by dynamic tomography. Excessive instability is treated by a posterior orthosis or an internal posterior stabilization procedure.

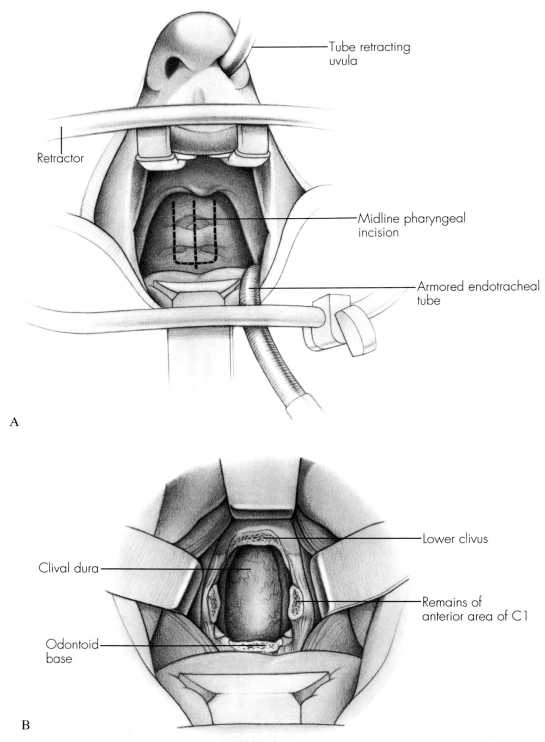

Figure 3-5. (A) Retractor positioning for transoral approach. **(B)** Exposure of the retroclival dura via the transoral approach. (*Figure continues.*)

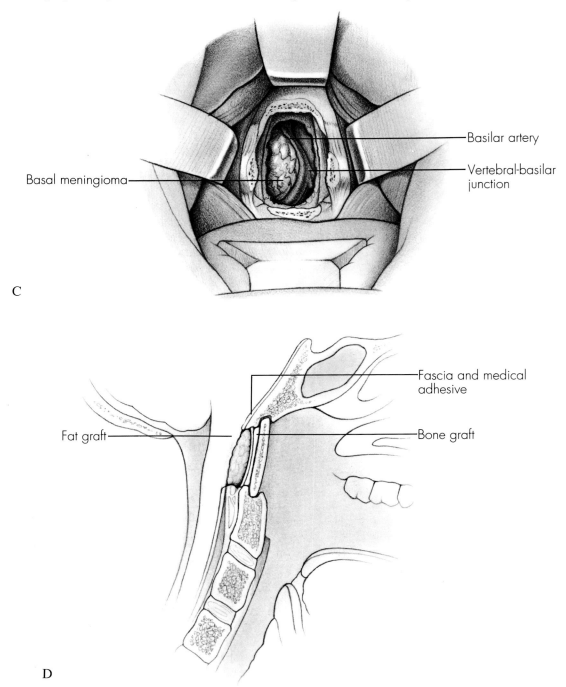

Basilar artery

Vertebral-basilar
junction

Basal meningioma

C

Fascia and medical
adhesive

Fat graft

Bone graft

D

Figure 3-5 (*Continued*). **(C)** Exposure of the meningioma. **(D)** Lateral view of closure for the transoral procedure.

REFERENCES

1. Albin MS, Bunegin L, Hirsel P et al: Intracranial pressure and regional cerebral blood flow responses to experimental brain retraction procedures. p. 131. In Shulman K, Marmarow A, Miller JD et al (eds): Intracranial Pressure IV. Springer-Verlag, New York, 1980
2. Butler VM, Dean L, Little J: Positioning of neurosurgi-

cal patient in the operating room: ''a team effort.'' J Neurosurg Nursing 16(2):89, 1984
3. Cabequdo JM, Carrielo R, Vognero S et al: Air embolism from pin type head holder as complication of sitting position: case report. J Neurosurg 55:147, 1981
4. Hallenhorst RW, Svien HS, Benoit CR: Unilateral blindness occurring during anesthesia for neurosurgical operations. Arch Ophthalmol 52:819, 1954
5. McCaig C: Review: positioning for neurosurgery. AORN J 28(6):1053, 1978

4 Supratentorial Craniotomies

Ivan S. Ciric
Szymon Rosenblatt

GENERAL PRINCIPLES

Positioning

The patient should be placed into a position that would be considered comfortable for by awake person. Slight flexion of the knees and elevation of the back of the table is generally preferable. Care should be taken to protect all dependent peripheral nerves from pressure points as well as the dependent eye when the patient is in a decubitus or prone position. The position of the head and neck should be such that there is no kinking of the carotid or vertebral arteries and no obstruction of the jugular veins. To that end, the surgeon should always palpate the superficial temporal artery pulses and observe the neck for jugular vein distension. When these principles are not observed a vascular occlusion can occur resulting in either cerebrovascular ischemia or congestion, respectively. The latter can make dural opening dangerous. Furthermore, during positioning, the surgeon must avoid any traction on the brachial plexus lest there be a postoperative brachial plexus traction injury. This is most likely to occur when the patient is supine and the head turned acutely toward one side. Appropriate padding and elevation of the shoulder to relax the brachial plexus will avoid such an injury. Position of the patient's head in relationship to the horizontal should also be such that the natural gravitational forces aid in the relaxation and retraction of

the brain from the skull base or the falx in accordance with the operative plan. A properly positioned head in this regard will diminish and at times obviate the necessity for any retraction of the brain during surgery.

When positioning the patient on the operating table, the vertex of the head should be flush with the upper margin of the table. This will ensure ease of positioning of the three-point fixation clamp once the headrest is removed. If the position of the pins of the three-point fixation clamp is not satisfactory, a different point of entry must be used for all three pins, since placement of the pin in any of the previously made holes can result in skull perforation when the screw is again tightened (Fig. 4-1). If penetration occurs, immediate exposure of the area should be carried out in order to debride the bony fragments and inspect the dura for any tears. While securing the three-point fixation clamp to the operating table, the lock attachment on the horizontal bar must be in a position where it is under no strain. This is best assessed by moving the lock along the horizontal bar until it is in a position where least resistance is felt before the lock is secured tightly across the bar. Failure to do so can result in metal strain and fracture of the lock with a potentially disastrous sudden change in the neck and head position during surgery (Fig. 4-2). When a footrest is used, it should not exert undue pressure on the soles of the feet in order to avoid overstretching of the Achilles' tendons. Egg

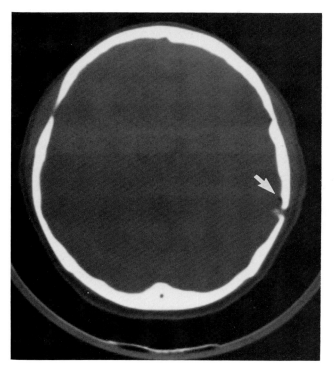

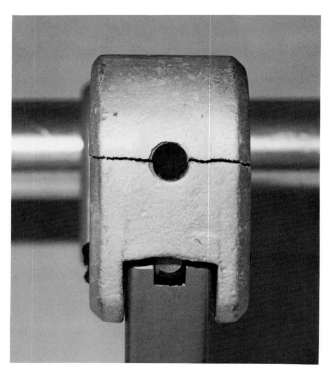

Figure 4-1. CT scan in a patient with depressed fracture and intracranial air caused by replacement and retightening of the three-point fixation clamp into the same hole in the skull (*arrow*).

Figure 4-2. Fracture of the lock device on the horizontal bar of the universal head holder due to metal strain during surgery.

crate pads should be used to support the patient when necessary instead of hard rolls or surgical towels. Eye protection during surgery is paramount. There are several good methods of protecting the eyes, such as placement of an ophthalmic ointment underneath the eyelids, placement of a layer of Vaseline over the eyelids, taping the eyelids shut, and placement of protective eye goggles. Greatest care should be exercised with the eye goggles, which can easily indent and cause pressure on the globe. Blindness due to improper positioning of goggles has been reported.[3] Thus a constant inspection of the goggles by the anesthesiologist throughout the procedure is mandatory. Goggles are usually in the way in patients requiring frontal and frontotemporal craniotomies.

Planning of the Craniotomy Site and Scalp Incision

The craniotomy site is dictated by the location of the lesion. A three-dimensional perception of the lesion within the head is obtained by studying carefully the axial and coronal computed tomography (CT)

slices as well as all three views of the magnetic resonance image (MRI). Gadolinium infused T_1-weighted MRIs should be used for planning of the surgical strategy. When indicated, cerebral angiogram is also useful in placing the craniotomy site.

The first step is to determine the location of the lesion within the relative sphere of the patient's head. This should be done in all three planes, namely, the coronal, sagittal, and axial planes. To accomplish this, relationships are established and distances calculated to various prominent surface landmarks such as the external ear canal, the superior or posterior margin of the ear, the glabella or occipital protuberance, the coronal and lambdoid suture, and so forth, and to such deep reference points as the anatomical midline, the tentorium, foramen of Monro, the lateral ventricles. For example, Figure 4-3 shows a glioblastoma multiforme situated above the right trigone. On the lateral surface of the head the center of this tumor (Fig. 4-3C, small arrowhead) projects 5 cm above the external ear canal or 3 cm above the top of the helix at the level of the posterior border of the ear lobe (Fig. 4-3B, arrow). The anteroposterior extent of the equator of the tumor projects on the surface of the head 5 to 9 cm anterior to the posterior midline (Fig.

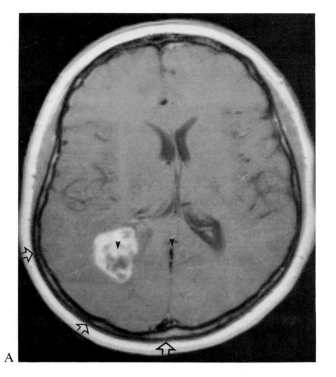

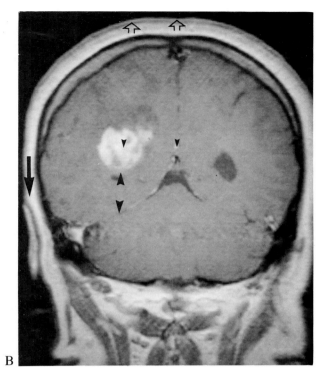

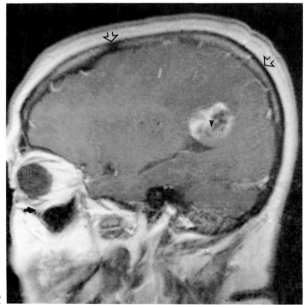

Figure 4-3. (A–C) T_1-weighted infused MRI from a patient with glioblastoma multiforme above the right trigone. Relationships and distances to various surface landmarks and deep reference points can be established and calculated precisely in all three planes (see text).

4-3A, open arrows). On the superior surface of the head, the center of the tumor projects 3 cm from the midline (Fig. 4-3B, open arrows). The projection of this tumor on the superior surface of the head at the approximate point of entry can also be determined in centimeters relative to a prominent bony landmark such as the coronal suture (Fig. 4-3C, open arrows). Relationships to deep reference points show that the center of this tumor is 3 cm from the anatomical mid-line (Fig. 4-3A, B, small arrowheads). The center of this tumor is also 3 cm above the tentorium (Fig. 4-3B, large arrowheads).

The distances can be calculated easily from the centimeter scale available on each image or by adding the distances in millimeters between consecutive slices from a reference plane (orbital roof, external ear canal, and so forth, in the axial plane, coronal suture in the coronal plane, and midline in the sagittal plane) to the plane of the tumor. When determining the distance from the midline, it is important to distinguish between the shortest distance from the midline and the actual distance projected on the head surface. Additionally, distinction should be made between the near distance, the distance to the center, and the distance to the outer margin of the tumor. When transferring the information from the CT scan or MRI it is important to view the head in a perfectly perpendicular fashion to the imaging study used without any parallax and to calculate the distance between the reference plane and the tumor parallel to the consecutive imaging slices used. If the relationship of the lesion to the surface of the patient's head is transferred correctly from the imaging study, the projection of the lesion on the surface of the head should be one and the same regardless of the imaging plane used. Similarly, distances from a lesion to a deep reference point should be one and the same on all three imaging planes regardless of the method of calculation used.

An angiogram can also be useful in determining the location of the lesion in relationship to various bony landmarks.[10] Care should be taken not to mistake a relatively low-situated posterotemporal lesion for a high parietal location due to the foreshortened image of the slanted portion of the skull on the lateral views of the angiogram.

Once the location of a lesion within the patient's head and its projection on the surface of the head has been determined, planning of the craniotomy site and of the operative approach will further require that the surgeon reviews in detail the relationships of the lesion to the cortical and/or basal ganglia anatomy, the ventricular system, the sylvian fissure, and the surrounding arterial and venous anatomy. In this respect, it is important to determine the relationship of the lesion to the opercular as well as the angular and supramarginal gyrus regions of the dominant hemisphere, the central gyrus, the insular and calcarine cortices. The relationship of the lesion to the ventricular system can be determined by both the CT scan and the MRI. The latter, however, is superior in recognizing the position of the lesion in relationship to the sylvian fissure. Relationship of a lesion, especially a tumor, to the surrounding arterial vessels is probably best appreciated on the gadolinium-infused T_1-weighted MRIs. The MRI can show better than an angiogram whether an arterial blood vessel in the vicinity of the tumor is displaced by the tumor, is straddled, or is actually engulfed by the tumor (Fig. 4-4). On the other hand, the cerebral angiogram is superior in determining the relationship of a tumor to the surrounding venous structures.

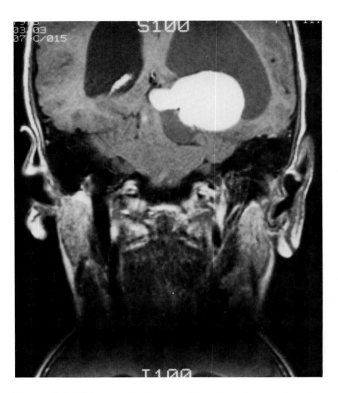

Figure 4-4. Trigone tumor, cystic astrocytoma, showing near circumferential straddling but not encasement of the lateral posterior choroidal artery and of the posterior cerebral artery.

Armed with the knowledge of the location of the lesion within the head and its relationship to the surrounding neurovascular structures, the point of entry on the brain surface and the avenue of approach to the lesion are chosen based on the proximity of the lesion to the brain surface, the presence (or absence) of an eloquent cerebral or critically important vascular structure, and the available sulcal avenues and parenchymal corridors to the lesion. For example, a lesion situated just above the trigone of the lateral ventricle in the dominant hemisphere is probably better approached through the sulcus between the superior and inferior parietal lobulus than from a more lateral approach, even though it may be closer to the cortical surface in the angular-supramarginal gyrus region.

With the planning of the craniotomy site completed, the exact placement of a scalp skull flap in the operating room can be further facilitated by a preoperative localizing CT scan or MRI although this is not always necessary. We prefer the MRI as our localizing imaging study. One or more vitamin E capsules, clearly visualized by the T_1-weighted MRI, can be placed on the scalp at the point of the planned entry to the lesion (Fig. 4-5). A rapid-sequence MRI is ob-

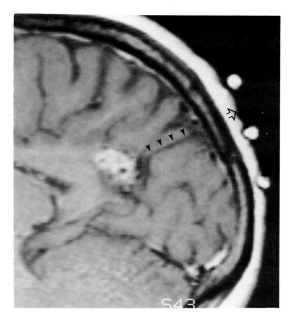

Figure 4-5. T₁-weighted infused localizing MRI from a patient with a cavernous angioma in the region of the splenium of the corpus callosum. Three vitamin E capsules were used as surface markers to localize the point of entry (*open arrow*). The avenue of approach was along the parietal-occipital sulcus (*small arrowheads*).

tained in one or two planes. The capsule can be shifted along the surface of the scalp until it is projected precisely over the desired point on the surface of the brain to be entered in the approach to the lesion. This area is marked and the mark kept in place until surgery. The scalp flap is then fashioned around the desired point of entry. At operation, a twist drill can be used to mark the skull underneath the scalp marker. From there the projection of the point marked on the skull onto the underlying dura and brain is easily determined. With this technique, surface and shallow subcortical lesions can be exposed quite precisely through relatively small flaps.

Approach to smaller and deep-seated lesions is probably best accomplished utilizing ultrasound guidance[13] or stereotactic craniotomies[6] with either CT scan or MRI. At our institution the latter has been the preferred technique (Fig. 4-6). Any of the three imaging projections of the MRI can be used alone or in combination. The point of entry is best calculated from the cortical surface, with the advantage that the exact location of a sulcus can be determined and vascular structures avoided. Any shift of the cortical surface in relationship to the target, which can occur after the dura is opened, would not amount to a significant change in the trajectory toward the lesion.

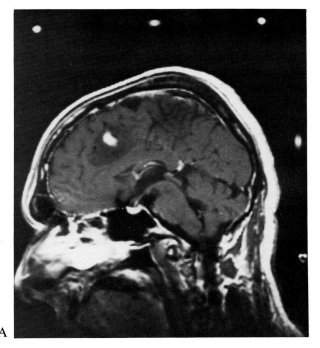

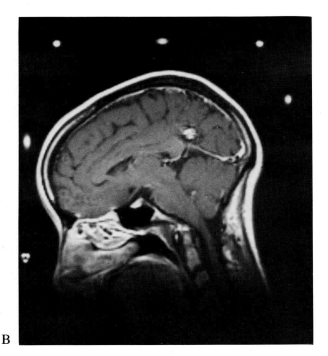

A

B

Figure 4-6. T₁-weighted MRI from a patient in the stereotactic frame for MRI-assisted and stereotactic-guided craniotomy to left posterior frontomedial anaplastic astrocytoma **(A)** and a cavernous angioma in the region of the splenium **(B)**, respectively. The patient in Fig. B was operated upon prone. The anterior part of the stereotactic frame must always be superior. The determination of coordinates must always proceed from the first localizing rod.

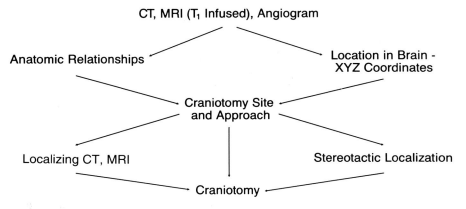

Figure 4-7. Craniotomy for intra-axial lesions: preoperative strategy.

Figure 4-7 summarizes our strategy in planning of the craniotomy site for a suprtentorial lesion. Due to an increased precision in localizing supratentorial lesions, the scalp incisions and craniotomy flaps have gotten generally smaller than in the past. Curvilinear, horseshoe-shaped, lazy S-shaped, or linear incisions are all acceptable, depending on the size and location of the lesion.

GENERAL TECHNICAL PRINCIPLES

We find that placement of mosquito hemostats for scalp hemostasis leads to less scalp damage and necrosis than the use of skin clips. While bipolar coagulation of scalp vessels is acceptable, discretion should be used not to coagulate too many vessels in order to avoid scalp necrosis. If bleeding from scalp margins is noted during surgery, it is preferable to apply additional hemostats rather than to coagulate more vessels in order to avoid scalp necrosis. When a horseshoe flap is carried out, its base should be toward the major blood supply (i.e., toward the base of the skull). The width of the base of the flap should be wider than its height. Consideration should be given to the blood supply of the scalp, and at least one of the major scalp arteries, namely, the supraorbital, the superficial temporal, the posterior auricular, or the occipital arteries, should be preserved at the base of the flap.[12] Relaxing incisions are permitted in areas of good blood supply and in a nonradiated scalp. A hot knife or laser should not be used for scalp incisions. Preferably the scalp flap is reflected together with the periosteum. When reflecting the scalp flap,

care should be taken to avoid kinking of its base in order to prevent necrosis of the scalp flap margins.[4]

With the scalp flap reflected and retracted with either special hooks or stay sutures and rubber bands, one, two, or several burr holes are placed circumferentially in the exposed cranium. In patients with extra-axial tumors that may be partially buried in the brain with a layer of brain interposed between the lesion and the skull, we prefer the hand-driven perforators. Vibrations from a powered instrument can transmit onto the underlying brain wedged between the extra-axial mass and the skull, resulting in a cerebral contusion or an epidural hematoma (Fig. 4-8). The number of burr holes will depend on the size and location of the craniotomy, the nature of the lesion, the patient's age, and the degree of adherence of the dura to the inner table of the skull. If the craniotomy is carried out to or across a major sinus, burr holes at shorter intervals will be necessary to avoid tearing the sinus. When a high convexity parasagittal craniotomy is carried out with the patient supine and the head elevated more than 20 degrees, exceptional care should be taken to prevent and watch for signs of air embolism. Under these circumstances the patient should be equipped with a central line and a precordial Doppler monitor. A preoperative routine cardiac echocardiogram should also be obtained to detect a possible septal defect that could lead to a paradoxical cerebral air embolism. Once the burr holes have been completed, separation of the dura should first proceed away from the great sinuses, leaving the sinus region for last. A right-angle dural separator should be used first. The burr hole is then undercut with a punch rongeur (Fig. 4-9A) along the projected path of

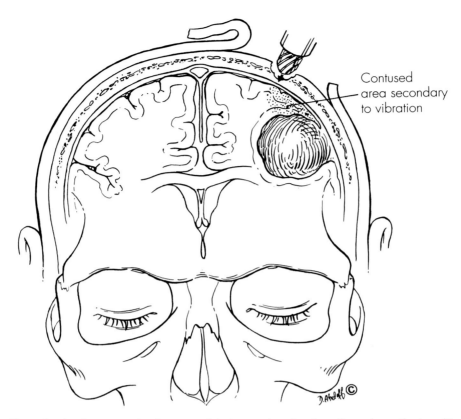

Contused area secondary to vibration

Figure 4-8. Since brain tissue can be interposed between two hard surfaces in patients with extra-axial tumors partially buried in the brain (tumor beneath and skull above), vibrations from power perforators can cause brain contusion. Hand-driven perforators may be preferable in such cases.

the separation before passing a curved dural separator. The angle of placement of the dural separator should be very much tangential to the inner surface of the skull and dura. This may be difficult to achieve at the beginning of the trajectory of separation. To facilitate this, a small amount of bone can be removed on top of the burr hole directly contralateral to the desired dural separation (Fig. 4-9B). This maneuver allows the dural separator to be placed more tangenitally at the very beginning of the dural separation. If the dura is torn at the beginning of the separation, further bone can be removed from the deeper part of the burr hole around the tear until intact dura is seen. Experience will eventually allow the surgeon to feel whether sideways motion or direct forward motion with the dural separator is preferable to avoid dural tears. In exceptionally thick skulls, when the dura appears unduly adherent to the inner table, additional burr holes will be necessary before using a dural separator. A high-speed microsurgical drill can also be used over the segment of adherent dura to

create a trough down to a paper-thin layer of the inner table, which can then be removed with the use of a small, thin-lipped punch rongeur (Fig. 4-9C).

Once the separation of the dura has been completed the burr holes are connected with the use of a craniotome. The choice of the power instrument is left to the surgeon's preference and comfort. Generally, instruments that have a lag in action once the power is disengaged should be avoided. The cutting surface should be angled in a crater-like fashion to avoid future sinking of the skull flap underneath the surface of the remaining skull. If a Gigli guide is used and it is seen at the exiting burr hole to be inside the dura, a second guide should be passed in the opposite direction so that it remains extradural (Fig. 4-10). When using a power instrument, an intradural position of the power instrument at the end of the cut will require the power instrument to be brought back toward the entering burr hole with the gears off. Bleeding from the bone and epidural space can be stopped by liberal application of bone wax over the finished

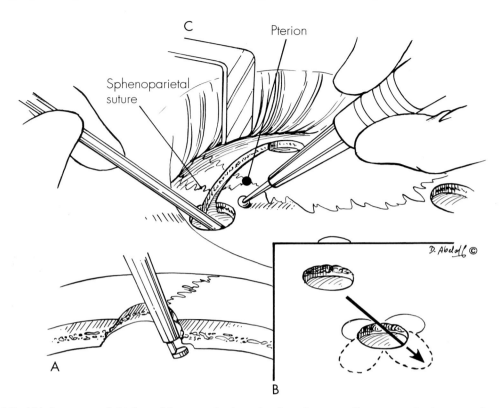

Figure 4-9. (A) In areas of thickened bone and when the dura is very adherent to the inner surface of the skull, a high-speed drill can be used under continuous irrigation/suction to create a trough in the outer table and the cancellous bone down to a thin layer of the inner table, which can then be rongeured away with a small, thin-lipped punch rongeur. **(B)** Undercutting the inner table at the burr hole facilitates placement of separating instruments between the inner table of the skull and the dura. **(C)** Removal of the rim of the burr hole opposite to the point of intended dural separation will facilitate tangential placement of separating instruments.

bony cut or by placement of Gelfoam underneath the bone if the point of bleeding is reachable.

Generally, we prefer free bone flaps over osteoplastic craniotomies, both techniques, however, being acceptable. With the bone flap reflected or removed, epidural bleeding should be stopped with the use of bipolar coagulation set at the lowest possible level and under continuous irrigation to avoid retraction and shrinking of the dura surface. Tacking sutures placed only under the outer layer of the dura, with or without Gelfoam placed underneath the bony margins, are also effective in stopping epidural bleeding. If tense and bluish discolored dura is encountered upon removal of the bone flap, a subdural hematoma secondary to a dural tear should be suspected. In that case, the dura should be immediately opened, the subdural hematoma flushed out, and hemostasis secured.

Frontal (Bifrontal) Craniotomy

Extra-axial or intra-axial frontal lobe and genu of the corpus callosum lesions and some frontobasal lesions anterior to the chiasm and the circle of Willis are approached via a frontal (Fig. 4-11A) or bifrontal craniotomy (Fig. 4-11B). The position of the head should be either straight up or slightly rotated to the side opposite the surgeon's handedness. The head should also be inclined about 10 to 20 degrees toward the operating room floor. The position of the head in space can be changed perioperatively as needed by changing the position of the operating table. Operating maneuvers along the frontobasal surface of the brain and in the region of the chiasm and the circle of Willis will require a greater inclination of the head toward the operating room floor, whereas maneuvers directed toward the bony skull base itself will require

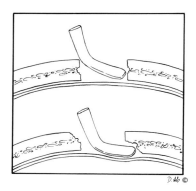

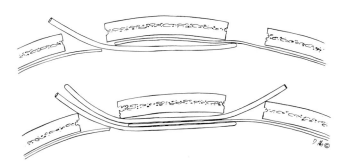

Figure 4-10. Proper placement of Gigli guides. If the first guide has penetrated the dura, the second one should be placed from the opposite burr hole.

a movement of the operating table in the opposite direction. Sideways rotations of the operating table should also be employed liberally during surgery as necessary to obtain the best possible view of the lesion.

When placing the key burr hole at the junction of the frontotemporal line and the zygomatic process of the frontal bone the position of the drill should be away from the orbital roof plane in order not to enter the orbit. Because of the change in the thickness of the skull between the frontal bone and the temporal squama in this region, one may reach the dura with the drill before the entire base of the burr hole is removed. Consequently, in patients with raised intracranial tension, especially if the lesion is a subfrontal extra-axial tumor with edema of the surrounding frontal lobe, a contusion may develop at the point of the impact of the drill against the dura. With this in mind, a hand-driven drill may be preferable to place this burr hole. If there is no need to cross the midline, the second burr hole should be placed immediately

adjacent to the most anterior part of the superior sagittal sinus.

In a bifrontal craniotomy the second burr hole should be at the level of the glabella, just above the crista galli. In a patient with a frontobasal tumor it is preferable to go straight through the frontal sinus, than to stay above the sinus, in order to avoid undue retraction of the frontal lobe. Again, a hand-driven drill may be preferable to open the anterior and posterior sinus walls separately. If properly placed, this burr hole will be perfectly in the midline. The midline is determined by the sloping of the frontomedial dura toward the most anterior part of the superior sagittal sinus, which is in a dural groove that deepens toward the crista galli. Consequently, if this burr hole is off to one side, only one dural slope toward the sinus will be visualized. When this is the case the drill should be redirected obliquely toward the opposite side to penetrate the inner table still covering the dura of the opposite frontal lobe.

Once both dural slops toward the midline groove are visualized, a midline bony ridge usually remains present covering the sagittal sinus. This bony ridge is best removed with a small, thin-lipped punch rongeur. If the exposed frontal sinus mucosa is intact it should be folded upon itself into the frontal sinus. If opened, it should be dissected away from the frontal sinus walls and collapsed into the bottom of the sinus.

The third burr hole will depend on the desired size and shape of the frontal (bifrontal) craniotomy. If a frontal craniotomy along the midline is planned, the third burr hole should be placed with its medial margin overlying the lateral one-third of the superior sagittal sinus at a distance from the second burr hole to be determined by the size and location of the lesion. If a bifrontal craniotomy is desired, two burr holes can be placed on either side of the midline. The final burr hole is then placed some 5 to 7 cm lateral to the third burr hole (and posterior to the first one). Burr holes away from the sinus should be connected first. Any change in the thickness of the skull and in the configuration and plane of the dural slopes may predispose to dural tears. Anticipating skull and dural anatomical details, many of which are constant, will decrease the potential for any dural or underlying brain injury. For example, the dura will adhere to the inner table of the skull at suture levels. The dura is especially thin adjacent to the most anterior portion of the superior sagittal sinus. When one connects the two anterior burr holes over the supraorbital ridge, it is better to pass the dural separator or to use the power instrument from lateral to medial since the

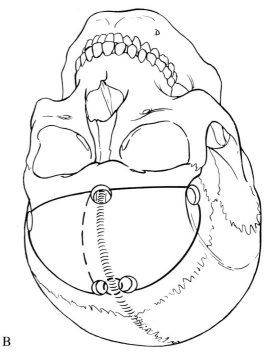

Figure 4-11. (A) Unilateral frontal craniotomy. **(B)** Bifrontal craniotomy. The bifrontal craniotomy can extend symmetrically into both sides or it can be predominantly on one side (*dashed line*).

curvature of the dura sloping downward toward the anterior part of the superior sagittal sinus is better negotiated when instruments are passed in that direction. In a similar vein it is easier to dissect dura away from the posterior medial burr hole toward the middle anterior burr hole than vice versa.

Frontotemporal (Pterional) Craniotomy

There are several principles that must be followed in skull base exposure. First, the bony exposure requires not only a low craniotomy down to the skull base but also additional removal of the skull base itself. Second, the brain should be slack. Slack brain is achieved by proper head position that utilizes gravitational forces, by lowering the PCO_2 with hyperventilation, by releasing the cerebrospinal fluid (CSF) from basal cisterns, and occasionally by the use of diuretics. Placement of a continuous spinal drainage catheter and rarely ventricular puncture are additional methods of releasing CSF.[19] Third, familiarity with the arachnoid anatomy and precise under-

standing of the relationship of the arachnoid to various skull base lesions cannot be overemphasized, since the arachnoid cisterns provide surgical avenues to the skull base and the arachnoid serves as a protective layer safeguarding neurovascular structures throughout the procedure.

A frontotemporal (pterional) craniotomy provides access to the pretubercular and retrotubercular regions, the suprasellar space, the anterior incisural space, as well as the sylvian fissure and the anterior temporal fossa. Consequently, this exposure is indicated for the majority of anterior and some posterior circulation aneurysms and for tumors in pre- and retrobercular regions, fronto-orbital tumors, sphenoid wing tumors, suprasellar and anterior incisural-petroclinoid tumors, as well as for tumors in the anterior temporal fossa. Intra-axial lesions in the anterior temporal lobe are also approached with this exposure. When properly positioned for a pterional craniotomy the head will be rotated about 20 to 30 degrees in the opposite direction, inclined about 20 degrees toward the floor, and slightly tilted toward the contralateral shoulder. The malar eminence should be the highest point in the skull in relationship to the horizontal. A scalp incision just behind and parallel to the anterior hairline is carried out toward the pre-auricular area, ending approximately 0.5 cm above the junction of the middle and posterior one-third of the corresponding zygomatic process. In doing so, the more posteriorly lying superficial temporal artery will be preserved. The incision should be placed no more than 1.5 cm anterior to the external auditory meatus in order to avoid the frontal branch of the facial nerve (Fig. 4-12).[11] When developing the scalp flap it is preferable to reflect the temporal muscle along with the scalp, since this will tend to preserve the frontal branch of the facial nerve. In contrast, if the skin incision is too low over the zygoma or too anterior and if the scalp flap is developed separately from the muscle flap, there is a greater chance of facial nerve injury.

When reflecting the scalp flap, one must be careful not to place pressure on the ipsilateral eye. Blindness can occur from an improperly placed scalp flap support due to compression against the globe. We prefer to put three to four layers of flatly folded gauze spanning between the malar eminence, the supraorbital ridge, and the bridge of the nose over which the scalp flap is reflected and held in this position by hooks or stay sutures.

The scalp flap should be developed to the supraorbital ridge, exposing also the zygomatic process of the frontal bone. When using the hot knife to divide the temporal muscle intermittent irrigation should be used to avoid overheating of the bone. The temporalis fascia and muscle can be incised in line with the scalp incision beginning inferiorly. The incision in the muscle can then be extended anteriorly to the zygomatic process of the frontal bone, leaving a cuff of fascia and muscle attached to the superior temporal line. At closure the temporalis muscle and fascia are reattached to this superior cuff of muscle and fascia, resulting in better temporalis muscle function and improved cosmetic appearance.[17]

The key burr hole is placed the same as in the frontal craniotomy. The second burr hole is placed approximately 2 cm medially and 4 to 5 cm above (posterior) the key burr hole. The third burr hole is placed 5 to 7 cm lateral to the second, and the fourth one, if necessary, in the temporal squama just above the roof of the zygoma (Fig. 4-13). When connecting the key burr hole with the burr hole in the temporal squama, resistance will be met where the greater wing of the sphenoid meets the temporal squama. Consequently, a bone cut in this region will have to be made with a high-speed microsurgical drill to create a trough in the skull, or the power instrument making the cut will have to loop around the greater wing of the sphenoid. When the bone flap is elevated, brisk bleeding may occur from a branch of the middle meningeal artery, which often runs through the bone at the junction of the temporal squama and the greater wing of the sphenoid. Hemostasis is ensured with the use of bone wax or by placing the ball of a nerve hook into the opening and coagulating the vessel with monopolar coagulation.

With the hemostasis secure, additional removal of the skull base will be necessary. The greater wing of the sphenoid, bony excrescences over the orbital roof, and, if necessary, part of the zygomatic process of the frontal bone are either rongeured away or drilled out with the use of a high-speed microsurgical drill under continuous irrigation-suction technique, preferably using the operating microscope. When a high-speed drill is used all cottonoids and sponges must be removed from the dura surface to prevent a high-velocity shearing effect of the cottonoid on the dura and underlying brain should the cottonoid begin to swirl with the drill bit action. Drilling of the bone should be carried out as far inferiorly and medially into the base of the skull until a small dura artery exiting the lesser wing of the sphenoid is encountered. This point is usually about 1 to 1.5 cm lateral to the anterior clinoid. This brings the surgeon in close proximity with the suprasellar region and avoids needless retraction of frontal and temporal lobes. As the greater wing is drilled way, it will be intermittently necessary to remove the lesser wing of the sphenoid with a fine, thin-lipped, single-action rongeur. Care must be taken during these maneuvers not to injure the dura and the underlying sylvian vessels. Exposure of the cavernous sinus region[1] will require an even more extensive drilling, with removal of the orbital roof, the lesser wing of the sphenoid, and the anterior clinoid with contiguous exposure of the periorbita, the dura of the superior orbital fissure, and the dura propria of the optic nerve canal.

Temporal and Posterotemporal Craniotomy

Temporal craniotomy (Fig. 4-14) can sometimes be combined with a frontotemporal craniotomy in patients with large skull base lesions involving the frontotemporal and temporal fossa regions. A relaxing incision extending posteriorly from the vertical segment of the frontotemporal incision and curving down toward the mastoid will allow for an additional temporal bone flap (Fig. 4-12 C, incision *b*). It has

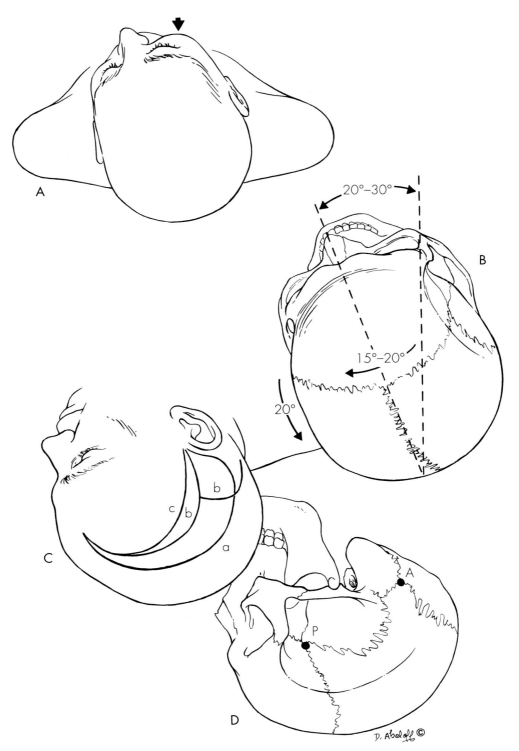

Figure 4-12. (A & B). Frontotemporal (pterional) craniotomy head position. **(C)** Scalp incisions: *a & b*, Modified frontotemporal incisions that allow for additional exposure of the petroclival region; *c*, standard pterional incision (see text). **(D)** Position of the pterion (*P*) and asterion (*A*).

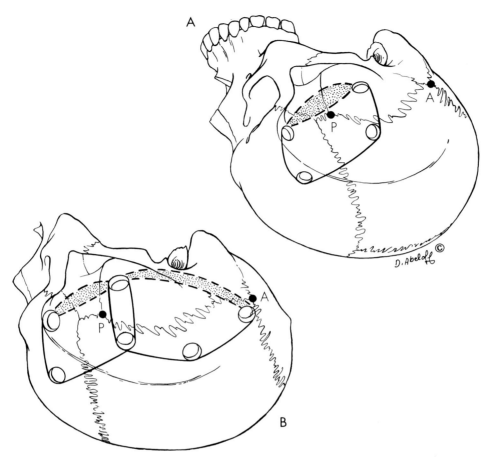

Figure 4-13. (A) Pterional craniotomy. **(B)** Frontotemporopterional craniotomy. The junction of the posterior limit of the sphenoparietal suture with the squamosal suture is the anatomical pterion. Additional bone removal at the base is necessary (*shaded area*) to reach into the skull base (see text).

Figure 4-14. Temporal craniotomy. When placing the burr hole over the asterion (junction of the mastoid portion of the temporoparietal suture with the lambdoidal suture) care should be taken not to injure the junction of the lateral and sigmoid sinuses or the point of influx of the great vein of Labbé into the lateral sinus.

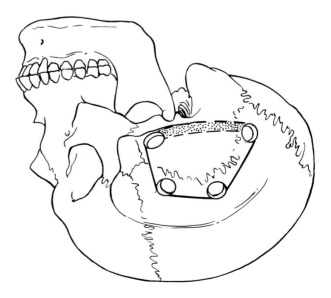

been our experience that such an incision is preferable to a deep question mark type of incision (Fig. 4-12 C, incision *a*). Combining a frontotemporal and temporal bone flap in this fashion will expose the entire supratentorial skull base, including the middle and posterior incisural spaces (Fig. 4-13B). Consequently, this exposure is indicated in large skull base tumors extending from the frontal fossa across the anterior into the middle and posterior incisural spaces.

A straightforward temporal craniotomy is the simplest to accomplish. The scalp flap is reflected in a semicircular fashion over the ear. Care should be taken during the exposure not to open the mastoid air cells. Opened mastoid air cells should be waxed thoroughly. The bony removal should reach as far down as the petrous ridge and superior margin of the lateral sinus. If the sinus is opened packing with thrombinated Gelfoam or a piece of temporal muscle will suffice to stop the bleeding. A major tear will require suture over either a piece of Gelfoam or muscle.

Tumors straddling the tentorial incisura and consequently presenting in the supra- and infratentorial compartment can be approached either through a temporal craniotomy with division of the tentorium posterior to the point of entry of the fourth cranial nerve or through a combined supra/infratentorial exposure. A temporal craniotomy is in such case combined with a suboccipital craniotomy with removal of the bone across the lateral sinus. In a majority of cases it will not be necessary to divide the sinus. If, however, sinus division is necessary it should be divided lateral to the point of entry to the vein of Labbé. A preoperative cerebral venogram is necessary in such case to demonstrate the presence of bilateral lateral sinuses and of a confluent torcula.

Occipital Craniotomy

Positioning of the patient is one of the most important aspects of performing an occipital craniotomy. We prefer to have the patient prone, placed over well-padded rolls made of surgical blankets or of egg crate spanned between the shoulders and the patient's iliac crest. The anterior thighs are supported by sloping foam rubber pads, the knees by foam rubber doughnut-type supports, and shins by folded pillows. The dependent peripheral nerves must be well padded with foam rubber. The arms are usually held extended alongside the body. The operating table should be flexed in such a way that the lumbar spine is not hyperextended. We prefer to have the head secured in a three-point fixation clamp rather than resting in a horseshoe-shaped head support, since the latter is more likely to leave pressure burns at the forehead, malar eminences, and so forth. The patient should be in a 20- to 30-degree reversed Trendelenburg position with the head slight flexed so that the chin is approximately two finger breadths away from the presternal notch (Fig. 4-15). Care must be taken to avoid any compression against the jugular veins. The scalp should be reflected toward the base of the skull along the nuchal lines, thus preserving the blood supply from the occipital artery. The scalp incision should cross the midline if the bony exposure is required to the midline. The burr holes should be placed at the junction between the torcula, the sagittal and lateral sinuses, and then at the junction of the lateral and sigmoid sinus, further, along the midline 5 to 7 cm above the torcula, with an additional burr hole 5 to 7 cm lateral to the last burr hole (Fig. 4-16).

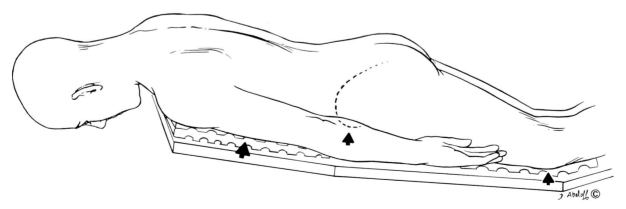

Figure 4-15. Position of patient for occipital craniotomy.

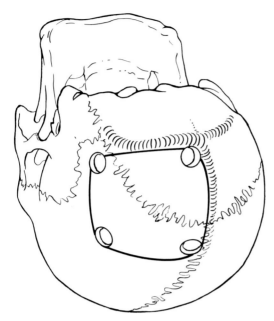

Figure 4-16. Occipital craniotomy. Midline burr holes should be close to or just over the lateral margin of the sagittal sinus with the inferior burr holes close to or just over the superior border of the lateral sinus. The sinus should not be completely exposed to prevent injury.

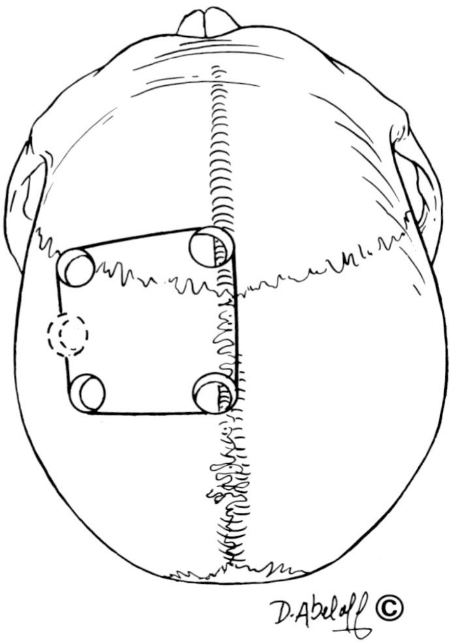

Figure 4-17. Parasagittal craniotomy. Midline burr holes should be close to or over the lateral margin of the superior sagittal sinus. The sinus should not be exposed completely in order to prevent injury or thrombosis. Laterally one or two burr holes could be made to complete the flap.

Parasagittal Craniotomies

The patient's position for anterior parasagittal craniotomies should be supine, with the patient's back and head slightly elevated (20 to 30 degree above the horizontal). In midparasagittal craniotomies, the patient's position is either decubitus or the back of the operating table is elevated 45 to 60 degrees. If the latter position is chosen, the patient should be equipped with a precordial Doppler monitor and a central venous line. In case of a suspected air embolism the patient should immediately be placed in Trendelenburg position and the operative field flooded with normal saline and covered with moist gauze. Any opening in the sinus should be controlled either with thrombinated Gelfoam or closed with a suture. Failure to observe these precautions can result in massive air embolism with a cardiac arrest.

Posterior parasagittal craniotomies are done with the patient either decubitus or prone. Scalp incisions are such that the flaps are reflected away from the midline. Alternative scalp incisions include coronally placed or lazy S-shaped incisions, especially if the exposure has to incorporate a previously placed incision from a stereotactic biopsy, burr hole, or some other procedure. Parasagittal lesions can generally be removed through relatively small skull flaps, espe-

cially since the advent of stereotactic approaches and the use of ultrasound localization. Along the midline the burr holes are placed in such a way as to expose the lateral margin of the superior sagittal sinus but not the entire sinus in order to prevent retraction injuries that can occur if the entire sinus is exposed and therefore retracted or kinked (Fig. 4-17). Occasionally, it is necessary to cross the midline because of a possible bilateral extension of a parasagittal lesion. In that case, burr holes should be placed on either side of the midline rather than directly over the midline.

Lesions that are along the falx can be approached with the same readiness with the patient supine and the back raised or with the patient in a decubitus position with the involved side dependent to allow for spontaneous retraction of the ipsilateral hemisphere by gravity. We have found the former position preferable.

Closure Technique

Important principles of the closure technique are meticulous hemostasis, avoidance of dead spaces, sealing off the opened paranasal sinuses, and maintenance of thorough asepsis. The dura should be closed in as water-tight a fashion as possible. Hemostasis from the epidural space is achieved by placing tacking sutures between the dura and the bony margins of the craniotomy. The sutures should be placed immediately beneath the craniotomy margin. Further dissection of the unexposed dura beyond the craniotomy margins is unwarranted and can result in epidural hematoma formation in spite of the tacking sutures. As many sutures as is necessary to achieve absolute hemostasis should be placed. The sutures should only go through the outer layer of the dura (Fig. 4-18). If the suture goes underneath both layers of the dura, the cortical veins or the cortex itself could be injured, resulting in a subdural hematoma. If there is even the slightest suspicion that this may have occurred, a small opening should be made in the dura adjacent to the suture to determine if this is the case. The suture should be placed through a small drill hole placed obliquely between the outer table and the cancellous bone. In places where the skull is thin the burr should go through the entire thickness of the skull. In this case, the dura must be protected with a brain retractor placed underneath the inner table of the skull. The dead space between the often flat dura and the convex bone flap can be obliterated partially by tacking the surface of the dura to the convexity of the skull flap. More than one suture is usually necessary to approximate the dura with the bone flap in a meaningful way. With the dura closed intermitted irrigation with a topical antibiotic solution is recommended.

At the completion of the procedure the opened frontal sinus is closed with a pericranial graft from the scalp flap (Fig. 4-19). A No. 15 blade knife is used to create a pericranial flap, leaving its base attached to the base of the scalp flap. The pericranial flap is reflected as tightly over the open frontal sinus and secured to the dura as close as possible to the bony margin of the craniotomy. The dural suture goes through the outer layer of the dura only with both ends of the suture placed through the pericranial graft in order to achieve a surface rather than a point contact with the underlying dura. This is carried out circumferentially until a tight seal has been accomplished.

Patients undergoing reoperation for brain tumors and other lesions will often have a leathery, taut dura rather than a thin and elastic one, which will make closure of the dura in a waterproof fashion difficult or impossible. Approximation of the dura may also be difficult following lengthy craniotomies, with dural margins retracting due to prolonged exposure to air or because the dura was unduly coagulated, resulting in its shrinkage. In either instance, a duraplasty will have to be done. We prefer a pericranial or galeal graft over a lyophilized cadvaer graft because of a postoperative meningeal irritation and graft rejection signs associated with the use of cadaver dura. We recognize the greater potential of adhesions between the cortical-pial surface and the graft when a pericranial or galeal graft is used. However, we find this preferable to the above-described rejection manifestations associated with a cadaver graft. Closure of scalp incisions in patients undergoing secondary or tertiary craniotomies, especially if they were previously radiated, can be associated with a higher incidence of scalp margin necrosis. Consequently, hemostasis, along the scalp margins at the time of the opening should be less vigorous. Slight bleeding from the scalp margins is preferable to a necrotic margin.

When the skull flap is not replaced or after it was secondarily removed for whatever reason, a cranioplasty plate will be necessary at a later date. If the skull flap was removed because of an infection, a minimum of 3 months should pass from the time the antibiotics have been discontinued. Methylmethacrylate plates are preferable for larger defects and for middle-aged to older patients. Autologous bone grafts fashioned from either a rib or the iliac crest are often used in children and in patients with smaller defects. A methylmethacrylate plate should never be used in the presence of infection and only with great reluctance in the presence of an opened frontal sinus or mastoid air cell.

Sinking of a replaced bone flap will be prevented by securing the flap sufficiently to the rim of the craniotomy with either nonabsorbable sutures or thin wire. If during the craniotomy more than one bony flap or fragment was removed in order to achieve

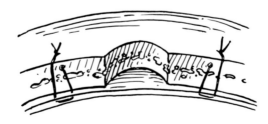

Figure 4-18. Tacking sutures should be placed only through the outer layer of the dura. There should be a surface contact rather than a point contact between the dura and the inner table of the skull.

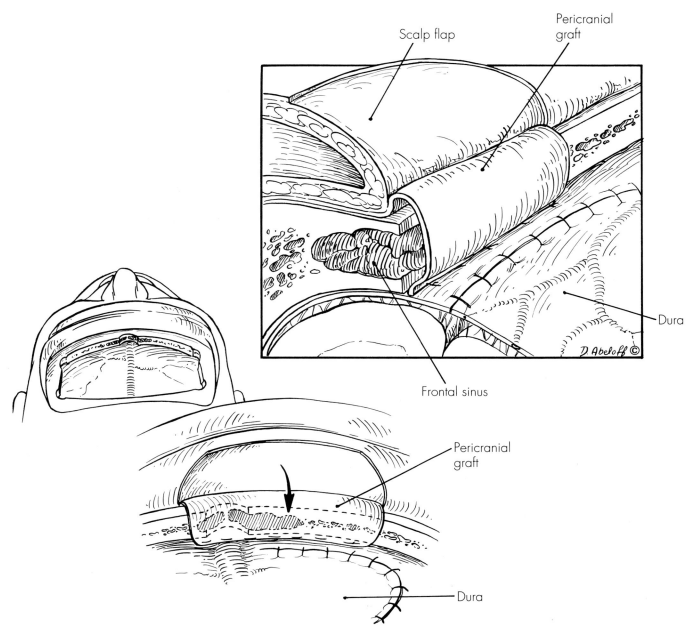

Figure 4-19. Closure of opened frontal sinus (*arrow*). Pericranial graft is fashioned, reflected over the frontal sinus, and sutured to the dura as close to the bony margins of the craniotomy as possible. Surface rather than point contact should be accomplished. A fat graft can be placed into the frontal sinus over the folded sinus mucosa.

exposure, these should be reconstructed meticulously prior to replacing the composite bone flap. The burr holes can be filled with bone dust or by using various types of synthetic plugs or by wire mesh. We prefer the use of the latter to cover the frontal burr hole if the frontal sinus was opened. Meticulous hemostasis of the temporal muscle is also necessary to avoid postoperative swelling of the scalp flap. The muscle should be sutured but not necessarily the temporal fascia. Most of the time the temporal muscle can be sutured back into place as far anteriorly as the key burr hole, which can therefore be covered.

The scalp is closed in one or two layers, both being acceptable. Generally, subgaleal drains are not necessary if meticulous hemostasis was achieved.

Generally, drainage techniques should be avoided. Intradural drains should not be used except in selected patients with subdural hematomas or intradural infections. The best way to avoid extradural drainage is to pay attention to meticulous hemostasis. When extradural drains are used they can be placed between the bone and the dura or above the bone in the subgaleal space. Flat drains with side perforations are preferable to round drains. Drainage tubing should be brought out through a separate incision. Intradural drains should drain into a closed system with the pressure regulated by gravity. Extradural drains can be attached to a suction mechanism.

MANAGEMENT OF COMPLICATIONS

The four most common complications associated with a supratentorial craniotomy are wound healing difficulties secondary to skin edge necrosis, postoperative hemorrhage, CSF leak, and infection. Other complications such as loss of sight, peripheral nerve injury, skin burn, decubitus ulcer, deep vein thrombosis, and so forth, are related to positioning, protection of the eye and peripheral nerves, pressure against prominent areas of the face as the scalp flap is reflected, kinking in the scalp flap, equipment failure, and length of surgery, many of which were already discussed.

Skin edge necrosis can be waited out for healing by secondary intention. However, it is preferable to revise the incision by excising the necrotic margins with secondary resuturing. A nonabsorbable monofilament or wire sutures may have to be considered if the plan is to keep the sutures in for a longer period of time.

Management of postoperative hemorrhage will depend on the location of the hemorrhage, its size, the presence or absence of any symptoms, and progression thereof. Subgaleal hematomas are better left alone unless there is a threat of wound dehiscence in which case it should be aspirated. Repeat aspirations are associated with a higher incidence of infections. As epidural hematoma if detected incidentally on the postoperative imaging study can also be left untreated as long as it is nonsymptomatic and does not increase in size on the follow-up imaging study, which should be obtained at regular intervals until the hematoma begins to show signs of resorption. In

this regard, it is preferable to obtain an early postoperative imaging study regardless of patient's condition, not only to assess the completeness of the operative procedure but also to establish the baseline as to the presence and appearance of a possible postoperative epidural, subdural, or intracerebral clot. Postoperative epidural hematomas after supratentorial craniotomy on the contralateral side have been reported either following a procedure in which the brain volume was drastically reduced or as an injury caused by the head rest.[14] Certainly, symptoms such as obtundation, progressive focal neurological deficit, and seizures call for an immediate imaging study. In case of a symptomatic, progressive epidural hematoma immediate evacuation is mandatory. In the case of a coagulopathy the same should be corrected in consultation with the hematology service. Postcraniotomy patients with coagulopathy who have no symptoms, signs, or imaging evidence of a hematoma must be monitored extremely carefully, for it is much more preferable to correct the coagulopathy before it causes hemorrhage than to treat the hemorrhage in face of a coagulopathy. Cerebellar hemorrhage as a complication after supratentorial craniotomy has been reported in patients with disturbed blood coagulation.[7]

The treatment of a postoperative infection will depend on its location and severity. A simple "stitch abscess" or superficial wound infection can be treated with moist warm compresses, betadine scrubs and showers, and topical and systemic antibiotics. A deep-seated infection with extension into the epidural space should be treated as an osteomyelitis of the skull flap until proven otherwise. One can attempt to treat such an infection with drainage and prolonged use of intravenous (IV) antibiotics initially. More often than not, however, the skull flap or any other foreign body found at the time of the wound revision will have to be removed. Routine placement of subgaleal or epidural drains postoperatively can be associated with a higher incidence of infections.[18] The use of drains can be avoided by meticulous and thorough hemostasis. Malis[8] reported zero infections of any kind in 1,732 neurosurgical cases with an antibiotic regimen including IV tobramycin and vancomycin supplemented by topical streptomycin solution. A prospective study on the benefit of prophylactic antibiotics in clean, noncontaminated cranial operations carried out over a period of 4 years at our hospital has shown an infection rate of 0.7 percent. This rate was considerably lower when compared with the incidence of infections occurring prior to this study, when prophylactic antibi-

Table 4-1. Supratentorial Craniotomy Complications During Certain Procedures

Positioning	Scalp Flap	Skull Flap	Hemostasis	Closure
Blindness	Necrosis due to inadequate blood supply, skin clamps, kinking, or postradiation	Cerebral trauma due to power instruments	Subgaleal hematoma	Postoperative hemorrhage
Neuropathy		Dural tears	Epidural hematoma	CSF leak
Pressure burn of decubitus		Sinus tears	Subdural hematoma	Dehiscence
Skull perforation by head clamping	Facial paralysis	Air embolism		Infection
Head clamp failure, fracture	Scalp anesthesia	Opened paranasal sinus, mastoid air cell		Sunken bone flap, burr holes
Increased intracranial pressure hemorrhage	Disfiguring scar			
Air embolism				
Deep vein thrombosis				

otics were given only at random or not at all. It was concluded therefore that prophylactic antibiotics are of benefit in lowering the infection rate in craniotomies. The regimen used was 2 g of nafcillin IV on induction followed by 1 g nafcillin q6h for the first 24 hours after surgery or longer if so indicated. In patients allergic to nafcillin, 1 g of vancomycin was given IV 30 minutes before induction followed by 500 mg of vancomycin q8h for the first 24 hours.

A CSF leak is a relatively rare complication of a supratentorial craniotomy. It is our impression that it occurs more often in patients in whom the lateral ventricle was opened during surgery. A CSF leak must be closed immediately along with a diversion technique. Whether the closure of the leak will only be in terms of scalp incision revision or will also involve an inspection and revision of the dural suture will depend on the surgeon's perception as to the site and extent of the leak. A revision of the scalp incision and/or dural suture line alone without a diversion technique is mostly unsuccessful. Consequently, a continuous spinal drainage for several days via a lumbar subarachnoid catheter should be done at the same time. If this proves unsuccessful in arresting CSF egress toward the epidural space, a ventriculoperitoneal or, less frequently, a subdural-peritoneal shunt will become necessary. Dural defects, especially over open paranasal and mastoid cavities, can be the source of accumulation of intracranial air,[16] which can lead to tension pneumocephalus.[15] We have not used tissue adhesives to seal a CSF leak following a craniotomy. This technique, however, should be part of the armamentarium in the treatment of a CSF leak with due consideration given to all aspects of preventive care associated with administration of blood products.[2] Extracranial repair of CSF fistulas of the

frontal sinus or the ethmoid-cribriform plate have been reported to have a high success rate combined with a low morbidity rate.[9] Table 4-1 summarizes complications of supratentorial craniotomies relative to positioning, opening (scalp and skull flap), and closure.

SUMMARY

The topic of avoidance and management of complications in supratentorial craniotomies is as broad as the number of patients operated upon by a surgeon in his or her lifetime. Individual variations from patient to patient are vast and consequently the possible pitfalls too numerous to list in one chapter. This chapter is but a mere glimpse into what most neurosurgeons intuitively already know and practice. We ask therefore for forgiveness if the reader perceives this chapter antiquated, redundant, and superfluous. This was far from our intent. This chapter was conceived as a compendium of cumulative experiences of knowledgeable and wise neurosurgeons, past and present, with a few personal contributions. We hope that this chapter will serve as a useful reference for all of our colleagues and especially so for those still in training. Attention to detail is the name of the game.

REFERENCES

1. Dolenc V: Anatomy and Surgery of the Cavernous Sinus. Springer-Verlag, New York, 1990
2. Drecker TB: Tissue adhesives in neurosurgery. p. 281. In Matsumoto T (ed): Tissue Adhesives in Surgery. Medical Examination Publishing Company, Flushing, NY, 1972

3. Hollenhorst RW, Svien HY, Penoit CR: Unilateral blindness occurring during anesthesia for neurosurgical operations. Arch Ophthalmol 52:819, 1954

4. Horwitz NH, Rizzoli HV: Postoperative Complications of Intracranial Neurological Surgery. Williams & Wilkins, Baltimore, 1982

5. Ishiguro S, Kimura A, Munemoto S et al: Epidural hematoma following craniotomy of a supratentorial lesion on the contralateral side. Report of three cases. Neurol Med Chir 26:245, 1986

6. Kelly PJ: Tumor Stereotaxis. WB Saunders, Philadelphia, 1991

7. Konig A, Laas R, Herrmann HD: Cerebellar haemorrhage as a complication after supratentorial craniotomy. Acta Neurochir 88:104, 1987

8. Malis L: Prevention of neurosurgical infection by intraoperative antibiotics. Neurosurgery 5:339, 1979

9. McCormack B, Cooper P, Persky M et al: Extracranial repair of cerebrospinal fluid fistulas, technique and results in 37 patients. Neurosurgery 27:412, 1990

10. Miyazaki Y: Method of superimposing the angiographically located supratentorial lesion on the scalp prior to craniotomy. No Shinkei Geka 4:673, 1976

11. Odom GL, Woodhall B: Supratentorial skull flaps. J Neurosurg 25:492, 1966

12. Rowe SN: Types and positions of some flaps for intracranial surgery. Clin Neurosurg 13:63, 1966

13. Rubin JM, Dohrmann GJ: Intraoperative neurosurgical ultrasound in the localization and characterization of intracranial masses. Radiology 148:519, 1983

14. Sato M, Mori K: Postoperative epidural hematoma— five cases of epidural hematomas developed after supratentorial craniotomy on the contralateral side. No Shinkei Geka 9:1297, 1981

15. Scherer R, Van Aken H, Lawin P et al: Spannungspneumozephalus. Eine haufig verkannte Komplikation nach neurochirur gischen Operationen. Neurochirurgia 27:59, 1984

16. Schramm VL, Maroon JC: Sinus complications of frontal craniotomy. Laryngoscope 89:1436, 1979

17. Spetzler RF, Lee KS: Reconstruction of temporalis muscle for the pterional craniotomy. Technical note. J Neurosurg 73:636, 1990

18. Wright RL: Septic complications of intracranial surgery. p. 93. In Guardjian ES (ed): Cranial and Intracranial Suppuration. Charles C Thomas, Springfield, IL, 1969

19. Yasargil MG, Kasdaglisk K, Jain KK et al: Anatomical observations of the subarachnoid cisterns of the brain during surgery. J Neurosurg 44:298, 1976

5 Use and Misuse of Instruments

Milton D. Heifetz

This chapter deals with some of the purely mechanical and technical aspects of surgery, primarily problems related to the use and misuse of surgical instruments.

GENERAL REMARKS

It is generally accepted that each surgeon should operate in whatever manner is most comfortable. This precept, I believe, has dangerous implications. It encourages resistance to change. Surgeons cannot assume that their approaches and the instruments they are accustomed to use are the most ideal. In all probabilities they are not. Continuous reevaluation is mandatory to surgical excellence and self-improvement.

It is important to appreciate the instrument as an extension of the hand. Each instrument should be studied away from the operating room to become thoroughly familiar with its function and how it handles. Manual dexterity and knowledge of instruments are intimately related. This is especially true when working with aneurysm clips.

There are several general principles that should be understood in the selection and use of instruments.

1. The shorter the instrument (near 5¼ inches long), the greater its precision.
2. A more delicate instrument will enhance the development of a lighter surgical touch. This will result in less tissue trauma.
3. Avoid using too many instruments. The instrument table should only contain the specific instruments that are to be used. When an instrument is no longer needed it

should be removed from the table so that there is no visual clutter for either the operating nurse or the surgeon.

I will now discuss specific principles of surgical technique with regard to instrument use and misuse as we move through the flow of a craniotomy.

HEADHOLDERS

Regardless whether one uses the Mayfield, Gardner, or Sugita headholder or any variation, there are several problems that can occur. One is slippage. This becomes especially dangerous if the self-retaining retractor system is attached to the surgical table instead of to the calvarium. The Sugita holder is least likely to slip since it utilizes a four-prong pin system.

The disadvantage of retractors attached to the skull by clasping the edge of the skull concerns the need to insert one prong of the clamp between the dura and the calvarium. This separates the dura from the inner surface of the skull with the possible development of epidural bleeding. It also necessitates a large craniotomy and may also impede movements of the hands. Its single real advantage is that if the head slips in the headholder, then the retractor moves with the head. Meticulous attention to detail should prevent this.

When using the Mayfield headholder, it is imperative when the joints are tightened that the teeth of the star joints are correctly meshed. Occasionally one will tighten the joint while the opposing teeth ride on top of each other. This can result in sudden slippage and possible rotation of the headrest (Fig. 5-1).

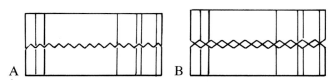

Figure 5-1. (A) Correct and **(B)** incorrect position of sunburst mechanism.

There are several problems that occur specifically with use of the pin headholder.

1. Infection can develop at the site of scalp perforation.
2. Air emboli can enter through the scalp perforation regardless whether the patient is in a supine or sitting position.[35]
3. The head can slip during surgery, not only surprising the surgeon and moving against a self-retaining retractor attached to the operating room table but also lacerating the scalp.
4. The pin headholder can penetrate the skull. This is especially true in the younger age group.
5. The headholder can puncture major scalp vessels or shunt tubes.

Fortunately there are also several methods to reduce complications associated with pin headholders.

1. Aside from using sterile technique, apply a large amount of Betadine or similar antibiotic ointment to the pins of the pin headrest before it is inserted. This will inhibit infection and reduce the chance of air emboli at the same time.
2. To avoid slippage, do not rely on the projecting pressure gauge at the knob controlling the insertion of the pin. The security of fixation must be checked by actual hand tension placed against the pin support.
3. Be certain that both pins of the rocker arm are firmly in place. The pins should insert at approximately 90 degrees to the scalp in order to be secure.
4. Try to place the single prong just above the mastoid and the double pronged arm at the temporalis insertion line or just above it when in the supine position. This will keep the protruding knob below the field of surgery; otherwise it may interfere with the self-retaining brain retractor frame.
5. Avoid placement of pins in temporalis muscle mass, frontal sinuses, mastoid bone, superficial temporal artery, or a shunt system. The pin headholder tends to be unstable when over the temporalis muscle, regardless of the spring tension reading on the bolt.
6. If the head position may need to be changed during surgery, it is advisable to use a non-pin support.

SCALP CLIPS

There is no ideal scalp clip. Clips that are associated with a crushing action, such as Adson or Michel clips, should no longer be used. The plastic Raney or the Leroy-Raney clips are excellent. The metal Raney clip has a tendency to imbed itself too deeply into the scalp edge during prolonged procedures, with occasional resultant ischemia, especially when placed on a thin scalp. The plastic clip is preferable for two reasons.

1. The clip edge is thicker than the metal clip and therefore there is less tendency for it to imbed itself.
2. Pierre Leroy's modification (Codman & Shurtleff Inc., Randolph, MA) using Delrin plastic loses some of its memory when the heat of the body penetrates the clip. This allows the clip actually to relax slightly after coagulation has had an adequate time to be complete. The chance of ischemia is reduced without loss of hemostasis.

A Delrin palstic scalp clip (Aesculap Corp., Burlingame, CA) has recently been presented that has the distinct advantage of easy application and very small protruding wings. The one possible drawback is that it may be difficult to apply on the edge of a scalp that has been injected with local anesthetic and is therefore thicker than normal.

SCALP REFLECTION

It is not uncommon for neurosurgeons to use heavy forceps with large teeth to handle the scalp. This is traumatic. The instrument to be used should be as delicate as a fine-toothed Adson or Brown-Adson forceps. The Brown-Adson forceps has excellent holding power. Its delicate teeth produce very slight tissue trauma.

When the scalp flap is to be reflected, one should be certain that the flap is not bent sharply at 180 degrees. There should be a soft curve to the fold to inhibit ischemia. Double fishhook retractors are less traumatic than single hooks or towel clips.

SUBPERIOSTEAL DISSECTION

Sometimes neurosurgeons use a round-tipped periosteal elevator such as a Cobb's elevator to lift up the galea above and the periosteum below the temporalis muscle. The round-tipped elevator acts like a pointed instrument due to its short radius. It is better to use a flatter periosteal elevator such as the Langenbach. This will result in less fragmentation, tearing, and shredding of the periosteum and the temporalis muscle when the muscle is elevated. If used in conjunction with a cottonoid pledget to push against the periosteum or galea one will produce cleaner and less traumatic dissection (Fig. 5-2).

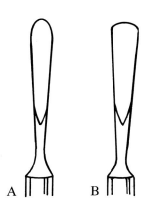

Figure 5-2. Periosteal elevators. **(A)** Too rounded, acts like a sharp point. **(B)** More desirable configuration.

Periosteal elevators should be sharp. When reflecting the scalp flap in the pterional approach, it is important to avoid the frontotemporal branch of the facial nerve. This passes along the surface of the arc of fatty tissue along the anterior aspect of the temporal fascia. Therefore, the surgeon should stay on top of the strongly striated temporalis fascia and use the sharp periosteal to scoot under this fat pad and thereby lift the facial nerve filament out of danger or incise the margin of the fat pad and use a periosteal to elevate it.

An acceptable alternative approach that essentially eliminates danger to the facial nerve filament is to reflect the temporalis muscle with the scalp flap.

BURR HOLES AND BONE FLAP

The most important danger in using a skull drill is the danger of plunging. A lesser danger is the tendency of drills to walk or slide on the calvarium as it begins to enter the outer table and possibly damage the surrounding tissue or wrap itself around a cottonoid or gauze pad.

There have been over 100 incident reports of plunging into and through the dura using the powered automatic skull perforator (Codman & Shurtleff Inc., personal communication), and for every reported incident there are probably 10 or more that have not been reported. A reasonable estimate is that there are at least 250 incidents of plunging per year, producing death or significant morbidity. Plunging through the dura can also happen with the standard Hudson drills. Regardless of which powered automatic stopping drill point is used, the spring mechanism that releases the rotating mechanism to stop the drill can fail. The disengagement mechanism can jam due to impurities or bone chips within the drill point. This can only be guarded against by cautious use or by using a power drill with a depth guard.

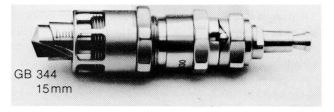

GB 344
15mm

Figure 5-3. Skull perforator with depth guard, nonwalking, and automatic stop. (Courtesy of Aesculap, Tuttlingen, Germany.)

A powered self-stopping drill point that cannot penetrate beyond a given predetermined distance is the Heifetz Skull Perforator, manufactured by Aesculap. This not only has an excellent automatic stop, but also presets the maximum distance one can possibly penetrate the skull. Because of this variable depth guard any incident of plunging into the brain is no longer a defensible accident. An additional advantage to the Aesculap drill point is its resistance to walking or slipping on the surface of the skull as the hole is started (Fig. 5-3).

Burr holes may also be made with safety by using the large acorn-shaped burr with the Midas Rex power system (Midas Rex, Ft. Worth, TX), but it is mandatory that cutting be done with the side of the burr. Drilling with the burr perpendicular to the skull could be catastrophic.

When developing a burr hole on or near a major sinus, one should never drill until the drill stops automatically. Regardless of whether one uses a Hudson brace or a power drill, one should drill in stages. As soon as an opening appears in the inner table, discard the drill and enlarge the opening with a curette, followed by a thin footplate, angled, 3-mm Kerrison bone punch to enlarge the base of the burr hole.

TURNING THE BONE FLAP

Several types of accidents can occur during the turning of a bone flap after the burr hole has been inserted. They include the following:

1. Laceration of the dura
2. Contusion of the brain
3. Laceration of a major sinus
4. Unwanted extension of fracture line

Laceration of the dura is especially common with improper use of the power router. To help prevent this problem, the surgeon should first be certain that the router blade is set to its proper depth. One should not rely on the nurse unless the nurse is experienced in the handling of the neurosurgical power instrument.

Among patients over 50 years of age the marked adherence between the dura and the inner table of the skull dictates that the router should not be used through a single burr hole and then moved across the proposed line of cut. Multiple burr holes should be made and the dura carefully dissected away from the inner table with a Hoen-like dura separator prior to the use of the router.

The dissector should not simply be inserted toward the neighboring burr hole. Dural separation should be done with a circular arc motion, sweeping the dissector laterally as one moves it along the line of intended bone cut.

If one penetrates the dura with a Davis guide, preparatory to using a Gigli saw, the guide should not be removed. Instead, a second guide should be inserted into the adjoining burr hole going in the opposite direction over both the intact dura and the first guide. Then the first guide is removed.

There is a tendency for the Davis guide to develop a deep curve that will compress and possibly contuse the brain. This becomes more pronounced when the burr holes are close together. The curve can be decreased by modifying the entrance and exit contours of the burr hole with a Kerrison bone punch to bevel the openings, as shown in Figure 5-4. This becomes especially pertinent when working close to the sagittal or lateral sinuses, where the push against the dura may tear a vein entering the sinus.

When cutting over the sagittal or lateral sinus with a power router be aware of the change in the contour of the inner table of the skull. This change demands a slight correction in the angle of the router. The tip of the router must be tilted slightly upward. If one is not aware of this maneuver, the sinus can be pinched and lacerated (Fig. 5-5).

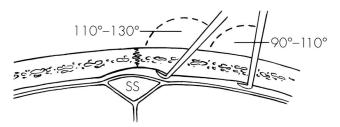

Figure 5-5. Angulation of router blade to prevent laceration of sinus. *SS*, sagittal sinus.

If the base of the bone flap is fractured as a final maneuver, one should be certain that the base or line of proposed fracture has been significantly weakened. The powered drill with a cutting burr works well to groove along the surface of the line of fracture. If a powered router is not available, a very narrow Kerrison rongeur can be used to section partially the base of the flap, or a Gigli saw can cut partially or completely through the base while the undersurface of the temporalis muscle is protected with a flat ribbon blade if the flap is to remain attached.

Once the bone flap is turned, the craniotomy bone edge should be waxed even if there is no evidence of blood, especially when in a sitting position. Air emboli can enter a "dry" bone edge.

EPIDURAL BLEEDING AND MISUSE OF SURGICEL AND GELFOAM

When the bone flap is removed, it is not uncommon to have significant bleeding along the edge of the dura-bone junction. Obviously tacking the dura up against the skull edge is advisable. All too often there is a tendency for neurosurgeons to insert Gelfoam, Surgicel, or Avitene under the bone—between the bone and the dura. This should not be done. It only invites further bleeding. The hemostatic material should be placed at the dura-bone junction. If necessary, dura tacking can then be used (Fig. 5-6).

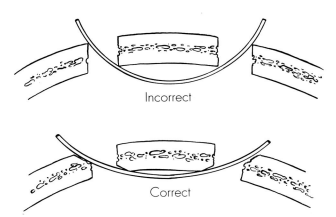

Figure 5-4. Technique for improving placement of the Davis guide using a bone punch to bevel the openings.

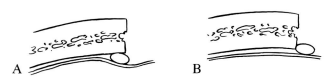

Figure 5-6. Placement of Gelfoam or Surgicel at dura-bone junction. **(A)** Incorrect. **(B)** Correct.

INSTRUMENTS AND TECHNIQUES FOR DURA PROCEDURES

Removal of Sphenoid Wing–Dura Protector

The lateral aspect of the wing is most easily removed with any straight narrow-bite bone rongeur. Recently Kobayashi et al.[19] described an instrument to protect the dura during removal of the medial aspect of the sphenoid wing while using the high-speed drill. I have used a narrow tapered brain spatula, but, although I have not used it, I believe Kobayashi's retractor is probably superior for this purpose. Aoki[1] has suggested that this retractor is also of value when drilling away the petrous bone over the junction of the lateral and sigmoid sinus.

Dura Pickup

Probably the finest dura pickup is a Castroviejo eye suture forceps with 0.9-mm forward projecting teeth. However, after the dura is incised, the edge of the cut dura should be held with a fine-toothed Adson forceps or with the Brown-Adson forceps.

Misuse of Bipolar Coagulation on the Dura

If the bleeding from the edge of the cut dura is from a large vessel, a clip or bipolar coagulation may be needed. However, much of the oozing from the cut dura usually can be controlled by simply squeezing the bleeding point several times with a small mosquito forceps. This would avoid unnecessary shrinkage of the dura caused by bipolar coagulation, which would inhibit tight closure of the dura.

One should not try to bipolar coagulate a partial sinus hole unless the opening is on the side of the sinus where the bipolar blades can approximate both edges of the sinus opening. Otherwise it will only increase the size of the opening.

Dura Retraction

To take full advantage of exposure through a curved cranial opening, the retracting suture should be placed through the line of the future chord line, which is the line of the dural fold, not through the edge of the dura flap. This will deflect and angle the chord line toward the bony edge and will permit another 2 to 3 mm of exposure (Fig. 5-7).

Arachnoid Nicks—Drainage of Cerebrospinal Fluid

As soon as the dura is open and even before it is reflected out of the way, it may be advisable to make two or three tiny nicks in the arachnoid. This will allow a surprising among of cerebrospinal fluid to drain out while one is getting ready to retract the brain. One may place a small cottonoid over this nick and suck on the cottonoid to increase the speed of removal of the spinal fluid. I have found this to be a helpful adjunct.

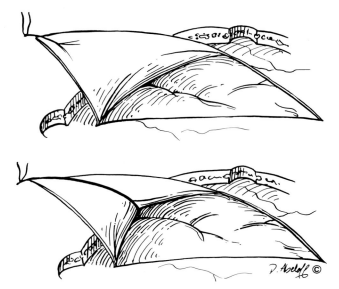

Figure 5-7. Brain exposure may be optimized by placing a tension suture at the fold of dura.

Protection of Brain Surface

The best brain covering is the dura; therefore, it should not be opened more than is necessary.

Several materials are used to cover exposed brain or are placed under brain retractors. Some are cotton, rayon (cottonoid), polyester (polycot), Gelfoam, Telfa, collagen sheet (Biocol), rubber sheeting, and latex covered pledgets. Choice depends on protective quality, ease of use, adherence tendency, and tissue reactivity.

The least adherent material is rubber, usually cut sections of surgical gloves. The disadvantage is that it is more difficult to manipulate, and one must carefully remove all powder particles, which may act as foreign bodies.

Cotton, rayon (cottonoid), and polyester (polycot) patties tend to adhere to the brain surface. Polyester is slightly less adherent than either cotton or cottonoid and theoretically less reactive to tissue than rayon (cottonoid). Pure cotton patties have a tendency to leave residual filaments that hopefully are eventually absorbed. Since the polyester (polycot) patty is thinner than either cotton or cottonoid patties, it is easier to handle. It is also less friable.

All three types of patties should be wetted and washed before using to remove any surface residue. All three are acceptable absorbers of laser energy when wet, but rayon tends to evaporate and polyester to melt. The blue polyester patty (manufactured by American Silk Sutures Inc., Lynn, MA), when wet, is a safer absorber of reflected laser energy.

Telfa is slightly stiffer and therefore less easy to handle than patties, but it has good release properties and good protective texture. Biocol (collagen sheet) has good releasing qualities, but is somewhat fragile and fairly expensive. Gelfoam is slightly adherent, but gives good protection. Gelfoam, designed for use as a prostate cone in prostate surgery, comes as a thin sheet. It is excellent to use, but will not resist the indenting edge of a brain retractor. Therefore, it is advisable to place a thin polycot patty under a brain retractor on top of the Gelfoam sheet.

When a surface covering is to be removed, it should not be simply picked up off the brain surface. It should be irrigated off.

There is a tendency to overuse and therefore misuse patties during the control of a bleeding surface, and multiple layers of patties on top of a layer of Gelfoam, Surgicel, or Avitene, should be avoided.

If after a tumor has been debulked there are numerous areas of slow bleeding, it is frequently best to line the surface with clotting material: pack the center of the tumor cavity with a cotton pattie. A common misuse of a pattie is to slide a wide cottonoid through a narrow opening into the tumor bed. It is better to roll a cottonoid into a tube, insert it into the center of the tumor bed, unroll it, and repeat the process until the pack is complete. Then wait 5 minutes by the clock, by which time most if not all oozing will have stopped. Then reroll the patties and remove them under irrigation.

BIPOLAR COAGULATION

There are two main principles underlying modern bipolar coagulating units. The old spark-gap bipolar equipment should no longer be used. A spark-gap instrument tends to cut through a vessel more readily than the new solid-state instruments. Of the modern instruments, the Malis (Codman & Shurtleff Inc., Randolph, MA) and the Radionics (Burlington, MA) bipolar instruments illustrate the two approaches.

The Radionics bipolar unit has a built-in sensing device that monitors the rise of impedance. When a certain point has been reached, the current is automatically shut off. This tends to prevent charring and sticking of coagulum to the forceps tip. Irrigation is therefore not mandatory. This is excellent in principle, but there is the danger of inadequate coagulation. The visual sign that coagulation is complete is diminished. Therefore, if this instrument is to be used, one should repeat the coagulation at least once, if not twice, to avoid surprises.

The Malis unit does not utilize this sensing element and therefore should be used with irrigation to prevent formation of coagulum on the forceps tip, but there is much less danger of inadequate coagulation of a bleeding vessel. Therefore one is much less apt to be surprised by a sudden spurt of blood.

The bipolar coagulating forceps is one of the most misused instruments in the neurosurgical armamentarium. Complications due to misuse are

1. Formation of coagulum at the tip
2. Adherence of the blood vessel to the tip of the forceps
3. Penetration of an aneurysm
4. Undesirable regional tissue damage due to grounding of current through the body[32]

General principles for the proper and most efficient use of the bipolar instrument include the following.

1. Do not start the current flow until the desired moment to coagulate a bleeder. If one blade of an open, noninsu-

lated bipolar forceps inadvertently touches tissue while the current is on, the current will try to ground through the tissue with possible resultant damage. This is especially true if the current is at a high setting.

2. Reduce the current setting when switching from a standard bipolar forceps to a fine-tipped forceps for microsurgery. The narrower the forceps tip, the higher current density for the same amount of current flow. Therefore, if the current flow is not reduced, there will be a greater tendency of the forceps to form coagulum, stick to the vessel, and even rupture the vessel.

3. Coagulate within a small pool of water. The interface between forceps tips and tissue should be wet. Suction irrigation is therefore advisable.

4. Pulsate (minimally open and close) bipolar forceps when on a blood vessel. Do not simply close forceps over a vessel and hold it in a closed position. Pulsate it approximately twice per second. Apply current in short bursts.

5. Set current as low as feasible. This will vary with the size of the forceps tips and the thickness of the tissue that has to be coagulated. If higher power settings are to be used it may be advantageous to use the insulated bipolar forceps.

6. When the forceps are being irrigated they should not be flooded. There should just be a small amount of solution at the coagulation site. If there is too much solution the current may flow between stems of the forceps as well as the tip and may shunt current away from the tip. Malis' well-designed new forceps (Codman & Shurtleff Inc., Randolph, MA), whose tips are slightly bent toward each other, thereby increasing the space between the blade stems, speaks to this problem.

7. Avoid forceps with rough or discolored tips.

8. Clean bipolar forceps tips immediately after use. One should not wait for coagulum to build up; clean before it is necessary with moist gauze. Do not wipe the tip with a rough surface or a knife blade.

Factors in Design of Bipolar Forceps

1. Forceps that are made in a straight line tend to shunt current between the stems of the forceps as well as the tip when immersed in saline. Therefore, not only should fluid be limited to cover only the tips but also the configuration of the forceps should be such that the tips are slightly bent toward each other so that the tips meet significantly sooner than the stems of the forceps unless the stems are insulated.

2. The tips of the forceps should be extremely smooth to inhibit adherence of coagulated tissue.

3. Develop the habit of using the bipolar forceps as a tissue plane dissector. Therefore the spring tension of the forceps should not be extremely low. It should allow dissection of tissue planes when the tips spread apart.

Specific Principles Regarding Bipolar Use

Arteriovenous Malformations

1. The vessels of arteriovenous malformations (AVMs) are extremely delicate. There is a tendency for the vessels to shear off during bipolar coagulation, and then one has to follow the end of that vessel into the AVM or gliotic tissue. To bipolar these vessels, the bipolar tips should be kept slightly open. Straddle the vessel and close the tips just enough for current flow to pass across the vessel. In essence, do not attempt to squeeze shut the small AVM vessels to stop the bleeding. As the current flows, pulsate the bipolar tips.

2. Avoid the dangerous tendency to use a stripping motion or pulling movement during the moment of coagulation. This is commonly done. To bipolar in a linear manner, walk the forceps. Do not slide it along the vessel. This action tends to pull the vessel.

Aneurysms

If at all feasible the aneurysm should first be softened by reducing the intra-aneurysmal pressure prior to bipolar coagulation by temporary occlusion of the proximal blood flow. After that is done one should use low current with short bursts.[36]

One can at times reduce the size of the fundus of the softened aneurysm by walking open-tipped forceps over the surface of the wall of the fundus. For this maneuver the standard bipolar rather than the fine-tipped microbipolar forceps should be used. This must be done with extreme caution, especially if the intra-aneurysmal pressure is not reduced. Outpouchings or lobules may also be collapsed with this technique.

The neck should not be coagulated until it has been completely exposed. The forceps tips must completely cross the neck; otherwise one may penetrate the side of the neck of the aneurysm as the forceps are closed. This has been stressed by Yasargil[36] and especially holds true if the intra-aneurysmal pressure has not been reduced. The walls should collapse when this is done. The forceps tips should not touch the parent artery. The coagulation area should be moistened and low intermittent current applied. Above all, one must avoid any tendency of the forceps to stick to the aneurysm. Low current monopolar coagulation may also be used to contract and thicken the aneurysm wall, but I have refrained from using it during the past 30 years.

MONOPOLAR COAGULATION AND CUTTING

One must ascertain before using the monopolar instrument that there is adequate contact between the skin and the ground electrode to avoid a burn of the skin. The major reason for accidental burns is the faulty attachment of the patient's ground plate either to the base of the unit or between the ground plate and the patient.[34] This is especially true when the patient is connected to multiple electronic devices.[3]

One must also avoid contact between the patient's body and metal parts of the operating table. Battery clamp types of connectors should not be used because of the lack of certainty of contact and the possibility that they may become disconnected.

If the cutting current is used to cut the temporalis muscles, one should move very slowly through the muscle. It is surprising how well the cutting current will also coagulate the small bleeders if the movement is slow.

Bayonet Forceps

Bayonet instruments should be reserved for use when visualization is hampered by a straight instrument. There is greater precision in use of a straight instrument. There are two basic types of bayonet instruments (Fig. 5-8).

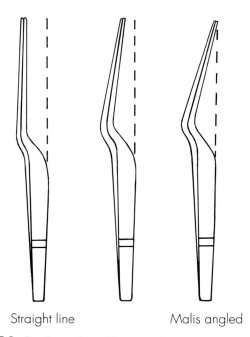

Straight line   Malis angled

Figure 5-8. Configuration of bayonet forceps with compromise design.

The angled bayonet forceps of Malis are theoretically more closely akin to a straight forceps, since the center of rotation of the handle is in line with the center of rotation of the tip. The disadvantage is the need to extend the hand slightly dorsoradially to accommodate the angle. This may be, for some surgeons, slightly uncomfortable. A useful modification may be a compromise between the straight line and the angled forceps by reducing the angle 50 percent.

BRAIN PUNCTURE

Ventricular needles can cause a fatal hemorrhage by disruption of a blood vessel along the path of insertion, and brain biopsy needles can cause fatal hemorrhage at the site of the biopsy. The risk in stereotactic biopsies ranges from almost 2.4 percent as reported by Chimowitz et al.[6] to 1 in 3,400 cases as reported by Apuzzo (personal communication).[13,17] This risk is higher if the biopsy is in a vascularized tumor.

There are three ways of reducing this risk (aside from better understanding of the underlying vascular configuration). They relate to needle design, technique of insertion, and flow studies. Needles that are sharply pointed can pierce a blood vessel whereas needles that have a flat tip can straddle and tear a fine blood vessel as the instrument is inserted. Therefore neither sharply pointed trocars nor flat-faced ventricular biopsy needles should be used. Stylettes or the needle itself should be trocar shaped, but blunt and rounded. This would eliminate the piercing potential and reduce the straddling tendency.

At the same time it may be warranted to rotate the needle slowly as one advances it into the brain. This would tend to roll a blood vessel to the side, which may be sitting exactly under the center of the needle.

Another approach is the use of a Doppler probe, as suggested by Gilsbach et al.[13] The tip of such a monitoring probe should have the contour of a smooth, round-tipped trocar.

BRAIN RETRACTION

Areas of Misuse

There is a tendency for the base of self-retaining retractors that are not bolted to the skull to be placed in a position that is inconvenient and at times dangerous. The main retractor support should be placed so that the proximal end of the retractor lies below the level of the opening of the calvarium. By keeping the retractor arm low and hugging the curve of the drapes and calvarium, there is less chance of accidental movement of the retractor stem during surgery. Spetzler[25] has recently described this maneuver using the Yasargil-Lelya retractor.

There is a tendency for flexible arm retractors to fall short of the intended retracting position after they are tightened due to a slight drift tendency. This can be overcome by slight pressure against the main retractor support in the direction opposite to the direction of retraction as the retractor arm is tightened. This will compensate for the slight drift of the retractor arm. The shorter the flexible retractor arm the less the drift.

Retractor Blade Factors: Areas of Concern

Occasionally it is difficult to identify the exact cleavage plane of the sylvian fissure, and there may be a tendency for one to attempt to retract on the temporal lobe inferiorly to help expose the groove. A simple and less traumatic technique to identify a hidden sylvian fissure is to insert a 25- to 30-gauge needle with 1 ml of air or saline under the arachnoid and inflate the arachnoid along the area of the sylvian groove. It is surprising how the arachnoid will suddenly balloon out and expose the sylvian line of demarcation.

Brain retraction probably should be released every 10 to 15 minutes during surgery for 3 to 5 minutes to reduce regional damage due to compression per se and to ischemia. Intermittent traction is safer than continuous traction.[16,22,38] This is especially important if the retractor is against a crucial structure such as the pons, medulla, or optic structures. There is much written about the need to maintain brain retractor pressure below 20 mmHg. But such numbers are not as important as the surgeon's technique, which should be

1. To retract only what is necessary
2. To retract only as far as is necessary
3. To release pressure intermittently
4. To realize that the retractor can often be completely removed or at least relaxed after the initial stages of a procedure

I have observed neurosurgeons who have a tendency to retract beyond what is necessary. One should not become enthralled with the exposure of intriguing anatomy. Excess retraction not only causes unwarranted compression, but also elongates perforating vessels and thereby may possibly induce spasm through mechanical irritation. During the residency training program it may be advisable to use pressure sensors on retractors so that an understanding of the amount of pressure that is exerted is gained.

The tendency to move the retractor position by sliding it along the brain is traumatic. This produces an unnecessary lateral vector that compounds the trauma of the needed vector. The retractor should be released and reapplied rather than slid laterally.

Multiple retractor blades may result in less retraction pressure than a single blade.[16] Many neurosurgeons use stiff, rigid retractor blades. Stiff retractors not only limit the ability to maneuver because one cannot bend the blade to the desired configuration, but also are more inclined to produce regional ischemia. The type of ribbon blade to use should pulsate slightly with movement of the brain and still maintain its position. Therefore the blade should be slightly flexible. Avoid using very thin blades whose edge may tend to cut the cortex. Ribbon blades should not be thinner than 1 mm (0.039 inch). All blades may cut into the cortex unless the cortex is protected.

One common misuse of the retractor blade is the tendency to bend the blade at right angles and then insert it into position. When this is done, the exposed portion of the blade, the horizontal section, is frequently 2 to 4 cm above the brain. This is obtrusive and may inhibit maneuvers. It is better to bend the blade in a curve to follow the contour of the brain and skull opening (Fig. 5-9).

At times the surgeon may improve exposure and reduce the force of retraction by utilizing retractor blades (Heifetz Brain Spatula, Aesculap, Tuttlingen, Germany), which can exert a double vector (i.e., to lift as well as perpendicularly displace the brain or the vascular structure). Curved-tip spatulas function as double vector blades.

One may retract to a certain point and then utilize the lifting vector to expose the area of interest more readily. This maneuver is of special value in situations such as exposing a posteriorly placed anterior cerebral artery or an aneurysm complex (Fig. 5-10).

The double vector blade is of help to lift benign tumors out of their bed or to support the edge of cystic cavities. It is of special value in dissecting an AVM out of its gliotic bed. The ability to lift as well as to retract a large vein draining an AVM or the AVM nidus frequently permits greater delineation of the gliotic bed (Fig. 5-11).

Tapered blades, both flat and curved, should be available for situations involving deep narrow retraction. Sugita has popularized the value of the tapered blade.[28–30] The tapered curved blade functions well to lift and retract small vessels, especially during the pterional approach to basilar aneurysms.

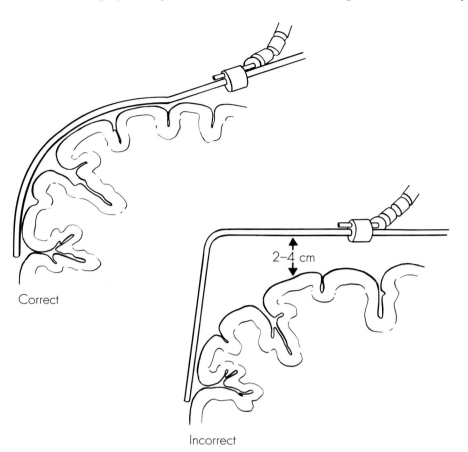

Correct

2–4 cm

Incorrect

Figure 5-9. Optimal manner of bending the brain spatula to reduce interference with surgical movements. The retractor blade is commonly misused by bending it to a 90-degree angle before positioning it, which will inhibit maneuvering.

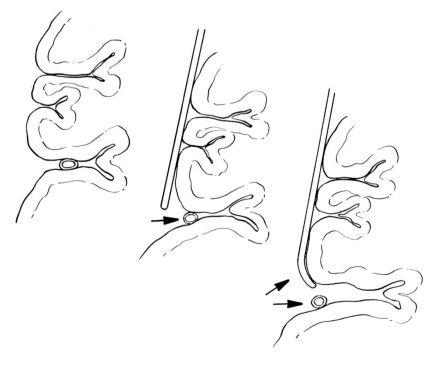

Figure 5-10. Diagrammatic depiction of the value of the double-vector brain spatula in exposing the suprachiasmic segment of anterior cerebral artery.

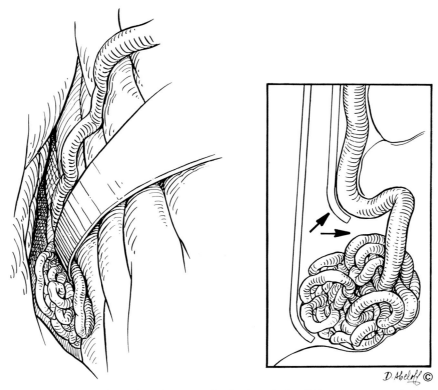

Figure 5-11. Use of the double-vector brain spatula for lifting segments of AVMs.

TUMOR-GRASPING FORCEPS

To try to grasp tumor tissue with a standard forceps such as Gerald forceps is frequently a waste of time, since this type tends to cut through the tissue rather than to hold it. There are three forceps that seem to work well: the Yasargil flat serrated ring forceps, the Heifetz cup serrated ring forceps, and the Hunt angled serrated forceps (Aesculap, Tuttlingen, Germany). They are all distributed by Aesculap Corporation and are all ringed formed forceps. The angled tip forceps of Hunt may be of special value to reach under the spinal cord or under the chiasm to grasp an edge of tumor.

The Sugita fork is also of value in retracting tumor tissue such as an acoustic neuroma or meningioma. Its blunt points are relatively atraumatic. This instrument holds very well.[30]

HIGH-SPEED DRILL: THE AVOIDANCE OF ACCIDENTS

The high-speed drill must be used with extreme caution. There are several specific areas for potential accidents.

1. Do not use the drill in the vicinity of a cottonoid or its tail. It can suddenly convert the cottonoid to a devastating whip.
2. Be aware that rotating bits have a tendency to walk or to skid to the side, especially when drilling at slow speed or with a dull bit. When drilling at a slow speed, added pressure is usually necessary. This will tend to increase the walking tendency. Therefore, the slower drills such as the electric drills should not only have variable speed but also be reversible. It is important that the rotation direction, the direction of its walk, should be away from crucial areas. Reversibility is only of value if there is a skidding tendency. This becomes much less pertinent when using high-speed (60,000 to 100,000 rpm) air drills. With high-speed air drills there is much less tendency to walk. The removal of bone is done in a brushing manner with light intermittent pressure. The motor should be started just prior to touching the bone; otherwise there will be an inclination to skid. Hold firmly, but use a light brushing type of touch. When using the electric drill, which has a greater tendency to walk because of its slower revolving speed, also start the drill point before touching the bone, but this must be held firmly and at the highest speed that the electric motor will run.
3. Cut with the side of the burr, and use the largest burr feasible. Do not use the tip of the drill to drill straight down, but bevel the hole.
4. When drilling near the end point adjoining soft tissues,

switch to a diamond burr, which may rub against soft
tissue with less trauma.
5. Significant heat is generated during drilling. Continuous
irrigation is necessary to cool the area.

CURETTES

It should be stressed that the curette is a two-
handed instrument. A dull curette must be avoided
because of its tendency to slip. One should use the
side of the curette when possible and always be
aware that the direction of force should be away from
any critical tissue.

ANEURYSM CLIPS

Of all the instruments used by neurosurgeons,
none are as misunderstood and mishandled as the
aneurysm clips. To correct this situation it is imperative that aneurysm surgeons study aneurysm clips
away from the operating room to become familiar
with their various angles and with the ways of manipulating the appliers. To operate on a patient with an
aneurysm without such prior study is a disservice to
the patient.

There is no ideal aneurysm clip system. It is necessary to have several clip systems available. To be
wed to a single system limits the surgical options and
therefore increases the risk to the patient.

The Hemoclip

Some neurosurgeons are inclined to use nonre-
movable clips like the hemoclip (Weck Corp., Research Triangle Park, NC). This is dangerous for
three reasons. First, it is not easy to correct the
placement if necessary. Secondly, there is a definite
scissoring tendency to the hemoclip which may cut
through a vessel or aneurysm neck. This occurs
when too much force is applied when closing the clip
(Fig. 5-12).

The scissoring problem could be reduced if the appliers had a built-in stop. One must be aware of the
degree of pressure necessary simply to close the clip
and not squeeze beyond that point. The third danger
is the tendency of the clip sometimes to stick within
the groove of the clip appliers.

Prior to clip placement it is advisable to be prepared to reduce intra-aneurysmal pressure.

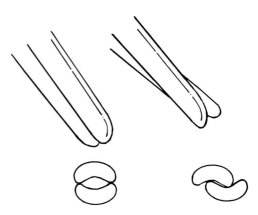

Figure 5-12. Diagrammatic representation of the scissoring potential of a hemoclip.

Reduction of Intra-Aneurysm Pressure

In anticipation of possible intraoperative rupture of
the aneurysm, temporary clips should be in their appliers ready for use. Standard aneurysm clips should
not be used for temporary occlusion, because they
will produce significant intimal damage. Instead clips
designed for temporary occlusion should be used.

Temporary clips are applicable for the distal carotid and basilar group of aneurysms, but, when operating on the more proximal carotid group (ophthalmic carotid, giant carotid, or carotid cavernous
aneurysms), proximal control demands control of
the carotid artery in the neck. The Heifetz carotid
occluder[14] allows the neurosurgeon or assistant neurosurgeon to have immediate on-off control of the
internal carotid circulation. This is safer than using
standard Selverstone type clamps or ligatures around
the internal or common carotid arteries, which are
then pulled up by the anesthesiologist (Fig. 5-13).

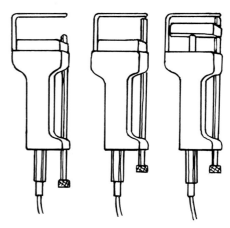

Figure 5-13. Device for instantaneous on-off control of
carotid blood flow.

Recently Batjer and Samson[2] described a technique to reduce intra-aneurysmal pressure of the proximal carotid group by isolating the carotid circulation and then inserting an 18-gauge catheter into the internal carotid artery connected to suction. This action deflates the aneurysm.

Flamm's technique[12] of decompressing an aneurysm by direct needle aspiration is also of value. However, one must be cautious that the needle position or needle support does not hamper movements.

There are several complications due to misuse of aneurysm clips.

1. Slippage of the clip off the aneurysm neck
2. Inadequate occlusion of the aneurysm neck
3. Occlusion of unseen perforating vessels
4. Avulsion of the aneurysm neck
5. Stenosis of the parent artery
6. Improper handling of an arteriosclerotic plaque with secondary tear of the neck wall
7. Incompatibility with the magnetic resonance image (MRI).

Slipped Clip Problem

There are several factors related to the slippage of clips off an aneurysm neck. Obviously a clip that is too weak in relation to the aneurysm neck turgor will be pulsated off the neck. It is not uncommon to think that the clip is properly placed only to find that aspiration of the dome reveals persistent blood flow into the aneurysm. This may hold true even if there is no apparent pulsation of the clip blades. Setting of the clip by squeezing the blades of the clip together with Gerald forceps may be adequate to stop the flow, but it would be safer to apply a stronger clip or a second clip in tandem.

The risk of slippage is also reduced by collapsing the aneurysm and therefore confirming the complete absence of blood flow into the aneurysm. Intra-aneurysmal pressure is a major factor producing slippage of a clip. Double clipping, or use of the very strong Sundt clip (Codman & Shurtleff, Randolph, MA) or the Sundt straddling clip, may be necessary.[31] If a standard clip is applied over another clip to squeeze the first clip blades together, one must be aware that it can slip off later. Metal riding on metal will tend to slide, especially on tapered blades. Sundt booster clips would be preferable. It is obvious that any suggestion of pulsation of the clip blades can cause a clip to slip.

It is imperative when handling cross-legged clips (Yasargil, Sugita, Sundt, and McFadden) that one does not repeatedly open and close the clips prior to

application. In fact the clip should never be opened to its full extent until the time to apply it. Repeat opening and closing these clips will weaken their spring action. As expressed by Yasargil,[37]

> Unnecessary, repetitive opening of the blades of aneurysm clips is to be absolutely avoided. . . . The first time an aneurysm clip should be widely opened is immediately before it is applied to an aneurysm.

This problem of repeatedly opening a clip does not apply to the Heifetz clip,[15] which functions in a different manner utilizing a coiled spring. This clip may be repeatedly opened widely without fear of losing force. With the development of clips with high closure pressure, such as the new Sundt clips, it would be extremely rare to need to utilize glue or adjunct suture to tie the tips of the clip blades together.

When a clip has slipped off the neck of an aneurysm it is not always because of a weak closing pressure of the clip. When the brain returns to its normal position after surgery it may exert pressure against the protruding head of the aneurysm clip. This may tilt the clip. The torque against the head of the clip, when combined with the pulsation against the clip from within the parent vessel, as well as by the brain itself, may be enough to move the clip slowly off the aneurysm neck. This is especially true if the fundus of the aneurysm has not been opened, collapsed, and bipolar coagulated after the clip had been applied. The bulbous coagulated aneurysm nubbin acts as a barrier to lateral slippage of the clip.

The ideal removable aneurysm clip would not have a protruding back end. The only clip with that attribute was designed by Iwabuchi.[18] Although very ingenious, it is not very practical.

In those circumstances in which there is a significant likelihood of force being applied to the clip by the returning brain, clips with small back ends, such as a Scoville or a Heifetz clip, should be used. Both were specifically designed to reduce the protrusion of the back end of an aneurysm clip. The area where pressure against the back end of the clip is most apt to occur is in the region of the carotid bifurcation and middle cerebral artery aneurysms.

I have observed repeated misuse of the bayonet-shaped aneurysm clip. This excellent design of Sugita enhances visibility of clip placement. The fact that it does so has enticed neurosurgeons to use it when standard clips would do as well with a little bit more effort. Not only is the length of the back end more prone to being pushed by the returning brain, but, if placed wrongly, the angulation or offset of the back end will tend to obstruct access to the lesion.

There is an aspect of clip placement that is frequently overlooked. As one considers the placement of the clip blades one must also be cognizant of how and where the back end of the clip will fall. Will it be supported by the surrounding tissue, or will the weight of the back end fall to cause unwanted traction or twist to the aneurysm neck?

Inadequate Occlusion of Aneurysm Neck

The single most important test to determine occlusion of the aneurysm neck is to perforate the fundus. The two main reasons for persistent blood flow, aside from the need of a stronger clip, are, one, that the clip is too short and, two, that the clip has been inserted too deeply when using a fenestrated clip. In this design the space proximal to the blades may allow blood flow.

Another aspect of inadequate occlusion is not obvious and not determined by aneurysm puncture. It is not uncommon to observe surgeons clipping a posterior communicating artery aneurysm, whose neck is partially hidden, with a straight clip. This frequently does not conform to the principle that the blades of the clip should lie against and thereby follow the curve of the parent vessel. Unless one is aware of the geometry shown in Figure 5-14 a straight clip may invite secondary aneurysm formation.

Occlusion of Unseen Perforating Vessels

There is no specific technique to avoid occlusion of unseen perforating vessels except for meticulous application of the aneurysm clip with visualization of the distal aspect of the aneurysm. An important aspect is to evaluate carefully the length of the clip. If the blades are too long, they can occlude hidden perforating vessels. Drake[8,9] has stressed this point. One of the most important advantages of collapsing and coagulating the clipped aneurysm is that it allows bet-

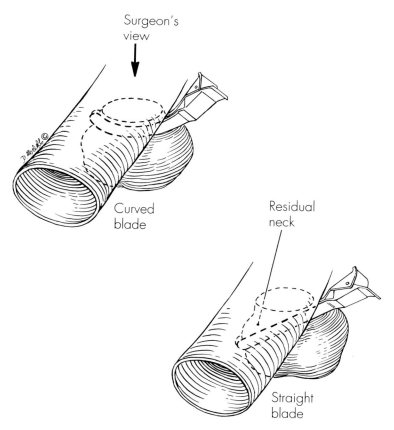

Figure 5-14. Diagrammatic depiction of a common cause of inadequate occlusion of the aneurysm neck: when a straight clip is used, the blades do not follow the curve of the parent vessel.

ter visualization of the dark side of the aneurysm. One may then rotate or elevate the collapsed aneurysm and detect inadvertent clipping of a perforator with much greater ease.

Aneurysm Neck Avulsion

Avulsion of the neck of an aneurysm is a serious accident. There are three crucial aspects to be considered in its prevention.

1. The contour of the parent artery and the relationship between the diameter of the aneurysm neck and the diameter of the parent artery and awareness of the long and short axis of the aneurysm neck opening
2. The degree of delicacy or thinness of the neck wall
3. The presence of a hard plaque at the neck-parent vessel junction

After the aneurysm is exposed, it is important to study not only the aneurysm but also the contour of the parent artery. For example, it is not unusual to note that the carotid artery may be widened over the orifice of a posterior communicating aneurysm (Fig. 5-15).

This contour should immediately alert the surgeon of a significant oval aspect to the aneurysm neck and the danger of applying a clip perpendicular to the parent artery, especially if the aneurysm neck appears fragile. With this contour the ability of the sides of the artery wall to be brought closer together and allow the aneurysm neck to collapse within the clip without significant tension is much greater than if one attempts to squeeze the aneurysm neck together along the longitudinal axis of the artery. To do so with a thin-walled aneurysm neck is an invitation to rupture of the neck or avulsion of the aneurysm.

Placing the blades parallel with the parent artery will reduce the shearing stress. Unless there are extenuating circumstances, the clip blade should lie as

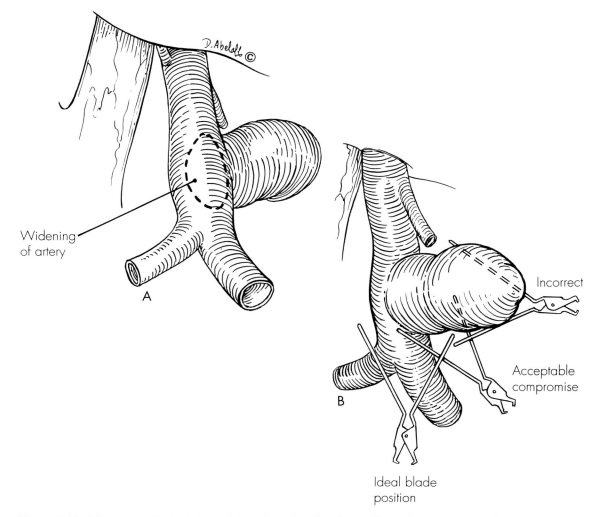

Figure 5-15. Diagrammatic depiction of the value of noting the configuration or contour of the parent artery.

close as possible along the longitudinal axis of the parent vessel.

If the aneurysm is large, very turgid with high intra-aneurysmal pressure, and associated with a broad neck that has a relatively thick wall, the strong Sundt clip, or a strong Sugita and Yasargil clip, may be ideal. The Scoville and Heifetz clip may not be strong enough under such circumstances, but if the neck of the aneurysm is extremely thin and delicate, then to use a narrow, strong-bladed clip (McFadden, Sugita, Sundt, or Yasargil) may be dangerous. A strong narrow clip may crush and tear the neck. This is the most specific indication to use the Heifetz clip. The width and the curve of the Heifetz clip blade was specifically designed to reduce the puckering and stretching of the neck of such a thin-necked aneurysm (Fig. 5-16). If avulsion does occur, it is then warranted to use the Sundt-Kees or Heifetz encircling patch clips.

Stenosis of Parent Vessel

The tendency of the clip to slip down and partially occlude the parent vessel can be annoying. This is especially true with broad-based aneurysms.

If there is any suggestion of accordion effect on the parent vessel, implying minimal stenosis, it is better to assume that there is significant stenosis intraluminally, especially if dealing with the middle cerebal group of aneurysms in which distal collateral supply is limited. There are several approaches.

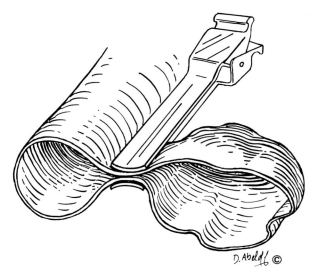

Figure 5-16. The curve and width of the Heifetz aneurysm clip blades prevent avulsion of aneurysms with thin-walled necks by reducing puckering.

1. Temporarily occlude the parent vessel, immediately place the clip, and decompress the aneurysm with fine-needle puncture of the fundus. Decompression of the aneurysm will usually allow the clip to retain its proper position unless the neck is bulbous. In such cases tandem clipping is frequently necessary.
2. One can allow the clip that has slipped down to a stenosing position to remain in place momentarily while a second clip is applied just distal to it with 1 to 2 mm space between them. The aneurysm is then punctured to relieve the pressure. The stenosing clip is repositioned, utilizing the space prepared for the shift. The distal clip may then be removed or replaced as an added support. A more persistent effort to align the clip blades parallel with the parent vessel also helps to reduce the stenosing tendency.

The Neck with an Arteriosclerotic Plaque

If a strong narrow clip is placed immediately distal to a hard plaque it can shear the wall of the aneurysm neck against the edge of the plaque. If the plaque is to be included in the blades of the clip, one must ascertain whether the plaque is soft or hard and what its configuration is. If it has a half circle formation, the clip should be placed parallel to the flatter aspect of the plaque, not in a position to bring the lateral edges of the plaque together unless the plaque is very soft. If the clip is to be placed distal to the plaque, because the plaque is circumferential and of hard consistency, there should be a space of approximately 1.5 mm between the plaque and the clip to prevent a shearing tear of the wall against the plaque itself. The same principle applies if one is to use a ligature. Under these circumstances, after the clip is in place, one can place two 0-silk sutures, snug but not tight, just proximal to and touching the clip. This hopefully will inhibit dilation of the residual neck between the clip and the plaque. A soft plaque can be compressed by a clip regardless of its contour.

MRI COMPATIBILITY

The problem of MRI compatibility has become very pertinent. Clips that can be moved by magnetic field are extremely dangerous during MRI study. The old Yasargil and Heifetz clips are now obsolete due to the metal that had been used. The new models are now excellent. The Mayfield clips that are made out of 300 series stainless are slightly magnetic and therefore not compatible with the MRI.

The clips that are compatible with the MRI are as follows:

1. Heifetz, Elgiloy
2. McFadden, MP35N
3. Sugita, Elgiloy
4. Sundt, MP35N
5. Yasargil, European "Elgiloy"

All of these clips are variants of cobalt-nickel-chrome alloys. The metals are nonreactive to magnetic fields and are of excellent stainless quality.

Every aneurysm tray should be prepared to handle the unexpected. Basic clips should be on the tray even though one may have a preference for one specific type. The basic set should include at minimum either the Sugita or the Yasargil system (which are very similar), the Heifetz system, and the high-force Sundt clip system. With this combination of aneurysm clips any aneurysm that can be clipped can be handled. Drake's superb concept of the fenestrated clip has been incorporated in these clips.

NERVE HOOKS—THEIR SIGNIFICANCE IN ANEURYSM SURGERY

In general, blunt dissection in hidden recesses should be avoided. The surgeon should use sharp dissection whenever possible under high magnification.

There are three sources of danger in the use of the nerve hook to dissect around aneurysms or to isolate the neck of the aneurysm. A sharp, pointed hook should be avoided because of the danger of perforation. The nerve hook with a ball tip also has the potential to harm. The ball end tends to inhibit the removal of the tip once it has been inserted into the area of dissection, because the tissue is inclined to constrict itself around the neck of the ball. As one attempts to remove it, the resistance can result in premature rupture of the aneurysm. Therefore the ball-tipped nerve hook should be avoided. Only the straight or the pear-shaped nerve hook should be used so that as one slides the hook out of the tissue plane there will be a smooth exit of the tip of the hook.

The third area of danger is lack of awareness of the position of the hook when it is hidden within tissue planes. Nerve hooks must have a finger indicator to be certain of the tip direction when the tip cannot be seen.

ULTRASONIC ASPIRATION—COMPLICATIONS SECONDARY TO MISUSE

In spite of the claim that ultrasonic aspirators tend to spare blood vessels, this is not altogether true. If one aspirates through to the opposite side of a tumor lying on a large blood vessel,[20] one can penetrate the vessel. Caution is necessary to remain "intracapsular" when debulking a tumor.

The ultrasonic probe has been used successfully for the removal of intramedullarly cord tumors,[10] but the studies of Flamm et al.[11] suggest that the ultrasonic probe can be dangerous to the spinal cord if held perpendicular to this sensitive structure even though separated by a body of fluid. Therefore the surgeon should be aware of the angle of attack when the device is used near the tumor-gliottic plane.

Another concern that has been reported is when the ultrasonic device is placed directly against the petrous bone. Transmission of the impulse may possibly damage adjacent cranial nerves.[22] I am not certain of the validity of this concern.

NERVE STIMULATORS AND ACOUSTIC NEUROMA

Sugita and Kobayashi[27] very aptly point out the possibility of misinterpreting the response of a nerve stimulator in acoustic neuroma surgery. If the stimulator is applied proximal to the area of surgery, one may find an absence of response. This does not necessarily mean that the stimulating tip is not on the facial nerve or that the nerve has been sectioned. The seventh cranial nerve may lose its response to stimulation if it has been traumatized, even if it is still intact.

SUCTION TUBES

Adherence to the suction tip by brain tissue, blood vessel, or aneurysm can be dangerous, but the suction tube should be capable of doing this when indicated. There are several aspects to this problem. In regard to suction force, one may use a low suction pressure system or a high suction pressure system with a large venting pore that can immediately negate any suction at the tip.

It is common for neurosurgeons to use standard Frazier suction tubes that do not have an enlarged finger vent in combination with strong suction pressure. This is dangerous. A suction tube without a vent or with a small vent that does not completely negate the suction effect should only be used with a low-pressure system. If a high suction pressure system is to be used, a finger vent that completely negates the suction force is mandatory.

The safety vent can be in the form of a large hole in relationship to the inside diameter of the suction tube, a pear-shaped or a linear slot, or a double or triple release hole. The principle is that the area of the safety vent should be significantly larger than the area at the tip of the suction tube. A double pore vent system works very well. When the proximal pore is closed a low negative pressure system is in effect. When both are closed, high suction pressure is produced, and when both are uncovered there is complete cessation of suction at the tip. This is also accomplished by a pear-shaped or linear slot but is not easily done with a single large round finger vent. Bondurant[4] has described the diameter of the venting hole desirable for a given size suction tube. I have been inclined to use a larger diameter vent or double vent system.

An area of misuse is the tendency to use a suction tube larger in diameter than necessary. It is unusual to need a suction tube larger than 9 F. A larger tube only inhibits visualization. One should use the slimmest tube possible to enhance visualization.

Various suggestions have been made regarding the design of suction tips. Slotted suction tips,[33] tips with projections,[24] and multipore tips are in use. Since 1950, I have intermittently used suction tips that have a slight angle to them in conjunction with high suction pressure and a large or double pore venting mechanism. The multipore tip suction tube is of special value when used for continuous stationary suction. The malleable multipore tube designed by Nishizaki and Wakabayashi[21] for this purpose has the added advantage of excellent variable control of suction force.

Another technique for stationary suction with a very atraumatic tip is to attach a section of Spetzler's Microvac suction tube[26] to a malleable metal tube whose safety pores can be partially or completely closed with bone wax.

The tendency to change the tip of the suction tube in the hope that it is less traumatic has led to two popular variations, both of which I believe to be of doubtful value (Fig. 5-17). If the outer edge of the tip of suction tube A is slightly buffed and therefore smooth, it will still not be advisable to use, but if it is smooth and almost fully radiused as in type B, there is no significant danger of damage due to the tip itself and visualization is maximized. Type C sacrifices visualization for the theoretical value of a more blunt type suction tube. The same is true for the design of type D, which, although potentially less traumatic than type B, in effect reduces the suction flow to correspond to the smaller inner diameter of the tip of the tube. Therefore one is actually using a larger tube in relationship to the amount of suction that is obtained. This has no advantage over type C; in fact it would be less desirable, since its main stem is larger than type C without gain in suction power.

Another area of danger is trauma to surrounding tissue by the inadvertent sudden lateral motion of the suction tube. This occurs when the twisting torque in the suction hose has not been negated. To avoid this accident, the suction tube should be allowed to fall free in the hand in the direction of use as it is attached to the suction hose. If it rotates to one side, it should be corrected before it is used. This will result in less fatigue fighting the torque and reduce the danger of inadvertent damage to surrounding tissue by a sudden lateral movement during moments of relaxation. Davidson and Rodgers[7] have logically suggested the use of a free-moving swivel proximal to the suction tip.[7]

Some of the problems with suction lie in the way the suction tube is used or rather misused. There are several principles involved.

1. The tube should rarely be placed perpendicular to the tissue.
2. One must dance along the tissue with one side of the tip slightly against it.

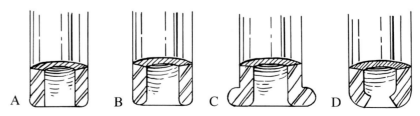

Figure 5-17. The configuration of suction tips dictates their traumatic potential. See text for explanation.

3. Never enter into a pool of blood or water beyond the surface of that pool. Stay on the surface and work down. It is safer and simultaneously removes floating debris.
4. Avoid the torque of the hose. Use a soft pliable hose and adjust the tube's position.
5. Occasionally there is a bleeding point that is hard to find. To squirt drops of water into the area to identify the bleeder may not be adequate. When this occurs rapidly fill up the cavity with several syringes of fluid to wash out and dilute the concentration of blood. One can then actually see the bleeding site in the bottom of the clear sea of water. Then suction from top down to the bleeding point. Avoid the tendency to overpack with cottonoids in such situations.
6. Avoid manipulating a thin-walled aneurysm or an aneurysm bleb with a bare suction tube. With such aneurysms it is best to place a tiny piece of cottonoid between the suction tube and the aneurysm. The cottonoid will adhere to the suction tip without completely reducing the suction effect.

THE LASER—ACCIDENTS DUE TO MISUSE

The major reason for accidents during laser surgery is the inadvertent activation of the laser, with resultant damage to tissues adjacent to the target or to personnel in the operating room. This is true especially with the hand-held laser. Inadvertent activation reflects lack of concentration. Laser surgery with or without the microscope demands deliberate precise movements. One must be certain of the path of the beam before the laser is activated.

The greatest danger to personnel in the operating room is damage to the eyes, although radiation to the skin can result in a third-degree burn. Protective glasses should be worn during laser work. Ordinary glass or plastic will inhibit CO_2 laser radiation, whereas special optical glass is necessary to block the argon, ruby, or neodymium-yag laser energy.

One must be certain that the CO_2 beam is aligned with the guiding beam. The laser beam can ignite flammable materials such as paper, flammable drapes, rubber, and plastic tubing. Flammable solutions such as alcohol, ether, and collodion, as well as volatile anesthetic gases, may also be ignited with disastrous consequences. Special care must be taken during transoral, transnasal, or anterior cervical surgery, when the beam may strike the endotracheal tube.[5] During these procedures plastic endotracheal tubes, especially if composed of polyvinylchloride, should not be used or at least heavily surrounded with wet gauge packing to cover the tubes.

As a general rule all tissue in the region of the target lesion should be protected with wet cottonoids. CO_2 laser energy is highly absorbed in water.

Inadvertent harm to tissue can also occur if the laser beam strikes a reflective surface. Metal objects in the operative fields such as brain spatulas should be covered with moist cottonoid or should be nonreflective. Nonreflective instruments are of two types. They either absorb the beam by having a blackened surface or they diffuse the beam by being sandblasted or glass beaded. Highly polished instruments are quite reflective and therefore must be used with caution. This applies to the forceps, retractors, nerve hooks, and suction tubes that are in the operating field.

Another source of hazard is the plume of smoke. This may blur the operating field, diffuse the beam, and carry viable neoplastic cells. The plume should be exhausted with a filtering system to avoid contamination of personnel.

During the debulking of tumor tissue one must be alert to the possible presence of an important vessel being embedded within the tumor, which may be inadvertently damaged. Motion of the brain can also be a problem during laser surgery. Solid fixation of the head and headrest should be routine, and cooperation between the surgeon and the anesthesiologist is mandatory. In crucial areas where motion should be at a minimum, the anesthesiologist may have to resort to very short-term apneic oxygenation to assist the surgeon in this area.[5] Rapid shallow respiration and high-frequency ventilation may be of value if motion is a problem.

In essence using the laser demands prior training, laboratory experience, and slow, deliberate movements. It is necessary to have experience and instruction to understand the appropriate settings to vaporize tissue without undue heating of the surrounding tissue and to coagulate tissue. In general it is better to reduce exposure time and increase wattage, but one has to be trained to understand these relationships depending on the type of tissue that has to be attacked.

THE CRANIOTOMY CLOSURE

One should use a fine-toothed Adson or Brown-Adson forceps to handle the dura. When closing the dura a continuous suture is appropriate, but all too often surgeons take a large "bite" through the edge of the dura. This captures too much dura. The needle insertion should not be more than 1.5 to 2 mm from the edge.

After the dura has been closed, if there is need to tack up the dura at the dura bone junction, the needle should be passed only through the outer layer of the dura. This is adequate for suture support and avoids the danger of puncturing a cortical vessel.

To secure the cranial flap with sutures, the usual technique is to insert a spatula or the foot plate of a drill guide between bone and dura to allow one to drill perpendicular to the skull without danger of striking dura. This tends to invite epidural bleeding. An alternative approach is to use the powered drill to drill at an angle. The surgeon inserts a hole through the cancellous bone parallel with the skull surface, then drills at an angle to meet this horizontal hole. To do so, first the drilling beings at 90 degrees to start the hole; then the drill is angled to exit between the inner and outer tables of the skull.

REFERENCES

1. Aoki N: Uses for dural elevator. J Neurosurg 72:834, 1990

2. Batjer HH, Samson DS: Retrograde suction decompression of giant paraclinoid aneurysms. Technical note. J Neurosurg 73(2):305, 1990

3. Battig CG: Electrosurgical burn injuries and their prevention. JAMA 204(12):91, 1968

4. Bondurant C: Alteration of suction tip pressure. Neurosurg 45:559, 1977

5. Cerullo LJ: Application of Lasers in Surgery. Yearbook, Chicago, 1988, p. 43

6. Chimowitz MI, Barnett GH, Palmer J: Treatment of intractable arterial hemorrhage during stereotactic brain biopsy with thrombin. J Neurosurg 74:301, 1991

7. Davidson RT, Rodgers C: Further modifications for the Frazier suction device. J Neurosurg 67:616, 1987

8. Drake C: Basilar aneurysms. Neurosurgery 3(2):141, 1978

9. Drake C: Giant intracranial aneurysms: experience with surgical treatment in 174 patients. Clin Neurosurg 26:12, 1979

10. Epstein F: The Cavitron ultrasonic aspirator in two surgeries. Clin Neurosurg 31:497, 1983

11. Flamm E, Rosohoff J, Wuchinich D, Broodwin H: Preliminary experience with ultrasonic aspiration in neurosurgery. Neurosurgery 2:240, 1978

12. Flamm ES: Suction decompression of aneurysms. Technical note. J Neurosurg 54:275, 1981

13. Gilsbach J, Mohadjer M, Mundinger F: A new safety device to prevent bleeding complications during stereotactic biopsy; the "stereotactic" Doppler sonography. Acta Neurochir (Wien) 89(1–2):77, 1987

14. Heifetz MD: Carotid control for intracranial aneurysms. J Neurosurg 69:142, 1988

15. Heifetz MD: A new intracranial aneurysm clip. J Neurosurg 30:753, 1969

16. Hongo K, Kobayashi S, Yokoh A, Sugita K: Monitoring retractor pressure in the brain. J Neurosurg 66:275, 1987

17. Horner NB, Potts DG: A comparison of CT-stereotaxic brain biopsy techniques. Invest Radiol 19:(5)367, 1984

18. Iwabuchi T, Suzuki S, Ebina K, Honma T: Memory clip for intracranial aneurysm surgery. J Neurosurg 42:733, 1975

19. Kobayashi S, Andrews T, Pitts L, Nakazawa S: A new dural elevator for use during removal of the sphenoid wing. J Neurosurg 69:793, 1988

20. Kudo T, Veki S, Kobayashi H et al: Experience with the ultrasonic surgical aspirator in a cavernous hemangioma of the cavernous sinus. Neurosurgery 24:628, 1989

21. Nishizaki T, Wakabayashi T: A self-retaining multipore suction tube. J Neurosurg 63:304, 1985

22. Riddenheim P, Von Essen CL, Zeterlund B: Indirect injury to cranial nerves after surgery with Cavitron ultrasonic surgical aspirator. Acta Neurochir (Wien) 89:84, 1987

23. Rosenhorn J, Diemer NH: Intermittent versus continuous brain retractor pressure as protective procedure against ischemic brain cell damage. p. 381. In Auer LM (ed): Timing of Aneurysm Surgery. Walter de Gruyter, New York, 1985

24. Shahbabian S, Modified suction tip. J Neurosurg 47:794, 1977

25. Spetzler RF: Two technical notes for microsurgery. BNI Q 4:38, 1988

26. Spetzler RF, Iversen AA: Malleable microsurgical suction device. J Neurosurg 54:704, 1981

27. Sugita K, Kobayashi H: Technical and instrumental improvements in the surgical treatment of acoustic neurinomas. J Neurosurg 57:747, 1982

28. Sugita K, Kobayashi S, Shintani P, Mutsuga N: Microneurosurgery for aneurysms of the basilar artery. J Neurosurg 57:615, 1979

29. Sugita K, Kobayashi S, Yokoo A: Preservation of large bridging veins during brain retraction. J Neurosurg 57:856, 1982

30. Sugita K: Microsurgical Atlas. Springer-Verlag, Vienna, 1985, p. 9

31. Sundt TM, Jr, Piepgras DG, Marsh WR: Booster clips for giant and thick based aneurysms. J Neurosurg 60:751, 1984

32. Vallfors B, Erlandson BE, Hanson HA, Wieck BO: Current leakage in bipolar electrocoagulation. Neurosurgery 13:111, 1983

33. Vallfors B, Hansson HA: Modified suction system for neurosurgery: slotted tubes better than with cotton pledgets. Surg Neurol 12:397, 1979

34. Wald AS, Mazzia VD, Spencer FC: Accidental burns associated with electrocautery. JAMA 217:916, 1971

35. Wilkins RH, Albin MS: An unusual entrance site of venous air embolism during operations in the sitting position. Surg Neurol 7:71, 1977

36. Yasargil MG, Fox JL, Ray MW: The Operative Approach to Aneurysms of the Anterior Communicating Artery. p. 143. In Advances and Technical Standards in Neurosurgery. Vol. 2. 1975

37. Yasargil G: Microneurosurgery. Vol. I. George Thieme-Verlag, Berlin, 1984

38. Yokoh A, Sugita K, Kobayashi S: Intermittent versus continuous brain retraction. An experimental study. J Neurosurg 58:918, 1983

6 Problematic Intraoperative Events

William F. Collins

The neophyte believes that surgical skills consist mainly of technical knowledge and manual dexterity, but a surgeon knows that, while both are important and not to be deprecated, additional skills are required for surgery, including knowledgeable preoperative evaluation and decision making, intraoperative problem solving, and comprehensive postoperative care. Good technical surgery for the wrong reason is of no value, and manual skill that can correct an event that should not have occurred during surgery can be a liability if it prevents the surgeon from learning not to allow the event to happen. It is better for a surgeon to have both problem-solving ability and dexterity, but my prejudice is that without problem-solving ability one cannot be a good surgeon. This chapter is about problem solving to control untoward intraoperative events and consists of a discussion of the means of keeping these events from occurring as well as a discussion of how to recognize and correct the events when they do occur.

Surgeons should plan to avert problematic events in surgery, and, if this is not possible, they should be prepared to limit their effect by having the means at hand for control of the situation. If the event is rare but not unexpected during the procedure being done, surgeons should always be ready to respond. An example of such an event is extensive hemorrhage during excision of a meningioma. If the event is not expected in the context of the surgery being done, one should still have the knowledge to consider the causes rapidly, since only with recognition of the cause can a rational response be initiated. An example is sudden onset of increased intracranial pressure (ICP) or swelling of the brain. In general, expected

and unexpected intraoperative problematic events can be classified under a few categories: problems in localization of pathology, unexpected pathology in an unexpected position that could cause unacceptable neurological deficit if it were approached or removed, finding no obvious pathology, unexpected or severe hemorrhage either from the lesion being approached or from vascular structures nearby, problems from anesthesia, and sudden changes in ICP, mainly marked increases in pressure.

PROBLEMS IN LOCALIZATION

Modern imaging techniques have lowered the rate of problems in localizing lesions and have decreased the need for using intraoperative exploratory techniques. They also, however, require the surgeon to be familiar with the type of imaging being used, including the persons doing the study and the techniques employed. To take maximum advantage of the various imaging techniques requires an ability to think in three dimensions, because much of the imaging and many imagers use techniques that have different angles of scanning or imaging, and the angle of the operative position of the head is almost always different from the imaging angle. Including roentgenographic opaque markers on the scalp while performing a computed tomography (CT) scan is one form of localizing assistance, but it can be a fleeting assistance once the drapes are in place unless some aspect of the exposure is related to the previously placed markers. A more traditional approach is to study the surface venous anatomy as shown on an arteriogram and to use recognizable patterns to localize the position of the exposure. One should not dismiss the use of intraoperative roentgenograms since they may clearly delineate that the assumed localization of the surgical approach is not in the area planned. A more accurate method is stereotactically to place the lesion in relation to extracranial points on the CT scan or magnetic resonance image (MRI), but the instruments necessary to do this interfere with the surgical approach when the approach and the external marking points are in the same operative field. As an additional intraoperative aid, if the lesion is not seen on the surface, ultrasound localization of the lesion can be very helpful.

The operative strategy to decrease the possibility of placing a craniotomy in the wrong position is to study the patient adequately, consider the relationship of brain, vascular, bony, and dural anatomy to the lesion, and, as the surgeon, be certain the information is known and accurate before the procedure is started.

UNEXPECTED PATHOLOGY

As with localization, modern imaging has decreased the possibility that no pathology would be found and has markedly improved the accuracy of preoperative diagnosis. Unfortunately, it has not eliminated either. If no pathology is seen upon opening the dura, the first thing to do is to determine if the craniotomy is in the correct position. There have been cases in which the surgery is performed on the incorrect side of the skull. One cause has been the mislabeling of the diagnostic studies, most commonly either CT or MRI. While this can be difficult to correct or to determine in the middle of surgery, a skull film that identifies the size of frontal sinuses or some aberration of the skull can identify the problem. Unfortunately dentition that was helpful in marking the side of the skull in air studies or arteriograms is of little use with CT and MRI, since in CT the angle of scanning is usually planned to miss the teeth and in MRI imaged dental anatomy is not clear.

Unexpected pathology can be a different lesion, a lesion in a different position, or both. An example of such a problem comes when what was thought to be an extracerebral meningioma turns out, at exposure, to be an intracortical lesion, possibly a glioma or a metastatic tumor. If localization of functional areas of the cerebrum was not considered preoperatively and if mapping of the somatosensory cortex is not available, a decision to enter a lesion that, for instance, appears to involve a portion of the speech

area is not easily made. On the other hand, not knowing the pathology because a biopsy specimen is not examined makes future decisions for therapy almost impossible to make. Generally a transverse gyral incision at the point where the lesion is closest to the surface is not likely to cause significant permanent deficit and allows exposure of the lesion and biopsy material. If the lesion is not an intrinsic tumor of the cerebrum the decision to remove it depends on the pathology, size, and position. If the lesion is an intrinsic glioma, excision is not usually of value if functional cortex would be sacrificed.

Another problem that can occur intraoperatively is the diagnosis based on frozen section material that appears to be at variance with the pre- and intraoperative information. It is important to know what is possible with frozen section material. For instance, it may not be possible to differentiate between peritumoral gliosis and a low-grade astrocytoma, or if significant information is not given to the neuropathologist an accurate diagnosis may not be possible. I prefer to drop out of surgery, leaving my assistant to continue and personally to discuss with the neuropathologist any problem that I as the surgeon am having with a diagnosis or lack thereof. The opportunity to look at the lesion under the microscope and to discuss directly with the neuropathologist the concepts of the surgeon has enabled me to continue to be familiar with intraoperative pathology and to give information to the neuropathologist that cannot be written on a laboratory request form.

For example, when operating near the midline the relative possibilities of a pituitary tumor, an intraventricular tumor, or an extracranially arising tumor can be difficult to differentiate histologically. Discussion of the surgeon's interpretation of the preoperative studies and where he believes anatomically the specimen was obtained can help to resolve some problems that are not resolvable without the kind of information that is emphasized in a face-to-face conversation over a pathology slide. Finally, the problem of differentiating an infectious process from neoplasia can at times be difficult macroscopically, and discussion with the neuropathologist as to the value of aspiration and smear of the lesion can help to make the decision to risk local contamination.

The operative mode of trying to maximize the effectiveness of a neuropathologist in contributing to intraoperative decisions is for the surgeon to know as much neuropathology as possible, to understand and appreciate what the neuropathologist in the institution can or cannot do, and to keep a continuous dialog with neuropathology in general. All of the above will improve problem solving in the operating room and decrease the significance of untoward intraoperative events that relate to neuropathology.

HEMORRHAGE

To prevent or control intraoperative problems caused by hemorrhage, the surgeon should anticipate what can happen. This is one situation in which a surgeon's optimism should not outweigh prudent caution. First, in any operative approach to the cranium one must have adequate access to the intravascular space and must have available adequate blood and fluid supply for volume replacement. In addition, if there is a significant chance that a rapid, severe blood loss may occur, as when a vessel is to be deliberately opened, intravascular volume should not be allowed to be compromised during other portions of the operation. Preservation of intravascular volume allows time to correct for a sudden loss of blood as a vessel is purposely or accidentally opened. In procedures that may require direct approach to a blood vessel, exposure or at least the possibility of exposure of the proximal feeding vessel should be considered. This exposure for control of arterial hemorrhage may be of the cervical vessels or in supratentorial surgery of the internal carotid arteries, within the skull or other major vessels (e.g., middle cerebral or anterior cerebral arteries). To be certain that the temporary occlusion of an intracranial vessel with a clip does not cause damage to the intimal surface of the vessel, clips with known minimally required hemostatic compressive forces should be available in the operative field and tested for their closing pressure before the operation starts.

Temporary clips also can be helpful when arteries or venous structure are opened either intentionally or accidentally during another portion of the procedure, such as opening the skull or exposing a border or portion of a lesion. One situation is the laceration of a dural sinus during opening or during removal of a lesion. A simple concept to control the bleeding is to consider what would be necessary if the opening were deliberate and planned. First is to be certain that exposure of the area is adequate to delineate all borders of the opening as would be obtained in a planned opening. If this is not present in the accidental opening, the first step is to obtain the necessary exposure.

Placing vascular clips blindly into an area of rapid bleeding is rarely if ever successful because inability to see may lead to the clips enlarging the opening by further tearing of the sinus. Obtaining adequate exposure cannot be stressed too much and includes using a technique to control the bleeding so the surgeon can see and can determine the edges of the opening. This is most easily done with direct pressure on the area. The area of applied pressure should be as small as possible in order to improve visualization but large enough to be effective. Removing skull anteriorly, laterally, and posteriorly to the suspected area of the dural opening will often allow more effective control of hemorrhage, because if local pressure is not adequate, cannulation of the sinus, particularly the sagittal sinus, with a small Foley catheter can be used to occlude the lumen by distending the balloon. It also can be used to form a bypass shunt if the lesion is long. Most important, the exposure often will allow determination if the opening can be approximated directly, requires grafting to preserve patency, or can be controlled by closing the lumen. Major venous sinuses can produce what appears to be an overwhelming flow of blood, but the surgeon should remember that venous pressure is low and can be lowered even more by elevating the patient's head.

Once the borders of the opening and the transverse and longitudinal anatomy of the sinus opening have been identified, the decision as to how to close the opening can be made. Most can be closed by using a running suture as an assistant keeps local pressure for hemostasis and exposes a little of the defect at a time. This technique can be used for direct closure of most venous sinus lacerations but may require, in addition, a graft when too much tissue is lost to preserve the lumen. Pericranium, galea, or temporalis fascia are all satisfactory sources for obtaining graft tissue. The use of a Foley catheter occlusion and/or shunt, as described above, may be required if the extent of the suturing will require considerable time and the lesion would be difficult to control with local pressure for the entire time. Most supratentorial sinuses, unless occluded slowly such as by a meningioma, cannot be occluded acutely without considerable risk. On the other hand, sinuses such as the parasellar, the anterior portion of the sagittal, and the sinuses along the tentorial edge, except for the transverse and straight sinuses, can be acutely occluded with little risk.

Another significant problem with venous bleeding can occur when a lesion has stripped the dura away from the skull. To attempt to control such bleeding by coagulation and/or Gelfoam or Surgicel is usually futile unless two other principles are observed. First, when the mass of clotted blood is removed, as in an arterial extradural hematoma, it should not be followed by more suction but rather by supporting the dura against the skull with stay sutures and mild pressure from the subdural space against the inner table of the skull. Second, progressing with this technique around the entire area of striping will provide hemostasis if the second part of rule one is not broken, that is, if the surgeon does not continue to remove with a sucker a clot that is formed in areas that have been supported by stay sutures. The rule that adequate exposure is required applies, as it does in all surgery.

The approach to lesions that are known to be vascular, such as arteriovenous malformations, meningiomas, or hemangioblastomas, should be via the adjacent subdural space or normal brain if at all possible. This allows the control of small surface vessels and often can identify major feeding vessels. If excessive hemorrhage occurs and the reason for the hemorrhage is the exposure of the surface of, or entrance of the dissection into, the lesion, and the bleeding cannot be controlled, then rapid excision of the lesion to obtain normal as possible perilesional surrounding brain may be an effective hemostatic technique. The judgment to take some risk by increasing the speed at which a lesion is being removed is something not easily learned and depends on many variables. The skill of the surgeon, the position of the lesion, the type of lesion, and the condition of the patient are some of the variables that have to be considered in the risk-benefit equation. Unfortunately, unlike surgery in other areas of the body, closing a bleeding wound over a drain is not an option if the patient is to survive functionally. If local blood flow control is either inadequate or not possible, another option is to decrease systemic blood pressure. At times this can be a life-saving temporary measure. The period of time and the extent of induced hypotension that can be employed to control bleeding is dependent on the age of the patient, the presence of vascular disease, suspected cardiac dysfunction, body temperature, and level of anesthesia at the time hypotension is induced.

In contrast to bleeding from a tumor or a vessel, generalized bleeding from exposed surfaces suggests a coagulopathy, either preexisting to operation or acquired during the operation. It is always difficult to stop an operation and study a problem, and most surgeons have a tendency to continue operating and to have the problem studied without interrupting the procedure. If the bleeding is a continuous surface oozing it is usually better to stop operating and determine the cause. If it is also deep and could cause compression or displacement of the brain, the surgeon may not have the choice of stopping without endangering the patient. Both situations may require laboratory studies to determine the cause, but a surgeon should always remember that uncontrolled or continued bleeding is most often caused by lack of

suitable or effective treatment of blood vessels and very rarely is caused by a coagulopathy.

When a search of the area does not reveal a cause for the bleeding, and, as implied above, that search should be a careful attempt to identify an open vessel or vessels, then the possibility of a coagulopathy must be considered. The most common causes for intraoperative coagulopathy relate to transfusions of blood bank blood or a preexisting coagulopathy. The problem, if related to transfused blood, usually is either from massive transfusions or a mismatched transfusion. The term *massive* means that more than 50 percent of the patient's blood volume has been replaced within 3 hours by blood bank blood or approximately 3,000 ml were transfused during that time period. Following a large transfusion of blood bank blood, the reasons for a problem in hemostasis are probably multifactorial, as the volume of transfused blood can cause dilutional thrombocytopenia with altered platelet function and deficiencies in factors V and VIII, the so-called labile factors, which, along with platelets, are depleted during storage of bank blood. However, even larger volumes of transfused blood given in a brief period usually can be tolerated with little alteration in clotting function; thus some other factors may also be involved. Transfusions of banked blood of greater than 5,000 to 6,000 ml in a few hours or when over many hours repetitive transfusions are almost certain to be required, platelet transfusion is probably indicated, even though it is difficult to get objective laboratory or clinical data to document this opinion. The dilutional effect causing a decrease in number of platelets and interference with individual platelet function are the basis for the use of platelet replacement.

To determine if a clotting problem has arisen during surgery, a simple test is to draw blood, place it into a clean glass tube, and time how long it takes to clot. If it clots in less than 10 to 12 minutes it is unlikely that there is a clotting problem. In addition, as a test for fibrinolysin activity, if the clot lyses within 20 minutes, then excess circulating fibrinolysin is present, which suggests intravascular coagulation.

To correct the factor V and VIII deficiencies that can occur with massive transfusions of blood bank blood, fresh frozen plasma (FFP) is effective. A problem that cannot be ignored is that FFP has both hepatitis and human immunodeficiency virus (HIV) infection risks and should be ABO antigen compatible. Cryoprecipitate also is effective in correcting factor V and VIII deficiencies as well as fibrinogen deficiency and probably has less chance of causing hepatitis and less HIV contamination risk. The other changes following transfusion that can cause clotting problems are a decrease in body temperature and alteration in calcium levels. Clotting is affected if the core temperature falls below 34°C. Rapid transfusion of cold blood, particularly if it follows rapid infusion of cold or room temperature crystalloid solutions, can easily cause this degree of drop in temperature and thus add altered clotting to a standard open vessel bleeding situation. A common concern of surgeons is that there may be a deficiency of calcium, an ion required in the clotting cascade, which has occurred because the transferred blood contains citrate. In my experience, although I know it is possible with very rapid replacement of the intravascular volume to decrease circulating calcium transiently, this is rare and thus it is equally rare that calcium will be required intraoperatively or that an infusion of calcium will correct a coagulopathy. Cardiac and/or blood pressure problems, however, can occur when there is elevated potassium in the presence of even mild hypocalcemia, which may occur transiently with rapid large volume transfusions. Even though potassium may be elevated in stored blood, there is usually some additional intrinsic cause for the potassium elevation, such as kidney failure, particularly if the elevation is prolonged.

Transfusion reactions are much more serious, and, while a coagulopathy may develop, they rarely present with diffuse bleeding as the initial symptom and more often tachycardia, hypotension, and hemoglobinuria precede it. If a mismatched transfusion is suspected of being the cause of the diffuse bleeding the transfusion should immediately be stopped, the tubing down to the needle or canula changed, and the blood checked for correct matching to the patient and the patient's blood type. The hypotension should be controlled as soon as possible, preferably with fluid to keep renal function adequate. If this is not possible because of ICP, mannitol or another solute diuretic can be used. In severe transfusion reactions, usually from a primary ABO mismatch, disseminated intravascular coagulation (DIC) may occur. The presence of DIC and hypotension after a mismatched transfusion is a grave sign, for severe DIC has usually been present only in fatal cases. Along with the fluid, FFP or cryoprecipitate may be required to replace the deleted clotting factors. The diagnosis of DIC can be confirmed by the presence of circulating fibrin split products. As mentioned above, checking blood in a clean glass tube for clotting time and clot dissolution can be helpful in recognizing severe and less severe cases.

If a patient has a congenital clotting problem, such as hemophilia, von Willebrand's syndrome, or a more rare clotting factor deficiency, except in emergency surgery where an adequate history often cannot be obtained, discovering such a condition in the middle of a surgical procedure usually means an adequate history was not taken. Other major causes of coagulopathy are most commonly related to medications with acetylsalicylic acid being a major contributor, with prolongation of bleeding time. Problems can also arise from coumarin therapy, which prolongs prothrombin time (PT), or from vitamin K deficiency with liver disease. Both problems should respond to intravenous vitamin K but in the former the response may be too slow and the latter patient may be unable to respond because of the liver disease. The most rapid way to correct the defect is to use FFP. I believe obtaining a platelet count, a PT, an activated partial thromboplastin time (PTT), and bleeding and clotting times is indicated when major intracranial surgery and probable transfusion are being considered. The inability of preoperative tests to pick up many of the coagulation deficits unless a major blood screen is done has caused many physicians to question the cost effectiveness of doing the tests. I recognize that many studies have indicated that careful family and personal histories are a better screening test, but in my experience too many patients in the stress of the preoperative period do not give complete histories.

A platelet count identifies the patient with thrombocytopenia. A bleeding and clotting time will also identify a majority of other platelet problems, congenital or acquired coagulopathies including von Willebrand's syndrome, qualitative platelet disorders, factor V deficiency, fibrinogen deficiency, and alterations in clotting from the use of acetylsalicylic acid

Table 6-1. Blood and Blood Products and Their Use

Product	Indications	Hepatitis/AIDS Risk
Whole blood	Replace loss of volume and red blood cells (RBCs)	+/±
Packed RBCs, washed or deglycerolized	Replace RBCs to raise hematocrit	+/±
Platelet concentrate	Thrombocytopenia or platelet dysfunction	+/±
Fresh frozen plasma	Deficits in labile factors vitamin K and fibrinogen	+/+
Cryoprecipitate	Same as fresh frozen plasma	±/±

Table 6-2. Coagulation Factors

Factor I	Fibrinogen
Factor II	Prothrombin
Factor III	Thromboplastin
Factor IV	Calcium
Factor V	Proaccelerin
Factor VII	Proconvertin
Factor VIII	Antihemophilic factor A
Factor IX	Plasma thromboplastin
Factor X	Stuart-Power factor
Factor XI	Antihemophilic factor C
Factor XII	Hageman factor
Factor XIII	Fibrin stabilizing factor

and similar drugs. The PT will detect deficiencies in factors II, V, VII, and X as well as deficiencies in fibrinogen. The PTT will, in conjunction with the PT, identify most deficiencies. If the PTT is normal and the PT prolonged, then deficiencies in factors II, V, IX, or fibrinogen may be present, whereas if the PTT is prolonged and the PT is normal then factor VIII, IX, XI, or XII may be deficient.

Blood and blood products commonly available that are often used and their major indications are summarized in Table 6-1. The clotting factors are given in Table 6-2.

ANESTHETIC PROBLEMS

Most supposed anesthetic problems are not caused by the anesthesia but by something else; however, it is well to keep in mind the various problems that can occur and that can mimic other problems. A serious problem that can appear early is malignant hyperthermia. It can be overwhelming in that potentially lethal fever can occur within a brief period of anesthetic induction. It can be difficult to recognize since the initial symptoms are variable, including the fever, which can be delayed. A physical symptom that is difficult to recognize in neurosurgical cases is muscle rigidity, since in craniotomies little muscle is available to display the symptom. The symptoms usually include tachycardia, hypertension, hypercarbia, hyperthermia, and cardiac arrhythmias as well as the muscle rigidity. This combination can cause increased intracranial pressure. While the syndrome usually appears in the early periods of anesthesia, such as at induction, it is well to consider the syndrome at any time the constellation of symptoms appears, since changes in anesthetic agents may be made by the anesthetist during a case. Rapid shifting from the drugs being used and to dantrolene can avert a fatal outcome if the situation is recognized

early enough to inhibit the increased muscle activity and hypermetabolism.

Intraoperative untoward events that relate to anesthesia are much less common since the development of modern anesthetics, anesthetic techniques, and intraoperative monitoring. Difficulties that can arise from anesthesia that can cause intraoperative problematic events usually relate to inadequate intracranial blood supply and oxygenation caused by relative changes in systemic blood pressure, circulating oxygen, and cerebral perfusion pressure. In addition, increased ICP from altered cerebral autoregulation, elevated circulating levels of carbon dioxide, and/or elevated central venous pressure can occur even with modern controlled neuroanesthesia. While problems are less common, one should not assume that they do not occur nor blame every untoward operative event on the anesthetist. However, incorrect positioning of an endotracheal tube can still be missed and the resulting increase in ICP will at first relate to the increased respiratory pressure required to keep the arterial oxygen within acceptable ranges and later to both the hypercarbia that may occur and the high respiratory pressure that can be needed. It is wise to stop and allow the anesthesiologist to determine the cause for the increased respiratory pressure and to be certain there is no obstruction in the passage of the anesthesia and oxygen to both lungs.

Another area that is not exactly an anesthetic problem but is usually monitored by the anesthesiologist is air entering the venous system. If the amount of air is large cardiac output will fall, and circulation failure, along with air emboli, can cause severe central nervous system damage. Air entering the heart can be detected with the use of a Doppler monitor, and one can stop the entrance of air by flooding the field with fluid and changing the position of the head. While this problem is not as common in supratentorial craniotomies as in posterior fossa procedures, which are more commonly done in the sitting position, it can occur whenever part of the venous system that may be opened is more than 6 to 8 cm above the heart, a not uncommon position for placement of the head when doing supratentorial craniotomies. It should always be considered as an explanation for a precipitous drop in blood pressure not related to blood loss. The presence of a venous access line in the right auricle of the heart can add a safety factor in the situation of intravascular air, when, along with flooding the wound and altering the position of the patient, aspiration of the right auricle to remove air is done.

Although the causes of gradual and sudden onset of intraoperative increased ICP will be discussed as a subject later in the chapter, the etiological factors relating to anesthesia should be considered in the context of this portion. Some of the factors that should be considered are elevated central venous pressure, elevated level of circulating blood carbon dioxide, excessive positive end tidal respiratory pressure or other causes of increased intrathoracic pressure, loss of autoregulation from the anesthetic, and hyperthermia. Elevated central venous pressure generally indicates central venous obstruction or heart failure, whereas elevated carbon dioxide indicates something wrong with the control of respiration or the anesthetic system or a block in the access of the anesthetic mixture to the lungs. Increased intrathoracic pressure also may be caused by the positioning of the endotracheal tube, prolonged positive pressure respirations, or acquired thoracic pathology such as pneumothorax. Loss of cerebral vascular autoregulation from an anesthetic is rare and even rarer as the cause of raised ICP, since usually the level of anesthesia to cause this is deep enough to lower rather than raise systemic blood pressure, and the cause of the increased ICP is that without autoregulation systemic blood pressure is directly transmitted to the brain. A possible rare case for the anesthetic to be the cause may be when the anesthetic is additive to some previous cerebral injury or during the short period as an anesthetic is lightened faster than the regulation recovers. The latter usually can occur only with inhalation anesthetics.

INCREASED ICP

Increased ICP that is present before surgery commences can cause untoward intraoperative events that require planning for their prevention or control. The gradual or sudden onset of increased ICP during supratentorial surgery or increased ICP that does not come under control when the planned surgery to control it has not been completed are untoward intraoperative events that are difficult to treat. The patient whose preoperative workup reveals increased ICP requires consideration of methods to reduce the pressure before undergoing even the premedications of anesthesia since the alterations in ICP that can occur with premedication for or induction of anesthesia may cause permanent damage to the brain before any surgery commences.

It is also mandatory that until the ICP is controlled cerebral perfusion pressure must be supported by adequate systemic blood pressure, usually a mild hypertension. If the pressure can be controlled by the use of preoperative corticosteroids, as is often the

case with malignant tumors with surrounding edema, it is worthwhile to delay surgery until the drug has had time to be effective. Another possible method of preoperative or intraoperative control of increased ICP when it is caused by an intraventricular block, such as a third or lateral ventricular tumor, is chronic drainage by internal shunting, prolonged external drainage by ventriculostomy, or acute ventricular drainage just before surgery commences. If none of these techniques can be used or none of the above situations are present other acute methods for control of ICP should be considered so that the changes that can occur with induction of anesthesia do not cause a problem. The most effective of these is the use of a solute diuretic such as mannitol or urea given intravenously as anesthesia is started. This is especially important if there is considerable shift of the intracranial contents along with the increased pressure. Because of the diuresis that occurs, a urinary catheter should be in place.

Problems that need to be averted include loss of cerebral perfusion pressure from a drop in systemic blood pressure with induction and the acute further elevation of ICP that can occur with an acute increase in systemic blood pressure either during induction or from the acute vasomotor response that can occur with intubation. Any of these phenomena can cause a marked increase in the shift of the brain, infarction of displaced or other poorly perfused brain, and then, with reperfusion of the infarcted areas, swelling and a further increase in ICP, making surgery even more difficult. These possible complications are now usually recognized and therefore usually prevented, but, to do this effectively, in addition to the surgeon being aware of the possible problems and how to control them, it is imperative that the surgeon discuss with the anesthesiologist the fact that an increase in ICP is present so the anesthesiologist can use techniques to minimize the untoward effects of the ICP.

If increased ICP appears when it is not expected, then a series of possibilities should be considered to explain the problem and to help indicate the therapy. Early in an operative case, that is, as the skull is opened, the unexpected finding of increased ICP should suggest that there may be problems with the position of the patient, the patient's head, or the blood CO_2 level. In addition, there is the possibility that an intraoperative hemorrhage has occurred either in a tumor being treated or from a vessel abnormality, such as an aneurysm or arteriovenous malformation (AVM) that is being treated. Other considerations include the possibility that excessive fluid was given before and during the early operative period, increased venous pressure from abdominal compression, excessive positive ventilation pressure, or the development of a pneumothorax or some other thoracic pathology. A problem with the use of mannitol or other solute diuretics to lower ICP is that the shift in the brain that they can cause may lead to a hemorrhage that causes more pressure than was originally treated. If hemorrhage appears to be the cause of the increased ICP it must be rapidly contained. If it is caused by an aneurysm or AVM that has ruptured, then a rapid approach to the area of the pathology or the feeding vessel is indicated. If the hemorrhage is in the brain, in a tumor, or in a cyst, evacuation of the hemorrhage and/or the tumor is required. If the cause is not apparent, then a diagnostic and therapeutic tap of a lateral ventricle is indicated. If there is considerable volume of fluid in the ventricle, it may indicate a block in the ventricles from either intraventricular blood or midline shift of the brain. Obstruction of the aqueduct can occur with a midline shift and incisural compression that is most commonly caused by herniation of the medial portion of the temporal lobe.

Ventriculostomy is the most efficacious treatment of the intraventricular block, while excision of the uncus or incision of the tentorial incisural border to enlarge the opening are effective means of relieving symptoms of an incisural herniation. While incisural herniation may occur in many situations it is most commonly seen during surgery for posttraumatic intracerebral hemorrhage and/or contusion. It should be considered if, after what appears to be adequate excision of a posttraumatic hematoma or a swollen contused area of brain, the ICP is not significantly decreased. In addition to the possibility of a ventricular or incisural block is the possibility of hemorrhage on the other side of the cranium. If a ventricular tap does not produce a significant amount of cerebrospinal fluid and reduction of pressure, then correction or excision of the medial temporal lobe herniation is necessary. If the tense brain makes middle fossa exposure difficult, as it often does, excision of the inferior portion of the temporal lobe can be helpful.

Another helpful technique that was used before incision of the incisural border was developed was to make an incision through the tentorium into the supracerebellar subarachnoid space. It often allows drainage of a considerable volume of trapped spinal fluid with relief of the intracranial pressure. The effect, however, is usually short lived and should not stop the neurosurgeon from correcting the herniation by reduction or excision.

As was mentioned above, the possibility of hemorrhage on the opposite side of the cranial cavity must also be considered. With modern imaging most neurosurgeons feel secure that the hemorrhage is confined to the operative area. The problem is that the tamponade of increased pressure can be removed with the surgery, allowing a previously compressed ruptured cortical vein or a cortical laceration to bleed. Previously, with inadequate imaging, both sides of the skull were draped into the field; although I must admit I rarely use it, I like to have access to the opposite side of the skull during posttraumatic surgery. While the exposure rarely allows adequate decompression it does allow rapid diagnosis and repositioning of the patient if the pressure cannot be controlled.

A problem of continued increased ICP that is also most frequently seen after trauma and for which there is no solution is when before operation there has been a significant period of loss of cerebral perfusion pressure and therefore cerebral blood flow so that a considerable volume of dead brain is without autoregulation or a blood-brain barrier. On opening the skull, the release of the calvarial support of ICP that has blocked perfusion allows reperfusion through the dead areas of brain. The combination of loss of autoregulation and absent blood-brain barrier causes marked swelling and intracerebral petechial hemorrhages. There is no therapeutic solution. Recognizing the situation can be difficult, and, when it is recognized, the patient is best handled by controlling systemic blood pressure, and excising contused brain to allow cosmetic dural and scalp closure, usually with a pericranial tissue dural graft, and a floating bone flap.

Ending this chapter with such a devastating situation puts too much of an emphasis on conditions with no treatment, so I will close with something that can mimic increased ICP but is not increased cranial pressure, and can be handled very simply. In an infant with a nonfused skull, the attaching of drapes that absorb fluid to the scalp can lead to pressure on the skull that causes the unfused bones to overlap and decrease the size of the intracranial cavity. This gives the appearance of increased ICP because the brain starts to herniate. Relieving the weight of the drapes stops the entire process and only requires that one think of the possibility or not use absorbent drapes when operating on infants.

7 Adverse Postoperative Events

Julian T. Hoff
H. Bushnell Clarke

As neurosurgeons, we strive for perfection in every operative case. Nevertheless, adverse postoperative events occur. Sometimes they are trivial, but sometimes they are not.

Many complications identified in the postoperative period are avoidable and can be attributed to a variety of mistakes made at the time of the operation. On the other hand, some complications seem to be inevitable, developing despite careful operative planning and execution.

This chapter concerns both avoidable and unavoidable complications of supratentorial surgery and how we and others have managed them. Careful preoperative planning, meticulous intraoperative technique, anticipation of complications, and diligent postoperative care are all essential measures required to avoid an adverse outcome. The surgeon's training, skill, and judgment provide the foundation upon which safe and competent surgical management is based.[2,39]

We focus on the management of some adverse postoperative events that develop in patients following supratentorial surgery. Our review is limited to common and often avoidable complications. Wound care, infection, hemorrhage, cerebrospinal fluid (CSF) obstruction/malabsorption/leak, raised intracranial pressure, cerebral ischemia, coagulopathies, metabolic disturbances, and systemic complications are discussed.

WOUND CARE

Planning the Incision

Knowledge of the vascular supply and nerve distribution in the scalp is a prerequisite for incision planning in supratentorial surgery. The integrity of the scalp, including potentially problematic scars, is an important consideration prior to incision. The general principle of "thinking ahead" is directly applicable, since mistakes made with incisions may lead to a postoperative wound problem. The incision should be planned with the expectation that a second or third operation in the same area will follow. If the surgeon consciously thinks beyond the present operation, anticipating a return to the same operative site, incision mistakes can be avoided. Traversing scars that have resulted from a poorly planned incision at a previous operation can create major difficulties with scalp healing in the postoperative period. The vascular supply of a flap that has been scarred from previous surgery is often unreliable and may be inadequate to support good wound healing in the postoperative period.

Protection of the incision edges and of the flap (if one has been made) throughout the procedure should be goals of every surgeon. Vigorous retraction of wound edges, forceful hemostatic clamps that create incision-edge ischemia, acute folds in the turn-back flap, excessive exposure to air allowing the reflected tissues to dry, coagulation burns of the skin resulting from hemostatic efforts, and excessive manipulation of tissue with sharp-toothed forceps are all conditions that may cause a wound problem in the postoperative period. Surgeons should regard the patient's tissue with respect and treat it as if it were their own.

Securing Hemostasis

Securing hemostasis in stages and layers during supratentorial surgery prevents intraoperative frustrations by the surgeon and postoperative adverse events in the patient. Scalp bleeding must be secured before proceeding to work with bone. Bone bleeding must be secured before proceeding to control epidural ooze. The dura should not be incised until hemostasis in all of the preceding stages and layers has been assured. Bleeding from scalp, bone, and the epidural space that continues during subsequent stages of the operation often provides major frustrations to the surgeon, clouding judgment and testing patience. Staged hemostasis inherent in good neurosurgical technique is fundamental even though it may be time-consuming.[56]

Closing the Wound

The dura should be closed carefully, as water-tight as possible. If a drain is placed in the subdural space, then complete closure is not possible, nor desirable. Interrupted sutures are usually better than a continuous running suture because of the binding effect of the latter. Interrupted sutures are particularly effective if the dural closure is tenuous. Patching areas of poor closure is also an effective means to secure a tight seal. Pericranium, muscle, fat, or other connective tissue can provide the needed patch without resorting to artificial substances.

Epidural hemostasis secured at the time of opening must be resecured at the time of closing. Spaced tack-up sutures to the craniotomy edges combined with hemostatic agents such as oxidized cellulose usually provide good hemostasis. Tack-up sutures from the dura to the craniotomy bone plate are also effective to reduce the dead space between the dura and the overlying bone. This is particularly effective if the bone plate is large.

The bone plate should be created with care so that it will fit well at the time of closure. Beveling the sawcuts prevents displacement inward during the postoperative period. A wide sawcut created by powered instruments may predispose the bone plate to inward displacement. Shims made from bone chips placed in the sawcuts is a good means to secure the bone plate tightly when wires or sutures are tied. Multiple wires or sutures are preferred to only a few in order to establish a tight fit.

The scalp incision should not lie directly over the sawcuts necessary to elevate the bone plate. Better healing occurs if the scalp incision is larger than the bone plate. Similarly, linear incisions overlying a burr hole or bone plate should be avoided in preference to a curvilinear incision that creates a well-placed, broad-based flap with normal scalp overlying the bone defect.

The scalp should be closed carefully with two layers of sutures. The galea should be approximated with sutures that provide anatomical approximation and also hemostasis. Failure to approximate the galea accurately results in a sunken skin incision caused by retraction of the unsecured galea beneath the healed epidermis. Scalp sutures and staples should be used simply to approximate the skin edges accurately for good healing and a cosmetically pleasing appearance.

The scalp is forgiving. Poorly planned incisions, rough handling of tissues, inaccurate reapproximation of the skin edges, and poor hemostasis may all be followed by a healed wound. On the other hand, adverse postoperative events may (and oftentimes do) follow the foregoing. If they do, it is the surgeon's responsibility.[22]

Draining the Wound

Some surgeons drain all craniotomy flap wounds from the subgaleal space. Others never drain wounds. Proponents of each approach are convinced that their results are better and that the rationale for each is beyond reproach. Facts indicate that wound infections are not prevented by the avoidance of drains, and postoperative subgaleal bleeding, hematomas, and scalp ecchymoses are not prevented by the use of drains. More often than not the use or avoidance of drains falls into the realm of lore rather than science. It is an established fact, nevertheless, that the use of drains in craniotomy wounds increases the incidence of postoperative infection if a drain remains for a prolonged period. There is no evidence that subdural drains, tumor bed drains, and subgaleal drains predispose the patient to postoperative seizures, long-term epilepsy, or both.

Dressing the Wound

Craniotomy wounds should be dressed with the same precision used to close the wound. Bacteriostatic ointments, nonadherent bandaging materials, and a snug headwrap that covers the wound and remains in place are all desirable. The ears must be protected so that they are not abraded or distorted. Dressing changes should be avoided if possible simply to reduce the contamination that is inevitable in postoperative recovery rooms, intensive care units, and open wards.

The Compromised Scalp

Patients who have scalp injuries from previous surgery or radiation are vulnerable to postoperative adversity if the incision necessary is poorly planned and the procedure poorly done. Mistakes are simply not permissible in the patient with a compromised scalp. The help of a plastic surgeon or head and neck surgeon is better than a poorly conceived operative plan, including an inappropriate incision.

Use of Scalp Lacerations as Part of the Scalp Incision

Sometimes scalp lacerations can be incorporated into the scalp incision necessary to expose the operative field.[34] The lacerations should be clean, and all layers of the scalp should be present. Avulsion/lacerations may also be used, but often require rotation flaps at the time of closure. Again, plastic surgery expertise may be required to do the job well. Scalp wounds should not be incorporated into the planned incision necessary to achieve good operative exposure if the compromise results in either poor exposure of the surgical field or poor wound healing.

INFECTION

Prevention of Postoperative Infection

"An ounce of prevention is worth a pound of cure." The old adage applies to surgery for supratentorial problems as it applies to most other avoidable complications in surgery.[4,31] The operative procedure must be done meticulously with good hemostasis, respect for tissues, precise dissection at the operative site, and minimization of needless plane development and dead space within the field. Surgery must be expeditious, taking no longer than absolutely necessary. There is a direct correlation with prolonged operation and postoperative infection.

Surgery should be avoided in patients harboring infections, either locally or systemically. Notorious sites for the source of postoperative infection include inadequately prepared skin, uncontrolled or smoldering upper respiratory infection, chronic pulmonary disease, and unrecognized urinary tract infections. Preoperative testing that detects potential infection is reason for surgery postponement. The patient should be as healthy as possible prior to any elective supratentorial procedure.[72] Postoperative infections may be preventable with the use of prophylactic antibiotics prior to, during, and briefly after operation.[23] If a foreign body is to be used as part of the procedure, antibiotic coverage should be routine. Foreign materials in a wound not only are a potential source of infection but also can be the site of infection after surgery.

Superficial Wound Infection

Most infections after supratentorial craniotomy develop in the scalp and subgaleal space.[28] The infection is often difficult to recognize immediately. In fact, infection may be undetectable for days to weeks after surgery. The usual clinical symptoms of an infected wound including tenderness and swelling are often absent in the scalp early on. The incision itself may not be erythematous, and drainage may not be obvious. Once fluid accumulation beneath the scalp flap (often present initially for a few days) remains unresolved or if the wound develops the classic signs of inflammation, then aspiration and culture of the fluid is necessary. Gram stain of the aspirate and cultures for anaerobic and aerobic organisms are required. Appropriate antibiotic management then follows. Occasionally, wound infections do not require open drainage if they are minimal and the antibiotic coverage is specific for the responsible organism.

If a superficial wound infection is recognized, then every effort should be made to clear it rapidly. Skull films should be obtained for comparison with later films to detect osteomyelitis of the bone plate if it develops. A computed tomography (CT) scan with bone windows is also helpful for comparison at a later time.

Occasionally, a wound that appears to be infected can be opened, drained, irrigated, and closed loosely over a drain without removal of the bone plate.[19] Whether the bone plate should be removed depends on the severity of the infection, the patient's overall condition, and the appearance of the wound itself. Rapid resolution of the infection and its clinical signs, including fever, are justification for an attempt to preserve the bone plate. In almost all instances, the wound infection can be eliminated by removal of the bone plate itself, providing a safe and effective alternative.

Bone Plate and Epidural Infection

Bone plate removal and drainage of the wound rapidly establish infection control. The dura must be closed. Whether the bone plate should be removed and discarded depends on the appearance of the wound and on the overall condition of the patient.[16,19] Removal of the bone plate commits the patient to a lengthy period of cosmetic deformity and to loss of the protection of the brain that the plate normally provides. Consideration for cranioplasty should wait for 6 to 12 months following clearance of such an infection.

When a craniotomy wound that was previously infected is reopened, precautions for reinfection should be intense. Material from the wound, as well as the bone plate if it remained in the wound, should be Gram stained and cultured. Smoldering infection, undetectable clinically, can be activated by manipulation of tissue planes and suture lines. Appropriate antibiotic coverage for the organism detected by Gram stain and by culture should be administered prior to, during, and after surgery for an extended period of time. When organisms are detected by Gram stain during reexploration of the craniotomy wound, drains should be placed in the epidural space, in the subgaleal space, or in both. They should not be removed until drainage has ceased and/or the patient is afebrile.

Epidural Infection

Epidural infections after craniotomy are usually confined to that space. If the dural closure was incomplete, then the infection must be assumed to be subdural as well. The presence of pus in the epidural space precludes successful preservation of the bone plate. Generally patients are not septic, though signs of inflammation in the wound and a febrile response are typical.

There is no evidence that use of a free bone plate, as opposed to an osteoplastic one, is associated with a greater infection rate. While resorption of bone may occur in the postoperative period in either circumstance, the radiographic appearance on both skull films and CT bone windows is different than that associated with osteomyelitis of the plate. Normal vascularized bone bordering the bone plate is rarely involved by infection within the subgaleal or epidural space.

Subdural Empyema

Subdural empyema is a rare postoperative event that may develop whether a subdural drain has been used or not. There is a direct correlation with the presence of infection at this site with the longevity of the drainage apparatus. Subdural drains are usually intended to remove accumulated blood and inevitably allow the escape of CSF as well. In most instances, subdural drains, whether for drainage of accumulated blood or for subdural pressure monitoring, should not be left in place longer than a few days. Antibiotic coverage during the time of drainage is imperative.[80] Drainage should be cultured daily when it occurs.

If subdural empyema is suspected on clinical grounds, including fever, seizures, wound drainage, and fluid accumulation documented by CT or magnetic resonance imaging (MRI), then it should be drained by reexploration of the wound (Fig. 7-1). The presence of subdural empyema demands not only drainage of the purulent material but also copious irrigation, removal of the bone plate, and a tight dural closure.[5] Drainage of the epidural and subgaleal space is then essential in the absence of the bone plate.

Cerebritis and Brain Abscess

While rarely the site of postoperative infection, brain may become involved. Imaging modalities, including CT and MRI, show edema, mass effect, and enhancement of tissue beyond that expected for a clean operative site.[88] The use of a foreign body at the time of operation, such as a ventricular catheter or a drain in the resection site, predisposes the patient to infection at this site.[67]

When nasal sinuses are traversed at the time of craniotomy, organisms within them may be responsible for the deep infection. Air cells from nasal sinuses and/or the mastoid processes are included in these

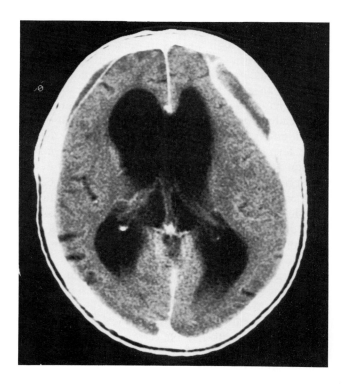

Figure 7-1. CT scans with intravenous contrast showing enhancing lentiform mass. Cultures of the semisolid pus yielded propionobacter species. Evacuation required a craniotomy.

potential sites for wound infection. If infection of the brain is suspected, its treatment includes an appropriate culture, often obtained by needle aspiration or possibly reexploration of the wound as well as appropriate intravenous antibiotics.[68] Topical antibiotics, while often used, provide little if any benefit. The scalp wound usually shows no evidence of the underlying infection process.

Meningitis

Postoperative meningitis is almost always pyogenic in nature.[70] The organism responsible is most often a skin contaminant, a contaminant of the instruments used, or of foreign bodies implanted. Fever, meningismus, seizures, and progressive neurological deterioration all signal uncontrolled infection in the ventricular system and/or the subarachnoid space.[15] Unanticipated bleeding from deep drains also suggests infection, prompting Gram staining and culturing of the drainage fluid.

Aseptic meningitis, occasionally occurring after posterior fossa exploration, is a rare event after supratentorial surgery. Hence pleocytosis of the ventricular fluid, as well as signs of meningismus, must be regarded as bacterial in origin from the beginning and treated appropriately.

Other Common Sites for Postoperative Infection

Urinary Tract

Chronic urinary tract infections obvious by routine urinalysis may be the source for organisms causing postoperative wound infections. Unless a supratentorial craniotomy is emergent, surgery should be delayed until appropriate antibiotic coverage has been established and the infection is controlled. Bladder drainage during and after craniotomy is essential to prevent reactivation of the infection during the postoperative period.[38]

Pulmonary System

Purulent sputum, whether accompanied by a febrile response in the patient or not, is a reason to delay elective surgery. Appropriate cultures and antibiotic coverage at the time of subsequent craniotomy are essentials.[27] Patients with chronic obstructive pulmonary disease are particularly prone to postoperative pulmonary infections and seeding to the operative site. The patient is also vulnerable if a foreign body has been placed in the craniotomy wound.

Nasal Sinuses

When nasal sinuses are traversed by the craniotomy wound and purulent sinusitis is encountered in the process of bone plate removal, surgery should be halted at that point and postponed until nasal infection has cleared. Gram staining and culturing of the sinus fluid allow selection of the appropriate antibiotics to clear the infection. The bone plate may be replaced in an effort to preserve it despite the nasal sinus infection. Craniotomy should be delayed for weeks to months until all signs of infection have cleared. When a craniotomy must be carried out despite the presence of nasal infection and open sinuses, the infection rate is clearly higher and appropriate prophylaxis for infection should be prolonged.

The use of nasogastric tubes and nasotracheal tubes at the time of operation and afterwards predisposes patients to nasal sinus infection if they remain in situ for a prolonged period. Unexplained fever in such patients should prompt evaluation of the nasal sinuses by radiographs, CT scans, and otolaryngological consultation. The transnasal tubes must be removed in these circumstances to allow drainage of the obstructed sinus.

Sepsis

Sepsis in the postoperative period can be attributed to any of the above infection sites. More commonly, however, systemic infection is the result of contaminated intravenous or intra-arterial infusion lines that have remained in place too long. In patients who require prolonged peripheral or central line infusion routes, lines should be replaced every 3 to 7 days and urgently in the presence of unexplained fever. Cultures of blood and intravascular catheter tips are essential steps in the diagnosis of intravenous or intraarterial line sepsis.[38]

Deep Venous Thrombosis

Deep venous thrombosis in the lower extremities is a common sequela of craniotomy and a source of unexplained fever in the postoperative period.[11] Often the thrombotic process is not readily detected clinically. Noninvasive vascular studies and venous angiography of the lower extremities may be required to establish the diagnosis. Once detected, then treatment must be either low-dose heparinization or placement of an inferior vena cava filter to prevent pulmonary embolism. Ambulation of the patient should not be allowed until one or the other treatments for deep venous thrombosis has been established and clinical evidence of resolution of the thrombosis is apparent.

HEMORRHAGE

Site of Hemorrhage

Subgaleal Hematoma

Most subgaleal hematomas can be prevented by careful hemostasis when the wound is first opened and again at the time of closure. Bleeders from deep muscle and uncontrolled ooze from the main scalp arteries, that is, supraorbital, superficial temporal, and occipital, are principal sources for large subgaleal collections. A two-layer closure is preferred for its hemostatic advantage. Galeal sutures placed at 1-cm intervals followed by firm hand compression of the partially closed site by the surgical assistant are good preventive measures. A hemostatic running lock suture provides excellent hemostasis for the skin edges. A snug dressing that completely covers the wound site is the final step. The bandage itself should not be removed for at least 24 hours in order to secure lasting hemostasis and a sealed wound.

Some surgeons routinely place drains in the subgaleal space. That measure, while traditional and preferred by many, is no substitute for good hemostasis and meticulous closure with a compressive and occlusive dressing. If drains are used routinely, then they should be removed within 24 hours to reduce the likelihood of superficial infection. It is rarely necessary to reexplore a wound because of a subgaleal collection except in children when blood loss is critical and hemostasis imperative.

Creation of unnecessary dissection planes at the time of opening increases the possibility of postoperative hematomas in one of the various layers created. Thus reflection of a scalp flap separate from reflection of the muscle flap is not desirable because the procedure simply increases the dead space available for hematoma collection and potential infection.

Epidural Hematoma

While a small amount of blood collects in the epidural space after every craniotomy, the volume should not be enough to depress the dura. The routine use of epidural tack-up sutures to surrounding bone edges or soft tissue is a necessary step to reduce the ooze from the epidural space. We prefer to use tack-up sutures and oxidized cellulose at the edges of the craniotomy to secure hemostasis further. A tack-up suture or several between the dura and the overlying bone plate through drill holes placed in the center of the bone plate can also be helpful to minimize the mass effect of epidural collection. Careful waxing of the bone edges is fundamental.

Postoperative studies, including CT scan, should show no depression of the dura in ideal circumstances. Large quantities of Gelfoam and other hemostatic agents should be avoided since they produce not only masses themselves but also unnecessary artifacts in the postoperative studies that often become necessary.

A significant dead space is occasionally created between the dura and the inner table at the bone plate by necessarily complicated dural closures. Serosanguineous fluid inevitably collects in the space.[39] In those rare circumstances, Gelfoam sufficient to just fill the dead space is advisable. The use of epidural and subdural drains or monitors increases the likelihood that epidural fluid collection may develop. While in some instances the fluid is simply CSF that has tracked through the drain site, in other instances it may be blood that not only collects in the epidural space but may further track into the subdural compartment. Thus the dural opening for the drain site should be snug though not occlusive by appropriate dural sutures.

Subdural Hematoma

Ideally, a subdural hematoma after craniotomy should not occur.[39] Thus hemostasis at the time of closure should be complete before the dura is closed. In rare instances when continued ooze cannot be satisfactorily controlled despite extra effort, subdural drains are often placed. They rarely drain the subdural space completely even though multiple drains may be used. Thus the surgeon can expect to have not only subdural foreign body mass effect but also some subdural hematoma collections.[2] How much subdural collection develops generally depends upon the surgeon's perseverance for adequate hemostasis at the time of closure. Subdural hematomas following ventriculoperitoneal shunts may require treatment in the event of progressive neurological deterioration (Fig. 7-2).

A subdural hematoma following craniotomy is usually detected with CT scan early after operation. If sufficient mass effect develops from a hematoma then clinical signs may follow. Usually, clinical deterioration from a postoperative subdural hematoma is obvious within the first few hours.

It is essential to study patients by CT if any unexpected neurological compromise is detected in the recovery room or in the intensive care unit. The CT scanner should be used liberally so that the amount of hematoma is determined early and thus its size can be followed objectively.

If a mass is sufficient to cause neurological com-

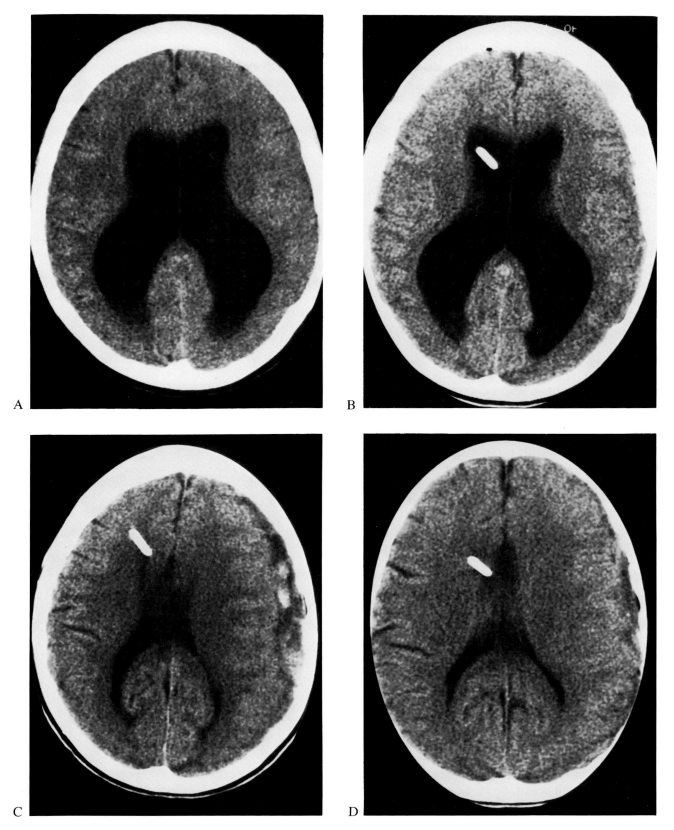

Figure 7-2. CT scan showing hydrocephalus from adult-onset aqueductal stenosis. **(A)** Preoperative CT scan prior to VP shunt. **(B)** CT scan 1 week after VP shunt. The hydrocephalus has resolved. **(C)** CT scan 4 weeks after VP shunt. A subdural hematoma has developed. **(D)** CT scan 6 weeks after burr-hole drainage and 4 weeks after craniotomy for subdural hematoma. The subdural hematoma is resolving.

promise and/or it enlarges by clinical or radiographic criteria, then reoperation is essential. Hemostasis must again be secured meticulously. The risk of wound infection and subdural empyema increases with additional surgery and prolonged exposure of the fresh operative site necessitated by a second craniotomy within a few hours or days following the initial event. Some subdural hematomas resolve spontaneously. If one is present after craniotomy and it is asymptomatic, then it may be followed by clinical and radiographic studies with the expectation that it will disappear. In rare instances, it may evolve into a chronic subdural hematoma.

When subdural drains have been placed at the time of initial craniotomy, their removal may cause additional bleeding in the operative site. Subdural drains rarely adhere to the brain or dura, though their removal can create fresh hemorrhage. The dural opening through which the drain passes can also provide access for bleeding into the subdural space from the subgaleal and epidural spaces.

Occasionally, a subdural hematoma develops in a remote area of brain without explanation.[39] This is particularly true in circumstances when the head has been elevated during operation. The sitting position, a well as the semi-sitting position for craniotomies in the occipital-parietal area, is notorious for remote hematoma development in the frontal region. The hematoma source is usually a torn bridging vein resulting from CSF drainage, parenchymal shrinkage, and brain sag created by the craniotomy site. Remote subdural hematomas usually are not sufficiently large to require removal.

Parenchymal Hematoma

An intracerebral hematoma usually develops after craniotomy at the site of maximum brain dissection or retraction. A hematoma in the bed of a resected tumor is the most common circumstance. CT scanning, as well as clinical examinations, determine whether the hematoma is clinically significant. If there is doubt, then a hematoma should be removed by reexploration and a second effort made to secure hemostasis better.

Many surgeons use hemostatic agents in the tumor bed at potential sites of hemorrhage to reduce the likelihood of a postoperative clot. The judicious use of the Valsalva maneuver by the anesthesiologist also can demonstrate potential sites of venous bleeding that require additional coagulation prior to closure. The use of hemostatic material such as Gelfoam or oxidized cellulose is not as reliable as good cauterization of bleeding sites, however. At the time of clo-

sure, irrigations of the wound with saline should be continued until the returns are completely clear. The wound itself should be filled to capacity with saline at the time of dural closure to fill the dead space and displace intracranial air that can be potentially problematic in the subdural space after surgery. Intracranial pressure monitors and subdural drains can also be the source of parenchymal hematomas.

Whether a hematoma in the brain requires removal depends on its size, mass effect, and influence on the patient's clinical condition. Edema inevitably develops because of the operative manipulation of brain tissue and the edemogenic properties of extravasated blood on underlying brain tissue. One can expect the initial hematoma to increase its mass effect over hours to days after it is initially detected (Fig. 7-3).

Ventricular Hemorrhage

Ventricular hemorrhage resulting from surgery is unusual unless the ventricle itself has been opened. When the ventricular system is opened, it should be isolated from the operative site to reduce pooling of

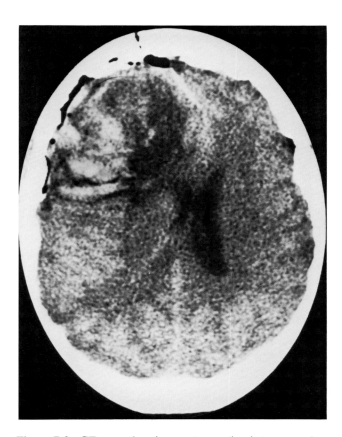

Figure 7-3. CT scan showing postoperative intraparenchymal hemorrhage after craniotomy for malignant astrocytoma.

blood within it.[86] Continued ooze into the ventricular system increases the probability of postoperative intraventricular hematomas and spillage of blood into the subarachnoid space through the ventricular system. Hydrocephalus may then be a later development in the postoperative period.[78]

When intraventricular lesions including vascular malformations and tumors are resected, hemostasis is imperative throughout the procedure. The foramina distal to the operative site should be packed off so that local bleeding does not fill the entire ventricular system. Drainage of the ventricles may be done if they have been entered. The drain should be brought out through the bone opening and through a separate stab wound in the scalp. The drain is useful for decompressing the ventricles and for monitoring intracranial pressure after surgery. CT scans in the early postoperative period assess the amount of hematoma in the ventricular systems initially. Subsequent CT scans show either resolution of the hematoma or the development of postoperative hydrocephalus resulting from subarachnoid hemorrhage or obstruction of distal ventricular outlets.

Timing of Hemorrhage

Early

Hematomas in all the sites mentioned above may develop during or early after closure. Failure of the patient to respond appropriately after operation is an absolute indication for return to either the operating room or the CT scan unit. While burr holes rarely are the source of major hematoma development, they can be if hemostasis is not absolute when they are made and closed.

Late

Late hematomas may develop in the parenchyma or subdural space after any intracranial procedure. They may appear at the operative site or may be remote.[2] Late hematoma development is particularly problematic in patients with traumatic injury who undergo early operation for lifesaving purposes. The coalescence of multiple contusions and small hematomas can then cause an additional mass effect that may require additional treatment.

Contributing Factors

Patients who require intracranial procedures should have documentation of good clotting capacity before operation.[35] Operation should be postponed if there is doubt about the ability of the patient to clot unless the procedure is highly emergent. Platelet counts should exceed 100,000. Screening tests for clotting factors, including prothrombin time (PT) and partial thromboplastin time (PTT), are additional preoperative essential tests. Other causes of coagulopathies that should be recognized and treated prior to operation are reviewed below (see *Metabolic Disturbances*).

Some intracranial procedures must be performed despite marginal coagulation parameters. Patients with depressed bone marrow because of chemotherapy for neoplasms, patients with severe multiple traumatic injuries, and patients with depressed immune systems are all potential victims of intracranial problems requiring operation.

Placement of ventricular catheters for intrathecal chemotherapy present special problems. When platelet counts are less than 50,000 and white blood cell counts are less than 2,000, catheters should not be placed because of the high incidence of intracerebral hematoma and infection, either or both of which may prove fatal.[18]

Craniotomies sometimes are necessary for severe traumatic injury. These patients occasionally have or develop disseminated intravascular coagulation. They can often be identified prior to operation or during operation by coagulopathy or screening, including an assessment of plasma fibrinogen and fibrin split products. Continued bleeding from numerous sites after operation is an obvious clinical clue that a disseminated coagulopathy has developed.

While blood screening today is highly effective in preventing transfusion reactions, such reactions still occur. Hemolysis can develop, accounting for difficulties in securing hemostasis. Consultation with a hematologist during surgery and in the early postoperative period is advisable to identify and correct the problem.[35] When massive transfusions are required to replace lost volume, hemostatic problems can develop. Again, consultation with a hematologist in the operating room may be imperative to identify the problem and correct it.

CSF OBSTRUCTION, MALABSORPTION, AND LEAK

Hydrocephalus

Generalized

Assessment of ventricular size prior to operation should establish a baseline for comparison with postoperative imaging studies. CT scans or MRIs are the principal tests used today for that purpose. In the postoperative period, CT scanning is particularly useful to determine whether CSF obstruction or malabsorption has developed because it is usually accessible without delay and at a moderate expense. If ventricular enlargement is detected, the problem is usually related to spillage of blood into the subarachnoid space and/or ventricular system because of inadequate hemostasis or undetected bleeding into the ventricles during operation.[86] Then postsubarachnoid hemorrhage hydrocephalus develops, probably related to malabsorption of CSF at arachnoid granulation sites.[78] Ventricular drainage, established through a coronal burr-hole entry site, effectively controls further dilatation, allowing return of intracranial pressure to normal.

Use of the Camino ventriculostomy system allows concomitant ventricular drainage and intracranial pressure (ICP) monitoring.[17] Drainage can be established to commence at any present threshold at the bedside. Securing the system to the patient's head with a Velcro headband is effective to establish stable and comparable pressures even though the patient is mobile in bed. Continuous drainage may be required for several days to control ICP. When drainage reduces in volume at pressures tolerable to the patient, then intermittent clamping and eventual closure for a day or so is routine prior to discontinuation of monitoring.

If ventricular drainage is required for more than several days, then a shunting procedure may be necessary. The sooner the decision for shunt is made the less likely will a systemic or shunt infection occur at the time of shunt placement. In general, ventricular drainage that requires more than a week in situ should be converted to a shunt or a new ventriculostomy placed on the opposite side. Anticipation of permanent shunting and the need for a healthy scalp site for it should accompany every ventriculostomy change. Incisions in the scalp should be made anticipating reopening of them for permanent shunting.

Infection of the CSF after operation may cause hydrocephalus.[38] In the presence of meningitis or ventriculitis, ventricular drainage controls pressure and drains the site of infection effectively. Daily cultures of ventricular fluid and Gram staining of the drainage fluid initially are essential to follow the infection. Prophylactic antibiotics that penetrate the blood-brain barrier readily, such as cefotaxime or cefuroxime, are preferred. Vancomycin and gentamycin are commonly used alternatives.

Ventricular obstruction may develop because of swelling in the operative site and secondary sealing of the outlets for CSF. The situation applies when surgery is done in or around the aqueduct and foramina of Monro.

When ventricular dilatation is evident by CT or MRI prior to operation, intraoperative drainage of CSF by ventriculostomy should be considered. We routinely place a coronal ventriculostomy prior to craniotomy in order to reduce intracranial pressure and vent CSF at the time of dural opening if ICP is elevated because of CSF retention. ICP monitoring after operation is done routinely if ventricular dilatation existed prior to craniotomy.

Focal

Focal hydrocephalus or a "trapped" ventricle can develop when surgery is undertaken near or through the foramen of Monro. Distortion of the midline and enlargement of one lateral ventricle heralds this complication. Drainage of the trapped ventricle obviates the problem, and it may be continued until swelling around the CSF outlet has resolved, allowing egress of trapped fluid (Fig. 7-4). The ventriculostomy drain may be required for several days or longer, in which case shunting is necessary.

Occasionally blood clots from the operative site or residual tumor are responsible for obstruction of the CSF outlets.[86] Clots usually absorb enough to allow egress of fluid around them, though tumor lodged in the foramen of Monro or aqueduct may not. Operation may be required to remove the obstruction or to convert a ventriculostomy into a ventriculoperitoneal shunt.

Pseudomeningocele

Pseudomeningoceles develop because the dura has been inadequately closed. CSF then tracks through the dural opening into the subgaleal space beneath or above the bone plate, resulting in a pocket of CSF beneath the scalp. If left untreated, a permanent communication may develop, establishing a pseudomeningocele. Pseudomeningoceles generally are not symptom producing except for the stretch sensation that patients feel when the scalp distends. Brain rarely herniates through the dural opening unless the hole is large.[39] Because a pseudomeningocele creates unsightly scalp swelling and often headache, patients usually require reoperation and closure of the leak (Fig. 7-5). Underlying hydrocephalus may compound the problem until CSF pressure is brought under control.

Subgaleal fluid is often apparent early after craniotomy. It resolves when CSF pressure beneath the dura normalizes in almost all instances. When CSF

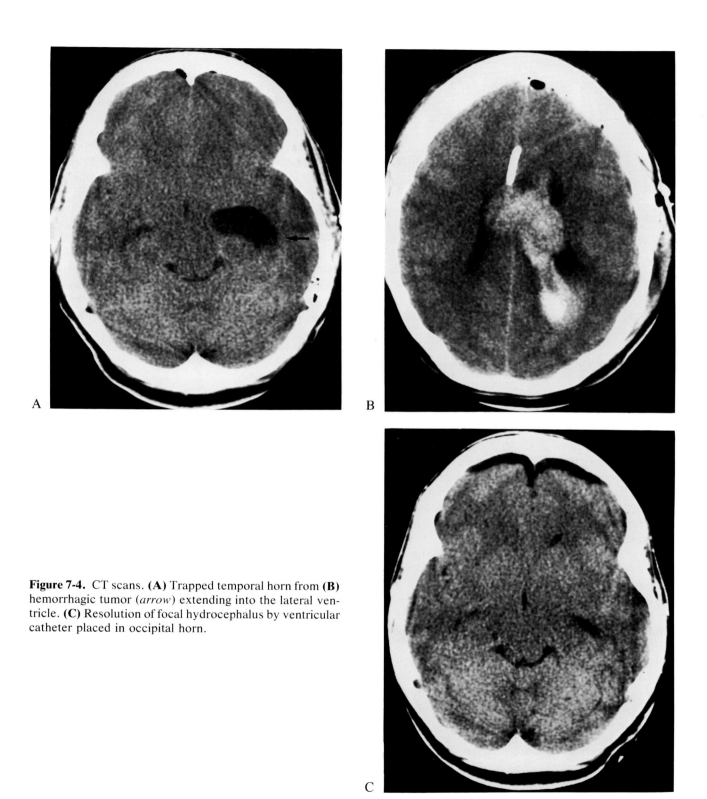

A

B

C

Figure 7-4. CT scans. **(A)** Trapped temporal horn from **(B)** hemorrhagic tumor (*arrow*) extending into the lateral ventricle. **(C)** Resolution of focal hydrocephalus by ventricular catheter placed in occipital horn.

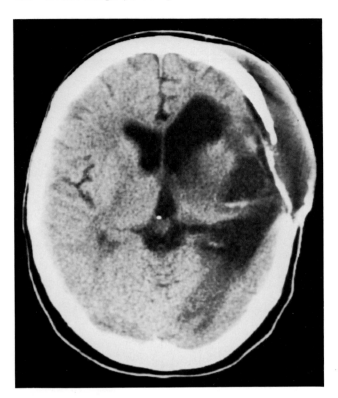

Figure 7-5. CT scan 1 week following craniotomy revealing pseudomeningocele from incomplete dural closure.

pressure fails to normalize, then pseudomeningocele may fail to resolve. A subgaleal fluid collection that persists after several days usually indicates the need for closure and/or shunting of pressurized CSF. Aspirating the fluid beneath the scalp and wrapping the wound tightly is rarely effective, though occasionally it may solve the problem.

The principal reason to prevent pseudomeningocele development early after operation is to protect the wound closure. Hence sutures should not be removed prematurely when fluid is noticeable beneath the scalp flap and the incision is stretched over it.

When pseudomeningoceles require repair, the surgeon should be ready to secure dural closure by any means necessary[74] The use of pericranial patches, dural substitutes, fascia lata, or, occasionally, cadaver dura grafts may be required. When the dura is friable or not tough enough to hold sutures, then patches are often effective. Muscle or fat is preferred. A tight dural closure does not mean the dura itself is closed but that a water-tight seal has been fashioned.

If the pseudomeningocele has been repaired and a two-layer scalp closure again effected, then the patient should be monitored for development of hydrocephalus. This situation is comparable to that seen in infants when myelomeningoceles are closed and hydrocephalus subsequently develops.

Subdural Hygroma

Fluid collection between the brain and dura after operation may be hematoma, hygroma, or pus. CT scans with and without intravenous contrast can generally differentiate one from the other. Hygromas (more accurately, subdural CSF) usually do not create significant mass effects and can be followed to resolution. If there is midline shift or deformity of the brain created by the fluid, its mass effect may be caused by loculation of the fluid. In that circumstance, drainage of the fluid by reexploration of the wound and subdural drainage through a scalp stab wound to a closed system resolves the problem. Subdural hygromas rarely require subdural-peritoneal shunting, though shunting for subdural hygromas is sometimes required in the pediatric population.

CSF Leak

Incision

If CSF leaks from the scalp wound, the wound should be reclosed. Occasionally oversewing obviates the problem, but more often the patient should be returned to the operating room and the wound closed in a better, more meticulous fashion. Infection remains the major problem that CSF wound drainage creates. Oversewing a scalp wound that leaks CSF should be done with minimal, if any, local anesthetic. Local anesthetic spilled or injected into the CSF can simulate the effects of a spinal anesthetic, resulting in respiratory distress and paralysis of motor units of cranial nerves.

Otorrhea and Rhinorrhea

When otorrhea or rhinorrhea develops after operation, the surgeon must consider those sites encountered during operation that could conceivably result in leakage of CSF to either site.[81] Otorrhea is rarely encountered, because the tympanic membrane seals off the middle ear from the outside world. Only if the tympanic membrane is open will CSF emerge unless the external canal itself has been violated. The mastoid air cells, exposed at the time of middle fossa exploration, are common sites of CSF leakage. Drainage of CSF into the middle ear will not occur unless there has been direct penetration of the air cells or the dural closure is insecure. Sealing the leak requires occluding the mastoid air cells with bone wax or muscle and reclosure of the dura if its integrity is tenuous. Occasionally, the dura on the floor of the middle fossa is violated during the course of a procedure in that area. In that circumstance, an onlay graft of fascia over the damaged or resected dura suffices. Other sources of CSF leak include air cells in the anterior clinoid processes that communicate directly with the sphenoid sinus and the various frontal sinuses exposed during frontal craniotomy.

CSF drainage by the lumbar route is an effective means to reduce CSF pressure and seal small leaks from the supratentorial compartment. Its use is limited, depending on the presence or absence of mass effect in the intracranial cavity. If mass effect persists after operation, then CSF drainage by the lumbar route cannot be used safely. If CSF drainage does not eliminate the leak after 3 to 4 days of its continuous use, then the wound demands reclosure.

Pneumocephalus

Occasionally, pneumocephalus develops if CSF drainage by the lumbar route or a ventricular catheter is excessive.[71] Air can be sucked into the intracranial cavity because of the low pressure in the system created by the lumbar drain. Effective treatment is elevation of the CSF pressure threshold required for fluid to escape through the lumbar catheter. When pneumocephalus is detected, the wound should simply be reexplored and reclosed to reduce the risk of infection.

Subdural air can almost always be detected in the supratentorial compartment by current imaging modalities after craniotomy. It resorbs within a few days and rarely causes problems from intracranial pressure or displacement of the brain. To minimize the amount of intracranial air persisting after operation, all craniotomy wounds should be filled "to the brim" with saline prior to final dural suture placement, securing a water-tight closure. In general, water-tight closures should be created from the most dependent site to the highest portion of the dural closure to minimize the air bubble that remains intracranially.

When a large amount of air is trapped intracranially, its expansion by increased temperature coupled with parenchymal swelling may create tension pneumocephalus. Removal of the air bubble by aspiration may be required. This is generally effective through one of the craniotomy burr holes. Additional air may escape into the intracranial cavity if there is a CSF leak and the patient is not cautioned to refrain from straining, such as during noseblowing (Fig. 7-6).

Treatment for tension pneumocephalus, in addi-

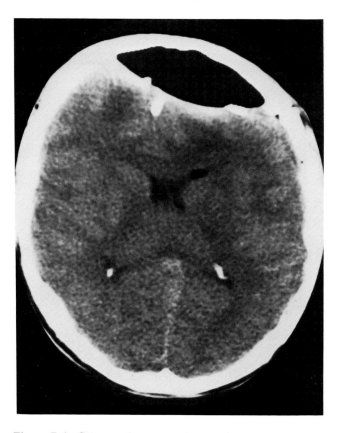

Figure 7-6. CT scan demonstrating tension pneumocephalus after frontal resection of esthesioneuroblastoma.

tion to aspiration of air that may be under pressure, is persistent dependence of the head so that CSF accumulates, thereby displacing the air from the intracranial cavity. Subdural air may require a substantially longer period of time to resorb than subarachnoid or intraventricular air that is displaced into the subarachnoid space and absorbed through the arachnoid villi and venous systems of the central nervous system.

RAISED ICP

ICP elevation occurs in many patients following intracranial supratentorial surgery. When it does, monitoring of that pressure can simplify clinical management and remove uncertainties that develop without it (Fig. 7-7). The surgeon can often predict which patients are likely to develop raised ICP and which will not at the time of surgery. When intracranial hypertension is not anticipated, the case goes smoothly, and the situation for which the operation is done is routine, then invasive monitoring by indwelling intracranial catheters is unnecessary.

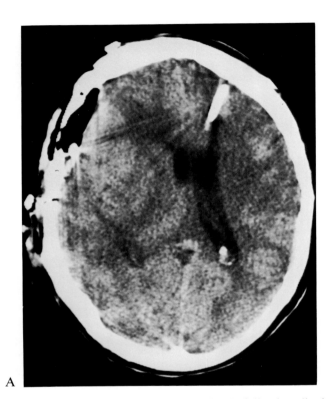

A

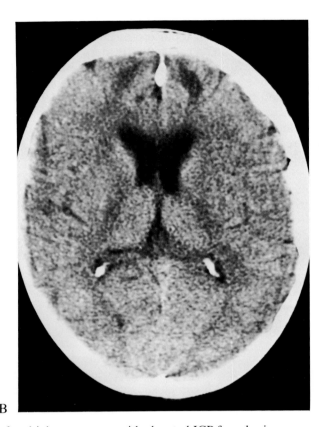

B

Figure 7-7. **(A)** CT scan immediately following clipping of multiple aneurysms with elevated ICP from brain swelling with midline shift. **(B)** CT scan 1 week later revealing resolution of brain swelling.

ICP Monitoring

There are three popular techniques for postoperative intracranial monitoring. The simplest is subdural pressure monitoring, which can be done with a soft catheter placed in the subdural space overlying the operative site. The catheter passes through one of the burr holes and a stab wound separate from the incision site. The catheter is then connected to a pressure transducer, the system filled with saline, and a waveform readily obtained. Pressure reliability of this system is good provided pressures are relatively low (<40 mmHg). The waveform and pressure values from it are recorded continuously as monitoring guidelines.

The second method is tissue pressure monitoring with a Camino device. The catheter is placed in parenchyma, the fiberoptic transducer at its tip records pressure of brain parenchyma (which is reflection of ventricular pressure), and adequate waveforms for monitoring are recorded continuously.

Both of these methods have the disadvantage that fluid cannot be aspirated from the intracranial cavity.

Thus neither method can be used to reduce ICP. Intraventricular monitoring by a simple ventricular catheter or by a more elaborate Camino device allows both pressure monitoring and CSF drainage when necessary to control ICP.

All three systems are reliable for clinical purposes, enabling the clinician to gauge therapy based on the values obtained. Generally, the pressure transducer should be placed at ear level so that head position does not influence transducer calibrations. Catheters may be left in situ for several days, but their presence should be accompanied by intravenous antibiotic administration.

Purpose of Monitoring ICP

The purpose of monitoring ICP is to ensure that cerebral perfusion pressure (CPP) is adequate at all times and homeostasis is approximated as best as possible. Abnormalities of ICP can often be detected before they become clinically obvious.

CPP should exceed 55 to 60 mmHg in order to maintain adequate perfusion of the cerebral capillary bed.[69] CPP normally exceeds 75 mmHg, assuming normal systemic arterial pressure (90 mmHg mean) and ICP (15 mmHg mean). CPP is not significantly influenced by head position unless the patient is hypovolemic or hypotensive and vulnerable to position change. Then head positions may lower blood pressure in excess of its effect on ICP, causing CPP to fall below critical levels.

Causes of Intracranial Hypertension After Operation

When ICP elevations occur, there must be a reason. The clinician must find that reason and eliminate it, if possible. The following causes of raised ICP after operation are generally correctable.

CO_2 Retention

Inadequate ventilation and retention of CO_2 rarely occurs in the intubated patient who has been carefully monitored throughout operation and in the recovery room. Still, hypoventilation does occur. When CO_2 rises, cerebral blood flow rises and ICP elevation follows. It is a simple measure to normalize PCO_2 and thereby to reduce ICP because hyperventilation causes vasoconstriction until $PaCO_2$ falls below 20 mmHg. Thus arterial blood gas monitoring soon after extubation and at intervals thereafter is critical to ensure adequate gas exchange. Because the intravascular volume in the brain at any moment is only about 75 ml, hyperventilation sufficient to cause vasoconstriction can reduce intracranial volume by only a part of that 75 ml. Still, space gained by vasoconstriction may be desperately needed with the net effect of ICP reduction.[85]

The effectiveness of hyperventilation to reduce ICP depends on the CO_2 reactivity of cerebral arterioles. If CO_2 reactivity of vessels is lost because of injury or vascular insult, then hyperventilation simply cannot achieve vasoconstriction and ICP reduction. Thus CO_2 retention after operation, while rarely encountered, should be considered first when ICP elevation develops.

Hyperthermia

When core temperature rises, cerebral blood flow and metabolism also rise.[55] ICP elevation follows. A febrile patient, particularly in the early postoperative period, may have raised ICP because of raised body temperature. The situation is correctable by reducing temperature. The cause of hyperthermia needs to be sought simultaneously.

Drugs and Anesthetics

Various drugs and anesthetics cause hyperthermia. Malignant hyperthermia is occasionally encountered during operation and may persist after operation for hours. There is no specific antidote except symptomatic treatment by hypothermia blankets, ice, antipyretics, and so forth. Anesthetics, particularly halothane, cause increased ICP because they cause vasodilatation and increased cerebral blood flow.[76] Nitroglycerine is also commonly associated with raised ICP, despite the arterial hypotension it produces.

Intracranial Hematoma

Raised ICP after operation is often caused by an intracranial hematoma. If pressure is elevated after operation in excess of that anticipated by the state of the brain at the time of closure, then urgent reexploration or CT scanning or both is essential. A retained hematoma in the bed of the operative site or in the subdural or epidural space demands evacuation if it is responsible for raised ICP. The hematoma may develop early or days later. Continuous monitoring of ICP may detect coalescence of a hematoma hours to days after surgery. It is thus desirable to continue ICP monitoring for several days after surgery if it has been instituted initially.

Hydrocephalus

Either generalized or focal hydrocephalus may raise ICP significantly. If a ventricular monitor is in place, CSF can be vented successfully. If the monitor is in the parenchyma or subdural space, then egress of CSF is not possible through the catheter system. Work-up for the cause of raised ICP includes CT or MRI, either of which can detect CSF flow disturbance and indicate appropriate treatment.

Intravascular Congestion

Swelling of the brain from intravascular congestion may occur after operation from a number of causes.[86] If major veins have been occluded by the surgeon at the time of operation, for example, the vein of Labbé, then brain swelling, particularly in the temporal lobe, can be anticipated. Raised ICP may then develop, heralding swelling of the temporal lobe and potential uncal herniation.

Venous return may also be compromised by head dressings that are too snug beneath the chin, compromising jugular veins, or by poor cardiopulmonary function and early congestive heart failure. Central venous pressure monitoring and/or Swan-Ganz catheter monitoring can help to determine the cause of impaired venous return.

Loss of Autoregulation

When autoregulation is lost, blood vessels do not respond to blood pressure change by automatic vasoconstriction or dilation. Thus they are in a state of vasomotor paralysis and only respond to blood pressure change by flow changes through them. Hypertension in the presence of vasomotor paralysis causes severe vascular congestion of the brain, whereas hypotension causes relative ischemia. Loss of autoregulation is particularly common in severe head injury but may also be noted in complex surgery involving arteriovenous malformations and other vascular lesions.

Reperfusion hyperemia develops in brain when flow has been restored after temporary occlusion.[87] This circumstance arises following carotid endarterectomy when occlusion has been required during plaque removal or shunting has been inadequate. When flow is restored, then reactive hyperemia develops in brain that was made relatively ischemic earlier. In that circumstance, brain swelling related to hyperemia is reflected by raised ICP.

Treatment of Raised ICP

The purpose of treating raised ICP is to maintain CPP as close to normal as possible.[85] Treatment requires finding its source first. The above causes are common reasons for raised ICP, though not the only ones. If no obvious source for raised ICP can be found, then therapy must be given empirically.

Hyperventilation is the first step to reduce ICP. It may be used chronically and supplemented by transient bursts of bag hyperventilation to lower PCO_2 further. Plateau waves of pressure may be aborted by this maneuver.

Osmotic diuretics, particularly mannitol, are commonly used to reduce ICP. Their effect is principally on brain that has an intact blood-brain barrier since this substance does not readily cross the barrier, exerting its osmotic effect by withdrawal of water from brain parenchyma. Hypothermia is also used to reduce ICP, since its metabolic depressant effect reduces blood flow and brain bulk. Sedation, particularly in the form of morphine, etomidate, or barbiturates, is also used to suppress cerebral metabolism and blood flow. Paralytic agents, such as lidocaine or pancuronium, can reduce raised ICP by reducing agitation and muscle exertion that are reflected in raised ICP in the postoperative period.

ISCHEMIA

Generalized

It is usually accepted that CPP must exceed 55 mmHg for brain blood flow to remain relatively undisturbed. Since CPP is the difference between arterial blood pressure and ICP, both ICP and arterial blood pressure must be monitored in order to calculate perfusion pressure. CPP becomes critically narrowed most often in patients with severe head injury. Uncontrolled ICP and failure of CPP to rise concomitantly means that perfusion is inadequate and generalized ischemia develops.[41] Prolonged CPP deficit, that is, below 55 mmHg, is likely to be followed by permanent neurological deficits or by brain death.

Sometimes blood pressure rises in response to rising ICP, a phenomenon known as the Cushing response. This reflex vasomotor activity, which is generated from brainstem circuits, is usually seen in moribund patients and is rarely beneficial.

Focal Ischemia

Focal ischemia after supratentorial craniotomy has many causes. Retraction pressure that is either excessive or prolonged can cause regional or focal ischemia in the arterial network downstream from the site of vascular compression. Retraction pressure measurements have demonstrated widespread disruption of the blood-brain barrier and subsequent development of edema in the region of retractor compression.[25] Excessive retraction pressure (including the common "towing-in" maneuver) can occlude relatively delicate, thin-walled, cerebral arteries, resulting in widespread ischemic effects in the area.[9]

Occlusion of arteries in the operative field may be done intentionally to secure hemostasis or unintentionally in the course of resection or repair of the pathological lesion (Fig. 7-8).[8] Temporary occlusion, often used now during aneurysm surgery, is accompanied by transient ischemia in the vascular bed. Regional ischemia is normally followed by vasogenic edema, breakdown of the blood-brain barrier, and swelling for days to weeks thereafter. Infarction may develop if the threshold for duration and severity of ischemia has been exceeded.

Embolic particles may be dislodged during the course of supratentorial surgery, particularly when atherosclerotic vessels or aneurysms are manipulated excessively.[79] Focal edema and/or ischemic infarction may occur after supratentorial surgery from retraction pressure, intentional or unintentional vascular occlusion, embolic phenomena originating in

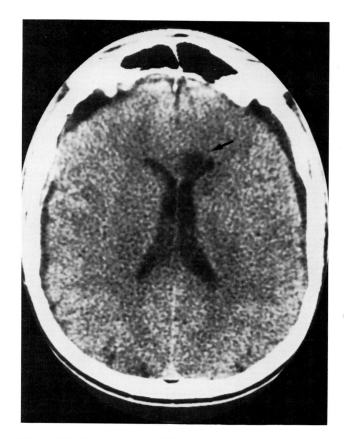

Figure 7-8. Postoperative CT scan following clipping of anterior communicating artery aneurysm. Occlusion of a small perforating branch of the artery resulted in a septal infarction (*arrow*) and recent memory loss.

normothermic brain can tolerate severe ischemia for only a few minutes without permanent ischemic change.

Treatment for focal or generalized cerebral ischemia thus is preventive in one sense with protective drugs and hypothermia and therapeutic in another sense that treatment is initiated after the ischemic event has occurred. Most protective drugs have little benefit if given after the ischemic event has taken place.

Maintaining CPP, normal blood gases and temperature, and adequate blood glucose and avoidance of extremes of arterial pressure are desirable goals.[49]

There is significant interest today in the use of hypervolemia to maintain maximal blood flow and vascular dilatation, particularly after neurovascular procedures in the supratentorial compartment.[43,64] Albumin, blood, and abundant intravenous crystalloid fluids are all commonly used to maximize volume expansion.[73] Coupled with hypertension therapy, blood flow can be increased in ischemic regions where cerebrovasospasm may be present (Fig. 7-9).[46] Cardiac output determinations with Swan-Ganz catheter monitoring and the use of the Starling curve for efficiency of cardiac contractility are common methods of gauging the effects of hypertensive/hypervolemic treatment of focal and generalized cerebral ischemia (Fig. 7-10).

COAGULOPATHIES

Expected Changes in Coagulation

The trauma of surgery causes increased coagulability. Platelets and damaged tissue release thromboplastin and vasoconstrictors. Acidosis and ischemia induced by surgery also shorten clotting time. This hypercoagulable state returns to normal within about 48 hours. Consequently, patients who undergo operations for supratentorial problems are subject to hypercoagulation throughout the body. As a consequence, deep venous thrombosis in the legs and pelvis becomes a threat, particularly in relatively immobile patients. The same threat applies to those undergoing other neurosurgical procedures.[58]

Prolonged operations with complicating factors, such as blood transfusions, poor hemostasis, and excessive tissue manipulation, increase the risk of complications from hypercoagulation. In addition, positioning of the patient during craniotomy, particularly when the semiprone or sitting position is used, subjects dependent extremities to venostasis and coagulation complications.[62]

The best prevention of complications from hyper-

atherosclerotic vessels, and the use of temporary occlusion that exceeds metabolic tolerance of the tissue.[84]

A number of measures are available to reduce the effects of focal and generalized cerebral ischemia produced during the course of supratentorial surgery.[51] Most are ineffective if given after the ischemic event has taken place, while some are probably effective if given before the onset of ischemia.

Barbiturates have been used with modest success.[3] Typically, pentobarbital or thiopental is given at the time of vascular occlusion or before if occlusion is anticipated.[37,42] Etomidate, a drug with cerebral ischemia protection properties and only modest sedative effects, is now preferred to other metabolic depressant agents.[7,53]

Hypothermia has also been used successfully, particularly when body temperature is maintained below 33°C. The duration of ischemia tolerance increases linearly with falling body temperature so that at a brain temperature of 5° to 10°C the brain can tolerate severe ischemia for up to 1 hour. On the other hand,

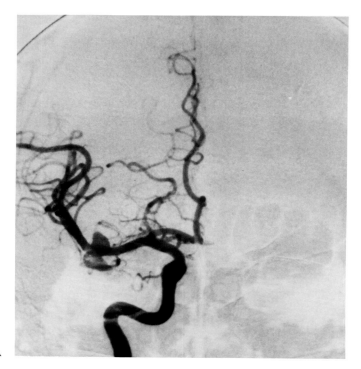

A

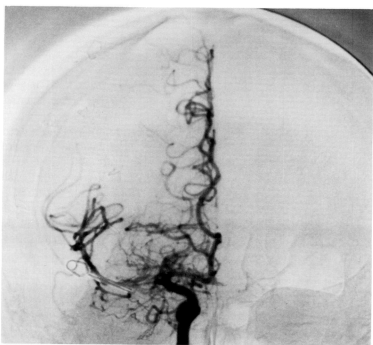

B

Figure 7-9. **(A)** Preoperative and **(B)** 2-week postoperative angiogram of asymptomatic patient with vasospasm of the middle cerebral artery.

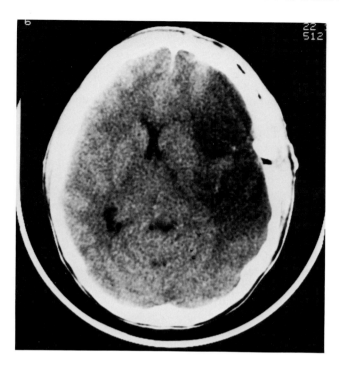

Figure 7-10. CT scan revealing an infarct from vasospasm in a patient with an unclipped intracranial anterior circulation aneurysm.

coagulation is the use of intermittent calf pumps placed on the patient before the operation begins.[11] Low-dose heparinization, to reduce the risk of hypercoagulation without concomitant increase in the risk of bleeding during the operation, is also a good preventive measure.[6]

Coagulopathy Induced by Massive Transfusions

While massive transfusions are rarely required during supratentorial surgery, they may be necessary.[59] As a general rule, more than 10 units of blood can induce an abnormality in the coagulation system. Hematology consultation in the operating room is advisable in these circumstances.[12] Altered platelet function and deficiencies of clotting factors V and VII are the most common causes of intraoperative bleeding secondary to massive transfusion.[21]

Other Coagulopathies

Bleeding intraoperatively that does not respond to simple compression and electrocauterization is most commonly the result of vitamin K deficiency, liver disease, coumadin administration beforehand, or

consumptive coagulopathy. Vitamin K deficiency due to dietary exclusion, biliary tract obstruction, malabsorption, or gastrointestinal sterilization with systemic antibiotics may also result in coagulopathy. The synthesis of prothrombin and factors VII, IX, and X, requires vitamin K for them to be active.

Virtually every hemostatic function may be impaired in a patient with severe liver disease.[24] All coagulation factors except factor VIII may be deficient. Hypofibrinogenemia also occurs, requiring cryoprecipitate administration to correct it transiently. Treatment of hemorrhagic complications in liver disease is initiated with fresh frozen plasma as well as parenteral vitamin K.

Coumadin antagonizes the action of vitamin K and thereby inhibits the activities of factors II, VII, X, and XI. Following cessation of coumadin, the prothrombin time gradually returns to normal, hastened by vitamin K administration. Administration of intravenous vitamin K (20 mg) returns the prothrombin time to normal within 6 to 12 hours. More rapid reversal is accomplished with fresh frozen plasma.[66]

Disseminated intravascular coagulopathy (DIC) is a syndrome still under investigation. It occurs most commonly in the setting of massive trauma from shock injury, sepsis, hemolytic transfusion reactions, and massive blood transfusions.[26] Two problems develop in DIC: depletion of coagulation factors due to consumption of them and activation of clot dissolution by fibrinolysis.[44] Outcome is determined by the dynamic interplay between fibrin deposition and fibrinolysis. Optimal therapy remains controversial, though fresh frozen plasma, cryoprecipitate, and platelet transfusions are standard therapy. The use of heparin and ε-aminocaproic acid remains controversial. Major clinical features of DIC are bleeding, shock out of proportion to blood loss, and acute renal failure.[52] Generalized ecchymosis with oozing or bleeding from previously intact venapuncture sites are commonly seen. Plasma fibrinogen, PT, PTT, platelet count, and presence of fibrin split products are the most important laboratory tests showing the abnormalities of DIC.

Patients with inherited coagulation deficiencies occasionally require neurosurgical procedures. Fresh frozen plasma is used to treat the rare congenital deficiencies of factors II, V, VII, X, and XI.

Management of Deep Venous Thrombosis—Pulmonary Embolus

Treatment options are limited when deep venous thrombosis is detected in the postoperative period after craniotomy. Heparin anticoagulation is not advisable until 2 weeks after the procedure has been completed.[6] Coumadin is similarly problematic and has little role in the acute phase of anticoagulation for thromboembolic phenomena postoperatively. A vena cava filter is probably the best option in the first 2 weeks following craniotomy, despite the complications it causes, including peripheral edema and post-thrombotic venous insufficiency in the legs.

Neurosurgeons must have a high index of suspicion of deep venous thrombosis in patients after craniotomy.[40] A combination of factors contributes to the problem of deep venous thrombosis and pulmonary embolus, including normal hypercoagulability for the first 24 hours and relative immobilization. Unexplained fever, even in the absence of pain, tenderness, and swelling in one or both legs may indicate deep venous thrombosis detectable readily by noninvasive Doppler studies and/or peripheral venous angiography.[77]

METABOLIC DISTURBANCES

Water/Electrolytes

Water and electrolyte imbalances after craniotomy are unusual in patients who are basically healthy. However, healthy circumstances do not always prevail. Some patients are predisposed to metabolic disturbances after an operation, manifested by water and electrolyte imbalances.[48] Patients who have been chronically dehydrated prior to operation may not be adequately hydrated before the surgery is performed because of the urgency of the procedure or because of an underestimation of the fluid debt.[50] They are then prone to fluid and electrolyte imbalances postoperatively. Similarly, patients on steroids chronically pose potential problems. A sodium/potassium imbalance is frequently encountered in patients requiring craniotomy for illnesses of the neuroendocrine system. Some drugs that are widely used, such as diuretics, cause chronic electrolyte depletion, which may create significant problems during anesthesia and in the early postoperative period.[82]

The most common electrolyte problem in postcraniotomy patients is caused by overhydration during surgery. Hyponatremia is the hallmark of excessive water replacement, most often seen in older patients whose hydration was suboptimal before surgery. It is masked by the use of mannitol or any other osmotic diuretic to reduce brain bulk during surgery. The net result may be good balance with hypovolemia early after surgery. Fluid overload with electrolyte-poor solutions then results in dilutional hyponatremia. Patients with normal kidneys secrete excessive fluid and correct their own sodium/potassium balance. If renal function is marginal or if the fluid overload is severe, however, then significant hydronatremia may develop. Seizures are the most common manifestation of severe hyponatremia, though obtundation and pulmonary edema may also develop.[13]

Anesthesiologists often have difficulties estimating blood loss and the need for fluid replacement during operation because of the liberal use of irrigating fluids by surgeons and the imprecise measurements of total fluid volumes used. Thus blood loss estimates and fluid requirements are often difficult to determine accurately.

Real problems such as diabetes insipidus and the syndrome of inappropriate antidiuretic secretion hormone (SIADH) are occasionally seen after supratentorial surgery.[20] Diabetes insipidus is best managed by replacement of vasopressin by nasal insufflation of 1-desamino-8-D-arginine vasopressin (desmopressin [DDAVP]).[75] The syndrome is encountered when surgery in and around the hypothalamus and pituitary axis is performed. SIADH, which in effect causes free water retention, may also develop, particularly in association with some tumors and infections.[54] Its management is essentially one of fluid restriction initially, osmotic diuretics such as mannitol secondarily, and hyperosmolar saline solutions as a last resort.[32]

Mannitol can cause acute tubular necrosis of the kidneys if used excessively. Serum osmolality exceeding 350 mOsm/L should be avoided to prevent this problem. Similarly, hypovolemia and hypotension for prolonged periods are accompanied by renal failure, which compounds water/electrolyte imbalance problems.

Glucose

Patients with diabetes mellitus should be managed intraoperatively and postoperatively by careful sliding scales of insulin, as well as serum and urinary glucose determinations. When a patient resumes oral intake after surgery, then the insulin schedule that existed prior to operation should also be resumed. Steroids commonly used by neurosurgeons during and after craniotomy increase serum glucose and exaggerate the glucose management problems in the postoperative period. Gradual reduction and early elimination of glucocorticoids is imperative in patients with insulin-dependent diabetes mellitus. The glucocorticoids may also unmask latent diabetes in some patients. There is evidence now that increased blood glucose aggravates focal cerebral ischemia by creating an acidotic state resulting from anaerobic metabolism that follows the ischemic event.[65] Thus high blood glucose levels should be avoided. Low blood glucose should also be avoided because glucose is the fundamental metabolic substrate of the brain.

Acidosis

Acidosis accompanies any low perfusion state whether induced by coagulation of vessels intraoperatively, by hypotension used during craniotomy for hemostasis, or by reduced CPP resulting from raised ICP following the procedure. The best management for cerebral acidosis resulting from low perfusion is improved perfusion either by reducing raised ICP or by raising arterial perfusion pressure. Buffers such as tromethamine (THAM) are currently used in some situations for cerebral acidosis.

Anesthetic Agents

The effects of some anesthetic agents may be prolonged in the postoperative period.[30] Nitroprusside, an effective hypotensive agent, may cause cyanide poisoning if used to excess.[14] Cyanide poisoning is readily detected by blood analysis and in effect is recognized as an hypoxic state. The problem is well known to anesthesiologists. Opiates commonly used by anesthesiologists during "balanced" anesthesia may account for the failure of some patients to awaken after operation. Intravenous naloxone reverses the narcosis produced by opiates.

Drugs/Alcohol

Patients who are alcoholics, whether recognized or unrecognized, may develop delirium tremens during the postoperative period. Fever, tachycardia, agitation, sweating, and other systemic responses of stress are readily observed. Treatment is generally with careful fluid support and sedation with such drugs as Librium or other analeptics.

Dilantin intoxication can also occur during the postoperative period.[63] It is commonly recognized by the presence of nystagmus, dysmetria, and ataxia. Blood sampling can detect the problem. Dilantin is also a common cause of postoperative erythematous rash over the entire body. The presence of a rash warrants discontinuance of the drug. In its most severe form, the Stevens-Johnson syndrome may develop, manifested by acute liver failure.

Steroid psychosis may be seen in the postoperative period in patients taking corticosteroids. Particularly affected are elderly patients who have been relatively immobile and unstimulated in their home environments. Rapid withdrawal of steroids is the best treatment.[63]

Antibiotic allergies are a common cause of fever and rash. They are generally used for prophylaxis during and after craniotomy. The fever and rash resolve quickly after their discontinuance.[63]

Mannitol excess in the postoperative period results in water/electrolyte imbalances. Furthermore, it may cause renal failure unless serum osmolality is carefully controlled.

Hypertension

Arterial hypertension after supratentorial surgery is an undesirable circumstance. Hypertension in a patient who did not have hypertension before may be an indication of an intracranial mass causing raised intracranial pressure. That possibility should be evaluated early. If no specific cause for hypertension is detected, then it should be treated to reduce pressure to normal ranges. Hypertension aggravates postoperative edema, particularly if mean arterial pressure exceeds 170 mmHg.[33]

Hypopituitarism

Hypopituitarism should be recognized prior to operation. Hypocortisolemia and hypothyroidism are particularly important to recognize since complications in the postoperative period frequently arise if the condition was not known before.[61] The complications that ensue are lethargy, coma, electrolyte imbalance, and fluid retention.

SEIZURES

Preoperative Seizures

Most patients who have preoperative seizure disorders are well medicated with anticonvulsants prior to surgery. The best prevention of postoperative seizure problems is establishment of therapeutic medication levels preoperatively.[60] Anticonvulsants should be continued throughout the procedure on a regular dose schedule and following operation. Surgery itself does not increase the risk of a postoperative event, and anesthesia protects the patient during the procedure itself. We believe anticonvulsants should be administered prior to operation on an elective basis whenever possible even though the patient has never had a convulsive disorder. Dilantin is the drug of choice, though it has known side effects, including hematopoietic suppression, rash, fever, and hepatic toxicity. Overdose with the drug causes significant disequilibrium characterized by nystagmus, dysmetria, and truncal ataxia.

Prevention of seizures after operation also includes an effort to keep the patient metabolically stable. Good water and electrolyte balance, prevention of hyperthermia, prophylaxis against infection, and careful and timely surgical techniques are all important prophylactic measures.[45]

Anticonvulsants

Anticonvulsants routinely used today include Dilantin, Tegretol, and phenobarbital. Each of these drugs has a good therapeutic effect to prevent generalized seizures. They are best used if given preoperatively, anticipating elective surgery. Adequate blood levels can then be ensured, providing the best protection for the patient. If the anticonvulsant has not been or cannot be given for a few days prior to surgery, then a loading dose at the time of surgery is preferred. Loading doses of Dilantin include 1,000 mg administered intravenously over 1 hour, then a maintenance level of 100 mg q8h until adequate blood levels are reached. Tegretol must be given incrementally, beginning with 100 mg q8h and then adjusting the dose over a few days to ensure a therapeutic level. Phenobarbital is rarely used as the only anticonvulsant prior to surgery because of its metabolic suppressant and soporific effects.

Dilantin has definite neurological toxicity.[60] Toxicity is almost always reversed when the drug is stopped. Worrisome side effects from Dilantin include hematopoietic suppression characterized by depressed white count, hemoglobin, and platelets. Cessation of the drug is usually followed by reversal of the hematologic problem. Hepatic toxicity is potentially more serious and can even be fatal if the Stevens-Johnson syndrome develops. Hepatic necrosis, when severe, cannot be reversed, and fatality may result. Dermatological problems are common, particularly generalized erythematous rash, oftentimes without pruritis. Cessation of the drug reverses the dermatological problem, though several days may elapse before the rash disappears. Side effects of Tegretol are much the same as Dilantin, though gastrointestinal upset is common when the patient is treated with medication orally. Patients often have changes in sensorium and thought processes with Tegretol, a phenomenon that may preclude its use. Phenobarbital, a drug of long-standing use, is effective to prevent convulsions despite its soporific effect. Usually, the soporific effect diminishes with time so that a maintenance dose of 30 mg q8h can be tolerated very well with good effect. Phenobarbital is usually the last resort as an anticonvulsant if the patient cannot tolerate Tegretol and/or Dilantin.

Predisposing Factors

Hyponatremia that often develops in the postoperative period after supratentorial surgery because of fluid overload and pituitary hormone imbalance is a predisposing factor for seizure disorders.[60] Patients with seizures prior to surgery continue to have them after operation. Patients who have had subclinical or occult seizures prior to surgery may develop overt seizures postoperatively during the stress of hyponatremia. The best treatment is correction of electrolyte imbalance and simultaneous improvement of anticonvulsant blood level. Hyperthermia also predisposes patients to seizure disorders, particularly if they have had them before. Every effort should be made to prevent hyperthermia in these patients. Usually hyperthermia is related to one of the many causes of fever after operation and is rarely a central nervous system problem.

SYSTEMIC COMPLICATIONS

This section focuses on the most common systemic complications that follow supratentorial surgery. Each of them is a problem in its own right. All contribute to the morbidity of patients after supratentorial surgery.

Cardiovascular

Myocardial infarction may occur during or after operation without warning, particularly in older patients. If the patient has had a myocardial infarction within 6 months of the procedure, the likelihood of a second infarction is significantly increased. Thus intraoperative and postoperative monitoring of cardiac function is essential. The preferred course is that craniotomy be postponed until myocardial function has stabilized for several months.

Cardiac arrhythmias develop in the postoperative period spontaneously or in the presence of metabolic disturbance, myocardial irritability, and drug effects. The host of arrhythmias possible is best detected by continuous monitoring of cardiac function in the postoperative period and consultation with appropriate specialists.

Similarly, congestive heart failure is frequently present prior to operation in older patients who require supratentorial surgery. Monitoring of central venous pressure and/or pulmonary artery and wedge pressure can detect problems before they become clinically apparent in this group of patients. Cardiac medications used prior to operation should be continued during and after the procedure to obviate the problem.

Patients are prone to pulmonary embolism because of their transient hypercoagulable state and relative immobility after craniotomy.[40] Often the craniotomy is lengthy, further predisposing the patient to deep venous thrombosis. Use of calf compression pumps during the procedure and, in some instances, low-dose heparin during and after reduces this likelihood. The development of chest pain, a friction rub, electrocardiographic changes of right heart strain, hypotension, tachycardia, and systemic hypoxia all herald pulmonary embolism. The problem is difficult to treat, particularly in the early postoperative period, because of the limited options available. Plication of the inferior vena cava or use of a Greenfield filter is the preferred treatment. Anticoagulation is not an option during the first 10 to 14 days following craniotomy.

Hypertension should be avoided in the patient who has undergone a supratentorial craniotomy, because it enhances vasogenic edema that follows manipulation of brain tissue. The additional insult of systemic hypertension enhances the process. Thus hypertension above a systeolic pressure of 170 mmHg should be avoided, even in patients who require hypertensive therapy to enhance perfusion.

Pulmonary

Patients are usually extubated soon after craniotomy. Laryngospasm or bronchospasm can develop in the recovery room in some patients. Reintubation is then essential. Occasionally, reintubation cannot be accomplished with ease, necessitating urgent tracheostomy.[10,29] Maintenance of an airway is fundamental in the postoperative period.

Patients who have undergone placement of monitoring lines, including subclavian and internal jugular vein catheters, may develop pneumothorax or hemopneumothorax during operation or afterwards (Fig. 7-11).[27] Generally, the lines should be placed prior to induction of anesthesia and their position, as well as

pulmonary inflation, confirmed by chest roentgenogram. Still, the presence of hypotension and hypoxia in the early postoperative period demands investigation of pulmonary function and detection of pneumothorax at an early time. A chest tube may be necessary to control the iatrogenic air leak.

Aspiration pneumonitis may develop after craniotomy if extubation has been poorly controlled and aspiration of gastric contents or mucous plugs has occurred. The use of prophylactic antibiotics and extended maintenance of steroids generally used for brain swelling are the best treatments. Oxygen inhalation, vigorous pulmonary toilet, and occasionally the use of a ventilator are necessary.

Atelectasis is the most common cause of pulmonary dysfunction after any general anesthetic. The problem is particularly common when patients are placed in the lateral decubitus position. The "down lung" is much less expandable by ventilation during operation, while the "up lung" is significantly easier to inflate. Thus, atelectasis is common in patients who have undergone lengthy procedures in this position. The prone position is less problematic and the supine position probably even less. The sitting position is good for lung function, but increases the risk of air embolus, negating its advantage for blood gas exchange.[1] Atelectasis also ensues if the endotracheal tube has been placed in one of the main stem bronchi, excluding the opposite lung. The net result is an atelectatic lung, not aerated during the procedure, and only detected in the recovery room after the procedure. Repositioning the endotracheal tube and positive pressure ventilation are effective treatments.

Gastrointestinal

Stress ulcer develops in patients who undergo craniotomy and who are on high doses of steroids for prolonged periods. Thus prevention of hyperacidity is essential. Use of H^+ suppression medications is preferred, in addition to liquid antacids given by the nasogastric route.

The nasogastric tube itself may be misplaced in an effort to administer calories or drugs into the gastrointestinal tract. The nasogastric tube can enter the floor of the cranial vault, penetrating the brain in patients who have had traumatic disruption of the nasopharynx. Nasogastric suction also reduces gastric acidity and decompresses the stomach in the early period after operation. Nasal tube feeding by way of a duodenal catheter (Dobhoff) is begun later when calorie intake must be resumed.

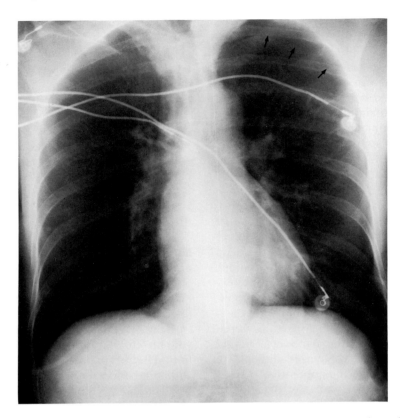

Figure 7-11. Left pneumothorax (*arrow*) following placement of a central venous catheter by the subclavian route.

Genitourinary

Most patients who undergo craniotomy require indwelling bladder catheters so that fluid volumes can be accurately measured. Catheters remain in place until the patient is able to void spontaneously. Usually by the second or third day after craniotomy the patient is ambulatory enough to allow removal of the catheter and spontaneous micturition. Prophylactic antibiotics for the bladder catheter are given commonly during its use and for 12 to 24 hours after catheter removal.

If a urinary tract infection predates the craniotomy, then it should be treated and the operation postponed until it is adequately controlled. Drugs that are used commonly by neurosurgeons in patients undergoing supratentorial surgery include osmotic diuretics, steroids, anticonvulsants, and antibiotics. Any or all may adversely affect renal function. Thus monitoring of renal function during the early postoperative period is essential to detect renal failure at the earliest moment.

Endocrine

Careful history taking, physical examination, and preoperative testing of hormone function when necessary can prevent postoperative adverse events related to endocrinopathy. Lesions in and around the pituitary fossa may cause panhypopituitarism, a condition readily detected by appropriate hormone studies and electrolyte balance measurements. Patients who have been on long-term steroids are subject to hypocortisolemia in the postoperative period unless appropriate adjustments are made in the dose of steroid used preoperatively. Patients with conditions such as rheumatoid arthritis, systemic collagen diseases, and other illnesses treated commonly by prednisone and hydrocortisone are good examples of those who develop complications frequently after surgery.

Hypothyroidism may be subtle prior to operation, only to become problematic in the postoperative period. Careful history taking and physical examination can preclude the problem. Rarely does hypothyroidism or hyperthyroidism become a problem after craniotomy in patients who have not had a clinically detected problem prior to operation.

Either excessive or insufficient ADH is responsible for major swings in sodium content and fluid volume after operation. Either is managed readily once detected by electrolyte water balance studies. Free water diuresis and additional salt administration correct the problem of SIADH. Conversely, the use of systemic antidiuretic hormone combats the problem of diabetes insipidus early after operation and later on if normal ADH production is not restored.

Some excessive hormonal responses are encountered in postoperative patients after supratentorial surgery. Severe and intractable systemic hypertension signals the possible presence of pheochromocytoma, whereas hyperthermia, hypertension, and tachycardia suggest hyperthyroidism.

Progressive Neurological Deficits

Mass Effects and Ischemia

Deficits that develop in a progressive fashion after craniotomy suggest accumulation of mass, reduced perfusion, or infection. All must be corrected with dispatch. The mass may be CSF, air, hematoma, pus, or swollen brain parenchyma. Each can be detected by imaging studies. If the progressive deficit is caused by increasing mass, then the problem must be corrected by controlling the mass effect.

If the deficit is related to ischemia, then the problem is more difficult to correct. The precise diagnosis is made with imaging techniques, including angiography and blood flow studies. Increased perfusion is the essential treatment. If increased perfusion demands reduction of mass, then that should be done. If increased perfusion means increasing blood pressure, then that must be done. If increasing perfusion means removing the obstruction to flow, then that must be done.

Positioning in the Operating Room

After surgery that has been performed carefully patients may awaken with major neurological deficits unrelated to the craniotomy itself. Some examples include quadriplegia in patients who have cervical spondylosis and have had hyperflexion or hyperextension of the neck to enhance operative positioning.[36] Avoidance of the problem demands careful positioning of the head and neck to minimize strain on the spinal cord and a compromised spinal canal.[47]

Abnormal postures of the head and neck should be avoided. Whenever possible, the surgeon should view the patient prior to draping with the thought that the patient should look "comfortable" in a position that will be maintained for a number of hours. If a twisted, hyperflexed position is used, it should be clearly justified and the only option in order to gain exposure of the operative field. The risk of head positioning and spinal cord compromise is significant enough that the surgeon must always ensure prior to scrubbing that the patient can maintain that posture for a prolonged period of time without difficulty.[83]

Other positioning problems that commonly plague anesthesiologists and surgeons in the postoperative period include pressure on the ulnar groove resulting in an ulnar neuropathy, a peroneal palsy because of compression around the fibular head by overhead tables or table rods, and sciatic nerve palsies related to prolonged periods of time in the sitting position. When patients are placed in the decubitus position, the greater trochanteric area can have excessive pressure if the procedure is prolonged. Decubitus ulcer can develop at that bony prominence. Other prominences that become problematic in the decubitus position are the ankles, knees, and shoulders.[57]

Patients who undergo supratentorial surgery in the prone position should be placed in three-point fixation skull tongs. The use of a horseshoe in the prone position increases the risk of orbital pressure and retinal ischemia, which can result in postoperative blindness. If a horseshoe rest is essential because of the skull shape or complicated scalp wounds, then the anesthesiologist and the surgeon should be aware of orbital ischemia prior to the procedure so that it can be prevented by proper positioning.

Sometimes three-point fixation devices penetrate the skull, causing epidural hemotomas or CSF leak. If the problem is simply a CSF leak, oversewing the site can stop the leak. If an epidural hematoma or skull fracture develops, then it should be corrected when it is recognized. Long-term problems with pin sites include epidural abscess, brain abscess, and osteomyelitis.

SUMMARY

Surgeons are obligated to see their patients through the operation and the postoperative period safely. A smooth, uncomplicated operation and postoperative course is universally sought and often occurs. Patients do remarkably well from major surgery, a tribute not only to the skill of the surgeon but also to the resilience of the patient. Surgery for supratentorial problems today is much better and more effective then ever before.

Complications do arise and should be anticipated. Some discussed in the preceding pages are commonly encountered and are readily treated. Some are missed, some are not treated well, and some adversely affect patient outcome. The purpose of this chapter has been to point out a few of the many complications that can arise and to suggest approaches to them. When complications become serious, surgical and medical consultants should be used without hesitation.

Neurosurgeons pride themselves on the ability to manage patients in the office, hospital, operating room, recovery room, and intensive care unit. Each situation demands different skills. Thus neurosurgeons must be trained extensively in the clinical skills that encompass all of those areas. Complications are a part of neurosurgery, and they always will be. Their effective management remains essential.

REFERENCES

1. Albin MS, Babinski M, Maroon JC, Jannetta PJ: Anesthetic management of posterior fossa surgery in the sitting position. Acta Anaesthesiol Scand 20:117, 1976

2. Allen MB, Johnston KW: Preoperative evaluation: complications, their prevention, and treatment. p. 833. In Youmans JH (ed): Neurological Surgery. WB Saunders, Philadelphia, 1990

3. Bailes JE, Spetzler RF, Hadley MN et al: Management morbidity and mortality of poor-grade aneurysm patients. J Neurosurg 72:559, 1990

4. Balch R: Wound infections complicating neurosurgical procedures. J Neurosurg 26:41, 1967

5. Bannister G: Treatment of subdural empyema. J Neurosurg 55:82, 1981

6. Barnett HG, Clifford JR, Llewellyn RC: Safety of minidose heparin administration for neurosurgical patients. J Neurosurg 47:27, 1977

7. Batjer HH, Frankfurt AI, Purdy PD et al: Use of etomidate, temporary arterial occlusion, and intraoperative angiography in surgical treatment of large and giant cerebral aneurysms. J Neurosurg 68:234, 1988

8. Batjer HH, Samson D: Intraoperative aneurysmal rupture: incidence, outcome, and suggestions for surgical management. Neurosurgery 18:701, 1986

9. Bennett MH, Bunegin L, Albin MS et al: Evoked potential correlates of graded brain retraction pressure. Stroke 8:487, 1977

10. Bennett RL, Lee TS, Wright BD: Airway-obstructing supraglottic edema following anesthesia with the head positioned in forced flexion. Anesthesiology 54:78, 1981

11. Black PML, Crowell RM, Abbott WM: External pneumatic calf compression reduces deep venous thrombosis in patients with ruptured intracranial aneurysms. Neurosurgery 18:25, 1986

12. Boral LI, Dannemiller FJ, Stanford W et al: A guideline for anticipated blood usage during elective surgical procedures. Am J Clin Pathol 71:680, 1979

13. Brigham KL: Pulmonary edema: cardiac and noncardiac. Am J Surg 138:361, 1979

14. Brown DF, Hanlon K, Crockard HA, Mullan S: Effect of sodium nitroprusside on cerebral blood flow in conscious human beings. Surg Neurol 7:67, 1977

15. Buckwold FJ, Hand R, Hansebout RR: Hospital-acquired bacterial meningitis in neurosurgical patients. J Neurosurg 46:494, 1977

16. Bullitt E, Lehman RAW: Osteomyelitis of the skull. Surg Neurol 11:163, 1979

17. Chambers IR, Mendelow AD, Sinar EJ et al: A clinical evaluation of the Camino subdural screw and ventricular monitoring kits. Neurosurgery 26:421, 1990

18. Chen JC, Hoff JT: Rickham reservoirs in patients with neoplastic meningitis. Surg Forum 36:500, 1985

19. Chou SN, Erickson DL: Craniotomy infections. Clin Neurosurg 23:357, 1976

20. Cobb WE, Spare S, Reichlin S: Neurogenic diabetes insipidus: management with dDAVP (1-desamino-8-D-arginine vasopressin). Ann Intern Med 88:183, 1978

21. Collins JA: Surgical problems of transfusion therapy, including cardiopulmonary bypass. p. 455. In Petz LD, Swisher SN (eds): Clinical Practice of Blood Transfusion. Churchill Livingstone, New York, 1981

22. Converse JM, Dingman RO: Surgical closure of scalp defects. p. 528. In Schneider RC, Crosby EC, Kahn EA, Taren JA (eds): Correlative Neurosurgery. 3rd Ed. Charles C Thomas, Springfield, IL, 1982

23. Dempsey R, Rapp RD, Young B et al: Prophylactic parenteral antibiotics in clean neurosurgical procedures: a review. J Neurosurg 69:52, 1988

24. Deren JJ: Postoperative liver dysfunction. p. 343. In Goldmann DR, Brown FH, Levy WK et al (eds): Medical Care of the Surgical Patient: a Problem-Oriented Approach to Management. JB Lippincott, Philadelphia, 1982

25. Donaghy RMP, Numoto M, Wallman LJ, Flanagan ME: Pressure measurement beneath retractors for protection of delicate tissues. Am J Surg 123:429, 1974

26. Feinstein DI: Diagnosis and management of disseminated intravascular coagulation: the role of heparin therapy. Blood 60:284, 1982

27. Gallagher TJ: Pulmonary care and complications. p. 765. In Youmans JH (ed): Neurological Surgery. WB Saunders, Philadelphia, 1990

28. Goodman SJ, Cahan L et al: Subgaleal abscess. A preventable complication of scalp trauma. West J Med 127:169, 1977

29. Grillo HC: Tracheostomy and its complications. p. 1986. In Sabiston DC Jr (ed): Textbook of Surgery: the Biological Basis of Modern Surgical Practice. 13th Ed. WB Saunders, Philadelphia, 1986

30. Grosslight K, Colohan A, Bedord RF: Isoflurane anesthesia—risk factors for increases in ICP. Anesthesiology 63:533, 1985

31. Haines SJ: Antibiotic prophylaxis in neurosurgery. Clin Neurosurgery 33:633, 1986

32. Hantman D, Rossier B, Zohlman R, Schrier R: Rapid correction of hyponatremia in the syndrome of inappropriate secretion of antidiuretic hormone: an alternative treatment to hypertonic saline. Ann Intern Med 78:870, 1973

33. Hatashita S, Hoff JT, Ishii S: Focal brain edema associated with acute arterial hypertension. J Neurosurg 64:643, 1986

34. Hennessy RJ, Persing JA, Morgan RF: Scalp injuries and their management. p. 2352. In Youmans JH (ed): Neurological Surgery. WB Saunders, Philadelphia, 1990

35. Henry DH: Clotting abnormalities in the surgical patient. p. 442. In Goldmann DR, Brown FH, Levy WK et al (eds): Medical Care of the Surgical Patient: a Problem-Oriented Approach to Management. JB Lippincott, Philadelphia, 1982

36. Hitselberger WE, House WSA: Warning regarding the sitting position for acoustic tumor surgery. Arch Otolaryngol 106:69, 1980

37. Hoff JT: Cerebral protection. J Neurosurg 65:579, 1986

38. Hoff JT, McGillicuddy J, Schaberg D: Infections: prevention and management. p. 151. In Wirth FP, Ratcheson RA (eds): Neurosurgical Critical Care. Williams & Wilkins, Baltimore, 1987

39. Horwitz NH, Rizzoli HV: Postoperative Complication in Neurosurgical Practice. Williams & Wilkins, Baltimore, 1982

40. Joff SN: Incidence of postoperative deep vein thrombosis in neurosurgical patients. J Neurosurg 42:201, 1975

41. Kassell NF, Boarini DJ: Postoperative care of the aneurysm patient. Contemp Neurosurg 6:1, 1984

42. Kassell NF, Peerless SJ, Drake CG et al: Treatment of ischemic deficits from cerebral vasospasm with high dose barbiturate therapy. Neurosurgery 7:593, 1980

43. Kassell NF, Peerless SJ, Durward QJ et al: Treatment of ischemic deficits from vasospasm with intravascular volume expansion and induced arterial hypertension. Neurosurgery 11:337, 1982

44. Kaufman HH, Moake JL, Olson JD et al: Delayed and recurrent intracranial hematomas related to disseminated intravascular clotting and fibrinolysis in head injury. Neurosurgery 7:445, 1980

45. Keränen T, Tapaninaho A, Hernesniemi J, Vapalahti M: Late epilepsy after aneurysm operations. Neurosurgery 17:897, 1985

46. Kosnik EJ, Hunt WE: Postoperative hypertension in the management of patients with intracranial arterial aneurysms. J Neurosurg 45:148, 1976

47. Kurze T: Quadriplegia following upright position in posterior fossa surgery. Proc Am Assoc Neurol Surg, Paper 75, Boston, April 9, 1981

48. Lester MC, Nelson PB: Neurological aspects of vasopressin release and the syndrome of inappropriate secretion of antidiuretic hormone. Neurosurgery 8:735, 1981

49. Ljunggren B, Säveland H, Brandt L: Causes of unfavorable outcome after early aneurysm operation. Neurosurgery 13:629, 1983

50. Maroon JC, Nelson PB: Hypovolemia in patients with subarachnoid hemorrhage: therapeutic implications. Neurosurgery 4:223, 1979

51. Martz RD, Hoff JT: Physiological protection against cerebral ischemia. p. 337. In Schverr A, Rigor BM (eds): Cerebral Ischemia and Resuscitation. CRC Press, Boca Raton, FL, 1990

52. Miner ME, Kaufman HK, Graham SH et al: Disseminated intravascular coagulation, a fibrinolytic syndrome following head injury in children: frequency and prognostic implications. J Pediatr 100:687, 1982

53. Moss E, Powell D, Gibson RM, McDowall EG: Effect of etomidate on intracranial pressure and cerebral perfusion pressure. Br J Anaesth 51:347, 1979

54. Nelson PB, Seif SM, Maroon JC et al: Hyponatremia in intracranial disease: perhaps not the syndrome of inappropriate secretion of antidiuretic hormone (SIADH). J Neurosurg 55:938, 1981

55. Nemoto EM, Frankel HM: Cerebral oxygenation and metabolism during progressive hyperthermia. Am J Physiol 219:1784, 1970

56. Owen CA Jr, Bowie EJW: Surgical hemostasis. J Neurosurg 51:137, 1979

57. Parks BJ: Postoperative peripheral neuropathies. Surgery 74:348, 1973

58. Pizzo SV: Blood coagulation. p. 369. In Wilkins RH, Rengacharry SS (eds): Neurosurgery. McGraw-Hill, New York, 1985

59. Plapp FV, Bayer WL: Blood transfusion. p. 372. In Wilkins RH, Rengacharry SS (eds): Neurosurgery. McGraw-Hill, New York, 1985

60. Porter RJ: Management of convulsive seizures. p. 1008. In Asbury AK, McKhann GM, McDonald WI (eds): Diseases of the Nervous System. WB Saunders, Philadelphia, 1986

61. Post KD, Cobb W: Perioperative endocrine management of patients with pituitary tumors. p. 868. In Wilkins RH, Rengacharry SS (eds): Neurosurgery. McGraw-Hill, New York, 1985

62. Powers SK, Edwards MSB: Prophylaxis of thromboembolism in the neurosurgical patient: a review. Neurosurgery 10:509, 1982

63. Prasad P, Albertson TE, Turner JE: Adverse drug reactions and interactions in neurosurgical patients. p. 752. In Youmans JH (ed): Neurological Surgery. WB Saunders, Philadelphia, 1990

64. Pritz MB, Giannotta SL, Kindt GW et al: Treatment of patients with neurological deficits associated with cerebral vasospasm by intravascular volume expansion. Neurosurgery 3:364, 1978

65. Pulsinelli WA, Waldman S, Rawlinson D et al: Moder-

ate hyperglycemia augments ischemic brain damage. Neurology 32:1239, 1982

66. Renaudin JW, George RP: Coagulopathies causing intracranial hemorrhage. p. 1518. In Wilkins RH, Rengacharry SS (eds): Neurosurgery. McGraw-Hill, New York, 1985

67. Rish BL: Analysis of brain abscess after penetrating craniocerebral injuries in Vietnam. Neurosurgery 9:535, 1981

68. Rosenblum ML, Hoff JT et al: Decreased mortality from brain abscess since advent of computerized tomography. J Neurosurg 49:658, 1978

69. Rosner MJ, Coley IB: Cerebral perfusion pressure, intracranial pressure, and head elevation. J Neurosurg 65:636, 1986

70. Ross D, Rosegay H, Pons V: Differentiation of aseptic and bacterial meningitis in postoperative neurosurgical patients. J Neurosurg 69:669, 1988

71. Ruge JR, Cerullo LJ, McLone DG: Pneumocephalus in patients with CSF shunts. J Neurosurg 63:532, 1985

72. Savitz MH, Malis LI: Prophylactic parenteral antibiotics in neurosurgery. J Neurosurg 70:150, 1989

73. Scandinavian Stroke Study Group: Multicenter trial of hemodilution in acute ischemic stroke. Stroke 19:464, 1988

74. Shaffrey CI, Spotnitz WD, Shaffrey ME: Neurosurgical applications of fibrin glue: augmentation of dural closure in 134 patients. Neurosurgery 26:207, 1990

75. Shucart WA, Jackson I: Management of diabetes insipidus in neurosurgical patients. J Neurosurg 44:65, 1976

76. Smith AL, Marque JJ: Anesthetics and cerebral edema. Anesthesiology 45:64, 1976

77. Valladares JB, Hankinson J: Incidence of lower extremity deep vein thrombosis in neurosurgical patients. Neurosurgery 6:138, 1980

78. van Gijn J, Hijdra A, Wijdicks EFM et al: Acute hydrocephalus after aneurysmal subarachnoid hemorrhage. J Neurosurg 63:355, 1985

79. Weir B: Aneurysms Affecting the Nervous System. Williams & Wilkins, Baltimore, 1987

80. Weisberg L: Subdural empyema. Arch Neurol 43:497, 1986

81. Westmore GA, Whittam DE: Cerebrospinal fluid rhinorrhea and its management. Br J Surg 69:489, 1982

82. Wijdicks EGM, Vermeulen M, Hijdra A et al: Hyponatremia and cerebral infarction in patients with ruptured intracranial aneurysms: is fluid restriction harmful? Ann Neurol 17:137, 1985

83. Wilder BL: Hypothesis: the etiology of midcervical quadriplegia after operation with the patient in the sitting position. Neurosurgery 2:530, 1982

84. Wilkins RH: Natural history of intracranial vascular malformations: a review. Neurosurgery 16:421, 1985

85. Wilkinson HA: Intracranial pressure. p. 661. In Youmans JH (ed): Neurological Surgery. WB Saunders, Philadelphia, 1990

86. Wilson CB, Stein BM (eds): Intracranial Arteriovenous Malformations. Williams & Wilkins, Baltimore, 1984

87. Wood JH, Kee DB: Hemorrheology of the cerebral circulation in stroke. Stroke 16:765, 1985

88. Yang SY: Brain abscess: a review of 400 cases. J Neurosurg 55:794, 1981

8 Infectious Complications

John M. Leedom
Paul D. Holtom

Infection is one of the most dreaded enemies of neurosurgeons and their patients. In this chapter, the causes and methods of prevention of infection in neurological surgery are discussed in some detail. Specific problems and their management are addressed, in addition to the general problem of approach to the patient with postoperative fever. There is also a discussion of a relatively new problem for the surgeon and his patient—the potential for spread of the blood-borne pathogen, the human immunodeficiency virus (HIV).

CONSIDERATIONS OF ASEPTIC TECHNIQUES

Authorities argue about whether the development of anesthesia or the dawn of understanding of the causation of wound infections by bacteria with consequent development of strategies for prevention of such infections was responsible for the rapid development of modern surgery.[18,49] Certainly, the development of the technique of antiseptic surgery by Lister, which stressed the treatment of the surgeon's hands with 1:20 carbolic acid, was a major advance.[55] Aseptic bloodless surgery utilizing meticulous technique to obviate hematomas and devitalized tissue was an even more cogent advance. Infection control during surgery now employs a combination of antisepsis, asepsis, and meticulous techniques. Despite these techniques, though, infections of surgical wounds or tissues of the cavities entered during surgery continue to occur. Reasonable estimates of the frequencies of such infections by risk category are[39]

1. Clean surgery (<5 percent)
2. Clean-contaminated surgery (5 to 15 percent)
3. Contaminated surgery (10 to 25 percent)
4. Dirty surgery (30 to 80 percent)

Asepsis and antisepsis are most important in reducing the incidence of surgical wound infections in the first two categories. However, adherence to their principles can be expected to decrease the frequencies of infections caused by specific nosocomial pathogens even in the last two categories of patients.

Broadly speaking, *asepsis* refers to procedures that will kill pathogenic microorganisms on instruments and objects that are in contact with the patient and the surgical wound as well as techniques that will prevent environmental microorganisms from contaminating the surgical wound. That ideal can be attained with inanimate objects like instruments that can be autoclaved. Prevention of environmental organisms entering the patient requires proper architectural design of the surgical suite and strict adherence to aseptic discipline by the surgical team. As recently stated by Laufman,[52] antibiotics, devices, and other means are not substitutes for scrupulous adherence to aseptic techniques by all personnel who work in the surgical suite or its vicinity.

Because the human skin cannot be sterilized in an autoclave, there has always been great interest in nontoxic chemicals that would be capable of removing resident or transient bacteria from the skin of patients undergoing surgery or operating-room personnel who directly touch the patients or the sterile instruments that are used in surgery. The topic of decontamination of the human skin, with a review of the pros and cons of various agents, has recently been reviewed by Laufman.[51] He points out that the human skin contains potentially harmful bacteria, not only on the surface, but also in the deeper layers of the skin that reach the surface as sweat and oil are secreted. He reviewed work that reported cultures of surgical glove sweat after use were positive, that treatment of the hands with antiseptic agents could reduce the bacterial numbers, and that dermatitis or skin abrasions caused by excessive scrubbing resulted in bacterial persistence despite treatment by antiseptic agents.[96] Walter (as also discussed by Laufman[50,51]) led the way for the elaboration of the modern components of skin antisepsis. These are (1) soap and water to wash away transient contaminants, (2) a rapid-acting antiseptic with broad-spectrum bactericidal activity, and (3) a long-acting, nonirritating broad spectrum bactericidal agent to kill organisms brought to the surface of the skin in sweat. Such treatment of the surgeon's hands is rendered necessary by the statistic that 30 percent of surgical gloves become perforated during operations.

Many different antiseptics have been used. A review of the pros and cons of each agent is beyond the scope of this chapter. The interested reader is referred to Laufman's review.[51] One group of excellent antiseptics is the alcohols. Three alcohols are particularly useful—ethyl, isopropyl, and normal propyl.[51] Alcohols must be diluted with water to denature proteins and kill bacteria. The best concentrations are from 70 to 92 percent by weight. The most usual concentration is 70 percent. This concentration causes less drying of the skin, and adding water reduces expense. Often an emollient is added to help prevent skin irritation and to prolong the bactericidal action of the alcohol, which is otherwise quite brief. Tincture of iodine is an excellent antiseptic, but it is quite irritating to the skin and causes a burning sensation when it contacts raw tissue. Iodophors have the iodine bound to polyvinylpyrrolidone or to a comparable compound. They are water soluble, less irrigating, and do not stain the skin. Iodophors act by releasing free iodine. They are not immediately active, requiring about 2 minutes of contact time to release free iodine. Tincture of iodine has essentially been replaced by iodophors. Povidone-iodine is the most frequently employed iodophor for surgical scrub. This substance has an iodine content of 7.5 percent, with 1 percent available as free iodine.

Another agent receiving wide use is chlorhexidine gluconate.[51] It is nontoxic. It has a broad range of antimicrobial activity, although it is somewhat more active against gram-positive than gram-negative bacteria. It is a good fungicidal agent, has only fair activity against tubercle bacilli, and has poor action against viruses. The onset of the antibacterial action of chlorhexidine is not as rapid as that of the alcohols, but it retains its activity for 5 to 6 hours. It remains active in the presence of organic materials, including blood. Chlorhexidine's activity is pH dependent, so it is capable of being neutralized by hard tap water, chemicals containing nonionic surfactants,

inorganic anions, and organic anions such as natural soaps. For these reasons chlorhexidine is sold in a detergent—as a 4 percent concentration or as a 2 percent liquid or foam. To combine the rapid action of alcohols with the persistent action of chlorhexidine gluconate, it is also sold as an alcohol-based hand rinse.[51,89]

These considerations have resulted in specific recommendations from the Association of Practitioners of Infection Control. These recommendations have been modified from Larson by Laufman.[51] Two alternative methods are recommended and are quoted verbatim from Laufman,[51] with permission.

1. Alcohol preparation
   a. Wash hands and arms and clean fingernails; dry.
   b. Apply alcohol solution containing emollient, rubbing until dry. Use approximately 3 to 5 ml per application; continue applications for approximately 5 minutes, using a total of 9 to 25 ml.
2. Traditional 5-minute scrub with an agent containing chlorhexidine or an iodophor.

Preparation of the surgeon's hands is only part of the problem. The patient's skin must also be rendered as bacteria free as possible. The same assortment of antiseptics are used for patients as for surgeons. Obviously, prior to the application of antiseptics, the patient's skin should be clean. Walter[97] and Cruse[19] demonstrated that infection rates were higher if an operative area were shaved many hours prior to surgery. Indeed, if feasible it is preferred that areas not be shaved at all; depilatories are preferred. If shaving is done, it should be done immediately prior to surgery. An electric razor is preferred. In studies quoted by Cruse,[18,19] the clean wound infection rate was 2.3 percent in patients shaved with a sharp razor, 1.4 percent in those shaved with an electric razor, and 0.9 percent in those with no form of hair removal. Seropian and Reynolds[84] reported a clean wound infection rate of 5.6 percent in patients shaved with a razor and 0.6 percent in those in whom a depilatory was used. It is presumed that bacteria grow in razor nicks.[37]

There are other important aspects of good aseptic technique. Proper draping should be employed. Operating suites should be properly designed architecturally, easy to clean, and have no dust-retaining niches. Clean nonrecirculated air should be available. Finally, all persons in the operating suite—surgeons, anesthesiologists, nursing personnel, messengers, orderlies, and even student observers—should maintain strict aseptic discipline at all times.

ANTIMICROBIAL PROPHYLAXIS

Background

Since the advent of anesthesia, the major impediment to progress in surgery has been postoperative infection. In general, surgical wound infection accounts for about 24 percent of all nosocomial infections encountered in the United States.[36] With the discovery of antimicrobial agents, there was a great interest in the use of those drugs to prevent infections in surgical patients.

In 1939, Jensen et al.[43] published a report on the use of topical sulfanilamide in open fractures. This resulted in a decrease in the incidence of postoperative infections from 27 percent to less than 5 percent, using historical controls. Meleney et al.,[61] in 1945, reported a massive nine institutional cooperative study on topical plus systemic sulfonamide to prevent infection in civilians with traumatic injuries. The results were negative. Indeed, the controls fared better than the treated patients.

These studies, as well as others performed early in the antibiotic era, concentrated on patients who had dirty wounds as the result of trauma or who had contaminated wounds. (The classification of surgical wounds is discussed in more detail later in this chapter.) Today, most students of infectious disease would term such usage of antimicrobials as *early treatment,* not *prophylaxis.* The remainder of this discussion concentrates on true prophylactic treatment: the use of antimicrobials to prevent the uncommon occurrence of infection in patients with clean or clean-contaminated wounds. With the exception of patients undergoing procedures for trauma or established infection, neurosurgical procedures are clean or clean-contaminated.

Early studies in animals showed that the period of time for prophylactic efficacy is brief.[12] Delaying administration of antibiotics for 3 to 4 hours after subcutaneous inoculation of bacteria in guinea pigs resulted in lesions identical in size to those of controls. On the other hand, giving antibiotics at, or shortly before, inoculation of the bacteria resulted in remarkable diminution in the sizes of the lesions. This has resulted in the principle that prophylactic antibiotics must be given before, during, and after the operation. Antibiotic prophylaxis has become routine for a large variety of surgical procedures.[46] The situation in neurosurgery is a little more murky, but, on balance, as reviewed by Haines[35] and discussed below, prophylactic antibiotics in neurosurgery are now accepted as valuable by most authorities. However, much re-

mains to be learned about optimal drugs, proper dosage levels from the point of view of efficacy and cost, and optimal duration of treatment.

There are general principles of antibiotic prophylaxis that arise out of many experimental and clinical studies[39,40]:

1. The risk of infection and/or its consequences must outweigh the adverse effects of therapy, not only on the patient receiving the therapy but also on other patients who may subsequently need treatment for infections due to resistant organisms shed into the environment as a result of widespread use of prophylaxis.
2. The antibiotic chosen must be effective against the most probable infecting organisms, and the dosing intervals should be chosen consonant with the pharmacokinetic profile of the agent so that effective levels will be present in the tissues at risk just before, during, and after the procedure.
3. The antibiotic must be present at a concentration sufficient to kill potential pathogens at the time the bacterial contamination occurs.
4. Prolonged antibiotic prophylaxis is no more effective than a short course and may result in bacterial or fungal superinfection.
5. If possible, antibiotics commonly used to treat established infections should not be used for prophylaxis, because their use as prophylactic agents may contribute to the emergence of resistant bacteria in the hospital.
6. Antibiotic prophylaxis is not a substitute for good aseptic and surgical techniques.

The Ideal Prophylactic Antibiotic

From the above considerations a profile of the ideal drug for neurosurgical prophylaxis emerges. The drug should be nontoxic and nonallergenic. It should have a relatively long half-life. It should attain levels in the skin, subcutaneous tissues, muscle, bone, dura, cerebrospinal fluid (CSF), and central nervous system tissue that are bactericidal for all likely contaminants. The antibiotic should not alter the patient's normal microflora or predispose to superinfection. There should be no selection of resistant mutants of potential pathogens to be carried by the patient and subsequently disseminated to the animate and inanimate environment. The drug should be so inexpensive that its widespread use as a prophylactic agent would have no impact on the cost of care. The cost-saving for the prevention of the rare infection should clearly outweigh the costs of administering the drug universally. Keep in mind that an infection rate of only 3.6 to 11.7 percent is expected in neurosurgery patients without any prophylaxis.[35] Thus prophylaxis with a drug 100 percent efficacious would be given to 88 to 96 patients to prevent 4 to 12 infections. Unfortunately, at this time no such "prophylaximycin" exists. All regimens have at least one disadvantage.

Microbiological Considerations

Dempsey et al.[22] reviewed seven published studies and tabulated the predominant causes of infection in postoperative neurosurgical infections. Gram-positive organisms predominated, with *Staphylococcus aureus* causing 49 percent of the infections and *Staphylococcus epidermidis* being isolated from 28 percent. Collectively, only 8 percent of the infections were solely due to gram-negative organisms. The remaining patients had problems due to mixtures of organisms, including anaerobes. One of the problems that might be anticipated from these data is that prophylaxis might predispose to gram-negative infections. To date, it appears that short perioperative courses of prophylactic antibiotics have not resulted in shifts toward gram-negative flora in neurosurgical wounds.[17]

Pharmacokinetic Considerations

Contamination occurring during surgery is usually low grade. As stated above, the organisms most commonly originate from the skin of the patient, although they occasionally come from the surgical team or from the environment. Antibiotics should be in the potentially contaminated tissues at the time the wound is made, remain at good levels in the tissue during surgery, and discontinued after the procedure. The regimens detailed below are commonly recommended for prophylaxis in neurosurgical procedures and have been designed with these principles in mind. They are taken from Conte.[17]

A combination of vancomycin and gentamicin is the most commonly used regimen.[17] Doses of 1.0 g of vancomycin and 80 mg of gentamicin IV are given just prior to surgery. For procedures lasting more than 6 hours doses are repeated. Clindamycin, 300 mg IV immediately preoperatively, repeated every 4 hours during surgery, is another common regimen. A third regimen is cefazolin, 1.0 g and gentamicin 80 mg IV just prior to surgery and repeated at 6 hours.

Prophylaxis in shunting procedures is often used, but its precise utility is controversial.[17] Recommended regimens for institutions with high infection rates are trimethoprim-sulfamethoxazole 160/800 mg every 12 hours for a total of four doses of oxacillin 200 mg/kg/day in six divided doses for 1 day.

Published Studies of Antimicrobial Prophylaxis in Neurosurgery

The efficacy of prophylactic antibiotics in neurosurgical procedures has been an area of controversy for many years. Despite the large number of published articles, very few controlled clinical trials have been done. The results of these trials have been difficult to interpret because of both the use of different antibiotic regimens among the trials and the relatively low infection rates that have been seen in the control groups. In addition, different types of neurosurgical procedures may have different rates of infection and thus require different approaches to prophylaxis.

A convenient way of classifying surgical wounds is to use the system proposed by the National Academy of Sciences–National Research Council, which defines four groups of wounds: clean, clean-contaminated, contaminated, and dirty.[67] The use of antibiotics in dirty wounds is in fact treatment rather than prophylaxis, and the same argument can be made for the use of antibiotics in patients with contaminated wounds. For neurosurgical procedures it is additionally helpful to distinguish between clean procedures and clean cases with the implantation of a foreign body.

Clean Neurosurgical Procedures

When a review of the literature regarding clean neurosurgical procedures was published in 1980,[34] no completed prospective controlled clinical trials had been reported. In 1989, Haines[35] reviewed the literature that had been published between 1980 and 1989. A number of uncontrolled series were reported during that decade, reaching contradictory conclusions on the efficacy of prophylactic antibiotics. Five controlled studies were covered in the review article and three more have been published since that time. One of these was a retrospective study,[63] and seven were prospective randomized controlled studies. Interpretation of the results of two of these studies is clouded because of a lack of statistical power[32] or because of the use of an unusual statistical design.[86] The remaining five studies[8,11,25,95,102] all showed a benefit from the use of prophylactic antibiotics. Table 8-1 shows a comparison of the results of these trials.

The results of these controlled trials support the evidence from many uncontrolled series suggesting that antibiotic prophylaxis in clean neurosurgical procedures lowers the infection rate. The choice of which antibiotic to use for prophylaxis is a more difficult question, and, because of the low postsurgical infection rate, it is unlikely that the question of which

Table 8-1. Infection Rates in Controlled Trials of Prophylactic Antibiotics

Investigators	Infection Rate (%)		Relative Risk
	With Prophylaxis	Without Prophylaxis	
Mollman and Haines[63]	NG	NG	5.6
Geraghty and Feely[32]	0.5	3.6	7.4
Shapiro et al.[85]	2.8	11.7	4.1
Young and Lawner[102]	1.0	3.8	3.9
Blomstedt and Kytta[8]	1.8	7.4	4.1
Bullock et al.[11]	2.1	5.9	2.8
van Ek et al.[95]	3.3	10.3	NG
Djindjian et al.[24]	0.6	4.9	NG

Abbreviations: NG, not given.
(Adapted from Haines,[35] with permission.)

antibiotic regimen is preferable can be effectively addressed in a randomized clinical trial. The studies mentioned above have used different antibiotic regimens for prophylaxis. The most studied one is the Malis regimen,[59] consisting of intramuscular gentamicin or tobramycin, intravenous vancomycin, and topical streptomycin. Other regimens have included clindamycin,[79] cefazolin and gentamicin,[102] single-dose vancomycin,[8] lincomycin,[80] piperacillin,[11] cloxacillin,[95] and oxacillin.[24] None of these regimens has been demonstrated to be superior to the others, and the choice of prophylactic regimen should be individualized to the patterns of infection and types of resistance of the organisms encountered at each individual institution.

Clean Procedures With Implantation of a Foreign Body

The implantation of intracranial devices is associated with a greatly increased risk of infection and of morbidity associated with the infection. The two circumstances in which large foreign bodies are implanted during cranial surgery are CSF shunts and cranioplasty plates.

CSF shunts have reported infection rates of 2 to 39 percent.[1,30,62,82] Although a number of the trials mentioned above for clean neurosurgical procedures included some patients with shunt placement, these patients were not analyzed separately. Shunt placement is generally associated with a much higher risk of infection than other clean procedures. Several studies have now shown that prophylactic antibiotics are

effective in lowering the infections rates in shunt placement patients. These studies have used preoperative trimethoprim-sulfamethoxazole[7,99,81] or oxacillin.[25]

It would seem logical that antibiotic prophylaxis would be of value in cranioplasty. Unfortunately no randomized clinical trials have been done to look at this question. However, prophylactic antibiotics have enjoyed wide clinical use in cranioplasties.

Clean-Contaminated Surgeries

Clean-contaminated wounds are "operative wounds in which the bronchus, gastro-intestinal tract or oral-pharyngeal cavity was entered, but without unusual contamination."[67] Certain neurosurgical procedures fall into this category, either because the paranasal sinuses or mastoid air cells are entered (such as low frontal craniotomy or retromastoid craniotomy) or because the oral cavity is entered (such as a transoral approach to the clivus). There has been divided opinion on the use of prophylactic antibiotics in these surgeries, since no controlled clinical trials are available to assess their efficacy.

The paranasal sinuses have long been considered sterile sites in patients without sinus infection. However, Brook[10] found anaerobes present in noninflamed maxillary sinus aspirates of 12 of 12 adults studied, as well as streptococci, *Streptococcus pneumoniae, Hemophilus parainfluenzae,* and *S. aureus* in some patients. Although there have been no controlled clinical trials to evaluate the use of prophylactic antibiotics in clean-contaminated neurosurgical procedures, studies found in the older otolaryngological literature do not support the use of prophylactic antibiotics in such surgeries. However, given the fact that recent studies have shown that antibiotic prophylaxis is efficacious in preventing postoperative infections in clean neurosurgical procedures, it would seem logical that the same would be true for clean-contaminated surgeries. Since no one regimen has been shown to be superior to any other, the choice again can be individualized to the institution.

NEUROSURGICAL INFECTIOUS PROBLEMS AND THEIR MANAGEMENT

Infections of Intracranial and Intravascular Devices

Over the last 40 years a number of different types of shunt devices have been used in the surgical treatment of hydrocephalus. During the same period a wide variety of infection rates with shunts has been reported,[47] ranging from 2 to 40 percent, with a gradual decline in incidence over the past 15 years. There has been no difference in infection rates between ventriculoatrial (VA) and ventriculoperitoneal (VP) shunts,[48] but lumbar-peritoneal (LP) shunt infection rates have been reported to be significantly lower[83] than the others.

There are four major routes of infection that have been described in the pathogenesis of shunt infections. The major one is introduction of organisms during the perioperative period. This is suggested by the clustering of shunt infections in the 2 months following surgery and the fact that the majority of organisms isolated from infected shunts are commensal skin organisms. Another pathogenic mechanism is direct extension from infected tissues adjacent to the shunt or from the breakdown of the surgical wound overlying the hardware. A third mechanism is the retrograde infection of externalized devices or the introduction of infection during diagnostic or therapeutic entries into the CSF via the device. A final mechanism, suggested by Shapiro et al.[86] is hematogenous seeding of VA shunts by transient bacteremias and ascending infection of the shunt.

The diagnosis of a shunt infection can be difficult because of the lack of reliable clinical signs and symptoms. Frank meningitis or ventriculitis is frequently not present. The most common symptoms are those resulting from the shunt malfunction that is caused by the infection: headache, nausea, lethargy, and alteration in mental status. Meningeal symptoms are not expected, since there is usually an absence of communication between the ventricles and the meninges either because of the original reason for shunting or secondary to aqueductal stenosis acquired after shunting.[28] Meningeal signs are three times more common in LP shunt infections than in VP shunt infections.[98]

Systemic signs and symptoms are often present and can be clues to the presence of a shunt infection. Fever is frequently but not uniformly present. Bacteremia is generally present in patients with VA shunt infections but is usually absent in those with VP shunt infections. Infections of VP shunts can lead to inflammation of the absorbing peritoneal tissues, resulting in a failure to absorb the shunted CSF with resultant fluid build-up and symptoms of peritonitis.[72] One well-recognized but uncommon complication of shunt infection is hypocomplementemic glomerulonephritis.[90]

Diagnosis thus cannot be made reliably on clinical criteria alone. Definitive diagnosis requires culturing of the shunt or of the fluid in and around it. Sampling the lumbar CSF in patients with ventricular shunts may not reflect the presence of infection in the ventricular fluid, as mentioned above. Cultures are usually positive in shunt infections, even in the absence of pleocytosis or changes in the chemistries.[66]

Considerations of Treatment of Infected Devices

Prescribing an antibiotic therapy for shunt infections depends on the most likely causative organisms. Infections caused by staphylococcal species account for more than two-thirds of all shunt infections.[47] Coagulase-negative staphylococci (such as *S. epidermidis*) are the most common species, followed by *S. aureus*. The next most common organisms are the gram-negative enteric bacteria (6 to 20 percent), while *Pseudomonas* species are relatively infrequent. In addition, patients with shunts appear to have an increased risk of infection from the bacteria that commonly cause meningitis in the general population,[88] such as *H. influenzae, Streptococcus pneumoniae,* and *Neisseria meningitidis*. In recent years there has been an increase in the reported number of shunt infections caused by diphtheroids.[86] This reported increase may not represent a true change in the incidence of diphtheroid infection, but rather the use of better culture techniques, as well as the widening understanding that diphtheroids are a true clinical entity not a mere cultural contaminant as earlier thought.

Treatment of an infected shunt includes removal of the shunt, antibiotic therapy with external drainage of CSF and replacement of a new shunt at a different anatomical location after a period of days or weeks. Early attempts to treat shunt infections were made using IV antibiotics alone and resulted in a very low success rate of 24 percent, with a high mortality rate among those who failed therapy.[48] Subsequent efforts to improve outcome utilized IV and intrathecal antibiotics, raising the success rate to 40 percent,[31] but patients required prolonged hospitalization for antibiotic administration. Immediate shunt replacement combined with IV antibiotics resulted in a treatment success rate of 75 percent.[98] The current therapy with IV antibiotics, immediate shunt removal, and placement of external ventriculostomy has resulted in successful treatment in greater than 90 percent of the cases.

All components of the infected shunt need to be removed because of both the likelihood that the entire shunt is contaminated and the ability of many organisms to adhere to prostheses and thus survive antibiotic therapy. The placement of an external shunt as part of the therapy results in quicker clearance of the ventriculitis.[42] Appropriate antibiotic therapy, based on the identified organism or on a consideration of the most likely etiological agents, should be continued for 10 days,[47] followed by a 3-day observation period off antibiotics to verify that the infection has been eradicated and not merely suppressed. Following this the patient can be reshunted. Intrathecal antibiotics are not usually necessary in the treatment of shunt infections.

Postsurgical Meningitis

Although the incidence of postsurgical bacterial meningitis is relatively low, it remains a major problem because of the serious morbidity and mortality associated with the diagnosis and because of the difficulty in differentiating bacterial meningitis from the far more common chemical meningitis that occurs postoperatively. The rate of postoperative bacterial meningitis varies by the type of surgery (clean or clean-contaminated). The literature reports rates of 0.5 to 0.7 percent in clean procedures[79,94] and 0.4 to 2.0 percent in clean-contaminated surgeries.[6,101] As discussed in the section on antimicrobial prophylaxis, the use of perioperative antibiotics has been shown to lower the rate of infection.

Postsurgical bacterial meningitis can result from colonization at the time of surgery, wound or skin breakdown, or hematogenous seeding. The most common source is colonization occurring at the time of surgery. Surgery usually occurs through the scalp, which is highly colonized with bacteria, or through the frontal, sphenoid, or mastoid air sinuses, which can be colonized in normal hosts.[10] Another access point for bacteria is through the wound in the dura, the closure of which is nearly always incomplete.

The type of organism causing postsurgical meningitis is dependent in part on the type of surgery performed. Overall, staphylococcal species are the most common. In procedures that enter the air sinuses, bacteria that are part of the respiratory flora need to be considered.

Symptoms of meningitis usually begin several days after the operation. Symptoms include fever, meningismus, nausea, vomiting, and occasionally altered mental states. Unfortunately, the diagnosis of postsurgical meningitis can be confounded by the more common syndrome of aseptic or chemical meningitis that develops after surgery. In one report up to 70 percent of children undergoing posterior fossa surgery developed chemical meningitis. The etiology is thought to be chemical irritation from the breakdown of blood introduced into the subarachnoid space during surgery, or from factors released by the dural substitutes.[13]

The differential diagnosis between bacterial and chemical postoperative meningitis can be difficult, and definitive diagnosis of bacterial meningitis requires isolation of an infectious agent from the CSF. The results of CSF analysis can be confusing, since postoperatively the CSF cell count and protein are almost always elevated and the glucose may be depressed. The Gram stain may be negative in up to 70 percent of cases of culture-positive postsurgical meningitis.[75]

Because of the difficulty in making the diagnosis of bacterial meningitis in postoperative patients and since serious morbidity and mortality can result from a delay in therapy, the recommended approach is to begin broad spectrum antibiotic therapy in all postoperative patients who have onset of symptoms suggestive of bacterial meningitis. CSF should be obtained for cultures before antibiotic therapy is started. If the CSF culture remains negative and the CSF cell count and chemistries do not suggest infection as a cause of the symptoms, then the antibiotics can be stopped and corticosteroids begun for presumed chemical meningitis.

Cranial Osteomyelitis

Cranial osteomyelitis is a relatively rare infection that is usually a complication of craniotomy or cranioplasty. Other causes include contamination of an open skull wound and extension from infection in contiguous sites, such as with otitis media or chronic sinusitis. In a series of 165 cases with compound depressed skull fractures, Braakman[9] found that 45 percent of patients developed cranial osteomyelitis. Hematogenous seeding has been reported but appears to be a very unusual cause of cranial osteomyelitis.

Symptoms of cranial osteomyelitis are usually local: pain, swelling, and tenderness. Systemic signs such as fever are infrequent and usually suggest underlying pus, such as a subdural empyema. Laboratory values such as the white blood count and erythrocyte sedimentation rate are frequently normal and thus offer no diagnostic assistance. Although the infection may be indolent, it often will result in spread into intracranial structures. Diagnosis can often be made on the basis of abnormalities on the skull roentgenograms, but these are usually negative early in the infection. Bone scans are very sensitive, but previous surgery or trauma may result in increased uptake without infection being present. Culture of purulent drainage from the wound may not reflect the actual causative organisms.

Effective therapy requires excision of the involved bone or removal of the alloplastic plate, with drainage of the area. Antibiotic therapy is an important adjunct to surgical therapy, protecting against spread of the infection, but it is ineffective without surgical excision of involved necrotic bone. Antibiotics should be directed against the causative organisms that are identified by intraoperative cultures. *S. aureus* is by far the most common organism, but, in cases associated with otitis and sinusitis, gram-negative organisms can also be involved.

Brain Abscess

A brain abscess can arise by any of four different mechanisms: (1) contiguous spread from a suppurative focus, (2) spread following cranial surgery or trauma with a break in the dura, (3) hematogenous spread, or (4) cryptogenic abscess with no primary source of infection found. The most common mechanism is contiguous spread from otitis media or frontal sinusitis via a direct extension from osteomyelitis or retrograde spread through the diploic or emissary veins. Hematogenous spread is often associated with chronic lung infection or bacterial endocarditis.

The etiological agents found in brain abscesses correlate with the primary source of infection. With otitis media and sinusitis the usual isolates are streptococci, *Bacteroides* species, and the Enterobacteriaceae, usually in mixed cultures. Abscesses following head trauma are often caused by *S. aureus*, streptococci, mixed cultures of Enterobacteriaceae, and *Clostridium* species.

The clinical course of a brain abscess can range from indolent to fulminant. Only a minority of patients will have the classical triad of fever, headache, and focal neurological findings. The most common symptom is a moderate to severe headache. Alteration in mental status, ranging from lethargy to coma, occurs in most patients. Fever only occurs in approximately one-half of the patients.[77] Focal deficits also occur in approximately one-half of the patients, with hemiparesis being the most common finding. Nausea, vomiting, seizures, and nuchal rigidity can be present, and other focal symptoms depend on the location of the abscess. In patients who have had recent trauma or cranial surgery, these symptoms and signs may be difficult to distinguish from those caused by underlying lesions.

The cornerstone of diagnosis is a CT scan of the head, which has a 95 to 99 percent sensitivity.[68] Unfortunately its specificity is not nearly that good, as other lesions such as neoplasms, cerebral infarctions, and resolving hematomas can present with similar CT scan findings. Results of the CSF studies are non-specific, with pleocytosis and increased protein occurring in over one-half of the cases. CSF sampling by a lumbar puncture is contraindicated because of the danger of herniation.

Therapy for brain abscesses requires a combination of medical and surgical management. Although there have been reports of early brain abscesses cured by medical therapy alone,[74] most patients require surgery for optimal therapy. In patients who are neurologically stable and whose CT scans show cerebritis, antibiotic therapy alone can be attempted.[73] Aspiration should be performed if the patient is stable and the abscess is accessible to make a specific bacteriologic diagnosis. If the lesion appears on the CT scan to be encapsulated, then aspiration should be performed.

The ideal type and timing of surgery remain controversial, with no prospective, controlled studies having been done to compare regimens. The two standard approaches are aspiration of the abscess through a burr hole and craniotomy with complete excision of the abscess. Current practice favors more conservative therapy with aspiration. Aspiration done with stereotactic CT guidance is a promising technique that appears to be effective and to have a low associated morbidity rate.

Antibiotic regimens that are commonly recommended are empirical, with no controlled clinical trials to evaluate the different regimens. Antibiotic therapy is directed against the most likely pathogenic organisms, depending on the identified primary site of infection. In neurosurgical patients with cranial trauma or following cranial surgery the most common organisms are *S. aureus*, Enterobacteriaceae, and *Clostridium* species, as mentioned above. The recommended therapeutic regimen would include an antistaphylococcal penicillin (such as oxacillin or nafcillin), a third-generation cephalosporin (cefotaxime, ceftriaxone, or ceftizoxime), and high-dose penicillin. For patients with sinusitis or chronic lung infections in which *Bacteroides* species may be present, metronidazole should be added. Aspirates of the abscess should be cultured for both aerobes and anaerobes; the results may help direct antibiotic therapy. Parenteral antibiotic therapy is usually continued for 4 to 6 weeks, often followed by prolonged oral therapy.

Subdural Empyema

LeBeau[53] has called the subdural empyema "the most imperative of all neurosurgical emergencies." Infection in the subdural space usually results in a rapidly spreading infection that can lead to herniation and death without immediate intervention.

In most cases of subdural empyema, the source is infection in the paranasal sinuses, middle ear, or mastoid air cells. Other sources include extension from cranial osteomyelitis (as discussed above), cranial trauma, surgical procedures, or infection of a subdural hematoma. Post and Modesty,[71] in a review of cases of subdural empyema in the literature, found that approximately 5 percent of the cases were related to intracranial surgery. Polymicrobial infections are commonly associated with sinusitis or otitis, usually with anaerobes present. Other organisms such as aerobic streptococci, *S. pneumoniae, H. influenzae,* gram-negative bacilli, and staphylococci can be recovered. In postsurgical infections *S. aureus* and facultative gram-negative bacilli are common.

Subdural empyema is usually a rapidly progressive infection. Initial symptoms include fever, focal headache, vomiting, and signs of meningeal irritation, although meningitis occurs in only 14 percent of cases. The infection spreads rapidly through the subdural space, resulting in the development of focal neurological signs such as hemiparesis, focal seizures, and aphasia. Without therapy progressive increase in intracranial pressure occurs, with resulting herniation. With subdural empyemas that occur postcraniotomy the development of symptoms may, in contrast to the usual presentation, be insidious and subacute.[71]

The diagnosis of subdural empyema should be considered in any patient with meningeal signs and focal neurological deficits. In patients with head trauma or who have just undergone surgery, the symptoms may be masked by their underlying disorders. Laboratory studies are often nonspecific. CSF changes are usually not helpful as purulent meningitis is rare and lumbar CSF sampling is contraindicated because of the danger of herniation. Magnetic resonance imaging (MRI) is the diagnostic procedure of choice,[64] as it gives better detail than CT scans. MRIs can detect empyemas that are not shown on CT scans.

Because of the rapidly progressive nature of the infection emergency craniotomy is indicated for drainage of empyema fluid. The fluid (as well as blood) should be sent for aerobic and anaerobic cultures. Intravenous antibiotic therapy should be directed toward the most likely causative organisms. In empyemas in which the paranasal sinuses or middle ears are the source of infection, an antistaphylococcal penicillin such as oxacillin or nafcillin should be used together with metronidazole. For subdural empyemas following cranial surgery, an antistaphylococcal penicillin should be used with a third-generation cephalosporin such as cefotaxime, ceftriaxone or ceftizoxime. Antibiotic therapy should be continued for at least 3 weeks.

Meningitis After Head Trauma

There is a significant incidence of acute bacterial meningitis following head trauma, with a reported incidence ranging from 0.2 to 17.8 percent. Although infection can occur following any degree of head trauma, the risk of infection is greatly increased when a CSF leak is present.[93] Infection can obviously occur by direct inoculation of organisms during a penetrating trauma or in a closed fracture adjacent to an infected air sinus. The development of a fistula with CSF leakage can also provide a point of entry for bacteria to the central nervous system.

The signs and symptoms of bacterial meningitis following head trauma are similar to those of acute bacterial meningitis due to other causes. However, symptoms such as headache, stiff neck, nausea, vomiting, confusion, and seizures may be difficult to interpret in the setting of acute head trauma, as they can be secondary to the underlying injury. A change in the physical or neurological examination should suggest the development of central nervous system infection.

A careful search must be undertaken for evidence of a CSF leak. Rhinorrhea and otorrhea are often difficult to detect acutely in trauma patients. Radiographic studies can suggest the presence of a basilar fracture with CSF leakage, but basilar fractures can be very difficult to detect. If a CSF leak is suspected, metrizamide cisternography with high-resolution CT scanning is the best test for defining the site of the leakage.

The differential diagnosis is often difficult because the underlying injury may preclude CSF sampling and because interruption of normal CSF flow is not uncommon in patients following trauma. Lumbar CSF samples may not accurately reflect changes in the ventricles or even in the basilar cistern. Similarly, a normal CSF sample taken from a ventriculostomy does not rule out the diagnosis of meningitis. Interpretation of the CSF results can also be difficult. CSF pleocytosis, hypoglycorrhachia, and increased CSF protein can be secondary to trauma with a subdural hematoma or to craniotomy as well as to acute bacterial meningitis. Latex agglutination or counterimmunoelectrophoresis (CIE) tests on the fluid may be helpful if positive for an organism, but are inconclusive if they are negative.

In patients with basilar skull fractures, the majority of cases of acute bacterial meningitis are due to *S.*

pneumoniae. Other bacterial causes include organisms that are resident flora of the upper respiratory tract, such as *H. influenzae, N. meningitidis*, and β-hemolytic group A streptococci. Staphylococci and gram-negative bacilli are rare causes of meningitis after basilar skull fractures, but are more common in patients who have had penetrating or open cranial wounds or who have been hospitalized for extended periods of time.

Since posttraumatic meningitis occurring in the early period after a basilar skull fracture is almost always secondary to *S. pneumoniae*, empiric therapy with high-dose penicillin (20 to 24 million units IV per day) is appropriate. If infection due to *H. influenzae* is suspected a third-generation cephalosporin such as cefotaxime, ceftriaxone, or ceftizoxime should be used instead. For patients with penetrating cranial wounds or who have had prolonged hospitalization therapy is needed for staphylococci and gram-negative bacteria. The combination of vancomycin and ceftazidime would be a reasonable choice in this situation. Whatever the initial antibiotic regimen chosen, it should be modified to more specific therapy when the results of the cultures become available.

EVALUATION OF POSTOPERATIVE FEVER

The neurosurgical patient is subject to numerous causes of postoperative fever—some of infectious origin and some of noninfectious origin. These conditions include atelectasis and pneumonia, "sterile" inflammatory responses, subgaleal collections of fluid, hematomas, urinary tract infections, wound infections, postsurgical meningitis, infection of an implanted foreign body such as a shunt or a monitoring device, thrombophlebitis, infected intravascular catheters, parotitis, and drugs. Fever of infectious or noninfectious cause can also be related to blood transfusions. These conditions are summarized in Table 8-2.

Causes of Fever by Time of Onset

In textbooks,[87] postoperative fever evaluation is traditionally discussed in terms of the time elapsed since surgery. The traditional wisdom[87] states that certain conditions should be sought by the surgeon or the consultant depending on the duration of the postoperative period prior to the onset of fever. It is important to remember that these time frame guidelines are only approximate and that complications may appear ahead of schedule or behind schedule.

During the first 24 hours postoperatively, the most likely causes of fever are atelectasis, aspiration, or a response to the surgery itself. From 24 to 72 hours, new fever is most likely related to atelectasis, bacterial pneumonia, or thrombophlebitis.

Possible causes become more numerous once the patient reaches 72 hours. They include pneumonia, pulmonary embolism, thrombophlebitis, intravenous catheter associated sepsis, surgical wound sepsis, urinary tract sepsis, and meningitis. Some of these conditions are discussed in more detail below. It is important to remember that the above comments about time frames are only approximate and that the cause of fever in a given patient may be off schedule. For this reason, Talbot and Gluckman,[91] in their discussion of the evaluation of the febrile postoperative surgical patient, advise the consultant that "since overdependence on such schemata may potentially lead to misdiagnosis, it is preferable to approach each patient individually. . . ." Each patient should be treated as though the febrile episode is due to a specific infectious or other treatable cause, and every effort should be made to arrive at a diagnosis. Optimal therapy is as specific as possible. Even empiric therapeutic trials should be made in such a way as to test a specific diagnostic theory. *Antibiotics should not be used as antipyretics.*

Table 8-2. Fever in Neurosurgical Patients

	Infectious Causes	Noninfectious Causes
Neurosurgically related	Posttraumatic meningitis (after open head trauma)	Central fever
	Postoperative meningitis (after clean surgery)	Meningismus (posterior fossa syndrome)
	Shunt infections	
	Wound infections	
Not neurosurgically related	Nosocomial and aspiration pneumonias	Drug fever
	IV line sepsis	Transfusion reactions
	Urosepsis	Atelectasis
	Hepatitis	Phlebitis
	Parotitis	Pulmonary embolus

Wound Infections

Wound infections usually become manifest at least 48 hours after surgery. They are generally caused by *S. aureus* or other skin flora such as *Staph. epidermidis*. Occasionally, *Strep. epidermidis* is involved. (The former organism is often carried in the nares or on the skin of the patient or persons in the operating suite; the latter is ordinarily a respiratory organism and may come from the patient's own flora or a nosocomial source.) Occasionally, wound infections may be caused by gram-negative aerobes such as *Escherichia coli* or *Pseudomonas aeruginosa*. These gram-negative organisms are especially apt to be present if the patient has had open head trauma. Wound infections are readily observable and diagnosable, and specimens for gram-stain and culture are easily obtained. An infected wound ordinarily shows the classical signs of dolor, rubor, and calor. One exception to this rule is the wound that is infected with a toxigenic strain of *S. aureus*. Toxigenic staphylococci may produce enough toxin to cause systemic illness with all or some of the manifestations of toxic shock syndrome before there has been enough local replication of the organisms for the clinician to realize that the wound is infected.

As implied above, local wound infections are usually easily diagnosed specifically. Antibiotic treatment should be tailored to the Gram stain and isolate. Because most infections are due to gram-positive cocci, a first-generation cephalosporin such as cefazolin is the usual initial therapy.

Meningismus

Some early febrile responses may be due to a sterile inflammatory reaction to blood spilled in the subarachnoid space.[2] Often, this response is mild and occurs during the first postoperative day as a rise in temperature of only 1° to 1.5°C. The patient will have mild stiff neck and pain in the operative site. Mild pain in the lumbar area and in the lower extremities may also be seen. More severe reactions generally occur later. The exposure of large areas of the central nervous system with manipulation or significant removal of tissue with subsequent areas of necrosis can produce similar reactions.[13,41] The temperature may rise as high as 41°C with local pain in the wound and signs of meningeal irritation. These reactions were first reported in children after the removal of cerebellar tumors and were termed *posterior fossa syndrome*.[13] It is now appreciated that such signs and symptoms may occur following any procedure that leaves blood in the subarachnoid space.[21]

At first glance, the patients may resemble those with postoperative bacterial meningitis. However, the inflammation usually does not appear as toxic. It should be emphasized that the diagnosis of this sterile meningitis is a diagnosis of exclusion. All patients with these symptoms should be evaluated for bacterial meningitis and sepsis. This evaluation should include a careful history and physical examination, complete blood count, cultures of blood and urine, other laboratory tests as indicated, and lumbar puncture.

The lumbar puncture in these patients is typically grossly bloody. The early inflammatory response to the blood and necrotic tissue is predominantly polymorphonuclear, but after a few days converts to a mononuclear predominance. The glucose is usually normal, but values in the low normal range (about 25 mg/dl) are occasionally encountered. Protein concentrations are quite variable and may range from 120 to 1,000 mg/dl. Sterile meningeal reactions usually run their courses within 3 weeks. They resolve without sequelae.

Ideally, the management of patients with meningismus is expectant. If the patient is not toxic and the fever and systemic signs and symptoms are mild, antibiotics may be withheld and the patient observed carefully. Often, even the experienced clinician will have difficulty in differentiating meningismus from bacterial meningitis. This difficulty is exacerbated if the patient has undergone a procedure that required the insertion of a foreign body or if the patient has an underlying condition or therapeutic program that confers immunosuppression. In case of doubt, it is better to err on the side of overtreatment. That is, start appropriate treatment for nosocomial meningitis, observe the patient carefully with repeated physical examinations and lumbar punctures, and truncate the antibiotic therapy if the clinical course seems incompatible with bacterial infection and CSF cultures are negative. The details of the antibiotic treatment of postoperative meningitis are given elsewhere in this chapter.

Atelectasis

Atelectasis is the most common complication of anesthesia. Some degree of atelectasis exists in as many as 70 percent of individuals who have received a general anesthetic.[2,70] Atelectasis is the collapse of one or more segments of the lung. It occurs when hypoventilation, inspissation of secretions, and absorption of alveolar gas causes loss of expanded volume. Neurological deficits and aspiration are also contributory causes. Normally, the unevenness of breathing in the waking state, with periodic sighing, helps to prevent this condition. Small areas of subsegmental atelectasis can occur without symptoms or signs. Larger atelectatic areas result in fever, tachypnea, and tachycardia. The PaO_2 is decreased, even in mild cases, but the $PaCO_2$ is usually normal except in severe cases when hyperventilation supervenes. In most cases, fever, tachypnea, and a few rales are the only physical signs. Diagnosis is made on the basis of a clinical suspicion that prompts a chest roentgenogram. In severe cases, with considerable areas of involvement, tracheal deviation, decreased chest expansion, flatness to percussion, and decreased breath sounds may also be present. Humidification of inspired air, encouragement of coughing and deep breathing, chest percussion, and suctioning are all preventive and therapeutic. Mobilization of respiratory secretions and the maintenance of clear airways are of the utmost importance. Dehydration, promoting the inspissation of secretions, is to be avoided. Intermittent positive pressure breathing and incentive spirometry are often used in an effort to promote alveolar expansion postoperatively. The precise utility of these modalities in the prevention and therapy of atelectasis remains controversial.

Nosocomial Pneumonia

Conditions that promote atelectasis also predispose to acquisition of pneumonia. Intubation, ventilator treatment, and prior antibiotic therapy are also risk factors. Neurosurgical patients are especially prone to macro- or microaspiration. Macroaspiration may involve the inhalation of enough particulate matter to occlude a bronchus. Irritation due to the foreign body may cause a chemical pneumonitis that becomes secondarily infected by organisms from the mouth and pharynx that entered the lung with the aspirate.

Microaspiration is a more frequent cause of aspiration pneumonia in the neurosurgical patient. Indeed, the degree of aspiration is often so small that it is not clinically evident. The usual diagnostic terminology used for postoperative pneumonia in the hospital is *nosocomial pneumonia*. Hospital epidemiologists classify a pneumonia as nosocomial if it has onset more than 48 hours after hospital admission. In a recent review,[60] the incidence was estimated at 0.6 percent of hospital admissions.

Pneumonias are caused by microbes residing in the mouth and/or oropharynx. In nonnosocomial aspiration pneumonia, anaerobic gram-negative rods, anaerobic cocci, and aerobic or microaerophilic gram-positive cocci are the most important etiologies. In patients hospitalized for more than 48 hours, gram-negative aerobic bacilli and *S. aureus* assume major roles, with the gram-negative aerobes having the most important role.

Classic studies by Johansen et al.[45] and Sanford[78] shed some light on the reason for this gram-negative aerobic predominance. These investigators documented that hospitalization predisposes to pharyngeal colonization with aerobic gram-negative bacilli. Among normal subjects, the frequency of carriage of gram-negative bacilli was 6 percent; in psychiatric patients it was 6 percent; in moderately ill patients it was 35 percent; and among patients judged to be moribund in the intensive care unit it was 73 percent. These hospital acquired gram-negative bacilli are thus available as etiologic agents if patients micro- or macroaspirate. In two recent series, reviewed by Maunder,[60] gram-negative aerobes caused 54.9 percent of the pneumonias in one and 73.2 percent of the cases in the other. Many of these pneumonias are caused by hard to treat species such as *P. aeruginosa* and *Acinetobacter* sp. Recent studies have also estimated that as much as 50 percent of the pneumonias occurring in intensive care units may be polymicrobial.[26,44]

Respiratory secretions or aspirations from nasotracheal tubes may yield potential pathogens that are colonizers and not invaders of the respiratory tissue. To minimize errors in interpretation of sputum cultures, the most serious consideration should be given to results from specimens whose gram stains, when examined at ×100 magnification, show more than 25 polymorphonuclear leukocytes and fewer than 10 epithelial cells per field.[65,78]

Blood cultures of pathogens obtained from patients with pneumonia yield highly significant results. Therefore, blood cultures should always be done. Unfortunately, they are usually negative, being positive in only 2 to 6 percent of patients with nosocomial pneumonia.[60]

One frequent therapy used in neurosurgical patients in intensive care units may predispose to nosocomial pneumonia. Stomach colonization with gram-negative aerobes has been associated with an increased risk of nosocomial pneumonia.[26,44,60] The use of H_2 blockers and/or antacids to prevent stress ulcers promotes this stomach colonization. Some reports have indicated that stress ulcers can be prevented by sucralfate. Since sucralfate does not destroy the gastric acid, which acts as a barrier to stomach colonization, the subsequent frequency of gram-negative pneumonia seems to be decreased compared with patients who have received antacids or H$_2$ blockers.[23,26,60]

Therapy of aspiration pneumonia should be directed at the most likely organisms. Obviously, if satisfactory laboratory specimens have established an etiology, those organisms should be targeted.

In community acquired aspiration pneumonia, therapy should be directed at the gram-negative anaerobes from the mouth and oropharynx as well as the gram-positive anaerobes and microaerophilic and aerobic streptococci. Acceptable regimens include intravenous ampicillin or penicillin G plus metronidazole or intravenous clindamycin. If the patient has recently been hospitalized, or has received a recent course of antibiotics, consider adding an aminoglycoside such as gentamicin or amikacin.

For the patient with nosocomial pneumonia, therapy is directed at hard to treat gram-negative aerobes such as *P. aeruginosa, Acinetobacter* sp., and so forth. The initial gram stain of the sputum should be carefully examined to verify that the predominant organism is a gram-negative rod. An acceptable regimen is a third-generation cephalosporin such as cefotaxime plus an aminoglycoside like gentamicin or amikacin. If *P. aeruginosa* is an important pathogen in the unit of institution caring for the patient, ceftazadime is the cephalosporin of choice. *S. aureus* should be treated with oxacillin or nafcillin if methicillin resistance is not documented or suspected. For methicillin-resistant strains, vancomycin is the drug of choice.

Sepsis Secondary to Intravascular Lines

Neurosurgical patients are often at risk for line sepsis. Lines for prolonged parenteral support and/or monitoring are often required. Infection is especially likely if lines are left in place for too long. Peripheral intravenous lines should be changed at least every 72 hours.[21] Arterial lines should not be left in place for more than 4 days, and central lines should be removed after a maximum of 7 days.[21]

Line sepsis is not always associated with obvious signs of phlebitis along the course of the involved catheter. The diagnosis is made by careful examination to exclude other causes coupled with proper cultures. Simultaneous blood cultures should be obtained through the suspected catheter and from an unaffected contralateral extremity. The suspected catheter should be removed and the tip cultured semiquantitatively by the technique of Maki and col-

leagues.[57,58] The diagnosis is confirmed if the culture tip yields a colony count of 15 or more of the same organism isolated from the contralateral unaffected extremity.[57,58] The most frequent pathogens encountered are *S. aureus* and coagulase-negative staphylococci. However, a variety of gram-negative aerobes and *Corynebacteria*, especially K strains, may also be encountered.[38] Patients on hyperalimentation are especially prone to sepsis caused by *Candida* sp.[38]

The single most important therapeutic maneuver is the removal of the offending intravascular device. As stated above, staphylococci are the most important pathogens. Coagulase-negative strains, which are often methicillin resistant, are frequently encountered. Therefore the usual empiric therapy is vancomycin. The least toxic, most effective drug on the basis of susceptibility tests should be chosen when laboratory results are available.

Urinary Tract Infection

Neurosurgical patients frequently have indwelling urinary catheters because they are unable to void or because close monitoring of urinary output is desired. Even with adherence to aseptic closed system drainage techniques the catheters and the urinary bladders become colonized with a variety of organisms over a period of time. After 2 weeks of indwelling catheterization, virtually all patients are bacteriuric.[20] Most episodes of short-term catheter-associated bacteriuria are asymptomatic, but a review by Warren[100] found that 10 to 30 percent of patients with catheter-associated bacteriuria develop fevers or other symptoms of urinary tract infection. About 1 to 5 percent develop clinical bacteremia.[100]

For short-term catheterization (<30 days), the most common infecting organisms are *E. coli, Klebsiella pneumoniae, Proteus mirabilis,* and *P. aeruginosa.*[100] Among patients catheterized for more than 30 days the flora colonizing the bladder tends to shift. *Providencia stuartii, Pseudomonas* sp. *E. coli, P. aeruginosa, Enterococcus* sp., and *Morganella morganii* are the most common.[100]

The diagnosis of urinary tract origin of fever is made on the basis of clinical findings plus laboratory data. There should be no other obvious cause of the fever. Bacteriuria and even pyuria may be local phenomena without systemic consequences. Finding casts on microscopic examination of the urine is diagnostic of upper tract involvement and supports, but does not prove, that fever and symptoms are due to urinary tract infection.

Evaluation for possible urinary tract infection should include a history and physical examination, a complete blood count, a urinalysis, and a quantitative urine culture. A Gram stain of the unspun urine is a good, quick screening test for significant bacteriuria ($>10^5$ colonies per milliliter of clean voided midstream urine). Finding one or more gram-negative rods per oil immersion field correlates very well with such colony counts.[16]

A third-generation cephalosporin such as cefotaxime is excellent therapy for urinary tract infections associated with a short duration of catheterization if the patient is not severely septically ill. If the patient is severely septic, therapy should be broader and should include agents effective against *P. aeruginosa*, *P. stuartii*, *Enterococcus* sp., and *M. morganii*. For those patients a combination of a ureido penicillin such as piperacillin and an aminoglycoside such as amikacin should be started empirically. Treatment should be changed to the most effective, least toxic drug after cultures and susceptibilities are reported.

Drug Fever

Neurosurgical patients received a large variety of drugs, many of which are capable of causing fever.[21] Drug fever should be considered after other infectious and noninfectious causes have been ruled out. Patients typically look better than their temperature curves. They are usually not toxic. The height and pattern of the temperature elevation is so variable that it is of no diagnostic assistance. Drug fever may be associated with a rash, so careful attention to the skin is warranted if this diagnosis is being considered. Likewise, mild eosinophilia and mild elevations of liver function tests may be present. If drug fever is suspected, all nonessential drugs should be discontinued. Essential medications should be changed to drugs of different chemical structure if at all possible. Elimination of the offending drug will usually result in cessation of the fever within 72 hours. For the neurosurgical patient, antiseizure medications, particularly barbiturates and phenytoin, are frequent offenders.

Central Fever

After all other infectious and noninfectious causes of fever are ruled out, fever of central origin should be considered. It is a diagnosis of elimination. Any pathology that affects the base of the brain or hypothalamus can result in temperature elevations.[21] The temperature regulatory center is located in the preoptic nucleus of the anterior hypothalamus. Any mass lesion, trauma, or circulatory disorder that impinges on this structure may result in fever. Typically, the fever is unrelenting and plateau-like. It is unaffected by antipyretics or antibiotics. There may, or may not, be a relative bradycardia. The absence of perspiration in such patients may be a valuable clinical clue. Central fevers may persist for days or weeks.

HIV-RELATED ISSUES

Acquired immunodeficiency syndrome (AIDS) was first described in 1981.[33] It soon became apparent that the virus could be transmitted by blood and blood factors. It was postulated that the disease was caused by an infectious agent, presumably a virus, that could be transmitted in a manner analogous to hepatitis B, that is, by the transferral of infected bodily fluids by activities such as sexual intercourse or by parenteral contact with infected blood and blood products as in therapeutic administration of such materials or by the sharing of contaminated needles by abusers of intravenous drugs. By 1983, the causative virus was discovered and named—the *lymphadenopathy-associated virus* (LAV) by one group[4] and the *human T-cell lymphotrophic virus III* (HTLV-III) by another.[29] This virus is now called the *human immunodeficiency virus type 1* (HIV-1). As expected, the virus was shown to persist indefinitely in the blood and other tissues of infected persons.

Surgeons are exposed to blood during the course of performing operations, not only from spurting vessels but also from blood soaking through gowns and other clothing. More importantly, during the course of surgical procedures, surgeons employ sharp instruments, sharp solid and hollow needles, and even wire and other materials that have the potential to become contaminated with blood from the patient, puncture rubber gloves and the surgeon's skin and inoculate infectious material if the patient is infected with HIV or other blood-borne agents. Obviously, these facts raise at least the theoretical possibility that HIV might be transmitted from an infected patient to a surgeon or to another member of the operative team during the course of a procedure. This clear possibility of hazard has caused anxiety among surgeons. During the remainder of this section we will examine the data regarding this risk and comment on protective measures.

HIV-infected individuals also may have the virus resident in the central nervous system tissue.[40,54] The theoretical hazard of this fact to the neurosurgeon is obvious. To date the U.S. Public Service regards 27 health care workers as having been infected with HIV in the course of their professional activities.[5,27]

None of these persons has been a neurosurgeon. The largest single group has been nursing personnel infected with deep needle sticks with contaminated hollow needles.[5,27] The current best estimate of hazard to medical personnel from deep needle sticks with hollow needles or other significant blood to blood exposure is 0.3 percent, or about 1/330 such exposures.[5]

If a significant exposure to blood or to possibly contaminated fluids occurs, each hospital should have procedures in place to record and handle the incident. The Centers for Disease Control (CDC) has recently issued specific guidelines for the management of occupational exposures to HIV.[14] Immediately following an exposure to blood and body fluids, whether the patient is known to be HIV positive or not, contaminated areas should be washed with soap and water and thoroughly rinsed. Ethanol kills HIV in vitro, so an ethanol rinse can also be used, although there are no clinical data that prove that it is efficacious. Conjunctival exposure should prompt flushing of that area with saline. If a deep needle stick or cut occurs, force blood from the wound and irrigate as above. Do not employ invasive procedures or debridement.

The exposure should be reported to the proper authority in that hospital. Details about the exposure should be recorded. The patient who was the source of the exposure should be asked for permission to test his blood for HIV antibodies. Hepatitis B serology should be done as well.

The injured person should be counseled and reassured that the risk of seroconversion is very low. HIV serology should be done immediately and at 6 weeks, 3 months, 6 months, and 12 months after the exposure. The injured person should employ barrier contraception during the period of evaluation.[14]

Zidovudine, an agent currently licensed for the treatment of HIV infection, has been advocated for prophylaxis by some. It has been shown to delay, but not to prevent, the onset of infection in animals with HIV or similar viruses.[76,92] However, the challenge doses have been high. Certainly, zidovudine prophylaxis does not always work. Three people thus treated have seroconverted.[14,49,56]

Finally, there is the question of whether HIV-infected health care workers performing invasive procedures might transmit the virus to their patients. There has been a recent report of a dentist with HIV infection who was the presumed source of secondary cases in three patients in his practice.[15] It is not clear whether the transmission occurred directly during procedures or whether it might have resulted from improperly cleaned contaminated instruments. The viruses from the dentist and the three patients showed a high degree of relatedness. Retrospective studies of 753 patients from the practices of three infected surgeons have failed to show any instances of transmission.[15] The experience with the dentist mentioned above remains the sole instance of possible transmission of HIV from a health care worker to a patient in 10 years of observation of the HIV epidemic.[15]

At present there are no recommendations for universal HIV testing of health care workers who perform invasive procedures, although such testing has been considered. Some have recommended that all health care workers performing invasive procedures be voluntarily tested and inform their patients of the results of those tests. Formal guidelines and even legal restrictions are likely to be enacted in the future. A *New York Times* article published April 5, 1991, discusses a draft of new federal guidelines being considered by the CDC. In that draft, it is recommended that physicians and dentists should obtain permission from local panels of experts if they continue to perform certain operations and invasive procedures.[3]

REFERENCES

1. Ajir F, Levin AB, Duff TA: Effect of prophylactic methicillin on cerebrospinal fluid shunt infections in children. Neurosurgery 9:6, 1981
2. Allen MB, Johnston KW: Preoperative evaluation: complications, their prevention and treatment. p. 8330. In Youmans JR (ed): Neurological Surgery. 3rd Ed. WB Saunders, Philadelphia, 1990
3. Altman LK: U.S. drafts guidelines on doctors with AIDS. New York Times, April 11, 1991
4. Barre-Sinoussi F, Chermann J-C, Rey F et al: Isolation of a T-lymphotropic retrovirus from a patient at risk for acquired immunodeficiency syndrome (AIDS). Science 220:868, 1983
5. Beekmann SE, Fahey BJ, Gerberding JL, Henderson DK: Risky business: using necessarily imprecise casualty counts to estimate occupational risks for HIV-1 infection. Infect Control Hosp Epidemiol 11:371, 1990
6. Black PM, Zervas NT, Candia GL: Incidence and management of complications of transsphenoidal operation for pituitary adenomas. Neurosurgery 20:920, 1987
7. Blomstedt GC: Results of trimethoprim-sulfamethoxazole prophylaxis in ventriculostomy and shunting procedures: a double-blind randomized trial. J Neurosurg 62:694, 1985
8. Blomstedt GC, Kytta J: Results of a randomized trial of vancomycin prophylaxis in craniotomy. J Neurosurg 69:216, 1988

9. Braakman R: Depressed skull fracture: data, treatment, and follow-up in 225 consecutive cases. J Neurol Neurosurg Psychiatry 35:395, 1972

10. Brook I: Aerobic and anaerobic bacterial flora of normal maxillary sinuses. Laryngoscope 91:372, 1981

11. Bullock R, van Dellen JR, Ketelbey W, Reinach SG: A double-blind placebo-controlled trial of perioperative prophylactic antibiotics for elective neurosurgery. J Neurosurg 69:687, 1988

12. Burke JF: The effective period of preventive antibiotic action in experimental incisions and dermal lesions. Surg 50:161, 1961

13. Carmel PW, Fraser RA, Stein BM: Aseptic meningitis following posterior fossa surgery in children. J Neurosurg 41:44, 1974

14. CDC: Public Health Service statement on management of occupational exposures to human immunodeficiency virus, including considerations regarding zidovudine post-exposure use. MMWR 39(RR1):1, 1990

15. CDC: Update: Transmission of HIV infection during an invasive dental procedure—Florida. JAMA 265:563, 1991

16. Cobbs CG: Presumptive tests for urinary tract infections. p. 43. In Kaye D (ed): Urinary Tract Infection and Its Management. CV Mosby, St. Louis, 1972

17. Conte JE Jr: Antibiotic prophylaxis in non-abdominal surgery. Curr Clin Top Infect Dis 10:254, 1989

18. Cruse P: Surgical infection: incisional wounds. p. 423. In Bennett JV, Brachman PS (eds): Hospital Infections. 2nd Ed. Boston, Little Brown, 1986

19. Cruse PJ: Wound infections: epidemiology and clinical characteristics. p. 429. In Simmons RL, Howard RJ (eds): Surgical Infectious Diseases. Appleton-Century-Crofts, East Norwalk, CT, 1982

20. Cunha BA, Beltran MD, Gobbo PN: Implications of fever in the intensive care setting. Heart Lung 13:460, 1984.

21. Cunha BA, Tu RP: Fever in the neurosurgical patient. Heart Lung 17:608, 1988

22. Dempsy R, Rapp RP, Young B et al: Prophylactic parenteral antibiotics in clean neurosurgical procedures: a review. J Neurosurg 69:52, 1988

23. Dirks MR, Craven DE, Celli DR et al: Nosocomial pneumonia in intubated patients given sulcrafate as compared to antacids or histamine type 2 blockers. The role of gastric colonization. N Engl J Med 317:1376, 1982

24. Djindjian M, Fevier MJ, Otterbein G et al: Oxacillin prophylaxis in cerebrospinal fluid shunt procedures: results of a randomized open study in 60 hydrocephalic patients. Surg Neurol 25:178, 1986

25. Djindjian M, Lepresle E, Homs JB: Antibiotic prophylaxis during prolonged clean neurosurgery: results of a randomized double-blind study using oxacillin. J Neurosurg 73:383, 1990

26. Fagon JY, Chastre J, Domart J et al: Nosocomial pneumonia in patients receiving continuous mechanical ventilation. Am Rev Respir Dis 139:877, 1989

27. Flexner C: Management of occupational exposures to HIV: an update. AIDS Med Rep 4:13, 1991

28. Foltz EL, Shurtleff DB: Conversion of communicating hydrocephalus to stenosis or occlusion of the aqueduct during ventricular shunt. J Neurosurg 24:520, 1965

29. Gallo RC, Salahuddin SZ, Popovic M et al: Frequent detection and isolation of cytopathic retroviruses (HTLV-III) from patients with AIDS and at risk for AIDS. Science 224:500, 1984

30. Gardner BP, Gordon DS: Postoperative infection in shunts for hydrocephalus: are prophylactic antibiotics necessary? Br Med J 284:1914, 1982

31. Gardner P, Leipzig T, Phillips P: Infections of central nervous system shunts: symposium on infections of the central nervous system. Med Clin North Am 69:297, 1985

32. Geraghty J, Feely M: Antibiotic prophylaxis in neurosurgery. A randomized controlled trial. J Neurosurg 60:724, 1984

33. Gottlieb MS, Schiroff R, Schanker HM et al: *Pneumocystic carnii* pneumonia and mucosal candidiasis in previously healthy homosexual men: evidence of a new acquired cellular immunodeficiency. N Engl J Med 305:1425, 1981

34. Haines SJ: Systemic antibiotic prophylaxis in neurological surgery. Neurosurgery 6:355, 1980

35. Haines SJ: Efficacy of antibiotic prophylaxis in clean neurosurgical operations. Neurosurgery 24:401, 1989

36. Haley RW, Culver DH, White JW et al: The nationwide nosocomial infection rate: a new need for vital statistics. Am J Epidemiol 129:159, 1985

37. Hamilton HW, Hamilton KR, Lone FJ: Preoperative hair removal. Can J Surg 20;269, 1977

38. Henderson DW: Bacteremia due to percutaneous intravascular devices. p. 2189. In Mandell GL, Douglas RG, Bennett JE (eds): Principles and Practice of Infectious Diseases. 3rd Ed. Churchill Livingstone, New York, 1990

39. Heseltine PNR, Leedom JM: Prophylactic antibiotics. p. 250. In: Maronde RF (ed): Topics in Clinical Pharmacology and Therapeutics. Springer-Verlag, New York, 1985

40. Hollander H, Levy JA: Neurologic abnormalities and recovery of human immunodeficiency virus from cerebrospinal fluid. Ann Intern Med 106:692, 1987

41. Horwitz NH, Ruzzoli HV: Postoperative Complications in Neurosurgical Practice. Williams & Wilkins, Baltimore, 1982

42. James HE, Walsh JW, Wilson HD et al: Prospective randomized study of therapy in cerebrospinal fluid shunt infection. Neurosurgery 7:459, 1980

43. Jensen NK, Johnsrud LW, Nelson MC: Local implantation of sulfanilamide in compound fractures. Surgery 6: 1, 1939

44. Jiminez P, Tores A, Rodriguez-Rosen R et al: Incidence and etiology of pneumonia acquired during mechanical ventilation. Crit Care Med 17:882, 1989

45. Johanson WG, Pierce AK, Sanford JP: Changing pha-

ryngeal flora of hospitalized patients. Emergence of gram-negative bacilli. N Engl J Med 281:1137, 1969

46. Kaiser AB: Postoperative infections and antimicrobial prophylaxis. p. 2245. In: Mandell GL, Douglas RG, Bennett JE (eds): Principles and Practice of Infectious Diseases. 3rd Ed. Churchill Livingstone, New York, 1990

47. Kaufman BA, Tunkel AR, Pryor JC, Dacey RG: Meningitis in the neurosurgical patient. Infect Dis Clin North Am 4:677, 1990

48. Keucher TR, Mealey J: Long term results after ventriculoatrial and ventriculoperitoneal shunting for infantile hydrocephalus. J Neurosurg 50:179, 1979

49. Lange MMA, Boucher CAB, Hollack CEM et al: Failure of zidovudine prophylaxis after accidental exposure to HIV-1. N Engl J Med 322:1375, 1990

50. Laufman H: Carl Walter's half century of achievement in asepsis. Am J Surg 148:565, 1984

51. Laufman H: Current use of skin and wound cleansers and antiseptics. Am J Surg 157:359, 1989

52. Laufman H: What's happened to aseptic discipline in the OR? Todays OR Nurse 12:15, 1990

53. LeBeau J, Creissard P, Harispe L et al: Surgical treatment of brain abscess and subdural empyema. J Neurosurg 38:198, 1973

54. Levy RM, Bredesen DE, Rosenblum ML: Neurological manifestations of the acquired immunodeficiency syndrome (AIDS): experience of UCSF and review of the literature. J Neurosurg 62:75, 1985

55. Lister J: On the aseptic principle in the practice of surgery. Lancet 1:741, 1867

56. Locke DFM, Grove DI: Failed prophylactic zidovudine after needlestick injury. Lancet 1:1280, 1990

57. Maki DG, Jarrett F, Saraffin HW: A semiquantitative method for identification of catheter-related infection in the burn patient. J Surg Res 22:513, 1977

58. Maki DG, Weise CE, Sarafin HW: A semi-quantitative method for identifying intravenous-catheter-related sepsis. N Engl J Med 296:1305, 1977

59. Malis LI: Prevention of neurosurgical infection by extraoperative antibiotics. Neurosurgery 5:339, 1979

60. Maunder R: Recognition and treatment of pneumonia in the intensive care patient. Infect Med 7(S):18, 1990

61. Meleney FL: A statistical analysis of a study of the prevention of infection in soft part wounds, compound fractures, and burns with special reference to the sulfonamides. Surg Gynecol Obstet 80:263, 1945

62. Merrill RE, McCutchen T, Meacham WF, et al: Myelomeningocele and hydrocephalus. JAMA 191:115, 1965

63. Mollman HD, Haines SJ: Risk factors for neurosurgical wound infection. A case control study. J Neurosurg 64:902, 1986

64. Mosely IF, Kendall BE: Radiology of intracranial empyemas, with special reference to computed tomography. Neuroradiology 26:333, 1984

65. Murray PR, Washington JA: Microbiologic and bacteriologic analysis of expectorated sputum. Mayo Clin Proc 50:339, 1975

66. Myers MG, Schoembaum SC: Shunt field aspiration. Am J Dis Child 129:220, 1975

67. National Academy of Sciences—National Research Council: Postoperative wound infections: the influence of ultraviolet irradiation of the operating room and of various other factors. Ann Surg 160(Suppl):22, 1964

68. New PFJ, Davis KR, Ballantive HT Jr: Computed tomography in cerebral abscess. Radiology 121:641, 1976

69. New York Academy of Medicine Working Group: The risk of contracting HIV infection during the course of health care. JAMA 265:1872, 1991

70. Owens GR: Postoperative pulmonary problems. p. 378. In Goldman DR, Brown FH, Levy WK et al: Medical Care of the Surgical Patient: a Problem-Oriented Approach to Management. JB Lippincott, Philadelphia, 1982

71. Post EM, Modesty LM: "Subacute" postoperative subdural empyema. J Neurosurg 55:761, 1981

72. Reynolds M, Sherman JO, McLone DG: Ventriculoperitoneal shunt infection masquerading as an acute surgical abdomen. J Pediatr Surg 18:951, 1983

73. Rosenblum ML, Hoff JT, Norman D et al: Nonoperative treatment of brain abscesses in selected high-risk patients. J Neurosurg 52:217, 1980

74. Rosenblum ML, Mampalam TJ, Pons VG: Controversies in the management of brain abscesses. Clin Neurosurg 33:603, 1986

75. Ross D, Rosegay H, Pons V: Differentiation of aseptic and bacterial meningitis in postoperative neurosurgical patients. J Neurosurg 69:669, 1988

76. Ruprecht RM, O'Brien LG, Rossoni LD, Nussinoff-Lehrman S: Suppression of mouse viraemia and retroviral disease by 3'-azido-3'-deoxythymidine. Nature 323:467, 1986

77. Samson DS, Clark K: A current review of brain abscess. Am J Med 54:201, 1973

78. Sanford JP: Lower respiratory infections. p. 285. In Bennett JV, Brachman PS (eds): Hospital Infections. 2nd Ed. Little Brown, Boston, 1986

79. Savitz MH, Malis LI: Prophylactic clindamycin for neurosurgical patients. NY State J Med 76:64, 1976

80. Savitz MH, Malis LI, Meyers BR: Prophylactic antibiotics in neurosurgery. Surg Neurol 2:95, 1974

81. Schmidt K, Gjerris F, Osgaard O, et al: Antibiotic prophylaxis in cerebrospinal fluid shunting: a prospective randomized trial in 152 hydrocephalic patients. Neurosurgery 17:1, 1985

82. Schoembaum SC, Gardner P, Shillito J: Infections of cerebrospinal fluid shunts: epidemiology, clinical manifestations, and therapy. J Infect Dis 131:543, 1975

83. Selman WR, Spetzler RF, Wilson CB et al: Percutaneous lumboperitoneal shunt: review of 130 cases. Neurosurgery 6:255, 1980

84. Seropian R, Reynolds BM: Wound infections after preoperative depilatory versus razor preparation. Am J Surg 121:251, 1971

85. Shapiro M, Wald U, Simchen E et al: Randomized clinical trial of intra-operative antimicrobial prophylaxis of infection after neurosurgical procedures. J Hosp Infect 8:283, 1986

86. Shapiro S, Boza J, Kleinman M et al: Origin of organisms infecting ventricular shunts. Neurosurgery 22:868, 1988

87. Sherman R, Ferguson CM, Lubin MF: Fever and infection. p. 453. In Lubin MF, Walker HK, Smith RB eds: Medical Management of the Surgical Patients. Batherworth Publishers, Stoneham, MA, 1988

88. Shurtleff DB, Chrisstie D, Flotz EL: Ventriculosauriculostomy-associated infection: a 12-year study. J Neurosurg 35:686, 1971

89. Smylie DG, Logie JRC, Smith G: From pHisoHex to Hibiscrub. Br Med J 4:586, 1973

90. Stickler GB, Shin MH, Burke EC et al: Diffuse glomerulonephritis associated with infected ventriculoatrial shunt. N Engl J Med 279:1077, 1968

91. Talbot GH, Gluckman SJ: Approach to the patient with postoperative fever. p. 482. In Goldman DR, Brown FH, Levy WK et al (eds): Medical Care of the Surgical Patient: A Problem-Oriented Approach to Management. JB Lippincott, Philadelphia, 1982

92. Taveres L, Ronecker C, Johnston K et al: 3'-Azido-3'-deoxythymidine in feline leukemia virus-infected cats: a model for therapy and prophylaxis of AIDS. Cancer Res 47:3190, 1987

93. Tenney JH: Bacterial infections of the central nervous system in neurosurgery. Neurol Clin 4:91, 1986

94. Tenney JH, Vlahov D, Salcman M et al: Wide variation in risk of wound infection following clean neurosurgery. J Neurosurg 62:243, 1985

95. van Ek B, Dijkmans B, van Dulken H et al: Antibiotic prophylaxis in craniotomy: a prospective double-blind controlled study. Scand J Infect Dis 20:630, 1988

96. Walter CW: Preoperative skin preparation. Hosp Top 1955

97. Walter CW: Disinfection of the skin [film]. Sponsored by American Medical Association, American Hospital Association, American College of Surgeons, American Nurses Association, and National League for Nursing, 1986

98. Walters BC, Hoffman HJ, Hendrick EB et al: Cerebrospinal fluid shunt infection: influences on initial management and subsequent outcome. J Neurosurg 60:1014, 1984

99. Wang EEL, Prober CG, Hendrick BE et al: Prophylactic sulfamethoxazole and trimethoprim in ventriculoperitoneal shunt surgery: a double-blind, randomized, placebo-controlled trial. JAMA 251:1174, 1984

100. Warren JW: Nosocomial urinary tract infections. p. 2205. In Mandell GL, Douglas RG, Bennett JE (eds): Principles and Practices of Infectious Diseases. 3rd ed. Churchill Livingstone, New York, 1990

101. Wilson CB, Dempsey LC: Transsphenoidal microsurgical removal of 250 pituitary adenomas. J Neurosurg 48:13, 1978

102. Young RF, Lawner PM: Perioperative antibiotic prophylaxis for the prevention of postoperative neurosurgical infections: a randomized clinical trial. J Neurosurg 66:701, 1987

9 Hematological Problems and Complications

Mark U. Rarick
Donald I. Feinstein

Hemostatic control in any surgical field is important, but, because of the confines of the rigid structure of the skull and the spinal skeleton, hemostatic control for the neurosurgeon is of utmost importance. Excessive bleeding either as the cause of the neurological emergency or perioperatively can result in devastating consequences for the patient. A basic understanding of the normal control of hemostasis and its perturbation can transform a potentially fatal complication into a satisfactory clinical outcome.

Hemostasis is controlled by three major factors. First, platelets circulating in an inactive state are essential for early hemostatic plug formation when the vascular integrity is interrupted. Plasma factors that also circulate in an inactive form are responsible for the conversion of fibrinogen to fibrin that acts as the cement that holds the platelets together. The third component of hemostasis is the vascular integrity itself. Once the vascular integrity is interrupted various factors, including the release of activators and exposure of collagen, initiate hemostatic plug formation and the activation of procoagulant proteins at the site of injury (Fig. 9-1).[22,31]

The majority of perioperative bleeding is secondary to vessel damage that is encountered pre- or postoperatively. However, it is still important to recognize the occasional preexisting bleeding tendency that may be either inherited or acquired. In this chapter the causes of bleeding in the neurological patient, both preexisting and perioperatively, are explored. With the availability of new factor concentrates, ease of obtaining platelet products, and inhibitors of fi-

brinolysis, most bleeding episodes can be controlled once an accurate diagnosis has been made (Table 9-1).

CLINICAL PRESENTATION

When possible, a rapid but thorough bleeding history should be obtained from the patients prior to neurological surgery. Inherited coagulation abnormalities can be distinguished from acquired disorders in relation to the duration and initial age of the bleeding problem. Patients with inheritable factor disorders, such as severe hemophilia A or B, will have a long history of bleeding, especially of the joints (hemarthoses) and muscles. Patients with inherited platelet disorders often will have mucosal bleeding, that is, epistaxis, gum bleeding, and menorrhagia. A history of surgical procedures or significant trauma in the past without significant bleeding, such as during wisdom teeth extraction and tonsillectomy, is strong evidence against the existence of an inherited bleeding disorder.

A drug history, especially of aspirin and other nonsteroidal anti-inflammatory agent use, is important, since they interfere with hemostatic plug formation and potentially can cause excessive intra- and postoperative bleeding. Antibiotics such as penicillins and cephalosporins can cause both platelet dysfunction and vitamin K deficiency, resulting in a bleeding tendency. Chronic liver disease resulting in decreased production of important coagulation factors

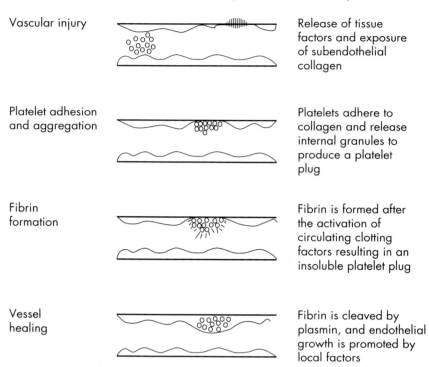

Vascular injury — Release of tissue factors and exposure of subendothelial collagen

Platelet adhesion and aggregation — Platelets adhere to collagen and release internal granules to produce a platelet plug

Fibrin formation — Fibrin is formed after the activation of circulating clotting factors resulting in an insoluble platelet plug

Vessel healing — Fibrin is cleaved by plasmin, and endothelial growth is promoted by local factors

Figure 9-1. Hemostasis control.

Table 9-1.   Blood Products for Clinical Use

Product	Indication	Hazards
Red blood cells		
Whole blood	Anemia with hypovolemia; massive trauma fresh blood may be used to avoid low 2,3-DGP in stored blood	Hemolytic transfusion reactions; volume overload, infection transmission (bacterial, viral, parasitic), citrate intoxication with massive transfusions, and (rarely) graft-vs-host disease
Packed red blood cells	Anemia, without hypovolemia	As above
Leukocyte-poor	Prevention of nonhemolytic febrile reactions; thrombocytopenic patients	As above, added cost
Leukocytes	Bacterial sepsis with severe neutropenia by antibiotics	High cost, short half life, hemolytic reactions, acute pulmonary insufficiency
Platelets	Thrombocytopenia with bleeding if caused by hypoproduction	Alloimmunization, graft-vs-host disease, infectious complications
Fresh frozen plasma	Coagulation factor (II, V, VII, IX, X, XI, XIII) deficiencies, massive blood transfusion, reversal of warfarin effect, thrombotic thrombocytopenic purpura	Hypervolemia, alloimmunization, infection transmission, noncardiogenic pulmonary edema
Cryoprecipitate	Factor VIII, fibrinogen deficiency; von Willebrand disease	Same as for fresh frozen plasma
Factor VIII and IX concentrates	Hemophilia A and B	Infection transmission, rare hemolysis; older factor IX concentrate can cause thrombosis
Albumin	Hypovolemia with hypotension, severe burns	Hypertension with rapid infusion
Immunoglobulin	Immune thrombocytopenia	Hypervolemia, fever, chest tightness, anaphylaxis in patients with IgA deficiency

Abbreviations: 2,3-DPG, 2,3-diphosphoglycerate.

and inhibitors of fibrinolytic proteins can result in excessive bleeding. Similarly, renal insufficiency can be the cause of prolonged bleeding in operative procedures.

The presence of a systemic hemostatic defect should be suspected when there is a previous history of abnormal bleeding; particularly after minor trauma or minor surgery such as wisdom tooth extraction or tonsillectomy. In addition, bleeding from multiple sites in a hospitalized patient should suggest a systemic defect. Thrombocytopenia and qualitative platelet disorders can result in petechiae, purpura, and ecchymoses. Mucosal bleeding can also be present. Hemarthoses and muscle hematomas often indicate plasma coagulation factor deficiencies. Delayed hemorrhage can be caused by disorders of the fibrinolytic system or factor XIII deficiency.

More complete coagulation studies should be obtained in particular cases. A bleeding time assesses qualitative platelet function in a patient with a normal platelet count. The protamine-sulfate test measures the presence of fibrin monomers after thrombin is generated and indicates the presence of disseminated intravascular coagulation (DIC).[9] Fibrin degradation products (FDP) and D-dimers are also elevated in cases of DIC. Fibrinogen levels can also be useful when one suspects DIC or accelerated fibrinolysis.

COAGULATION FACTOR DEFECTS

Inherited

Hemophilia A, or classic hemophilia, results when there is a decreased production of (and/or the production of a defective) factor VIII molecule.[6] Classically this is inherited as an X-linked genetic disorder. Patients may have mild, moderate, or severe deficiency, and the degree of bleeding will parallel the factor VIII level. Normal hemostasis occurs when the factor VIII level is greater than 30 percent of control level.

Neurosurgeons often become involved in the care of hemophiliacs because of traumatic or spontaneous intracranial hemorrhage. Children with hemophilia A can present with subarachnoid or intracerebral bleeds. Treatment can be quite successful, with aggressive factor replacement therapy keeping the factor VIII level near normal and neurosurgical intervention when needed.

The treatment of patients with mild hemophilia and minor bleeding problems can be easily controlled with desmopressin acetate (DDAVP) and antifibrinolytic agents such as ε-aminocaproic acid (AMI-

CAR).[8,23,37] Patients with moderate or severe hemophilia and significant bleeding will require specific factor VIII concentrates. If the patient has no evidence of chronic hepatitis or human immunodeficiency virus (HIV) infection, then highly purified factor VIII concentrates with low risk for transmission of these agents should be utilized. Patients with chronic hepatitis or HIV infection can be successfully treated with heat-treated factor VIII concentrates. Frequent factor VIII levels guide the amount of factor concentrates that are needed.

Hemophilia B (Christmas disease) results from decreased factor IX activity (patients present similar to those with classic hemophilia).[1,5] As with hemophilia A, factor replacement is important to control bleeding. The factor IX product available at this time may result in the paradoxical complication of thromboembolism because of the presence of activated factors in the concentrate. New products that have purified factor IX with very low levels of activated factors are currently undergoing clinical trials. Preliminary studies reveal the risk of thromboembolism to be much lower with these purified factor IX concentrates.

Deficiencies of factor XI may also result in a bleeding tendency but usually only after trauma or surgery.[36] Factor XI deficiency is particularly common in the Jewish population.

Acquired

Vitamin K deficiency may result in a bleeding tendency secondary to the decreased synthesis of vitamin K–dependent factors, which include factors II (prothrombin), VII, IX, and X.[10,32]

Vitamin K deficiency may be due to decreased intake, antibiotic use, malabsorption, or use of the anticoagulant warfarin. The most common cause of vitamin K deficiency in the neurosurgical patient is a lack of intake combined with the use of antibiotics. Since stores of vitamin K are limited, vitamin K deficiency may occur fairly rapidly, particularly in the postoperative period. A sensitive laboratory marker for vitamin K deficiency is a prolonged prothrombin time (PT). In the absence of concomitant liver disease, the response to intravenous vitamin K is rapid, with the PT shortening significantly within 4 to 12 hours.

Liver Disease

The liver is the site of synthesis of the great majority of the plasma clotting factors, including the vitamin K–dependent factors and factor V.[27] Therefore, significant liver dysfunction can be associated with a bleeding tendency. Coagulation laboratory abnormalities include a prolongation of both the PT and partial thromboplastin time (PTT).

Splenomegaly that occurs in patients with liver disease causing thrombocytopenia, a frequently associated qualitative platelet defect, and both coagulation and fibrinolytic defects place patients with liver disease at great risk for bleeding. Acute or chronic subdural hematomas can often be a difficult diagnostic dilemma in patients with alcoholic liver disease who fall and have lapses of memory of the traumatic event.

Treatment of patients with severe liver disease requiring surgery can be extremely complex and should be under the supervision of a hematologist. Patients who have significant ascites may not respond to fresh frozen plasma because of the large volume of distribution secondary to third spacing. When thrombocytopenia is present and requires platelet transfusions, platelet count increments (5,000 to 10,000/mm^3 for each platelet pack) may not occur due to sequestering of the platelets in the spleen. Patients with liver disease also may have increased fibrinolysis due to decreased hepatic synthesis of specific fibrinolytic inhibitors. Increased fibrinolytic activity should be suspected in a patient who has achieved immediate hemostasis but subsequently has bleeding from a surgical or venipuncture site. In these cases increased fibrinolytic activity can be detected by obtaining a dilute whole blood clot lysis time and/or a euglobulin clot lysis time (Fig. 9-2).

Disseminated Intravascular Coagulation

The coagulation cascade ultimately is dependent on the formation of thrombin from the inactive protein prothrombin. Once the thrombin is formed fibrinogen is cleaved to fibrin, with subsequent stabilization of fibrin polymers to obtain an insoluble clot. With normal hemostasis this reaction takes place on the vascular endothelium or platelet surface. However, if excessive thrombin is generated in the intravascular space, fibrin can form and lead to intravascular thrombosis.[9,24] The generation of excess thrombin is known as disseminated intravascular coagulation (DIC) and can result in extensive thrombosis and/or excessive bleeding due to consumption of hemostatic factors. DIC can be associated with a variety of disorders, including massive trauma, sepsis, thermal injury, disseminated neoplasm, and head injuries (including gunshot wounds). The brain has high levels of tissue thromboplastin, which can activate the extrinsic blood coagulation system (Fig. 9-3).

Laboratory abnormalities that commonly are found in patients with DIC include prolongation of both the PT and the PTT, the presence of fibrin monomers as demonstrated by a positive protamine-sulfate paracoagulation test, and the presence of fibrin degradation products (or D-dimers). In addition, thrombocytopenia is a consistent finding in DIC and is frequently associated with depressed fibrinogen levels.

The most important aspect of the treatment of DIC is to identify and treat the underlying cause if it is still present. For example, if the patient has a serious infection, then intravenous antibiotics should be given immediately; if the patient has an underlying malignancy, then the malignancy should be treated as clinically indicated as soon as possible. One of the most common problems in neurosurgery associated with DIC is gunshot wounds to the brain. In these cases, tissue thromboplastin is released from the injured brain and triggers intravascular coagulation. However, by the time the patient usually reaches the physician the thrombin generated has been neutralized and active DIC is no longer present. However, the patient frequently has low levels of hemostatic factors because of the previous consumption. Thus, if a patient is deemed salvageable and requires surgery for intracranial debridement or other types of

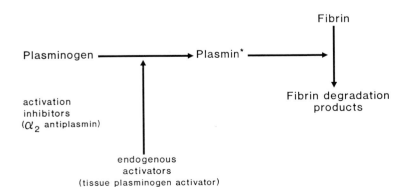

Figure 9-2. Fibrinolytic system. *, degree of activity measured by the dilute whole blood clot lysis time and euglobulin lysis time.

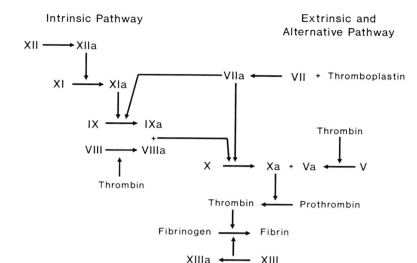

Figure 9-3. Coagulation cascade.

trauma, low fibrinogen levels should be corrected by the transfusion of cryoprecipitate (one bag usually will increase the fibrinogen level by 5 to 10 mg/dl, and the fibrinogen level should be at least 150 mg/dl prior to surgery), and thrombocytopenia should be corrected with platelet transfusions (one random-donor, nonapheresed platelet concentrate will raise the platelet count by 5,000 to 10,000/μl, and the platelet count should be 100,000/μl prior to surgery.

Coagulation Factor Inhibitors

Specific coagulation factor inhibitors are a rare but potentially serious cause of bleeding. The inhibitors usually are immunoglobulins of the IgG variety that either can arise after replacement therapy, as seen in patients with congenital factor deficiencies, or spontaneously.[12,16] Patients clinically present with bleeding either spontaneously or postoperatively. Depending on which factor is inhibited, the coagulation tests are markedly prolonged without correction by a mixture of normal plasma and the patient's plasma. Treatment can be difficult in these patients and includes massive specific factor replacement (in order to neutralize the offending antibody), immunosuppressive medications such as prednisone and cyclophosphamide, and plasmapheresis.

Heparin can also be the cause of an insidious acquired bleeding disorder, especially in hospitalized patients when heparin is used as an anticoagulant for indwelling vascular catheters to prevent thrombosis and for treatment of venous thrombosis. Therapy for heparin-induced bleeding involves stopping the heparin and, if rapid reversal is required, neutralizing the heparin with protamine sulfate.

PLATELET DISORDERS

Thrombocytopenia

Depressed platelet counts are seen in a variety of medical disorders. Specific therapy will depend on the etiology. Therefore, prior to any surgical procedure the precise etiology of the depressed platelet count is important to establish.

Immune thrombocytopenia may occur in various clinical settings, including HIV infection, lymphoproliferative disorders, and collagen vascular diseases. The most common form is not associated with any identifiable underlying disease (idiopathic). In patients with immune thrombocytopenia, especially that due to intracranial hemorrhage, the morbidity rate in this group of patients can be significant.[30] The standard treatment for these patients includes corticosteroids and, if there is no response, splenectomy. For the acute control of severe bleeding in patients with immune thrombocytopenia, intravenous IgG and platelet transfusions are frequently helpful.[15]

A multitude of drugs can cause thrombocytopenia via immune mechanisms (Table 9-2) or depression of production in the bone marrow. A careful drug history is important to obtain from every patient with thrombocytopenia. Heparin-induced thrombocytopenia can result in a rapid onset of thrombocytopenia associated with paradoxical thrombosis. The cause of the thrombosis is thought to be secondary to antibodies formed in the presence of heparin, resulting in spontaneous platelet aggregation.[20] The thrombosis may be venous and/or arterial. Treatment involves cessation of heparin therapy and the substitution of an oral anticoagulant to achieve anticoagulation.

Table 9-2. Drugs Causing Immune Thrombocytopenia

Analgesics	Anticonvulsants
Acetominophen	Valproic acid
Aspirin	Diphenylhydantoin
Antibiotics	Miscellaneous
Rifampin	Cimetidine
Penicillins	Chlorothiazide
Cephalosporins	Heparin
Sulfonamides	Gold salts
Cinchona alkaloids	Arsenical helminthics
Quinidine	
Quinine	

Infectious complications both pre- and perioperatively may also cause increased consumption of platelets and therefore thrombocytopenia. In addition, infection can trigger DIC and result in increased consumption of platelets and significant thrombocytopenia. Patients with massive injuries requiring prolonged operative procedures may have thrombocytopenia caused by increased consumption of the platelets at the operative site, along with massive infusion of blood products that contain few platelets.

Treatment of the thrombocytopenia must consider the underlying etiology. If the thrombocytopenia is caused by inadequate bone marrow production and platelet counts are less than 75,000/mm^3, increased perioperative bleeding may occur. With hypoproduction, platelet counts less than 20,000/mm^3 may result in an increased risk of spontaneous bleeding and when less than 5,000/mm^3 there is a high incidence of spontaneous intracranial bleeding. Random-donor platelets or a platelet pheresed product should be given to patients with surgery or trauma in order to keep the platelet count above 100,000/mm^3.

Qualitative Platelet Defects

Inherited qualitative defects of platelets are rare but treatable disorders that clinically manifest with a history of mucosal bleeding. Patients can have increased epistaxis and gum bleeding, and females often will have increased menorrhagia. Platelet counts usually are normal unless there is another underlying cause for thrombocytopenia. The most common qualitative platelet defect is Von Willebrand disease. These patients often will have a prolonged PTT and abnormal bleeding times. Because von Willebrand factor is involved in platelet adherence to vascular surfaces there is excessive bleeding tendency. Treatment of these patients usually can be easily controlled by the use of DDAVP or cryoprecipitate.[23,28]

Glanzmann thromboasthenia and the Bernard-Soulier syndrome are rare inheritable defects of

platelet receptors. These patients may undergo surgical procedures with the support of platelet concentrates.

Acquired qualitative platelet defects can occur in a variety of medical disorders. The most common is probably the ingestion of aspirin and other nonsteroidal anti-inflammatory agents, including indomethacin and ibuprofen.[38] A careful history must be obtained from patients, since many do not consider aspirin as a medication.

Patients with elevated gammaglobulin levels, especially in multiple myeloma and macroglobulinemia of Waldenström, may have platelet dysfunction secondary to platelet coating by the paraprotein.[19] Patients with a variety of myeloproliferative disorders may have a variety of qualitative defects. These defects may result in thrombosis and/or excessive bleeding, and often both may occur simultaneously.

The treatment for patients with acquired platelet qualitative defects depends on the underlying etiology. If an elective procedure is being performed on patients with a history of aspirin ingestion, postponement of the procedure until the bleeding time is normal is probably prudent. For the patient with qualitative defects secondary to an underlying medical disorder, platelet support with platelet concentrates is indicated. Lowering the offending paraprotein in patients with lymphoproliferative disorders will often result in an improvement in the bleeding time.

Patients with renal failure often have a prolonged bleeding time due to a poorly defined qualitative defect. This may result in excessive bleeding after surgery. If the bleeding time is prolonged and the patient needs an invasive intracranial or intraspinal procedure, the bleeding time can be corrected by a variety of therapeutic strategies, including the administration of high-dose estrogen for several days prior to surgery,[34] the administration of DDAVP 25 μg/kg 30 minutes prior to surgery, or by raising the hemoglobin level to approximately 10 to 12 g/dl by blood transfusion[11] or recombinant human erythropoietin (epoetin-alfa) administration.[26] On occasion the administration of cryoprecipitate may also be useful.[18]

ANEMIA

Preoperative Anemia

The evaluation of patients with anemia prior to the surgical procedure is important to assess the need for blood replacement to maximize oxygen-carrying capacity and also wound healing capabilities. Blood loss due to traumatic injury must be assessed and can present either in the gastrointestinal tract or be compartmentalized in the lung, abdomen, muscles, or even intracranially. Traumatic bleeding usually is obvious by the history and physical examination results.

Vitamin deficiencies, including those of iron, folate, and B_{12}, can cause anemia and need to be correctly diagnosed because the treatment can be simple and effective. Patients presenting with iron deficiency will often have microcytic red cells (MCV <80). Laboratory abnormalities in iron deficiency include depressed serum iron levels, along with a high total iron-binding capacity and low percent saturation of transferrin. Ferritin levels are low and reflect absent body stores of iron.[17] The cause of iron deficiency in adults is usually due to blood loss, and thus a source of chronic blood loss should always be sought in these patients. Megaloblastic anemias are usually caused by vitamin B_{12} or folate deficiency. The megaloblastic anemias can also cause leukopenia and thrombocytopenia. The latter occasionally may be so severe that the patient may have excessive bleeding.

Patients with hemolytic anemias, either acquired or congenital, will often have elevated indirect bilirubins levels, reticulocytosis, and elevated lactate dehydrogenase (LDH) levels. The precise cause of the hemolytic anemia is important to establish in order that treatment be given appropriately.

The anemia of chronic disease is common and is associated with a wide variety of disorders. It is often seen in patients with malignancy, collagen vascular disease, and both acute and chronic infections.[21] The patient's hemoglobin level is frequently about 10 g/dl, with a peripheral blood smear showing very few changes in the red blood morphology. Often the iron studies reflect a low serum iron level with low iron-binding capacity and mildly depressed percent saturation. In these patients ferritin levels are often normal or elevated.

Splenomegaly results in a redistribution of the cellular elements of blood into the enlarged splenic bed, resulting in varying degrees of pancytopenia. In these patients it is important to realize that transfusions of blood products will not raise the hemoglobin or platelets to the level expected.

Intra- or Postoperative Blood Loss

The most common cause of anemia in this patient group is from blood loss due to vascular injury. In the central nervous system postoperative bleeding can result in a rapid and dramatic decline in mental status. Patients with central nervous system bleeding also will often have wide fluctuation in blood pressure. When an acute anemia occurs, a computed tomography (CT) scan of the brain should be obtained. An aggressive approach to the patient should be undertaken to ascertain the cause of the bleeding (Table 9-3) in order to treat the anemia effectively.

Gastrointestinal blood loss secondary to gastritis and/or peptic ulcer disease is often seen in the patients with traumatic intracranial processes. Neurosurgical patients are frequently treated with corticosteroids in order to treat brain edema. Corticosteroids are frequently associated with the development of active ulceration or gastritis. This can occasionally be prevented by the use of carafate and the histamine antagonists (cimetidine, ranitidine, and famotidine).

Treatment

Patients with mild, stable anemia may not require therapy. More severe anemia, especially that which compromises cardiovascular function or oxygen-carrying capacity, needs immediate attention. The precise definition of anemia with respect to hemoglobin levels and/or hematocrit level varies widely. Transfusion of blood products to correct a laboratory value should be discouraged. Once one has established that treatment of the anemia is important there are many options. Whole blood or packed cells and colloid should be used if expansion of intravascular volume is indicated, for example, for the severely traumatized patient. Packed red blood cells are the treatment of choice for patients in whom volume expansion is not needed. Patients with identifiable vitamin deficiencies, such as of B_{12} or folate, can easily be managed with supplementation by the appropriate vitamin. Iron deficiency can be treated with oral supplementation or, if needed, intravenous iron.

The risk of transmittable infectious agents in the blood supply have been greatly reduced with the stringent screening procedures that are performed, but there is still a risk of transmission of rare agents. The risks of transmission of HIV, hepatitis B virus, hepatitis C virus, and the human T-cell leukemia virus type I have been minimalized since serologic testing is done for these agents. Epoetin-alfa has been shown in early clinical trials to increase the yield of autologous blood donation. Many states now are requiring that the physician counsel the patient prior to any elective surgical procedures on the use of autologous and directed donor blood donations. It behooves the physician to understand the different

Table 9-3.   Uncontrolled Surgical Bleeding

Cause	Laboratory Values					Actions
	PLTS	F	BT	PT	PTT	
Vascular	→	→	→	→	→	Control vessel bleeding
DIC	↓	↓	↑→[a]	↑	↑	Establish cause, protamine-sulfate, paracoagulation test to confirm diagnosis; platelet infusions, F replacement with cryoprecipitate to keep >100 mg/dl
Thrombocytopenia						
Immune	↓	→	↑→[a]	→	→	Corticosteroids, intravenous gammaglobulin, splenectomy in selected cases
Decreased production	↓	→	↑→[a]	→	→	Established cause, platelet infusions to keep count, >100,000/mm³
Excessive heparin	→	→	→	↑→[b]	↑	Stop heparin infusions, if immediate reversal required, protamine sulfate
Inherited factor VIII, IX, or XI deficiency	→	→	→↑[c]	→	↑	Replace with deficient factor, with monitoring of factor level
Vitamin K deficiency	→	→	→	↑	↑→[d]	Establish cause, vitamin K infusion, FFP if correction required rapidly
Liver disease	↓→[e]	↓→	↑	↑	↑	Treatment difficult; FFP and platelets may be needed for serious bleeding; excessive fibrinolysis occurs in 50% of patients
Excessive fibrinolysis	→	↓→	→	↑→[f]	↑→[f]	Establish diagnosis with DWBCLT and EGCLT, ε-amino caproic acid if DIC not present
Von Willebrand disease	→	→	↑	→	↑→	Establish diagnosis, cryoprecipitate and/or DDAVP
Qualitative platelet defect	→	→	↑	→	→	Establish diagnosis, platelet infusions

Abbreviations: DIC, disseminated intravascular coagulation; FFP, fresh frozen plasma; PLTS, platelets; F, fibrinogen; BT, bleeding time; PT, prothrombin time; PTT, partial thromboplastin time; DDAVP, 1-deamino-8-D-arginine vasopressin (desmopressin); DWBCLT, dilute whole blood clot lysis time; EGCLT, euglobin clot lysis time; ↑, increased; ↓, decreased; →, within the normal range.
[a] With platelet counts <100,000/mm³, BT may be prolonged.
[b] High levels of heparin may prolong the PT.
[c] May be markedly prolonged in the presence of platelet inhibitor, such as aspirin.
[d] With severe deficiency.
[e] With splenic sequestration.
[f] Can be slightly prolonged.

transfusion options available for patients and also to be aware of the possibility of autologous donation with or without epoetin-alfa supplementation.

POLYCYTHEMIA

Primary Polycythemia

Primary polycythemia results from an uncontrolled proliferation (neoplastic) of hematopoietic stem cells that is clinically manifested as an increased hemoglobin or hematocrit level. Patients often will have a ruddy appearance. There is frequently a leukocytosis and an increase in platelet count. These patients are at risk for thrombotic complications (including stroke), especially when the hematocrit is over 60 percent.[3] Treatment of these patients consists of frequent phlebotomies to reduce hematocrit level to less than 45 percent.

Secondary Polycythemia

Numerous medical conditions may produce a secondary polycythemia due to qualitive tissue hypoxemia. Residence at high altitude is probably one of the most common causes of secondary polycythemia. To counter the reduced oxygen tension in high altitudes there is a secondary erythropoietin response with resulting increase in red cell mass. Chronic hypoxemic states including chronic tobacco use, chronic pulmonary disease, congenital cardiovascular disorders, and abnormal hemoglobins can produce a polycythemic state. Rarely, these patients may have symptomatic polycythemia requiring occasional phlebotomy.[35]

HYPERCOAGULABLE STATE

Hereditary

Recently, identifiable hypercoagulable states have been attributed to inheritable deficiencies in plasma anticoagulant proteins or defects in fibrinolysis. Patients with deficiency of antithrombin III, a cofactor responsible for inactivation of thrombin, can result in venous thrombosis, occasionally involving the sinuses of the central nervous system.[33] Treatment consists of high doses of heparin or, more recently, the use of purified antithrombin III concentrates.

Protein C is a vitamin K–dependent factor that in the presence of thrombomodulin and protein S, another vitamin K–dependent factor, results in the inactivation of factors V and VIII. Individuals who are heterozygotes for protein C or S deficiency may experience venous and rarely arterial thromboses.[4,7]

Acquired

Patients with disseminated solid tumors can have unusual arterial thrombosis (Trousseau syndrome). Marantic endocarditis can also be seen in these patients and can result in systemic arterial emboli.[29] Myeloproliferative disorders, especially essential thrombocythemia with platelet counts above 1,000,000/mm³ may result in thrombosis and/or bleeding.[2]

Thromboembolism is a common complication in the surgical patient due to venous pooling secondary to immobility of the patient and a relative hypercoagulable state postoperatively (increased procoagulant activity and decreased anticoagulant activity along with decreased fibrinolytic activity). The development of impedance plethysmography and color Doppler duplex scans for the detection of deep vein thrombosis along with radionuclide ventilation-perfusion scans to detect pulmonary embolism allow for rapid diagnosis.[13,14]

Pneumatic compression of the lower extremities in the perioperative and postoperative period is a safe and effective measure of preventing venous thromboembolism in the neurosurgical patient. In addition, low-dose, low-molecular-weight heparin or regular heparin may be given safely without excessive bleeding.[25]

REFERENCES

1. Aggeler PM, White SG, Glendenning MB et al: Plasma thromboplastin component (PTC) deficiency: a new disease resembling hemophilia. Proc Soc Exp Biol Med 79:692, 1952
2. Bellucci S, Jan vier M, Tobelem G et al: Essential thrombocythemias. Clinical evolutionary and biological data. Cancer 58:2440, 1986
3. Berk PD, Goldberg JD, Donovan PB et al: Therapeutic recommendations in polycythemia vera based on polycythemia vera study group protocols. Semin Hematol 23:132, 1986
4. Bertina RM: Hereditary protein S deficiency. Haemostasis 15:241, 1985
5. Biggs R, Douglas AS, Macfarlane RG: Christmas disease: a condition previously mistaken for hemophilia. Br Med J 2:1373, 1952
6. Brinkhous KM: A study of the clotting defect in hemophilia. The delayed formation of thrombin. Am J Sci 198:509, 1939
7. Broekmans AW: Hereditary protein C deficiency. Haemostasis 15:233, 1985
8. Casper CK, Dietrich SL: Management of haemophilia. Clin Haematol 14:507, 1985
9. Colman RW, Robboy SJ, Minna JD: Disseminated intravascular coagulation: a reappraisal. Annu Rev Med 30:359, 1979
10. Furie B, Furie BC: The molecular basis of blood coagulation. Cell 53:505, 1988
11. Gotti E, Mecca G, Valentino C et al: Renal biopsy in patients with acute renal failure and prolonged bleeding time. Lancet 2:978, 1984
12. Green D, Lechner K: A survey of 215 non-hemophilia patients with inhibitors to factor VIII. Thromb Haemost 45:200, 1981
13. Hirsch J: Diagnosis of venous thrombosis and pulmonary embolism. Am J Cardiol 65:45c, 1990
14. Huisman MV, Bueller HR, ten Cate JW et al: Unexpected high prevalence of silent pulmonary embolism in patients with deep venous thrombosis. Chest 95:498, 1989
15. Karpatkin S: Autoimmune thrombocytopenia purpura. Semin Hematol 22:260, 1985
16. Kasper CK: Incidence and course of inhibitors among patients with classic hemophilia. Thromb Diath Haemost 30:263, 1973
17. Jacob RA, Sandstead HH, Klevay LM, Johnson LK: Utility of serum ferritin as a measure of iron deficiency in normal males undergoing repetitive phlebotomy. Blood 56:786, 1980
18. Janson PA, Jubelirer SJ, Weinstein MS, Deykin D: Treatment of bleeding tendency in uremia with cryoprecipitate. N Engl J Med 303:1318, 1980
19. Lackner H: Hemostatic abnormalities associated with dysproteinemias. Semin Hematol 10:125, 1973
20. Laster J, Cikrit D et al: The heparin-induced thrombocytopenia syndrome: an update. Surgery 102:763, 1987
21. Lee GR: The anemia of chronic disease. Semin Hematol 20:61, 1983
22. Macfarlane RG: An enzyme cascade in the blood clotting mechanism and its function as a biological amplifier. Nature 202:498, 1964
23. Mannucci PM: Desmopressin (DAVP) for treatment of hemophilia. Prog Hemost Thromb 8:19, 1986

24. Marder VJ: Microvascular thrombosis. Sci Pract Clin Med 6:230, 1980

25. Mohr DN, Ryu JH, Litin SC, Rosenow EC: Recent advances in the management of venous thromboembolism. Mayo Clin Proc 63:281, 1988

26. Moia M, Vizzotto L, Cattaneo M et al: Improvement in the hemostatic defect of uraemia after treatment with recombinant human erythropoietin. Lancet 2:1227, 1987

27. Olson JP, Miller LL, Troup SB: Synthesis of clotting factors by the isolated rat liver. J Clin Invest 45:690, 1966

28. Perkins HA: Correction of the hemostatic defects in von Willebrand's disease. Blood 30:375, 1967

29. Rohner RF, Prior JT, Sipple JH: Mucinous malignancies, venous thrombosis and terminal endocarditis with emboli: a syndrome. Cancer 19:1805, 1966

30. Shulman NR, Jordan JV Jr: Platelet Immunology. p. 452. In Colman RW, Hirsh J, Marder VJ, Salzman EW (eds): Hemostasis and Thrombosis. JB Lippincott, Philadelphia, 1987

31. Sixma JJ, Wester J: The hemostatic plug. Semin Hematol 14:265, 1977

32. Suttie JW: Vitamin K dependent carboxylation. CRC Crit Rev Biochem 8:191, 1980

33. Thaler E, Lechner K: Antithrombin III deficiency and thromboembolism. Clin Haematol 10:369, 1981

34. Vigano G, Marchesi E, Remuzzi G, Mecca G: Conjugated estrogens (CE) to reduce bleeding in uremics. Thromb Haemost 58:81, 1987

35. Wallis PJW: Effects of erythropoiesis on pulmonary haemodynamics and oxygen transport in patients with secondary polycythemia and cor pulmonale. Clin Sci 70:91, 1986

36. Ragni MV, Sinha D, Seaman F et al: Comparison of bleeding tendency, factor XI coagulant activity and factor XI antigenic levels in 25 factor XI deficient kindred. Blood 65:719, 1985

37. Walsh PN, Rizza CR, Matthews JM et al: Epsilon-aminocaproic acid therapy for dental extraction in haemophilia and Christmas disease: a double blind controlled trial. Br J Haematol 20:463, 1971

38. Wisloff F, Godal HC: Prolonged bleeding time with adequate platelet count in hospital patients. Scand J Haematol 27:45, 1981

10 Seizures

Christopher M. De Giorgio
Adrian L. Rabinowicz

Seizures are commonly seen in neurosurgical practice. The morbidity resulting from seizures ranges from none to sudden death. Seizures significantly impact a patient's physical and psychological health and economic security. For example, a single seizure may result in loss of driving privileges, with severe economic impact to the patient. Employers, frequently ignorant of the disorder, are hesitant to hire individuals with epilepsy. The death rate in those experiencing a single seizure is twice the control population and is highest within the first 2 years.[11] Given these sobering data, seizures are more than just a nuisance. Neurosurgeons should have a strong grasp of issues such as prophylaxis, the drugs of choice and the use of drugs other than phenytoin or phenobarbital, the treatment of status epilepticus, and when to withdraw treatment. The goal of this chapter is to identify those variables that increase the risk of seizures and to communicate the latest information in seizure management in order to minimize the morbidity associated with seizures in neurosurgical practice.

NEUROSURGICAL SETTINGS ASSOCIATED WITH SEIZURES

Trauma

Every year over 420,000 individuals are hospitalized for head trauma, 5,000 to 30,000 of whom develop posttraumatic seizures.[15,35] Overall 2 percent of individuals with traumatic brain injury develop chronic epilepsy.[1,2,15] Early studies such as those by Jennet[18] introduced the concept of early and late posttraumatic seizures. Early seizures present within the first week posttrauma and correlate with the presence of depressed skull fractures, focal neurological deficits, and intracerebral hemorrhage.[13,18] Late seizures typically occur within the first year and correlate with the same factors plus the presence of early-onset seizures and posttraumatic amnesia lasting more than 24 hours.[2,18] The incidence of early seizures has been reported to be 2 to 14 percent, whereas late seizures occur in up to 27 percent after 2 years.

Prophylaxis in Head Trauma

Prophylaxis (usually with Dilantin) has been the standard of practice for years, with the intended goal of preventing posttraumatic seizures and chronic epilepsy.[30] Early studies provided a basis for the use of prophylactic antiepileptic drugs; however, prospective studies in the 1980s, particularly that of Young et al.[41,42] failed to demonstrate any benefit of antiepileptic drugs in the prevention of posttraumatic epilepsy. Temkin et al.,[35] in an important recent study, demonstrated that prophylactic phenytoin in the high therapeutic range decreased the risk of early (1-week) seizures threefold compared with placebo but failed to improve the incidence of late seizures and epilepsy (see Table 10-1).

Brain Tumor

Seizures associated with tumors could be due to the neoplasm itself, craniotomy, acute or chronic radiation change, edema or increased intracranial pres-

Table 10-1. Prophylaxis in Head Trauma: Summary of Two Recent Key Studies

Year	Authors	No.	Type of Study	Conclusions
1983	Young et al.[42]	244	Prospective	Prophylactic phenytoin does not reduce early posttraumatic seizures
1990	Temkin et al.[35]	404	Prospective	Prophylactic phenytoin does not reduce the incidence of posttraumatic epilepsy, but does decrease the incidence of early seizures

sure.[13] The incidence of seizures associated with supratentorial tumors range from 20 to 80 percent.[21,40] Lund popularized the concept that seizures are inversely correlated with the severity of the tumor.[21] This has been confirmed by later investigators (see Table 10-2).

Among benign brain tumors, meningiomas are highly epileptogenic, with seizures the presenting symptom in up to 91 percent of the cases depending on the location.[14,33] It is clear that histology and location are primary determinants of postoperative seizures in brain tumors.

Infection

Subdural empyemas and brain abscesses are extremely epileptogenic.[3,6,19,20] Although antibiotics diminish the rate of complications, seizures remain a frequent sequelae in 50 to 60 percent and up to 80 percent in intracerebral abscess. Abscesses may require treatment for prolonged periods, as seizures may present several years after presentation.

Aneurysms

The incidence for seizures following subarachnoid hemorrhage (SAH) due to ruptured aneurysms ranges from 3 to 26 percent.[4,5,17] Aneurysms located at the middle cerebral artery (MCA) and posterior

Table 10-2. Incidence of Seizures as a Presenting Symptom in Brain Tumors

	Incidence of Seizures as a Presenting Symptom (%)	
Tumor Type	Lund[21] (1952)	Youmans and Cobb[40] (1982)
Metastasis	19	26
Glioblastoma	42	30
Astrocytoma	66	40
Oligodendroglioma	81	50

cerebral artery (PCA) are associated with the highest incidence of seizures, especially when associated with intracerebral hemorrhage.[31] The incidence of seizures following surgery for unruptured aneurysms has been found by our group to be 15.7 percent.[28] We identified perioperative complications and temporal lobe retraction as risk factors in this population. The data suggest from this small study that most patients could be successfully tapered off antiepileptic drugs within 12 months after surgery for unruptured aneurysms.

Arteriovenous Malformations

The incidence of seizures as a major presenting symptom in arteriovenous malformations (AVMs) is about 17 percent. The vast majority of patients actually present with hemorrhage. Epilepsy as a sole presenting symptom without hemorrhage or neurological deficit is rare. Only 6 percent of patients who present with hemorrhage had epilepsy prior to diagnosis.[9]

Several factors increase the risk of epilepsy. For those AVMs diagnosed but not treated surgically, there is an approximate 1 percent/year risk of developing epilepsy. For those treated surgically, the risk is much higher for the first 5 years postoperatively and then levels off to about 1 percent/year. In patients treated surgically, the 10-year risk of epilepsy is 47 percent versus 11 percent in conservatively treated patients. Ninety percent of patients who do develop epilepsy postoperatively do so in the first 5 years. Large superficial AVMs carry the highest risk of hemorrhage, and, in those patients treated surgically, surgery in the frontal and parietal lobe is associated with the highest risk of epilepsy.[9]

Craniotomy

The incidence of postoperative seizures after craniotomy has been extensively studied, as has the issue of prophylaxis. North et al.[24] demonstrated an 8 percent incidence of postoperative seizures in those treated with phenytoin versus 16.7 percent in those untreated. Interestingly, this risk seems related to the type of procedure and pathology. Sbeih et al.[32] reported that the incidence of postoperative epilepsy following aneurysm surgery was only 3 percent and that phenytoin did not affect the development of epilepsy. North et al.[25,26] did report that meningioma, metastasis, and head injury presented a higher risk for postoperative seizures compared with other surgeries, such as sellar surgery.

Several additional risk factors have been identified, which include the surgical approach,[7] presence of preoperative seizures, pre- and postoperative deficits, the anesthetic agent, and antibiotics. Michenfelder et al.[23] documented an increased risk of seizures since the introduction of isoflurane in 1982. They noted that the incidence of seizures postoperatively doubled from 4 to 8 percent after the introduction of isoflurane. Zaccara et al.[43] recently echoed this correlation, noting that most anesthetics are epileptogenic, especially enflurane.

Recently, Michenfelder et al.[23] reported that the intraoperative and early postoperative use of antibiotics (penicillins, especially nafcillin) nearly tripled the incidence of postoperative seizures from 1.8 to 4.7 percent. Other antibiotics, such as cephalosporins, imipenim, flagyl, and some of the antitubercular agents have also been reported as increasing the risk of seizures.[43]

The type of craniotomy impacts the risk of seizures. Michenfelder et al.[23] reported no postoperative seizures in 323 suboccipital craniotomies despite the use of antibiotics. North et al.[25,26] reported that sellar surgery was associated with a lower risk than other craniotomies, despite the subfrontal approach. Temporal lobe retraction is notoriously correlated with postoperative seizures.

Prophylaxis

No absolute consensus guides the initiation of prophylactic anticonvulsants or the duration of treatment. Deutschman and Haines[11] in their excellent review identify patients at risk who should be considered for prophylaxis. They believe those patients with a risk of seizures of 10 to 15 percent to be candidates for prophylaxis. At particular risk are patients with posttraumatic intracerebral hematomas, depressed skull fractures, subdural empyema, and abscess.

MANAGEMENT OF SEIZURES AND EPILEPSY IN NEUROSURGERY

Preoperative, Perioperative, and Postoperative Management With Phenytoin

Phenytoin (Dilantin) is the most commonly used antiepileptic drug in neurosurgical practice. Dilantin is available in intravenous (IV) or oral (PO) form, can be given in a loading dose, and, because of its relatively long half-life, can be administered orally once every 24 hours, which is an advantage in patients having to be NPO or undergo long procedures. In the preoperative patient, therapeutic levels can be reached rapidly through either IV or oral loading. Dilantin oral loading may be accomplished by giving 20 mg/kg in three to four divided doses (Table 10-3), and, because of slower absorption (3 to 12 hours after a single dose), it is safer. IV loading results in much more rapid peak blood levels, but may result in hypotension, skin infiltration and necrosis, electrocardiographic (ECG) conduction disturbances, arrhythmias, and, rarely, respiratory depression, usually from excessively rapid IV loading. Dilantin cannot be hung and infused without careful monitoring, so it is recommended to infuse by slow IV push, 25 to 50 mg/min, flushing the IV line with normal saline, with careful ECG and blood pressure monitoring. Infusion rates should be reduced in the elderly, in those with cardiac disease, and in those who have already been loaded with other anticonvulsants (pentobarbital, phenobarbital, lorazepam). Patients with subtherapeutic levels can be bolused to achieve the desired blood level (see Table 10-3).

If achieving a rapid blood level is not essential, such as in patients scheduled for elective surgery, Dilantin should be initiated at 5 mg/kg either in two divided doses or once daily, and a trough (prior to a dose) plasma level should be drawn at 5 to 7 days in order to allow sufficient time for steady state to be determined. If the level is subtherapeutic it may be a result of (1) patient noncompliance, (2) a fast metabolizer, (3) interactions from other drugs (inducers of metabolism such as phenobarbital), (4) poor gastrointestinal absorption (tube feedings, vomiting, diarrhea), and (5) failure to achieve steady state. Due to saturation or zero order kinetics, large changes in Dilantin dose (e.g., 100 mg), except in those with very low Dilantin levels, may result in Dilantin toxicity, including ataxia, incoordination, nystagmus, nausea/vomiting, and lethargy. For example, if a patient has a Dilantin level of 9 and the dose is in-

Table 10-3.   Oral Loading With Dilantin

Previously untreated patients

1. Determine body weight in kilograms

2. Calculate the mg/kg loading dose:
   a. Oral: 20 mg/kg (1–1.5 g) in three to four divided doses separated by 2-hour intervals
   b. IV: 15 mg/kg slow IV push at a rate of <50 mg/kg, flushing with normal saline. Monitor ECG and blood pressure frequently

3. Start maintenance Dilantin dose in 24 hours

Patients with subtherapeutic levels

1. Obtain a preloading Dilantin level

2. Determine desired blood level (between 10 and 25 μg/ml)

3. Determine body weight in kilograms

4. Calculate the mg/kg loading dose:
   a. IV loading dose (mg/kg) = 0.7 × [desired plasma level − observed plasma level]. Infuse as above
   b. Oral loading does (mg/kg) = 0.7 × [desired plasma level − observed plasma level] + 10%

5. Start maintenance Dilantin dose in 24 hours

(From Right Dose Card Dosing Guidelines Dept. of Pharmacy, Thomas Jefferson Hospital, with permission.)

creased by 100 mg, the resulting steady-state level may be reached. Adjust Dilantin dose in 30 to 60 mg increments or consider using a nomogram for calculating doses (Fig. 10-1).[29]

Adverse Effects

Aside from acute effects from rapid loading, Dilantin may cause serious adverse effects such as rash, especially in the first 10 days of treatment, which may occasionally progress to a Stevens-Johnson reaction. In a recent study of Dilantin prophylaxis for head trauma, rash was the most common idiosyncratic reaction in those treated with Dilantin (12 percent), 68 percent of whom were discontinued from Dilantin (Table 10-4).

Alternative Drugs

Three major alternatives to Dilantin are carbamazepine, valproic acid, and phenobarbital. Alternatives may be necessary when an intolerable or idiosyncratic reaction develops, when there is a history of allergy or intolerance in the past, or if there is clear lack of efficacy of Dilantin even at the maximum tolerated dose.

The landmark Veterans Administration[22] cooperative trial demonstrated no difference in efficacy be-

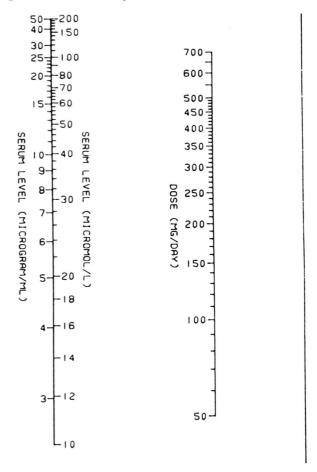

Figure 10-1. Nomogram for calculating phenytoin dosage. Given a single reliable serum level on a given daily dose of phenytoin, the dose required to achieve a desired serum level can be predicted. A line is drawn connecting the observed serum level (left-hand scale) with the dose administered (center scale) and extended to intersect the right-hand vertical line. From this point of intersection, another line is drawn back to the desired serum level (left-hand scale). The dose required to produce this level can be read off the center scale. Note that this nomogram will give misleading predictions if the serum level measurement is inaccurate, if the patient's compliance is in doubt, or if a change in concurrent treatment has been made since measurement of the serum level. (From Rambeck et al.,[29] with permission.)

tween phenytoin, carbamazepine, or phenobarbital in the treatment of tonic-clonic seizures. However, the study did demonstrate that carbamazepine was significantly better in controlling partial seizures, the primary seizure disorder in neurosurgical patients. Forty-five percent of those with partial seizures were controlled by carbamazepine versus 26 percent for phenytoin.

Table 10-4. Early Idiosyncratic Adverse Reactions to Dilantin

1. Morbilliform rash (measles-like) with/without fever: frequently in the first 10 days, usually within 30 days
2. Systemic hypersensitivity: 10–30 days. Fever, rash, lymphadenopathy, eosinophilia, liver function elevation or hepatitis—may occur alone or in combination:

Rash	100%
Fever	90%
Leukocytosis	66%
Hepatomegaly	65%
Jaundice	55%
Bleeding disorder	40%
Spenomegaly	35%

3. Hepatitis—usually associated with systemic hypersensitivity

(From Parker and Shearer,[27] with permission.)

Unfortunately, valproic acid was not included in this clinical trial. Turnbull et al.[39] did report that valproic acid was equally efficacious to phenytoin in adults with tonic-clonic or partial seizures. Likewise, Callaghan et al.[8] found phenytoin, carbamazepine, and valproic acid to be equally effective in partial and generalized tonic-clonic seizures (Tables 10-5 and 10-6).

Initiation and Maintenance

Valproic Acid (Depakote)

Valproic acid (Depakote) is now more commonly used for patients with partial seizures. We have used valproic acid effectively in several neurosurgical patients, especially those who have idiosyncratic side effects to other antiepileptic drugs. The incidence of rash is lower than the other antiepileptic drugs, which makes valproic acid a good alternative because of the frequent cross-reactivity of phenytoin, carbamazepine, and phenobarbital.[8]

Adverse effects of valproic acid include nausea, diarrhea, and abdominal discomfort, especially with nonenteric coated depakene. These side effects are

Table 10-5. Pharmacology of the Major Antiepileptic Drugs

Drug	Peak (h)	Half Life (h)	Time to Steady State (days)
Phenytoin	3–12	22–24	5–7
Carbamazepine	2–8	12–17	2–4
Valproic acid	1–4	5–20	2–4
Phenobarbital	8–12	48–144[a]	21–28

[a] Average = 96.

Table 10-6. Antiepileptic Drugs: Therapeutic Ranges

Drugs	Range (μg/ml)
Phenytoin	10–20
Carbamazepine	4–12
Phenobarbital	15–40
Valproic acid	50–100

reduced with enteric coated Depakote. Weight gain and tremor are two common side effects, and alopecia is occasionally encountered. Thrombocytopenia is the most common hematological side effect.

Hepatotoxicity and pancreatitis are the most severe adverse effects of valproic acid. Fatal hepatotoxicity most commonly occurs in infants and children less than 2 years old and is highly correlated with polytherapy.[13] The rate of valproic-associated hepatotoxicity is 1 in 500 in children less than 2 years. This risk is significantly reduced in children less than 2 years who are on monotherapy (1 in 7,000). In children older than 2 years on monotherapy, the incidence is 1 in 45,000, while in the same age group on polytherapy the incidence is 1 in 12,000. The overall incidence of hepatotoxicity is 1 in 10,000. There have been no reports of fatal hepatotoxicity above age 10 years in monotherapy patients. Pancreatitis has been recently reported, occurs in the first 6 months of treatment, and is not age related. Fatal pancreatitis has been reported, and pancreatitis should be considered in patients with either significant abdominal pain or vomiting. Amylase level determinations are helpful and should be drawn in patients with abdominal pain or vomiting.

Depakote (enteric coated valproic acid) is initiated at 10 to 15 mg/kg in three divided doses. Steady state should be achieved in 2 to 4 days. Therapeutic levels are 50 to 100 μg/ml. The dose can be increased by 5 to 10 mg/kg at weekly intervals. The maximum recommended dose is 60 mg/kg, which is rarely necessary and which may be associated with greater sedation.

Carbamazepine (Tegretol)

Carbamazepine (Tegretol) is also an effective alternative antiepileptic drug. As noted previously, its efficacy in tonic-clonic seizures is similar to that of phenytoin and valproic acid, and the VA cooperative study demonstrated greater efficacy against partial (focal) seizures than phenytoin or phenobarbital.

Carbamazepine gained popularity because of reports that it caused less cognitive impairment than phenytoin or phenobarbital, but recent data suggest that this difference is less than initially reported. A reevaluation by Dodrill and Troupin[12] of their original data showed that differences between phenytoin and carbamazepine were largely a function of blood level.

The most common side effects of carbamazepine are drowsiness, diplopia, and ataxia (especially at high doses and 2 to 4 hours after the dose). Rash may occur with similar frequency to phenytoin (5 to 10%). Idiosyncratic reactions such as the Stevens-Johnson reaction have been reported. Hyponatremia and syndrome of inappropriate antidiuretic hormone secretion (SIADH) have been commonly reported.

Aside from idiosyncratic allergic reactions, the most feared adverse effects are bone marrow suppression and aplastic anemia. The incidence of aplastic anemia and agranulocytosis is five to eight times more common than in the general population. Though carbamazepine frequently causes mild decreases in white and red blood cells and platelet counts, severe bone marrow suppression is actually rare. A survey of the literature by Sobotka et al.[34] demonstrated that a benign decrease in white blood cells to 4,000/mm^3 occurs in 12 percent of children and 7 percent of adults, and a frequent decrease in total white blood cells by 25 percent is common, especially in the first 3 months of treatment. The leukopenia usually resolves but may persist without adverse effects. Problematically, when aplastic anemia or agranulocytosis occur, it is rapid. Table 10-7 summarizes the most recent monitoring recommendations (from Ciba Giegy and Sobotka et al.[34]).

For those over 12 years of age, the manufacturer recommends an initial dose of 200 mg bid. The dose may be increased up to 200 mg/day at weekly intervals, with an average maintenance dose of 800 to 1,200 mg/day. Carbamazepine induces its own metabolism, so the half-life does decrease in the first few weeks of treatment. After initiation of treatment, blood levels should be checked in 3 to 4 weeks to ensure a stable steady state. Some patients may experience nausea, diplopia, or ataxia at even these dosages, and in these individuals initiation of carbamazepine at a lower dose and at a slower rate may be necessary.

Status Epilepticus

Status Epilepticus is a common medical emergency, with mortality rates of about 1 to 10 percent.[10,16] About 50,000 to 60,000 new cases occur yearly.[16] The incidence of status epilepticus is particularly high in patients with acute cerebral lesions such as trauma or neoplasm.[16] Status epilepticus is commonly preceded by drug withdrawal or acute neurological insults such as stroke, trauma, infection, and brain tumors. Diazepam, lorazepam, phenytoin, phenobarbital, and pentobarbital are the most commonly used drugs, but the short elimination of diazepam and the long infusion times and hypotension associated with phenytoin have led to the common use of lorazepam (Ativan) as an initial therapy for status epilepticus.[36] Treiman et al.[37] prospectively compared lorazepam to phenytoin for the initial management of status epilepticus and found lorazepam to be effective in 79 percent of the 39 patients who received it as the first drug. Phenytoin was effective as the initial drug in 59 percent who received it as the initial drug. Multiple studies have demonstrated lorazepam to be effective in 68 to 96 percent of patients in status epilepticus.[36] Table 10-8 summarizes a recommended treatment protocol for the effective management of status epilepticus. Treiman et al.[36–38] have clearly shown that an organized protocol approach with sequential infusions of antiepileptic drugs is superior to a haphazard random approach.

Withdrawal of Treatment

A decision to withdraw treatment must take into consideration the type of craniotomy, the pathology, the presence of preoperative seizures, the seizure-free interval, and the window within which seizures usually present postoperatively. For example, with

Table 10-7.   Carbamazepine Hematological
Monitoring Recommendations

Manufacturer recommendations (Ciba Geigy, Tegretol)

1. Obtain complete pretreatment hematological testing data as a baseline

2. Periodic hematological evaluations at the physician's discretion

3. Discontinuation should be considered if any evidence of bone marrow suppression occurs.

Sobotka et al.[34] recommendations (1990)

1. All patients should have a pretreatment complete blood count, differential, and platelet count

2. Monitor those patients with low normal and subnormal white blood cell count and neutrophil counts every 2 weeks for the first 1–3 months. If the white blood cell count falls below 3,000/mm^3 or the absolute neutrophil count falls below 1,000 mm^3, decrease dose or discontinue carbamazepine

3. Hematological side effects are best monitored by early recognition of signs, including fatigue, fever, infections, ecchymosis, and mucous membrane bleeding

4. The maximum risk is primarily during the first year of treatment.

Table 10-8. Treatment Protocol for Generalized Convulsive Status Epilepticus

1. Make diagnosis by observing one additional seizure in a patient with a history of recent acute seizures or impaired consciousness, or by observing continuous seizure activity for more than 30 minutes

2. Call EEG technician and start recording continuous EEG ASAP. Do not delay treatment unless EEG is necessary to verify the diagnosis

3. Establish IV catheter with normal saline

4. Draw blood for serum chemistries, CBC, and antiepileptic drug levels

5. Give thiamine 100 mg followed by 50 ml of 50% glucose IVP

6. Give lorazepam (Ativan) 0.1 mg/kg IV push at less than 2 mg/min

7. If status does not stop, start phenytoin 20 mg/kg slow IVP (<50 mg/min) directly into IV port nearest to patient. Monitor blood pressure and ECG closely during infusion

8. If status does not stop after 20 mg/kg, give an additional 5 mg/kg and, if necessary, another 5 mg/kg until a maximum dose of 30 mg/kg is reached

9. If status persists, intubate patient and give phenobarbital 20 mg/kg by IV push (<100 mg/kg)

10. If status still persists, induce coma with a barbiturate. Give pentobarbital 5 mg/kg slowly as initial IV dose to induce an EEG burst suppression pattern. Continue 0.5–2 mg/kg/h to maintain burst suppression pattern. Slow the rate of infusion every 2–4 h to see if seizures have stopped. Monitor blood pressure, ECG, and respiratory function closely

(Adapted from Treiman,[36,38] with permission.)

empyema or abscess, treatment may need to be continued for several years because of the high incidence of late seizures. However after routine craniotomy, North et al.[24–26] found that 75 percent of those who did develop postoperative seizures did so in the first month, and they concluded that prophylaxis should continue for 3 to 4 months postoperatively. Rabinowicz et al.[28] found that most patients could be successfully weaned off antiepileptic drugs within 12 months. Tapering of antiepileptic drugs should always be performed, whenever possible, over several months.

CONCLUSION

Seizures are a common sequelae of neurosurgical procedures and are associated with the very conditions for which neurosurgeons frequently are referred. A rational, informed approach to the management of seizures, an awareness of the pharmacology and toxicity of the major antiepileptic drugs, and a knowledge of the management of status epilepticus

Table 10-9. Summary Recommendations for the Management of Seizures in Neurosurgical Practice

1. Prophylaxis in head trauma does not clearly reduce the long-term risk of epilepsy

2. Prophylaxis for craniotomy should be selective, and consideration should be given to prophylax those patients at highest risk, especially those with hemorrhage, depressed skull fracture, and infection

3. After craniotomy, anticonvulsants can generally be discontinued in seizure-free patients after 1 year, except in patients with significant risk factors, breakthrough seizures, or a previous history of seizures

4. In patients with postoperative seizures, treatment may be withdrawn after a seizure-free period of 2 years, unless there is a medical or social reason precluding withdrawal

5. Monotherapy should be used whenever possible

6. Be wary of idiosyncratic side effects, especially early in treatment

7. Unless it is a medical emergency, withdrawal of anticonvulsants should be done slowly, generally over a few months

8. Be aware of agents used perioperatively that may increase the risk of seizures, especially intraoperative antibiotics such as penicillin and anesthetics such as iso/enflurane

9. When treating status epilepticus, use a logical sequence such as is contained in this chapter. Consider Ativan in the initial treatment of status epilepticus

are essential to neurosurgical practice. Table 10-9 provides an overall summary to the management of seizures in neurosurgical practice.

ACKNOWLEDGMENTS

This work was supported by the Garnier Endowment for Epilepsy Research.

REFERENCES

1. Annegers JF, Grabow JD, Groover RV et al: Seizures after head trauma: a population study. Neurology 30:683, 1980
2. Annegers JF, Grabow JD, Kurland LT et al: The incidence, causes and secular trends of head trauma in Olmsted County, Minnesota, 1935–1974. Neurology 24:921, 1974
3. Bannister G, Williams B, Smith S: Treatment of subdural empyema. J Neurosurg 55:82, 1981
4. Bartholow R: Aneurysms of the arteries of the base of the brain: their symptomatology, diagnosis and treatment. Am J Med Sci 64:373, 1972
5. Biller J, Godersky JC, Adams HP: Management of aneurysmal subarachnoid hemorrhage. Stroke 19:1300, 1988

6. Borzone M, Capuzzo T, Rivano C et al: Subdural empyema: fourteen cases surgically treated. Surg Neurol 13:449, 1980

7. Cabral R, King TT, Scott DF: Epilepsy after two different neurosurgical approaches to the treatment of ruptured intracranial aneurysms. J Neurol Neurosurg Psychiatry 39:1052, 1976

8. Callaghan N, Kenny RA, O'Neill B et al: A prospective study between carbamazepine, phenytoin, and sodium valproate as monotherapy in previously untreated and recently diagnosed with epilepsy. J Neurol Neurosurg Psychiatry 48:639, 1985

9. Crawford PM, West CR, Shaw DM, Chadwick DW: Cerebral arteriovenous malformations and epilepsy: factors in the development of epilepsy. Epilepsia 27:270, 1986

10. Delgado-Escueta AE, Wasterlain C, Treiman DM, Porter RJ: Management of status epilepticus. N Engl J Med 306:1337, 1982

11. Deutschman CS, Haines SJ: Anticonvulsant prophylaxis in neurological surgery. Neurosurgery 17:510, 1985

12. Dodrill CB, Troupin AS: Neuropsychological effects of carbamazepine and phenytoin: a reanalysis. Neurology 41:141, 1991

13. Dreifuss FE, Santilli N, Langer DH et al: Valproic acid hepatic fatalities: a retrospective review. Neurology 37:379, 1987

14. Foy PM, Copeland GP, Shaw MD: The incidence of postoperative seizures. Acta Neurochir 55:253, 1981

15. Hauser WA: Prevention of post-traumatic epilepsy. N Engl J Med 323:540, 1990

16. Hauser WA: Status epilepticus: epidemiologic considerations. Neurology 40(Suppl 2):9, 1990

17. Heidrich R: Subarachnoid hemorrhage. p. 68. In Vinken PF, Bruyn AW (ed): Handbook of Clinical Neurology. Vol 12. American Elsevier, New York, 1972

18. Jennet B: Epilepsy after Non-missile Head Injuries. 2nd Ed. WM Heinemann Medical Books, London, 1975

19. LeBean J, Creissard P, Harispe L et al: Surgical treatment of brain abscess and subdural empyema. J. Neurosurg 38:198, 1973

20. Legg NF, Gupta PC, Scott DF: Epilepsy following cerebral abscess: a clinical and EEG study of 70 patients. Brain 96:259, 1973

21. Lund M: Epilepsy in association with intracranial tumors. Acta Psychiatr Neurol Scand 8(Suppl):1, 1952

22. Mattson RH, Cramer JA, Collins JF et al: Comparison of carbamazepine, phenobarbital, phenytoin and primidone in partial and secondarily generalized tonic-clonic seizures. N Engl J Med 313:145, 1985

23. Michenfelder JD, Cucchiara RF, Sundt TM: Incidence of intraoperative antibiotic choice on the incidence of early postcraniotomy seizures. J Neurosurg 72:703, 1990

24. North JB, Hanieh A, Challen RG et al: Postoperative epilepsy. A double blind trial of phenytoin after craniotomy. Lancet 1:384, 1980

25. North JB, Penhall R, Haneih A et al: Phenytoin and postoperative epilepsy: a randomized double blind trial. J Neurosurg 58:272, 1982

26. North JB, Penhall RK, Hanieh A et al: Phenytoin and postoperative epilepsy: a double blind study. J Neurosurg 58:672, 1983

27. Parker WA, Shearer CA: Phenytoin hepatotoxicity: a case report and review. Neurology 2:175, 1979

28. Rabinowicz AL, Ginsburg DL, Gott PS et al: Unruptured intracranial aneurysms: seizures and antiepileptic drug treatment. J Neurosurg (in press).

29. Rambeck B, Boenigk HE, Dunlop A et al: Predicting phenytoin dose—a revised nomogram. Ther Drug Monogr 1:325, 1979

30. Rapport RL, Penry JK: A survey of attitudes toward the pharmacological prophylaxis of post-traumatic epilepsy. J. Neurosurg 38:59, 1973

31. Rose FL, Sarner M: Epilepsy after ruptured intracranial aneurysms. Br Med J 1:18, 1965

32. Sbeih I, Tamas LB, O'Laoire SA: Epilepsy after operation for aneurysms. Neurosurgery 19:784, 1986

33. Shaw MD, Foy P, Chadwick D: The effectiveness of prophylactic anticonvulsant following neurosurgery. Acta Neurochir 69:253, 1983

34. Sobotka JL, Alexander B, Cook BL: A review of carbamazepine's hematologic reactions and monitoring recommendations. DICP Ann Pharmacother 24:1214, 1990

35. Temkin NR, Dikmen SS, Wilensky AJ: A randomized, double blind study of phenytoin for the prevention of posttraumatic seizures. N Engl J Med 323:497, 1990.

36. Treiman DM: Pharmacokinetics and clinical use of benzodiazepines in the management of status epilepticus. Epilepsia 30(Suppl 2):S4, 1989

37. Treiman DM, DeGiorgio CM, Ben-Menachem E et al: Lorazepam vs. phenytoin in the treatment of generalized convulsive status epilepticus. Report of an ongoing study. Neurology 35(Suppl 1):284, 1985

38. Treiman DM: Status epilepticus. p. 38. In Johnson RT (ed): Current Therapy in Neurological Diseases. 2nd Ed. BC Decker, Philadelphia, 1987.

39. Turnbull DM, Rawlins MD, Weighthan D, Chadwick DW: A comparison of phenytoin and valproate in previously untreated adult epileptic patients. J Neurol Neurosurg Psychiatry 45:55, 1982

40. Youmans JR, Cobb CA: Glial and neuronal tumors of the brain in adults. p. 2759. In Youmans JR (ed): Neurological Surgery. WB Saunders, Philadelphia, 1982

41. Young B, Rapp RP, Norton JA et al: Failure of prophylactically administered phenytoin to prevent early post-traumatic seizures. J. Neurosurg 58:231, 1983

42. Young B, Rapp RP, Norton JA et al: Failure of prophylactically administered phenytoin to prevent late post-traumatic seizures. J Neurosurg 58:236, 1983

43. Zaccara G, Muscas GC, Messori A: Clinical features, pathogenesis and management of drug-induced seizures. Drug Safety 5(2):109, 1990

11 Perioperative Cardiopulmonary Considerations

David T. Kawanishi

The success of a neurosurgical procedure may at times be compromised by a cardiopulmonary complication. Avoidance of such complications is preferable to emergent management after they occur. The anticipation of potential problems and the management planning necessary to avoid difficulties requires accurate preoperative diagnosis and timely assessment of patient status. Likewise, during and after surgery steady vigilance and evaluation of the patient based on constantly updated data are essential to provide support at a level sufficient to prevent serious complications or to deal with them quickly and appropriately should they occur. Although general screening and perioperative management guidelines have been helpful in providing a conceptual framework, they cannot be a substitute for close, individualized patient care when there are known underlying cardiopulmonary disorders in the neurosurgical patient.

There have been a number of reviews of noncardiac surgery in the cardiac patient.[27,57] The subject of perioperative management of patients with neurological disease also has been reviewed.[30] However, few data are available regarding cardiopulmonary management of the neurosurgical patient specifically. In general, the process of management involves a preoperative assessment of the patient with some form of assignment of risk for complications and a weighing of the risk : benefit ratio for proceeding with anesthesia and surgery. If the need for surgery is emergent, then the cardiopulmonary disorders must be managed in as supportive a manner as possible. If the surgery is elective, then steps may be taken to prepare the patient for surgery such as by obtaining control of hypertension or by stabilizing the patient with angina. As with all surgery, the earlier the medical disorders are recognized the more easily and completely they can be brought under control. Anticipation of the stress of the neurosurgical procedure and the institution of corrective or prophylactic measures to minimize the impact on the patient inherently involves some preoperative risk assignment.

Probably the most widely recognized formulation of preoperative cardiac risk from noncardiac surgery is the cardiac risk index (CRI) developed by Goldman et al.[16] By comparing preoperative characteristics with the incidence of life-threatening or fatal postoperative cardiovascular complications, this index provides one basis for identifying types of patients at higher or lower risk. The patients studied underwent a wide variety of anesthetic and surgical procedures. The features of the history, physical examination, and laboratory testing that comprise this index are shown in Table 11-1. The incidence of life-threatening complications was found to increase as the point total for any given patient increased from a low of 1 percent in class I patients ($=0$ to 5 points), to 7 percent for class II (6 to 12 points), to 14 percent for class III (13 to 25 points) and 78 percent for class IV (≥26 points). Likewise the cardiac death rate increased from 0.2 to 2, 2, and 56 percent, respectively, for classes I, II, III, and IV. Fully 53 percent (10 of

Table 11-1. Components of the Cardiac Risk Index

Components	Points
History	
Age over 70 years	5
Myocardial infarction within past 6 months	10
Physical examination	
Third heart sound or jugular venous distention	11
Significant aortic stenosis	3
Electrocardiogram	
Rhythm not sinus or presence of premature atrial complexes	7
More than five premature ventricular complexes per minute	7
General condition	
PO_2 <60 or PCO_2 >50 mmHg	
K^+ <3.0 or HCO_3 <20 mEq/L	
Blood urea nitrogen >50 or creatinine >3.0 mg/dl	
Abnormal SGOT (serum glutamic oxaloacetic transaminase)	
Chronic liver disease	
Bedridden patient	3
Type of operation	
Intraperitoneal, intrathoracic, or aortic	3
Emergency surgery	4
Total possible	53

(Adapted from Goldman et al.,[16] with permission.)

19) of all cardiac deaths in the 1,001 patients studied occurred in the class IV group. It should be noted that many of the points in this index are associated with remediable conditions.

Prospective application of this method of preoperative risk assessment has largely confirmed its validity.[21,56,59] These prospective studies also suggest that the physical status classification of the American Society of Anesthesiologists (ASA) may have similar predictive capabilities. In fact, a correspondence rate of 69 percent in terms of risk assignment between the two methods was observed.[56] The more recent studies have shown a lower incidence of cardiac events in the high-risk class IV patients, and it has been proposed that identification of these patients leads to better pre- and postoperative care with consequent improvement in outcome.[59] A more detailed review of the ASA classification is included in the anesthesiology chapters in this text. The data strongly support that careful preoperative evaluation and treatment of cardiac problems can lead to reduced complications.

Another important implication of studies of prospective application of the CRI is that cardiac risks can differ depending on specific surgical procedures. For example, patients undergoing abdominal aortic surgery have a significantly elevated risk of cardiac complication despite a low predicted risk based on the CRI.[21] The fact that the patients identified as being at high risk did indeed have a high rate of complications suggests that the CRI correctly identified patient-related factors that increased the risk of complication. However, during an abdominal aortic procedure, there is a high risk even to patients who would otherwise be considered at low cardiac risk for noncardiac surgery in general. This was attributed to a higher incidence of cardiovascular disease in patients undergoing this procedure. Patients with vascular disease of the central nervous system may be another similar group[30,49,52]; they may also have a higher incidence of associated cardiovascular disease and more careful preoperative evaluation and treatment may be warranted. There are no prospective studies on any neurosurgical procedures available at this time to document that such is the case.

There are other patient subsets in which the CRI may fail to identify those at increased risk of cardiac complications for noncardiac surgery. People over age 65 years appear to belong to one such group. A prospective evaluation of the CRI and the ASA classification in 120 patients aged 65 years or older who underwent intra-abdominal or intrathoracic noncardiac surgery found that the inability to do 2 minutes of supine bicycle exercise and increase heart rate to over 99 beats/min were the best independent predictors of perioperative cardiac complications.[12] Importantly, this study population was asymptomatic, and failure of the CRI to predict complications may have been a result of the lack of any patients falling into either CRI class I or IV. Though known to be subjective, nonspecific, and poorly reproducible, all the patients having perioperative complications were in ASA class III or IV. These data suggest that for patients over age 65 years a more conservative preoperative classification than the CRI may be more able to identify the tendency toward cardiac complications. Alternatively, or as an adjunct to management, preoperative exercise testing endurance may be helpful.

These classification systems do appear to be generally useful for stratifying a preoperative patient population into those groups with less or greater risk of perioperative cardiac complications. Until prospectively applied to specific surgical procedures and patient subsets, it would be hazardous to overextrapolate these data, however, Specifically, when lacking information regarding neurosurgical patients in particular, care must be used in assigning preoperative risk. Application of the current guidelines for the preoperative assignment of relative risk of cardiac complications may be helpful as a frame of reference.

Successful management of the individual patient, however, still depends on skill and judgment in tailoring general principles of pathophysiology and therapeutics to the needs of each patient.

GENERAL CONSIDERATIONS

Anesthesia and surgery are associated with hemodynamic and metabolic stresses that may increase the demands on an already impaired cardiovascular system. The patient undergoing a neurosurgical procedure may be subjected to perioperative pain, loss of intravascular volume, the stress of surgery itself, and possibly alterations of autonomic function that may provoke an increase of circulating catecholamines. The catecholamine stimulus should result in an appropriate compensatory tendency to conserve water, to maintain or increase cardiac output, and thus to maintain the circulation and perfusion of vital organs. However, the increased peripheral vascular resistance and increased intravascular volume, though usually well tolerated in normals, may lead to deleterious effects in patients with cardiac disease. These physiological changes usually result in an increased myocardial oxygen demand. If this demand exceeds the amount of oxygen that the coronary arteries can supply, then myocardial ischemia results. The more severe the underlying coronary disease, the less is the reserve and the less stress is required before the demand exceeds the supply. Manifestations of myocardial ischemia include angina, congestive heart failure, myocardial infarction, and electrical instability resulting in arrhythmias. In the presence of altered mental status, the usual early indicators of ischemia such as discomfort, weakness, angina, or dyspnea may not be appreciated, and this problem is the basis for careful monitoring of the electrocardiogram (ECG) and of intracardiac pressures and cardiac output in these patients.

The presence of a structural cardiac abnormality also may limit the ability to accommodate the demands of increased peripheral resistance, increased intravascular volume, and tachycardia associated with the attempt to respond to the stress of anesthesia and surgery. The presence of a stenotic valvular lesion will severely curtail the ability of the heart to increase output despite all these compensatory mechanisms, and congestive failure may result. A regurgitant lesion similarly may worsen in the face of increased vascular resistance. With dilation of the left ventricle, whether chronic because of cardiomyopathy or resulting from acute myocardial failure such as that due to ischemia, mitral regurgitation may newly appear or worsen. Left ventricular hypertrophy with attendant stiffening of the ventricles will increase the tendency to elevation of left atrial pressure in response to increased volume.[33] Again, congestive heart failure may be easily provoked. Finally, myocardial changes such as dilation, hypertrophy, fibrosis, or scarring whether in the ventricles or atria, may predispose to arrhythmias with increased sensitivity to the arrhythmogenic effects of catecholamines and metabolic abnormalities.

In the perioperative management of coronary disease, the goal is to minimize myocardial oxygen demand while avoiding any compromise of coronary blood flow or oxygen content. In the setting of valvular or myopericardial disease, intravascular volume and peripheral resistance changes must be carefully regulated. Attention to the underlying cardiac disorder and modulation of the catecholamine response may be helpful in managing a tendency toward arrhythmias.

It is known that the rates of cardiovascular complications and mortality do not differ according to whether regional or general anesthesia is used.[37,42] Regional anesthesia may be associated with less myocardial dysfunction and respiratory depression. However, the effects of marked changes in vascular tone resulting from regional anesthesia may be deleterious in some cardiac disorders. For example, in aortic valvular stenosis or hypertrophic cardiomyopathy with left ventricular outflow tract obstruction, the heart cannot accommodate a marked reduction in peripheral arterial resistance, as there is a structural limitation to left ventricular outflow. Severe hypotension may therefore result. Excessive dilation of the systemic veins likewise may be poorly tolerated if the right ventricle is diseased and critically dependent on adequate venous return for maintenance of right ventricular output. The choice of anesthesia should be made by the anesthesiologist with consideration of the particular nature of the cardiac disorder.

ISCHEMIC HEART DISEASE

Among patients undergoing noncardiac surgery after recent myocardial infarction, a decrease in perioperative reinfarction occurs as the interval between initial infarction and surgery increases (Table 11-2).[47,50] The precise reason for this is not clear. There has been a trend toward a reduced reinfarction rate in the more recent studies than in the older studies.[36,58] In one of the recent ones, perioperative invasive hemodynamic monitoring was aggressively applied. Also, newer cardiac drugs such as β-blockers,

Table 11-2. Perioperative Reinfarction Rate

Author	Year of Study	Reinfarction Rate Time of Surgery After First Infarction		
		(0–3 mo)	(4–6 mo)	(>6 mo)
Tarhan et al.[50]	1967–1968	37	16	4–5
Steen et al.[47]	1974–1975	27	11	5
Wells and Kaplan[58]	1981	0	—	—
Rao et al.[36]	1983	6	2	—

dopamine, and intravenous nitroglycerin had become available. These observations suggest that, although delay of surgery for 6 months after prior infarction reduces reinfarction rate, aggressive management with invasive hemodynamic monitoring may now permit earlier operation with risk comparable to that achieved by waiting in the past.

For an individual patient, the extent of left ventricular dysfunction and residual myocardial ischemia following the infarction may also contribute to the risk of reinfarction with surgery. For example, following an uncomplicated acute infarction, the 1-year mortality rate increases from approximately 2 percent in those without severe left ventricular dysfunction and no provokable ischemia on exercise testing to 25 percent in those who have severe left ventricular dysfunction.[8] One component of the increased surgical risk in these patients may be the tendency for patients with known heart failure preoperatively to develop perioperative pulmonary edema.[17] Additionally, the presence of residual myocardium at risk of ischemia in patients with recent infarction should always be considered a possibility. The improved outcome of patients undergoing surgery early after an acute infarction in the more recent trials suggest that current aggressive management is more successful in preserving a favorable balance between myocardial oxygen supply and demand, although this remains an unproven hypothesis.

Patients with unstable angina are probably at equal, or greater, risk of infarction and cardiac complications than patients with recent infarction if the urgency of the procedure does not allow for coronary arteriography and revascularization.[19,53,57] When coronary artery bypass graft surgery (CABG) can be successfully accomplished, the risk of perioperative reinfarction appears to be low.[11,28] Use of the intra-aortic balloon pump improves coronary flow and also provides reduction of peripheral resistance and thereby reduction of myocardial oxygen demand. Ischemia is often relieved, but there is a reported risk

of vascular complications of up to 18 percent.[10,41] Newer equipment with smaller diameter sheaths may reduce this complication rate. Revascularization through percutaneous transluminal coronary angioplasty (PTCA) may be an alternative to coronary bypass surgery. There are currently five randomized trials underway comparing PTCA to CABG in patients with unstable angina, recent myocardial infarction, and severe stable angina.[38] Although none will study the effect of PTCA on perioperative complications, there may be implications regarding the adequacy of reperfusion by PTCA. In patients in whom PTCA produces complete revascularization, there would appear to be no disadvantage as regards risk for neurosurgical procedures compared with revascularization by CABG.

Patients who have stable exertional angina only appear to be at relatively low risk for cardiac complications with noncardiac surgery.[14] Perioperative mortality may be reduced from 2.4 to 0.9 percent by having CABG prior to the noncardiac surgery. However, in the Coronary Artery Surgery Study, this was achieved only at the expense of a 1.4 percent operative mortality from the CABG procedure so that the overall mortality remained the same as medical management.[11] PTCA may have a lower mortality rate than CABG and may be a preferable alternative to either CABG or medical management alone, but this has not yet been proven.

As the prior discussion suggests, careful management of hemodynamics via invasive monitoring may facilitate maintenance of an adequate balance between myocardial oxygen supply and demand. As heart rate is a primary determinant of demand, its control is important. Also the maintenance of adequate, but not excessive, filling pressures may be critical.

The medication regimen available for control of myocardial ischemia for the perioperative patient usually must be limited to parenteral or topical routes of delivery. Nitroglycerin is available for either parenteral or transdermal delivery. Of the β-blockers, the short-acting agent esmolol can be used intravenously, usually for control of transient increases of heart rate. The longer acting metoprolol also can be given intravenously, as can propranolol, and either is preferable to the short-acting agent for angina control. At present, of the calcium channel blockers only verapamil is available in parenteral form.[32] It has found specific usage for control of intraoperative coronary artery spasm. Although nifedipine may be given sublingually, probably its major route of absorption is via gastrointestinal absorption.

Since most postoperative myocardial infarctions occur at 2 to 5 days after surgery, the patient must be closely followed for at least this length of time. The consultant should also be aware that up to 61 percent of such infarctions occur without angina.[47] The importance of adhering to the general principles of management of ischemic heart disease cannot be overstated.

HYPERTENSION

Few studies exist that may serve as a basis for establishing guidelines for management of hypertension in the perioperative neurosurgical patient. As a rule, for noncardiac surgery there is apparently no benefit derived in terms of reduced cardiovascular complications by preoperatively controlling hypertension to below a diastolic pressure of 110 mmHg.[15] Also independent of the level of preoperative control, hypotension or hypertension can be expected to occur perioperatively in 25 percent of patients known to be hypertensive.[15,35] Neither of the available studies included or specifically evaluated neurosurgical procedures, however.

The cerebrovascular system is known to be fairly tightly autoregulated. The range of pressures through which flow can be maintained may be elevated as a consequence of prolonged poorly controlled hypertension, however. Perhaps of special significance for the neurosurgical patient, it has been noted in some of the studies that the responses to anesthesia and surgery were such that the lowest systolic blood pressure observed intraoperatively tended to be higher in patients with a history of hypertension and concomitant renal or cerebrovascular complications. This was independent of the in-hospital preoperative level of systolic pressure.[15] It was not clear, however, whether this resulted from a conscious attempt by the anesthesiologist to maintain blood pressure at higher levels in these patients. Since those patients with heart failure or ischemic heart disease did not

have significantly different pressures from those of patients with uncomplicated hypertension, the data suggest that hypertensive patients with renal or cerebrovascular complications have more inherent resistance to lowering of pressure in the perioperative setting. Important also is the observation that patients with persistent hypertension preoperatively tend to have a greater absolute decrease of pressure intraoperatively than their more tightly controlled counterparts.[15,35] If autoregulation of cerebral blood flow is adjusted to significantly higher pressures, such decreases would tend to argue in favor of gradual preoperative reduction of pressures to avoid provoking cerebral ischemia.

Patients with heart failure or ischemic heart disease had intraoperative systolic blood pressure nadirs that did not differ from those of patients with uncomplicated hypertension. The inference that perioperative blood pressure lability is more a function of a patient's inherent vascular characteristics rather than a reflection of pharmacological modification of those characteristics was further supported by the data showing that new hypertensive events in the perioperative period were more common in patients with a history of severe increases prehospitalization regardless of the success of tight preoperative control of the blood pressure.[15] In practice, it would appear that there is little to be gained by over-rigorous attempts to obtain tight regulation of blood pressure preoperatively or reduction to below a diastolic pressure of 110 mmHg, at least in regard to the effect of such treatment on intraoperative lability of the pressures. Untreated or inadequately treated hypertensives do have a greater absolute fall in pressure intraoperatively, however, and may need closer and more careful anesthesia management to avoid myocardial ischemia resulting from intraoperative hypotension.[15]

The type of operative procedure also can have an impact on intraoperative pressure. There is a strong correlation of abdominal aortic aneurysm resection and peripheral vascular procedures, particularly carotid endarterectomy, and perioperative hypertension. This was independent of cardiovascular complications of the hypertension.[17] The maximum pressures appear 2 to 3 hours postoperatively.[55] There are no data specifically on neurosurgical procedures and perioperative blood pressure.

Perioperative cardiovascular complications are not strongly influenced by the presence of hypertension, the extent of hypertension control, or the severity of prior hypertension.[16,17] Hypertensives subjected to 50 percent or more reduction of pressure intraoperatively or to a reduction of 33 percent for more than 10 minutes do have increased rates of intraoperative and postoperative cardiac complications[15,35] and perioperative myocardial ischemia.[29] Although there are certain procedures known to be accompanied by hypertensive episodes, none in particular are associated with lower pressures. This may reflect the effectiveness of close surveillance and treatment by the anesthesiologist more than the pathophysiology of patient or operation, however, as fluid challenges or adrenergic agents tend to be used more frequently for those types of procedures that might be associated with hypotension: 39 percent of abdominal aortic aneurysm resections, 25 percent of peripheral vascular operations, and 14 percent of other procedures.[15] In a series of 676 operations, one of the anesthetic agents commonly used, halothane, particularly when combined with nitrous oxide, had a particularly hypotensive effect by way of decreasing cardiac output.[15,34] Patients with known cardiac disease and coronary artery disease in particular should be closely monitored and any perioperative hypotension quickly corrected.

Preoperatively, patients fare better if their antihypertensive medications are continued up to the time of operation.[15,35] Withdrawal syndromes with rebound hypertension and sympathetic overactivity have been recognized after discontinuation of methyldopa[20] and clonidine.[1,6,7,20] The hypertension rebound with clonidine might be exaggerated in the presence of β-blockade, which leaves the α-vasconstrictors unopposed.[1] Clonidine is available in a transdermal patch preparation, but, since therapeutic steady-state levels require 48 to 72 hours to be reached, it should be started well in advance of the surgery.

Among the other antihypertensive agents, abrupt withdrawal of a β-blocker in patients with ischemic heart disease is generally not advised. Metoprolol is available in an intravenous preparation. There appear to be no true withdrawal syndromes associated with either the angiotensin-converting enzyme inhibitors or the calcium channel antagonists. Among these, the calcium channel antagonist verapamil and diltiazem are available in intravenous form.

A most critical period for complications in the cardiac patient or hypertensive person is during intubation and anesthesia induction, when reflex stimulation of the autonomic system results in potentially marked increases in blood pressure and heart rate. At this and other times intraoperatively, hypertension may be treated either with increased depth of anesthesia or intravenous medications such as nitroprusside, hydralazine, nitroglycerin, α-methyldopa, or phentolamine. Hypertension associated with volume overload should improve with intravenous diuretic administration.

Postoperative hypertension usually occurs soon after discontinuation of artificial ventilation or in the recovery room. Provocative factors include volume overload, anxiety, pain, and hypoxemia. Management can include diuretics, pain medications, and supplemental oxygen. Parenteral agents such as nitroprusside, parenteral hydralazine, or methyldopa for its delayed effects at 4 hours may be useful for tiding the patient over this period of postoperative stress.

VALVULAR HEART DISEASE

Patients who have valvular heart disease and who undergo anesthesia and noncardiac surgery are at risk for both general problems associated with diminished cardiac reserve and special problems such as infection (endocarditis), tachycardia, embolization, and acute pulmonary edema or sudden death. The pressure-overloaded chambers associated with valvular stenosis and the volume-overloaded chambers associated with regurgitant lesions tolerate volume overload poorly. Because of the obligate diminution of flow rate associated with a narrowed valve orifice, patients with valvular stenosis cannot accommodate tachycardia well either. These patients are prone to congestive heart failure, and, as might be expected, worse outcomes are associated with worse preoperative functional class.[16,45] Patients with clinically evident congestive failure should be treated and brought into a compensated state, if at all possible. For patients with a severe valve lesion who are to undergo an elective procedure, surgical valve repair or replacement first should always be considered an option. For aortic stenosis, percutaneous balloon valvuloplasty may be an option to allow stabilization of the patient in order to tolerate noncardiac surgery better.[18,24,26,40] Results of percutaneous balloon commissurotomy for mitral stenosis have been even more long-lasting than for aortic stenosis and may not only allow stabilization of the patient but also result in definitive treatment.[25] Patients with severe regurgitant lesions may require valve surgery before an elective noncardiac operation. Medical management of valvular regurgitation with afterload reduction and careful titration of the preload may result in sufficient improvement to allow noncardiac surgery.[48]

Patients with prosthetic heart valves pose a special problem because of their chronic anticoagulation therapy. Discontinuation of chronic anticoagulation during the perioperative period usually can be accomplished with minimal risk of thrombosis on a normally functioning prosthesis. Factors that tend to increase risk include location of the prosthesis, abnormal function of the prosthesis, presence of atrial fibrillation, presence of other cardiac disease such as congestive heart failure due to myocardial dysfunction, or associated noncardiac problems such as carotid or other peripheral artery disease or chronic venous stasis. At least one study found that overall risk was low: coumadin was discontinued an average of 2.9 days preoperatively in 159 patients and resumed 2.7 days postoperatively with no thromboembolic complications.[54] The influence of valve location is indicated by the findings of another study in which no thromboemblic complications occurred in 25 patients with an aortic valve prosthesis and in 2 of 10 patients with a mitral prosthesis.[22] More recent studies suggest the possibility of identifying patients at higher risk of thromboembolism formation using transesophageal echocardiography to visualize sluggish intracardiac flows.[3]

In individuals thought to be at greater risk of thromboembolism formation than the average person, an alternative management approach is to begin intravenous heparin therapy at some time after discontinuation of oral anticoagulants until about 6 hours before the operation. Then heparin may be resumed postoperatively at 36 to 48 hours or when the risk of hemorrhage at the surgery site is deemed to have sufficiently decreased, and the patient subsequently may be converted back to treatment with oral anticoagulants.

Antibiotic prophylaxis against endocarditis is usually performed in conjunction with the guidelines of the American Heart Association.[44] Use of antibiotics is recommended whenever the surgical procedure can result in transient bacteremia in the presence of damaged or abnormal valves, prosthetic valves, or

Table 11-3. Prophylactic Antibiotic Regimens for Endocarditis

	Oral	Parenteral
Dental/respiratory tract procedures		
Standard	Penicillin V 2.0 g 1 h before 1.0 g 6 h after	Aqueous penicillin 2 × 10 6 units IV or 1 h 30–60 min before 1 × 10 6 units 6 h after
Special First: (e.g., prosthetic valves)		Ampicillin 1–2 g 1 hr or + Gentamicin 1.5 mg/kg 1 hr 30 min before
Then, either	Penicillin V 1 g 6 h after or	Repeat above medication 8 h after
Penicillin allergic	Erythromycin 1.0 g 1 h before 500 mg 6 h after	Vancomycin 1 g IV 1 h before
Gastrointestinal/genitourinary procedures		
Standard		Ampicillin 2 g 1 h or IV + Gentamicin 1.5 mg/kg 1 h or IV 30 min before Repeat 8 h later
Special	Amoxiciliin 3 g 1 h before 1.5 g 6 h after	
Penicillin allergic		Vancomycin 1 g IV 1 h before Gentamicin 1.5 mg/kg IV or 1 h before May repeat 8–12 h after

(Adapted from Shulman et al.[44])

congenital anatomical defects, with the exception of isolated secundum type of atrial septal defects. Included in the indications for antibiotic prophylaxis are patients with ventriculoatrial shunts for hydrocephalus, as bacterial endocarditis in them has been reported.[44] Recommendations for use of prophylactic antibiotics for patients with mitral prolapse is not clear from the data because the rate of bacterial endocarditis in these patients is very low. Routine use of antibiotic is generally not recommended; instead such use is currently reserved for patients in whom the presence of mitral regurgitation has been documented.[4,9,31]

The type of antibiotic used is generally dependent on the type of bacterial exposure expected from the surgical procedure (Table 11-3). Patient-related factors, especially allergies, need also to be considered.

CONGESTIVE HEART FAILURE/CARDIOMYOPATHIES

In neurosurgical patients with congestive heart failure, perioperative risk and management will be based on the underlying etiology. Heart failure, if severely decompensated, will increase the risk of surgery as described in the preceding sections.[16,17] If at all possible, the coronary disease (or the valvular lesion) in such severe cases may need definitive correction. If the patient can be brought to a compensated state with medical therapy, careful monitoring of intracardiac (filling) pressures, oxygenation/ventilation, and arrhythmias may allow the neurosurgical procedure to proceed safely without correcting the underlying lesion, as described above.

Among the cardiomyopathies, the hypertrophic cardiomyopathies associated with idiopathic hypertrophic subaortic stenosis (IHSS) are characterized by dynamic obstruction of the left ventricular outflow tract.[5,13] Thus obstruction to outflow and therefore a drop in cardiac outflow and systemic pressures tend to occur whenever there is a stimulation of cardiac contractility. Since any event that results in a compensatory sympathetic response will produce such a response, vasodilation, hypovolemia (which also worsens the situation by decreasing cardiac chamber volumes and thereby enhancing outflow tract obstruction further), hypotension, hypoxia, and pain must be avoided. Direct inotropic stimulation using drugs such as digitalis also would be counterproductive in such cases. In one series of 56 patients, intra- or postoperative hypotension requiring vasoconstric-

tor therapy occurred in less than 10 percent of cases.[51]

CONGENITAL HEART DISEASE

Patients with congenital heart disease should have the same precautions taken with regard to antibiotic prophylaxis against bacterial endocarditis as described above for those who have valvular heart disease. Those patients who have cyanotic congenital heart disease, that is, an appreciable right-to-left shunt, may have considerable polycythemia. They are at risk of intra- or postoperative bleeding due to associated coagulopathies and thrombocytopemia. This risk can be reduced by phlebotomy.[46] Some authors suggest, however, that the risk of hypotension, which would worsen the right-to-left shunt and possibly lead to shock, may be excessive and that phlebotomy really is not justifiable unless the hematocrit exceeds 70 percent.[27]

Patients with cyanotic congenital heart disease in whom by definition there is already a large right-to-left shunt tolerate systemic arterial vasodilation and/or hypotension poorly. This circumstance creates a decrease in systemic resistance, which favors the right-to-left shunt, thereby allowing more venous blood to pass into the arterial system, bypassing the pulmonary circulation. Occasionally, vasoconstrictive agents may be necessary to reduce shunt flow in these patients. They are also at risk for paradoxical emboli so that meticulous surgical technique must be used to avoid allowing air and solutions into the venous system, which then can inadvertently enter the arterial system.

ARRHYTHMIAS

To the extent that many arrhythmias occur in conjunction with some underlying heart disease, both ventricular and atrial arrhythmias appear to represent a risk factor for the development of cardiac complications in noncardiac surgery.[16] However, patients with premature ventricular contractions (PVCs) in the absence of underlying heart disease appear to have a normal prognosis for cardiac disease and may not be at any increased risk.[23] Therefore there is currently no data to support the routine aggressive suppression of asymptomatic PVCs perioperatively.

Supraventricular tachyarrhythmias in the postoperative period may occur less frequently in patients receiving digitalis, or, if they do occur, the heart rate may be slower than in patients not receiving digitalis.[2,17,43] Parenteral β-blockers or diltiazem may produce similar rate control.[39] Patients who are particularly prone to supraventricular arrhythmias, such as the elderly or those with valvular stenosis, should be considered for preoperative therapy if they are not already taking digoxin or some other antiarrhythmic drug.

Patients with conduction defects such as complete heart block may not derive sufficient chronotropic response from their secondary rhythm. Either temporary or permanent pacing should be considered before such patients undergo any procedures that might place increased demands on the cardiovascular system. In patients with lesser degrees of heart block, prophylactic pacing is usually not necessary. The exception is in those patients with second-degree arteriovenous block type II (non-Wenckebach type) or bifascicular block who also have a history of syncope or intermittent third-degree block. Any patient who develops new bifascicular block in the perioperative period, including early postoperatively, might also be considered for temporary pacing.

Patients with devices such as permanent pacemakers or automatic implantable cardiac defibrillators may be given antibiotic prophylaxis for endocarditis, although there are no data to support the need or benefit. Electrocautery in the vicinity of permanent pacemakers or the leads should be avoided.

CHRONIC LUNG DISEASE

In general, patients with chronic lung or airways disease can be brought through noncardiac surgery without complications. Preoperative pulmonary function testing and blood gases should be done, and any reversible parameters should be optimized. Bronchodilators, adequate hydration, and training in use of incentive spirometry and good pulmonary toilet may be helpful and certainly beneficial to patient education. In the presence of acute pulmonary infection, the surgical procedure should be delayed, if possible. Bullous lung disease patients are at risk of pneumothorax with positive pressure ventilation. Patients with severe pulmonary hypertension are particularly at risk of decreased cardiac output or ventricular fibrillation with hypovolemia. Such patients also appear to be at higher risk of atrial arrhythmias, particularly multifocal atrial tachycardia.[27] Preoperative optimization of the patient and careful perioperative monitoring to minimize perturbation of hemodynamics and oxygenation/ventilation, as with the

cardiac disorders described above, should minimize the risk of complications in these patients.

REFERENCES

1. Bailey RR, Neale TJ: Rapid clonidine withdrawal with blood pressure overshoot exaggerated by beta-blockade. Br Med J 1:942, 1976
2. Bergh NP, Dotturi O, Malmberg R: Prophylactic digitalis in thoracic surgery. Scand J Respir Dis 48:197, 1967
3. Black IW, Hopkins AP, Lee LCL, Walsh WF: Left atrial spontaneous echo contrast: a clinical and echocardiographic analysis. J Am Coll Cardiol 18:398, 1991
4. Bor DH, Himmelstein DV: Endocarditis prophylaxis for patients with mitral valve prolapse. Am J Med 76:711, 1984
5. Braunwald E, Lambrew CT, Rockoff SD et al: Idiopathic hypertrophic subaortic stenosis. I. A description of the disease based upon an analysis of 64 patients. Circulation 30(Suppl):3, 1964
6. Brodsky JB, Bravo JJ: Acute postoperative clonidine withdrawal syndrome. Anesthesiology 44:519, 1976
7. Bruce DL, Croley TF, Lee JS: Preoperative clonidine withdrawal syndrome. Anesthesiology 51:90, 1979
8. DeBusk R, Blomquist C, Kouchoukos N et al: Identification and treatment of low-risk patients after acute myocardial infarction and coronary artery bypass graft surgery. N Engl J Med 314:161, 1986
9. Durack DT: Current issues in prevention of infective endocarditis. Am J Med 78(Suppl 68):149, 1985
10. Foster E, Olsson C, Rutenberg A et al: Mechanical circulatory assistance with intraaortic balloon counterpulsation for major abdominal surgery. Ann Surg 183:73, 1976
11. Foster E, Davis K, Carpenter J et al: Risk of noncardiac operation in patients with defined coronary artery disease: the Coronary Artery Surgery Study (CASS) Registry experience. Am Thorac Surg 41:42, 1986
12. Gerson MC, Hurst JM, Hertzberg VS et al: Cardiac prognosis in noncardiac geriatric surgery. Ann Intern Med 103:832, 1985
13. Glancy DL, Shepherd RL, Beiser GD, Epstein SE: The dynamic nature of left ventricular outflow obstruction in idiopathic hypertrophic subaortic stenosis. Ann Intern Med 75:589, 1971
14. Goldman L: Cardiac risks and complications of noncardiac surgery. Ann Intern Med 98:504, 1983
15. Goldman L, Caldera DL: Risks of general anesthesia and elective operation in the hypertensive patient. Anesthesiology 50:285, 1979
16. Goldman L, Caldera DL, Nussbaum SR et al: Multifactorial index of cardiac risk in noncardiac surgical procedures. N Engl J Med 297:845, 1977
17. Goldman L, Caldera D, Southwick F et al: Cardiac risk factors and complications in non-cardiac surgery. Medicine 297:845, 1977

18. Hayes SN, Holmes DR, Nishimura RA et al: Palliative percutaneous aortic balloon valvuloplasty before non-cardiac operations and invasive diagnostic procedures. Mayo Clin Proc 64:753, 1989

19. Horowitz R, Morganroth J, Levy W: Evaluation and management of the surgical patient with coronary artery disease. p. 87. In Goldman D (ed): Medical Care of the Surgical Patient. JB Lippincott, Philadelphia, 1982

20. Houston M: Abrupt cessation of treatment in hypertension: consideration of clinical features, mechanisms, prevention and management of the discontinuation syndrome. Am Heart J 102:415, 1981

21. Jeffrey CC, Kusman J, Cullen DJ, Brewster DC: A prospective evaluation of cardiac risk index. Anesthesiology 58:462, 1983

22. Katholi RE, Nolan SP, McGuire LB: Living with prosthetic heart valve. Subsequent noncardiac operations and the risk of thromboembolism or hemorrhage. Am Heart J 92:162, 1976

23. Kennedy HL, Whitlock JA, Sprague MK et al: Long-term follow-up of asymptomatic healthy subjects with frequent and complex ventricular ectopy. N Engl J Med 312:193, 1985

24. Kulick DL, Kawanishi DT, Reid CL, Rahimtoola SH: Catheter balloon valvuloplasty in adults, part I: Aortic stenosis. Curr Probl Cardiol 15:355, 1990

25. Kulick DL, Kawanishi DT, Reid CL, Rahimtoola SH: Catheter balloon commissurotomy in adults, part II: mitral and other stenoses. Curr Probl Cardiol 15:399, 1990

26. Levine MJ, Berman AD, Safian RD et al: Palliation of valvular aortic stenosis by balloon valvuloplasty as preoperative preparation for noncardiac surgery. Am J Cardiol 62:1309, 1988

27. Logue B, Kaplan JA: The cardiac patient and noncardiac surgery. Curr Probl Cardiol 7:1, 1982

28. Mahar L, Steen P, Tinker J et al: Perioperative myocardial infarction in patients with coronary artery disease with and without aorta-coronary artery bypass grafts. J Thorac Cardiovasc Surg 76:533, 1978

29. Mauney FM, Ebert PA, Sabiston DC Jr: Postoperative myocardial infarction: a study of predisposing factors, diagnosis and mortality in a high risk group of surgical patients. Ann Surg 172:497, 1970

30. Merli GJ, Bell RD: Preoperative management of the surgical patient with neurologic disease. Med Clin North Am 71:511, 1987

31. Mills P, Rose J, Hollingsworth J et al: Long-term prognosis of mitral valve prolapse. N Engl J Med 297:13, 1977

32. Nussmeier NA, Slogoff S: Verapamil treatment of intraoperative coronary artery spasm. Anesthesiology 62:539, 1985

33. Peterson KL, Tsuji J, Johnson A et al: Diastolic left ventricular pressure-volume and stress strain relations in patients with valvular aortic stenosis and left ventricular hypertrophy. Circulation 58:77, 1978

34. Prys-Roberts C, Foex P, Green LT et al: Studies of anesthesia in relation to hypertension. IV: The effects of artificial ventilation on the circulation and pulmonary gas exchanges. Br J Anaesth 44:335, 1972

35. Prys-Roberts C, Meloche R, Foex P: Studies of anesthesia in response to hypertension. Br J Anaesth 43:122, 1971

36. Rao T, Jacobs K, El-Etr A: Reinfarction following anesthesia in patients with myocardial infarction. Anesthesiology 59:499, 1983

37. Rogers MC: Anesthetic management of patients with heart disease. Modern Concepts of Cardiovascular Disease 52:29, 1983

38. Rouben GS: Status of percutaneous transluminal coronary angioplasty. Curr Probl Cardiol 15:723, 1990

39. Roth A, Harrison E, Mitani G et al: Efficacy and safety of medium- and high-dose diltiazem alone and in combination with digoxin for control of heart rate at rest and during exercise in patients with chronic atrial fibrillation. Circulation 73:316, 1986

40. Roth RB, Palacios IF, Block PC: Percutaneous aortic balloon valvuloplasty: its role in the management of patients with aortic stenosis requiring major noncardiac surgery. J Am Coll Cardiol 13:1039, 1989

41. Sanfelippo P, Baker N, Ewy HG et al: Experience with intraaortic balloon counterpulsation. Ann Thorac Surg 41:36, 1986

42. Sapala J, Arkins R, Tinker J: Perioperative myocardial infarction. Semin Anesth 1:253, 1982

43. Selzer A, Walter RM: Adequacy of preoperative digitalis therapy in controlling ventricular rate in postoperative atrial fibrillation. Circulation 34:119, 1966

44. Shulman ST, Amren DP, Bisno AL et al: Prevention of bacterial endocarditis: a statement for health professionals by the committee on rheumatic fever and infective endocarditis of the Council on Cardiovascular Disease in the Young. Circulation 70:1123A, 1984

45. Skinner JF, Pearce ML: Surgical risk in the cardiac patient. J Chronic Dis 17:54, 1964

46. Sommerville J, McDonald L, Edgill M: Postoperative hemorrhage and related abnormalities of blood coagulation in cyanotic congenital heart disease. Br Heart J 27:440, 1965

47. Steen P, Tinker J, Tarhan S: Myocardial reinfarction after anesthesia and surgery. JAMA 239:2566, 1978

48. Stone JG, Hoar PF, Calabro JR et al: After load reduction and preload augmentation improve the anesthetic management of patients with cardiac failure and valvular regurgitation. Anesth Analg 59:737, 1980

49. Sundt TM, Sandok BA, Whisnant JP: Carotid endarterectomy: complications and preoperative assessment of risk. Mayo Clin Proc 50:301, 1975

50. Tarhan S, Moffitt E, Taylor W, Givliani E: Myocardial infarction after general anesthesia. JAMA 220:1451, 1972

51. Thompson RC, Liberthson RR, Lowenstein E: Perioperative anesthetic risk of noncardiac surgery in hypertrophic obstructive cardiomyopathy. JAMA 254:2419, 1985

52. Thompson JE, Putman RD, Talkington CM: Asymptomatic carotid bruits: long term outcome of patients having endarterectomy compared with unoperated controls. Ann Surg 188:308, 1978

53. Tinker J, Noback C, Vliestra R, Frye R: Management of patients with heart disease for noncardiac surgery. JAMA 246:1348, 1981

54. Tinker JH, Tarhan S: Discontinuing anticoagulant therapy in surgical patients with cardiac valve prosthesis. JAMA 239:738, 1978

55. Towne JB, Bernhard VM: The relationship of postoperative hyptertension to complication following carotid endarterectomy. Surgery 88:575, 1980

56. Waters J, Wilkinson C, Golman M et al: Evaluation of cardiac risk in noncardiac surgical patients, abstracted. Anesthesiology 55(Suppl 3A):A343, 1981

57. Weitz HH, Goldman L: Noncardiac surgery in the patient with heart disease. Med Clin North Am 71:413, 1987

58. Wells PH, Kaplan JA: Optimal management of patients with ischemic heart disease for noncardiac surgery by complementary anesthesiologist and cardiologist interaction. Am Heart J 102:1029, 1981

59. Zeldin R: Assessing cardiac risk in patients who undergo non-cardiac surgical procedures. Can J Surg 27:402, 1984

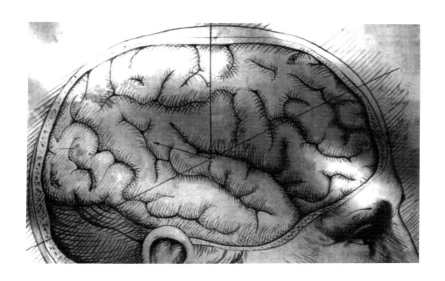

Supratentorial Procedures

Part 2: Neoplastic Disorders

12 General Considerations

Charles B. Wilson

As later chapters in this volume cover the major categories of supratentorial tumors, most of my general considerations regarding the potential complications of brain surgery concern supratentorial tumors approached through the cranium. Only in a final and brief section will I comment on the transsphenoidal approach to primarily intrasellar neoplastic conditions. Pituitary adenomas, although supratentorial tumors in the strict sense, are customarily excluded from the category.

To place the following chapters in perspective, I reviewed all serious postoperative complications for supratentorial tumors treated at my own institution during the years 1984 through 1990. Excluded were the transsphenoidal procedures and operations in which removal of tumor was not the primary objective. This retrospective provided a frame of reference in which to determine the frequency of complications and their relationships to operations on particular tumors. During the period so defined, 1,771 craniotomies were performed. The relative frequency of any particular complication changes from year to year and it appears that serious complications may be less frequent today than they were a decade ago as a consequence of improvements in medical care generally. For these reasons, the postoperative complications occurring in the 346 patients undergoing craniotomies for brain tumor performed during 1990 were selected for separate analysis as representing contemporary experience (Table 12-1).

Postoperative complications, whether fatal or not, have a profound effect on the results of surgery for supratentorial tumors. Among 346 patients undergoing craniotomy during 1990 (Tables 12-1 and 12-2), for example, 35 patients had 40 serious complications, for a case incidence of 10 percent. Most of the complications (25 of 40) were directly attributable to the operation, whereas a smaller number (15 of 40) were related indirectly to the operation. Stated simply, 1 of 10 patients undergoing a craniotomy for a supratentorial tumor suffered a complication that had a significant effect on recovery and the ultimate outcome of the procedure.

For the purposes of this discussion, I have separated the fatal and the nonfatal complications. This distinction is to some degree artificial because certain fatal complications might have been nonfatal complications if management were improved, and similarly almost any nonfatal complication, managed inappropriately, could result directly or indirectly in a fatal outcome. Nonetheless, as a format for discussing the avoidance and management of complications, the distinction seems justified.

The 37 deaths occurring among the 1,771 patients reviewed represent a mortality rate of 2.1 percent (Table 12-3). Unexpected tumors harbored by patients who died were pituitary adenoma, lymphoma, sarcoma, craniopharyngioma, and colloid cyst (Table 12-4), which are relatively less common tumor types. The added risks associated with advanced age and reoperation account for the deaths in some cases, and for unknown reasons a high proportion of deaths in this group related indirectly to the operation.

FATAL COMPLICATIONS RELATED DIRECTLY TO THE OPERATIVE PROCEDURE

Herniation

Herniation was responsible for the majority of the deaths related to surgery, and two-thirds of those deaths were caused by edema. Excluding brain

Table 12-1. Supratentorial Brain Tumors among 346 Patients Undergoing Craniotomy and 126 Undergoing Adenomectomy during 1990

Tumor	Patients (No.)	(%)
Astrocytoma	142	41.0
Meningioma	67	19.4
Glioblastoma	54	15.6
Craniopharyngioma	18	5.2
Metastatic	15	4.3
Oligodendroglioma	11	3.2
Ependymoma	6	1.7
Colloid cyst	5	1.5
Other	28	8.1
Total	346	100.0
Pituitary adenoma	126	100.0

edema attributable to anesthesia and desiccation of the surface of unprotected brain, the principal causes of postoperative edema are three: excessive retraction, interference with venous drainage, and cerebral infarction.

Excessive retraction is most likely to occur when the brain is full, although excessive retraction pressure can also be applied to a well-relaxed hemi-

Table 12-2. Postoperative Complications in 35 Patients among 346 Undergoing Craniotomy for Supratentorial Brain Tumors[a] during 1990[b]

Complication/Status	Patients (No.)	(%)
Direct relation to operation		
Neurological deficit	9	2.6
Wound infection	4	1.2
Hematoma	5[c]	1.5
Cerebrospinal fluid leak	2	0.6
Diabetes insipidus	2	0.6
Aseptic meningitis	2	0.6
Negative biopsy	1	0.3
Total complications	25	7.2
Indirect relation to operation		
Deep venous thrombosis	6	1.7
Pneumonia	3	0.9
Sepsis, drug toxicity, hyponatremia, urinary tract infection, IV site infection	1	0.3
Pulmonary embolism	6	1.7
Total complications	15	4.3

[a] Pituitary adenomas excluded.
[b] Case incidence = 10%.
[c] Epidural in one patient, subdural in one, tumor bed in three.

Table 12-3. Cause of Death among 1,771 Patients Undergoing Craniotomy for Resection of Supratentorial Brain Tumors

	Patients (No.)	(%)
Pulmonary embolism	8	0.5
Herniation	13	0.7
Edema	(7)	
Hemorrhage	(6)	
Sepsis	5	0.3
Myocardial infarction	3	0.2
Intraoperative hemorrhage	2	0.1
Intraoperative brain injury	2	0.1
Pneumonia cytomegalovirus	2	0.1
Aspiration	1	0.06
Gastrointestinal hemorrhage	1	0.06
Total	37	2.1

sphere—often because the line of operative approach is inappropriate. Excessive retraction of a tight brain inflicts trauma, the most common expression of which is brain edema. More than once I have abandoned an operation, before or after opening the dura, when I have encountered a tight brain that could not be relaxed by tapping the ventricular system or by opening an accessible subarachnoid cistern. The problem of retraction injury arises primarily when dealing with either deep or basal exposures. When it is known to be safe beforehand, the introduction of a lumbar subarachnoid catheter before the procedure begins is a useful adjuvant. More often than not, I cannulate the lateral ventricle because this step has the advantage of relieving tension while providing a means of reexpanding the ventricle at the end of the procedure, a route for irrigating the basilar cisterns if they become contaminated with chemically irritating

Table 12-4. Deaths by Type of Tumor in 1,771 Patients Undergoing Craniotomy for Resection of Supratentorial Brain Tumors

Tumor	Patients (No.)	(%)
Astrocytoma and glioblastoma	18	1.0
Meningioma	7	0.4
Metastatic	4	0.2
Pituitary	1	0.06
Lymphoma	2	0.1
Sarcoma	2	0.1
Craniopharyngioma	2	0.1
Colloid cyst	1	0.06
Total	37	2.1

material, and an ideal means of monitoring and controlling postoperative intracranial pressure.

Of equal or perhaps even greater importance as a cause of edema is impairment of venous drainage, either permanently by purposely interrupting or allowing spontaneous occlusion of major draining veins, or transiently during the course of the operation by interrupting flow through a critical draining vein by means of stretching or direct compression. Sustained venous hypertension leads inexorably to edema and when acute and extreme, venous overload causes infarction and petechial hemorrhage. Exposed draining veins must be protected, with meticulous attention to avoiding desiccation, by placing strips of wet Gelfoam along the course of the vein, and to avoiding interruption of flow caused by distortion or compression of the vein. I am convinced that the most frequent cause of morbidity during operations on meningiomas is related to impairment of venous drainage, usually by damage to the bridging veins in the course of removing parasagittal tumors. Less often, catastrophe results from interrupting flow through a vein bridging from the sylvian fissure to the sphenoparietal sinus or the vein of Labbé.

The third cause of edema is cerebral infarction. Less common than venous infarction, but clearly important, is the ischemic infarct that represents interruption of an artery. Usually, there is a tearing of an artery, which results in brisk bleeding, and then, as the surgeon tries to repair the tear using bipolar coagulation or a clip, the torn artery is damaged and subsequently closes by thrombosis. More will be said about this complication in discussing intraoperative hemorrhage in the next section.

When detected in its incipient stages, herniation of brain caused by edema can be reversed by nonsurgical means, including the use of high-dose steroids and the induction of hyperosmolarity and hyperventilation. The surgical options—increasing the available space for swelling by opening the dura, with or without replacing the bone flap and with or without removing edematous brain—may be life saving. Fatal herniation related to a hematoma occurs in far fewer cases.

Postoperative hematomas requiring reoperation complicated 24 (1.4 percent) of the 1,771 craniotomies (Table 12-5) and yet only two of these, both originating in the tumor bed, proved fatal. These numbers can be explained by two factors: first, hematomas are readily recognized, are usually suspected clinically, and are confirmed by computed tomography. Moreover, surgeons in general are inclined to operate immediately on a patient with incipient herniation resulting from hematoma, whereas, in a similar

Table 12-5. Postoperative Hematoma[a] Requiring Reoperation among 1,771 Operations for Resection of Supratentorial Brain Tumors

Location of Postoperative Hematoma	Patients		Meningioma	
	(No.)	(%)[b]	(No.)	(%)[b]
Epidural	13	0.7	7	0.4
Subdural	3	0.2	2	0.1
Tumor bed[c]	8	0.5	3	0.2
Total	24	1.4	12	0.7

[a] Incidence = 1.4%
[b] Percentages are rounded.
[c] Fatal in two cases, one of anaplastic astrocytoma and one, meningioma.

clinical situation with brain edema uncomplicated by hematoma, most surgeons are inclined to procrastinate. Second, reoperations for postoperative hematomas have a high likelihood of success. The measures taken to avoid postoperative hematoma will be described later in this chapter (see *Postoperative Hematomas Requiring Reoperation*).

The frequency of significant postoperative hematomas can be reduced substantially by adhering to well-established practices and certain rules. During the course of an operation, a surgeon follows the principle that bleeding from a tumor can be stopped most effectively by removing the tumor. This association between bleeding and remaining (or retained) tumor carries over into the postoperative phase, especially in cases of malignant glioma, in which postoperative hematoma is a significant cause of morbidity and mortality.

Intraoperative Hemorrhage

With rare exceptions, fatal intraoperative hemorrhage has an arterial origin. Although I have no statistical basis for an opinion, I believe that the most common cause of massive intraoperative hemorrhage is the tearing of a normal artery caused by stretching the artery intraoperatively. The injured parent vessel is almost always vital and of large caliber, and typically such tears occur at a branching—the carotid bifurcation, the anterior communicating complex, or the internal carotid artery at the anterior clinoid process. In each of these cases, the usual situation in which normal vessels are overstretched is when retraction is used in the course of removing a large meningioma. Simply the awareness of this possibility is sufficient impetus for appropriate precautionary measures.

When such a vessel is torn, traction should be eliminated to the extent possible while still retaining adequate exposure, and closure of the tear should proceed with a firm resolve to retain flow through the vessel if this is at all possible. As soon as a tear is recognized and traction on the injured vessel is lessened, a cottonoid patty should be placed directly over the tear while the surgeon plots reparative maneuvers and prepares the rest of the operating team to execute the proposed plan. A permanent patch can be fashioned using muscle, muslin, or even cotton, and it is a rare tear that cannot be repaired with a patch, gentle pressure, and patience.

Less effectively managed is a tear in a vessel weakened by tumor. Such cases are almost always one of two types. The vessel either is found coursing within a malignant glioma or else it is a large artery enveloped by a meningioma. In the most frequent cases, a glioblastoma has surrounded the middle cerebral or pericallosal arterial complex and, when the artery is exposed within the tumor, it literally disintegrates. The weakened wall is extremely difficult to repair, although the same measures described earlier for closing a tear in a normal artery should be tried. Too often it is ultimately necessary to occlude either a major branch or the trunk of the middle cerebral artery to stem the hemorrhage. A high-resolution magnetic resonance image (MRI) obtained preoperatively will indicate unequivocally the course of major arteries in relation to a parenchymal tumor. The issue then becomes one of simply avoiding the immediate vicinity of the major branches.

In another instance, a meningioma involves an abnormal vessel wall. Meningiomas often displace major arteries, such as the sylvian vessels, but when the same tumor recurs, direct involvement of the same arteries is a distinct possibility. Subfrontal meningiomas often displace the anterior cerebral–anterior communicating artery complex, but if the tumor engulfs these structures, direct involvement of the arterial wall sometimes causes a rent in the artery or avulsion of a branch while it is being dissected free from the tumor. In cases of parasellar meningioma that surrounds the internal carotid artery, the artery is vulnerable during the attempt at radical tumor removal. A tear in an artery, whether the vessel is normal or abnormal, has a dual risk: one of causing significant intraoperative loss of blood; and one of major distal infarction in the event of temporary or permanent occlusion of the injured artery.

The damage to arterial walls just discussed does not entail a causative role for instruments. Three instruments—the unipolar cutting loop, the laser, and the ultrasonic aspirator—have the potential for direct injury to an arterial wall. The unipolar cutting loop is an instrument with great potential for producing damage to any normal structure and must be handled at all times with the utmost care. A laser can be used in the immediate vicinity of a major artery if the artery is protected properly. It is unusual for arterial injury to be caused by the ultrasonic aspirator, but very definitely possible.

Intraoperative Injury to the Brain

Brain damage is seldom a direct cause of immediate or delayed death. In the great majority of cases in which the brain is damaged, the result is morbidity rather than death. When a patient is rendered hemiplegic by an operation and later dies of pneumonia or pulmonary embolism, the illness just preceding death is incidental to the actual cause of death, which is the brain damage sustained as a direct outcome of a surgical procedure.

Functioning neural structures can be damaged in a number of ways, some of which were delineated earlier in discussing fatal brain herniation caused by edema. Because of the wide range of potential for damaging brain, I find it difficult to make any useful general statements and, instead, I offer three approaches that I consider valuable in avoiding damage to functioning or potentially functioning brain:

1. Obtain a detailed knowledge of the function and anatomy of the operative field, establishing and reinforcing a three-dimensional concept *before* the operation with standard texts and models.
2. Use cortical mapping when appropriate.
3. Rely on an acquired sense (called judgment) of how far to go and when to stop. Clearly, judgment is in part a matter of experience, both good and bad, but it is well to remember that *you can always come back to do more on another day, but you can't come back and do less.*

FATAL COMPLICATIONS INDIRECTLY RELATED TO THE OPERATIVE PROCEDURE

Fatalities indirectly caused by craniotomy account for slightly more than one-half of all postoperative deaths in the 1,771 patients evaluated. Heading the list is fatal pulmonary embolism (Table 12-6). Pulmonary embolism was documented in 17 patients (1 percent), of whom six (35 percent) harbored meningiomas. In 8 of the 17 cases, the pulmonary embolism was fatal—a mortality rate of almost 50 percent. Prevention of deep venous thrombosis effectively eliminates the risk of pulmonary embolism, but despite our practicing a broad range of contemporary prophylactic measures, deep venous thrombosis con-

Table 12-6. Postoperative Pulmonary Embolism among 1,771 Craniotomies for Resection of Supratentorial Brain Tumors

Cases	Patients	
	(No.)	(%)
Documented	17	1.0
Meningioma	6	0.3
Fatal	8	0.5

tinues to occur. Most effective in our hands has been the use of intermittent compression stockings, early ambulation, and aspirin.

Once pulmonary embolism is strongly suspected or documented, the most effective therapeutic measure is full anticoagulation. Although caval filtration devices reduce the incidence of subsequent pulmonary embolism, we prefer immediate anticoagulation. Because pulmonary embolism almost always occurs more than 48 hours after operation, anticoagulation can be commenced as early as 48 hours postoperatively in the absence of a known *active* source of intracranial bleeding. A pulmonary embolus is fatal in almost one-half of cases. The likelihood that an anticoagulant-induced hematoma will be fatal is less than 10 percent, assuming timely diagnosis and treatment.

The other causes of death indirectly related to the operation were sepsis, myocardial infarction, cytomegalovirus pneumonia, aspiration, and gastrointestinal hemorrhage. Sepsis can be the fatal consequence of a seemingly benign infection at the site of an intravenous line, but more often serious sepsis occurs in a disabled patient who concurrently has bacterial pneumonia. Two fatal cases of cytomegalovirus pneumonia reflect the recent emergence of this entity on postoperative wards. Postoperative aspiration occurs only rarely and in most instances is avoidable. A falling hematocrit may be the first and only indication of potentially fatal gastrointestinal hemorrhage, even in a patient who is fully alert. Once suspected, gastrointestinal hemorrhage becomes an emergency.

NONFATAL POSTOPERATIVE COMPLICATIONS

Postoperative Hematomas Requiring Reoperation

In regard to the 24 craniotomies that were followed by postoperative hematomas requiring reoperation (incidence, 1.4 percent) (Table 12-5), more than half

of the postoperative hematomas were epidural (13 of 24) and more than half of all epidural hematomas (7 of 13) followed operations for meningiomas. Less frequent, and accounting for exactly one-third of the total (8 of 24), were hematomas within the tumor bed. The only two fatalities in this group of patients resulted from hematomas within the tumor bed, one in a patient with bleeding into an incompletely removed anaplastic astrocytoma, and the other with bleeding into the bed of a totally excised meningioma. Three of the eight hematomas involved the bed of a meningioma. Subdural hematomas were relatively infrequent, and two of the three cases involved patients with meningiomas.

The evolution of postoperative epidural hematomas is subacute and the bleeding is arterial, originating from muscle, bone, or the outer surface or cut edge of the dura. Accepting these sources of bleeding, the corresponding prophylactic measures involved are:

1. Precise coagulation of arterial bleeders in the incised and reflected temporalis muscle.
2. Use of either a free bone flap or an osteoplastic flap attached only by pericranium, the muscle being detached using a broad periosteal elevator. The pericranial attachment will prevent absorption of the bone flap while at the same time temporarily devascularizing it.
3. Liberal use of bone wax on the bone edges and meticulous coagulation of all dural vessels.
4. Firm tenting of the dura along the bone edges with sutures to pericranium or holes drilled into the bone edge; attaching the midportion of the dura to the bone flap with a final suture passed through paired drill holes.

To incur bleeding into a tumor bed is a particular risk in cases of incompletely removed malignant gliomas, in part because of their vascularity but more importantly because the vessels within such a tumor have abnormal walls that are difficult to seal firmly with bipolar coagulation. Any artery with a diameter greater than 1 mm, whether the artery is stretched over the surface of a meningioma or entering a glioma, should be sealed by coagulation for a distance of 3 to 5 mm from the open end. Arteries much larger than this should be coagulated and then clipped. One patient in the series suffered devastating but nonfatal delayed bleeding into the tumor bed from an artery 1.5 mm in diameter that was coagulated instead of coagulated and clipped.

At the conclusion of tumor removal, whether it is a meningioma that has been completely removed or a glioblastoma removed subtotally, the full surface of the tumor bed must be visualized. First, all adherent clots should be removed by gentle irrigation and traction, and saline used to fill the cavity should remain clear. This is a requisite step in the operation, and any compromise on this point is fraught with a serious risk of delayed bleeding within the tumor bed. After removal of all clots, as well as adherent hemostatic material such as Gelfoam and Surgicel, the anesthesiologist is asked to raise intrathoracic pressure (and indirectly intracranial venous pressure), a maneuver that greatly reduces the likelihood that venous bleeding will be started again by the predictable abrupt rises in intrathoracic pressure that follow extubation and coughing during the early postanesthetic period. Essential also is the return of blood volume and blood pressure to normal levels while the surface of the tumor bed is still under direct vision. Having satisfied all of the foregoing tests of complete hemostasis, I like to line the cavity with one or more strips of Surgicel, the one exception being a cavity that opens into the lateral or third ventricle, which has the potential for a foreign body to become impacted in the third ventricle or aqueduct.

Subdural hematomas occur relatively infrequently. They are likely to arise when the patient has undergone an operation in an erect or semierect position, particularly if drainage of large ventricles causes the cortex to fall away from the vertex, thereby stretching and tearing bridging veins. In any situation in which the brain can fall away from a venous sinus to which veins course in the subdural space, there exists the same opportunity for a subdural hematoma to develop. In theory, reexpansion of the hemisphere by returning ventricular fluid through an indwelling catheter lessens the possibility that abrupt movements of the head postoperatively, for example with violent coughing, will cause tearing of a bridging vein postoperatively.

Postoperative Cerebrospinal Fluid Leak

A postoperative cerebrospinal fluid (CSF) fistula complicated 9 of the 1,771 craniotomies, for an incidence of 0.5 percent (Table 12-7). Of the nine cases, seven involved operations for meningiomas. Three CSF leaks occurred into the ethmoid sinus and six through a scalp incision.

Cerebrospinal Fluid Fistula

Although the frontal sinuses are opened in a great many neurosurgical procedures, postoperative leakage through the frontal sinus is relatively rare. There were no such cases in this series, reflecting the ease with which the sinus can be excluded from the subarachnoid space by one of several effective means.

Table 12-7. Postoperative Cerebrospinal Fluid Leak among 1,771 Operations for Resection of Supratentorial Brain Tumors

Location of Postoperative CSF Leak	Patients	
	(No.)	(%)
Subfrontal tumor, opening into ethmoid sinus	3	0.2
Scalp[a]	6	0.3
Total	9[b]	0.5

[a] Two cases occurred after irradiation.
[b] Seven cases involved meningiomas.

CSF can leak into the middle ear through air cells in the temporal bone, but the rarity of this complication indicates the effectiveness of bone wax applied under direct vision. Most CSF fistulas involving the paranasal sinuses follow operations for removal of basal meningiomas with dural attachments to the cribriform plate, planum sphenoidale, and tuberculum sellae. Dural repair after removal of these midline meningiomas are considered elsewhere in this volume (*see* Ransohoff and Patterson sections of Ch. 13). With the use of autologous fibrin glue, which is now routine on our service, I predict that CSF leaks from this source will become diminishingly rare.

Why drainage of CSF through a scalp incision complicated operations on meningiomas can be explained by several factors. First, often when a portion of involved dura is removed and a dural patch is used, the patch is not sewn well enough to become water tight. Second, the brain invariably swells to a degree paralleling the size of the removed meningioma and, in addition, CSF flow over the affected convexity is often impaired—a situation that becomes intensified postoperatively, resulting in a somewhat excessive amount of intracranial CSF. In the case of a porous dura, a subarachnoid space that communicates with the subdural space, and impaired CSF absorption, CSF readily accumulates in the subgaleal space and, under pressure, it stresses the suture line. The most effective management, once this occurs, is prophylactic spinal drainage through one or a series of spinal punctures. In two of the six fistulas involving the scalp in this series, a meticulous two-layer closure of the scalp was complicated by tissue damage from prior irradiation.

Aseptic Meningitis

For our present purposes, aseptic meningitis (Table 12-8) is defined as symptomatic meningeal inflammation requiring either prolonged hospitalization, or

Table 12-8. Aseptic Meningitis[a] in 1,771 Patients Undergoing Craniotomy for Resection of Supratentorial Brain Tumors

	Patients	
Location	(No.)	(%)
Parasellar cisterns	8[b]	0.5
Lateral ventricle	1[c]	0.06
Total	9	0.5

[a] Symptomatic inflammation requiring prolonged hospitalization, steroid therapy longer than 4 weeks, or both.
[b] Five were meningiomas.
[c] Invaded by glioblastoma.

steroid therapy for longer than 4 weeks, or both. In this series, nine patients had aseptic meningitis, for an incidence of 0.5 percent. Eight of the nine cases involved operations in or near parasellar cisterns, and five of the tumors were parasellar meningiomas. When operating in the basal cisterns, it is essential to close the entry into any opened cistern using cottonoid patties or Gelfoam. Actually, the surgeon can almost entirely avoid the seepage of blood into opened basal cisterns by carefully packing off the operative field. When managing either blood or the chemically irritating contents of a cyst, such as a craniopharyngioma or an epidermoid cast, I add Solu-Cortef to the fluid used for irrigation and then I use irrigation liberally. After operations on the basal cisterns, I like to irrigate the cisterns slowly by injecting saline (without preservative) into an in-line ventricular catheter.

There was only one instance of aseptic meningitis, originating from an operation that involved the lateral ventricle. When a lateral ventricle is entered, as in a transcallosal approach to a colloid cyst, the body of the lateral ventricle should be occluded gently with one or more cottonoid patties during subsequent manipulation on the tumor—although rarely is this operation complicated by significant bleeding. Frequently in the course of removing the deep portion of a large glioma, the ventricle is entered. In that event, the ventricle should be packed off to prevent the ingress of blood and debris. Because significant contamination of the ventricular fluid is most likely to occur when operating on gliomas, and as steroids may be continued for extended periods of time after operation, for those tumors the true incidence of aseptic meningitis related to an opened ventricle is no doubt higher than it would appear.

Negative Biopsy

There was one case of a negative biopsy in this series of craniotomies. This volume is not a forum for argument regarding stereotactic needle biopsy as opposed to open biopsy, and clearly there is a place for both approaches. A negative biopsy, whether the procedure is done by stereotactic or nonstereotactic technique, reflects one or more of several possible errors:

1. Faulty selection of a patient for the procedure based on clinical, radiographic, and probable pathological criteria.
2. A sampling error meaning that misleading or nondiagnostic material is obtained.
3. Incorrect technique—and in this category I would include misinterpretation of intraoperative ultrasonic localization and an error in calculating stereotactic coordinates.

Intraoperative Injury of Cranial Nerves

The cranial nerves injured most frequently are the olfactory (cranial nerve I) and optic (cranial nerve II). Cranial nerves III, IV, V, and VI are injured less often, and when they are injured it is usually because of their involvement by basal tumors, the details of which are considered elsewhere in this volume (see Chs. 13, 15, 20, 22, 23, 60–62, and 82–88).

Deep retraction of one frontal lobe to gain exposure of the parasellar region very often disrupts the olfactory tract or avulses the olfactory bulb. I prefer to divide the tract purposely just behind the bulb and then carefully dissect the contralateral olfactory tract from its groove along the gyrus rectus. In addition, opening the interhemispheric fissure rostral to the genu allows me to displace one frontal lobe without, at the same time, displacing the unretracted frontal lobe. These two maneuvers, freeing the olfactory tract from its attachment to the undersurface of the frontal lobe and separating the frontal lobes from one another by dividing arachnoid attachments between their medial surfaces, should provide optimal protection of the intact olfactory bulb and tract. Patients with huge bilateral subfrontal meningiomas are usually anosmic preoperatively. Almost all meningiomas of the planum sphenoidale and tuberculum sellae can be removed through a unilateral approach, which for a right-handed surgeon is beneath the right frontal lobe. Because these patients are not rendered anosmic by their tumors, every effort should be made to protect the left olfactory tract.

There are several types of basal tumors that displace or compress the optic nerves and chiasm, and avoiding injury involves meticulous technique and enormous care to prevent any additional traction or stretching of these sensitive structures. In the case of meningiomas, this means devascularizing the tumor initially as it is detached from its dural base and then removing the central portion of the tumor piecemeal before dissecting it away from the optic nerves and chiasm.

As a cause of postoperative morbidity, injury to the optic nerves ranks high in all series of operations for supratentorial tumors. The optic nerves are often at risk of injury, and, unfortunately, their capacity for recovery from traumatic damage is quite limited. The optic nerves demand reverent respect.

COMPLICATIONS OF TRANSSPHENOIDAL SURGERY

This subject is covered expertly and in detail in Chapter 14 and in the transsphenoidal surgery section of Chapter 15 for the removal of both pituitary adenomas and craniopharyngiomas. I restrict my comments to practices that I find important in avoiding the complications I have either encountered myself or observed following transsphenoidal operations performed by my colleagues.

First and foremost, I advocate a direct midline approach. I think it makes little difference whether the procedure is done entirely by the neurosurgeon or in conjunction with a rhinologist. The important principle is to approach the sella in the direct midline, to maintain unequivocal orientation and have equal access to both sides of the sella.

Almost routinely, I insert a lumbar subarachnoid catheter following the induction of anesthesia because this gives me complete control over both the intracranial pressure and the subarachnoid space. The one disadvantage to this use of the catheter is the predictable incidence of headaches characteristic after lumbar puncture. An autologous epidural blood patch can be used to close a spinal dural opening with 95 percent certainty. The advantages of the lumbar subarachnoid catheter in surgery for suprasellar tumor, and in the event that the subarachnoid space is entered, far outweigh the modest morbidity rates associated with it.

Although high-resolution MRI of the brain is, in my opinion, invaluable in planning and conducting operations for all supratentorial tumors, it is a *sine qua non* for transsphenoidal procedures. The detailed anatomy of the sella and of the tumor and its relation to surrounding structures requires high-resolution, thin-section images; anything less is a compromise that may lead to an avoidable complication.

With MRI in hand and possessing a thorough knowledge of the relevant anatomy, the surgeon enters the sphenoid sinus and obtains an exposure of the entire anterior wall of the sella, drilling away bone in an incompletely pneumatized sphenoid sinus as is required to view the horizontal portion of the sellar floor. For optimal visualization of the sellar contents, the dura must be exposed over to the medial edge of each cavernous sinus, well up to the tuberculum, and down to the junction of the anterior wall and floor of the sella. This area of the dura is then excised with an incision 1 to 2 mm from the bone edge, and the dural edges are coagulated with a right-angle forceps to give full access to the sella and its contents. Such an exposure avoids either overlooking residual tumor or damaging compressed anterior lobe that is displaced laterally against the wall of the cavernous sinuses. When the tumor is confined to the sella, and if the cavity does not communicate with the subarachnoid space, I use absolute alcohol to fill the dry cavity for a total exposure of 6 to 10 minutes in order to destroy any remaining microscopic nests of tumor cells. Although the alcohol presumably penetrates the exposed surface of the normal gland, the depth of penetration seems to be negligible and I have observed no detrimental effect on pituitary function.

The complication of secondary hypopituitarism can be avoided first by identifying the location of the residual anterior lobe on the preoperative MRI and second by identifying the residual anterior lobe and protecting it during the operation. Hypopituitarism can also result from damage to the pituitary stalk, whose position can be defined accurately on the MRI. In the case of large tumors with a major suprasellar component, the stalk is flattened against the upper dorsum sellae and angulated sharply over its upper surface. The delicate connective tissue covering the stalk should not be disturbed for fear of permanently injuring the portal vessels on the stalk's surface.

Perhaps the most frequent complication of transsphenoidal surgery is a postoperative CSF fistula. If I encounter CSF during the course of the operation, I take the following steps:

1. Through the indwelling lumbar subarachnoid catheter, the anesthesiologist injects saline (without preservative) at my request in order to maintain a slight positive pressure and to prevent ingress of air into the subarachnoid space.

2. After removing the tumor, I take subcutaneous fat from the right lower abdomen and gently pack it into the sella, folding it into place with a backing of Surgicel.
3. I reconstitute the anterior wall of the sella by slipping a graft of septal cartilage (or septal bone) beneath the dural edges; lacking a septal graft, I fashion a piece of titanium mesh of the appropriate dimensions.
4. I cover the operative field with autologous fibrin glue.
5. I attach the lumbar subarachnoid catheter to a drainage bag maintained at the level of the right atrium for a period ranging from 48 to 72 hours.

Rarely have I encountered delayed visual loss caused by downward traction of the optic chiasm into a large empty sella through the mechanism of an adherent suprasellar capsule. Such a complication is highly unlikely if the sella is packed with subcutaneous fat, and I do this irrespective of the presence or absence of a CSF leak.

13 Meningiomas

Convexity, Parasagittal, and Parafalcine Meningiomas

Robert G. Ojemann
Christopher S. Ogilvy

Parasagittal meningiomas involve the sagittal sinus and adjacent convexity dura and falx. Only the lateral wall of the sinus may be involved, or the tumor may grow to occlude the sinus partially or completely.

Falx meningiomas arise in any area of the falx inferior to the sagittal sinus but are more common anteriorly. They are often bilateral but usually grow asymmetrically into the cortex of the medial aspect of each cerebral hemisphere. When they are large, the superior and inferior sagittal sinuses may be involved, and they may project into the corpus callosum.

Convexity meningiomas may arise from any area of the dura over the cerebral convexities. The most common sites of occurrences are in the parasagittal region, along the coronal suture, and at the frontal-temporal junction, where they have been referred to as anterior sylvian or pterional meningiomas.

Of all supratentorial meningiomas, approximately one-third are parasagittal and falx and one-third are located over the cerebral convexities. Various aspects of the clinical presentation, radiographic studies, preoperative evaluation, operative technique, and results of treatment of these meningiomas have been described.[1–32] Cushing's classic two-volume text[7] clearly defines the anatomic locations of meningiomas for purposes of description of symptoms, surgical approach, complications and results.

LITERATURE REVIEW

Operative Technique

Operative experience with these meningiomas has been described in the past by Cushing,[6,7] Gautier-Smith,[8] Hoessly and Olivecrona,[14] Kempe,[16] Morley,[24] Northfield,[25] and Poppen.[29] More recent publications include those of Guthrie et al.,[11] Logue,[18] Long,[19] MacCarthy et al.,[20] Maxwell and Chou,[21,22] and Ojemann.[26] Bonnal and Brotchi[2] have described techniques for replacing or repairing the sagittal sinus when removing parasagittal meningiomas.

Results and Complications

The results of surgery for all meningiomas have improved over the past two decades. Chan and Thompson[4] and Horwitz and Rizzoli[15] have reviewed the published results and complications of surgery for meningiomas.

In my series of parasagittal, falx, and convexity meningiomas operated on between 1968 and 1982, the operative mortality was 2.5 percent (two deaths in 79 patients).[26] In the last 10 years the perioperative mortality in my series of these meningiomas has been zero. Logue's series[17] reports mortalities of 2.4 percent for convexity meningiomas, 4.4 percent for parasagittal meningiomas, and 2.4 percent for falx meningiomas. Horwitz and Rizzoli[15] noted similar results. In the Mayo Clinic series[11] the mortality of all meningiomas operated on from 1970 to 1975 was 2.9 percent. Even patients over 70 years of age now have a low perioperative morbidity and mortality.[23]

Complications of surgery for meningiomas include transient and permanent increase in neurological deficits, seizures, hemorrhage (extradural, subdural, and intracerebral), air embolus, wound infection, cardiopulmonary problems, and thrombophlebitis. Patients who have parasagittal meningiomas arising from the middle or posterior third of the sagittal sinus or falx or convexity meningiomas over eloquent cortex may have an increase in neurological deficit in the immediate postoperative period but this usually clears gradually over several weeks to a few months.

In my series of 23 patients with total removal of benign parasagittal or falx meningiomas,[26] there was no evidence of late recurrence. At the first operation in two patients with middle third parasagittal meningiomas, tumor was left growing into the wall of an open sagittal sinus. When the tumor recurred and occluded the sinus, a total removal could be done. In two other patients with subtotal removal of middle third lesions, there has been no regrowth in one and the other died of a postoperative myocardial infarction.

There was only one recurrence in my series of 51 patients with convexity meningiomas,[26] in a patient with an atypical meningioma; this tumor has not recurred after the second operation. In 48 of the 51 there was a good result, 2 had a fair result, and 1 died of a pulmonary embolus. Some patients require long-term anticonvulsant therapy. In earlier reported series, the recurrence rate in patients who had a total removal of a convexity meningioma was also low.[15]

PREOPERATIVE PREPARATION

Preparation for the operation begins when the neurosurgeon first meets the patient. The decision for operation will be based on an evaluation of the patient's history, examination, radiographic findings, and an assessment of the benefits and risks of the treatment options. At times these decisions are difficult, but spending time to make sure that an operation is the best treatment recommendation is the first step in avoiding complications.[27]

As part of this initial evaluation inquiry is made about any important medical problems. What drugs is the patient taking? Are there any important cardiopulmonary problems that need further evaluation? Is there any history to suggest diabetes that may be aggravated with steroids?

In planning the operative procedure adequate radiographic studies are essential. Magnetic resonance imaging (MRI) with and without gadolinium enhancement gives the most precise information on the size and configuration of the tumor, the degree of edema in the adjacent brain tissue, and the relationship of major blood vessels to the tumor.[10] In 60 to 70 percent of patients with gadolinium-enhanced MRI, a thickened enhanced linear structure or "tail" is seen in the dural surface adjacent to the tumor mass (Fig. 13-1A&B). Goldsher et al.[10] have summarized the literature on this subject. This is a highly specific feature of meningiomas. The problem is that there have been a limited number of pathology studies of the "tail," with the finding of reactive connective tissue and blood vessels in many, but tumor invasion in some. Surgical preparation must include the "tail" in the exposure. If information is needed about the status of the bone of the skull, a computed tomography (CT) scan with bone windows is indicated.

We rarely use angiography in convexity meningiomas unless the tumor is very large and embolization might be considered. We know the blood supply comes from the meningeal arteries, and these can be occluded early in the course of the operation. In parasagittal and falx meningiomas angiography is indicated to determine the status of the sagittal sinus, the location of cortical veins, and the relationship of the anterior cerebral arteries to the tumor (Fig. 13-1C&D).

The use of preoperative embolization has become increasingly available with advances in endovascular techniques. There have been reports documenting the use of this technique in large convexity meningiomas.[12,13,31] While there is the risk of serious neurological complications from brain edema or embolic material, such complications were not seen in parasagittal, falx, or convexity meningiomas reported by Hieshima et al.[13] (five patients) or by Richter and Schachemmayr[31] (23 patients). The neurosurgeon must also be sure that the scalp arteries to the skin flap being planned are patent, since scalp necrosis has been reported due to the combined loss of blood supply from surgery and embolization.[1,4]

The timing of embolization in relation to surgery is important in avoiding potential complications from increased cerebral edema. We prefer to proceed with surgery within 48 hours of the embolization so new collateral circulation does not have time to develop. In some patients who already have significant edema, surgery will be planned on the same day. We rarely use embolization in these meningiomas since feeding arteries in the dura can be readily occluded early in the operation in parasagittal and convexity meningiomas and rarely is there other arterial supply that can be safely embolized.

Cerebral edema associated with meningiomas is usually well controlled with the use of steroids. There appears to be no relationship to the degree of edema with respect to meningioma location although the larger the meningioma, the more likely there is to be edema.[9,28] However, significant edema can occur with small tumors as well.[3] Every patient with meningioma receives steroids for at least 48 hours prior to operation (methylprednisolone or decadron). If there is significant cerebral edema it may be wise to give steroids for up to a week before surgery. On the evening prior to surgery and on the morning of surgery, higher doses of steroids are given intravenously.

OPERATIVE TECHNIQUE

Preparation at Time of Surgery

The possibility of a complication is reduced if the neurosurgeon has appropriate help and equipment. An anesthesiologist who is familiar with neurosurgical techniques and positioning is essential. The operating room used should be dedicated to neurosurgical procedures and the surgeon should be provided with trained personnel, operating microscope, bipolar coagulator, laser, and ultrasonic aspirator. During the postoperative period the patient should be observed in a recovery room or intensive care unit staffed with personnel familiar with neurosurgical procedures and potential problems.

When the patient initially arrives in the operating room, a radial artery catheter is inserted for continuous monitoring of blood pressure and evaluation of blood gases. Thigh-high alternating compression air boots are placed and their use started. An antibiotic, usually a cephalosporin, is administered and is continued until 24 hours after surgery. Following a

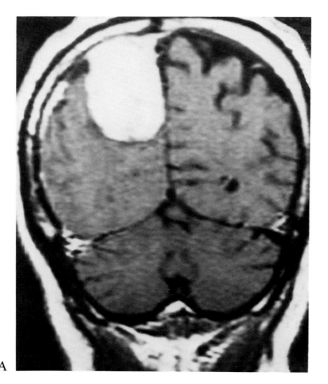
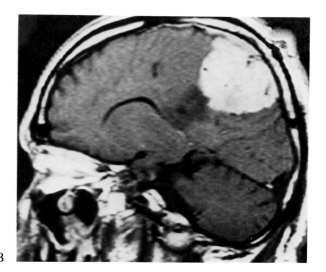

A   B

Figure 13-1. Parasagittal meningioma—junction of middle and posterior third of sagittal sinus. **(A)** Coronal and **(B)** sagittal T$_1$-contrast enhanced MRIs. The coronal view shows the tumor growing into the lateral wall of the sagittal sinus but the sinus is open. Note the linear enhancement or "tail" extending anteriorly on the cortical surface of the sagittal view and over the superior surface of the sinus on the coronal view (see text). (*Figure continues.*)

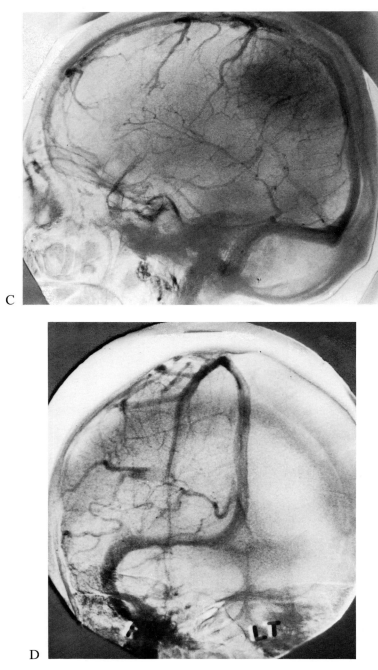

Figure 13-1 (*Continued*). **(C)** Lateral venous phase of angiogram shows the tumor stain and the large cortical vein at the anterior margin of the tumor. This vein will have to be carefully preserved. This view suggests that the sagittal sinus is open but it does not fill quite as well over the tumor area. **(D)** Oblique venous phase of angiogram clearly shows the status of the sagittal sinus.

smooth induction of anesthesia an in-dwelling Foley catheter is inserted. Once flow of urine is confirmed, 10 to 20 mg of furosemide is given intravenously. During the preparation and exposure of the dura, a 20 percent solution of mannitol is given in a dosage of 1 to 1.5 g/kg over 20 to 30 minutes.

The key point to remember in positioning the patient for parasagittal and convexity meningiomas is that the scalp over the approximate center of the tumor should be the highest point on the head. For falx meningiomas the planned area of exposure along the falx should be the highest point. This will allow maximum benefit from reduced venous pressure, take advantage of gravity in avoiding compression of the brain against the edge of the dura, and allow the surgeon to have full access to the tumor with minimal brain retraction.

Once the patient's body is positioned and adequate padding of all exposed bony prominences is done, the head is positioned to avoid any potential for poor venous outflow from the head. Careful attention is paid to the neck in order to ensure that there is no undue pressure on the jugular veins. If the head needs to be well elevated or if a semisitting position is planned, a central venous pressure line is placed in the right atrium with x-ray confirmation of the correct location. The head is held with a three-point skeletal fixation head rest. Both surgeon and anesthesiologist should agree on the final position. The extra time spent in planning the position and taking care to check all of the details cannot be overemphasized in avoiding potential complications.

Surgical Management of Parasagittal Meningiomas

Some type of magnification (either loupes or the operating microscope) is used for the entire operation. In planning the surgical management it is useful to divide these tumors according to the area of the sinus from which they arise, into anterior, middle, and posterior third.[7,22,26] Careful evaluation of the preoperative radiologic studies is done to determine the relationship of the anterior cerebral arteries, the position of and direction of flow in the cortical veins, and the status of the sagittal sinus (Fig. 13-1). Tumor involvement of the sinus can be estimated by careful study of the coronal sections on the MR study (Fig. 13-1A). An oblique view of the venous phase of the angiogram will help determine the patency of the sagittal sinus (Fig. 13-1D). The anterior cerebral artery branches are usually displaced inferiorly and laterally

and will be encountered in the deepest part of the tumor dissection.

Position and Skin Incision

The planned skin incision must allow for full exposure of the tumor and adequate removal of surrounding dura. Blood supply to the scalp flap must be adequate, and a wide enough base must be left to provide sufficient vascularization. The cosmetic result of the scar and bone flap should be considered.

Anterior Third of Sagittal Sinus

For meningiomas located anterior to the coronal suture, the patient is placed supine with the head slightly elevated (Fig. 13-2). This places the tumor at the highest point in the operating field and allows the surgeon to have the widest view angles from either side. The head should be angled posteriorly enough so the surgeon can look down the anterior portion of the tumor capsule to have direct visualization of the major branches of the anterior cerebral arteries. A bicoronal skin incision is used (Fig. 13-2, inset). Often the incision on the side opposite the tumor does not need to be extended as far inferiorly. The incision is placed well behind the posterior limit of the tumor as defined on the radiographic studies and is always behind the hairline. In most patients the temporalis muscle can be left attached to the superior temporal line on both sides of the head. The pericranial tissue is kept intact and serves nicely as a dural graft at the conclusion of the operation.

Middle Third of Sagittal Sinus

For tumors at the coronal suture, in the middle third of the sagittal sinus, and for some at the junction of the middle and posterior third, the patient is placed in a supine or semilateral position with the head well elevated so that the scalp over the center of the tumor is uppermost (Fig. 13-3A).

A horseshoe-shaped incision is used, extending approximately 2 cm across the midline, with the anterior limb well behind the tumor (Fig. 13-3A, inset). For some tumors centered at the coronal suture, the skin flap may be turned forward rather than laterally as shown in Figure 13-8, where the only difference would be placing the incision about 2 cm to the opposite side as shown. The scalp and underlying tissue including the pericranial tissue are carefully elevated together.

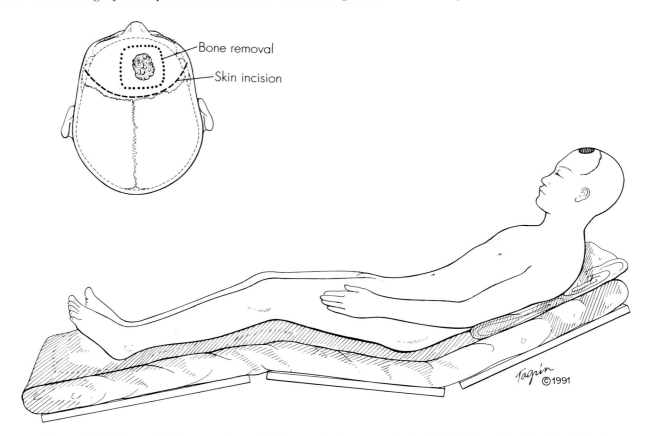

Figure 13-2. Parasagittal, convexity, and falx meningiomas—anterior third. The patient is placed in the supine position with the head elevated. The scalp over the area of the center of the tumor is uppermost. This allows the surgeon to work around the tumor from all angles with minimal brain retraction. **(Inset)** A coronal incision is used. The free bone flap extends about 2 cm across the midline to the opposite side from the tumor.

Posterior Third of Sagittal Sinus

For meningiomas located in the posterior third of the sagittal sinus the patient is placed in the lateral position. The head is well elevated and turned at least 45 degrees toward the floor to bring the center of the tumor to the highest point (Fig. 13-4A). The skin incision is horseshoe-shaped, extends about 2 cm across the midline, and is based in the posterior temporal-inferior occipital region (Fig. 13-4B).

Craniotomy Opening

A free bone flap will allow wide, expeditious exposure of tumor and can be easily enlarged if necessary. Burr holes are placed as needed around the periphery of the planned free bone flap including both sides of the sagittal sinus. The dura is then separated from the overlying bone using Penfield dissectors. The separation over the sinus is done last when all the other bone cuts have been made; thus, if there is any evidence of air embolus, the bone flap can be readily elevated. If the patient is elderly, the dura does not separate easily between burr holes or if there is a large area of sagittal sinus to be exposed, the bone flap can be taken in two parts. The first place is taken on the side of the tumor with the medial cut approximately 1 cm from the midline. Then the dura over the sinus can be separated under direct vision and the second part of bone flap can then be safely removed. As the bone flap is elevated, Gelfoam and cottonoids are placed directly over the sagittal sinus. Bleeding from meningeal arteries is controlled with coagulation and from meningeal venous sinuses with Gelfoam, Surgicel, and cottonoids. If an air embolus is detected by a reduction in end tidal CO_2 or if air is heard on the precordial Doppler, the patient's head can be lowered by using the Trendelenburg control on the operating table. Once the opening is covered and vital signs are stable, the patient can be returned to the original position. The dura is held to the inner table of bone along the craniotomy opening with sutures placed from the superficial layer of dura into

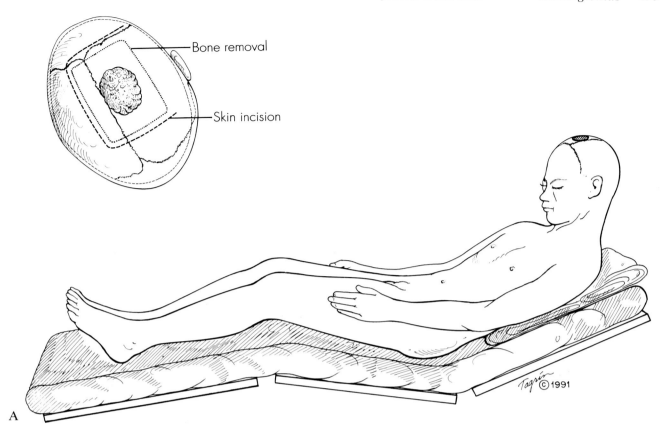

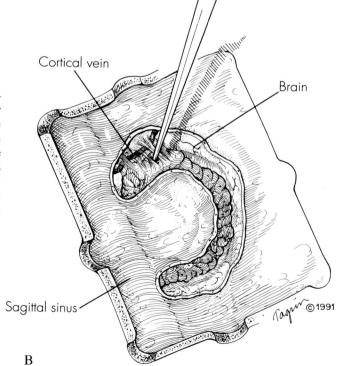

Figure 13-3. Parasagittal and convexity meningiomas—middle third. **(A)** The patient is placed in either a supine or semilateral position with the head elevated to bring the scalp over the center of the tumor uppermost. **(Inset)** The skin incision and bone flap extend about 2 cm across the midline. Multiple burr holes may be needed if the dura is very adherent. **(B)** The dura is cut around the tumor, staying about 1 cm from the tumor attachment. Cortical veins may be adherent along the anterior or posterior edge of the tumor and need to be carefully separated. (*Figure continues.*)

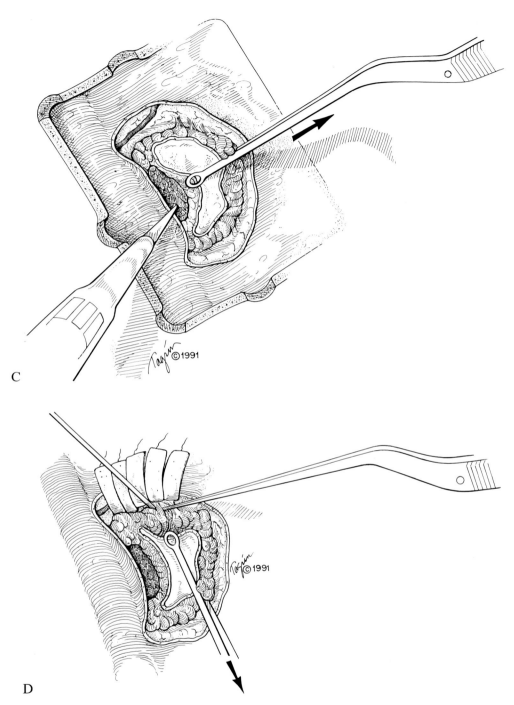

C

D

Figure 13-3 (*Continued*). **(C)** The dural cut is completed circumferentially, cutting through tumor along the medial area. If significant retraction on the brain is required to expose the tumor capsule, an internal decompression is done and most of the retraction placed on the tumor capsule. **(D)** The dissection of the tumor capsule is done in a circumferential fashion gradually deepening the dissection. The surgeon stays on the tumor capsule in the gliotic tissue adjacent to the capsule with the use of bipolar forceps and fine suction. As brain tissue is freed it is covered with moist cottonoids. (*Figure continues.*)

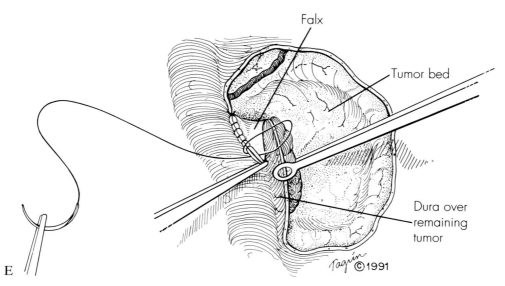

Figure 13-3 (*Continued*). **(E)** If the tumor only involves the edge of the sinus, as may be the case in some parasagittal convexity meningiomas, the edge of the sinus is gradually opened, held with a forceps, and sutured. If the tumor involves the sinus wall extensively and the sinus is open, the tumor is removed as close to the wall as possible.

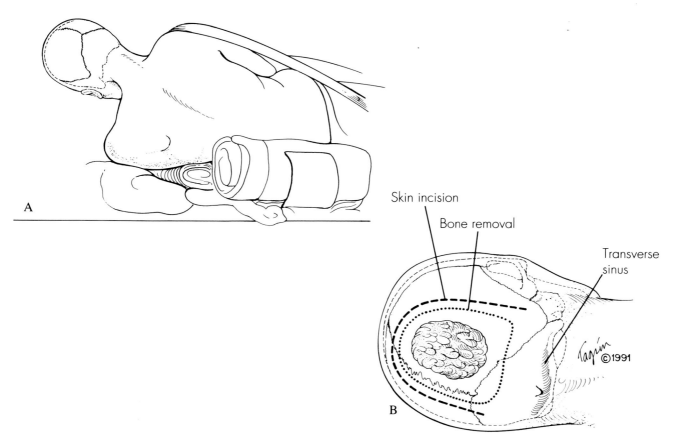

Figure 13-4. Parasagittal and convexity meningiomas—posterior third. **(A)** The patient is placed in the lateral position with a foam rubber roll in the axilla. The head is elevated and turned to the opposite side to bring the center of the tumor uppermost. **(B)** For parasagittal meningiomas, the skin incision goes across the midline for approximately 2 cm and the skin flap is based over the region of the transverse sinus. For convexity tumors, the incision is at or within a centimeter of the midline.

holes drilled at intervals in the edge of the craniotomy opening or occasionally into pericranial tissue.

If tumor has grown through the dura to involve the inner table of the bone, the abnormal area is removed with a high-speed air drill. If there is extensive involvement of an area of bone, particularly if the tumor is growing through the bone, it may be wise to leave an area of bone attached to the tumor and elevate the bone flap around it. The involved bone can then be removed by ronguers and bleeding controlled after each bite. On occasion the bone is left attached to the tumor if control of bleeding is difficult.

Dural Opening

When opening the dura the surgeon should always try to expose as little normal brain as possible, especially when the brain is full because of the presence of a large tumor. However, the dural incision should be about 1 cm from the tumor attachment. All dura attached to the tumor is eventually removed, but in convexity and parasagittal meningiomas it is wise to leave dura attached to the tumor to help in retraction.

The dural opening is usually started laterally or anteriorly. For parasagittal tumors, the tumor can often be palpated through the dura. The incision curves around the tumor near the edge of the sagittal sinus anteriorly and posteriorly (Fig. 13-3B). The dura is left attached to the tumor. As the dura is opened, great care is taken to avoid injury to the veins draining the cerebral hemispheres.

In the anterior third of the sagittal sinus and draining cortical veins can be occluded as they enter the sinus. This part of the sagittal sinus can be excised without complication and it should be removed with these tumors even if it is still patent to give the best chance for complete removal. In middle and posterior third tumors the sinus is excised if it is occluded. To remove the sinus the dura is opened around the tumor to the edge of the sinus both anteriorly and posteriorly. Then the dura is opened on the opposite side about 1 cm parallel to the sinus and at each end the incision is curved to the edge of the sinus opposite the cuts on the tumor side. The falx just beneath the sinus is exposed with retractors. Two 0-silk sutures are passed through the falx and edge of the dura next to the sinus posterior to the tumor (Fig. 13-5). In anterior third tumors, if it is known that the sinus is open, the sutures are tied and the sinus divided. If the sinus is occluded by tumor, the sinus is opened first to be sure a tongue of tumor has not grown beyond the point of ligation. If this is the case, this tumor is removed and then the sinus ligated and cut. If the falx can be easily divided down to its free edge or around

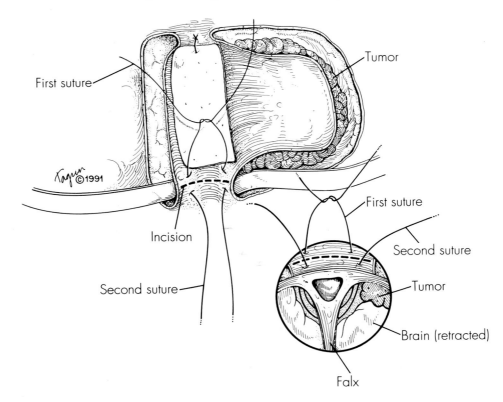

Figure 13-5. Technique for ligation of sagittal sinus. The sagittal sinus is ligated with two 0-silk sutures placed through the falx and the edge of the dura adjacent to the sagittal sinus so they will not slip. See text for details.

the tumor, this is done because this will allow gentle outward traction to be placed on the entire tumor mass through the attached dura. The assistant can retract the tumor gently posteriorly as the anterior cut is made in the falx and gently anteriorly as the posterior cut is made either to the free edge of the falx or around the tumor attachment. A Metzenbaum scissors or No. 15 knife is used to cut the falx. If the falx cannot be clearly visualized this is done later after internal decompression of the tumor.

If the sagittal sinus is open and cannot be removed in middle and posterior third tumors, we prefer to complete a circumferential dural cut by cutting through the dura and tumor parallel to the sagittal sinus (Fig. 13-3C). The tumor is then transected from its medial attachment doing whatever internal decompression is necessary to accomplish this. This also has the advantage of interrupting blood supply from the falx.

Tumor Removal

The junction between the tumor and adjacent cerebral cortex is then opened, dividing arachnoid and vascular attachments and staying on the tumor capsule. If draining cortical veins are adherent to the meningiomas in the middle and posterior third, they must be carefully dissected from the tumor capsule (Fig. 13-3C). Everything is done to minimize retraction or removal of adjacent brain tissue. Gentle pressure is placed against the capsule of the tumor along with mild traction on the dural attachment to help define the plane with adjacent brain tissue while working circumferentially. Cerebral tissue is carefully separated from the capsule of the tumor using bipolar forceps or fine dissectors (Fig. 13-3D). As blood vessels between the capsule and brain tissue are encountered they are coagulated with bipolar coagulation and cut with microscissors. As the cerebral cortex is separated it is protected with moist cottonoids. When the bulk of the tumor prevents retraction of the tumor capsule to define the plane of separation, internal decompression is done, usually with the ultrasonic aspirator or cautery loops in very firm tumors (Fig. 3E). Bleeding from within the tumor will often cease spontaneously, but bipolar coagulation or intermittent packing with Surgical may be used. As the tumor is decompressed, the capsule can be reflected away from surrounding brain tissue. Working in this manner, the surgeon can predict the extent of tumor removal possible at the next lower depth. Often, as the walls of the capsule are involuted, small focal areas of tumor extension into the brain are encountered.

Caution must be exercised as the deep portion of the tumor is reached. It is during this part of the dissection that the anterior cerebral branches are often displaced and may be adherent to tumor capsule. These vessels should be preserved and gently separated from the tumor.

Once the bulk of the tumor is removed, attention is directed to the removal of the residual tumor on the falx and sagittal sinus. If it appears that only a small portion of the lateral edge of the sagittal sinus is involved, it may be possible to resect the edge of the sinus with the tumor (Fig. 13-3E). Beginning at one end, the lateral edge of the sinus is opened and the tumor and walls of the sinus excised. After cutting 2 to 3 mm the two leaves of the sinus are held with a forceps and the edge closed with a running suture of a material such as Neurolon or Prolene. This maneuver is repeated until the attachment has been completely divided and the tumor removed. An alternative method is to use fine, curved hemostats.[16,21] The assistant can then use two tumor forceps on the dural attachments to suspend the tumor capsule carefully in the air while the final, deepest part of tumor is dissected from brain.

If there is extensive involvement of the sagittal sinus wall with tumor but the sinus is still patent, in the middle and posterior third meningiomas tumor is left in the wall of the sinus because of the risk of venous infarction. We do not believe the risks involved with placing a graft in this area of the sagittal sinus are warranted.

Once the tumor is removed, a good deal of time is spent ensuring that there are no bleeding points. Small vessels to the tumor capsule that do not appear to go to normal brain should be coagulated and divided as they are encountered during dissection. If these small vessels are avulsed, they may retract into the surrounding brain tissue and be unnoticed at the surface of the brain tissue adjacent to the tumor. Once it is certain that adequate hemostasis has been achieved, the exposed surfaces of brain are lined with Surgicel. The blood pressure can be elevated up to 140 mmHg systolic to see if any sites of bleeding can be identified.

Closure

The dura is closed by taking a large piece of pericranium from the back of the scalp flap and sewing it into the dural defect. The dura and graft are usually covered with Gelfoam. The bone flap is replaced and held with several No. 28 wire sutures placed through drill holes. These do not interfere with subsequent imaging studies. Where appropriate a wire is placed across each burr hole and the holes are filled with acrylic cranioplasty material. If bone removal due to tumor will leave a cosmetic deformity, a cranioplasty is done.

Surgical Management of Falx Meningiomas

It is important to study the preoperative MR images and angiogram to determine the relationship of the tumor to the sagittal sinus, access to the tumor in relationship to the cortical veins, and location of anterior cerebral artery branches (Fig. 13-6).

As with parasagittal meningiomas, these tumors can also be considered in relationship to the anterior, middle, and posterior thirds of the falx. The positions, incisions, and bone flaps are essentially the same as those used for parasagittal meningiomas in these locations.

The dura opening is made parallel to the sagittal sinus about 1 to 2 cm from the lateral edge of the sinus (Fig. 13-7). Exposure of the tumor is aided by the use of dehydrating agents, control of PCO_2, and position of the head. It may be necessary to divide a number of Pacchionian granulation attachments to gain access to the falx. It is only necessary to retract the medial cerebral cortex no more than 1 to 2 cm from the falx to expose the tumor capsule. In some cases a cortical vein can be freed from the cortex for a few millimeters to give the necessary exposure.

The anterior and posterior margins of the tumor capsule next to the falx are defined. The capsule is opened and a segment of tumor is removed so that the lateral mass of the tumor is separated from the falx. Great care is taken as the deep portion of the capsule is dissected because of the possible adherence of the anterior cerebral branches. Once the lateral mass of tumor is free, it is gradually brought into the area next to the falx, alternating internal decompression and dissection of the capsule. A sharp pointed instrument placed in the tumor with gentle medial pressure can be very helpful. This technique avoids putting excessive retraction on the adjacent brain.

After the lateral bulk of the tumor is removed, attention is turned to the residual tumor in the falx. The falx is opened with a sharp knife a few millimeters away from the tumor attachment and divided around the tumor. The inferior sagittal sinus can be occluded

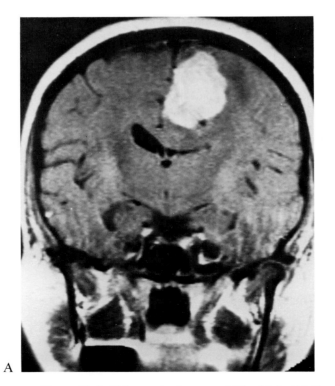

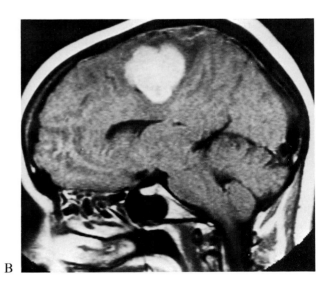

A   B

Figure 13-6. Falx meningioma—middle third. **(A)** Coronal and **(B)** sagittal T_1-weighted MRIs with contrast enhancement. The configuration of the tumor is precisely outlined. The inferior portion of the tumor is starting to indent the corpus callosum. On the coronal view an anterior cerebral artery branch is displaced laterally. (*Figure continues.*)

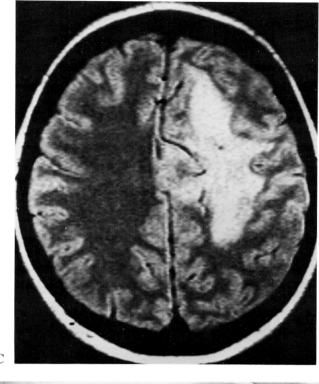

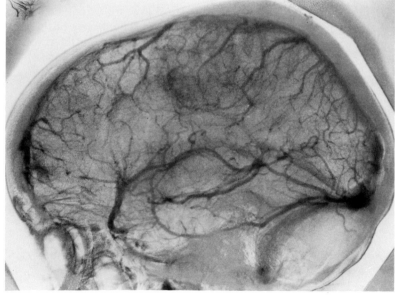

Figure 13-6 (*Continued*). **(C)** Axial T$_2$-weighted MRI through the inferior portion of the tumor. A large area of edema is seen in the adjacent white matter. The lateral displacement of the anterior cerebral branch is clearly seen. **(D)** Lateral venous phase of the angiogram. The tumor stain is seen in relationship to the cortical veins. In planning the approach, the surgeon needs to be prepared to expose the tumor anteriorly, directly over the tumor, or posteriorly. In this patient the large anterior vein came over the tumor as it reached the midline and then turned parallel to the sagittal sinus and was densely adherent to the sinus over a distance of about 2 cm. The tumor was completely removed from an approach anterior to this vein.

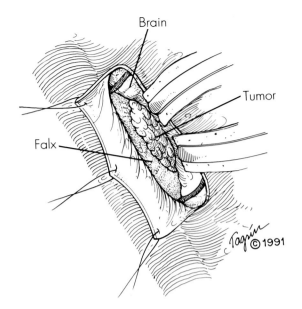

Figure 13-7. Falx meningioma. The incision in the dura is made between 1 and 2 cm parallel to the sagittal sinus. Only enough tumor needs to be exposed to separate it from the falx and to have room to do an internal decompression. The capsule can then gradually be withdrawn into the area of decompression.

when indicated. In many patients the extension of the tumor into the opposite hemisphere can be removed through this opening. In large bilateral falx meningiomas it will be necessary to expose both medial cerebral hemispheres. In anteriorly placed large falx tumors it is often helpful to take the sagittal sinus as described for parasagittal tumors to aid in the total removal.

Surgical Management of Convexity Meningiomas

Nearly all convexity meningiomas can be removed totally and the patient cured. Most of the principals outlined for parasagittal lesions apply to convexity meningiomas.

In positioning the patient the scalp overlying the central portion of the tumor is placed at the highest level if this is possible. Usually a horseshoe-shaped incision is used. For parasagittal convexity meningiomas the position of the patient and skin incisions are the same as those outlined for parasagittal meningiomas. For tumors centered on the coronal suture, the patient is usually placed in the semilateral position and the skin flap is turned anteriorly (Fig. 13-8). For frontal-temporal meningiomas a pterional skin incision is used. The pericranial tissue is preserved with the skin flap and is taken at the end of the resection to replace the excised dura.

A free bone flap is planned so that it is large enough to allow for adequate excision of dura around the tumor. The details of the craniotomy opening are the same as those outlined for parasagittal meningiomas.

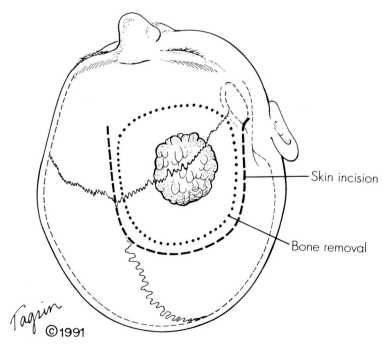

Figure 13-8. Convexity meningioma—coronal suture. The patient is in a semilateral position with the head well elevated and the scalp over the tumor uppermost. The skin flap is turned forward.

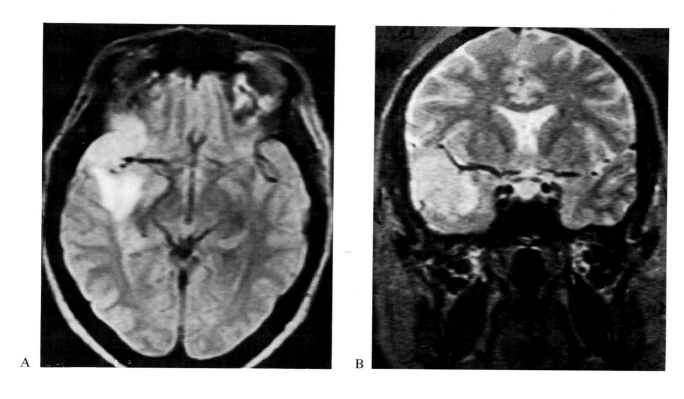

A

B

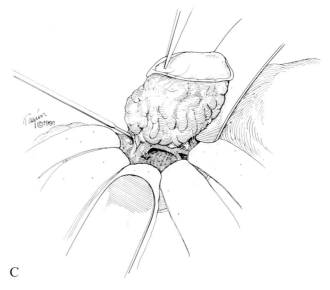

C

Figure 13-9. Frontal-temporal convexity (pterional) meningioma. **(A)** Axial and **(B)** coronal T$_2$-weighted MRIs. The middle cerebral artery is seen next to the medial posterior capsule of the tumor. On the axial view there is edema in the brain just posterior to the tumor. **(C)** Gentle traction is placed on the tumor through the dural attachment. The middle cerebral artery branches are carefully freed as the medial surface of the capsule is dissected.

Gentle palpation will usually give a good indication of the edge of the tumor. The dura is opened circumferentially around the tumor, occluding meningeal arteries as these are encountered, staying about 1 cm from the tumor attachment but exposing as little normal brain as possible. The dura is left attached to the tumor and used to apply gentle outward traction. The plane between the tumor capsule and arachnoid and surrounding brain is carefully opened around the tumor. Then, working circumferentially, retracting the tumor capsule, placing gentle traction on the dural attachment, and using bipolar forceps and dissectors to separate brain tissue, the tumor is gradually separated. Moist cottonoids are placed on the brain as it is separated. Smaller tumors may be removed intact. In large lesions it is best to do an adequate internal decompression as the plane between the tumor and brain is developed. This will allow most of the pressure needed to define the plane to be placed on the tumor capsule without displacing tumor into brain on the opposite side from which one is working and using only minimal retraction or no retraction on the adjacent brain. Closure is the same as described for parasagittal meningiomas.

A special circumstance occurs when the tumor arises over the frontotemporal junction (Fig. 13-9). There are two anatomical points to be kept in mind in order to avoid complications. First, the middle cerebral artery branches may be adherent to the medial capsule, and great care must be exercised in removing this tumor. The degree of involvement of this artery with the tumor may be predicted from the preoperative MRI. Second, some of the dural attachments may extend over the floor of the anterior fossa, sphenoid wing, and anterior wall of the middle fossa. This area of dural involvement must be removed, sometimes even into the lateral edge of the superior orbital fissure. The dural defect can often be repaired by sewing the graft directly to the edge of the remaining dura. After the intracranial dura is sewn, the graft can be tented along the bone edge and then the convexity margin of the dura closed. When the medial dural edge is too fragile to sew, the dural graft can be sewn through multiple drill holes along the craniotomy margin.

POSTOPERATIVE COMPLICATIONS

Early Complications

As the patient awakens from anesthesia, intravenous agents are used to control blood pressure tightly. A portable monitor is used to follow blood pressure and heart rate as the patient is transported to the recovery room or intensive care unit. Close observation in an intensive care unit setting is indicated for at least the first postoperative night. Steroids are continued for several days and then gradually tapered. Anticonvulsants are continued.

As the patient recovers from anesthesia, vital signs are monitored and an initial neurological evaluation is done. If there is a neurological deficit, the neurosurgeon will need to evaluate the situation carefully. Are there any associated vital sign changes? Was there an intraoperative event that likely explains the disability? Is the problem related to the finding of a brief increase in neurological deficit often seen and apparently related in some way to the effect of the anesthetic agents? Could a hematoma be developing? A short period of observation usually clarifies the problem. If the patient is not rapidly improving or is clearly worsening, then either an immediate CT scan or return to the operating room is indicated to look for a hematoma. The other problems that may be seen in the recovery room relate to cardiopulmonary complications.

During the first week the patient may show a delayed increase in neurological deficit. This is usually due to cerebral edema. CT scan evaluates this problem and also will show any evidence of a delayed hematoma. Rarely is hydrocephalus a problem in this group of patients. These symptoms usually respond to an increase in steroids. In some patients, intermittent mannitol is used to keep the osmolarity above 300 (25 g IV every 6 hours is the usual dose).

Toward the end of the first week is the time when one may begin to see problems with wound infection and thrombophlebitis. A superficial cellulitis may respond to antibiotics. Major wound infections usually require removal of the bone flap. Thrombophlebitis is treated with heparin and coumadin after the first week. During the first week a vena cava filter is used. The place of prophylactic subcutaneous heparin has not been established. During this time anticonvulsant levels are monitored. If they are adequate, seizure is rarely a problem, but on occasion additional medication is needed, usually for focal seizures when the tumor involves the motor-sensory cortex.

Late Complications

Late problems relate primarily to disabilities from neurological deficits that were either present preoperatively or resulted from the operative procedure. An active rehabilitation program may be needed. Anticonvulsants are continued for at least 3 months and longer if there was a history of a seizure.

Olfactory Groove and Planum Meningiomas

Joseph Ransohoff
Russ P. Nockels

Throughout our written and living history, generations of neurosurgeons have displayed a fascination with meningiomas that arise from the olfactory groove and planum sphenoidale. Our earliest records as skillful observers of integrated neurological anatomy and symptomatology reveal a select reverence for these tumors. Cushing, for instance, stimulated by his initial five cases, chose these tumors as the topic of the famous Macewen Memorial Lecture of 1927.[38] Another cherished patient with a subfrontal meningioma prompted Foster Kennedy's first description of the ophthalmologic syndrome that bears his name.[48] In fact, the first meningioma ever removed successfully was an olfactory groove tumor by Durante in 1885.[41] By virtue of his patient's amply documented long survival (at least 20 years) and postoperative cerebrospinal fluid (CSF) rhinorrhea, olfactory groove meningiomas also possess the dubious distinction of acquiring the longest history of operative complications.[41,45]

Elucidation of technical principles for the successful management of these tumors was to await the further observations of Cushing and Henderson—who contributed the standard frontal approach.[38,39,45] Through the years, the prevention of postoperative mishaps has become the focus of increasing surgical endeavor. Today, this historical experience is complemented by modern technical strategies to ensure both maximal safe removal and long-term tumor-free survival—with an associated progressive decline in the complication rate (Table 13-1).[44,57,58,62,63,66] This experience, along with that of the senior author's, is described in this chapter, paying special attention to postoperative difficulties. As a result of these efforts, today we enjoy an era in which patients with olfactory groove and planum tumors fare better and savor a longer duration of good-quality survival than those with most other supratentorial meningiomas.[37]

Constituting between 8 and 13 percent of all intracranial meningiomas,[37,57,62,63,66] these tumors occur in the midline in the region of the olfactory groove or planum sphenoidale and slowly expand in a bilateral fashion, elevating and compressing both frontal lobes. Occasionally, they arise unilaterally from one olfactory groove and can be somewhat asymmetrical, but even in this situation, they eventually compress the falx and appear on CT scan or MRI as bilateral lesions.

Olfactory groove meningiomas are generally of significant size before their associated symptoms are attributed to a subfrontal tumor. It has been known since the time of Cushing that the earliest recognition of these tumors usually comes from the astute ophthalmologist or neurologist, who recognizes the im-

Table 13-1. Complications and Mortality in Olfactory Groove and Planum Meningiomas

Author	Year	No. of Cases	Complete Removal (%)	Mortality Rate (%)	Anterior Cerebral Artery Injury	CSF Leak	Infection	Postoperative Seizures	Visual Loss
Cushing et al.[39]	1938	22	59.1	22.7	9	1	1	—	—
Olivecrona[58]	1967	75	93.3	17.3	—	—	—	—	—
Bakay et al.[33]	1972	25	76.0	12.0	3	1	0	4	1
Symon[63]	1977	18	100.0	0.0	—	—	—	—	—
Yamashita et al.[66]	1980	30	56.7	20.0	—	—	—	—	—
Solero et al.[62]	1983	98	93.8	17.3	5	3	3	6	7
Ojeman et al.[57]	1985	10	100.0	0.0	0	1	1	—	—
Hassler et al.[44]	1989	11	100.0	9.1	0	0	0	0	0
Ransohoff	1991	33	93.9	6.1	1	0	0	2	0

Table 13-2. Olfactory Groove and Planum
Meningiomas: Clinical Summary of 33 Patients

Male : female ratio	1 : 2
Mean age (range)	61 years (17–81)
Mean follow-up period (range)	6.4 years (0.5–11)
Mean duration of symptoms (range)	22 months (0.5–120)

Initial Symptoms/Signs on Presentation	
Altered mental status	12/15
Visual acuity loss	9/14
Seizures	10/—
Headache	2/—
Papilledema	—/2
Anosmia	1/29

portant but infrequent combination of personality dysfunction, visual loss either from optic nerve compression or papilledema, and anosmia.[39,42,46] The mental symptoms are generally those of a vague flattening of personality, short-term memory loss, and loss of initiative—symptoms that in the elderly patient are often attributed to aging and depression. The visual changes are characteristically insidious in nature, with a variety of presentations including scotomata, uni- or bitemporal field cuts, acuity loss, and papilledema. Infrequently, the tumors present with an apoplectic visual change.[52] On other occasions, severe headaches or a generalized seizure may be the first recognized symptom of these tumors; however, in retrospect, the patient and/or family will always be aware of some subtle personality change that has occurred over a period of months to years. Rarely, intranasal extensions of the tumor present first with epistaxis, or prompt recognition of their intracranial

site following biopsy.[59] It is interesting that whereas the sense of smell is almost always absent on careful examination, it is rarely a primary complaint of the patient.

The senior author's experience with these tumors in the post-CT era is summarized in Table 13-2. All patients operated on between 1979 and 1990 on whom complete follow-up information could be obtained were included in this series of 33 patients. They share the common profile of patients harboring meningiomas at this site: generally a third of patients first present with psychological symptoms, a third with seizures, and a third with visual deterioration. Visual impairment, present in 14 (42 percent) of 33 patients, was severe upon presentation (<20/200 in at least one eye) in 11 (79 percent) of these 14 patients. Seizures were invariably generalized in nature, and augered well for the patient if they preceded visual or mental deterioration.

Complications arising from the surgical removal of these tumors have remained fairly uniform since Cushing's time, and fall under five main headings (see Table 13-1): (1) CSF leak and infection, (2) postoperative seizures, (3) anterior cerebral artery (ACA) injury, (4) visual loss, and (5) recurrence. Mortality given the advances in medical care and operative technology, has declined dramatically since the time of Cushing (see Table 13-3), from 22.7 to 6 percent and less.[39,44,62] Prior causes of operative death, such as diencephalic dysfunction, have been virtually eliminated since the introduction of corticosteroids and the operating room microscope. Other factors, such as patient age (>55 years, 21.4 percent mortality rate versus 15.7 percent for <55 years) and tumor size (>3 cm) 14,[46,62] have also been reported to in-

Table 13-3. Causes of Postoperative Mortality in Olfactory Groove Meningiomas

Author	Year	No. of Cases	Mortality Rate (%)	Anterior Cerebral Artery Injury	Infection	Cerebral Edema	Postoperative Hematoma	Systemic	Total
Cushing et al.[39]	1938	22	22.7	2	1	2	—	—	5
Bakay et al.[33]	1972	25	12.0	3	—	—	—	—	3
Yamashita et al.[66]	1980	30	20.0	—	—	—	—	—	6
Solero et al.[62]	1983	98	17.3	6	2	4	1	5[a]	17
Hassler et al.[44]	1989	11	10.0	—	—	—	—	1 PE	1
Ransohoff	1991	33	6.1	1	—	—	—	1 PE	2

Abbreviation: PE, pulmonary embolus.
[a] Two myocardial infarct, one each Cushing's ulcer, bronchopneumonia, sepsis.

crease risk of perioperative death. Tumor size alone may not be as important as the ensuing encasement of the anterior cerebral vessels, which Kadis et al.[46] found to be present in all 10 cases of postoperative death in their series of 105 planum and tuberculum tumors. Since 1983, however, in series reporting patients solely operated upon by modern microsurgical techniques, the combined mortality rate approaches 5 percent (see Table 13-1).[44,57,62]

OPERATIVE PROCEDURE

Diagnostic Measures

Whereas in the recent past, CT scan with and without contrast has been the initial diagnostic measure, today MRI followed by an MRI with gadolinium enhancement is becoming far more common. Triaxial MRI scan, however, is essential even if the patient carries a CT scan diagnosis unless contraindicated because of the presence of cardiac pacemakers or other metal in the patient's body (Fig. 13-10). The sagittal MRI is invaluable in demonstrating the relationship of the tumor to the optic nerves and chiasm, which are rarely encased in the tumor unless there is dural spread of the meningioma posterior to its site of origin (Fig. 13-11). The coronal plane is particularly helpful in distinguishing those tumors that influence the sphenoid jugum and ethmoid bone by hyperostoses from the less common ones that produce erosion. Such erosion and extension into the subfrontal sinuses has been reported in up to 15 percent of cases.[40] Although this seems high in comparison with our experience, it does underscore the need for multiplanar imaging, either with CT or MRI, to assess the need for skull base reconstruction and to define operative tactics to ensure total tumor removal

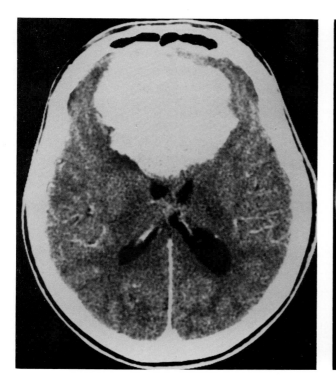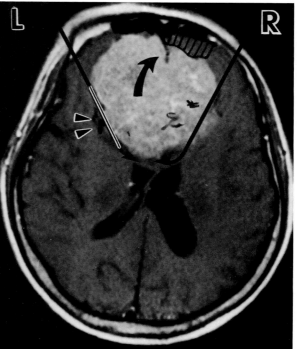

Figure 13-10. Comparison of contrast-enhanced CT and MRI of an olfactory groove meningioma. These preoperative images of a patient with a typically large olfactory groove meningioma highlight the differences between each study (the scans have been reversed to emphasize the operative perspective). CT is consistently better at imaging bone. A noncontrast CT scan in the coronal plane is particularly helpful to define areas of skull base hyperostoses or destruction. The MRI is superior in demonstrating all nonosseous structures, including the signal void of cerebral vessels along the perimeter of the tumor (*arrowheads*) and the falx (*curved arrow*). Note the area of the right frontal pole to be resected (*hatched area*) during initial uncapping of the tumor. The planned bifrontal craniotomy allows greatest access to the posterior pole of the tumor and optimizes the plane between tumor capsule and the left cerebral arteries (*white line*).

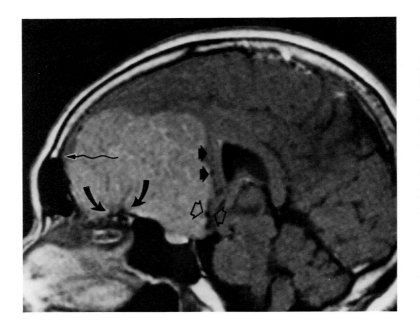

Figure 13-11. Gadolinium-enhanced sagittal MRI of the same patient as in Fig. 13-10. This view of the MRI defines the relationship of the tumor to the skull base and displaced cerebral structures. The tumor's vascular pedicle is seen emanating from the frontal base (*curved arrows*). Note in particular the posterior pole of the tumor, torquing the genu of the corpus callosum and compressing the optic chiasm and anterior cerebral artery (*open arrows*). The need to expose the frontal sinuses is further illustrated, as the level of the sinuses (*wavy arrow*) is far above that required for a sufficiently low craniotomy. Compare this image with the cerebral angiogram of the same patient in Fig. 13-14.

(Figs. 13-12 and 13-13). CT scan is somewhat better than MRI in demonstrating this bony abnormality. Cerebral angiography is of value in preoperative planning, both to demonstrate the relationship of the anterior cerebral arteries to the tumor as well as to reveal the external carotid supply, which is nearly always from the ethmoidal and ophthalmic arteries, reaching the tumor through perforations of the bony floor of the anterior cranial fossa (Fig. 13-14). Preoperative embolization is rarely possible, as these feeders are small and multiple and the risk of an embolus entering the ophthalmic artery rarely warrants this procedure. It must also be noted that as MRI angiography becomes more available, as it undoubtedly will in the next few years, one may avoid formal angiography altogether.

Preoperative Evaluation

The patient should undergo a general medical evaluation, including cardiac and pulmonary functions. MRI should be evaluated for the presence of chronic frontal or ethmoidal sinusitis, which, if present, may require preoperative drainage and appropriate antibiotic therapy for several weeks prior to elective surgery. This is particularly true as the bone flap will inevitably expose the frontal sinuses, and the potential for postoperative infection can be minimized by these precautions. If the patient has experienced seizures as a result of the tumor, anticonvulsant therapy will already have been initiated. If not, the patient

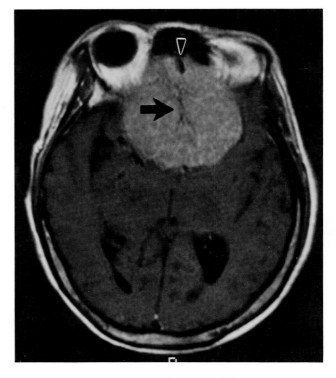

Figure 13-12. Gadolinium-enhanced axial MRI of the same patient as in Figs. 13-10 and 13-11. The intratumoral vascular supply (*black arrow*) is again identified as signal voids within the body of the tumor. Calcification of the cribriform plate is seen in the midline (*arrowhead*). Note that this axial view is inadequate to define the tumor's relationship with the infracranial sinuses, necessitating a coronal study.

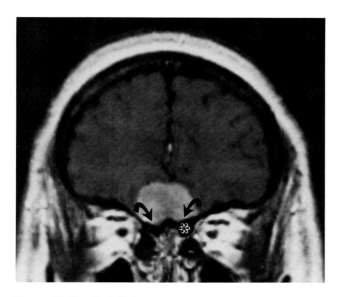

Figure 13-13. Gadolinium-enhanced coronal MRI of an olfactory groove meningioma. By defining the relationship of the tumor to the skull base and underlying ethmoidal sinuses (*asterisk*), the surgeon can preoperatively evaluate the need for skull base reconstruction, and subsequent risk of CSF fistula.

should receive phenytoin for several days prior to admission followed by serum confirmation that therapeutic levels have been obtained. If the patient has significant peritumoral edema or if papilledema is present, it is wise to premedicate for several days prior to surgery with adequate doses of corticosteroids. Dexamethasone 4 mg qid is appropriate for

this regimen, and is supplemented the night before surgery with intravenous corticosteroids. It is also wise to advise the patient to shampoo vigorously for several days prior to admission. This is particularly true for women in whom the coronal incision can be made well behind the hairline and a frontal tuft of hair allowed to remain for cosmetic purposes. Patients with diabetes are placed on sliding scale insulin coverage based on urinary sugar estimations as soon as corticosteroids are initiated. The night before surgery, the patient is placed on Solu-Medrol (Upjohn Co., Kalamazoo, MI) 250 mg IV every 6 hours. Phenobarbital is added to the anticonvulsant regime, usually 240 mg in two divided doses on the night before surgery, and another 45 mg IM upon call to the operating room. Once in the operating room, following the appropriate placement of arterial and venous lines for fluid and blood replacement and anesthetic monitoring, the three-pin Mayfield head holder is placed in an appropriate position to avoid interference with the bicoronal skin incision. Pneumatic compression boots are placed on the lower extremities presuming that the patient has been fully ambulatory prior to surgery. If the patient has been on bed rest before surgery, Doppler studies are essential to evaluate the venous drainage of both lower extremities. The presence of any suggestion of venous obstruction contraindicates the use of the compression boots. If the patient has been chronically ill, it is probably wise to consider the placement of a vena cava umbrella to prevent postoperative pulmonary emboli.

Figure 13-14. Lateral internal carotid angiogram of patient in Figs. 13-10–13-12. The vascular supply of the tumor is seen arising from ethmoidal branches (*curved arrows*) of a large ophthalmic artery (*straight arrow*). The posterior displacement of the internal carotid artery and superior and posterior bowing of the ACA are characteristic for subfrontal tumors (*arrowheads*).

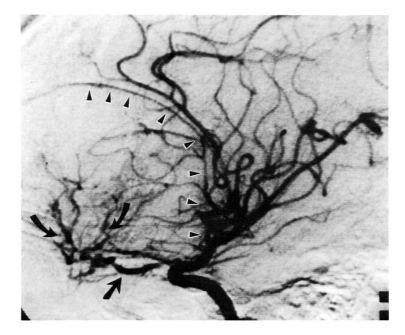

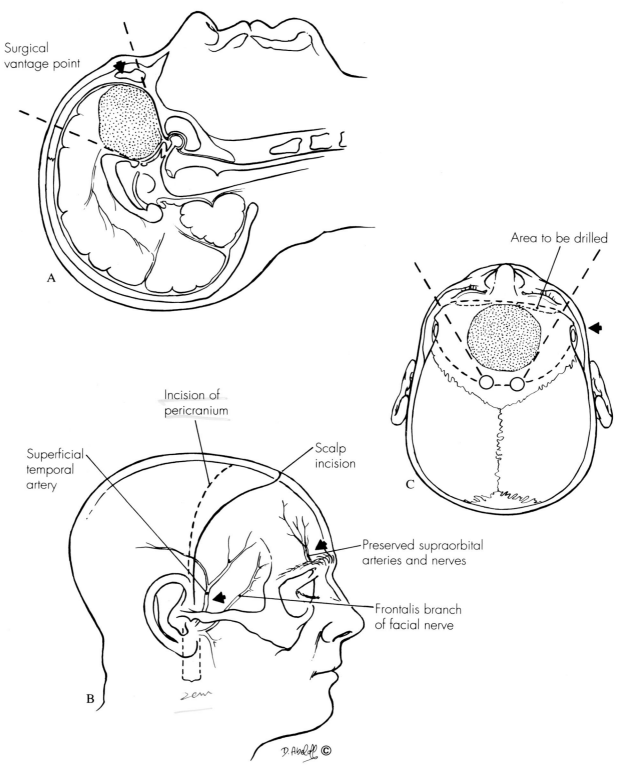

Figure 13-15. **(A)** Operative position and surgical exposure. Note that mild head extension brings the sloping frontal skull base into the surgical vantage point and that the frontal lobes will tend to fall away from the cranial floor. In the majority of patients, the frontobasal craniotomy will enter the frontal sinus. **(B&C)** Scalp incision and bony opening. The standard Soutar skin incision is used and the underlying pericranium is spared. The pericranium is incised separately after retracting the scalp posteriorly, affording a larger poten-

Operation

As always, adequate exposure of the tumor is linked to proper patient positioning. In this case, maximal midline exposure of the anterior cranial fossa is required (Fig. 13-15A). The patient is positioned supine with the knees slightly gatched, and the head is positioned "straight up" and slightly higher than the rest of the body. For optimal head position, the Mayfield sprocket must be perpendicular to the floor, allowing maximal degrees of freedom during final adjustment. The head is extended approximately 30 degrees, in such a way that the frontal lobes following craniotomy will tend to fall away from the floor of the anterior fossa. This maneuver is crucial for minimizing the need for retraction of cerebral tissue, which is to be avoided at all cost. The anesthesiologist should have ready access to the operating table controls, as minor intraoperative adjustments in head extension and rotation can be carried out in this way. Prior to scrubbing and prepping the scalp, the eyes are protected with waterproof drapes. In men, an area of scalp is shaved in order to permit a bicoronal skin incision just behind the coronal suture, whereas in women it is perfectly acceptable to shave an area for several inches both anterior and posterior to the incision line, preserving a frontal tuft of hair.

Following prepping and draping, the standard Soutar or bicoronal skin incision is developed. The incision begins just anterior to the ear at the level of the root of the zygoma. This is in order to avoid the extracranial seventh nerve, which is sometimes found within 1 cm of the external auditory meatus (EOM) at this level. In addition, the superficial temporal fascia must be incised within this 1-cm distance of the EOM and reflected with the scalp anteriorly to avoid postoperative weakness of the frontalis branch of the facial nerve.

If extensive covering of the frontal sinuses or anterior cranial fossa is expected during closure, the pericranium is spared with the skin incision, and incised as a separate layer 2 cm posteriorly to allow for an adequate graft (Fig. 13-15B). The loose connective tissue between the galea and the pericranium swells when irrigated with saline, aiding dissection along this plane with blunt scissors. The skin flap is carried down to the orbital rims bilaterally, caution being taken to avoid damage to the supraorbital nerves as they exit from the supraorbital foramen. By carefully remaining within the connective tissue plane between the galea and pericranium, these nerves are spared in the superficial layers. The pericranial flap is then sandwiched between two sponges and kept moist with saline during the procedure. The bone flap is outlined with the cutting current to extend from one sphenofrontal suture to the other, just at the point of the frontal process of the zygoma (the anatomic "keyhole"). The anterior boundary of the craniotomy should be placed as low as possible, just avoiding transgression of the orbital roof. Burr holes are placed bilaterally at these points, and an additional two burr holes are placed on either side of the midline just anterior to the coronal suture, allowing a small ridge of bone to protect the longitudinal sinus. Recently, it has been easier to open the frontal sinuses with a small acorn attachment on the high-speed drill (Fig. 13-15C). By shaving the bone along the frontal base, the mucosa of the frontal sinus can be exposed in its entirety, and the posterior wall of the sinus removed through a greater opening. The posterior wall is then removed with either the drill or a Kerrison punch to expose several centimeters of dura on either side of the midline. This makes fracture of the nasal portion of the sinus with the hand-held perforator and tearing of the dura with the craniotome footplate along the irregularities of the bony posterior wall of the frontal sinus less likely. The somewhat more extensive resulting frontal defect is easily restored using methyl methacrylate during closure.

Attention is turned to the two posterior burr holes and the bone is again rongeured from the subadjacent dura and longitudinal sinus. The dura is then stripped with dural elevators as far as possible between the various burr holes. Once this has been achieved, the craniotome is utilized to develop the bone flap. The bone flap is then elevated from posteriorly to anteriorly, being careful to strip the longitudinal sinus and adjacent dura from the undersurface of the bone. Bleeding from the exposed dura covering the longitudinal sinus and adjacent pacchionian granulations can be controlled with bipolar cautery and thin strips of thrombin-soaked Gelfoam, which are suctioned dry through a cotton patty.

To prevent epidural stripping and postoperative epidural collections, perforations are developed at

tial pericranial graft. Note that the scalp incision starts just anterior to the tragus to avoid injury to the frontalis branch of the facial nerve. The bony exposure must provide access to the posterior pole of the tumor by incorporating burr holes behind the frontal process of the zygoma. Note the area along the frontal base to be drilled in order to expose and adequately obliterate the frontal sinuses.

this stage along the margins of the exposed skull in order to place dural retention sutures. These holes will also be placed in adjacent areas of the bone flap and utilized to wire the bone flap in place at the termination of the procedure. Attention is now turned to the exposed frontal sinuses, where the same acorn drill bit can be used to remove the mucosa of the frontal sinus completely, exposing the frontal ostia. Dry oxidized cotton impregnated with dry bacitracin is now packed into the sinus. Muscle is harvested from the temporalis muscles, soaked in cyanoacrylate or biological fibrin glue, and placed into the ostia of the frontal sinus. The muscle is then covered with a layer of oxidized cotton, completely sealing the frontal sinuses in order to prevent postoperative spinal fluid leakage. At the end of the procedure, the pericranium will be utilized as a vascular pedicle to cover the frontal sinuses.

We are now ready to turn our attention to the dural opening (Fig. 13-16). It is reassuring at this point to utilize the ultrasonic localizer to be certain that the posterior limit of the bone flap is large enough to visualize the posterior extent of the tumor. The dura is now opened initially on the nondominant side (usually right), the initial incision being made parallel to the anterior margin of the bone flap. Here one must be careful to leave an adequate margin for eventual dural closure, as this is an important technical measure to minimize the risk of CSF leakage. The dural opening is carried laterally to the extent of the craniotomy, then posteriorly for 3 to 4 cm, and then sharply toward the midline. The dura is reflected medially to expose the falx and its junction with the longitudinal sinus. Attention must be directed to any bridging veins, which must be exposed and coagulated. A cottonoid is now placed between the frontal lobe and falx to prevent any accumulation of blood while our attention is turned to the left frontal area. The dural incision on the left side is made similar to that on the right, exposing once again the falx and longitudinal sinus. Any bridging veins in the area are coagulated and sectioned. This dural incision, however, is not carried further posteriorly, avoiding undue exposure of the dominant frontal lobe.

The next step of the procedure is to ligate the longitudinal sinus, as it is exposed between the two anterior dural incisions (Fig. 13-16A&B). The frontal lobes are gently retracted laterally from the area of the sinus by the operator and first assistant. Silk sutures (3-0) are placed beneath the sinus, through the falx and back to perforate the dura on either side just lateral to the sinus, and are tied. This technique is designed to prevent slippage of these sutures once the sinus has been sectioned. These sutures are not cut as they will be utilized at the termination of the procedure to reoppose the dura in the midline. The longitudinal sinus is now sectioned with a No. 11 blade between the two sutures, and any bleeding is coagulated with the two-point cautery. At this point one may see the upper surface of the meningioma as it is indented by the falx. It is important to section the falx completely down to, and at times even into the body of the tumor. Once this is achieved, the posterior falx and sinus are gently retracted posteriorly and held in place with a mosquito clamp placed on the suture, which has been used to ligate the sinus. The anterior falx is retracted anteriorly in a similar fashion.

In general, we wish to avoid the use of brain retractors throughout the operative procedure. Retraction of edematous brain that is chronically compressed by the underlying mass frequently leads to postoperative edema, infarction, and intracerebral hemorrhage. For this reason, we prefer to carry out a polar resection of the right frontal lobe electively, uncapping the superior surface of the meningioma (Fig. 13-16C&D). This resection is carried to the midline and laterally to the area of the sphenoidal ridge, just lateral to the margin of the meningioma. Cottonoids are now placed over exposed surface of the meningioma, sweeping the subadjacent frontal lobe from the superior and lateral surfaces of the tumor. At this stage in the operative procedure, the microscope has been brought into the field and is utilized intermittently during the remainder of the tumor removal. Here the microscope enables one to identify the arachnoid plane over the tumor and examine the surface of the meningioma, coagulating any intrinsic vessels on the capsule.

The typically large subfrontal meningioma forbids the exposure of the dural base of the tumor. As an initial step, therefore, one begins debulking the tumor in stages, utilizing the ultrasonic surgical aspirator and bipolar cautery (Fig. 13-17A&B). Beginning with the most anterior aspect of the tumor, the resection is directed toward the base from which the blood supply of the tumor is arising. As the resection is carried to the skull base, the surgeon will expose the perforating arterial vessels supplying the tumor and coagulate them with the two-point cautery. The degree of tumor removal can be documented at this and any subsequent stage with the ultrasonic localizer. After 60 to 70 percent of the bulk of the meningioma on the right side has been removed, the surgeon begins to retract the capsule of the tumor gently on the right side toward the midline and anteriorly. This retraction is initiated along the most lateral aspects of the tumor and will provide a valuable perception as

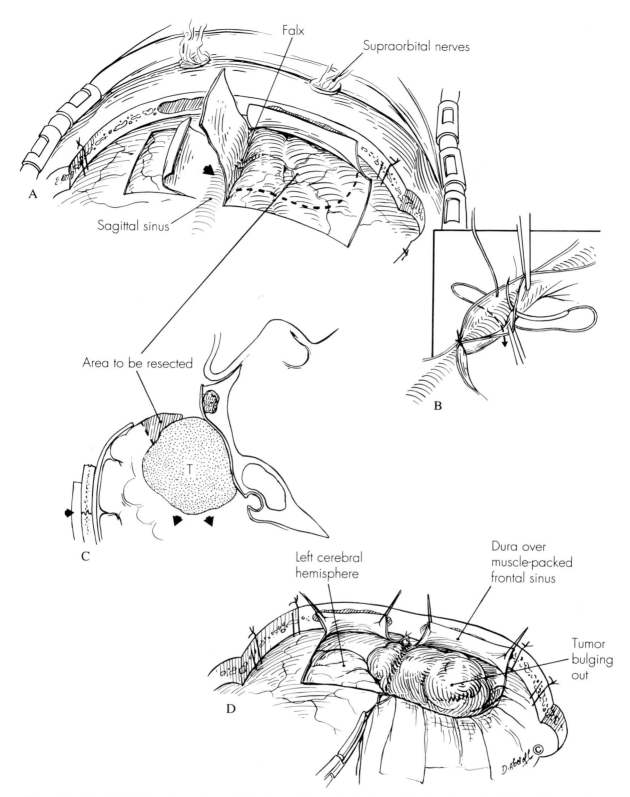

Figure 13-16. (A&B) Dural opening and ligation of the sagittal sinus. The dural opening is based upon the midline, with the right exposure slightly greater than the left. Note that a 1-cm dural flap remains at the base to be utilized at closure. After the sagittal sinus is ligated as shown, the dura can be reflected superiorly, exposing the tumor and compressed frontal lobes. **(C&D)** Polar resection of the right frontal lobe. Initial exposure of the tumor (*T*) often requires resection of the right frontal pole (see hatched area). Saline-moistened cotton pledgets are used to protect exposed cerebral structures before beginning intratumoral decompression.

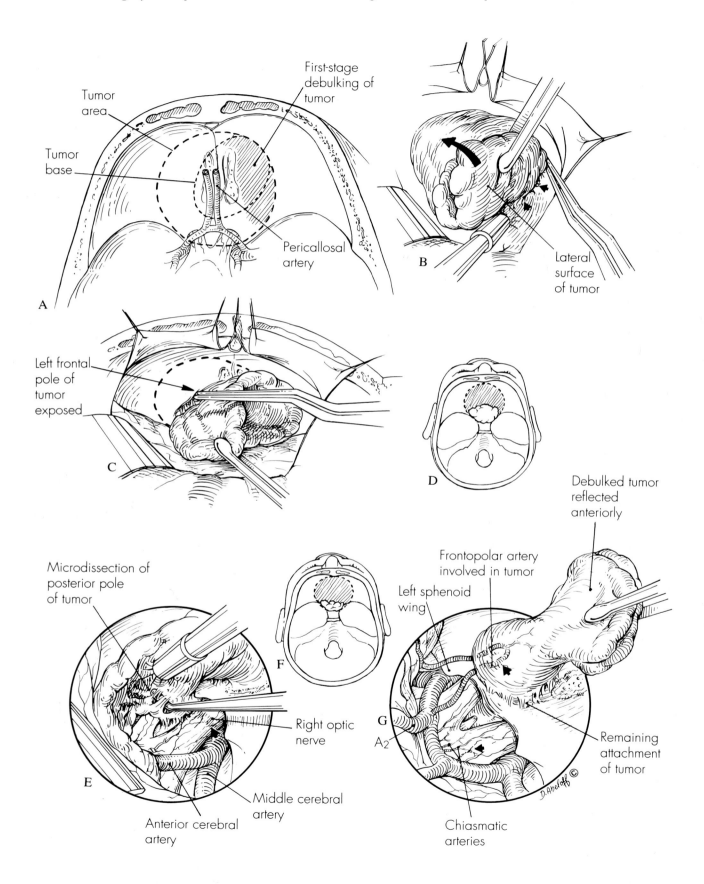

Tumor area

Tumor base

First-stage debulking of tumor

Pericallosal artery

A

Lateral surface of tumor

B

Left frontal pole of tumor exposed

C

D

Microdissection of posterior pole of tumor

Right optic nerve

Anterior cerebral artery

Middle cerebral artery

E

F

Debulked tumor reflected anteriorly

Frontopolar artery involved in tumor

Left sphenoid wing

Remaining attachment of tumor

Chiasmatic arteries

A2

G

D.Abeloff ©

to the adherence of the meningioma to the underlying brain. As one approaches the midline with this retraction, one will begin to visualize the superior surface of the meningioma underlying the opposite left frontal lobe; caution is exercised here to prevent injury to the brain on that side.

Attention is returned to the skull base, where, with the use of the ultrasonic aspirator, the most inferior portion of the tumor on the left side is debulked, exposing the left perforating feeding vessels to coagulation and hence, further devascularizing the tumor (Fig. 13-17C&D). It is important to work anteriorly and laterally toward the left side, avoiding the most posterior aspect of the tumor capsule. It is reassuring at this stage to note the egress of CSF from the basal arachnoidal cisterns, which signals that an adequate debulking of the tumor has been achieved.

The most important maneuver in the successful removal of these tumors is now ready to be carried out. One swings the microscope well laterally to the right side and begins to explore the most posterior aspect of the capsule, working towards the midline. This maneuver is critical to identify the posterior attachment of the tumor, which is almost always anterior to the optic nerves and chiasm (Fig. 13-17E&F). One is eventually able to identify this posterior pole, and probe the base of the skull and exposed dura anterior to the optic nerves and chiasm just posterior to the attachment of the meningioma, which may in this region be associated with an area of hyperostosis. This dissection must be carried well across the midline to ensure protection of both optic nerves.

One now begins the final phases of capsular removal, turning attention once again to the superior and posterior aspect of the tumor. Via gradual retrac-tion on the capsule of the tumor and periodic intracapsular debulking, one reduces the remainder of the bulk of the tumor on the right side as well as toward the left, always working in this right to left fashion. Eventually, one will visualize the most lateral aspect of the tumor on the left side in the region of the sphenoid wing.

By this stage, a small fragment of tumor still remains attached to the skull base at its most posterior limit, with a midline segment extending into the region of the anterior cerebral vessels. Utilizing the operating microscope, the tumor is progressively retracted forward from both the left and right sides, visualizing and taking advantage of the arachnoidal plane, which usually exists between the tumor and major branches of the anterior cerebral artery, including the frontal polar branches. One should take care during this stage in the microdissection to preserve the chiasmal blood supply (superior hypophyseal or chiasmal arteries), which bridges the internal carotid artery or the anterior communicating artery complex and the chiasm in the subarachnoid space (Fig. 13-17G). At times small perforating vessels from the branches of the ACA will enter the tumor and will be coagulated and sectioned with microsurgical technique.

Finally, one reaches the posterior and most inferior limit of the tumor. Working again from the right side, the most posterior attachment of the tumor is excised from the skull base. As the final bulk of tumor is delivered, one often experiences troublesome venous oozing from the most inferior medial aspects of both frontal lobes. This is best controlled by bipolar cautery under direct vision. Any denuded cortical areas and exposed white matter are now covered

Figure 13-17. (A&B) Initial tumor removal. The first stage of tumor removal involves intracapsular debulking of the right anterior quadrant (see hatched area). Note the relationship of the debulked tumor to the skull base and tumoral vascular supply. Following this initial removal of tumor, the tumor capsule can be drawn anteromedially into the area of decompression, allowing separation of the lateral tumor surface from the medial and inferior right frontal lobe. **(C&D)** Further tumor devascularization and removal. Removal of the tumor progresses across midline, alternating between intracapsular debulking and cauterization of the basal blood supply. This allows further dissection of the tumor capsule by retracting it into the area of tumor decompression and away from the left frontal lobe. Note that at the termination of this initial stage of removal, the posterior pole of the tumor remains. **(E&F)** Microsurgical dissection of the posterior pole of the tumor. The operating microscope is now used as the residual posterior pole of the tumor is drawn forward, allowing microdissection from the optic nerves and chiasm. As this is performed, further meticulous intracapsular removal of tumor may be necessary, with the eventual goal being the exposure of the left sphenoidal ridge and complete separation of the posterior tumor capsule from the optic apparatus. **(G)** Microsurgical dissection of the ACA. Following identification of the entire optic nerve and chiasm, the ACA can now be safely dissected from the final portion of tumor capsule. Every attempt should be made to spare the chiasmal blood supply, which may originate from the undersurface of the anterior communicating artery and requires meticulous separation from the tumor capsule. Note that the frontopolar branch of the ACA may be adherent to the tumor capsule.

with a thin sheet of oxidized cotton and protected with cottonoids while attention is turned to the dural attachment at the skull base. The entire dura serving as the attachment of the meningioma must be removed, either with sharp dissection or with the CO_2 laser, which, in our experience, has been a simple and effective way of achieving total removal down to exposed bone. Also, it is advisable to remove the area of hyperostosis with the high-speed drill or ron-geur only after protecting the chiasm and anterior circulation vessels with cotton pledgets. The amount of bony removal must be limited to true areas of bony intracranial extension. Great caution is utilized to avoid perforation of the skull base, which may lead to postoperative spinal fluid rhinorrhea through the underlying ethmoidal sinuses.

After the dural attachment has been completely removed, one must explore this area with a sharp dental tool or similar instrument to be certain that the skull base is intact. If areas of dehiscence are found, they must be sealed with pledgets of muscle soaked in cyanoacrylate or biological glue. Finally, following the careful removal of all cottonoids, the area of the optic nerves and chiasm is inspected to be certain that no hematoma has seeped into this area.

Attention is now turned to the dural closure (Fig. 13-18). It is important to make every attempt to achieve a watertight closure of the dura to avoid leakage of spinal fluid through the exposed frontal sinus. The traction sutures that were placed in the cut ends of the longitudinal sinus are used to approximate the sinus as an initial step in closure. The dura can be

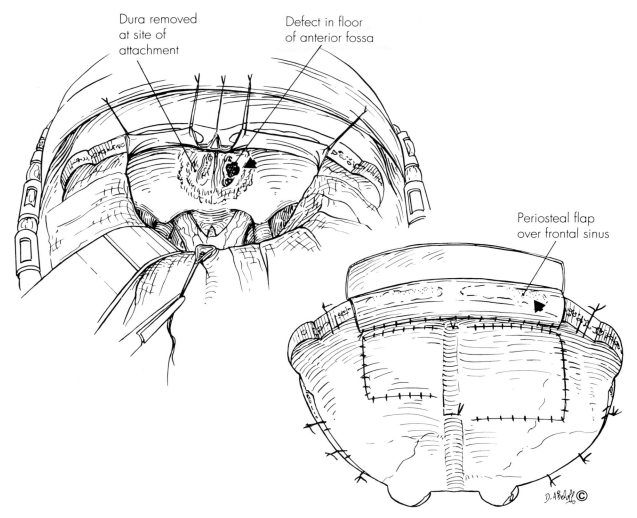

Figure 13-18. Closure. All areas of hyperostoses along the skull base are removed after protecting the optic and arterial structures. The skull base is probed to detect areas of bony dehiscence, which may require repair with pericranium and biological fibrin glue. Following meticulous dural closure, the pericranial graft is trimmed and sewn to the basal dura, covering the muscle-packed frontal sinuses.

easily stripped from the superior surface of the orbit using a flat dissector, permitting relaxation of the inferior dural extent in this area to permit a more satisfactory reapproximation. Once this has been achieved, the pericranial flap is now placed over the exposed frontal sinuses and tacked to the dura anterior and inferior to the line of the dural closure, thus further isolating the frontal sinuses from any potential area of CSF leakage. An alternate method involves gluing the pericranium to the exposed skull base epidurally as a vascularized pedicle. This technique is particularly helpful when the frontal sinuses are extensive, and allows a broader base of adherence than that resulting from dural suturing.

The bone flap is now wired utilizing 3-0 stainless steel everywhere but along the base of the flap, where the pericranial graft should be left uninterrupted. Margins of the bone flap and burr hole defects are coated with a layer of semihardened acrylic to provide a smooth cosmetic effect. The scalp is closed with interrupted inverted galeal sutures and skin staples. A Jackson Pratt drain enters the subgaleal space through a separate stab incision near the posterior aspect of the surgical wound, the majority of its perforations lying along the superior orbital rim to prevent fluid accumulation in this area.

Postoperative Management

Whereas this procedure generally requires between 4 and 6 hours, it may well be that the patient has received sufficient anesthetic agent to make extubation in the operating room ill-advised. We much prefer to allow the patient to recover consciousness entirely before extubation and often have the patient in the recovery room for several hours before the endotracheal tube is removed. One must alert patients preoperatively that this may be the case to avoid a sense of panic during their progressive recovery of consciousness.

If the patient's recovery appears to be delayed, it is advisable to carry out a noncontrast CT scan prior to extubation to be certain that the patient has not developed an early postoperative hematoma or massive brain edema. If the surgeon has carried out an adequate frontal debulking of the right frontal lobe and has avoided undue retraction of brain, these problems rarely arise. In the recovery room an additional intravenous dose of phenytoin 200 mg, Solu-Medrol 250 mg, and intramuscular phenobarbital 60 mg should be administered if the surgery exceeded 6 to 8 hours and these drugs were not already given during the operative procedure.

With regard to prophylactic antibiotics, it has been our practice in recent years to administer a single cephalosporin, such as defazolin 1 g IV 1 hour before skin incision and every 6 hours for the duration of the procedure and 48 hours postoperatively.

Other than postoperative hematoma or infection, postoperative seizures represent the major risk in the early management of these patients. If the patient has experienced seizures preoperatively, one obviously returns to the pharmacological regime that best controlled the seizures prior to surgery. In the patient who has not experienced seizures, following several days of both phenytoin and phenobarbital as described above, we would discontinue one or the other of these drugs. Of course, one confirms an adequate blood level prior to discharge. We prefer to use phenobarbital as the sole agent in the older patient, because of concern over the sedative effects of phenytoin in this population. In general, the patient is thereafter kept on anticonvulsants for 1 year, and if no seizures have been experienced one can then withdraw further anticonvulsant medication.

The patient is generally out of bed in a chair the day following surgery and is progressively ambulated thereafter. The pneumatic compression boots are removed once ambulation has been initiated. High elastic stockings are substituted for the compression boots until the patient is discharged in order to inhibit further the development of postoperative deep venous thrombosis. The skin staples are removed 1 week after surgery, the average length for inpatient stay averaging between 7 and 10 days. The patient is seen postoperatively in 1 month to 6 weeks and a postoperative CT scan with and without contrast material obtained at that time. MRI early after surgery demonstrates a multiplicity of postoperative artifacts and can be more misleading than helpful. In terms of long-term follow-up, MRI 6 months after surgery is a valuable baseline for evaluating the potential of any residual or recurrent tumor. This study is thereafter carried out 1 year following surgery and, if entirely negative, a final image is obtained 2 years later.

COMPLICATIONS

Olfactory groove, planum meningiomas, occurring as they do in an area of maximal intracranial tolerance, present at a time when their posterior extent may certainly involve the optic nerve, chiasm, and ACAs to some degree. The main operative considerations, therefore, center around avoiding injury to these vital structures during delivery of this pole of tumor. Cushing,[39] without yet envisioning intraoperative magnification, hoped future recognition of these tumors would occur before their growth included these structures. As this has not been realized, some lack of uniformity has developed over a standard approach to this portion of the tumor. Many authors have continued to base their operative techniques on the experience of Henderson and Cushing, using bifrontal craniotomies followed by tumor devascularization and debulking, and lastly by dissection of the remaining posterior capsule of tumor.[39,45,51,57] Others favor a unilateral right frontotemporal craniotomy, especially in smaller tumors, because it obviates concern about entry into the frontal sinus, and spares the dominant hemisphere to exposure.[43,44,47,50,62] Certainly the low rate of frontal sinus complications in the modern era (see below), however, does not support surgical maneuvers that focus primarily on this issue. Today's focus is upon maximizing neurological outcome subsequent to tumor removal; in this regard, the bifrontal craniotomy has the advantage of minimizing retraction injury to the frontal lobes. In order to reduce cerebral retraction through the unilateral craniotomy, some have further recommended a limited right frontal lobectomy to uncap the anterior pole of the tumor.[43,45,58,62] Retraction injury, in fact, is Logue's[50] primary objection to the bifrontal technique. We have found, however, that the best exposure is via a bifrontal craniotomy *combined* with a limited right frontal lobectomy, affording the greatest possible options in dissecting the posterior pole while eliminating the need for prolonged retraction.

CSF Leak and Infection

Postoperative cerebrospinal fluid leak can result from any craniotomy that violates the frontal or ethmoidal sinus; likewise, the theoretical risk of meningitis is increased by any exposure of sinus mucosa. Both conditions are potentially serious, and have resulted in the development of a number of techniques to diminish their appearance, and if necessary, to successfully manage their postoperative occurrence.

Any barrier to CSF egress through the frontal sinus is contingent upon meticulous removal of all frontal sinus mucosa. Once the sinus ostia have been exposed in this way, a variety of sealing techniques can be employed. A particularly helpful strategy involves sealing the sinus with biological or cyanoacrylate glue, followed by scar tissue (muscle) and a vascularized layer (pedunculated pericranium). One must also be aware that the ethmoidal sinuses too, can serve as a potential pathway for CSF rhinorrhea, es-

pecially after enthusiastic removal of overlying hyperostotic bone. Ojemann and Swann[57] recorded a transethmoidal CSF leak following removal of an olfactory groove meningioma that eventually required operative repair, although this is probably avoidable in most cases of hyperostoses if removal of the involved bone is limited. Derome and Guiot[40] point out that in some cases, the frontal bone can be thinned rather than hyperostosed, making inadvertent entry into the ethmoidal sinuses a serious concern as well. Proper preoperative imaging in the coronal plane should alert the surgeon to the type and extent of frontal bone alteration, and allow adequate preparation for more extensive cranial base reconstruction should sinus entry occur. For this reason, we prefer harvesting a large pericranial graft during the initial stages of the operation, which can subsequently be used along with temporalis muscle to repair almost any size floor defect. With these modern techniques of sinus repair, postoperative CSF leak occurs in about 2 percent of cases (Table 13-1).

Two factors appear to contribute to the development of postoperative infection following bifrontal craniotomy: contamination through the paranasal sinuses, and use of cranioplasty materials. Specific recommendations concerning antibiotic prophylaxis following sinus entry are lacking, primarily because procedures that transgress a mucosal sinus are classified as "clean-contaminated," and are often excluded from retrospective analyses of craniotomy-related infection rates. The risk of bacterial spread from the sinus mucosa in fact, led Symon[63] to recommend removal of the bone flap in any case in which the frontal sinus is entered. In his series of transcranial procedures for pituitary adenoma, however, Ray and Patterson[61] recorded an infection rate of less than 2 percent following entry into the frontal sinus and a postoperative 10-day course of antibiotics. The author's preference is to administer a single cephalosporin intraoperatively for repeated doses every 6 hours and for 2 days postoperatively. Additionally, it is also our policy to culture the nasopharynx of any patient in whom the frontal sinus may be encountered. For patient comfort, this can be performed just following anesthetic induction. The occasional patient will harbor a somewhat resistant organism, such as *Haemophilus* species, and recognition of this may allow expectant treatment of this flora should meningitis become symptomatic, necessitating antibiotic therapy before positive CSF cultures are available.[55] Packing the frontal sinus with bacitracin probably reduces this risk further.

In evaluating additional factors responsible for infection, Tenney et al.[64] also implicated the use of cranioplasty, although this risk even in the absence of intraoperative antibiotics was less than 5 percent. In 26 patients with methyl methacrylate cranioplasties randomized in a study of antibiotic prophylaxis by Young and Lawner,[67] no infections were found in patients with or without therapy. Certainly, the treatment of any patient with a culture-proven postoperative wound infection that does not clear with a prolonged course of antibiotics mandates the removal of all cranioplasty materials. Employing the techniques described, none of the patients in our series developed CSF rhinorrhea or meningitis. In broader terms, mortality caused by infection following craniotomy for olfactory groove meningiomas is less than 1.5 percent, with none in reported cases since 1983 (Table 13-2).[39,62]

Seizures

Basofrontal tumors, because of their intimacy with the epileptogenic median frontal lobes, kindle preoperative seizures in about 25 percent of patients. Records of a generalized seizure as the initial symptom of an olfactory groove, planum meningioma agree with this figure, and amplify the importance of adequate anticonvulsant therapy.[33,63] In such high-risk patients, 1 week of preoperative phenytoin therapy (5–6 mg/kg/day) appears necessary.[56] The author's preference is to add phenobarbital (30 mg three times daily after a loading dose of 240 mg) to the perioperative regimen, tapering the drug over a 1-week course following surgery. Seizures recur in the early postoperative period in about 11 (6 percent) of 176 cases in reported series noting seizure phenomenon.[33,63] Early recognition and control of these seizures is critical, as prolonged fits may induce a severe reduction in postoperative neurological function.

Seizure control is best when therapeutic levels are maintained in the postoperative period, and the influence of steroids, anesthetic agents, and other drugs must be considered. Of the two patients experiencing postoperative seizures in our series, both had subtherapeutic levels of phenytoin in the recovery room and responded well to additional intravenous supplementation (50 mg/min to a total dose of 18 mg/kg). Occasionally, a patient with resistant status epilepticus may require reintubation and a potent barbiturate, such as thiopental, although this is rare.

Long-term elimination of seizures following removal of olfactory groove meningiomas appears favorable, although this must always be weighed against the converse surgical risk of developing de novo fits. Foy[43] reported that 5 (55 percent) of 9 pa-tients with preoperative seizures were cured following removal of their basal meningiomas, while 5 (19 percent) of 26 patients developed de novo epilepsy. Ramamurthi et al.[60] likewise reported that 7 (58 percent) of 12 patients with preoperative fits and ''frontal'' tumors were relieved of their seizures postoperatively, while 6 (16 percent) of 38 developed new postoperative epilepsy. Others note similar success, and emphasize the epileptogenic character of these tumors, along with the potential for curing epilepsy following tumor removal.[37]

Arterial Injury

A strategy must be developed for the safe removal of that portion of tumor that extends between the optic chiasm and may involve branches of the ACA. In fact, adherence of tumor to these vessels is the most common reason for failure to remove these tumors totally.[33,39,63] Here, the importance of the relationship between the tumor and branches of ACA cannot be underemphasized. While intraoperative hemorrhage resulting from ACA injury has become less common in the age of microsurgery, postoperative ACA territory infarction remains a serious threat. Fortunately, the subarachnoid space is frequently preserved around these vessels, allowing separation of the tumor capsule from the main ACA and its branches during the final phase of tumor removal. However, one is occasionally faced with a tumor-vessel interface that is densely adherent and not dissectable. Either sacrifice of the encased vessel or incomplete tumor removal is then required.

The fate of any individual in whom such a dilemma exists appears to rest upon the vascular anatomy involved. Solero et al.,[62] in the course of treating their series of 98 patients with olfactory groove meningiomas, clipped 16 anterior cerebral arteries. Of these patients, four (25 percent) died, six (38 percent) had new or worse postoperative deficits, and six (38 percent) were clinically unchanged. One must conclude that this is due to the inherent variation in the perfusion territory of these vessels. Hence, any patient in whom a main branch of the ACA is sacrificed subsequently depends upon a collateral network to supply important brain areas. This of course should be avoided at all cost. However, occlusion of the smaller branches, such as frontopolar arteries, is usually well tolerated.[57,62] Two patients in our series required sacrifice of frontopolar arteries to achieve complete tumor removal, and this was without subsequent neurological sequelae. Perhaps because of the earlier experiences with ACA injury, some authors recommend leaving tumor behind if one cannot safely dissect it from the ACA.[63] While this is true for the main ACA, such involvement of the frontopolar arteries should not serve as justification for incomplete tumor removal.

Visual Loss

Any postoperative deterioration in visual acuity or fields must be the result of surgery. Manipulation of an attenuated optic apparatus during delivery of the midline posterior pole of tumor can result both in direct injury to the optic nerve and chiasm, or injury to the chiasmal blood supply.

Visual loss following removal of olfactory groove tumors is recorded as 8 (12 percent) of 67 patients in Finn and Mount's series,[42] and 7 (20 percent) of 35 in Solero et al.'s[62] series of large (>4 cm) olfactory groove meningiomas. Additionally, adherence of tumor to the optic apparatus is sometimes cited as a cause for incomplete removal.[57] The prospects for improving vision are good, about 40 percent in Solero et al.'s[62] series and 58 percent in Finn and Mount's,[42] although this is probably dependent upon the degree and duration of preoperative visual impairment.[46]

One cannot overemphasize the importance of microsurgical dissection in this area. Perhaps less appreciated than the integrity of the optic nerve itself is the chiasmal blood supply, which, if interrupted, may lead to an otherwise unexplainable postoperative visual deficit.[54,65] The decussating fibers of the chiasm are entirely dependent upon an inferior and superior group of vessels that arise from the internal carotid artery (ICA), the superior hypophyseal arteries, and ACA complex.[35] Known as the chiasmal arteries, these vessels may rest over the posterior capsule of the tumor, bridging the gap between the chiasm and ACA complex. Some of these vessels continue posteriorly to supply areas of the hypophysis and hypothalamus, perhaps explaining the postoperative appearance of diabetes insipidus and fatal hyperthermia seen in older series.[39,58] Great care should be exercised in this area, using gentle traction on the decompressed capsule of tumor, exposing and gently stretching these vessels in the subarachnoid space, allowing their meticulous dissection from the tumor capsule.

Recurrence

Meningiomas of similar histopathology recur as a function of their degree of removal. Modern techniques permit the total removal of olfactory groove and planum meningiomas in over 90 percent of cases. Typically, removal of these tumors can be catego-

rized as macroscopically complete, with removal or coagulation of the dural attachment. Despite this, Miramoff et al.[53] found olfactory groove meningiomas to be the only exception to the logical conclusion that total removal is associated with the lowest recurrence rates, with 9 (41 percent) of 22 recurring after 10 years of follow-up. However, the majority of reports convey a much lower recurrence rate, on the order of 5 percent.[33,58,63] Boker et al.'s[36] series of 29 olfactory groove tumors failed to observe a single recurrence in over 5 years of follow-up.

Derome[40] and others have cautioned that intraosseous tumor within areas of hyperostoses may serve as a nidus of recurrence. In an effort to combat this risk, and to remove any significant bony intracranial mass, a variety of approaches have developed. While bony removal is favored by some,[40,44] others consider that the risk of entering the underlying ethmoidal sinuses is considerably greater than the risk of recurrence.[33,57,63] We conclude that removal of hyperostotic bone should be performed in a prudent manner, so as not to risk entry into the ethmoidal sinuses. Certainly, an aggressive resection of the anterior skull base is apropos to the treatment of any frankly malignant meningioma with evidence of skull base invasion. However, in our hands, the recurrence of benign meningiomas of the olfactory groove and planum sphenoidale appears to be uninfluenced by aggressive removal of bone.

The low rate of recurrence associated with these tumors overall indicates that while many intraoperative maneuvers appear to prevent recurrence reasonably well, none are ideal. The endothermic treatment of the dural base, either with bipolar, monopolar, or, most recently, laser sources following complete tumor excision appears to strike a favorable balance between effectiveness and safety. The only recurrence in our series involved a tumor with histopathological characteristics of malignancy, which is a far more significant harbinger of recurrence. In about 5 percent of cases, tumor must be left because of involvement with the optic apparatus or main ACA branches. Despite modern technical advances, this is sometimes unavoidable, and we find it advisable to further treat these patients with radiation therapy if a threat to their visual pathways is present.[49] More aggressive means of focusing treatment in this area, either with radiosurgery or basal I[125] seeds have yet to be proved; however, they have strong theoretical grounds.

CONCLUSIONS

The senior author has carried out slightly over 800 craniotomies for meningioma since the advent of CT scanning, with a significant percentage represented by the tumor described in this chapter. The decision tree for the removal of these tumors is relatively standard as it has been developed over the years. The modern management of these tumors carries with it the expectation of a low mortality and morbidity, with long-term prevention of recurrent disease. Table 13-4 outlines basic considerations in accomplishing these goals. In spite of the large and threatening appearance of these tumors preoperatively, the surgical results have indeed been gratifying.

Table 13-4. Keys to Successful Management of Olfactory Groove and Planum Meningiomas

Preoperative diagnostic measures to determine tumor extent (especially coronal imaging)
Adequate operative exposure (bifrontal craniotomy)
Minimize brain retraction (right frontal lobe resection)
Proper treatment of frontal sinus
Adequate pre- and postoperative anticonvulsant therapy
Preservation of main anterior cerebral artery and chiasmal feeding vessels
Prudent resection of planum hyperostoses

Parasellar Meningiomas
Russel H. Patterson, Jr.

Complications in surgery around the sella are for the most part derived from five different sources (Table 13-5). These include cerebral edema, usually from excessive retraction; damage to important blood vessels, chiefly arteries; injury to cranial nerves; and injury to the hypothalamus. Other considerations are surgically induced CSF fistulae, infection, and cerebral compression by retained intracranial air or subdural fluid.

Reducing these complications to a minimum in the surgery of parasellar meningiomas requires attention to detail and a few simple principles; it need not be complicated.

Table 13-5. Complications of Surgery for Parasellar Meningiomas and How To Avoid Them

Complication	Prevention and Treatment	Complication	Prevention and Treatment

Postoperative brain swelling	Position the head for gravity retraction
	Bone removal flush with base
	Spinal fluid drainage and mannitol
	Split sylvian fissure
	Gentle retraction
	Unilateral exposure
	Not too many patties
	Resect brain if all else fails
		Neural structures
		  Olfactory tract
		
		  Optic nerves
		
		  Oculomotor nerves
			? Dissect the tracts free
			Unilateral exposure
			Handle with care
			Think of a straight frontal approach
			Short nerves—remove tuberculum
			Weigh merits of cavernous sinus surgery

Vascular injury	For MCA, split the fissure Watch out for CUSA and the laser Remember the Sundt-Kees clip Save the veins	Hypothalamus	Not a common problem Don't overtreat diabetes insipidus (DI) DI and adypsia a bad combination
		CSF leaks	Plug holes with fat ± pericranium
		Postoperative infection	IV antibiotics for 24 hours Soak bone plate in antibiotic solution
		Postop. hematoma/collections	Surgicel on raw brain Motorized drainage system

Abbreviations: MCA, middle cerebral artery.

RETRACTION

Many of the most serious and fatal complications of surgery around the sella are due to excessive retraction of the brain in the process of gaining exposure. There are many things that the surgeon can do to develop exposure without much retraction, even in young patients with a full brain. These are listed below.

Head Position

The head needs to be positioned with the neck extended so that the nose and chin are approximately on the same level. This will put the roof of the orbit at an angle of about 45 degrees, which means that the undersurface of the brain is also tipped back about 45 degrees. In this position, the brain will tend to fall back from the floor of the frontal fossa. Gravity is a safer retractor than stainless steel and should be employed whenever possible.

In contrast, if the head is positioned so that the undersurface of the frontal lobes and the roof of the orbits are vertical, then the brain, being a semisolid structure, will tend to sink down over the optic nerves and chiasm. In this position, the brain needs a substantial amount of retraction to gain exposure. Tipping back the head for subfrontal surgery is analogous to operating on angle tumors with patients positioned supine or in the park bench position and their head horizontal, which allows the cerebellum to fall out of the way.

Having the floor of the frontal fossa angle back at 45 degrees is quite convenient for a surgeon operating with a microscope while sitting down. This holds true whether the approach is straight frontal, over the roof of the orbit, or along the pterion. Most of the time, the head will need to be rotated to the side opposite to the craniotomy so that the line of sight to the chiasm is in the prime meridian rather than at the oblique angle that would be required if the head were square to the floor. Rotation for the pterional approach would be about 15 degrees more than it would be for an approach over the roof of the orbit (Fig. 13-19).

Bone Removal

It is most important that any saw cut in the frontal bone be flush with the roof of the orbit so as to minimize retraction. Surgeons are often tempted to make the saw cut in the frontal bone high enough to avoid the frontal sinuses, but then the price paid is excessive brain retraction to get exposure. The frontal sinuses can easily be dealt with at the end of the case by turning a small flap of pericranium over the open sinus. This effectively prevents a CSF leak and minimizes postoperative morbidity; in fact, the low saw cut reduces morbidity.

This principle of removing bone low near the base of the skull is embodied in the pterional craniotomy in which the outer part of the sphenoid ridge is removed to provide an additional centimeter of exposure without retraction. Recently, some surgeons have advocated even lower exposures such as are attained by removing the brow and roof of the orbit or by dividing the zygoma and turning down the temporal muscle. These extended exposures are not often necessary, but the tenet on which they are founded is an important one.

Splitting the Sylvian Fissure

Better retraction of the frontal lobe can be realized by dividing the arachnoidal adhesions at the inner end of the sylvian fissure. A good way to start is to place a self-retaining retractor along the fissure on the side of the frontal lobe to put the arachnoid on a mild stretch. Then incise the arachnoid with a knife. It may take a bit of guess work to decide where the fissure is and where the knife cut should be made, especially in young patients who have no cerebral atrophy. After the knife cut, a probe of some kind can be used to separate small blood vessels from the arachnoid before cutting the arachnoid with microscissors. Sometimes a small artery will be present that, if followed, will lead the way into the fissure to the main trunks of the middle cerebral artery. Another trick is to open up the presumed fissure for a short distance and then try to pry the fissure apart by allowing the forceps to spread under their own power or by using two probes.

The amount of fissure that needs to be split depends on the case. For a 20-g tumor on the tuberculum, perhaps the innermost portion is all that is necessary. For a large sphenoid ridge tumor, perhaps the split will have to extend well around on the convexity of the hemisphere with freeing of the temporal lobe from the incisura of the tentorium. Time spent getting exposure without retraction is well worth while.

Occasionally, the large veins that drain the sylvian region will overlie the fissure. However, it is almost always possible to work under or around them.

The most important part of opening the fissure is to open the medial end around the optic nerve and carotid artery. This includes extending the arachnoid

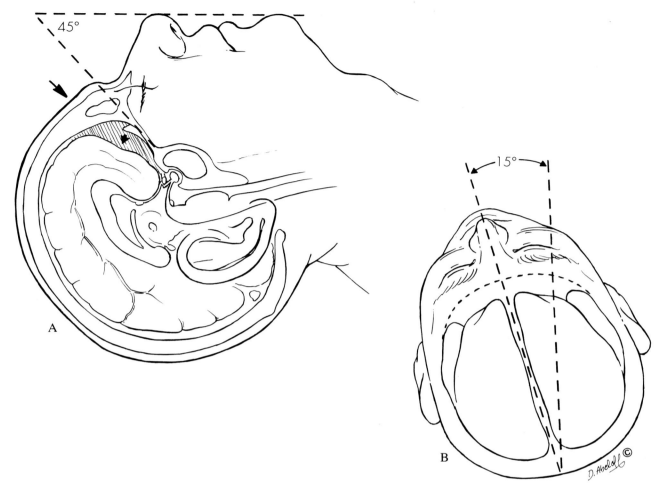

Figure 13-19. Position of the head. **(A)** The head should be tilted backward so that the roof of the orbit is at about a 45-degree angle to the horizontal. This allows the brain to fall back from the roof of the orbit in the sphenoidal ridge. **(B)** The head should be rotated to the opposite side. Fifteen degrees is about right for an approach over the orbit, and 30 degrees would be more appropriate for a pterional approach.

incision from the region of the optic nerve, across the front of the chiasm to the opposite nerve. In the case of a tumor, such as a meningioma of the tuberculum, the chiasm may be sufficiently elevated that it cannot be exposed without excessive retraction. About the best that can be accomplished at the beginning is to expose about a centimeter of the tumor and the ipsilateral optic nerve. As tumor is removed, exposure will progressively improve.

Besides helping with retraction of the frontal lobe, splitting the sylvian fissure plays a useful role in the surgery of sphenoid ridge meningiomas. A wide split of the fissure allows early identification of the middle cerebral artery and a view of how the artery relates to the tumor. If the fissure is split and the tumor debulked, it is quite convenient to follow the lateral branches of the middle cerebral artery medially to

where the artery might lie in a groove in the tumor or even be encased by tumor. It is much easier to free the artery from this perspective than by coming at the artery through the tumor from underneath.

Pterional and Subfrontal Approaches Compared

The pterional approach has the great advantage that it is the shortest route from the surface of the skull to the parasellar region. This is particularly advantageous in operating on aneurysms of the anterior circle of Willis. Its main disadvantage is that the carotid artery and optic nerves are between the surgeon and the pituitary zone. To remove a tuberculum sellae meningioma, pituitary tumor, or particularly a craniopharyngioma, the surgeon must operate through or around the optic chiasm, which exposes the chiasm to injury. The subfrontal approach over the roof of the orbit is a longer reach, but it gives a much better exposure of the pituitary zone between the optic nerves. However, for an aneurysm of the carotid artery at the level of the posterior communicating artery, the pterional approach provides a far better view of the neck than the view obtained by going over the orbital roof. Since more of the boundary zone between the frontal and temporal lobes is exposed, the pterional approach lends itself best to the wide splits of the sylvian fissure that are so useful in the surgery of sphenoid ridge tumors and most aneurysms (Figs. 13-20 and 13-21).

Spinal Drainage

The drainage of cerebrospinal fluid by the lumbar route during surgery provides more space in which to operate than any other strategy. While proper positioning and the use of diuretics and mild hyperventilation certainly are effective up to a point, the space obtained by letting out 50 to 100 ml of CSF is much greater. Usually the best practice is to let out CSF until the brain is relaxed and CSF is not welling up into the surgical field around the chiasm.

It is best not to drain out all the fluid so that any blood that runs back along the clivus is partly blocked from filling up the subarachnoid spaces by the remaining CSF. The drainage of fluid should not

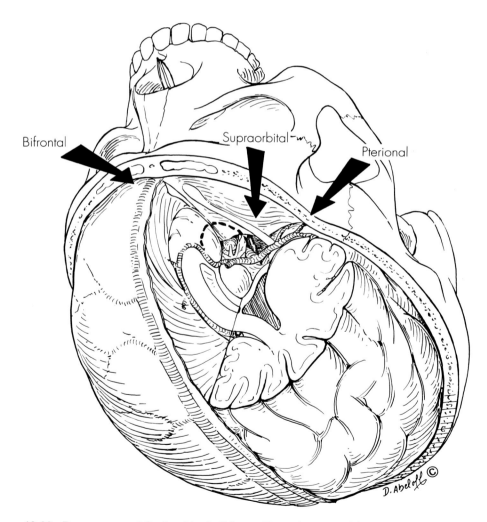

Figure 13-20. Bone removed flush with skull base. Frontal, supraorbital, and pterional approaches.

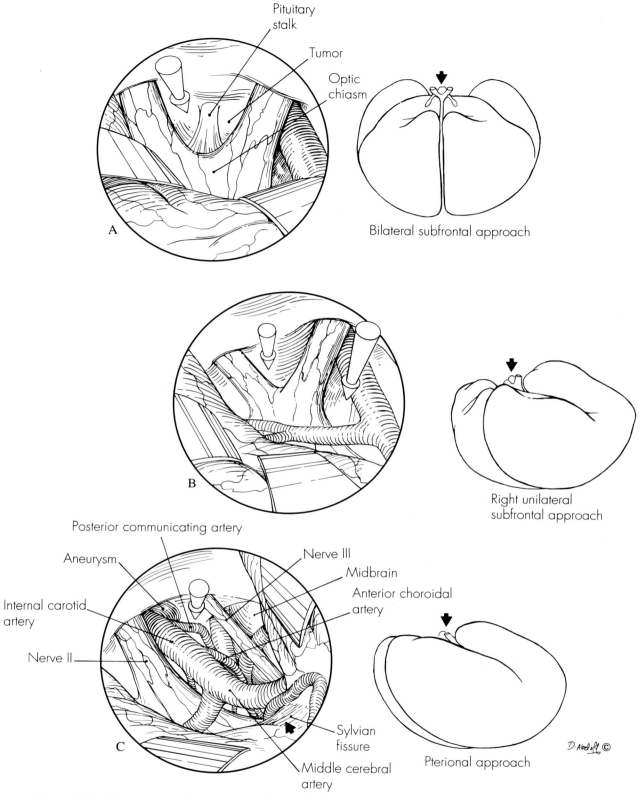

Figure 13-21. The anatomy changes depending on how much the head is rotated. **(A)** In a straight frontal approach, the optic nerves straddle the pituitary stalk, which is clearly visible. The two carotid arteries are equally well seen. **(B)** In an approach over the orbit, the right optic nerve is the first structure encountered. The right carotid artery is rotated anteriorly, and the left carotid artery is rotated posteriorly. The stalk is more difficult to see. **(C)** In a pterional approach, access to the suprasella region is impeded by the optic nerve, carotid artery, third nerve, and related structures.

be started until after the bone plate is removed so that if an intracranial vein is inadvertently torn by a saw cut, then blood will not have an opportunity to fill the head. In addition, as the fluid drains, cotton pledgets should be placed strategically to prevent blood that is spilled from filling the subarachnoid spaces. Fortunately, in many cases the arachnoid membranes guarding the basal cisterns will remain intact and keep the cisterns free of blood. The major exception is around the carotid artery and optic nerve after the sylvian fissure has been split.

The CSF that has been drained during surgery can be kept sterile and returned to the patient at the end of the case if it is not too bloody. This acts like a reverse flush in cleaning an automobile radiator and pushes air and blood out of the CSF pathways up into the surgical wound for easy aspiration. Any CSF that is xanthochromic or blood-stained should be discarded rather than replaced through the lumbar needles.

Retractor

Retraction is best done by a self-retaining retractor. These retractors usually depend on a segmented flex bar, which is a good thing because the retractor usually cannot put extreme pressure on the brain: the flex bar joints tend to loosen rather quickly. A case can be made for using a narrow retractor most of the time, perhaps one that is 1 cm in width. This is narrow enough that the surgeon will have to reposition the retractor periodically to see various parts of the operative field. The benefits are that at any one time much of the frontal lobe is not under the retractor and that no part of the frontal lobe is retracted continuously.

Brain damage from retractors depends on the force of the retraction, the duration of the retraction, and how large a cortical area is retracted. A large retractor, over a large cortical surface, for a long time, with heavy pressure, is the worst situation for the brain.

We currently use a piece of gauze impregnated with Vaseline as protection for the brain from the impact of the retractor. The material, which is readily available in most operating rooms as a dressing for burns and for skin graft donor sites, is quite thin, absolutely does not stick to the brain, and seems to offer adequate protection from superficial retractor trauma.

Unilateral Exposure

Some neurosurgeons feel that there are advantages to a bifrontal craniotomy in most surgery for tumors around the sella and certainly in the surgery of a large, bilateral, subfrontal meningioma. The benefits, proponents say, include better exposure and the ability to spread apart the frontal lobes rather than retract them. My experience suggests that these advantages are slight and that they are outweighed by some disadvantages.

In the case of large olfactory groove meningiomas of tuberculum sellae tumors, bilateral exposure leads to some kind of retraction or manipulation of both frontal lobes with consequent injury to both lobes. Even the largest of these tumors can always be removed unilaterally (Fig. 13-22). If the head is positioned as outlined earlier and rotated to the side opposite the craniotomy, the tumor on both sides of the falx is readily available after the falx is divided above the crista galli. The advantage is that after the tumor is separated from the floor of the frontal fossa and freed from any connections to the anterior cerebral arteries, the residual tumor on the far side of the falx easily lifts out with minimal trauma to the opposite frontal lobe and certainly with no retraction. The happy result is a smoother postoperative course for the patient.

In the case of chiasmal tumors, such as tuberculum sellae meningiomas, pituitary adenomas, and craniopharyngiomas, a unilateral exposure is just as satisfactory as a bilateral exposure and spares one frontal lobe from manipulation. In addition, the chances of saving olfaction are greater with a unilateral craniotomy. Dissecting out the olfactory tracts in a bilateral exposure is often, but not always, successful in preventing anosmia.

Brain Resection

Sometimes, even after all the strategies listed above have been tried and despite high-dose steroids and osmotic diuretics, the brain still will be too tight to reach the chiasm safely. This might happen during an acute operation for the repair of a ruptured aneurysm. It is often the case in patients with a large olfactory groove meningioma.

The first thing to do when encountering a tight brain is to make sure that nothing is amiss with the anesthesia. If all is well and if the strategies outlined above have failed, then the choice lies between abandoning the operation or resecting some brain to get the needed exposure. Resecting brain is preferable to excessive retraction. Excessive retraction will cause postoperative cerebral edema, which may be fatal, and the brain under the retractor may infarct anyway. Better to resect the brain and get the needed exposure with minimal retraction.

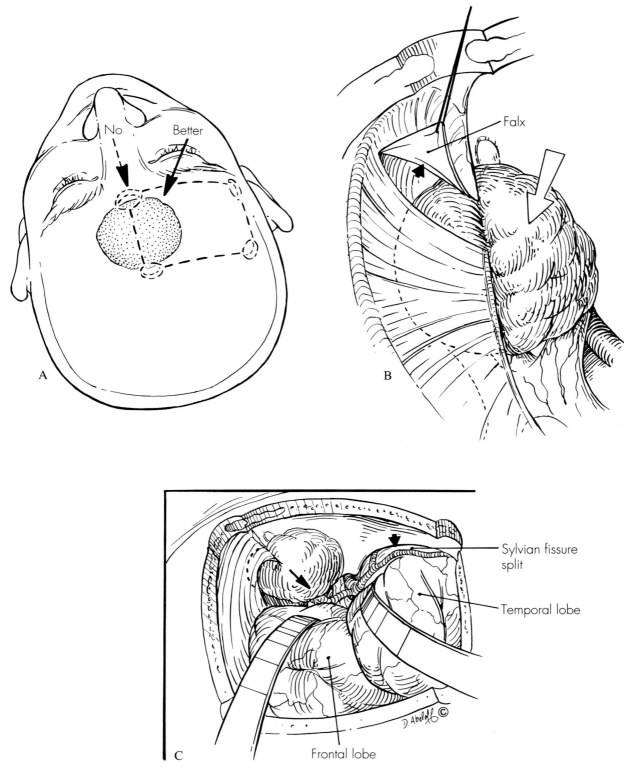

Figure 13-22. Meningioma of the olfactory groove or planum sphenoidale. **(A)** These tumors can be removed through a craniotomy situated above the right eye and reaching to but not passing the midline. **(B)** Exposure of the tumor on the left side is easily achieved by dividing the falx. Traction of the left frontal lobe is unnecessary. **(C)** Splitting the fissure will often enhance exposure. If the tumor is large, a few grams of the undersurface of the frontal lobe must be resected.

BLOOD VESSEL INJURY

It is axiomatic that every effort should be made to preserve the cerebral arteries and veins during surgery. However, it is in the neurosurgical lore that the veins at the tip of the temporal lobe and veins draining the anterior third of the frontal lobe can be taken without any consequence. This is no doubt true in many instances, but not always. If the brain is edematous from the effects of a subarachnoid hemorrhage or a tumor, then dividing these veins can add to the edema, with serious consequences such as postoperative depressed consciousness or worse. If possible, preserve the veins. Veins can be dissected from the surface of the brain and from the pia in order to work underneath them or to allow a degree of retraction of the brain from the falx and sagittal sinus.

With respect to arteries, of all the chiasmal tumors the most trouble comes with meningiomas, which stretch the arteries as they grow, then become grooved by the arteries, and finally encase the arteries. This is particularly true of meningiomas of the inner third of the sphenoid ridge, which tend to have an intimate relationship to the carotid and middle cerebral arteries.

The best approach, particularly in large tumors of the inner end of the sphenoid ridge, is to identify the affected arteries where they are free, which is proximal and distal to the tumor, and work toward the portion of artery in the middle that is encased. This can be difficult proximally if tumor surrounds the carotid artery as it leaves the cavernous sinus. However, it is always possible distally. It just requires splitting the sylvian fissure and tracking the middle cerebral artery proximally.

The search for the arteries should be delayed until the tumor has been debulked, which allows more room for the hunt. Debulking, in the case of a large meningioma, can be done with a cutting loop, recognizing that the loop is a potentially dangerous tool. The heat spreads perhaps 10 mm from the wire, so it should not be used to cut tumor close to the brain. It should not be used anywhere near a major cerebral artery for fear of dividing the artery. However, it will cut any meningioma no matter how firm, whereas the ultrasonic aspirator is best suited for softer tumors.

During the process of repeating hollowing of the tumor and collapsing it away from the brain it is tempting to insert patty after patty into the developing space between the tumor and the brain. Eventually, the mass of cotton begins to equal the amount of tumor that has been removed. All these patties are at the least unnecessary and at the most damaging to the brain. Patties are only needed from time to time

to cover a bleeding point to help with bipolar coagulation. It is better to obtain hemostasis as the operation progresses and leave the patties on their tray.

In the removal process, the surgeon should keep in mind that the principal blood supply to the tumor comes from the external carotid artery through the meningeal arteries. Blood loss is reduced if the base of the tumor is dealt with first. The base will no doubt be bloody, but once the major blood supply is taken, the rest of the tumor will be relatively avascular. Some additional blood supply will be evident coming from saprophytic cortical vessels, but the blood supply from the brain is generally much smaller than the meningeal supply.

Angiograms often do not add a great deal to meningioma surgery because the blood supply to the meningioma is so stereotypical. However, if the hospital has an interventional angiographer who can embolize the blood supply to the tumor, operating time for a vascular meningioma can be reduced by preoperative embolization.

The surgeon needs to remember that the important perforating vessels that supply the brain take origin from the side of the artery that normally faces the brain. Try to dissect on the side of the artery that faces the subarachnoid space to preserve these vessels. Often it is possible to slide two tiny dissectors, like a Rhoton No. 6, along the artery into the tumor and spread the dissectors to free the artery. Sometimes the project is hopeless, and fragments of tumor must be left on the artery in the interest of avoiding brain infarction.

Needless to say, all this surgery around the sella is made easier by use of the operating microscope. The surgeon needs to remember that most large arteries and veins on the capsule of the meningioma are not new vessels spawned by the tumor. They are arteries and veins that serve the brain and as such should be dissected free of the tumor and preserved, if possible. In years gone by, it was easy for a neophyte to mistake a thinned and stretched major artery, such as the middle cerebral artery, as an artery of no consequence. Coagulating and dividing such an artery led, of course, to a major cerebral infarction. The use of the microscope has gone a long way to preventing such errors.

One precautionary note: it is tempting to believe that the ultrasonic aspirator, which is so useful in the surgery of gliomas, can remove fragments of tumor from a cerebral artery without damaging the artery. This is not always the case; the device can tear a cerebral artery as well as coagulate it due to the heat generated by the vibrating tip.

In large subfrontal tumors, the anterior cerebral

artery and its pericallosal branch are more likely to be free of the tumor than is the first branch of the pericallosal artery, the frontobasilar artery. The frontobasilar artery supplies the gyrus rectus and orbital surface of the frontal lobe. Taking this artery has no obvious consequences, perhaps because these parts of the brain have already been rendered nonfunctional due to the effects of the tumor.

Sphenoid ridge meningiomas and meningiomas around the clinoid process are often extremely fibrous, which increases the difficulty of removing them. Suction, even suction with the ultrasonic aspirator, is inadequate, and a cutting loop near the carotid artery is out of the question. Meningiomas can be reduced in size by repeatedly coagulating small bits of tumor with a bipolar forceps and then cutting free the charred bits. This is tedious work, and one way to speed up the process is to use a *laser*. This is faster, but the laser introduces a whole new set of problems. The laser beam bounces off retractors and is likely to singe neural structures that are not covered up. The dura at the edge of the craniotomy is likely to be shriveled by the heat, which adds a small roadblock when the time comes to close. The worst danger is the risk of burning a hole in the encased carotid artery. The surgeon is better off abolishing any thought that he or she will simply stop when the artery is sighted; by then it may be too late since the first sight of the artery may be a jet of blood from a perforation. The laser, properly used, is a useful, though rarely needed, tool. However, the surgeon needs to be particularly careful about using it to remove tumor from an encased major artery.

Meningiomas that wrap around the carotid artery are also likely to track proximally and invade the cavernous sinus. Tumor in the sinus can be removed by dividing the dura over the anterior clinoid and removing the clinoid and adjacent bone around the optic nerve, tuberculum, and posterior orbit. Then it is a question of dissecting proximally on top of the carotid artery into the cavernous sinus and removing the tumor. This may be extremely tedious if the tumor is fibrous, and it may not be in the best interests of the patient if the nerves to eye muscles are functioning well at the time of surgery. Many of these tumors are slow-growing, and their growth rate can be slowed even further with radiation therapy. Whether or not surgery that places eye motility at risk is worthwhile must be decided in each case. Sometimes it certainly will be, and the surgeon needs to have the technique in his or her bag of tricks.

Sometimes, even with careful dissection, the surgeon may be unfortunate enough to put a hole in a major artery, such as the carotid. It is rarely neces-

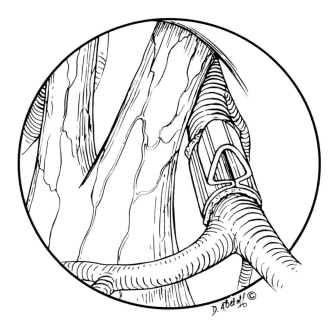

Figure 13-23. Repair of injury to the carotid artery using a Sundt-Kees encircling aneurysm clip.

sary to ligate the artery to stop the hemorrhage. While it may be possible to clip the vessel temporarily and repair the rent with sutures, a better strategy may be to make the repair with a Sundt-Kees encircling aneurysm clip (Fig. 13-23). This has worked well on the carotid in the subarachnoid space and also in the floor of the middle fossa. It can be used to salvage a pericallosal or middle cerebral artery as well.

If the perforated artery is mostly buried in tumor, the bleeding will often stop with simple tamponade. However, tamponade alone is not enough in the long run because the artery may leak again a few hours later. Some sort of mechanical backup is required for safety's sake. This can be a suture through the tumor or even cyanoacrylate glue, as a last resort. Tamponade alone is adequate for a torn vein, but it is not enough for a substantial hole in something like the carotid or basilar artery.

INJURY TO NEURAL STRUCTURES

Olfactory Tract

The olfactory tract is likely to be torn on the side of the craniotomy by the weight of the brain falling back from the roof of the orbit. It is possible to save the tract by dividing the adhesions that bind it to the undersurface of the frontal lobe. This exercise does not always succeed in preserving olfaction and may be more trouble than it is worth in unilateral exposure. In a bifrontal craniotomy with division of the falx, it is constructive to try to save both olfactory tracts because some patients are distressed by anosmia. However, bifrontal craniotomy is almost never needed to remove a subfrontal or chiasmal tumor, as was discussed above.

Optic Nerves

The perilous part of any operation for a parasellar tumor is the removal of the tumor next to optic nerves, which are more vulnerable to irreversible injury than the neighboring carotid artery. The problem is that the nerves are often covered by tumor and not visible in the beginning. Fortunately, there is a layer of arachnoid between tumor and nerves, so a time will come during the case when a bit of tumor is pushed to one side and the nerves are sighted. The question until that time is, "where are the nerves?"

The first thing to remember is the orientation of the head. If the head is rotated to the left and the surgeon is operating along the roof of the right orbit, then the right optic nerve is closer to the surgeon than the left, and the left carotid artery is rotated to a position that is seemingly medial to the left optic nerve and deep to the tumor.

One useful landmark is the insertion of the falx into the base of the skull between the two crista galli. In the first place, there is no optic nerve anterior to the free edge of the falx, so the surgeon can remove tumor quickly in this area without having to worry about injuring an important structure. The next point is that the falx points between the two optic nerves, so one can use the falx as a pointer and proceed posteriorly in the line of the falx coagulating and cutting free the base of the tumor. There is no danger to either the optic nerves or carotid artery in following the line of the falx across the planum sphenoidale and over the diaphragm sellae towards the posterior clinoid.

As the base of the tumor is freed and the mass of the tumor is debulked, it will become easier to separate the tumor from the frontal lobes and roll the tumor forward, which will lead to the first sighting of an optic nerve.

Normal optic nerves will tolerate a moderate amount of manipulation without ill effect. Optic nerves that are stretched and distorted by a mass stand manipulation poorly. The worse the vision in the eye, the less well will the nerve tolerate surgical trauma. Optic nerves are likely to be bumped when

the surgeon is operating in the region of the sella between the two nerves, such as when unroofing the optic nerve or removing bone to get into the cavernous sinus, perhaps for the repair of an aneurysm. This is not the case if the nerves are stretched by a mass and a degree of vision has already been lost. Some nerve fibers are gone, and others are on the verge of going. The blood supply to the elongated optic nerves is equally drawn out and probably marginal. All handling of these nerves stands a chance of reducing vision even further. It is easy to jostle the optic nerves repeatedly with an instrument when removing a tumor such as a tuberculum sellae meningioma. The trick is to design a strategy that will minimize this movement. For example, if the approach is along the sphenoid ridge, the surgeon is forced to operate around and over the nerves if the tumor is located between the nerves. Often a straight frontal approach is safer.

In the case of a tumor such as craniopharyngioma, which is often associated with short optic nerves, it may be appropriate to remove the tuberculum sellae and push the tumor down into the sphenoid sinus rather than pull lumps of tumor out through the small space available between the nerves. If the tumor is large enough to fill a good part of the third ventricle, an approach to the third ventricle through the corpus callosum may be a safer choice than a subfrontal operation. At times, even large tumors can be removed via the third ventricle with surprisingly little in the way of unwanted side effects. Going through the lamina terminalis and the sphenoid sinus is also satisfactory for smaller tumors restricted to the front of the third ventricle.

If a tumor is densely adherent to the optic nerves, it is a better choice to leave tumor fragments on the nerves rather than to strip the nerves clean. The difficulty is that the vascular supply to the nerves may be stripped away along with the tumor, leading to infarction of the nerves and resultant blindness. This general principle applies to all chiasmal tumors; stretched and distorted nerves that function poorly before surgery are intolerant of surgical trauma.

Hypothalamus

The hypothalamus is not usually in jeopardy in the surgery of meningiomas around the sella. Tumors of the tuberculum characteristically have a layer of arachnoid between the tumor and the pituitary stalk and hypothalamus. This tumor "capsule" is derived from the arachnoid that normally envelopes the optic nerves and chiasm. The tumor originates between the arachnoid and dura of the tuberculum, and the enlarging mass, covered by arachnoid, stretches the nerves and displaces the pituitary stalk posteriorly. After the tumor is removed, the stalk, covered by arachnoid, is visibly pushed posteriorly near the dorsum sellae. The stalk is recognizable as a reddish-brown band of tissue 1 or 2 mm wide running between the hypothalamus and the pituitary gland. The longitudinal, purplish striations that represent the pituitary portal system are a distinguishing feature.

Since in meningiomas, in contrast to craniopharyngiomas, the hypothalamic structures are protected by the arachnoid from invasion by tumor, diabetes insipidus and other manifestations of hypothalamic dysfunction are not a frequent complication of meningioma surgery.

Diabetes insipidus, when it does occur, is usually overtreated by house staff who are unfamiliar with the condition. It is best looked upon as nothing more than a nuisance for the patient rather than as a life-threatening disorder. The patient is unhappy because it causes excessive urination, the sensation of thirst, and much drinking of water. It is a mistake to try to replace the urine output with intravenous fluids unless the patient is stuperous or otherwise unable to drink. Doctors sometimes guess wrong and overhydrate the patient, which can lead to cerebral edema. It is safer to let the patient's own osmoreceptors lead the way to proper fluid balance.

Since great thirst and frequent urination are distressing for the patient, the condition, even though not dangerous, often needs to be treated. It is the volume of fluid exchange that is unpleasant for the patient, and the measurement of urinary output is the easiest parameter by which to judge when to give vasopressin. Urinary output is much more informative than measuring urinary specific gravity, which is of dubious value. One way is to follow urinary output hourly if a catheter is in place or, if not, the time and amount of voiding. If the urinary output is more than 200 ml/hr for 2 to 3 hours, the condition should be treated with vasopressin given intranasally or parenterally.

Rarely in meningioma and more often in craniopharyngioma of the hypothalamus, thirst sensation will be absent in addition to diabetes insipidus. Adypsia is the result of extensive hypothalamic damage that has disabled the osmoreceptors. This is a most serious condition since the serum osmolality may change rapidly as reflected by changes in the serum sodium, ranging between 120 and 180 mEq/L. Twice-daily vasopressin and careful monitoring of the patient's fluid balance is about the best that can be done.

THE SKULL BASE AND CSF LEAKS

Meningiomas arising from the skull base obviously involve the dura at the base and may involve the bone itself. In most cases, all that is required for a cure is to remove or coagulate the affected dura heavily, and coagulate the bone. Sometimes (not often) the tumor will penetrate the skull base to such a degree that something more must be done.

This is true when the preoperative images reveal tumor in an ethmoid sinus. It may be that after the tumor is removed, the base of the skull is seemingly intact; this should be no surprise if one remembers that the skull can be seemingly intact even though a calvarial tumor has infiltrated through the skull into the scalp. Whether or not the skull base is intact, the tumor is certainly there, and so the sinus must be opened with some combination of chisel, punches, and high-speed drill, and the tumor extracted.

Another reason to open a sinus is if a tumor is hidden behind short optic nerves. In this case, it may be best to remove the tuberculum and anterior wall of the sella to gain access to the retrochiasmal space. In either case, a hole into the sphenoid and ethmoid sinus may be the result. If the hole is not too large and particularly if the mucosa is intact, a piece of temporal muscle can be stuffed into the hole along with some Gelfoam and held with a few sutures placed to keep a sneeze from dislodging the plug. Larger holes can be repaired with fat taken from the thigh or abdomen.

If a very large hole is anticipated (one on the order of magnitude required by a carcinoma of the sinuses invading the skull base), we have found a large pericranial flap alone to be an adequate closure. A high coronal scalp incision is made, the incision being carried down through the galea, but not the pericranium. The scalp and galea are turned down towards the brow leaving the pericranium attached to the skull. Finally, the pericranium is divided as far high and posteriorly under the scalp as possible and turned down as a separate layer. This large flap of pericranium is adequate to repair even large defects in the skull base and prevent CSF leaks. Bone grafts or acrylic are not necessary to repair the skull base.

The frontal sinuses will often be opened during the course of a frontal craniotomy. An open sinus needs to be covered with a pericranial flap unless the opening is small and the sinus mucosa has not been torn. A large opening with a shredded mucosa is an invitation to a CSF leak unless it is repaired with a pericranial flap or perhaps a big piece of fat. Gelfoam will not do the job.

POSTOPERATIVE INFECTION

Wound infection after a craniotomy for a tumor near the sella is rare, and when it does occur, it usually is an infection of the bone plate with a slowly growing bacterium of low virulence, such as *Staphylococcus epidermatis*. The infection characteristically only shows up months or even years after the operation.

Adherence to the principles of sterile technique and the administration of intravenous antibiotics for 24 hours during and after the surgery will prevent most of the infections. However, a free bone plate can insulate bacteria from the brief exposure to intravenous antibiotics and serve as the reservoir for a delayed bone plate infection. To prevent airborne bacteria and skin contaminants from taking up residence in the bone plate, it is a good idea to store the bone plate in a basin filled with an antibacterial agent, such as bacitracin, during the interval between its removal and replacement. The agent percolates through the bone and stays there long enough to kill any staphylococci that might have found their way into the interstices of the plate.

As mentioned earlier in this chapter, it is important to close any paranasal sinuses that may have been opened during the course of the operation. The immediate problem with an unclosed sinus is CSF leak, but this is often followed by an infection, particularly a bone plate infection in the case of the frontal sinuses.

Sterile meningitis is a postoperative complication of meningioma and some other tumor operations, notably those in the posterior fossa. The usual scenario is that soon after leaving the hospital, the patient develops fever, possibly associated with a stiff neck and nausea. Questioning usually reveals that the corticosteroid dose was reduced substantially a day or two before the onset of symptoms. In this setting, it is safe to tell the patient to increase the steroid dose and to start the taper again; symptoms should clear within 12 hours after the patient takes an extra 4 to 8 mg of dexamethasone or its equivalent.

A physician who is unfamiliar with the syndrome is likely to hospitalize the patient, perform a lumbar puncture (which reveals many white cells in the CSF), and start massive antibiotics while awaiting the results of the cultures; this is unnecessary since the meningitis is a sterile meningeal inflammation secondary to blood and other proteins in the CSF as the result of the surgery. Bacterial meningitis after craniotomy is rare.

POSTOPERATIVE HEMATOMA AND OTHER AIR/FLUID COLLECTIONS

After bleeders in the tumor bed have been coagulated, it is a good idea to cover all the raw areas in the brain with a single layer of Surgicel. This will go a long way to prevent a postoperative hematoma in the tumor bed. The Surgicel should turn a dark brown. If any red blood is seen under the Surgicel, then the Surgicel should be removed, the bleeding point found and coagulated, and the Surgicel replaced.

Retained air, blood, and CSF in the craniotomy wound account for a substantial proportion of postoperative morbidity. In the case of frontal or pterional craniotomies, the patient is likely to collect fluid under the flap and to have swelling and eccymoses around the eye. More importantly, retained air and some postoperative leakage of blood and serum in the intracranial or epidural space can compress the brain, resulting in headache, drowsiness, or stupor. Bloody spinal fluid increases the chances of symptomatic sterile meningitis as the dose of steroids is tapered.

The likelihood of the patient having a smooth postoperative course without bruising, minimal headache, and an alert state of consciousness can be greatly increased by the use of a proper drain.

We currently favor a motorized drain widely used in orthopedic surgery (ConstaVac, the Stryker Corp). Drains that depend on gravity or suction applied by a silicone rubber "hand grenade" do not do the job. The plan is to leave an opening in the dura about 1 cm in diameter under a burr hole. This allows any CSF, blood, or gas that accumulates in the head free access to the space between the scalp and the bone plate. The drain is put in through a stab wound into the subgaleal space and left in place overnight. Typical drainage is 250 to 500 ml during this interval. The main concern, that the chances of a bone plate infection are increased, has not materialized.

Tentorial, Torcular, and Paratorcular Meningiomas
Leonard I. Malis

In order to limit the discussion in this section, I have classified as tentorial meningiomas only those tumors that have their largest attachment to the tentorium regardless of other attachments. Since the tentorium is so extensive, this leaves six groups: the parasellar or cavernous meningiomas; the petroclivotentorial meningiomas; the tentorial leaf meningiomas; the falcotentorial meningiomas; the torcular meningiomas; and the angle meningiomas. The approaches differ widely; thus, while many techniques to avoid complications are the same, others are quite different. While I would consider the meningiomas of the cavernous sinus as tentorial by my definition, I am omitting them in this section since they are well covered in another part of this book.

ANATOMY

All of the tentorial meningiomas arise from the dura, which is perhaps more complex than it appears but must be understood to deal with these tumors. The dura of the posterior fossa sweeps up the posterior surface of the suboccipital area, then has the lateral sinus as its demarkation from the occipital region, and then turns forward as the inferior wall of the lateral sinus to continue as the tentorial lower surface. Laterally the same dura of the posterior fossa sweeps up the posterior surface of the petrous bone to the superior petrosal sinus and apex of the petrous pyramid and then turns as part of the same tentorial undersurface, going medially to the straight sinus, which is within its apex as it joins the falx. The upper layer of the tentorium is the dura of the occipital and temporal areas, which medially becomes the upper surface of the straight sinus, and continues upward as the falx. The incisural area is really the fold where these two dural layers, the posterior fossa dura and the cerebral dura, are seen to be continuous. One could say the dura of the lateral surface of the calvarium crosses the middle fossa skull base up to the incisura, then turns 360 degrees and goes back to the lateral surface of the posterior fossa. This forms the two layers of the tentorium, which may be readily separable or fairly tightly fused. The incisural folded edge goes forward to the anterior clinoid process where it is attached. However, the two layers of the dura of the tentorium open and separate to form the cavernous sinus, with the inner layer (which is the continuation of the posterior fossa dura) being applied to the outer lateral surface of the sphenoid sinus while the continuation of the temporal dura forms the lateral wall of the cavernous sinus. There are folds that form the petroclinoid ligament to the posterior clinoid process, but there is no real tentorial edge attachment to the posterior clinoids as this fold is down close to the bone and turns around.

The gasserian sheath is an evaginated glove-like projection of the posterior fossa dura beneath the temporal dura. As noted above, the medial dura of the cavernous sinus is actually an extension of the posterior fossa dura as the underside of the fold of the tentorium. The gasserian sheath of the first division fuses with the lower margin of the cavernous sinus in its lateral wall, while the third and fourth nerves run in the lateral wall at the superior margin of the cavernous. The sixth nerve of course, enters the cavernous sinus lateral to the carotid artery through Durello's canal. By this definition, the cavernous sinus lies within the tentorium.

PATIENT SELECTION

Since all of the tentorial meningiomas, with the possible exception of some of those of the tentorial leaf, can be reasonably difficult, patient selection for surgery is quite important. Quality of life to be expected after surgery as well as surgical necessity in terms of the age and life expectancy of the patient require critical evaluation. A slow-growing meningioma that has changed very little over several years in a patient who is in the seventies with cardiac disease probably offers no good justification for removal unless the tumor itself is so large that it is immediately threatening. The same might be true of a relatively small tumor in a fairly young patient who has another serious disease that has limited life expectancy so that the chance of the tumor causing damage during the limited future survival is not great.

Many of these tumors are not totally resectable without producing damage, which may not be a reasonably acceptable outcome. For example, a patient presented with mild intermittent diplopia. The CT scan demonstrated a small parasellar tentorial meningioma, which could certainly be readily approached. However, the bone window CT of this lesion indicated hyperostosis of the bony lateral wall of the sphenoid sinus. The tumor therefore must have extended entirely through the cavernous sinus. In this patient, total resection of the cavernous sinus would almost certainly be required to achieve a cure, with a high probability of a complete ophthalmoplegia of the affected side even if the carotid artery could be spared or replaced. The choice between simple delay and observation versus radiation treatment was offered; the patient preferred observation. It has now been 3 years with no progression clinically or by CT scan. The patient remains well with a useful eye.

OPERATIVE CONSIDERATIONS

The adequacy of diagnostic studies contributes tremendously to the safety of the procedure. Unfortunately, all too often the quality of imaging studies, adequate for tumor diagnosis, is far from optimal for preoperative planning. CT scans are done on older machines with inadequate resolution, slice thickness is too great, field of view is too large, and coronal sections are not done. Between governmental interference and difficulties in obtaining certificates of need to replace antique machines as well as financial considerations (the charge for a poor study on an outmoded machine is the same as that for an excellent study on state of the art equipment), (expensive) repetition of poor data, with all of its complications, may really be indicated. The same problem may occur with MRI, particularly with insufficient magnetic field strength, less computer power, or modern surface coils. Even with the best imaging techniques yet available, one may still require the most precise angiography to demonstrate involvement of essential vessels and failure of collateral as well as venous drainage. Personally I have preferred digital carotid compression during angiography to demonstrate adequacy of cross-circulation rather than the use of invasive balloon studies with their slight but possible risk of vascular injury.

Particularly difficult tumors require a thoroughly experienced surgical team with all the facilities to deal with the procedure including a fairly large case volume of this type of tumor. The team should include a medical colleague who can adequately evaluate the patient's medical state and understand the stresses of the procedure and the techniques that are to be used; neuroanesthesiologists who are thoroughly familiar with the techniques to be used and who regularly use them; and a nursing team of considerable knowledge and skill. A dedicated, completely well-equipped operating room with proper microscopy is also required.

Preoperative care of the patient helps to prevent many complications. For example, patients who have been on aspirin are at a relatively significant risk for intraoperative or postoperative bleeding not correctable by other drugs. Accordingly, unless one is dealing with an emergency, we operate on no one who has had aspirin in the prior 10 days. The use of nonsteroidal anti-inflammatory drugs is also contraindicated, although the platelet inhibition of these drugs is generally reversible.

I use hypotensive anesthesia with a mean blood pressure of approximately 70 mm for virtually all cases, maintained by the use of nitroprusside. However, nitroprusside has a significant incidence of rebound due to renin release after discontinuation; this can lead to immediate postoperative surges of high blood pressure and hemorrhage. Accordingly, all patients (with the exception of severe asthmatics) are given a β-blockade, usually 200 mg of propranolol during the 24 hours before surgery. I believe that the use of fentanyl and nitrous oxide anesthesia, with the patient deeply curarized and under full respiratory control by the anesthesiologist, offers the greatest degree of safety and maintenance of appropriate PO_2 and PCO_2 levels. I do not use forane or ethrane anesthesia because they appear to cause some postoperative excitement and agitation as the patient awakens, which has caused serious blood pressure surges and possible bleeding. I also avoid the use of barbiturates because I want the patients to awake and be communicating at the time they leave the operating room, which in my experience is difficult to achieve with a barbiturate of any significant dosage.

I avoid ventricular puncture, spinal drainage, or shunting. I prefer to achieve the necessary space to permit the opening by dehydration techniques. I prefer the use of urea rather than mannitol because it puts less fluid into the patient. It is critically important to ensure that the anesthesiologist (unlike the requirement in general surgery) does not replace the fluid brought out with the urea so that the patient remains at least 800 to 1,000 ml behind in intake-output balance.

After exposure, additional space is achieved by local opening of the arachnoid. I avoid spinal drainage; when it was used early in our series, even slight amounts of intraoperative bleeding went into a relatively empty subarachnoid space and therefore could not be lysed by the presence of CSF; this led to postoperative adhesions and sealing of the subarachnoid pathways. The need for postoperative shunting has been greatly decreased since spinal drainage was eliminated.

I have mentioned operative and postoperative bleeding a number of times. A particular risk can occur with the use of heparin, which, given as a bolus to keep arterial lines open, can cause a marked increase in bleeding lasting just a few minutes even if the total heparin dosage over the course of hours is too trivial to cause any problem. While such bleeding may be handled during surgery, if it occurs in the intensive care unit postoperatively it can indeed be catastrophic. Accordingly, if a small amount of heparin is used to keep the lines open, we see to it that no flushing with heparin is done as a bolus. Bolus flushing is done with saline and then the very low concentration heparin is returned to the line.

Infection Prevention

It goes without saying that infection prevention requires strict asepsis and a consciousness of sterility on the part of the entire operating room team. Nevertheless, carriers may appear in the operating team; they must be identified if infections occur, and they must be barred from the operating room while they are carrying dangerous organisms. Particle shedding is much greater in men than in women, so carriers of skin and hair staphylococci, a serious problem, are more likely to be male. It again goes without saying that bathing and hair washing each morning prior to starting the work day is an absolute essential. In most institutions we still have strange ways of preventing true cleanliness. Hand washing as one goes from bed to bed remains relatively rare. There are even dress codes requiring neckties, and physicians make rounds wearing woolen suits. I strongly believe that no unwashed clothing should be worn by personnel who go from patient to patient within an institution. A necktie is never washed and it hangs out near the patient. Any organisms that are sprayed onto it are carried from one patient to the next. Woolen suits are equally bad. Dry cleaning, occasionally done, is not a good sterilizer. Jeans and T-shirts would be far safer. Many hospitals forbid staff to go around in scrub suits, which are actually much cleaner and better because they are changed regularly and constantly washed so they do not contaminate a patient pre- or postoperatively. If a scrub suit is worn while roaming through the floors and dirty staircases, one expects

that it will be changed when the wearer goes to the operating room. If that kind of consciousness of sterility is not available there is little hope for any other type of asepsis. It is far safer for the families to visit regardless of dress, as they only see one patient.

Despite the best of techniques, without prophylaxis there still appears to be a certain infection rate. Culture plates put out in operating rooms still regularly show appreciable numbers of colonies under the best of conditions. The intraoperative prophylactic antibiotic regimen that I have been using for the past 16 years has given us virtual immunity from infection. Jannetta has reported that in microvascular decompression procedures before using the Malis antibiotic regimen, in 500 operations he had six wound infections with two cases of bacterial meningitis. Since using the Malis regimen (more than 2,500 operations), the only infection after a microvascular decompression was in a woman who had a delayed leak of CSF through her wound after discharge from the hospital.

Positioning the Patient

Patient positioning is critical to reasonable exposure. Regardless of what position is to be used I always employ a pinned head rest, which supports the patient so that microsurgical procedures can be carried out without movement or displacement and compression of venous drainage can be completely avoided by the original placement, which is then not altered. The horror of "malignant edema" reminiscent of 35 or 40 years ago was almost certainly due to the twisting of the patient's neck and the compression of the jugular venous drainage in an era when patients had major craniotomies on little doughnut pads.

I operate on the parasellar, tentorial, and cavernous meningiomas through the pterional approach in the supine position with the patient's head rotated perhaps 45 degrees and slightly flexed so as to have a fully soft set of neck vessels. I do most of the suboccipital and petrosal approaches in the semisitting position. The advantages of the semisitting position are lowered venous pressure and ease of external drainage of fluids, irrigation, bone dust, and debris. This position requires additional special attention. The danger of venous air embolism can be very real. We place the Doppler monitor over the right atrium in every patient and we have an endocardiac venous catheter in the right atrium to measure the venous pressure and to permit aspiration of any air that might enter. The position of the Doppler monitor is confirmed by injecting a tiny bolus of saline (2 or 3 ml) rapidly into a peripheral vein. As this bolus goes through the atrium, the sound it makes is unmistakable if the Doppler is correctly positioned. We also constantly measure end-expiratory CO_2. The Doppler will pick up trivial amounts of air, while end-expiratory CO_2 will give a clear indiction of severity and the need for major change if the source cannot be found readily. The patients are supported in the Mast pressure suit, which is not inflated unless there is a question of air embolization, in which case the pressure is raised and the patient is tilted somewhat head down while the source is corrected. We have had no injury due to air embolization in the past 15 years using this technique.

Spinal cord injury in the sitting position has been reported with patients who have awakened quadriparetic after procedures that could not have caused spinal injury in and of themselves. Review of these cases indicates that this has happened mainly in young healthy patients. It is my contention that this occurs because of stretching the ventral surface of the cord over the flexible spine of the young individual in hyperflexion. In the older arthritic individual, damage to the cord would be far more likely to occur in hyperextension, and if there is severe hypertrophic cervical stenosis the greatest risk would occur during extension for intubation regardless of the position that the patient would later be in for the surgery. For many years we have used somatonsensory evoked potentials during patient positioning to demonstrate that no cord injury is being caused in placing the patient semisitting with moderate flexion. The latency measurements must remain the same from the supine prepositioning state to the positioned flexed semisitting state. If the latency of the evoked potential increases at all, the flexion is decreased, which would regularly correct the problem. The avoidance of traction forward into flexion makes this type of correction almost never necessary, but nevertheless I would still not be willing to position a patient without using the somatosensory evoked potential, even with the precaution of checking the patient awake to see how well any degree of flexion is tolerated.

Microscope Use

In our hands, all these operations are done under the microscope, with perhaps somewhat higher magnification than average. After orientation with a field diameter of 36 mm, I generally work with a magnification such that the visual field is about 24 mm in diameter, occasionally raising the magnification so the field is reduced to 14 mm. Special precaution is always required to ensure that the instruments stay within the visualized area. Microtechnique is a visual approach with the rubric ''never out of sight, never out of light.'' It is totally hemostatic. It is essentially subarachnoid and transfissural when possible. It is carried out with self-retaining retractors with pressures not higher than 20 torr, with dual instrumentation to avoid tissue traction and with sharp anatomical division.

High-Speed Drills

The use of high-speed drills has become an essential part of work in the skull base; they require special training and the development of skills. It is important when one is working in and around delicate neural structures that the drill be well irrigated and that its direction can be reversed to prevent running the wrong way. It has to be a very high speed drill and it has to work by wiping away bone rather than pressing on the drill. It is critically important to remove all cottonoids from the wound before using the drill because a cottonoid caught in the end of the drill bit becomes a devastating whirling propeller. Also, the drill should never be brought out of the wound without being turned off to avoid unintended damaging contact.

Mastoid cells are frequently opened in drilling out the petrous bone. The original Horsley bone wax was impervious to CSF, and could be used to seal mastoid cells intradurally or extradurally with an incomplete dural closure. This was also true of the Ethicon bone wax until 10 years ago. At that time the Ethicon wax processing was altered, so that it now crumbles in CSF, allowing leaks into the mastoid cells. I still wax the mastoid process air cells, but close the posterior fossa dura precisely. Intradural mastoid cells, opened with the high-speed burr in the petrous bone, were well sealed with the old wax, but the newer wax cannot now prevent leaks. I close all intradural mastoid cells with fat, packing each open cell with a small fat segment, and then suturing a larger fat piece to fill the whole drilled-out area. With this technique, neither tissue adhesive nor postoperative spinal drainage has been required. Openings of the nasal cavity or paranasal sinus require precise repair, but this topic is beyond the scope of this chapter.

PETROCLIVOTENTORIAL MENINGIOMAS: THE PETROSAL APPROACH

The petroclivotentorial tumors do not actually arise from the tentorium but from the apex of the petrous pyramid and clivus. As such, they involve the tentorial attachment along the incisura. They tend to grow to quite a large size before detection, rarely produce much ataxia, and do not alter eye movements until they extend forward into the cavernous sinus. Often their first sign is a hearing deficit, when they have grown large enough to push downward into the region of the internal auditory meatus and stretch the auditory neurovascular complex. Some patients have presented with facial numbness or facial pain, and a few have originally given the symptoms of typical trigeminal neuralgia. These tumors are approachable either by a purely posterior fossa lateral approach, or by a subtemporal approach, but neither technique has been completely effective. The most anterior part of many of these lesions simply cannot be gotten to from below, while dealing with them by a subtemporal approach carries the great danger of occlusion of the vein of Labbé and its consequences. Of all the superficial veins of the brain, the only one that almost invariably produces catastrophic damage is the vein of Labbé, for which there is almost no collateral and almost no substitute drainage. Occlusion of the vein of Labbé at surgery will generally produce hemorrhagic infarction of much of the temporal lobe. Preservation of the vein of Labbé while lifting the temporal lobe can be carried out by dissecting the vein of Labbé in the arachnoid back into the temporal lobe, but this can be followed by late occlusion a day or so after the surgery.

For the past 20 years I have been using a combined subtemporal-suboccipital approach whenever possible to deal with this group of tumors, both to provide a much more reasonable visualization of the entire tumor and to preserve the vein of Labbé undamaged. The absolute essential for this procedure is demonstration by preoperative angiography that there is adequate communication from the lateral sinus of the involved side across the torcula and down through the lateral sinus of the opposite side into the jugular system. The vein of Labbé of the operated side will then drain across the lateral sinus and down the opposite side. If either lateral sinus is defective, either anatomically because of congenital abnormality or because of disease, this approach cannot be carried out. Such patients may be operated on in stages from above and below but with the risk to the vein of Labbé markedly increased. I have had to reject 8 patients of 84 candidates for this approach because of defects in the venous drainage of which 6 were demonstrated angiographically. Two were angiographically uncertain, but at surgery had cerebellar swelling on test occlusion, so that ligation was not carried out.

The operation begins with a curved incision coming from the area posterior to the pterion upward, then backward above the ear, and then downward just posterior to the mastoid process. This large scalp flap is reflected downward almost to the external auditory canal, and then a suboccipital craniectomy is carried out including the entire mastoid process exposing the sigmoid sinus to the flat of the petrous pyramid and then carrying the craniectomy upward over the lateral sinus (Fig. 13-24). After this much exposure has protected the sinuses, the high-speed craniotome can be used to carry the flap to the pterion and down into the temporal base. The bone flap is turned just along the temporal floor. Using the high-speed cutting burr the lateral portion of the petrous pyramid is carved away superficial to the external auditory canal and vestibule. The posterior fossa dura is then opened by a semicircular incision with its base medially, and a relaxing incision is made superior-laterally up to the junction of the lateral sinus and the sigmoid sinus. The temporal dura is now opened in a flap from above the pterion down to parallel the temporal floor to the superior surface of the lateral sinus. Silk ligatures (0) are now passed around the junction of the lateral and sigmoid sinus through the tentorium. These ligatures lie above the entrance of the superior petrosal sinus and below the entrance of the vein of Labbé to the lateral sinus. After the two suture ligatures are secured, the sinus is divided between them (Fig. 13-25A).

The self-retaining retractor blade is now placed beneath the lateral sinus and used to support the tentorium as it is divided along the petrosal sinus (Fig. 13-25B) up to the point where the tumor invades the tentorium (Fig. 13-26). If this area is more anterior, the division line is turned somewhat medially to avoid the fourth nerve as the tentorial edge is divided at the incisura. Now the subtentorial retractor can be used to provide about 1.5 cm of elevation of the tentorium lifting up the posterior temporal and occipital lobe with it, carrying the vein of Labbé upward with the lateral sinus into which it drains so that there is no tension or separation of the vein of Labbé (Fig. 13-27). The retractor pressure used to support this area is maintained below 20 torr, which is more than adequate to support the weight of the structures and provide the necessary exposure (Fig. 13-28). A second self-retaining retractor can now be placed along the temporal floor particularly if the sylvian fissure has been opened with an exposure forward to the pterion, and the temporal lobe can be elevated to the same degree also without danger of venous damage (Fig. 13-29). The anterior sylvian venous drainage has regularly been taken in the course of sylvian fissure exposures, particularly for posterior aneurysms, without deficit. I do have one patient in whom the sacrifice of these veins appears to have caused a sig-

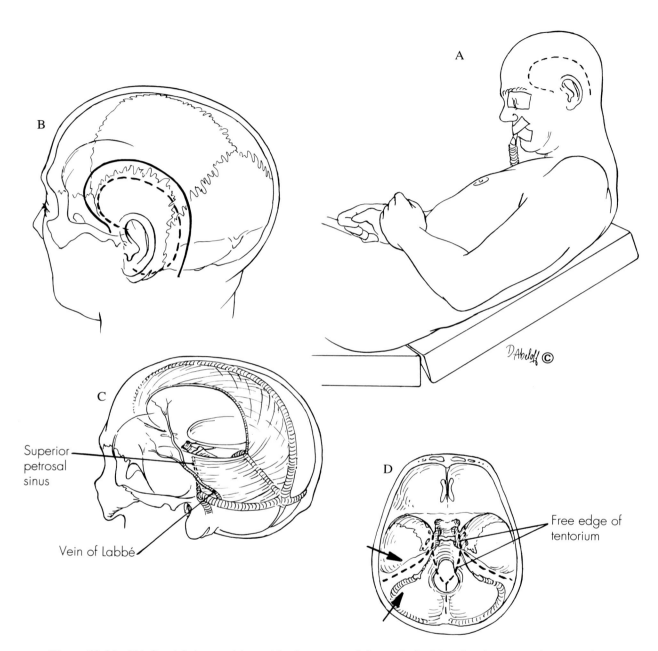

Figure 13-24. **(A)** Semisitting position with placement of the scalp incision for the petrosal approach. **(B)** Bone resection for the suboccipital craniectomy and mastoidectomy and the temporal pterional bone flap. **(C)** The falx and tentorium join to form the straight sinus. The superior petrosal sinus runs along the petrous apex, entering the junction of the lateral and sigmoid sinuses. The vein of Labbé drains into the lateral sinus above this junction. **(D)** The petrosal approach combining the subtemporal and posterior fossa directions.

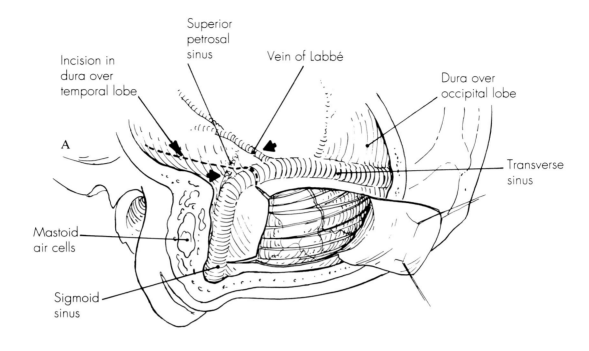

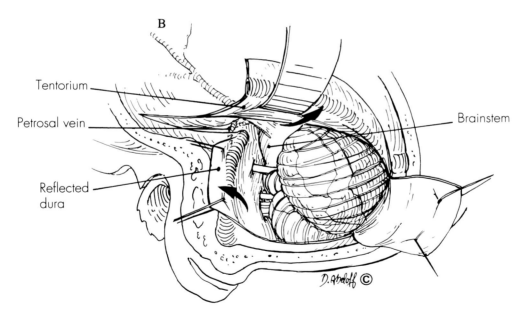

Figure 13-25. **(A)** The dura of the posterior fossa has been opened with a closable flap hinged medially and relaxing incision carried laterally. The dashed line shows the line of the temporal dural opening and the line where the lateral sinus will be ligated and divided above its junction with the sigmoid sinus. The vein of Labbé enters the lateral sinus medial to the point of ligation, and the superior petrosal sinus enters the junction below the point of ligation. **(B)** The temporal dura has now been opened, the sinus divided, and cutting of the tentorium is now proceding forward parallel to the petrosal sinus as the tentorium is supported with the retractor blade.

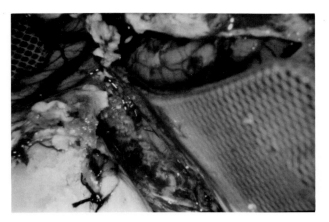

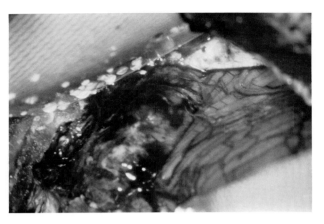

Figure 13-26. Left petrosal approach, field diameter 24 mm. Vertex is up, occiput is to the right. The posterior retractor supports the cerebellum in the plane of the petrous. The retractor seen in the left upper corner is against the temporal lobe, and the tentorium is being cut along the superior petrosal sinus.

Figure 13-27. Left petrosal approach, field diameter 36 mm. The left upper corner retractor is lifting the tentorium with the temporal lobe. The right lower corner retractor is supporting cerebellum a bit backward from the petrous surface. The meningioma can be seen lying on the apex of the petrous pyramid.

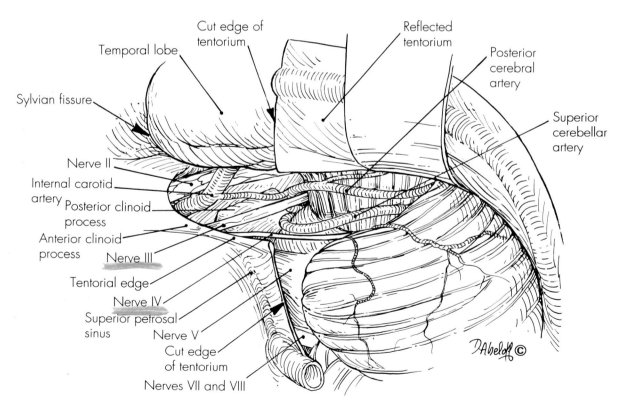

Figure 13-28. Left side, vertex up. After dividing the junction of the lateral sinus and the sigmoid sinus, the tentorium has been cut medial to the superior petrosal sinus at the petrosal apex. The retractor beneath the tentorium supports the temporal lobe, allowing the vein of Labbé to drain medially. The exposure permits visualization from the optic nerve to the foramen magnum.

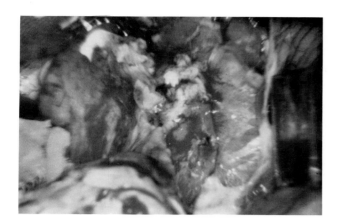

Figure 13-29. Left petrosal approach, field diameter 24 mm. The petrous pyramid can be seen in the lower left corner, the retractor supports the cerebellum to the right, and the tumor invading the cut petrous margin of the tentorium fills the center of the photograph.

nificant edema of the temporal lobe followed by an encephalomalacic picture on the CT scan with accompanying disfunction. On the other hand, these veins have been taken more than 200 times in the treatment of pterional and sphenoid ridge lesions without difficulty in my own experience. If necessary, a third retractor can be placed posteriorly in the plane of the petrous pyramid as it would be for an approach to angle tumors thus making the area available all the way down to the foramen magnum (Fig. 13-30).

The exposure thus available covers a range of about 120 degrees horizontally, actually considerably

more than is needed. Vertically the angle is very small but since the microscope ocular access is horizontal this does not interfere with adequate stereoscopic visualization nor with a two-handed approach. The resection of the tumor is carried out in the same manner as in the other tentorial tumors, coring first, then bringing the capsular surface into view, and finally clearing the dural base. The upper surface of the gasserian sheath may have to be resected. While most of these tumors do not involve the entire sheath, some involve the temporal dura and the upper layer of the gasserian sheath as well (Fig. 13-31 to 13-33).

Extension forward into the cavernous sinus is not unusual. Here resection is nothing like the risky process of dealing with arterialized channels as in a carotid cavernous fistula; instead, one finds merely the extension forward of meningioma surrounded by multiple separate venous channels, quite unlike a meningioma extending into the sagittal sinus or the lateral sinus. It is only necessary to push Gelfoam or Surgicel around the tumor as the dissection is carried forward to control bleeding and to protect the third and sixth nerves and the carotid artery (Fig. 13-34). In this group of tumors, unlike some of those that have their origin more anteriorly, the carotid artery is almost never invaded, and this portion of the tumor can be stripped away without having to ligate or replace the carotid artery as may be required in tumors of the temporal base or inner sphenoid ridge. Hyperostotic bone is rarely encountered in tentorial menin-

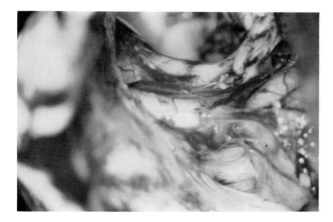

Figure 13-30. Left petrosal approach, field diameter 24 mm. The view is from the posterior aspect. The retractor can be seen in the right side of the photograph. The tumor has been largely removed above, and nerves V, VII, VIII, IX, X, and XI can be seen where they were all crowded downward together by the pressure of the previous tumor.

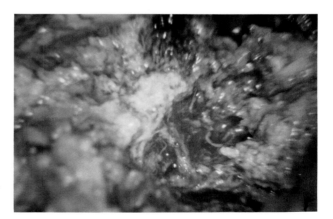

Figure 13-31. Left petrosal approach, field diameter 24 mm. A fungating meningioma surrounds many of the vessels and neural structures. As coring is carried out these may or may not be possible to free, and some tumors of this sort are unresectable. Fortunately this tumor had not invaded the vessels and it was possible to resect it completely.

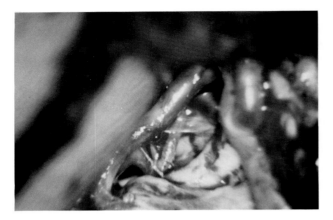

Figure 13-32. The removal of the tumor seen in Fig. 13-31 has been completed. Field diameter 24 mm. The retractor fills the left upper part of the field and supports the tentorium and temporal lobe. The right posterior clinoid is seen at the bottom of the field from the left exposure and the right third nerve can be seen just posterior to the apex of the right posterior clinoid. The basilar artery runs upward at the right side of the field and the superior cerebellar and posterior cerebral arteries branch off to the left of the photograph.

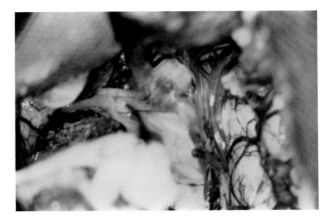

Figure 13-34. Left petrosal approach, field diameter 36 mm. A retractor is to the right supporting and covering the cerebellum. To the left of the retractor is the brainstem, and in front of the brainstem the basilar artery travels upward. In the left upper corner a retractor supports the anterior tentorium and temporal lobe. In the left lower corner the cut margin of the tentorial attachment to the superior petrosal sinus is seen with a ligature on the sinus. The third nerve lies almost in the center of the picture and goes downward, deeply cupped over the posterior cerebral artery. Just above the petrous pyramid anteriorly extending to the left there is a strip of Surgicel that is the remnant of the portion placed in the cavernous sinus.

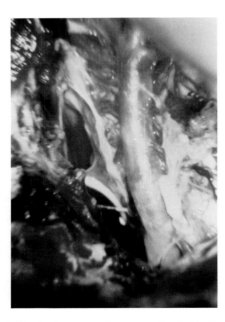

Figure 13-33. Left petrosal approach, field diameter 24 mm. The view is from the pterional region looking downward and backward. The meningioma has been removed. The basilar artery is visualized all the way down to the origin of the anterior inferior cerebellar arteries. The apex of the basilar artery can be seen just beneath the retractor dividing into the posterior cerebral and superior cerebellar arteries. The right sixth nerve can be seen to the left of the basilar artery in the lower third of the photograph.

gioma attachments but may occur in the petrous ridge.

Unlike conventional wisdom I routinely carry out a watertight closure of the posterior fossa dura if possible, as it nearly always is. On the other hand, watertight closure of the temporal dura is fairly frequently not feasible. Here I simply cover the opening with a sheet of Gelfoam. The craniotomy bone flap is replaced and sewn into position through drill holes made in its margin and in the margin of the calvarium. The large posterior fossa bone defect I now close by using a sheet of titanium mesh fitted into a groove cut in the diploe around the margins of the craniectomy, except of course in the area of the mastoid. The titanium mesh is then imbedded by smearing acrylic cranioplasty material into it and smoothing it to match the edges of the bony opening to provide a complete closure without any decompression. The absence of the decompression avoids the chance of brain damage on the edge of a bony opening if intracranial pressure were to go up but also requires that intracranial pressure be properly monitored and that adequate measures be taken to keep it within the normal range postoperatively. These measures have already been discussed at the beginning of this section.

MENINGIOMAS OF THE TENTORIAL LEAF

Tentorial leaf meningiomas form a small group because the tumors are small or they extend into the clival or petrosal areas and are then classified with those tumors. For those tumors arising mainly in the parasellar area from the tentorium adjacent to the cavernous sinus, I have used a pterional approach, opening the sylvian fissure widely. The exposure is much like that for aneurysms of the posterior communicating or basilar arteries (Figs. 13-35 to 13-37).

The posteriorly placed tentorial leaf meningiomas are a quite different group. I have preferred to operate on these from below the tentorium, in general doing a craniectomy along the lateral sinus, sometimes carrying it across the torcular and the other lateral sinus to give a bit more room. The craniectomy extends above the lateral sinus about 1 cm and downward over the cerebellar hemisphere about 2 cm. The dura is then opened in a straight line below and parallel to the lateral sinus and the upper margin is drawn upward by traction sutures so as to elevate the lateral sinus somewhat upward toward the edge of the bony involvement. Draining veins supporting the cerebellum are then sealed with the bipolar coagulator, and the cerebellum is allowed to drop. I do

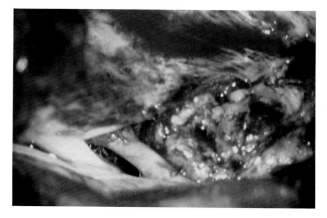

Figure 13-36. Same case in position as in Fig. 13-35. The incision has been made through the tentorial leaf into the surface of the tumor, and coring of the tumor has begun.

these in the sitting position so that no retraction is ordinarily necessary on the cerebellar surface. If the tumor is quite small it can be now separated from the tentorial surface with the cutting bipolar sharp forceps making a plane against the tentorium and allowing the tumor to drop free. Usually it is somewhat larger, in which case the tumor is first cored using the bipolar cutting ring forceps to reduce its bulk without significant bleeding. After the tumor has been debulked, the separation is carried with the bipolar cutting current and sharp bipolar forceps. As a final step, the dura is incised posterior to the attachment of the tumor and is divided around the periphery of the tumor using the bipolar forceps to seal the tentorial vessels as the cut is made progressively, finally resecting the entire dural attachment of the tumor.

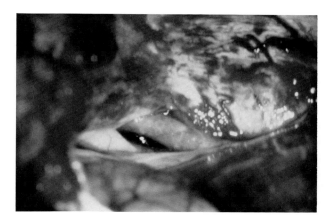

Figure 13-35. Right pterion approach, field diameter 36 mm. Tentorial leaf meningioma. Vertex is down. Anterior is to the left. The sylvian fissure has been opened. Sphenoid ridge fills the left upper corner. The retractor is in the right lower corner supporting the anterior temporal lobe. The sylvian fissure has been opened. The optic nerve and carotid artery are seen between the sphenoid ridge and the retractor, and the surface of the tumor fills the right upper corner. The uninvolved anterior portion of the tentorial edge crosses the carotid artery and optic nerve toward the sphenoid ridge.

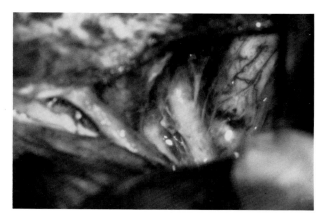

Figure 13-37. Same patient as in Figs. 13-35 and 13-36. The tumor has been removed, and the tentorium has been resected with the tumor. Behind the carotid artery, the basilar artery and the cerebellum are visualized.

Here again the arachnoid at the anterior end of the incisura usually is intact and protects the veins of Rosenthal and the vein of Galen. Occasionally this arachnoid is involved and so as a final step in the dissection, the arachnoid is removed under high magnification so as to separate it precisely from these vital venous structures.

FALCOTENTORIAL MENINGIOMAS

Falcotentorial tumors arise from the region abutting the straight sinus through the tentorial surface of the falx or directly from the lateral wall of the straight sinus. Most of them have occluded the straight sinus completely by the time they produce their first symptomatology and are usually quite large. The area where they are growing as they extend upward has few draining veins to the sagittal sinus and until the tumor reaches a size large enough to compromise the calcarine gyrus, symptoms may be minimal. I have usually approached these lesions through a posterior approach with the patient in the semisitting position but with the head not nearly as inclined forward as it is for the suboccipital region. The eye/ear line in these is usually set at about 15 degrees upward. Many scalp flaps have been used for this group of tumors. I have preferred a flap beginning above the ear coming directly up to the vertex and then turning down parallel to the midline on the opposite side of the midline to about 1 or 2 cm down below the occipital protuberance. This provides a flap with a very broad base and yet gives a complete exposure from the lateral sinus area upward and along the sagittal sinus. I turn the bone flap on the side of the lesion, stopping 1 cm from the sagittal sinus. I then generally dissect epidurally under direct vision from the lateral approach across the sagittal sinus, separating the dura so that the sinus will not be injured and will drop down away from the calvarium. I then cut a 3-cm free bone flap across the sinus, parallel to the sinus. This provides an exposure of the entire sagittal sinus without endangering the sinus, as can occur when burr holes are placed on the sinus or cuts are carried across it without first visualizing and separating. I generally open the dura with an incision parallel to the anterior, inferior, and posterior edges of the craniotomy, hinging it upward at the sagittal sinus. It can be done, of course, in a reverse direction, hinged downward. I am not really convinced that there is a good reason for the rationalizations requiring either technique. In any case there are few veins and none of great significance along the medial edge of the occipital pole. If there is a vein draining there it may

ordinarily be sacrificed without swelling or compromise. Now separation between the medial surface of the occipital lobe and the falx is carried out and at the same time the occipital lobe is separated from the tentorial surface going over the lateral margin of the sagittal sinus and the superior margin of the lateral sinus. Now the self-retaining retractors are placed on both sides of the separation along the falx. The falx and sagittal sinus can be retracted 0.5 cm or so to the opposite side without obstructing sinus flow, thus providing an easier visualization down the space between the occipital lobe and the falx. This can also be done using dural traction sutures to draw the sagittal sinus laterally. The occipital lobe can be retracted with another blade of the self-retaining retractor, achieving as a rule about 1.5 cm of space all the way down to the straight sinus while still keeping retractor pressure no greater than 15 torr. The surface of the tumor is generally reached well before this point. As soon as the surface has been reached I have preferred to begin the separation of the arachnoid from the occipital lobe side just enough to make sure that any branch of the posterior cerebral artery that may have been lifted out of the fissure is protected. I then begin the coring of the tumor along the falx and progressively empty the tumor, generally using the cutting loops of the bipolar coagulator and then bringing more of the lateral tumor medially toward the falx so as not to increase the amount of retraction. As these tumors are infiltrating along the tentorium as well, the same procedure is carried out along the tentorial surface; finally the tumor thickness on its lateral surface and the surface beneath the occipital lobe is brought into view sufficiently to allow dissection of the capsule from the adherent occipital lobe. This can regularly be done without perforating the pia and, despite the arachnoidal dissection, without resecting any significant arterial vessels. The tumor supply is virtually always from the dura, with branching vessels of the occipital artery coming in through the bone and down, and along the tentorium from the tentorial meningeal arteries, rarely from anteriorly along the falx where the anterior meningeal artery may be elongated. Using the cutting bipolar as the coring device, the vessels supplying from deep to the tumor offer very little in the way of problems since each coring bite frees the tissue without bleeding so that when the coring is completed the feeding vessel anteriorly can be coagulated in the dura without having to retract particularly and without having had to deal with excessive bleeding throughout the procedures. While I rather carefully seal the middle meningeal artery in sphenoid ridge meningiomas or in parasagittal meningiomas early in the case, I rarely find it necessary to be concerned about the tentorial meningeal arteries in these posterior tumors.

After the tumor has been cleared essentially down to its dural attachments, the resection of the dura may be carried out. Many of these tumors extend through the falx to the opposite side and then have been worked on through the side of the much larger tumor, since they are rarely symmetrical. The space available after the main bulk has been removed permits the incision through the falx to be carried around outside the margin of the tumor attachment; then the tumor of the opposite side can be delivered into the cavity on the primary side, separating nearly always with preservation of the arachnoid as well as all of the vessels from the opposite side. It is rarely necessary to expose separately between the opposite occipital lobe and the falx. While there should be little possibility of vascular damage or cortical damage to produce a hemianopic defect, the presence of such a defect can be fairly well compensated for, while a bilateral hemianopsia is of course an absolute and total catastrophe. Finally, the straight sinus would require resection in most of these tumors and so the incision must go through the tentorium lateral to the attachment of the tumor across the midline posterior to the involvement of the straight sinus through remaining patent venous structure. For this area I also first incise the tentorium of the opposite side and bring the incision there around to meet the opposite side of the straight sinus to permit its secure clipping or ligation before dividing it. A cut through the occluded straight sinus in the tumor would only be beneficial if additional room were needed to see the rest of the straight sinus, which ordinarily does not occur. Therefore the division is made through what would be the patent portion of the straight sinus except for the fact that it has been clipped. Opening the patent posterior straight sinus without clipping it can lead to abrupt sudden and massive air embolism and should of course be avoided. At the anterior end of the straight sinus of course the attachments to the vein of Galen and to the veins of Rosenthal must be preserved since the collateral from the vein of Galen may well go through the vein of Rosenthal and shunt to the cavernous region (Fig. 13-38). Even with the best of angiography all of the collateralization may not be visualized. Sometimes the shunting goes into the inferior sagittal sinus and then the drainage may be in a complex of anterior neovascularization.

Complete resection of involved dura is the best preventative of recurrence. However, when this has been particularly difficult to achieve for one reason or another, I have used the bipolar coagulator with one blade on one side of the dural layer and the other blade on the other side and coagulated the dura through and through. Using this technique I have not had a recurrence from dura, which I am sure would have otherwise provided tumor regrowth. I first began using this technique in some of the spinal cord meningiomas, where I was reluctant to excise dura of the ventral surface of the canal. After it worked out well there for many years I began to use this method elsewhere and have not been disappointed in the results. I have even used it within the wall of the sagittal sinus. Stroking the surface of the dura with the bipolar or even the Bovie unipolar current can not kill all the cells at levels of heating that I would consider satisfactory. On the other hand, when the bipolar is used with one blade on each side of the dura, the coagulum formed contains no living tissue (Fig. 13-39). Additionally, there is no need to replace any portion of the resected falx or tentorium, but again, if the tentorial margin has been preserved at the notch and this strip of dura is narrow, there is risk of injury by herniation of neural tissue over that strip, and accordingly the edge should also be resected.

TORCULAR MENINGIOMAS

Torcular meningomas are a particularly difficult group of tentorial tumors. A true torcular meningioma may occlude the actual torcula so that there is really no possible circulation through it from any direction. If the patient has reached that stage with survival, a good collateral has occurred spontaneously. Other lesions may partially occlude the torcula at the junction of the straight and the sagittal sinuses in which case total removal cannot be achieved without sacrificing these sinuses while they still have required flow. This is not an acceptable possibility since up to this time successful replacement of a totally resected sinus has not been achieved with any significant consistency, though it has been possible to replace the sinus successfully in animal studies.

Therefore complication avoidance after demonstration of the meningioma by CT or MRI requires, for me at least, angiographic demonstration of the venous drainage pattern. The choice may then be between a partial removal or a delay to wait for collateral development; this choice may be made on the basis of growth rate and age of the patient. In a very young patient the growth rate may be so fast that the chance of collateral is small by the time the tumor has created a major neurological deficit because of its size, while in an older patient the tumor may grow very slowly and have a great deal of time for develop-

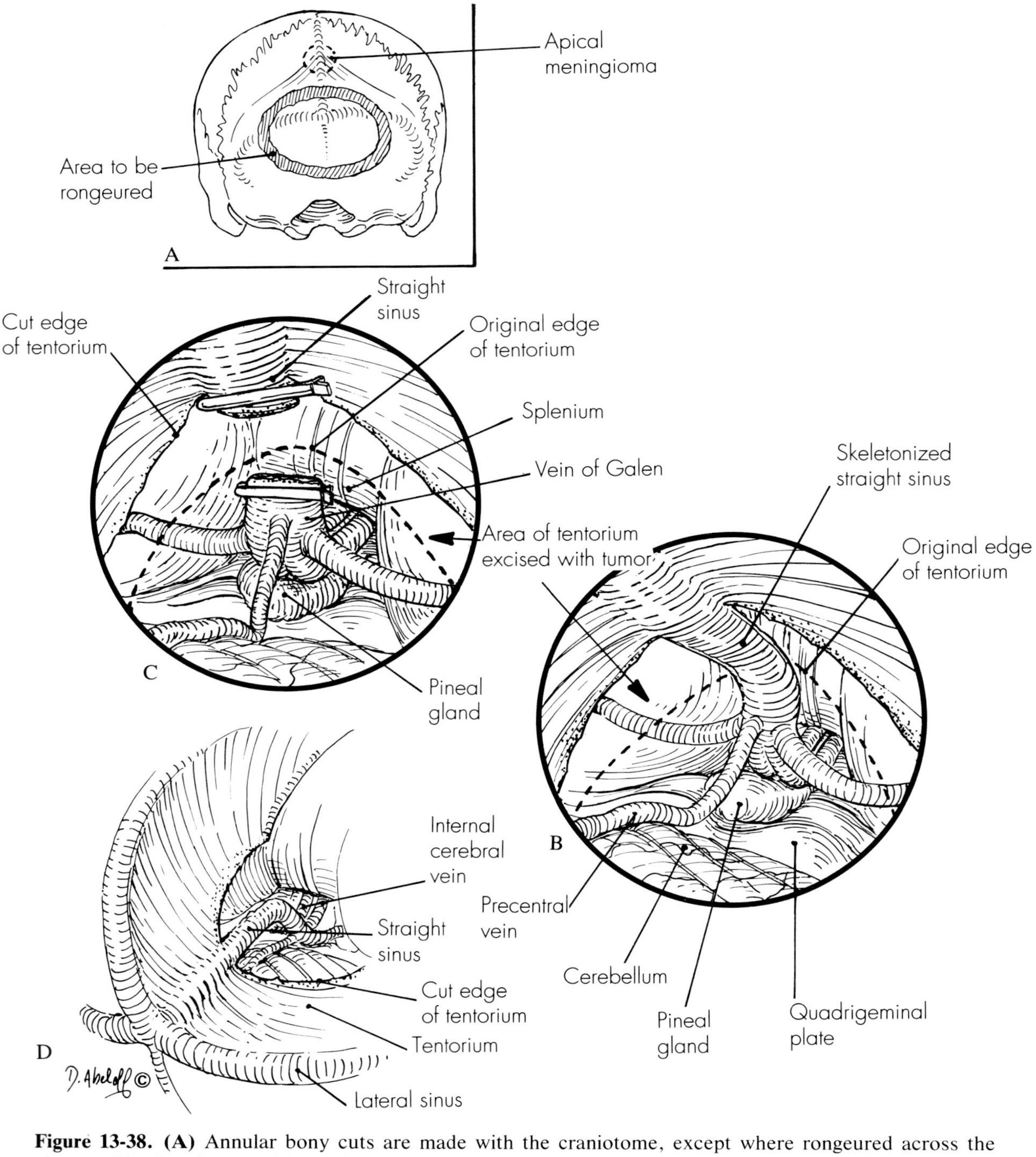

Apical
meningioma

Area to be
rongeured

A

Cut edge
of tentorium

Straight
sinus

Original edge
of tentorium

Splenium

Vein of Galen

Area of tentorium
excised with tumor

Pineal
gland

C

Skeletonized
straight sinus

Original edge
of tentorium

B

Internal
cerebral
vein

Straight
sinus

Cut edge
of tentorium

Tentorium

Lateral sinus

Precentral
vein

Cerebellum

Pineal
gland

Quadrigeminal
plate

D. Abeloff ©

D

Figure 13-38. (A) Annular bony cuts are made with the craniotome, except where rongeured across the sinuses. The dura is opened from sinus to sinus through the annular segments, markedly decreasing the dural blood supply to the central area and permitting removal of this remaining bone. **(B)** Infratentorial view of apex of tentorium, showing vein of Galen, straight sinus, veins of Rosenthal, precentral cerebellar vein, and the pineal. **(C)** Same view as in Fig. B. The straight sinus has been clipped, divided, and coagulated. **(D)** Supratentorial view of falcotentorial junction.

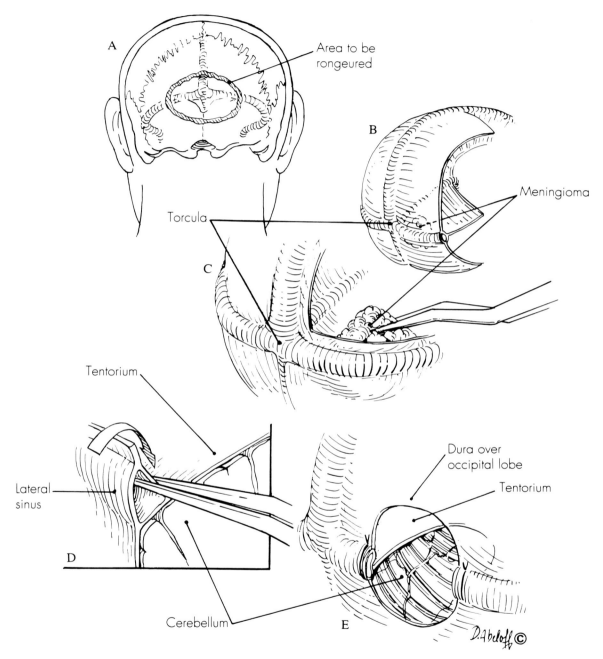

Figure 13-39. Paratorcular tumor invading tentorium and lateral sinus. **(A–C)** Resection of lateral sinus, adjacent dura, and tentorial segment. **(D&E)** Through and through bipolar coagulation of involved sinus wall if sinus is not resectable. One blade of forceps is inside the sinus, the other outside.

ment of collateral. I have been able to resect totally tumors of the torcula that had both lateral sinuses, the end of the sagittal sinus, and the straight sinus all totally occluded by tumor, with a major collateral distributed forward through the petrosal sinuses to the cavernous and through the sylvian veins, as well as accompanied by retrograde flow in the sagittal sinus draining forward into the frontal venous connections to the cavernous, as well as down the facial veins.

One of my patients with a tumor about 3 cm in diameter involving the junction of the sigmoid and lateral sinuses extending almost equally below the tentorium and above the tentorium was studied angiographically and found to have no significant lateral sinus on the opposite side, with all of the drainage from the sagittal sinus coming into the involved lateral sinus through the partially invaded area and down the remainder of the sigmoid sinus. I felt that resecting this tumor would require removal of all other drainage available to the sagittal sinus and would of course be fatal. I considered the possibility of partial removal, but since the tumor was only 3 cm in diameter and the syndrome not terribly threatening I elected to wait and do repeated studies. Over the course of a 10-year period the patient developed only slight mild increase in her ataxia without enough difficulty to keep her from working, and the tumor slowly increased to 4 cm in diameter. Finally, after a 10-year period, angiography demonstrated that she had now developed an adequate collateral flow through the previously absent lateral sinus of the uninvolved side as well as several other collateral vessels on the cerebellar surface and that the sinus itself in the area of the tumor had become completely occluded. Accordingly, radical resection could be carried out without the risk of the catastrophe that would have occurred earlier. Many possible problems can occur in such management. The patient may be psychologically unable to contend with this state of affairs. Again, the tumor may grow rapidly without repairing the circulation, forcing the issue under less than favorable circumstances. Without reasonably close observation the patient might develop chronic papilledema so that even after successful removal, postpapilledema atrophy would supervene. Accordingly, this is not a course to be followed casually.

Resecting torcular tumors requires the unroofing of all three posterior sinus areas into the normal zone. I have preferred to do this with a bone flap technique that I have used for more than 20 years for tumors requiring a bilateral craniotomy extending across the sagittal sinus. I turn a unilateral flap by standard technique with the craniotome, ending about 0.5 cm from the sagittal sinus. The dura is then separated from the calvarium across the sagittal sinus from the side under direct vision. After the sagittal sinus has been brought down from the calvarium for the whole extent of the flap from front to back, the bone flap of the other side is cut as a free flap starting from the margins of the previous cut and crossing the sagittal sinus laterally. At the end of the procedure drill holes in the two bone flaps are used to join them together. This is done only with 2-0 Nurolon, which has been completely adequate with quite satisfactory healing across the bone flaps.

For those tumors extending caudal to the lateral sinuses I have first done a craniectomy of the posterior fossa and then separated upward. If the tumor extends into the bone of the torcula and is clearly a vascular lesion, I have then used a doughnut-type of double incision in the bone. The first incision is made as close to the tumor as seems feasible using the craniotome and coming completely around the cephalad end of the tumor except for the area at the sagittal sinus. A second parallel incision is made in the same manner about 1 cm lateral to the first incision, and then these two strips of bone, one on each side, are removed. Under direct vision the dural separation is carried across the sinus and then the segment over the sinus is resected. When the dura is opened in this doughnut-shaped incision the arterial supply coming up from both sides in the dura to the tumor is interrupted and it is now possible to dissect the invaded bone off the tumor with minimal bleeding (Fig. 13-38A). At that point collateral veins previously identified on the angiographic picture will be separated from the attachments so that they can drain anteriorly to the sagittal sinus or laterally to the lateral sinuses, and then the sinuses can be ligated posterior to the last draining vein. Fortunately there are few such veins draining the occipital areas. The straight sinus must of course be known to be totally occluded if the torcula is to be resected in this manner (Fig. 13-38B).

MENINGIOMAS OF THE CEREBELLOPONTINE ANGLE

In the last 100 meningiomas of the cerebellopontine angle in my personal series, only 9 have actually invaded the dura of the tentorium. Many others have reached the superior petrosal sinus, but even those that lay against the inferior surface of the tentorium were not actually attached to it. This is partly due to classification, since a large number of tumors that might have been classified this way were actually grouped as clivopetrotentorial because of their extension. The entire matter of statistics is suspect because the largest series are nearly always related to a specific referral pattern. We do not yet have a reasonably adequate statistical base in neurosurgery for the classification of our lesions.

I have approached the angle meningiomas in the same manner as the acoustic neuromas, with a far lateral craniectomy completely exposing the sigmoid sinus and then drawing the sigmoid out of the wound over the cut surface of the mastoid with traction sutures. This procedure avoids the need for significant cerebellar retraction and certainly the need for any cerebellar resection (Fig. 13-40). A full discussion of the angle lesion resection is beyond the scope of this section, but the tentorial involvement requires some elucidation. Virtually all tumors that extend into the tentorium involve the superior petrosal sinus and the vein of the lateral recess as well as the petrosal vein. I have never seen any difficulty resulting from the resection of these three structures in these tumors. Collateral appears to be quite adequate.

I have generally preferred to incise the tentorium from below after the removal of the major mass of the tumor and then to cut around the tumor attachment on the tentorial undersurface, separating from the overlying occipital and temporal lobes and carrying the dissection over to the petrosal sinus (Fig. 13-41). As the petrosal sinus may have some residual tumor, it is coagulated with the bipolar forceps and then resected as well, exposing the petrosal apex. This may carry forward to the trigeminal sheath as it goes in under the temporal dura as the invaginated posterior fossa dura, which forms the gasserian sheath. Few of these tumors actually extend forward in this area along the gasserian sheath, but this approach allows this portion to be resected as well. The bipolar coagulator is used on the dural margins as the cut is carried around so that arterial supply coming from the tentorial meningeal or other vessels in the dura may be sealed without bleeding.

It has not been necessary to reconstruct the dura of the tentorium or to replace the tentorial edge when it is resected; however, I have not been willing to allow the remnant of the tentorial margin at the tentorial notch to remain in place as a thin band since the possibility of this band causing cerebral or cerebellar trauma if there should be any displacement seems at least theoretically possible. Accordingly, when the dural resection approaches the hiatal margin I have resected the margin with the segment of tentorium. Occasionally a small venous sinus anteriorly on the tentorial notch draining into the cavernous sinus is best clipped to be more certain of the seal.

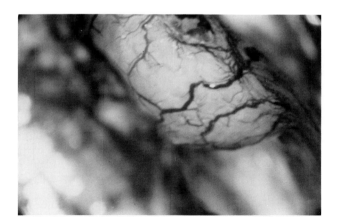

Figure 13-40. Right cerebellopontine angle, superior approach, field diameter 24 mm. Meningioma of the tentorial leaf protruding into the upper part of the cerebellopontine angle. The view is from behind. Vertex is up. The cerebellum has been dropped away from the tentorium without the need for retraction, and the surface of the tumor can be seen attached to the tentorium in the right upper corner of the photograph.

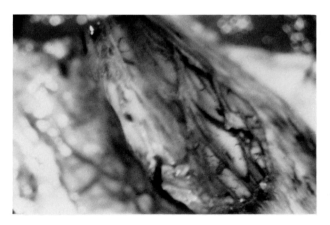

Figure 13-41. Same case as Fig. 13-40. The tumor has been removed. The cerebellum remains in the lower left third of the photograph. The tentorium has been resected around the margins of the tumor so that the exposed undersurface of the occipital lobe is visualized.

Sphenoid Wing Meningiomas

Manuel Cunha e Sa
Donald O. Quest

Meningiomas predominantly arise from areas of dural thickening or folding, being derived microscopically from the arachnoid cap or cluster cells in close intimacy with the dura mater. At the skull base some of the more common locations for these tumors are around the bony orifices, which allow the exit of vascular and nervous structures from within the skull, as well as along areas of dural duplication or folding related to the bony anatomy. Meningiomas of the cranial base, like most other meningiomas, are slow-growing neoplasms that tend to displace or distort rather than invade and destroy the nervous and vascular structures in close proximity. Planning how aggressive to be in the resection of the tumor is a complex matter. A decision is reached after balancing on the one hand the preoperative clinical condition and the possible progression of the disease left untreated as opposed to a more or less radical early intervention and the associated morbidity.[117] Referring to the surgeon's dilemma, Francis Grant[116] once wrote: "Think of the patient first; . . . remember that meningiomas in general are much like the little girl in the nursery rhyme who had a little curl, and when she was good she was very, very good; but when she was bad she was horrid.[1] And meningiomas at the base of the brain can be quite horrid."

Sphenoid wing meningiomas constitute nearly one-fifth of intracranial meningiomas.[107] Under this designation all the meningiomas that occur along the bony ridge formed by the ala magna and parva, which demarcates the boundary between the anterior and middle compartment of the cranial fossa, are included (Fig. 13-42A). The lesser wing makes up the inner two-thirds of the ridge and the greater wing the outer third. Stretching from the anterior clinoid process near the midline and reaching laterally to the low temporal convexity at the pterion, this anatomical ridge presents a wide variety of problems in surgical strategy. Add to this the known variability in histological type and morphology of tumor growth as well as the extent of invasion of the bone and meninges, and the span of the possible surgical problems can be ascertained. Planning for resection of a meningioma of the sphenoid wing will necessarily be thorough.

Meningiomas of the sphenoid wing have traditionally been separated into three categories, the inner, medial, and outer third sphenoid wing tumors, according to the classification of Cushing and Eisenhardt[107] in their monograph on meningiomas published in 1938. Inner third sphenoid wing meningiomas, also called clinoidal meningiomas, present most of the problems associated with parasellar tumors in general. In fact, the distinction between these meningiomas and those arising from the wall of the cavernous sinus or the suprasellar meningiomas growing out and inferiorly onto the floor of the middle cranial fossa is sometimes tenuous.[103,115] They tend to insinuate around the carotid artery and its branches, stretching, encasing, or (rarely) invading these vessels.[81] The optic nerve is also in jeopardy from direct pressure and the constricting effect of the tumor invading the dura and bone of the optic foramen and canal.[92,96,110,126,140,144,145] The other cranial nerves (III, IV, V, VI) traversing the parasellar region can also be involved by the meningioma, and their preservation certainly remains one of the main technical difficulties for the surgeon attempting excision of the tumor.[87,88,135,137] Midline structures of vital importance, such as the pituitary stalk and the hypothalamic/infundibular area, can be affected by mass effect, and any adherence of the tumor to these structures represents a major hazard during surgery. On the other hand, outer third or pterional meningiomas represent much less of a surgical challenge due to ready accessibility from the convexity. Middle third tumors are a much rarer entity, most of them representing the lateral or medial extension of a clinoidal or pterional meningioma, respectively.

Meningiomas grow for the most part as globular masses with a more or less wide base of attachment at the dura, although the so-called en plaque varieties occur often enough, 6.9 percent of operated meningiomas in Guiot and Derome's series[130] and 4 percent in Olivecrona's series.[101] Resection of en plaque meningiomas can present increased difficulty because of extensive invasion of the floor as well as the "hyperostosing" effect produced in the bone. A wide resection of the involved bone has been recom-

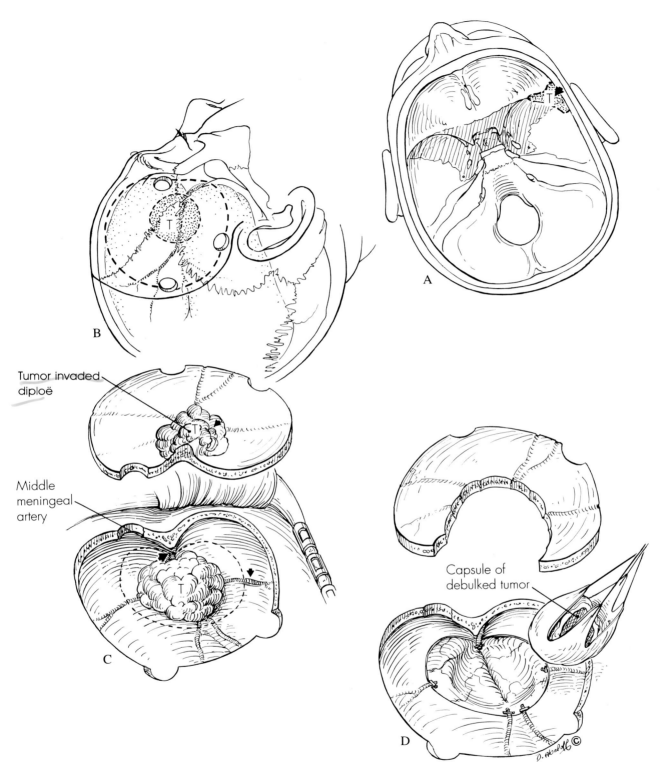

Tumor invaded
diploë

Middle
meningeal
artery

Capsule of
debulked tumor

Figure 13-42. **(A)** Skull base viewed from above showing sphenoid wing and cranial fossae. **(B)** Craniotomy site showing planned skin incision. **(C)** Tumor attached to bone flap and dural incision circumscribing tumor (*T*). **(D)** Separation of tumor capsule from brain and internal decompression.

Table 13-6. Sphenoid Wing Meningiomas—Mortality

Author	Year	No. of Patients	Type	Percent
Castellano et al.[101]	1952	15	En plaque	13
Guyot et al.[118]	1967	50	All	32
Fischer et al.[112]	1973	25	All	24
Dolenc[109]	1979	10	All	20
Bonnal[96]	1980	29	All	10
Pompili[130]	1982	49	All	4
Jan et al.[120]	1986	40	All	17.5
Fohanno et al.[113]	1986	44	All	23
Probst[131]	1987	40	Sellar	12
Sekhar et al.[137]	1989	16	Cavernous	0
Brotchi et al.[100]	1991	82	All	8.3
Al-Mefty[89]	1991	24	Clinoidal	8.3

mended based on microscopic studies demonstrating that the bone may be invaded by the tumor rather than just being thickened by the hyperostosing effect of the tumor. A large resection of the bone and dura at the base of the skull presents the need for the reconstruction of the floor; dead spaces should be avoided and, most importantly, a watertight closure of the dural defects is necessary in order to prevent CSF leak.

Meningiomas are benign tumors, and malignant varieties occur only rarely.[141] The surgical cure of a meningioma entails the complete excision of the tumoral mass, along with the involved meninges.[84,93,124,125,138] Determining the extent of dural infiltration may not be simple, as demonstrated by Borovich and Doron,[98] who showed that involvement is microscopically more disseminated than what is readily obvious surgically. This explains many of the recurrences of operated meningiomas, that is, regrowth of incompletely resected tumors. The aggressiveness of resection of the meningioma and the chance of a surgical cure, which remains problematical for the inner third tumors, does not apply to the pterional variety, which are of easy surgical access. Surgery for medial sphenoid wing meningiomas has some of the highest incidences of morbidity and mortality in the surgery of meningiomas[89,97,100,109,112,113,118,120,130] (Tables 13-6 and 13-7). Early series contemplated only partial removal, or even no surgery at all for certain more invading en plaque varieties. The introduction of microsurgical techniques and sophisticated electrophysiological monitoring has made possible a much more radical attitude toward these neoplasms. A profound knowledge of the anatomy of the skull base and its structures as well as techniques for reconstruction is absolutely necessary. This has been the domain for recent advances in skull base neurosurgery.

SURGICAL TECHNIQUE AND AVOIDANCE OF COMPLICATIONS

This section gives a detailed description of the multiple steps involved in the surgical approach to meningiomas of the sphenoid wing, consideration being given to the various nuances and stratagems that become necessary for tumors differing in location and morphology along the ridge. Careful preoperative planning in anticipation of the likely as well as the unlikely difficulties that the surgeon may encounter during the course of the operation is essential. All measures must be taken, pre- and intraoperatively, to reduce the possible morbidity of surgery.

Meningiomas can produce edema or swelling in adjacent areas of the brain, at times spreading extensively along the white matter, deforming or even obstructing the ventricular system, and greatly contributing to the increase in the intracranial pressure produced by the mass of the tumor.[111] It is therefore

Table 13-7. Comparative Mortality Rates for Different Varieties of Sphenoid Wing Meningiomas (No. of deaths/No. of patients operated)

Author	Year	Inner	Medial	Outer	En plaque	Entire Wing
Castellano[101]	1952				2/15	
Guyot[118]	1967	11/23		5/51	0/6	
Fischer[112]	1973	2/6	1/4	1/6	0/4	2/5
Dolenc[109]	1979	2/5		0/3		0/2
Bonnal[96]	1980	3/17	0/2	0/6	0/17	0/17
Pompili[130]	1982	1/9	0/6	0/16		1/15
Fohanno[113]	1986	27%		17%		
Jan[120]	1986	6/19		1/12		
Sekhar[137]	1989	0/16				
Al-Mefty[89]	1991	2/24				
Brotchi[100]	1991	5/28	0/9	0/13	0/17	0/15

of paramount importance that high-dose steroids, to reduce edema, be administered to the patient before the operation. Depending on the size of the tumor and the presence of associated hydrocephalus, a ventriculostomy may be necessary, although this is not usually the case with meningiomas growing in the sphenoid wing area. During surgery all brain retraction should be kept at an absolute minimum; the use of spinal drainage is advantageous. In cases with known increased intracranial pressure, intravenous mannitol is infused over a short period of time: around 15 minutes in a dose from 1 to 2 g/kg, starting at the time of the skin incision. Hyperventilation to maintain a low end-tidal PCO_2 is routine and so is the intraoperative administration of anticonvulsive agents such as dyphenylhydantoin and phenobarbital. It might be advisable to use both drugs at least transiently after the operation when a resistant preoperative tumor-related seizure disorder is present or when intraoperative conditions might indicate an increased risk for the occurrence of seizures in the postoperative period, such as when venous structures have been sacrificed during tumor resection. Prophylactic intravenous antibiotics (oxacillin or vancomycin in cases of a known penicillin allergy) are administered before the incision is made and repeated every 4 hours during the operation. They are discontinued on the second postoperative day.

The patient is placed in the supine decubitus position, and the head is held fixed in position with the use of the Mayfield three-pin head clamp. The head should be raised above the level of the right atrium to decrease venous pressure, with a 30- to 45-degree rotation away from the side of the tumor and a slight degree of extension so as to leave the malar process of the zygomatic arch parallel to the floor of the operating room; dropping the head at the vertex about 15 to 30 degrees provides enough extension to allow the temporal lobe to fall away from the floor of the middle cranial fossa, thereby minimizing the need for retraction. It may be necessary to use a small sandbag under the ipsilateral shoulder. All pressure points need to be carefully padded. Intermittent compressive leg sleeves are utilized to reduce the occurrence of intra- and postoperative deep venous thrombosis. A limited area of the scalp is then shaved. A Betadine scrub is routinely used on the skin followed by the customary three-application Betadine paint prepping (Fig. 13-43).

The surgical microscope is balanced prior to the start of the operation. The 275-mm lens is routinely used at an angle of about 60 degrees to the plane of the operating room floor. The Leyla bar holder and bar are routinely mounted on the operating room table at the time of the draping, to provide support further along in the operation either for the scalp flap and/or the Greenberg self-retaining apparatus.

The size of the skin and bone flap depends to some extent on the size of the tumor. A curvilinear skin incision of the type used for the pterional craniotomy is used, sometimes bringing it behind and above the ear lobe and more superiorly over the convexity for larger tumors. The incision should be kept behind the hairline, starting very low at the level of or immediately above the zygoma, about 5 mm anterior to the tragus, avoiding both the superficial temporal artery and the branches of the facial nerve, and being carried anteriorly just off the midline to the hairline on the forehead (Fig. 13-44). Michel clips can be used on the skin edges as they provide excellent hemostasis and are not cumbersome when compared to Raney or Dandy clamps. For the fronto-orbito-zygomatic approach a bicoronal, Soutar skin incision may be more advantageous.

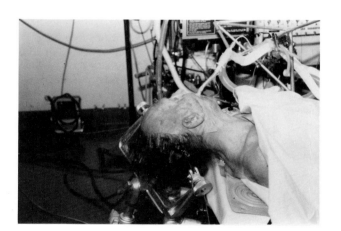 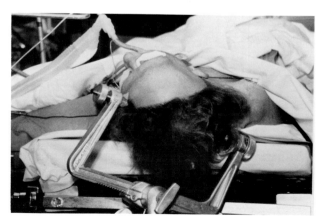

Figure 13-43. Operative photographs showing head position and scalp prepared for surgery.

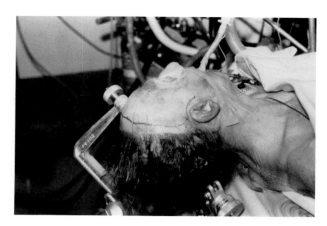
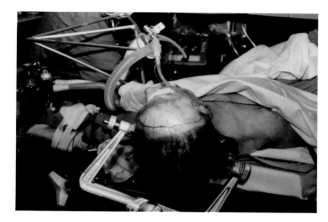

Figure 13-44. Operative photograph showing planned skin incision.

The scalp is elevated in a separate layer. The temporalis fascia is then divided in the same line as the skin incision, with a cutting cautery down through the muscle to the bone and the muscle with fascial attachment flapped back, hinged against the base of the skull leaving a small cuff of fascia on the superior temporal line in order to improve the reapproximation of the muscle at the time of the closure and to reduce the degree of postoperative atrophy. The flap is sutured back and held against the drapes with rubber bands to flap the muscle and skin back efficiently, as low as possible to provide access to the skull base.

A free bone flap is elevated with the use of the high-power drill and craniotome, one small hole drilled in the temporal squama posteriorly and inferiorly in an area covered by muscle with caution ex-

erted not to injure the middle meningeal artery on the surface of the dura. Alternatively, a Gigli saw can be used to cut the bone in between burr holes, one drilled in the temporal squama, one toward the vertex, and one on the temporal side of the attachment of the zygoma to the frontal bone (Fig. 13-42B). About 20 ml of CSF is removed from the spinal drain prior to the use of the craniotome. As the operation proceeds and as judged necessary, more CSF may be drained, usually to a maximum of 100 ml. The bone flap should encompass the whole pterional area, extending into the parietal and frontal bones according to the size of the tumor. For pterional meningiomas the flap should always include at least the whole area of its base of attachment (Fig. 13-45). For the clinoidal varieties the size of the mass as well

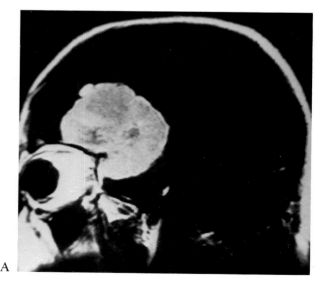
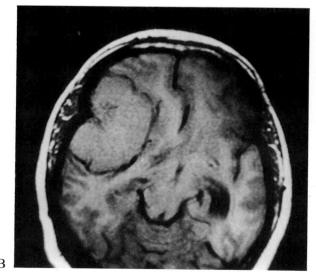

A

B

Figure 13-45. (A) Sagittal and **(B)** axial MRI of pterional-based sphenoid wing meningioma.

as its extension in the parasellar region from the anterior clinoid, to the cavernous sinus and back along the clivus may determine a more extensive approach such as the fronto-orbito-zygomatic approach.[86,87,119,122,129] This more anterior and inferior exposure provides a wider angle of attack to work on the more medial structures concealed or engulfed by the tumor mass—carotid artery, optic nerve, pituitary stalk, and infundibulum. In every case and even with a regular pterional flap, *it is necessary to reach low on the floor of the middle and anterior cranial fossae* because these tumors arise and get their blood supply from this area. In order to accomplish this, after the turning of the free bone flap the cutting burr should be used to drill extensively down the area of the wing medially and inferiorly toward the superior orbital fissure as much as the tumoral growth will allow (Fig. 13-42C). Bone wax should be used to stop all bone bleeding.

The resection of the zygoma is a variant that can be used to reach even lower on the cranial base (Fig. 13-46). The skin incision needs to be brought down to the inferior level of the tragus to the periosteum of the zygoma posteriorly immediately in front of the tuberculum articulare. Subperiosteal dissection is carried anteriorly over the lateral and medial surfaces of the zygoma, avoiding injury to the branches of the facial nerve. On the inferior aspect of the zygomatic arch posteriorly the capsule of the temporomandibular joint has to be dissected away, being careful not to avulse it, in order to reduce postoperative jaw pain and dysfunction of the temporomandibular joint. The zygoma is then divided anteriorly and posteriorly with the use of the drill or the Gigli saw (Fig. 13-47A). Staying low on the floor enables early access to the tumor base and its blood supply and also widens the

angle available to approach the tumor, reducing the need for retraction on the temporal lobe.

If an orbitotomy is necessary, the orbital rim and the entire zygomatic process of the frontal bone are subperiosteally exposed. A small hole is drilled just behind the zygomatic process of the frontal bone. Another hole is necessary near the glabella, medial to the inner angle of the orbit. If the frontal sinus is entered, the hole should be taken through the posterior wall in order to allow the use of the craniotome. Once the flap is turned, the sinus should be exenterated, packed with muscle, and sealed with pericranium before opening the dura. To avoid violating the periorbita when the orbital rim is divided, inferior retraction of the orbital contents with the use of a brain retractor is necessary; the Gigli saw or a small oscillating saw is used to connect both holes anteriorly. The supraorbital nerve is freed from its notch with use of the drill, and the trochlea is left untouched. After the zygomatic process has been divided and the craniotomy taken posteriorly across the frontal and temporal bones and inferiorly just above the floor of the temporal fossa, the bone flap including the orbital rim, the anterior part of the orbital roof, and the superior part of the lateral orbital wall are elevated in one piece (Fig. 13-48).

For the pterional tumors, elevation of the bone flap can constitute the most cumbersome and difficult part of the operation when extensive invasion of the underlying dura or of the bone itself exists. In these cases violation of the dura at the time of the flap elevation may be inevitable; it is imperative that the bone be rapidly freed from the dura and tumor in order to avoid blood loss, which may become copious especially when the middle meningeal artery, which is usually a main feeder to these laterally placed tumors, has been lacerated during the elevation of the flap. For tumors that extensively invade the bone it may not be safe to try to elevate the bone flap; drill holes should be placed and connected around the area of bone invasion, elevating the flap and leaving this area of invaded bone attached to the tumor (Fig. 13-42C).

The opening of the dura is another step in the operation that, although seemingly simple, remains of importance. For tumors that arise from the dura at the pterion, it might be wise to incise the dura in such a way as to circumscribe its base of attachment near the convexity (Fig. 13-42C). For all other tumors the dura should be incised in a curvilinear fashion, leaving a cuff inferiorly wide enough to prevent possible seeping of blood into the operative field. The dural cuff is held on stretch by sutures tented to the muscle (Fig. 13-47C). Moistened Bicol patties are used to

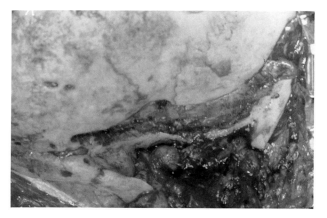

Figure 13-46. Operative photograph showing zygoma removed to allow greater access to cranial base.

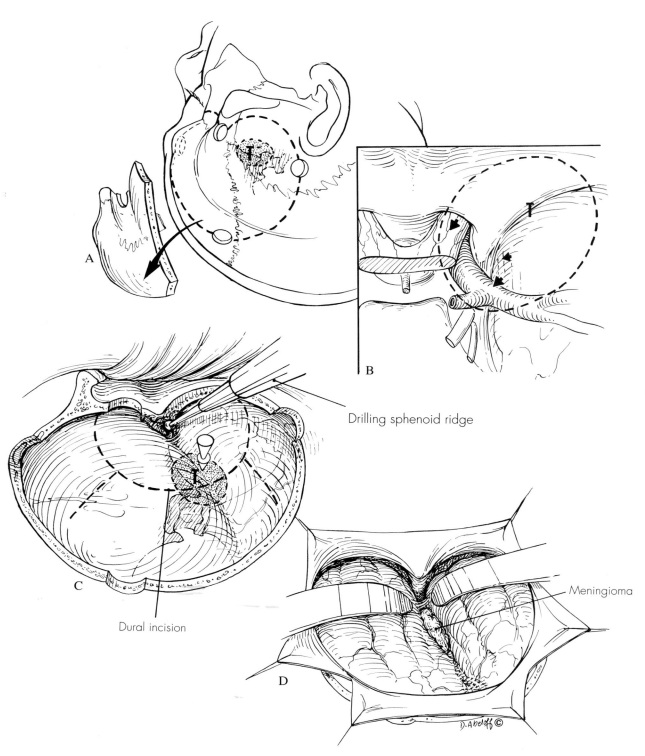

Figure 13-47. (A) Portion of zygoma to be removed. **(B)** Anatomy around cavernous sinus, which may be involved by medial sphenoid wing meningiomas. **(C)** Dural incision encompasses the sylvian fissure region. Sphenoid wing removal by drill toward superior orbital fissure. **(D)** Dural cuff tented inferiorly.

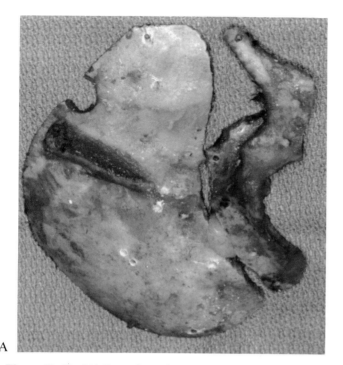 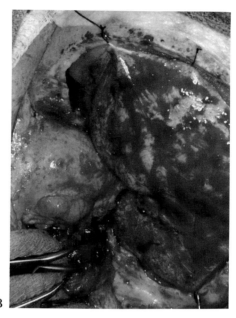

Figure 13-48. **(A)** Bone flap with part of zygoma. **(B)** Operative exposure after zygoma removal and orbitotomy completed showing frontal lobe, temporal lobe, and periorbita.

cover the exposed surface of the dura to prevent drying. Telfa rectangles are laid on the exposed brain for protection and always under the retractors. The Greenberg self-retaining retractor is usually assembled at this stage of the operation. A spinal needle connected to an arterial line tubing and a large syringe filled with saline is set on one of the arms of the retractor so as to provide an unobtrusive mode of continuous irrigation during the operation.

From here on the operation proceeds with the identification of the tumor mass by gentle retraction and separation of the sylvian fissure. One should initially come across the base of the tumor, attempting to devascularize it as much as possible. For outer sphenoid wing meningiomas, for which exposure does not constitute a problem, this can be accomplished in most cases with ease. A cuff of dura is left all around the base of implantation of the tumor, the capsule is coagulated to facilitate the dissection from the brain, and the tumor is internally debulked (Fig. 13-42D). For middle and inner third sphenoid wing tumors the size of the mass may become an obstacle when trying to proceed along the ala parva, and certainly at this stage debulking the tumor if it is not extremely vascular should be undertaken. Three different strategies may be undertaken in exposing the tumor mass and initiating the process of its devascu-

larization and debulking: a subtemporal progression along the floor of the middle cranial fossa, cauterizing all bridging veins to prevent them from tearing during retraction is useful for meningiomas growing outwards along the temporal floor; a transsylvian approach, opening the fissure as distal as necessary to expose the tumor mass should be utilized for tumors of large size that expand laterally and superiorly stretching the temporal lobe and sylvian region out, thereby preventing the possibility of initially proceeding along the floor (Figs. 13-47D and 13-49A&B); and finally, a direct approach along the ala parva identifying the optic nerve and the carotid artery early on in the operation can be the tactic of choice for the clinoidal meningiomas that do not extend laterally along the ridge. A combination of any or all of these surgical avenues can and very frequently is used, especially for the larger tumors.

The ultrasonic aspirator is useful for the intracapsular debulking of these neoplasms. Only for the deeper portion of the tumor may the instrument's handle become too cumbersome and hinder proper view. Some more fibrous types of meningiomas may be too tenacious for the aspirator, in which case one may have to debulk the tumor by cutting pieces of it. The monopolar loop is not recommended because it develops intense heat. Cauterization of any obvi-

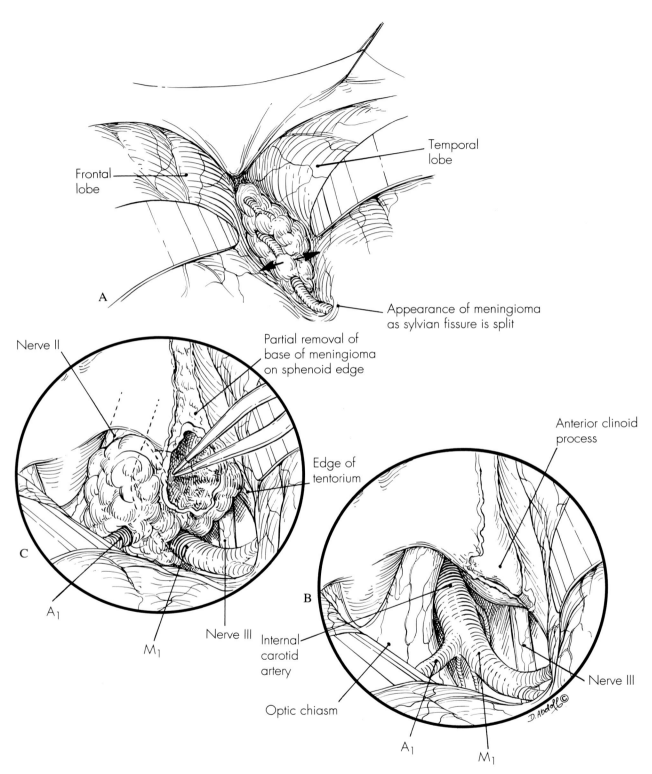

Figure 13-49. (A) Approach to tumor through the sylvian fissure. (B) Paraclinoid anatomy. (C) Tumor engulfing optic nerve and carotid artery.

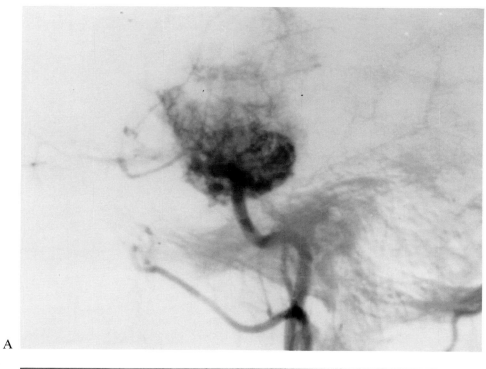

A

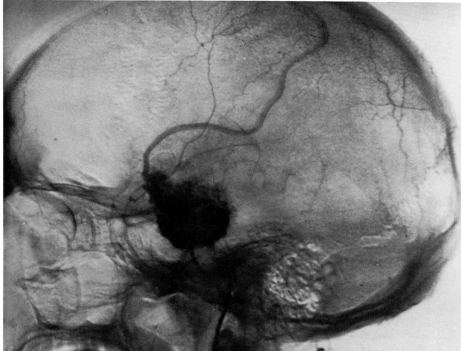

B

Figure 13-50. **(A&B)** Anteroposterior (AP) and lateral angiograms showing nonfilling of carotid artery distal to tumor blush. (*Figure continues.*)

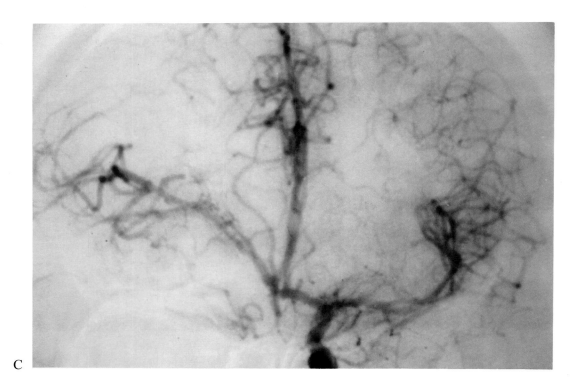

C

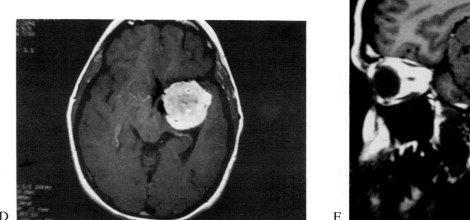

D

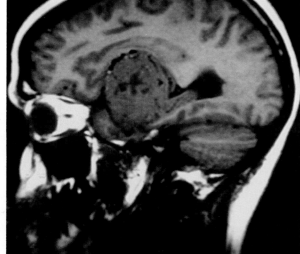

E

Figure 13-50. (*Continued*). **(C)** AP angiogram showing filling of distal middle cerebral artery from contralateral carotid artery. **(D)** Axial MRI showing vessel encasement. **(E)** Sagittal MRI showing vessel encasement. (*Figure continues.*)

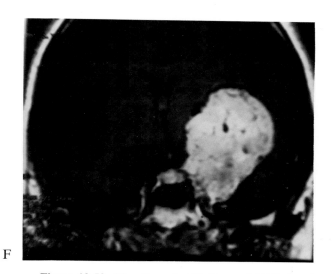

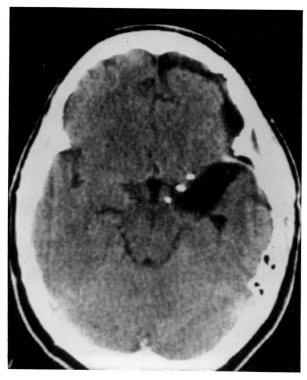

F

G

Figure 13-50. (*Continued*). **(F)** Coronal MRI showing vessel encasement. **(G)** Postoperative CT scan showing area of tumor removal and embolized vessels.

ously bleeding points should be undertaken interspersed with the use of the aspirator. The irrigating cautery is a useful instrument to avoid the sticking of the cautery tips with charred tissue, which all too frequently interrupts the work of the surgeon. The debulking should remain within the capsule boundaries but proceed aggressively so as to avoid having to retract or unduly manipulate the brain around the tumor. An en bloc technique of tumor resection[105] is strongly not recommended. Extreme care should be taken when proceeding deeply with the debulking when preoperative imaging studies (particularly MRI) suggests encasement of the carotid artery or its branches[99,146] (Figs. 13-50 and 13-51). This is more often the case with the large inner third sphenoid wing meningiomas, which typically grow around the branches of the circle of Willis. Spontaneous thrombosis of the carotid artery occurring in the postoperative period has also been reported.[128] For these tumors the strategy may have to differ. Debulking of the outer portion of the tumor and coming across its base remain the first steps. In these cases opening the sylvian fissure in order to expose the surface of the tumor and initiate its gutting is the initial stage of the operation.

Proceeding along the floor should not, at least initially, be taken all the way deep along the ala parva, in order to avoid damaging both the optic nerve and the proximal carotid artery, which may be engulfed by the tumor mass. Reducing the volume of the tumor allows better definition of these anatomical structures, and dissection from the investing meningioma is usually left for a later stage of the operation. The more distal branches of the carotid artery encased by tumor, usually middle cerebral artery (MCA) branches, should be deliberately sought; once they are identified they should be followed proximally, leading to the main carotid trunk (Fig. 13-49A). The dissection of these vessels from the tumor can be more or less difficult depending on the adhesiveness to or invasion of the vessel wall by the tumor. Nonetheless in most cases, a fine arachnoid plane can be developed around the arteries that greatly facilitates dissection. Great caution should be exerted in order to preserve every artery, even the small perforators stemming from the proximal MCA, ACA and posterior communicating artery (PCoA), because of the importance of their territory of vascularization but also because inadvertent manipulation of the tumor around these vessels may lead to avulsion at their

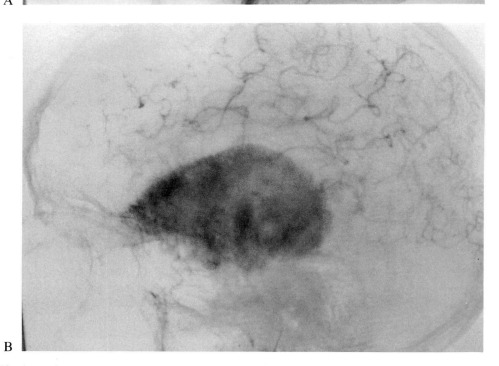

Figure 13-51. (A&B) AP and lateral angiograms showing vascular encasement and tumor blush. (*Figure continues.*)

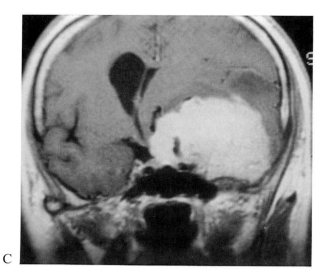

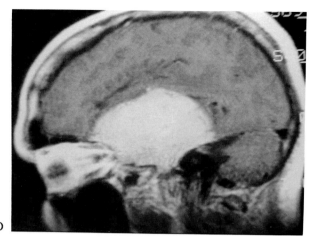

Figure 13-51. (*Continued*). (**C**) Coronal MRI showing encased vessels. (**D**) Sagittal MRI showing tumor extent.

origins, making it difficult to control bleeding. In the case of laceration of a major cerebral artery, if the vessel is not irreparably damaged, microsurgical reconstruction should be performed. Microclips are applied at each end of the segment to be repaired and with use of 10-0 prolene suture the tear is repaired. Bipolar cautery should be used with great care when dissecting the arteries, avoiding the vessel wall and irrigating continuously to prevent immediate or delayed thrombosis of the vessel[128] from either direct contact or heat spread. An insulated irrigating cautery is of great utility. The microscope should be used for all of this dissecting work. Gentle dissection is paramount as one gets deep into the tumor. With reference to the angiogram one can ascertain whether the vessels are encased by the tumor, enfolded in the capsule, or simply displaced by the tumor, which is the situation most of the time. With microdissection and appropriate microscopic illumination and magnification, one can identify the vessels and their branches and preserve them as one retracts the tumor away from them, cauterizing tumor capsule to shrink it and then gutting the tumor to remove it. Great care must be taken on the medial surface of the tumor near the hypothalamus and basal brain structures as well as the optic nerve, which can be considerably thinned by the tumor. Hollowing of the tumor mass will allow its walls to fall in. Cauterization of the capsule firms it, thereby facilitating dissection from the surrounding brain. Telfa rectangles are laid on the brain as the dissection proceeds.

The final stage of the operation deals with the tumor around the anterior clinoid, the carotid, and the optic nerve (Fig. 13-52). The meningioma frequently insinuates itself between the carotid artery and the optic nerve (Fig. 13-49C). Manipulation of the nerve should be avoided, and the fine blood vessels on its surface must be left untouched. In the same manner, when progressing posterior to the carotid artery, the third nerve has to be identified and protected, as even gentle manipulation may cause prolonged postoperative palsy. Even though the oculomotor nerve is frequently stretched or kinked by the tumor, it can be identified in most cases, whereas this proves to be much more difficult for the trochlear nerve, which is much smaller. This nerve is also frequently in jeopardy at the time of dissection along the tentorial notch, where the nerve is embedded at least for part

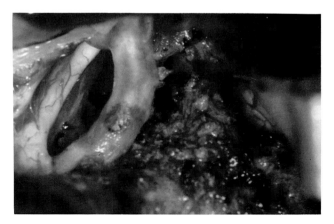

Figure 13-52. Operative photograph showing tumor dissected off of optic nerve and carotid artery and its branches.

of its course. The abducens is deeper and also enters the region of the cavernous sinus more posteriorly, making it less likely for it to be injured at least at this stage of the operation. If the tumor grows posteriorly toward the apex of the petrous pyramid, the trigeminal nerve and its ganglion within the dural sleeve of Meckel's cave may be involved. Just lateral and slightly inferior to it the intrapetrous carotid should be watched for, especially when there is bony erosion (Fig. 13-47B).

When the cavernous sinus is invaded by the tumor, one should be extremely careful when progressing with the debulking medially along the floor of the middle cranial fossa, so as not to enter the sinus inadvertently. In these cases the external dural layer of the sinus may not be identifiable due to the tumor invasion and continuing medially will risk damaging the third and fourth cranial nerves in the wall of the sinus. Warning bleeding from the sinus also may not occur due to tumor invasion. If it does, it is easily controlled by packing with Surgicel. What in most cases determines the fate following surgery of the cranial nerves that traverse the parasellar region is the extent of invasion of the cavernous sinus and its dural wall and the degree of aggressiveness in the resection of these tumors.[121] In general, when the oculomotor nerve has been left in continuity, the palsy tends to be transitory and in most patients the nerve will regain function at least partially. The trochlear nerve due to its decreased diameter and longer course is at greater risk; morbidity, however, is much less important due to the capacity that most patients have to compensate for the fourth nerve palsy. For patients with no symptoms referable to cavernous sinus invasion, a more expectant surgical attitude regarding that portion of the tumor in the cavernous sinus has been recommended.[131] If an aggressive resection, attempting a surgical cure, is decided upon, then proximal control of the carotid artery, either by exposing it in the neck or by skeletonizing its intrapetrosal segment, should be obtained. It is also mandatory to know whether the carotid artery involved by the tumor can safely be sacrificed if needed. An occlusion test, with balloon inflation and xenon cerebral blood flows, is the safest way of obtaining this information. If the patient does not tolerate the occlusion, bypass of the petrous carotid with the interposition of a saphenous vein graft should be considered.[136,142] Medial to the carotid the tumor has to be freed from the pituitary stalk, superiorly from the infundibular region and the hypothalamus. Indirect damage can also be caused to these structures by compromising their vascular supply.

The sphenoid wing tumors blend into those that affect the olfactory groove, the tuberculum sellae, the anterior clinoid process, the cavernous sinus, and the diaphragma sellae. These tumors can nearly always be totally removed unless they invade the cavernous sinus or proceed out the optic foramen or superior orbital fissure.

En plaque meningiomas grow by extensively invading not only the dura but the bone as well (Fig. 13-53). Patients tend to present with symptoms produced by distortion of the normal anatomy created by this thickening of the bone. Proptosis, decreased visual acuity, and oculomotor paresis may all occur due to the intraorbital growth and/or narrowing of the optic canal and superior orbital fissure. The surgical cure of these patients may require a radical bone excision.[95,106,123] Extradural removal by drill of the roof and lateral wall of the orbit, the ala parva progressing toward the anterior clinoid as much as the tumor will allow, finally unroofing the optic canal and the superior orbital fissure, might be attempted initially in the procedure. The tumor is then removed from within the orbit and also intradurally, and all the involved dura is resected. Care should be taken to avoid entering the ethmoid air cells in the body of the sphenoid bone medial to the anterior clinoid as this can become the source of a postoperative CSF leak.

Once the tumor has been removed the whole tumor bed should be copiously irrigated and meticulously inspected for any bleeding points. Induced hypotension is not used at any time during the operation, and at the end of the procedure the arterial blood pressure should be close to the preoperative value to check hemostasis. Surgicel is a useful hemostatic agent.

After the tumor mass has been resected it is necessary to determine the degree and extension of the dural involvement and resect it. By so doing, dural defects of varying size are created in the floor of the cranial fossa. This situation, along with the bone removal and the possible existence of other areas of erosion of the bone, contributes to the possibility of postoperative CSF leakage. It may therefore be necessary to reconstruct these areas of the floor, eliminating areas of dead space where fluid may collect, and ensuring a watertight closure of the dural defect. This should be achieved with the use of the patient's own tissue, preferably pericranium, frontalis and temporalis fascia, or tensor fascia lata graft harvested from the thigh. Reconstruction of the bone removed should be accomplished with the use of autologous bone in order to decrease the risk of infection.[108] The use of fibrin glue deserves consideration in improving the sealing of the dural or fascial edges. Other non-

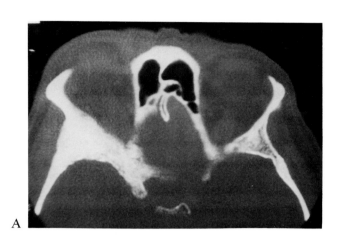

A

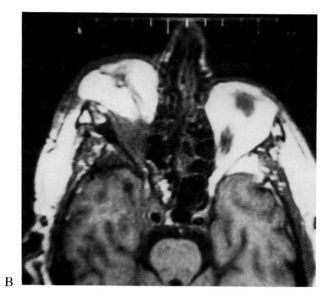

B

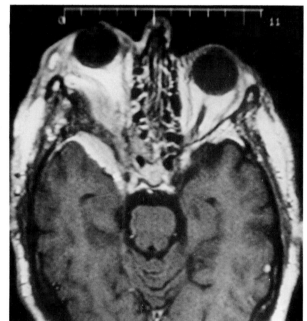

C

Figure 13-53. **(A)** Axial CT scan of en plaque meningioma showing hyperostosis of sphenoid wing. **(B)** Pregadolinium axial MRI showing extension of en plaque meningioma into orbit and middle fossa. **(C)** Postgadolinium MRI showing en plaque tumor extent.

autologous dural substitutes are best avoided in order to prevent infection and inflammatory reactions.[85,91,104,139]

Closure of the operative wound is carried out in the standard fashion. The bone flap is wired in place and the central tenting suture is tied. A Hemovac drain is placed under the muscle, to be left overnight, and the temporalis and its fascia are then approximated with interrupted 3-0 Vicryl sutures. This same closure is used for the galea, and skin staples are routinely applied. The head is dressed and the spinal drain is removed in the operating room, or left in for postoperative continuous draining when a CSF leak is possible.

MANAGEMENT OF POSTOPERATIVE COMPLICATIONS

At the end of surgery the patient should be able to be extubated. Prolonged anesthesia for operations that tend to be rather lengthy should not be used to justify the failure of the patient to awaken or be extubated. Other causes need to be ruled out, namely, eminently treatable conditions such as a rare but possible hematoma. The patient should be scanned immediately; other conditions such as edema, which can occur from excessive retraction or tumor manipulation, and may also contribute to the patient's obtundation, will also be clearly demonstrated. Areas of brain infarction can initially have a CT signal similar to parenchymal edema; serial CT scans will be necessary to distinguish one entity from the other when the patient's focal neurological deficit is not clearing. Hyperventilation, osmotic diuresis, and high-dose steroids are used when there is brain swelling. Ventricular drainage is used to relieve hydrocephalus. The age of the patient is another important factor in determining the surgical outcome, especially for meningiomas of the base for which surgery-related morbidity and mortality rates are higher.[90]

Postoperative hematomas are a rare complication of the surgery of meningiomas. An intracerebral, subdural, or epidural hematoma may be found, and evacuation may be necessary depending on size and location and whether it is felt this is contributing to the patient's neurological deficit. In some cases an incipient coagulopathy results from increased fibrinolytic activity caused by the tumor.[94,127,143] Venous infarction of areas of the brain where the venous drainage has been compromised can present as areas of hemorrhage, although generally with a typical patchy distribution on CAT scan. Significant edema with increased intracranial pressure may be associated with the infarction.

Seizures can occur de novo in the postoperative period, but they are more likely in patients who have had a seizure disorder before the operation.[132] Meningiomas at the base of the skull such as the sphenoid wing varieties are less frequently associated with the occurrence of seizures both pre- and postoperatively, compared with meningiomas in other intracranial locations.[102,114,132] Seizures are usually clinically obvious, but at times an electroencephalogram (EEG) may be necessary to rule out continuous or intermittent subclinical epileptic activity. In the immediate postoperative period seizures can become highly refractory to the medication; it is therefore recommended that anticonvulsants be kept at good therapeutic levels, with single or multiple drug regimens. Anticonvulsants are prescribed for a 1- to 2-year period after surgery, after which, if the patient has been seizure free, they may be discontinued.

Deep venous thrombosis and pulmonary embolism tend to occur more frequent in patients operated on for meningiomas. Although there had not been much statistical evidence to corroborate this contention, recent studies seem to indicate that it is in fact true and is not necessarily related to conditions such as hemiparesis which were thought to increase the occurrence of this complication.[133,134] Intermittent compressive leg stockings are obligatory peri- and postoperatively and early ambulation is desirable. Subcutaneous heparin should be administered starting 72 hours after the operation in patients who have severe paresis or who are bedridden.

REFERENCES

Convexity, Parasagittal, and Parafalcine Meningiomas

1. Adler JR, Upton J, Wallman J et al: Management and prevention of necrosis of the scalp after embolization and surgery for meningioma. Surg Neurol 25:357, 1986

2. Bonnal J, Brotchi J: Surgery of the superior sagittal sinus in parasagittal meningiomas. J Neurosurg 48:935, 1978

3. Challa VR, Monly DM, Marshall RB et al: The vascular component in meningiomas associated with severe cerebral edema. Neurosurgery 7:363, 1980

4. Chan C, Thompson GB: Ischemic necrosis of the scalp after preoperative embolization of meningeal tumors. Neurosurgery 15:76, 1984

5. Chan RC, Thompson GB: Morbidity, mortality and quality of life following surgery for intracranial meningiomas. A retrospective study in 257 cases. J Neurosurg 60:52, 1984

6. Cushing H: The meningiomas (dural endotheliomas): their source, and favoured seats of origin. Brain 45:282, 1922

7. Cushing H, Eisenhardt L: Meningiomas: Their Classification, Regional Behaviour, Life History and Surgical End Results. Charles C Thomas, Springfield, IL, 1938

8. Gautier-Smith PC: Parasagittal and Falx Meningiomas. Appleton-Century-Crofts, East Norwalk, CT, 1970

9. Gilbert JJ, Paulseth JE, Coutes RF et al: Cerebral edema associated with meningiomas. Neurosurgery 12:599, 1983

10. Goldsher D, Litt AW, Pinto RS et al: Dural "tail" associated with meningiomas on Gd-DTPA-enhanced MR images: characteristics, differential diagnostic value, and possible implications for treatment. Radiology 176:447, 1990

11. Guthrie BL, Ebersold MJ, Scheithauer BW: Neoplasms of the intracranial meninges. p. 3250. In Youmans JR (ed): Neurological Surgery. 3rd Ed. WB Saunders, Philadelphia, 1990

12. Hekster REM, Matricall B, Luyendijk W: Presurgical transfemoral catheter embolization to reduce operative blood loss. J Neurosurg 41:396, 1974

13. Hieshima GB, Everhart FR, Mehringer CMJ et al: Preoperative embolization of meningiomas. Surg Neurol 14:119, 1980

14. Hoessly GF, Olivecrona H: Report on 280 cases of verified parasagittal meningiomas. J Neurosurg 12:614, 1955

15. Horwitz NH, Rizzoli HV: Postoperative Complications of Intracranial Neurological Surgery. p. 85. Williams & Wilkins, Baltimore, 1982

16. Kempe LG: Operative Neurosurgery. Vol. 1. Cranial, Cerebral and Intracranial Vascular Disease. Springer-Verlag, New York, 1968

17. Logue V: Parasagittal meningiomas. p. 171. In Krayenbuhl H (ed): Advances and Technical Standards in Neurosurgery. Springer-Verlag, New York, 1975

18. Logue V: Surgery of meningiomas. p. 128. In Symon L (ed): Operative Surgery: Neurosurgery. Butterworth, London, 1979

19. Long DM: Atlas of Operative Neurosurgical Technique. Vol. 1. Cranial Operations. p. 218. Williams & Wilkins, Baltimore, 1989

20. MacCarty CS, Piepgras DG, Ebersold MJ: Meningeal tumors of the brain. p. 2936. In Youmans JR (ed): Neurological Surgery. 2nd Ed. WB Saunders, Philadelphia, 1982

21. Maxwell RE, Chou SN: Parasagittal and falx meningiomas. p. 563. In Schmidek HH, Sweet WH (eds): Operative Neurosurgical Techniques. 2nd Ed. Grune & Stratton, Orlando, FL, 1988

22. Maxwell RE, Chou SN: Convexity meningiomas and general principles of meningioma surgery. p. 555. In Schmidek HH, Sweet WH (eds): Operative Neurosurgical Techniques. 2nd Ed. Grune & Stratton, Orlando, FL, 1988

23. McGrail K, Ojemann RG: The management of benign intracranial tumors in patients 70 years of age and older. (In press)

24. Morley TP: Tumors of the cranial meninges. p. 1388. In Youmans JR (ed): Neurological Surgery. 1st ed. WB Saunders, Philadelphia, 1973

25. Northfield DWC: The Surgery of the Central Nervous System. A Textbook for Postgraduate Students. p. 229. Blackwell Scientific Publications, London, 1973

26. Ojemann RG: Meningiomas: Clinical Features and Surgical Management. p. 635. In Wilkins RH, Rengachary SS (eds): Neurosurgery. McGraw-Hill, New York, 1985

27. Ojemann RG, Black PMcL: Difficult decisions in managing patients with benign brain tumors. Clin Neurosurg 35:254, 1987

28. Phillippon J, Foncin JF, Grob R et al: Cerebral edema associated with meningiomas: possible role of secretory-excretory phenomenon. Neurosurgery 14:295, 1984

29. Poppen JL: An Atlas of Neurosurgical Techniques. WB Saunders, Philadelphia, 1960

30. Quest DO: Meningiomas: an update. Neurosurgery 3:219, 1978

31. Richter HP, Schachemmayr W: Preoperative embolization of intracranial meningiomas. Neurosurgery 13:261, 1983

32. Simpson D: The recurrence of intracranial meningiomas after surgical treatment. J Neurol Neurosurg Psychiatry 20:22, 1957

Olfactory Groove and Planum Meningiomas

33. Bakay L, Cares HL: Olfactory meningiomas. Acta Neurochir (Wien) 26:1, 1972

34. Barbaro NM, Gutin PH, Wilson CW et al: Radiation therapy in the treatment of partially resected meningiomas. Neurosurgery 20:525, 1987

35. Bergland R, Ray BS: The arterial supply of the optic chiasm. J Neurosurg 31:327, 1969

36. Boker DK, Meurer H, Gullotta F: Recurring intracranial meningiomas, evaluation of some factors predisposing for tumor recurrence. J Neurosurg Sci 29:11, 1985

37. Chan RC, Thompson GB: Morbidity, mortality, and quality of life following surgery for intracranial meningioma. J Neurosurg 60:52, 1984

38. Cushing H: Meningiomas arising from the olfactory groove and their removal by aid of electrosurgery. Lancet 1:1329, 1927

39. Cushing H, Eisenhardt L: The olfactory meningiomas with primary anosmia. p. 250. In Cushing H, Eisenhardt L (eds): Meningiomas. Charles C Thomas, Springfield, 1938

40. Derome PJ, Guiot G: Bone problems in meningiomas invading the base of the skull. Clin Neurosurg 25:435, 1978

41. Durante F: Estirpazione di un tumore endocranio. Arch Soc Ital Chir 2:252, 1885

42. Finn JE, Mount LA: Meningiomas of the tuberculum sellae and planum sphenoidale, a review of 83 cases. Arch Ophthalmol 92:23, 1974

43. Foy PM: The meningiomas: hemangioblastoma. p. 273. In Miller JD (ed): Northfield's Surgery of the Central Nervous System. 2nd Ed. Blackwell Scientific Publications, Edinburgh, 1985

44. Hassler W, Zentner J: Pterional approach for surgical treatment of olfactory groove meningiomas. Neurosurgery 25:942, 1989

45. Henderson WR: The anterior basal meningiomas. Br J Surg 26:124, 1938

46. Kadis GN, Mount LA, Ganti SR: The importance of early diagnosis and treatment of the meningiomas of the planum sphenoidale and the tuberculum sellae, a retrospective study of 105 cases. Surg Neurol 12:367, 1979

47. Kempe LG: Operative Neurosurgery. Vol. 1. p. 104. Springer-Verlag, New York, 1968

48. Kennedy, F: Retrobulbar neuritis as an exact diag-

nostic sign of certain tumors and abscesses in the frontal lobes. Am J Med Sci cxlii:355, 1911

49. Kupersmith MJ, Warren FA, Newall J et al: Irradiation of meningiomas of the intracranial anterior visual pathway. Ann Neurol 21:131, 1987

50. Logue V, Symon L: Surgery of meningiomas. p. 273. In Symon L, Thomas DGT, Clarke K (eds): Operative Surgery (Neurosurgery). Butterworths, London, 1989

51. MacCarty CS, Piepgras DG, Ebershold NJ: Meningeal tumors of the brain. p. 2936. In Youmans J (ed): Neurological Surgery. 2nd Ed. WB Saunders, Philadelphia, 1982

52. Marano SR, Sonntag VKH, Spetzler RF: Planum sphenoidale meningioma mimicking pituitary apoplexy: a case report. Neurosurgery 15:859, 1984

53. Mirimanoff RO, Dosoretz DE, Linggood RM et al: Meningioma: analysis of recurrence and progression following neurosurgical resection. J Neurosurg 62:18, 1985

54. Morello G, Frera C: Visual damage after removal of hypophyseal adenomas: possible importance of vascular disturbances of the optic nerves and chiasm. Acta Neurochir (Wien) 15:1, 1966

55. Neihart RE, Hodges GR, Papasian CJ et al: Nosocomial hemophilus influenzae type C meningitis in an adult. Diagn Microbiol Infect Dis 6:69, 1987

56. North JB, Penhall RK, Hanieh A et al: Phenytoin and postoperative epilepsy, a double blind study. J Neurosurg 58:672, 1983

57. Ojemann RG, Swann KW: Surgical management of olfactory groove, suprasellar and medial sphenoidal ridge meningiomas. p. 536. In Schmidek HH, Sweet WH (eds): Operative Neurosurgical Techniques, Indications, Methods and Results. 2nd Ed. Grune & Stratton, Orlando, FL, 1988

58. Olivecrona H: The surgical treatment of intracranial tumors. In Olivecrona H, Tonnis W et al (eds): Handbuch der Neurochirurgie. Bd. IV/4. Springer-Verlag, Berlin, 1967

59. Persky MS, Som ML: Olfactory groove meningioma with paranasal sinus and nasal cavity extension: a combined approach. Otolaryngology 86:714, 1978

60. Rammamurthi B, Ravi R, Ramachandran V: Convulsions with meningiomas: incidence and clinical significance. Surg Neurol 14:415, 1980

61. Ray B, Patterson R: Surgical treatment of pituitary adenomas. J Neurosurg 19:1, 1962

62. Solero CL, Giombini S, Morello G: Suprasellar and olfactory meningiomas, report of a series of 153 personal cases. Acta Neurochir (Wien) 67:181, 1983

63. Symon L: Olfactory groove and suprasellar meningiomas. p. 67. In Krayenbuhl H (ed): Advances and Technical Standards in Neurosurgery. Vol. 4. Springer-Verlag, New York, 1977

64. Tenney JH, Vlahov D, Salcman M et al: Wide variation in risk of wound infection following clean neurosurgery. J Neurosurg 62:243, 1985

65. Udvarhhelyi GB, Walsh FB: Complications involving the optic nerves and chiasm during the early period after neurosurgical operations. J Neurosurg 19:51, 1962

66. Yamashita J, Handa H, Iwaki K et al: Recurrence of intracranial meningiomas with special reference to radiotherapy. Surg Neurol 14:33, 1980

67. Young RF, Lawner PM: Perioperative antibiotic prophylaxis for prevention of postoperative neurosurgical infections; a randomized clinical trial. J Neurosurg 66:701, 1897

Tentorial, Torcular, and Paratorcular Meningiomas (Suggested Readings)

68. Bisaria K: Developmental defects of the tentorium cerebelli. J Neurosurg 58:402, 1983

69. Grisoli F, Vincentelli F, Fuchs S et al: Surgical treatment of tentorial arteriovenous malformations draining into the subarachnoid space. J Neurosurg 60:1059, 1984

70. Guidetti B, Ciappetta P, Domenicucci M: Tentorial meningiomas: surgical experience with 61 cases and long-term results. J Neurosurg 69:183, 1988

71. Jannetta P: Microvascular decompression of the trigeminal nerve root entry zone. p. 201. In Rovit R, Murali R, Jannetta P (eds): Trigeminal Neuralgia. Williams & Wilkins, Baltimore, 1990

72. Malis LI: Tumors of the parasellar region. Adv Neurol 15:281, 1976

73. Malis LI: Prevention of neurosurgical infection by intraoperative antibiotics. Neurosurgery 5:339, 1979

74. Malis LI: Surgical resection of tumors of the skull base. p. 1011. In Wilkins RH, Rengechary SS (eds): Neurosurgery. McGraw-Hill, New York, 1985

75. Malis LI: Surgical approaches to tentorial meningiomas. p. 399. In Wilkins RH, Rengechary SS (eds): Neurosurgery Update I. McGraw-Hill, New York, 1990

76. Mayberg MR, Symon L: Meningiomas of the clivus and apical petrous bone. J Neurosurg 65:160, 1986

77. Ojemann RG: Meningiomas: clinical features and surgical management. p. 635. In Wilkins RH, Rengechary SS (eds): Neurosurgery Update I. McGraw Hill, New York, 1990

78. Ono M, Ono M, Rhoton AL Jr et al: Microsurgical anatomy of the region of the tentorial incisura. J Neurosurg 60:365, 1984

79. Sakaki S, Shiraishi T, Takeda S et al: Occlusions of the great vein of Galen associated with a huge meningioma in the pineal region. J Neurosurg 61:1136, 1984

80. Sekhar L, Jannetta P: Cerebellopontine angle meningiomas. J Neurosurg 60:500, 1984

81. Sekhar L, Jannetta P, Maroon J: Tentorial meningiomas: surgical management and results. Neurosurgery 14:268, 1984

82. Sekhar LN, Schramm VL Jr, Jones NF: Subtemporal-preauricular infratemporal fossa approach to large lateral and posterior cranial base neoplasms. J Neurosurg 67:488, 1987

83. Sekhar LN, Sen CN: Anterior and lateral basal approaches to the clivus. Contemp Neurosurg 11:24, 1989

Sphenoid Wing Meningiomas

84. Adgebite A et al: The recurrence of intracranial meningiomas after surgical treatment. J Neurosurg 58:51, 1983
85. Adgebite A, Paine K, Rodzilsky B: The role of neomembranes in formation of hematoma around silastic dura substitute. J Neurosurg 58:295, 1983
86. Al-Mefty O. Approach selection in juxtasellar surgery. p. 57. In Al-Mefty O (ed): Surgery of the Cranial Base. Kluwer, Boston, 1989
87. Al-Mefty O: Surgical technique for the juxtasellar area. p. 73. In Al-Mefty O (ed): Surgery of the Cranial Base. Kluwer, Boston, 1989
88. Al-Mefty O: Management of cavernous sinus involvement. p. 91. In Al-Mefty O (ed): Surgery of the Cranial Base. Kluwer, Boston, 1989
89. Al-Mefty O: Clinoidal meningiomas. p. 427. In Al-Mefty O (ed): Meningiomas. Raven Press, New York, 1991
90. Awad I et al: Intracranial meningiomas in the aged: surgical outcome in the era of computed tomography. Neurosurgery 24:557, 1989
91. Banerjee T, Meagher J, Hunt W: Unusual complications with use of silastic dural substitute. Am Surg 40:434, 1974
92. Basso A et al: La chirurgie des tumeurs spheno-orbitaires. Neurochirurgie 24:71, 1978
93. Beks W, deWindt H: The recurrence of supratentorial meningiomas after surgery. Acta Neurochir (Wien) 95:3, 1988
94. Bodin D et al: Coagulopathie de consommation et meningiome. Ann Fr Anesth Reanim 5:308, 1986
95. Bonnal J, Castermans A, Stevenaert A, Brotchi J, Van Wijck R: Les meningiomes des étages anterieurs et moyens de la base du crane. Conduite à tenir vis-à-vis des envahissements osseux et des prolongements dans les cavités de la face. Neurochirurgie 18:441, 1972
96. Bonnal J, Sedan R, Paillas J: Problèmes cliniques évolutifs et thérapeutiques soulevés par les meningiomes envahissants de la base du crane. Neurochirurgie 7:108, 1961
97. Bonnal J et al: Invading meningiomas of the sphenoid ridge. J Neurosurg 53:587, 1980
98. Borovich B, Doron Y: Recurrence of intracranial meningiomas: the role played by regional multicentricity. J Neurosurg 64:58, 1986
99. Bradac G et al: Cavernous sinus meningiomas: an MRI study. Neuroradiology 29:578, 1987
100. Brotchi J, Bonnal J: Lateral and middle sphenoid wing meningiomas. p. 413. In Al-Mefty O (ed): Meningiomas. Raven Press, New York, 1991
101. Castellano F, Guidetti B, Olivecrona H: Pterional meningiomas ''en plaque''. J Neurosurg 9:188, 1952
102. Chan R, Thompson G: Morbidity, mortality and quality of life following surgery for intracranial meningiomas. J Neurosurg 60:52, 1984
103. Cioffi F et al: Cavernous sinus meningiomas. Neurochirurgia (Stuttg) 30:40, 1987
104. Cohen A, Aleksic S, Ransohoff J: Inflammatory reaction to synthetic dural substitute. J Neurosurg 70:633, 1989
105. Cook A: Total removal of large global meningiomas at the medial aspect of the sphenoid ridge. J Neurosurg 34:107, 1971
106. Cophignon J et al: Limits to radical treatment of spheno-orbital meningiomas. Acta Neurochir (Wien), suppl. 28:375, 1979
107. Cushing H, Eisenhardt L: Meningiomas of the sphenoidal ridge. A. Those of the deep or clinoidal third. p. 298. In Cushing H, Eisenhardt L (eds): Meningiomas: Their Classification, Regional Behaviour, Life History and Surgical End Results. Charles C Thomas, Springfield, IL, 1938
108. Derome P, Guiot G: Bone problems in meningiomas invading the base of the skull. Clin Neurosurg 25:435, 1978
109. Dolenc V: Microsurgical removal of large sphenoidal body meningiomas. Acta Neurochir (Wien), suppl. 28:391, 1979
110. Elsberg C, Dyke C: Meningiomas attached to the medial part of the sphenoid ridge with syndrome of unilateral optic atrophy, defect in visual field of the same eye and changes in sella turcica and in shape of interpeduncular cistern after encephalography. Arch Ophthalmol 12:644, 1934
111. Fine M et al: Computed tomography of sphenoid wing meningiomas: tumor location related to distal edema. Surg Neurol 13:385, 1980
112. Fischer G, Fischer C, Mansuy L: Prognostic chirurgical des meningiomes de l'arête sphenoidale. Neurochirurgie 19:323, 1973
113. Fohanno D, Bitar A: Sphenoidal ridge meningiomas. Adv Tech Standards Neurosurg 14:137, 1986
114. Foy P, Copeland G, Shaw M: The incidence of postoperative seizures. Acta Neurochirur (Wien) 55:253, 1981
115. Grant F: Intracranial meningiomas, surgical results. Surg Gynecol Obstet 85:419, 1947
116. Grant F: The surgery of meningiomas at the base of the brain. Clin Neurosurg 5:25, 1958
117. Guthrie B, Ebersold M, Scheitauer B: Neoplasms of the intracranial meninges. p. 3250. In Youmans JR (ed): Neurological Surgery. 3rd Ed. WB Saunders, Philadelphia, 1990
118. Guyot J, Vouyouklakis D, Pertuiset B: Meningiomes de l'arête sphenoidale. A propos de 50 cas. Neurochirurgie 13:571, 1967
119. Hakuba A, Liu S, Nishimura S: The orbitozygomatic infratemporal approach: a new surgical technique. Surg Neurol 26:271, 1986
120. Jan M et al: Devenir des meningiomes intracraniens chez l'adulte. Neurochirurgie 32:129, 1986
121. Lesoin F et al: Management of cavernous sinus meningiomas. Neurochirurgia (Stuttg) 28:195, 1985

122. Lesoin F et al: Intérêt de la voie d'abord orbito-fronto-temporo-malaire dans l'exérèse de certains meningiomes de l'arête sphenoidale. Neurochirurgie 32:154, 1986

123. MacCarthy C: Meningiomas of the sphenoidal ridge. J Neurosurg 36:115, 1972

124. Melamed S, Sakhar A, Beller A: The recurrence of intracranial meningiomas. Neurochirurgie 22:47, 1979

125. Mirimanoff M et al: Meningioma: analysis of recurrence and progression following neurosurgical resection. J Neurosurg 62:18, 1985

126. Newell F, Beaman T: Ocular signs of meningioma. Am J Ophthalmol 45:30, 1958

127. Oka K et al: Meningiomas and hemorrhagic diatesis. J Neurosurg 69:356, 1988

128. Oppido P, Delfini R, Santoro A, Missori P: Intra-extracranial thrombosis of the internal carotid artery associated with meningioma. Neurochirurgia 32:195, 1989

129. Pellerin P et al: Usefulness of the orbitofrontomalar approach with bone reconstruction for frontotemporosphenoid meningiomas. Neurosurgery 15:715, 1984

130. Pompili A et al: Hyperostosing meningiomas of the sphenoid ridge—clinical features, surgical therapy, and long-term observations: review of 39 cases. Surg Neurol 17:411, 1982

131. Probst C: Possibilities and limitations of microsurgery in patients with meningiomas of the sellar region. Acta Neurochirur (Wien) 84:99, 1987

132. Ramamurthi B, Ravi R, Ramachandran V: Convulsions with meningiomas: incidence and significance. Surg Neurol 14:415, 1980

133. Sawaya R, Ramo J: Systemic and thromboembolic effects of meningiomas. p. 137. In Al-Mefty O (ed): Meningiomas. Raven Press, New York, 1991

134. Sawaya R, Zucarello M, El-Kalliny M: Brain tumors and thromboembolism: clinical, hemostatic and biochemical correlations, abstracted. Ann Meeting AANS, Washington, 1989

135. Sekhar L: Operative management of tumors involving the cavernous sinus. p. 393. In Sekhar VS (ed): Tumors of the Cranial Base: Diagnosis and Treatment. Futura, Mt. Kisco, 1987

136. Sekhar L, Sen C, Jho H: Saphenous vein graft bypass of the cavernous internal carotid artery. Neurosurg 72:35, 1990

137. Sekhar L et al: Surgical treatment of intracavernous neoplasms: a four-year experience. Neurosurgery 24:18, 1989

138. Simpson D: The recurrence of intracranial meningiomas after surgical treatment. J Neurol Neurosurg Psychiatry 20:22, 1957

139. Spaziante R, Cappabianca P, Del Basso de Caro ML, de Divitiis E: Unusual complication with the use of lyophylized dural graft. Neurochirurgia 31:32, 1988

140. Stern WE: Meningiomas in the cranio-orbital junction. J Neurosurg 38:428, 1973

141. Strenger S, Huang Y, Sachdev V: Malignant meningioma within the third ventricle: a case report. Neurosurgery 20:465, 1987

142. Sundt T et al: Saphenous vein bypass grafts for giant aneurysms and intracranial occlusive disease. J Neurosurg 65:439, 1986

143. Tsuda H et al: Tissue-type plasminogen activator in patients with intracranial meningiomas. Thrombosis and hemostasis 60:508, 1988

144. Ugrumov V et al: Parasellar meningiomas: diagnosis and possibilities of surgical treatment according to the place of original growth. Acta Neurochir (Wien), suppl. 28:373, 1979

145. Uihlein A, Weyand R: Meningiomas of anterior clinoid process as a cause of unilateral loss of vision. Arch Ophthalmol 49:261, 1953

146. Young S et al: MR of vascular encasement in parasellar masses: comparison with angiography and CT. AJNR 9:35, 1988

14 Pituitary Adenomas

General Considerations

George T. Tindall
Eric J. Woodard
Daniel L. Barrow

Technical innovations during the last 30 years have helped make the transsphenoidal approach the procedure of choice in the operative treatment of most pituitary adenomas.[17] Low risk and effectiveness are primary reasons for the popularity of the procedure. Fortunately, complications are relatively uncommon with transsphenoidal surgery, averaging approximately 4 percent in series from institutions where a large volume of pituitary surgery is performed.[41] Severity ranges from minor, self-limited annoyances to potentially devastating hematomas or death. The prudent surgeon can avoid many problems and complications by carefully evaluating the patient preoperatively, and by developing a familiarity with potential pitfalls of the operation.

In some cases, however, the transsphenoidal approach is contraindicated, and a transcranial procedure is warranted. These situations include dumbbell configuration, anterior and/or middle cranial fossa extension, and sphenoid sinusitis. The operative risks associated with the transcranial approach are similar to those of other intracranial surgery and are discussed in a subsequent chapter.

PREOPERATIVE EVALUATION

As with any surgical procedure, a thorough patient assessment is necessary prior to undertaking transsphenoidal surgery. This includes evaluation of general medical health, endocrine function, and visual fields, as well as radiological study of sellar and parasellar anatomy.[19]

Careful assessment of the cardiovascular, respiratory, renal, and hepatic systems is routine for determining a patient's tolerance of general anesthesia.[41] Information regarding allergies, medications, and prior anesthesia should also be sought. Patients with an endocrinopathy may demonstrate unique medical problems that can affect anesthetic management. For example, patients with acromegaly and Cushing's disease frequently have associated medical conditions such as cardiomyopathy, congestive heart failure, coronary artery disease, hypertension, diabetes mellitus, and/or thyroid dysfunction. Prior consultation with a cardiologist or endocrinologist can help to ensure optimal medical status for these patients.[41]

A complete endocrine evaluation is mandatory be-

269

fore surgery. Endocrine testing confirms the diagnosis in cases of hyperfunctional tumors and allows documentation of endocrine deficiency states before and after surgery.[42] Routine tests for assessment of pituitary hormone reserve should be obtained in all patients with a sellar mass (Table 14-1). Patients with a particular clinical endocrinopathy may require specific testing for further diagnosis and evaluation (Table 14-2).

Patients with hypopituitarism before surgery are usually already receiving steroid replacement therapy and may require large doses of corticosteroid in the perioperative period.[19] Our patients with normal adrenal function routinely receive intravenous hydrocortisone both immediately before and during surgery. Hydrocortisone is then administered either by mouth or intravenously every 8 hours thereafter, beginning in the recovery room and continuing through the second postoperative day. Steroid administration is tapered and subsequently discontinued according to the patient's individual needs based on endocrine testing.[41] Should the patient suffer from significant pituitary-thyroid insufficiency preoperatively, efforts should be made to normalize thyroid function in anticipation of surgical stress.[19]

Preoperative radiological evaluation includes a plain lateral skull film and either a high-resolution contrast-enhanced, coronal computed tomography (CT) or a contrast-enhanced magnetic resonance imaging (MRI) study. The lateral skull x-ray film provides useful information for the operative approach by assessing the size and configuration of the sella, by determining the degree of sphenoid sinus pneumatization, and by detecting significant bony abnormalities.[42] A high-resolution CT or MRI can usually define the precise size and configuration of adenomas larger than 3 mm, and clearly outlines their relationship to the normal pituitary, surrounding CSF spaces, and parasellar structures,[17] which is obviously valuable in preoperative planning. MRI, especially with gadolinium enhancement, appears to be more sensitive than CT for detecting subtle tissue differences within the sella. MRI may also be better for detecting extrasellar extension of tumor and cavernous sinus invasion than CT, making it the diagnostic procedure of choice in current practice.[30,42]

Table 14-2. Specific Endocrine Testing

Acromegaly
  GH levels
  Somatomedin-C levels
  Glucose suppression
  TRH test
  GHRF levels
Cushing's syndrome (disease)
  Urinary free cortisol
  Dexamethasone suppression, low/high dose
  Metyrapone test
  ACTH levels
  Petrosal sinus sampling for ACTH
Prolactinoma
  Serum prolactin levels × 2
  Chlorpromazine (CPZ) test
  TRH test

Abbreviations: ACTH, adrenocorticotropic hormone; GH, growth hormone; GHRF, growth hormone-releasing factor; TRH, thyrotropin-releasing hormone.
(Adapted from Tindall and Barrow,[42] with permission.)

SURGICAL COMPLICATIONS

Surgical complications associated with the transsphenoidal management of pituitary adenomas may be categorized according to the anatomical structures involved (Table 14-3).

Parasellar Complications

Postoperative cerebrospinal fluid (CSF) rhinorrhea is one of the more common complications of transsphenoidal surgery for pituitary adenomas. Although reported in as many as 9.6 percent of patients,[15] rates in most large, modern series average approximately 3 percent.[4,5,7–9,34,36,38,46] Surgical experience and various characteristics of the intrasellar tumor are primary factors that determine the risk of developing a leak.[41] CSF leakage is a major complication because of the potential for serious sequelae, such as meningitis or tension pneumocephalus,[6,37,41] and because a significant number of patients may require a second operation to repair the leak.[5,38]

Table 14-1. Assessment of Pituitary Hormone Reserve

Target Organ	Tests of Pituitary Reserve
Adrenal	AM cortisol, cosyntropin stimulation
Thyroid	T₄ (total or free)
Gonadal	LH, FSH, testosterone (males), estradiol (females)
Prolactin	Baseline prolactin
Growth hormone	Not recommended
ADH	Urine volume, serum electrolytes

Abbreviations: ADH, antidiuretic hormone; FSH, follicle-stimulating hormone; LH, luteinizing hormone.
(Adapted from Tindall and Barrow,[42] with permission.)

Table 14-3. Operative Complications of Transsphenoidal Surgery

Parasellar
　CSF rhinorrhea
　Hypopituitarism
　Diabetes insipidus
　Cavernous sinus damage
　　Hemorrhage
　　Cranial nerve injury
　　Internal carotid artery injury
　　　Hemorrhage
　　　Carotid cavernous fistula
　　　False aneurysm
Intracranial
　Hemorrhage
　Hypothalamic damage
　Meningitis
　Visual loss
　Cerebral ischemia (vasospasm, embolization, carotid
　　occlusion)
Nasal/Sphenoidal
　Sinusitis
　Mucocele
　Palate/cribriform plate fracture
　Septal perforation
　Nasal deformity
　Epistaxis
　Denervation/devascularization of teeth

(Adapted from Tindall and Barrow,[41] with permission.)

CSF rhinorrhea may occur intraoperatively, perioperatively, or as a delayed phenomenon, appearing several months or even years after transsphenoidal surgery.[5] Intraoperative leaks result from surgical disruption or tumor erosion of the diaphragma sellae and/or adjacent dural structures. Clear CSF is usually obvious in the operative field once the subarachnoid space has been entered. Postoperative rhinorrhea occurs following inadequate repair of intraoperative leaks or with small occult tears in the diaphragm or dura, which are not noted intraoperatively. Patients with a congenitally large diaphragmatic aperture may also develop postoperative rhinorrhea because of delayed prolapse and rupture of arachnoid diverticula into the tumor resection bed.[21]

Specific factors that may affect the incidence of postoperative CSF leakage include (1) large tumor size, (2) prior surgical or radiation treatment, (3) presence of a preoperative leak, and (4) occurrence of an intraoperative leak.

Patients with macroadenomas (>10 mm) have a greater risk of developing postoperative leakage than those harboring microadenomas.[5,7,46] Large adenomas commonly expand the sella and erode the adjacent meninges, resulting in attenuation or violation of these barriers to the CSF space. Patients who have undergone prior surgical therapy (transsphenoidal or transcranial) are also at greater risk for postoperative CSF rhinorrhea after a subsequent transsphenoidal procedure.[2,9] Laws et al.[20] cite postoperative scarring, adhesions, abnormal vascularity, and distortion of anatomy as factors that complicate repeat transsphenoidal surgery. Although the effect of preoperative radiation therapy on the risk of CSF leakage is not clear, Laws suggests that radiation therapy may thin the parasellar bone and thereby predispose to postoperative leakage.[20] The presence of rhinorrhea preoperatively or a leak noted intraoperatively makes postoperative CSF leakage more likely.[38,39,41] In one series, 21 of 158 patients who had undergone prior therapy for a pituitary lesion were operated upon solely because of a CSF leak; repair was successful in only 75 percent.[20]

Diagnosis of postoperative CSF leakage is usually straightforward. Significant CSF rhinorrhea results in steady dripping of clear fluid from the nose, especially when the patient's head is placed in a dependent position.[41] If an adequate amount of fluid can be collected for quantitative analysis, a glucose or chloride determination may aid in the diagnosis.[5,41]

Prevention of rhinorrhea involves avoiding the creation of intraoperative leaks as well as delayed leaks. Because intraoperative CSF leakage is commonly iatrogenic, attention to technique is essential. If the dural opening performed during exposure of the pituitary is carried too far superiorly, inadvertent entry may be made into the anterior recess of the suprasellar cistern. Similarly, care must be taken to recognize and protect the blue diaphragma sellae during tumor removal, especially when resecting the anterior-superior aspect of the tumor. Recognition of the diaphragm may be especially difficult in repeat transsphenoidal surgery due to scarring. Despite taking precautions in handling the diaphragm and dural structures, occult CSF leaks may still occur. Some surgeons use the Valsalva maneuver to ensure that occult leaks are detected before closure.[13,43]

Adequate closure is also important for preventing CSF rhinorrhea, especially when an intraoperative leak has been recognized. Various techniques and many different materials have been used for this purpose with no single method appearing universally superior (Table 14-4). Of the packing materials described, autologous fat offers advantages of availability, ease of handling, and a long duration of viability.[32,38] Use of a fat graft, however, does require a second incision and may lead to graft site complications in as many as 4.1 percent of patients.[9,12] With significant intraoperative CSF leakage, a water-tight

Table 14-4.   Materials Used for Sellar Closure

Material	Advantages	Disadvantages
Fat	Availability Ease of handling Hemostatic Minimal shrinkage	Requires second incision
Muscle	Availability Ease of handling Hemostatic	Rapid necrosis/shrinkage Requires second incision Postoperative pain
Lyophilized dura	Strength Availability	Devitalized tissue Poor sealing characteristics Cost
Fascia lata	Strength Availability	Requires second incision Poor sealing characteristics Poor viability
Microfibrillar collagen	Hemostatic	Difficulty in handling Foreign body
Oxidized cellulose	Bacteriocidal Hemostatic	Coagulates due to low pH (<1) Cannot use with fibrin adhesive Difficulty in handling Foreign body
Gelatin sponge	Ease of handling Hemostatic	Foreign body Delayed resorption
Bone	Strength in repairing the sellar floor Usually available	Difficulty in handling Devitalized tissue Poor sealing characteristics
Cartilage	Strength in repairing the sellar floor	Difficulty in handling Poor viability Poor sealing characteristics May cause nasal deformity/perforation
Ceramic plate	Strength in repairing the sellar floor	Foreign body Poor sealing characteristics
Cyanoacrylate adhesive	Strength of seal/adhesion Ease of application	Potential carcinogen Poor long-term sealing characteristics Foreign body
Fibrin adhesive	Strength of seal/adhesion Ease of application Biocompatible Hemostatic Promotes wound healing	Requires relatively dry surfaces for application Potential for infection transmission unless autologous adhesive is used
Marlex mesh	Strength	Foreign body

closure is desirable; it can be facilitated by lumbar drainage of CSF during sellar packing.[41]

Pitfalls to be avoided during sella repair are related primarily to the creation of an intrasellar mass by overpacking, swelling of packing material (such as oxidized cellulose),[31] or migration of the graft.[22] Regardless of the type of material, the graft should be kept loose, taking care not to force excessive packing into the tumor resection bed. Our approach to sellar closure involves packing the tumor resection bed loosely with an autologous fat graft regardless of the size of the adenoma,[5] and then reconstructing the sellar floor. To prevent graft migration and ensure complete hemostasis, the fat graft may be secured with fibrin adhesive.[45] A small piece of bone (such as from the perpendicular plate of the ethmoid) is then wedged over the sellar opening between the dura and bony margins, and may be reinforced with fibrin adhesive.

Treatment of postoperative CSF rhinorrhea is initially conservative, with head elevation and/or lumbar CSF drainage.[41] Although Spaziante et al.[39] claim that only 1.5 to 2 percent of patients will require an operative repair of a leak, up to 15 percent of patients with postoperative rhinorrhea have been reported to fail conservative therapy.[5] Rhinorrhea persisting beyond 3 days of CSF diversion usually requires operative repair by repacking the sella and sphenoid sinus. Rarely, persistent rhinorrhea may be due to communicating hydrocephalus, which may be confirmed by CT scan and treated with a shunting procedure.[41]

Hypopituitarism

Impairment of pituitary function following selective removal of a pituitary adenoma results from damage to or removal of the normal adenohypophysis. Impairment may be partial or complete, transient or permanent. Estimates of the overall incidence of new pituitary hypofunction following pituitary adenomectomy vary considerably among different surgical reports.[27,28,34,46] Faria and Tindall,[12] however, studied the effect of selective pituitary surgery on endocrine status in 97 women with prolactinomas and concluded that 4 percent of patients would incur permanent damage to one or more pituitary endocrine axes after transsphenoidal surgery. Several studies suggest that the risk of creating new endocrine deficits after selective transsphenoidal surgery correlates with increased tumor size and the presence of a preoperative endocrine deficit, especially panhypopituitarism.[27,28]

Adequate recognition and preservation of normal pituitary tissue during adenomectomy is essential to minimize endocrine impairment following transsphenoidal surgery. Large adenomas frequently thin the gland and flatten it against the posterosuperior aspect of the sella. With experience, the normal gland can be distinguished from neoplastic tissue by its red-orange surface, striated by a fine capillary network. The toughness of the normal gland also allows its distinction from tumor, as it resists easy removal by suction or gentle curetting.[41]

Transient or permanent diabetes insipidus (DI) occurs because of damage or swelling of the neural lobe and/or proximal pituitary stalk. It remains one of the most frequent complications of transsphenoidal surgery, with permanent DI occurring in less than 3 percent[5,22,34,46] and transient DI in up to 60 percent of patients.[12]

Diagnosis of DI is relatively simple to establish. Patients have polyuria, polydipsia, and a urine specific gravity below 1.005. Plasma osmolalities are elevated, averaging 295 ± 15 mOsm/kg, and the serum sodium is elevated above 145 mEq/L. If subjected to a water deprivation test for 6 to 8 hours, the patient is unable to concentrate urine to greater than 200 mOsm/kg, and plasma osmolality may rise as high as

320 to 330 mOsm/kg.[41] True DI must be distinguished from a normal early postoperative diuresis resulting from intraoperative fluid administration. In this situation plasma sodium and osmolalities are normally regulated despite apparent polyuria.

Significant DI is treated by administration of aqueous pitressin during the peak period of ADH insufficiency. Often, an alert patient can maintain normal serum tonicity via a normal thirst mechanism. After nasal packing has been removed, and if the nasal mucosa appears intact, intranasal administration of desmopressin acetate (DDAVP) is a convenient and effective treatment for prolonged DI.

Prevention of postoperative DI requires recognition and preservation of remaining normal posterior pituitary tissue. In large tumors the remnants of normal gland are frequently quite attenuated. Careful handling of both the normal gland and stalk should minimize the degree of surgical trauma to the posterior lobe.

Cavernous Sinus

Hemorrhage from the cavernous sinus during selective adenomectomy may be brisk and troublesome. Rarely, a transsphenoidal procedure must be aborted because of excessive cavernous sinus bleeding.[11,15,21,36,44] Entry usually occurs when attempting to remove lateral extensions of tumor that impinge upon or invade the cavernous sinus. Venous hemorrhage can also result after entering abnormally large intersinus connections in the anterior sellar dura.[17,33] Dural venous bleeding is generally controlled by cauterizing the edge of the sinus opening. Sinus bleeding situated more laterally, out of direct view, may be controlled by gentle packing with microfibrillar collagen, autologous fat, or oxidized cellulose. The surgeon should refrain from overly vigorous packing, as damage to the internal carotid artery and its branches or intracavernous cranial nerves may occur. Air embolism is an additional complication of venous sinus entry, especially if the patient's head is significantly elevated.[29] Close attention should be given to even slight sinus bleeding and proper patient positioning.

Cranial Nerve Injury

Intracavernous cranial nerve dysfunction after adenomectomy is usually transient and self-limited. It results from direct injury by instrumentation during removal of lateral tumor extensions or from overly aggressive packing for control of cavernous sinus bleeding.[41] The frequency of cranial nerve injury after transsphenoidal surgery ranges between

0.4 and 2 percent, with the third and sixth nerves being most commonly involved.[9,22]

Arterial Injury

Although uncommon, intracavernous carotid artery injury can cause significant hemorrhage leading to severe disability or death. Carotid injury may occur with aggressive intracavernous instrumentation that tears the artery or avulses a small intracavernous arterial branch.

Other types of arterial injury can result if abnormalities of the vascular anatomy are not recognized preoperatively. The carotid siphons may occasionally bulge into the sella and obstruct a direct approach to the pituitary.[33] A persistent trigeminal artery,[23] abnormal carotid anastomoses,[40] and internal carotid aneurysms[21] have all been reported to lie within the sella. Suspicion of arterial anomalies on preoperative CT or MRI should prompt a full arteriographic study to define the precise anatomy of the parasellar arterial structures and thus avoid hemorrhagic complications.

Once encountered, arterial bleeding within the sella may be difficult to control. A small piece of microfibrillar collagen or autologous fat placed over the bleeding site will usually effect adequate hemostasis. As the intracavernous carotid is a relatively immobile structure, however, vigorous packing may enlarge any tear in the structure. Mild induced hypotension may help stop the bleeding during attempts at achieving hemostasis.[41] False aneurysms,[41,44] carotid cavernous fistulae,[44] carotid occlusion,[21] and vasospasm[3,21,22] are additional rare complications of intracavernous arterial injury.

Avoidance of internal carotid artery complications requires an awareness of normal and abnormal vascular anatomy in the sellar and parasellar area. Use of MRI in preoperative pituitary tumor evaluation helps to distinguish vascular abnormalities from pituitary tumors.[42] As with many complications, direct injury to the carotid artery may be avoided by adhering to meticulous surgical technique.

Intracranial Complications

Hemorrhage

Intracranial hemorrhage is a rare major complication that accounts for a significant proportion of operative deaths reported with transsphenoidal surgery. Hemorrhages may be parenchymal, subarachnoid, epidural, or intrasellar with secondary intracranial extension.[21,35] Occasionally, parenchymal hemorrhage is seen in patients with large tumors having significant extrasellar extension. Hemorrhage results from blind instrumentation in the suprasellar area and/or residual bleeding of the tumor resection bed. Subarachnoid hemorrhage may occur with direct injury to branches of the circle of Willis, which has the potential to result in delayed vasospasm.[3,21,22] Significant intrasellar hemorrhage occurs in 0.4 to 3 percent of cases[5,22,46] and may be a cause of early postoperative visual worsening.[3] Steps to minimize intrasellar bleeding include complete tumor removal, assurance of adequate hemostasis, and avoidance of cavernous sinus entry.

Treatment of intracranial hematomas following transsphenoidal surgery is similar to that with hematomas from other causes. Symptomatic clots in accessible areas should be considered for evacuation.

Hypothalamic Damage

Damage to the hypothalamus is a rare complication, which is frequently lethal. Surgical trauma, ischemia, or trauma from a secondary hematoma may result in hypothalamic injury. The clinical course is characterized by fever with a depressed level of consciousness.[17,41] Hypothalamic injury occurs most often in patients with large tumors with significant suprasellar extension.[21] Suprasellar tumor should be resected gently under direct vision. This may be facilitated by infusion of saline through a lumbar catheter, which in turn depresses the diaphragm into the sella.

Meningitis

Meningitis can occur following the direct inoculation of bacteria into the CSF space either at the time of surgery or secondarily through a CSF fistula.[21] Although generally uncommon, it is reported in 0.2 to 2 percent of cases and is a frequent cause of death after this procedure.[5,21,44,46] Meningitis in the postoperative period is heralded by symptoms of fever, meningismus, headache, and mental status changes approximately 2 to 3 days after surgery. Frequently, there is an associated CSF leak.[5] Meningitis may indeed be the first indication of delayed postoperative CSF rhinorrhea.

The use of prophylactic antibiotics in transsphenoidal surgery is somewhat controversial. Several authors have abandoned the use of perioperative antibiotic coverage and noted either no change or a reduction in subsequent rates of meningitis.[17,43,44] It appears that the use of perioperative antibiotic prophylaxis has either little impact on the rate of postoperative infection or may paradoxically increase the risk of meningitis after transsphenoidal surgery. The mechanism may relate to alteration of the normal flora of the nasopharynx. By its nature, however, the transsphenoidal approach to the pituitary is a nonsterile procedure. Because of the theoretical risk of contamination, we use an intraoperative dose of a second-generation cephalosporin with activity against *Haemophilus influenzae,* and discontinue the antibiotic once the nasal packing is removed.

Visual Worsening

Vision loss after a transsphenoidal procedure is a rare yet potentially devastating event. It may involve immediate or delayed injury to the optic nerves, chiasm, or optic tracts. Mechanisms of injury include direct operative trauma, secondary compression (e.g., hematoma formation or overpacking of the sella), ischemia, or chiasm prolapse.[3] Often, visual worsening accompanies another complication such as suprasellar hematoma formation. Barrow and Tindall[3] reviewed posttranssphenoidal visual loss and cited several potential risk factors associated with this complication. These included (1) large tumor size, (2) dumbbell tumor configuration, (3) preoperative visual deficit, (4) prior treatment, and (5) technical factors.

Vision loss after transsphenoidal surgery almost exclusively involves macroadenomas. Large tumors, especially those with suprasellar extension, usually are in close contact with the optic nerves or chiasm. Removal requires peeling tumor and/or tumor capsule from the undersurface of these structures, which may cause direct damage to the optic apparatus or interruption of its blood supply.[21] Tumors with a dumbbell configuration from a diaphragmatic constriction are difficult to remove by the transsphenoidal route without risking visual compromise.[3,41] The suprasellar portion does not easily descend into the sella for safe removal, so that blind curetting, suction, or vigorous manipulation of the diaphragm are necessary for complete resection. The existence of a preoperative visual deficit in a patient with a pituitary tumor implies some degree of optic nerve or optic chiasm compromise, which may render the visual apparatus more susceptible to intraoperative insult.[3] Patients who have had prior therapy for their tumors may also be at greater risk for postoperative visual loss. This is especially true in cases that have undergone preoperative irradiation.[1,3,26]

In contrast to the above risks for visual complications, several technical factors are potentially avoidable causes of vision loss. Optic canal fracture and optic nerve injury can occur if the self-retaining speculum is opened too vigorously after its tips have been advanced into the sphenoid sinus.[41] Overpacking of the sella or migration of graft material has been discussed in the section on CSF leaks. Failure to leave a "prop" in the resection bed after tumor removal may lead to downward traction on the chiasm into the sella, although the validity of this mechanism of visual dysfunction has been disputed.[1,26] Chiasmapexy has been shown to benefit visual recovery in select cases.[3]

Once a new postoperative visual deficit is suspected, prompt diagnosis of its cause should be made by CT or MRI. This is primarily to rule out the presence of a treatable lesion such as a postoperative hematoma or a misplaced sellar graft. Reoperation can reverse these deficits in some instances.[3,44]

Nasal/Sphenoidal Problems

Primary reasons for the popularity of the transsphenoidal approach are its comfort and safety for the patient. Although nasal/sphenoidal problems rarely cause major complications, related to this operative exposure, they can be troubling or disfiguring.

Sinusitis can occur with obstruction of paranasal sinus drainage from postoperative mucosal edema. It is usually self-limited or easily treated with a course of an appropriate culture-specific antibiotic. Postoperative use of a decongestant such as pseudoephedrine sulfate may help reduce sinus obstruction.[41]

Mucoceles are cysts resulting from redundant or scarred mucosal tissue. They are reportedly more common with the transethmoidal approach to the pituitary and theoretically are prevented by sphenoid sinus mucosal exenteration.[5,17,21]

Fractures of the hard palate or cribriform plate result from overspreading of the nasal speculum during the approach to the sella. This may also fracture the medial orbital wall and compromise the optic canal.[3] Some authors refrain from advancing the speculum into the sphenoid sinus to avoid this complication.[5] Adequate resection of the anterior wall of the sphenoid sinus usually obviates the need for excessive speculum opening. Because nasal deformities can occur with extensive removal of septal cartilage,[16] we do not routinely use cartilage for sella reconstruction. After packing the sella and reconstructing its floor, the speculum is withdrawn and the septum, which has been displaced laterally during the approach, is manually replaced in its midline position along the bony nasal spine.[41] This helps to prevent gross septal deformity and nasal obstruction.[16] It is also important to minimize removal of bone along the anterior nasal spine, which can result in a deformity or even nasal collapse.[16]

Septal perforations may be annoying when associated with persistent crusting, pain, whistling, or nasal obstruction from secondary scarring (synechiae).[16] They are reported in up to 8 percent of patients,[9,15,36] and are related to operative or infectious damage to the mucoperichondrium.[16,36] Simple packing of the nares at the end of the procedure will usually suffice in reapproximating the mucosa to the septum.[41]

Minor epistaxis after transsphenoidal surgery is normal in the immediate postoperative period. Significant hemorrhage, however, usually indicates damage to the mucosal blood supply. Bleeding is frequently self-limited or may require transient nasal packing. Extreme abrupt hemorrhage should prompt investigation of a carotid injury.

Excessive removal of bone along the rim of the pyriform aperture can damage distal branches of the alveolar nerves and/or superior alveolar artery, which may desensitize or devitalize the upper teeth or gums.[9,16,41]

CONCLUSIONS

The transsphenoidal approach is well established as a safe and effective procedure for the surgical treatment of pituitary adenomas. The successful outcome of this surgery is primarily related to preoperative preparation, surgeon's operative experience, and individual characteristics of the patient. Familiarity with the complications of this approach, as well as their avoidance and treatment, is essential for successful surgical management of patients with pituitary adenomas.

Pituitary Microadenomas
Jules Hardy
Ian E. McCutcheon

The transsphenoidal approach to pituitary microadenomas is, like any surgical procedure, accompanied by complications that may jeopardize the safety of the patient and the success of the treatment. The many hazards and pitfalls of these operations are understood best when approached in a systematic way. Most can be anticipated by those with a thorough knowledge of the anatomy of the nasal cavities, sphenoid sinus, sella turcica, and juxtasellar structures. Recognition of the consequences of damage to each of these structures and familiarity with the regional variability often encountered supplement the surgeon's manual skills and allow removal of tumors with a minimum of adverse sequelae. The ability to treat complications once they have occurred is equally important in attaining a satisfactory operative result.

The transsphenoidal approach to the pituitary gland was first used in the early years of this century and was originally performed only for the debulking of massive pituitary tumors. The major complications reported by the pioneers Hirsch[60] and Cushing[51] in that preantibiotic era were CSF fistulae and infection. Microsurgery of the pituitary gland was introduced in the early 1960s and the development of its techniques has allowed the selective removal of microadenomas for the treatment of endocrine disorders of the pituitary.[56] The modern approach to the sella turcica is very similar to that described originally by Cushing.[51] Although a strict midline oronasal rhinoseptal approach is most commonly used, both the lateral endonasal or the combined oronasal-lateral submucosal approaches are suitable in some patients. The advantages and limitations of each method should be considered before selecting one procedure for routine use and before choosing a modified operation for individual cases.

One of us (J.H.) has used the classical oronasal midline rhinoseptal approach in the majority of cases in a series of over 2,000 transsphenoidal operations. Unilateral submucosal dissection and deflection of the nasal cartilage to the other side as reported by

Tindall et al.[73] is also used occasionally, but without specific purpose since the extra step in their procedure results in a midline approach once the vomer bone has been reached. The lateral endonasal approach is used most often in patients with large nostrils such as acromegalics. Occasional use of this approach in patients with small nostrils has resulted in disruption of the margin of the nares; this can be prevented by the modifications suggested by Griffith and Veerapen,[54] such as an external incision into the upper lip, which leaves a discreet but visible scar.

STANDARD TRANSSPHENOIDAL APPROACH

The transsphenoidal approach has already been described in detail elsewhere.[57] It will be reviewed here with special emphasis on the difficulties and complications that may be encountered. Some have been experienced by the authors or described to them by colleagues; others have been reported in the neurosurgical literature.

Positioning

Proper positioning of the patient is crucial for adequate surgical exposure and ultimate operative success. Patients should be placed supine with the head firmly secured in a head rest. If three-point fixation is not used, care must be taken to tape the head tightly to avoid intraoperative movement. The head is fixed in a "sniffing" position with the neck flexed inferiorly and slightly extended superiorly to allow the surgeon an angled view of the nasal septum and sphenoid sinus 15 degrees above the horizontal (Fig. 14-1A&C). It is important as well to flex the neck 20 degrees laterally to allow adequate room for the surgeon to stand (Fig. 14-1B). The large amount of cervical manipulation and the relatively high degree of strain placed on the paracervical muscles and ligaments may cause neck pain postoperatively. If no abnormality is visible on plain x-ray films, the symptoms generally clear in 1 to 2 weeks with local heat, anti-inflammatory drugs, and a soft collar.

Fluoroscopic control is used only as needed during the operation. Proper placement of instruments requires only a few seconds of irradiation at each stage of the procedure. The image intensifier is switched on and off with a foot pedal controlled by the surgeon or by an assistant. Television input from the microscope and fluoroscopy from the image intensifier can be monitored on two separate channels of a video recorder.

Preparation

The nasal cavity, gingival surface, and lower face are cleaned with Hibitane or a similar noncaustic antiseptic agent. Some surgeons place intranasal pledgets soaked in a dilute solution of cocaine to promote vasospasm in the nasal mucosa and reduce blood loss from submucosal dissection. Infiltration of the upper lip and anterior maxillary gingival surface with 1 percent xylocaine and epinephrine (1 : 200,000) is then carried out, as well as infiltration of the inferior nasal spine, floor of the pyriform apertures, and cartilaginous nasal septum where dissection will occur. This makes dissection easier in those planes and reduces the incidence of mucosal tearing.

DIFFICULTIES AND COMPLICATIONS

No detailed statistics have been compiled on the incidence of complications in transsphenoidal surgery for microadenomas. An international survey of neurosurgeons experienced in the treatment of pituitary tumors has suggested a general mortality for this approach of 0.5 percent and a morbidity of 3.6 percent.[72] In these combined series death was confined mainly to patients in whom "unusual or extenuating circumstances" contributed to their demise. The most frequent nonfatal complication reported is still CSF fistula.[48,62,63,77] As most series contain significant numbers of patients with macroadenomas in whom a higher risk of complications might be expected, they probably overstate the risks for the surgical excision of microadenomas. Only Zervas,[79] who tallied complications from 80 neurosurgeons, has assessed results separately for microadenomas. He adduced a mortality of 0.27 percent and found the most frequent nonfatal complication of significance to be CSF rhinorrhea (1.3 percent), with permanent oculomotor palsy and visual loss running a distant second (0.1 percent each). Unfortunately, his definition of microadenoma (by hormonal levels instead of size) makes these figures difficult to interpret.

Difficulties and complications in the surgical management of pituitary microadenomas are summarized in Table 14-5.

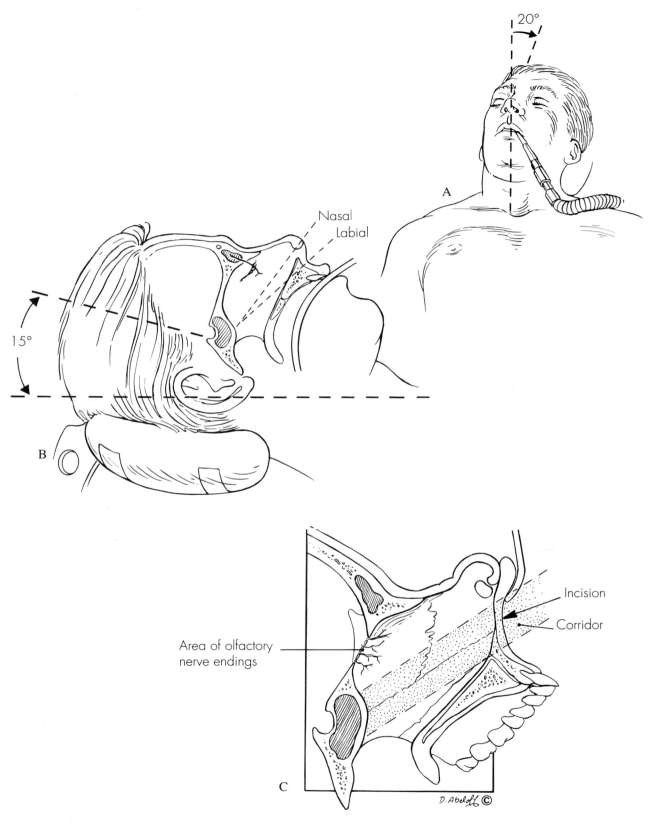

Figure 14-1. Position of the patient's head on the operating table. **(A)** In a semi-sitting position the neck is tilted 20 degrees toward the left shoulder. **(B)** The head is placed on a horseshoe headrest and slightly flexed 15 degrees upward. **(C)** The corridor leading to the sphernoid sinus from an oral inferior rhinoseptal approach.

Table 14-5. Pituitary Microadenomas: Difficulties, Pitfalls, and Complications Encountered during Management by Transsphenoidal Surgery

	Oral-Nasal	Sphenoidal	Sellar
Intraoperative difficulties: *anticipated*	Acromegaly: big nose Acromegaly: deep operative field Septal deviation	Misplacement of bivalve speculum inside sinus: fracture of skull base Bleeding from sphenopalatine artery Thick sphenoid floor Nonpneumatized sphenoid sinus Varieties of sphenoid septation and associated difficulties of approach	Hemorrhage: arterial Hemorrhage: venous CSF leak Encasement of carotid by tumor Closure of sellar floor

Hazards and pitfalls: *unexpected*	Mucosal tear
	Septal perforation
		Intrasphenoidal injury of the carotid artery	Unidentified aneurysms
			Problems specific to microadenomas
			    Tumor localization
			    Tumor consistency

Postoperative complications	Numbness of upper lip Tooth necrosis Septal perforation (delayed) Mucosal atrophy Nasal crusting Airway obstruction Anosmia Recurrent epistaxis Chronic rhinitis Cosmetic deformity: collapse of tip Cosmetic deformity: saddle nose	Abscess Sinusitis Mucocele	Persistent venous bleeding Hematoma Arterial bleeding (carotid/sphenopalatine) Carotid spasm Carotid thrombosis False aneurysm formation and rebleeding Carotid-cavernous fistula Delayed CSF fistula Meningitis

Nasal Problems

The incision into the upper gum should be made approximately 1 cm above the gingival margin and should not extend further laterally than the insertion of the canine tooth on either side (Fig. 14-2A). This reduces the incidence of upper lip numbness reported by some patients. Blackening and necrosis of the maxillary anterior teeth have been reported and are produced by a low incision too near the tooth sockets, which damages the anterior superior alveolar nerve and artery.[74] Postoperative peri-incisional numbness is common and will improve during the first 6 months after surgery.

After elevation of the soft tissue and periosteal layer of the upper maxilla, the nasal pyriform bony orifice is exposed. It is often too narrow and requires enlargement by rongeuring the upper maxillary rami on either side to provide a wider space for the opening of the bivalve speculum (Fig. 14-2B). Initiation of the submucosal dissection is facilitated first by elevating the mucosa from the floor of the nasal cavity and then by making an incision into the fibrous band that anchors the mucosa in the inner corner (Fig. 14-2C). Dissection of the mucosa along the subperi-

chondral space along the nasal cartilage is carried out deeply until the periosteal elevator reaches the vomer bone (Fig. 14-2D). It should not extend too high on the perpendicular plate of the ethmoid, or permanent anosmia will be produced by detachment of the olfactory nerve endings (Fig. 14-2E).

If a unilateral approach is chosen, the base of the cartilaginous septum is separated next. By detaching it with a blunt dissector and deflecting it to the other side, a cavity is made between nasal mucosa on one side and the tilted cartilaginous septum on the other side. If a bilateral approach has been chosen, the nasal mucosa is also dissected from the opposite side of the nasal septum. Often a deviation of the septum is encountered that may interfere with the nasal airway. It is therefore separated, fractured, and removed using a swiveled knife. The knife is introduced horizontally to detach the inferior portion of the septum until it reaches the posterior aspect, where it is swiveled upwards and returned anteriorly in order to resect the inferior portion of the septum, which is approximately 2×2.5 cm in size.

During the preparation of the nasal mucosa, it is infiltrated with xylocaine containing epinephrine. An injection of approximately 40 ml of fluid allows initia-

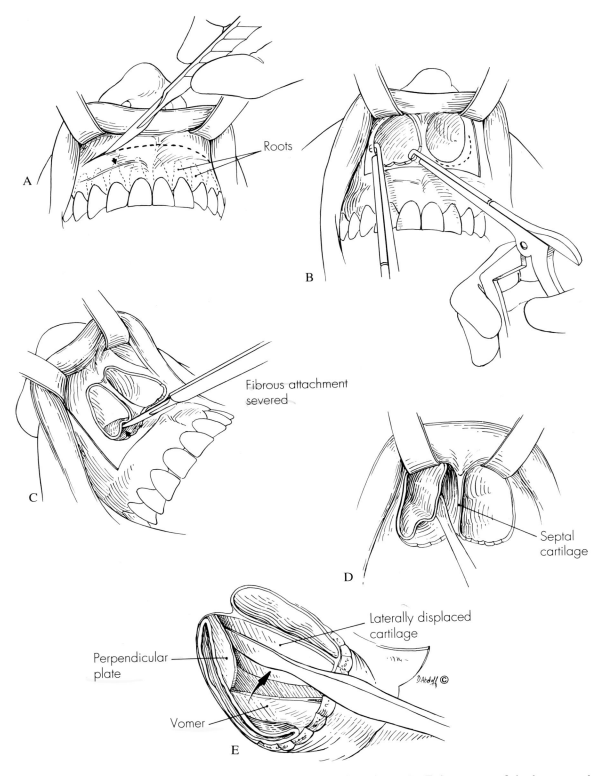

Figure 14-2. (A) Gingival incision 1 cm above the gingivolabial sulcus. **(B)** Enlargement of the bony nasal orifice by rongeuring the ascending branches of the maxillary bone. **(C)** Elevation of the mucosa from the floor of the nasal cavity, and incision of the fibrous band in the inner corner of the septal attachment. **(D)** Elevation of the septal mucosa from the subperichondral plane of cleavage. **(E)** Reaching the perpendicular plate of the ethmoid.

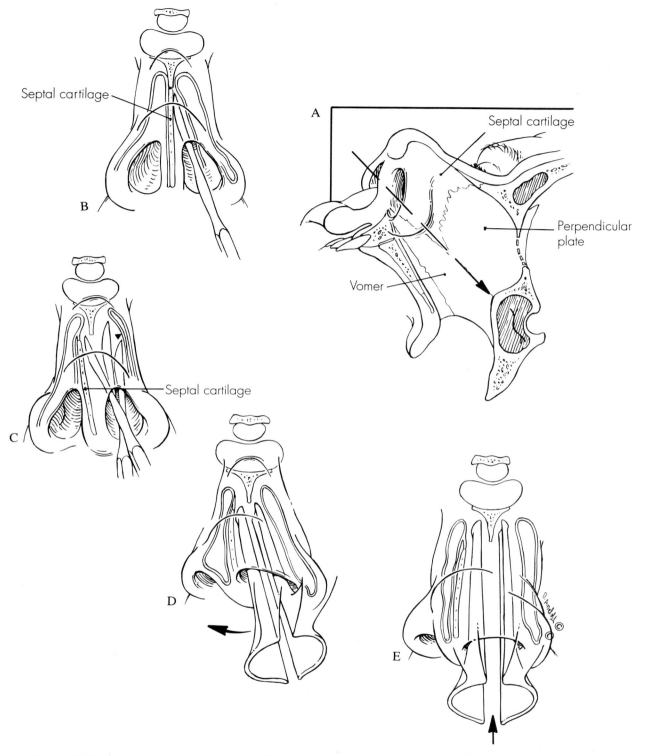

Figure 14-3. Lateral endonasal approach (in acromegalic patients or those with large nostrils. **(A)** The corridor through the right nostril. **(B)** Vertical incision in the posterior nasal mucosa on the right side. **(C)** Mucosal elevation and deflection of the cartilage to the opposite side. **(D)** Introduction of the speculum on either side of the vomer bone. **(E)** Reorienting the speculum on the midline, tilting the nose tip to the left side, and opening the valves to expose the sphenoid rostrum.

tion of the dissection and elevation of the mucosa on either side. When properly infiltrated the mucosal dissection is easily carried out. Occasionally the mucosa stays adherent to the cartilage despite adequate infiltration, and therefore a mucosal tear is produced. A small tear on one side only is of no postoperative consequence; if it occurs on both sides a postoperative septal perforation may be produced. Such septal adherence may be caused by primary allergic mucosal atrophy of the septum. The presence of such atrophy makes it difficult to achieve a plane of cleavage under the mucosa. Also, the absence of septal cartilage as a consequence of a previous operation may result in adhesion between the mucosae, which makes it difficult to reopen through the same approach. In such patients a lateral endonasal approach may be used, which is also recommended for a second or even a third operation should one become necessary.

In patients with large nostrils (such as acromegalics), a right lateral endonasal approach can be used instead of the midline rhinoseptal approach (Fig. 14-3). After preparation of the nasal mucosa, the bivalve speculum is readily introduced into the nasal cavity and opened. A vertical incision is carried out in the posterior nasal mucosa near the tip of the vomer bone. Then, with a movement forcing the septum to separate from the vomer, it is displaced to the other side. The mucosa is then elevated from either side of the vomer and the nasal speculum is introduced more deeply and is opened widely. The rest of the procedure is carried out as described above.

In the approaches described the most common postoperative complication is nasal septal perforation resulting in chronic or intermittent minor bleeding or crusting; this requires daily nasal washing to avoid adhesion of the crusts to the rim of the perforation. A very large septal perforation may not be symptomatic, nor are most small perforations.[64] A small perforation is better treated by enlarging it to approximately 1.5 cm^2 than by correction with a plastic prosthesis.

After the bivalve nasal speculum (Codman & Shurtleff, Inc., Randolph, MA) is introduced, the tips are applied against the lateral edge of the vomer and the valves are opened before the vomer is removed. If it is inserted after the sphenoid is opened, misplacement into the sinus cavity risks serious complication. Opening the valves into the rim of the sphenoid window and spreading the pterygoid apophysis can produce a distant fracture of the frontal base of the skull (Fig. 14-4). Maxillary or sphenoid fractures are common sequelae to overzealous spreading of the speculum and may cause permanent facial numbness (particularly in areas supplied by V_1 and V_2) if the

fracture disrupts these trigeminal branches as they traverse the skull. As only gentle pressure is required, there is no need for a dilator instrument to force the opening of the valves. If extra force is required it means that the nasal orifice is not wide enough and should be enlarged as described above (Fig. 14-2B). When too strong a force is applied, fractures of the upper maxillary rami may occur, giving postoperative bony defects in the lateral edge of the nose.

Sphenoidal Problems

After a periosteal elevator is introduced into the lateral orifice down to the anterior wall of the sphenoid sinus, a punch rongeur or Luke forceps is used to remove the vomer bone in one or two pieces. Further enlargement of the resulting opening of the sphenoid floor with a punch rongeur gives a wide access to the sphenoid sinus. During this maneuver the sphenopalatine artery may be avulsed at the inferior and lateral corners of the floor (Fig. 14-5). Since this artery is not visible and retracts toward the maxilla when torn, it can only be reached with a right-angle coagulator.

Varieties of Sphenoid Sinus

Once the floor of the sphenoid sinus has been opened and the sinus cavity exposed, several varieties of sinus can be encountered.[67,71] In 85 percent of cases the sinus is a large empty cavity in which the bulging floor of the sella turcica and the anterior wall of the clivus are readily identified. In the other 15 percent wide variations in sinus morphology can provoke misguided actions and serious complications (Fig. 14-6A–C). In extreme cases the sinus is an obscure labyrinth in which identification of the floor of the sella turcica is impossible.

A thick vomer bone and sphenoid floor is encountered in acromegalic patients and may require opening with a hammer and chisel or a diamond-tipped air drill. A sharp cutting blade is ineffective and is not recommended. Often in children the sphenoid sinus is not pneumatized and is then described as concha. In such patients the air drill should be used to create a tunnel. Its path should be guided by televised fluoroscopic monitoring in order to avoid a wrong trajectory, either too high (anterior to the tuberculum sellae) or too low (below the floor of the sella turcica towards the clivus) (Fig. 14-6D). A partially pneumatized or ''presellar'' sinus may be present anterior to the sella floor and identification and opening of the floor should be guided in such cases by fluoroscopy.

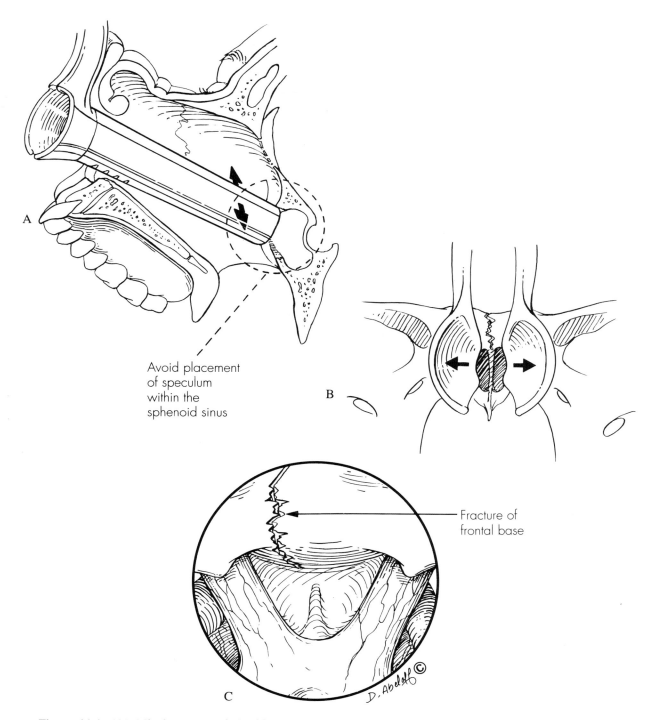

Avoid placement
of speculum
within the
sphenoid sinus

Fracture of
frontal base

Figure 14-4. (A) Misplacement of the bivalve speculum inside the rim of the sphenoid sinus window. **(B)** Spreading of the bivalve tips results in a fracture of the frontal base. **(C)** View of the fracture from the intracranial aspect: injury to the optic nerve may also occur.

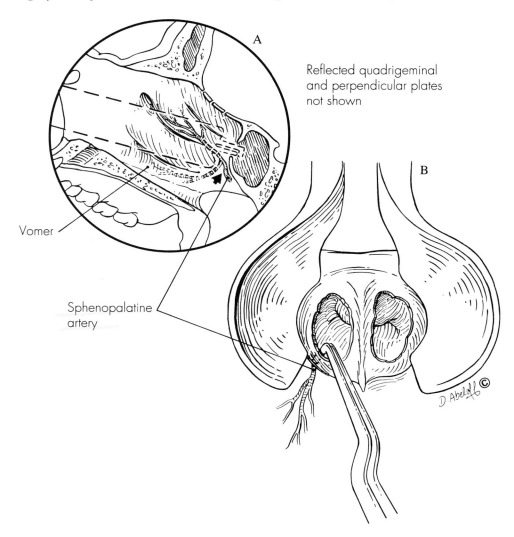

Reflected quadrigeminal
and perpendicular plates
not shown

Vomer

Sphenopalatine
artery

Figure 14-5. Avulsion of the sphenopalatine artery during the opening of the sphenoid rostrum. **(A)** Sagittal view: the artery is located in the hidden inferior corner of the sphenoid sinus. **(B)** Frontal view. Coagulation of the artery with a right-angled instrument (bipolar forceps or coagulating suction tube).

Sphenoid Septation

A midline septum dividing the sinus into two cavities (Fig. 14-7A) is usually readily identified and can be removed easily by breaking the thin bone with a Jensen-Middleton rongeur. The detachment of the last upper portion of the septum where it connects with the roof of the sphenoid may initiate the opening of the sellar floor. Multiple oblique septa dividing the sinus into three chambers (Fig. 14-7B) are also encountered and should be identified and removed carefully because some oblique septae go toward the lateral corner of the sella where only a thin layer of bone covers the carotid artery. Removal of that shell may create a small bone chip, which can lacerate the carotid wall.

One configuration in particular is very misleading: two vertical septa (Fig. 14-7C) located symmetrically on either side of the midline. Using one of these septa as a landmark may make it appear (falsely) that the procedure is being carried out on the midline and directed to the sella. A deviation to one side during the opening of the floor of a sphenoid sinus containing several septa may give the impression that the sinus is small and is divided only by one medial septum. Removal of only one septum leads surgeons incorrectly towards the lateral corner and brings them to the region of the cavernous sinus and the carotid

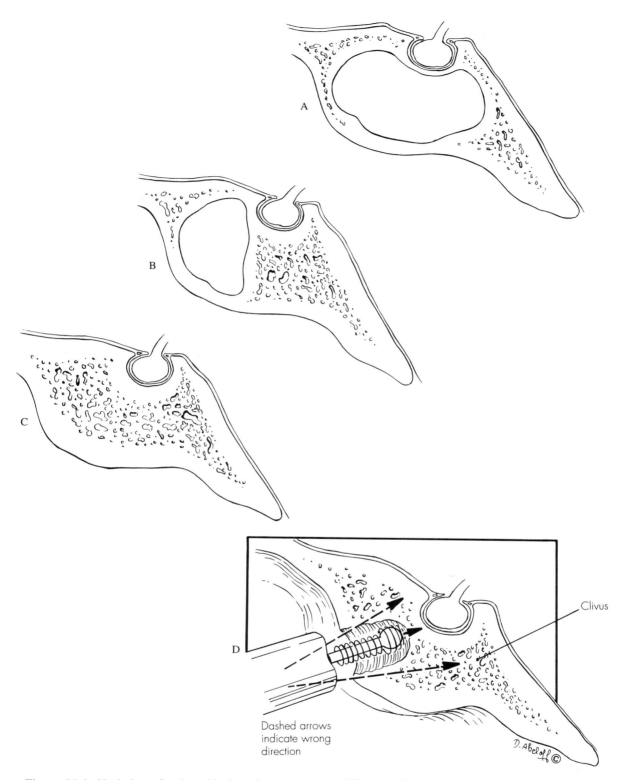

Clivus

Dashed arrows
indicate wrong
direction

D. Abeloff©

Figure 14-6. Varieties of sphenoid sinus increasing the difficulty of the approach to the sella turcica. **(A)** Completely pneumatized sinus (85 percent): no difficulty. **(B)** Presellar sinus with cancellous bone partially occluding its inferior portion and preventing clear identification of the sellar floor (10 percent) requires localization by lateral fluoroscopic control. **(C)** Nonpneumatized (conchal type) sinus (5 percent): extreme difficulty due to complete obliteration of the sinus by cancellous bone. **(D)** Use of the diamond-tipped air drill to chisel a tunnel into the cancellous bone of a nonpneumatized sinus should be monitored by lateral fluoroscopy.

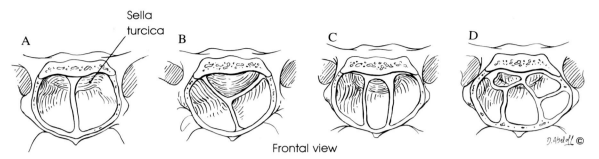

Figure 14-7. Varieties of septation in the sphenoid sinus. **(A)** Midline, **(B)** multiple oblique, **(C)** two vertical septae, and **(D)** honeycomb pattern.

artery. In patients with this honeycomb configuration of multiple septa surgeons must be careful to remove all septa before exposing the sella turcica (Fig. 14-7D).

Carotid Bulging into Sphenoid Sinus

In no case have we seen a bulging carotid artery within the sphenoid sinus; this is in contradiction to the findings in cadavers by Renn and Rhoton,[69] who described a carotid bulge in 71 percent of cases and little or no bony covering over the artery in two-thirds of the specimens they examined. In 4 percent

they saw no covering at all other than the sinus mucosa. However, such autopsy series may overemphasize the chance of carotid proximity as they contain many aged subjects with tortuous, arteriosclerotic vessels and an increased incidence of anomalies in the cerebral arteries at the skull base (Fig. 14-8). Nevertheless, the nearness of artery to sinus and the possibility that it may lie unprotected beneath a blanket of mucosa make careful placement of instruments mandatory to prevent them from straying from a midline course.

Similarly Renn and Rhoton[69] described the course of the inferior portion of the optic canal in the right

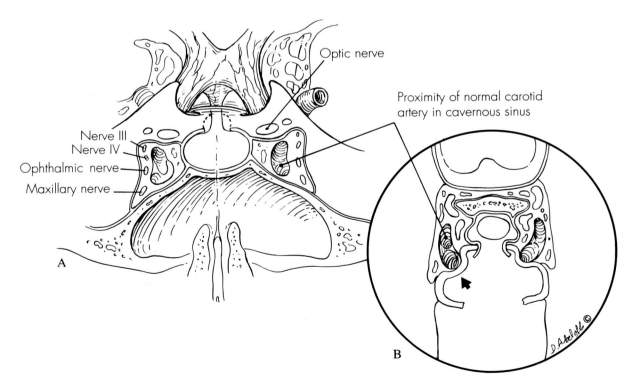

Figure 14-8. **(A)** Coronal section of the anatomy of the sellar and parasellar structures showing the proximity of the normal carotid artery in the upper lateral recesses of the sphenoid sinus. **(B)** Horizontal section showing a tortuous carotid artery bulging into the right upper posterior recess of the sphenoid sinus.

and left upper corner of the sphenoid sinus where its wall comprises a thin layer of bone that may be avulsed during transsphenoidal exposure. The optic canals, however, are too far lateral to be seen with the usual opening of the sellar floor. Overzealous maneuvers with curved instruments in this region may theoretically injure the optic nerves, but such maneuvers and such complications can obviously be avoided by limiting placement of instruments to a central corridor leading to the sella.

Chronic sphenoidal infection or abscess is very infrequent since prophylactic antibiotics are given routinely in patients before transsphenoidal operations. Should an infection occur, prophylaxis should be reassessed; a sphenoid abscess requires reopening and drainage of the cavity. A few patients develop sinusitis, which usually resolves with decongestants and a 2-week course of broad-spectrum oral antibiotics.

Sellar and Parasellar Problems

Once the floor of the sella turcica is exposed, and the posterior wall of the sphenoid sinus is outlined on the fluoroscopic monitor, only bone and dura remain between the pituitary gland and the surgeon's instruments. However, functionally important structures are located lateral to the sella turcica, notably the cavernous sinuses containing cranial nerves III, IV, V, and VI as well as the carotid arteries and several of their branches.

In the surgical management of pituitary microadenomas the entire operative procedure should remain within the anatomical boundaries of the sella turcica itself, and no surgical maneuver should be performed outside the sella either laterally, posteriorly, or superiorly. Adherence to this standard will minimize complications associated with surgery confined strictly to the sella itself.

In patients with microadenomas the sella floor is often normal in size and configuration. Occasionally a thinner floor on one side shows the surgeon where to begin the opening with a small blunt dissector that is pushed gently into the sella. Then piecemeal removal of the floor is done using sellar punches. It can be more difficult and delicate to perform a selective removal of a microadenoma than to remove an enclosed macrodenoma because of the minute operative field used with the former. The floor opening should extend from one side to the other and measure approximately 12 to 14 mm in width and 8 mm in height. More experienced surgeons can limit the opening to the side where the microadenoma is located, if preoperative radiographic clues or petrosal sinus sampling permit.[65]

Once the dura is exposed, small venous channels visible in the double layers of the aponeurosis may be coagulated with the bipolar forceps. The opening is made with a cruciform incision extending obliquely from the right upper corner to the left lower corner and from the left upper corner to the right lower corner, which produces four small dural flaps (Fig. 14-9A). These are retracted by coagulation. At this step venous bleeding frequently occurs from the intercavernous sinus or from a medial expansion of the cavernous sinus that may be located within the frame of the sellar bone opening (Fig. 14-9B&C). Various methods have been proposed to control this, either by clip application with a right-angle applier or by bipolar coagulation. These temporary methods are generally unsuccessful, and the only satisfactory method is tamponade with a piece of Surgicel and cottonoid. Further bipolar coagulation on the sinus may only increase the size of the opening and cause further bleeding, and should be avoided.

Difficulties in Microadenoma Localization

Pituitary microadenomas smaller than 5 mm are usually located either in the middle third of the gland, as is most frequently encountered in Cushing's disease, or more laterally if they secrete growth hormone or prolactin. In the absence of surface characteristics identifying the location of the tumor, the surgeon may direct the search to those sites. Lateralization of tumor or petrosal sinus sampling done before surgery in radiographically equivocal cases may prompt removal of 40 percent of the gland (on the lateralizing side) if strong biochemical evidence for tumoral secretion exists but no tumor can be identified at the time of operation. In Cushing's disease such practice has produced normal levels of serum cortisol postoperatively in 80 percent of patients (Oldfield EH: personal communication).

The removal of a microadenoma protruding from the surface of the gland presents little difficulty. The use of a microenucleator to circumscribe the lesion into a well-delineated nodule may allow excision of the tumor in one piece.

Anterolaterally placed microadenomas are least amenable to easy removal when they extend anteriorly into the hidden recess of the sella (Fig. 14-10). A right-angled long shaft microcurette has been devised specifically for scraping away any tumor tucked into this region. This maneuver may result in more profuse venous bleeding from detachment of capsular venous drainage entering into the cavernous sinus nearby. Coagulation may be ineffective and even increase the oozing of blood and should not be used.

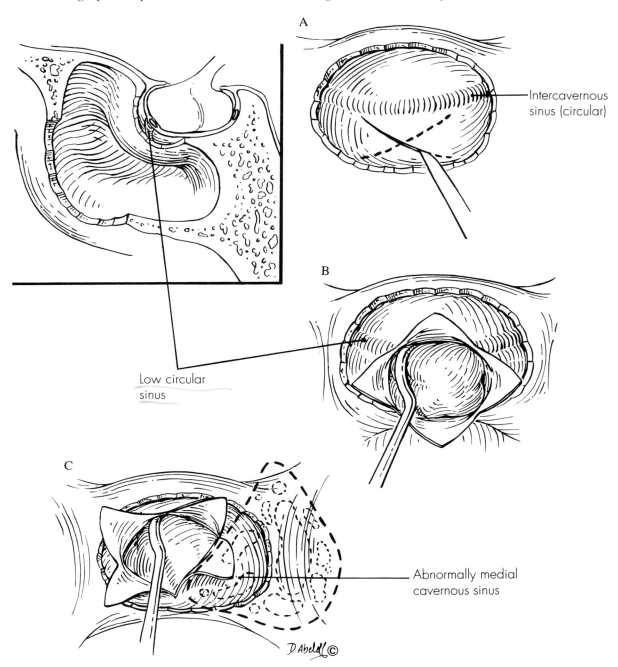

Figure 14-9. **(A)** Cruciate incision of the dura at the upper portion of the sellar window: the intercavernous (circular) sinus is seen in its normal position. **(B)** Abnormally low position of the intercavernous sinus in the central area of the sellar window requiring incision through the sinus. **(C)** Medial expansion of the cavernous sinus requiring eccentric opening of the dura above.

Only packing with Gelfoam or muscle will allow complete hemostasis. Hemorrhage from a small incision accidentally or intentionally made into the cavernous sinus can be stopped by occluding the opening with one of these substances.

Prolonged treatment of prolactin-secreting microadenomas with dopaminergic agonists over a period of 6 months or more may cause fibrosis of the tumor and adhesions to the pituitary capsule and the lateral walls of the sella turcica.[52] This loss of the plane between normal gland and tumor increases the risk of leaving neoplastic tissue behind. In such cases the pseudocapsule should be peeled away from the margin of normal gland beneath it (Fig. 14-10B).

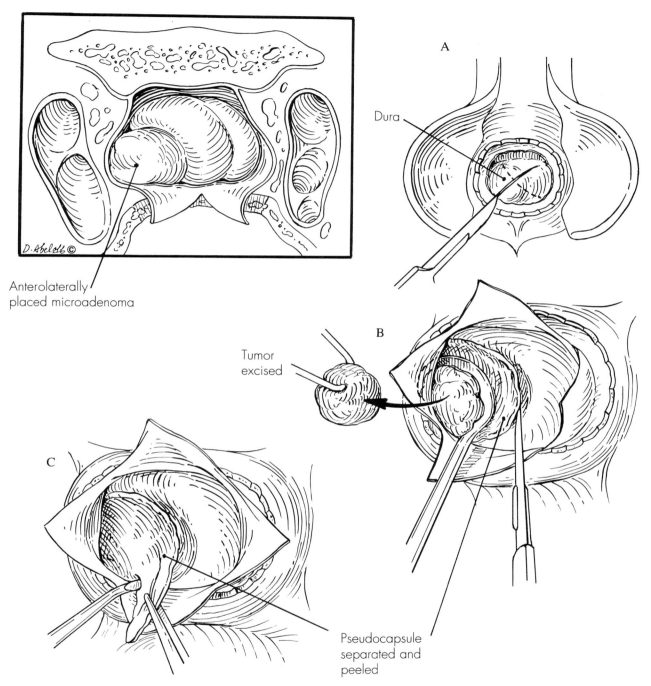

Figure 14-10. Stepwise removal of a microprolactinoma located anteriorly in the gland. **(A)** Cruciate incision of the dura. **(B)** Scooping out the microadenoma with a microenucleator. **(C)** Removal of remaining tumor from the anterolateral corner of the sella.

Tumors located posteriorly and deep within the pituitary parenchyma are less readily excised (Fig. 14-11). In anterolaterally placed microprolactinomas a vertical incision is made in the gland and the anterior portion of the lateral wing is first excised either with an enucleator or by suction (Fig. 14-10A–C). It is useful to preserve this normal piece of tissue for histological control by immunostaining methods. The tumor is usually found posteriorly as a greyish-purple or whitish, milky soft nodule. An enucleator or blunt ring curette is used to start the dissection, but this instrument is not accurate enough to finish it.[70] Com-

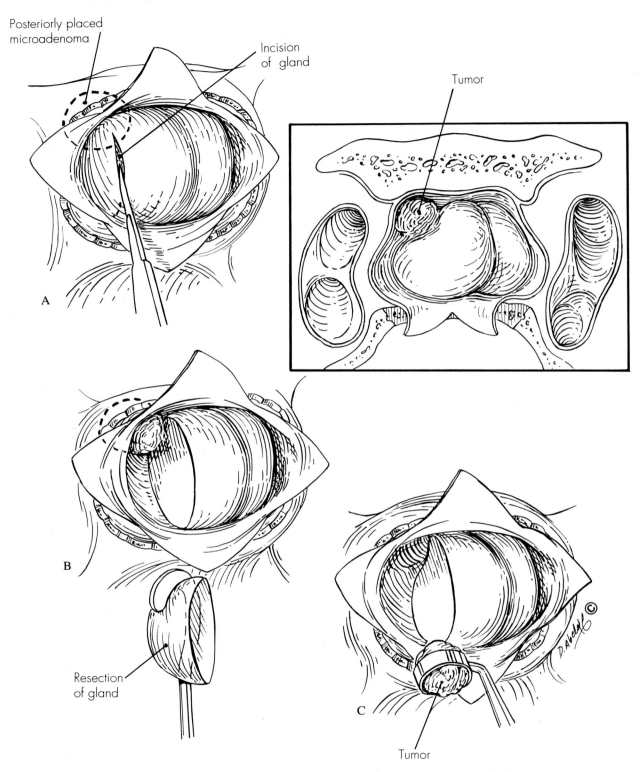

Figure 14-11. Removal of a posteriorly placed microprolactinoma. **(A)** Vertical incision of the gland. **(B)** Removal of the anterior portion of the lateral wing. **(C)** Scooping out the microadenoma with a sharp ring curette.

plete removal requires a sharp ring curette, which can be used to scrape off the remaining neoplastic tissue and separate it from the normal gland. At higher magnification (20×), careful inspection of the tumor cavity allows the surgeon to verify total removal of tumor from its yellow-orange margin of normal gland. If doubt exists, a small layer of normal gland can also be excised without producing further pituitary deficit. Consecutive removal of the anterior portion of the lateral wing, the tumor, and the margin of the normal gland has been called a "graded partial lobectomy."[59]

Studies of the microvascular supply of the pituitary have shown that the inferior hypophyseal artery supplies blood to the posterior lobe, the pituitary stalk, and the lower aspect of the infundibulum and also gives a collateral branch to the margin of the lateral wing of the adenohypophysis.[55,78] The main trunk of this artery emerges from the inferolateral corner of the sella. If it is damaged, ischemia to these regions may result in permanent diabetes insipidus. This can be avoided by removing the posterior part of the microadenoma by gentle suction on the tumor itself without peeling off the pituitary capsule.

A laterally placed microadenoma may appear as a well-circumscribed, protruding, and pulsating structure because of its proximity to the inner wall of the carotid syphon or to an intrasellar arachnoid invagination. In such cases a puncture with a small (e.g., 27-gauge) needle may reveal a thin jet of blood from a carotid artery mesially placed or even from a rare berry aneurysm protruding into the sella turcica.[76]

Anterior Lobe of Pituitary Gland

Removal of a pituitary microadenoma can usually be achieved without damaging the functional ability of residual normal gland. Some removal or contusive damage of normal tissue is common, however, and if extensive enough may impair one or more of the endocrine axes. A personal series compiled by one of us (J.H.) included 300 prolactinomas, of which 196 were microadenomas. Two-thirds of these measured less than 5 mm and were not visible at the surface of the gland; 32 such patients had a partial resection of the lateral wing of the pituitary before the microadenoma was found. In the total group of 300 patients two deficits in the adrenal axis occurred, three in the thyroid axis, and seven in the gonadotropic axis, most of which arose in patients with large tumors.[58] Preservation of endocrine function after transsphenoidal surgery has also been studied by Tindall and his colleagues; they reported permanent new damage in 4 of 97 patients with prolactinomas,

70 of which were microadenomas.[53] The thyroid axis is most likely to require long-term replacement therapy: deficits in the gonadal axis tend to recover spontaneously.

Cavernous Sinus and Carotid Artery

Normally no vascular structures (other than the rarely seen hypophyseal arteries) are found in the sella turcica in patients with prolactin- or adrenocorticotropin (ACTH)-secreting microadenomas. The carotid artery is outside the boundaries of the sella turcica; only faulty placement of instruments will result in bleeding from the carotid artery within the cavernous sinus. In aged subjects and in acromegalic patients with a long history, however, a tortuous carotid loop may protrude into the sella turcica and even extend to the midline (Fig. 14-12). Renn and Rhoton[69] reported an intercarotid distance as small as 4 mm in one specimen. In rare instances the two carotid arteries can anastomose within the sella and present obvious dangers to the surgeon who explores without adequate preoperative radiographic evaluation.[61] Demonstrating the presence of these vascular anomalies is mandatory before operation. Standard computed tomography (CT) and magnetic resonance imaging (MRI) studies will readily detect such carotid loops, and surgical complications can thereby be prevented. Their presence is not a contraindication to transsphenoidal surgery provided the procedure is performed by an experienced surgeon.

The dural incision should be performed with a No. 15 scalpel blade (not with a No. 11 pointed blade) to avoid blind penetration into the sella and injury to the carotid wall. Once the intrasellar contents are exposed, gentle suction of the tumor from around the carotid artery with angled suction tips is readily done. In acromegalic patients the carotid wall is rather thick and not easily entered by the dissectors. However, the known presence of a tortuous carotid artery within the sella always presents the hazard of arterial bleeding. One should be prepared to control in the following manner the profuse bleeding that results from any carotid disruption.

Immediate tamponade with a piece of Surgicel covered with a muscle plug applied with moderate pressure will reduce the profuse bleeding produced by a carotid laceration. Additional compression of the common carotid artery in the neck reduces considerably the local systolic pressure, allowing the surgeon enough time to pack the sella turcica with muscle. In five of our patients in whom carotid bleeding into the sella turcica occurred, immediate satisfactory control by sellar packing was achieved without the need for

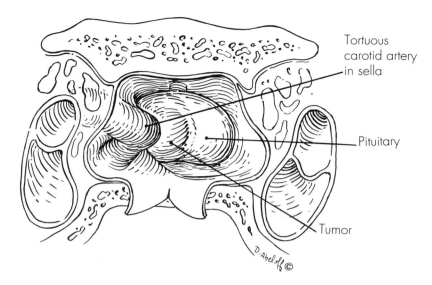

Tortuous
carotid artery
in sella

Pituitary

Tumor

Figure 14-12. A tortuous carotid artery bulging into the sella and encased by a microadenoma expanding laterally into the cavernous sinus.

other, more drastic measures. Persistence of bleeding despite this initial attempt requires further maneuvers such as ligation of the carotid in the neck or of the proximal carotid artery intracranially. The more recent methods of carotid occlusion by placement of a navigable intracarotid balloon has also been used successfully.[49]

Despite adequate early control of bleeding, the later development of an aneurysm from the traumatized carotid wall may produce sudden delayed episodes of profuse arterial bleeding and epistaxis, which may be fatal. Therefore any patient who has a carotid laceration during surgery should be studied immediately postoperatively by arteriogram to detect early defects in the wall of the artery and predict the possible development of an aneurysm within the next few weeks or months. Repeat angiography may be indicated if a suspicious or equivocal image is seen on the first postoperative study. Should an aneurysm develop it should be dealt with by the above-mentioned techniques of carotid occlusion as a prophylactic measure to prevent sudden, unexpected hemorrhage.[50] Delayed carotid-cavernous fistulae may also form after an injury to the artery and are detected and treated in a similar fashion.[68]

CSF Fistula

Even during the removal of the microadenomas, cerebrospinal fluid may leak into the sella turcica because of an opening of an arachnoid sheath prolapsing through a congenitally large diaphragmatic ori-

fice. This part of the procedure cannot be avoided in some cases. In others a small cottonoid pledget applied against the arachnoid may prevent intraoperative leakage of CSF. Nevertheless, in such instances the prevention of postoperative rhinorrhea should be undertaken by applying a piece of lyophyllized dura or fascia lata to the arachnoid opening followed by packing of the sellar cavity with muscle, fat, or Gelfoam impregnated with fibrin sealant (Tisseel). Further watertight closure of the sellar window can be accomplished by sealing a cartilaginous graft with this sealant (Fig. 14-13).

Despite adequate surgical closure a postoperative CSF rhinorrhea occasionally occurs due to uncapping of the cartilage by strenuous effort from the patient; any sustained valsalva maneuver with its attendant increase in intracranial pressure can reopen small, imperfectly occluded arachnoid tears in the first 2 or 3 days after surgery. Even an immediate CSF rhinorrhea may not be evident until the third postoperative day (when the intranasal tampons are usually removed) and in rare instances is discovered much later than that.

The discovery of a CSF rhinorrhea may be treated initially by continuous lumbar spinal drainage and restriction of the patient to bed rest. Diverting the fluid in this fashion promotes healing of the fistula and allows closure without reoperation in 80 percent of patients. Broad-spectrum antibiotics should be given prophylactically while the tube remains within the thecal sac. Drainage is continued for 2 to 3 days before the tube is clamped and the patient gradually

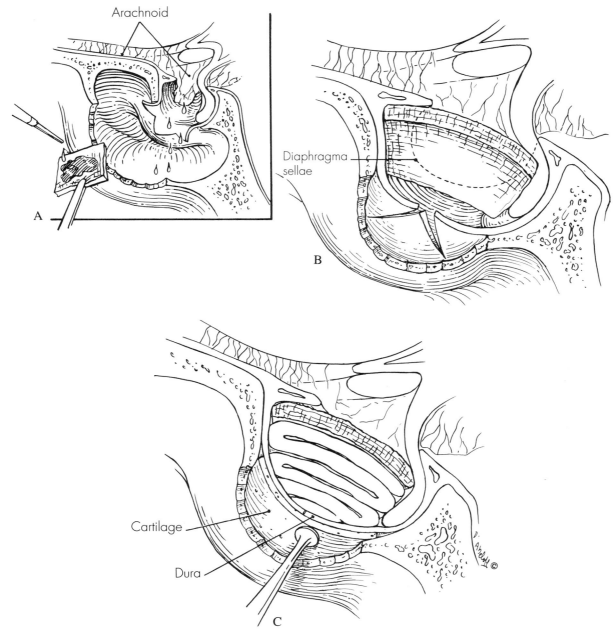

Figure 14-13. Closure of CSF fistula with lyophyllized dura, fibrin sealant (Tisseel), and cartilage. **(A)** Fibrin sealant is placed on the lyophyllized dura. **(B)** Dura is placed beneath the torn arachnoid at the diaphragma sellae to obliterate the leak. **(C)** The sella is packed further with muscle, fat, or lyophyllized dura. The sellar window is closed with a piece of cartilage from the nasal septum.

brought to a sitting position. In those patients who still show evidence of a leak, reopening with replacement of the dural graft by a larger piece and repositioning of the cartilaginous graft in the sellar window may achieve adequate permanent closure of the fistula. If a piece of cartilage from the nasal septum is not available because of previous operation, other materials may be used: these include a piece of bone, or a silicone plate that is snapped into the sellar window. This is not, however, watertight closure, and a further layer of fibrin sealant should be added. We prefer to reopen immediately those patients in whom a fistula is found, on the grounds that early direct closure minimizes the risk of meningitis.

Complications in the Wall of the Cavernous Sinus

The inner and outer walls of the cavernous sinus comprise the two layers of an aponeurosis containing the third, fourth, and sixth cranial nerves and the ophthalmic and maxillary divisions of the trigeminal nerve. During the removal of laterally placed microadenomas, placement of a right-angled curette to remove the last fragments of tumor in the anterior angle of the sella may induce temporary stretching of the sixth nerve, resulting in postoperative diplopia. As this does not disrupt the anatomical continuity of the nerve, the diplopia is most often transient and disappears within a few weeks after surgery. It has also occurred after attempts to coagulate with bipolar forceps in this region. Functional disturbance due to heating of the sixth nerve recovers quickly. Overpacking of a laterally placed resection cavity may induce similar cranial nerve pressure and dysfunction. Extensive scratching and scooping of tumor invading the wall of the cavernous sinus may result in further damage to all the cranial nerves it contains and may cause a partial or complete ophthalmoplegia. In patients with an invasive tumor, this is an anticipated complication that may also be produced by the packing needed to control profuse bleeding that occurs during the excision of such invasive tumors.

Intracranial Problems

Since all pituitary microadenomas are located within the sella turcica below the diaphragma sellae, direct damage to intracranial structures should not occur. However, diabetes insipidus can be produced by stalk traction causing functional disturbance of the infundibulum and hypothalamic nuclei, or by ischemic changes in the neurohypophysis and stalk that result from manipulation of the inferior hypophyseal artery. Diabetes insipidus, if present, occurs within 24 hours of surgery after existing stores of vasopressin in the neurohypophysis are depleted. It is diagnosed by close monitoring of urine output and serum and urine electrolyte concentrations and osmolality. In most cases intraoperative traction on the stalk (rather than transection) is the cause, and the condition is transient, requiring treatment for 3 months or less and usually only for a day or two.

Proper treatment requires not only vasopressin (given as DDAVP, 0.3 ml IV or SC, q12h as needed to control urine output) but also institution of a fluid restriction and ml for ml replacement of urine output to avoid dehydration and wide swings in serum sodium concentration. Once the amount of vasopressin needed to regulate urine volume has been established in those patients in whom the diabetes insipidus does not clear, intranasal vasopressin is started, and if necessary may be continued after the patient leaves the hospital. If the stalk is anatomically transected, standing orders for vasopressin should be instituted immediately after surgery.

Meningitis and its sequelae are uncommon after operation for microadenomas because the diaphragma sellae is not usually breached during the removal of completely intrasellar tumors. If it occurs it usually does so within 2 weeks of operation and should be treated aggressively with antibiotics chosen on the basis of bacterial sensitivities established by culturing CSF from the patient. If vasospasm occurs, it should be treated in an intensive care unit with the usual measures designed to maintain and increase intravascular pressure. Very rarely patients develop vasospasm after transsphenoidal surgery without proof of a concomitant infectious meningitis; in such instances subarachnoid bleeding from disruption of suprasellar vessels must be suspected and treated in the same way.

The diaphragma sellae may be congenitally deficient or absent in some patients and so open the way to the inadvertent introduction of instruments into the suprasellar region. However, the surgeon who guides the placement of instruments with fluoroscopic monitoring will avoid such accidents. Contusion injury of the optic nerve or chiasm may occur and results in postoperative visual disturbance. Similarly, lesions of the carotid artery above the sella turcica or of the anterior cerebral artery should not occur because of their distance from an intrasellar microadenoma.

In patients with a deficient diaphragma sellae, the cavity created by tumor removal may on very rare occasions allow postoperative prolapse of the optic chiasm into the sella.[75] Such patients present with sudden onset of visual field defects of an unpredictable nature, usually in the first 2 weeks after operation. This frightening complication has been successfully treated by us by lowering the patient's head into a recumbent or reverse Trendelenburg position. This maneuver allows the chiasm to resume its normal position by gravity and relieves the traction that produced the visual dysfunction. If no improvement ensues, the surgeon may elect reoperation by the transsphenoidal route to perform a chiasmapexy.[66] In some of these patients the chiasm will be found in its normal anatomical position; in these a diagnosis of ischemic damage to the optic system must be entertained.[47]

Deficiency of the diaphragma sellae is associated with the "empty sella" phenomenon even in the absence of surgery. After operation a resection cavity will in many patients be gradually filled by prolapsing arachnoid and give the radiographic appearance of an empty sella if the cavity is not packed with muscle or fat. However, the pituitary dysfunction associated with a symptomatic empty sella syndrome does not generally occur in patients after removal of a microadenoma.

CONCLUSIONS

Safe performance of transsphenoidal procedures requires a knowledge both of normal sphenoidal and sellar anatomy and of the variations that endocrine disease can cause. The removal of microadenomas is less perilous than surgical attack on larger tumors with a suprasellar component. Nevertheless, complications lie in wait for the unwary in the nasal, sphenoidal, sellar, and parasellar regions. They are all the more devastating in view of the unwarranted aura of safety that patients (and less experienced surgeons) attach to an operation that leaves no externally visible scar. The surgeon can maximize the chances of removing the tumor in its entirety, and of shepherding the patient through the procedure intact, by following established planes of dissection on his way to the sella, and by staying within the confines of the sella during his search for the tumor. An "intrasellar exploration" should be just that, and no more.

Pituitary Macroadenomas

William T. Couldwell
Martin H. Weiss

Large pituitary tumors often pose difficult management dilemmas, and may present formidable lesions to remove technically as they progressively impact upon low midline neural and vascular structures. In planning management strategies for larger tumors, it should be borne in mind that the two objectives in the treatment of pituitary tumors are relief of signs and symptoms attributable to mass effect, and correction of endocrine abnormalities (hypo- or hypersecretion of adenohypophyseal hormones).[91] When nonsecreting tumors are specifically considered, correction of endocrine abnormalities may be of lesser consequence than is hormonal excess, but it is important to realize that continued growth of the lesion may precipitate hypopituitarism.

The role of surgery in the management of macroadenomas must be individualized depending upon the nature of the particular underlying endocrine abnormality, and any respective available medical therapy. In this regard, a thorough endocrine evaluation is mandatory. This should include separate assay for all adenohypophyseal hormones, and appropriate stimulation studies prompted by the suspicion of any particular endocrinopathy from history or physical examination. Radioimmunoassay has revolutionized the diagnosis and management of pituitary tumors; in conjunction with advances in radiographic imaging and electron microscopy, the detection, diagnosis, and definition of these lesions has been greatly enhanced. It has further served to extend our understanding of the nature of the production and secretion of pituitary hormones.[84]

CLINICAL AND ENDOCRINOLOGICAL DIAGNOSIS

The definition of a pituitary macroadenoma is a lesion greater than 10 mm in diameter. While tumors that secrete any of the anterior pituitary hormones may grow to sufficient size to become macroadenomas, nonfunctioning adenomas more frequently present with symptoms of larger lesions, such as headache, visual failure, or hypopituitarism. Statistically, null cell tumors are the most common type of adenoma found in the pituitary, and present more frequently later in life than secreting tumors. The classic visual triad produced by larger tumors is characterized by optic disc pallor, early loss of central visual acuity, and visual field defects (bitemporal hemianopsia).[133]

In the endocrinological evaluation of the patient suspected of harboring a pituitary tumor, an important diagnostic pitfall to be avoided is the misdiagnosis of a prolactin-secreting tumor. Larger adenomas comprised of cells other than lactotrophs may produce a mild to moderate hyperprolactinemia from the so-called "stalk-section effect" (disconnection hyperprolactinemia-stalk compression causing loss of dopaminergic inhibition to tonic prolactin release),[116] which must be distinguished from a true prolactinoma (Table 14-6). Under such circumstances, it is rare to see prolactin levels in excess of 100 ng/ml, at most 250 ng/ml. Consequently, large tumors (>2 cm in size) associated with prolactin levels <250 ng/ml (certainly those <100 ng/ml) should be suspect of being nonfunctional when planning management strategies, and one would not expect such lesions to respond physically to chemical reductions of serum prolactin. Very high levels of serum prolactin (>1,000 ng/ml) are usually indicative of an invasive tumor, an important consideration when contemplating the likelihood of surgical cure (see below).[124] Nonsecreting pituitary adenomas may be defined as those that demonstrate no *apparent* clinical or biochemical abnormality indicating hormonal excess,[108] although it must be recognized that the potential for the secretion of an as yet undetectable hormone or its precursor exists, or an identified hormone may be synthesized in insufficient quantities to be detected by immunoperoxidase methods.[109] Indeed, the term "nonfunctioning" has been considered a misnomer by some for this reason.[80] To be distinguished from the true nonfunctioning tumors are those that secrete the α-subunit, common to all of the glycoprotein hormones; in these cases the α-subunit may be detected immunohistochemically in tumor specimens and biochemically in the urine, but, as it possesses no biological activity, it is of no endocrinological consequence if secreted. However, the *exclusive* secretion of the α-subunit may be difficult to determine if each of the glycoprotein hormones has not been independently assayed. For example, thyroid-stimulating hormone (TSH) secreting tumors may secrete excessive quantities of the α-subunit.[125]

With macroadenomas, varying amounts of hypopituitarism may be present, produced by compression of the gland by tumor, or from interference with

Table 14-6. Potential Endocrinologic Diagnostic Pitfalls

Prolactin stalk-section effect
False-positive low-dose overnight dexamethasone suppression
  test for Cushing's disease
Acromegalic with normal basal growth hormone level

blood supply leading to infarction of normal functioning gland. The normal anterior pituitary gland receives blood supply from two portal systems, with no certain direct arterial blood supply;[97] this likely results in less tissue perfusion pressure and increase in incidence of ischemic loss of function with intrasellar masses.[81] Reports of reversibility of hypopituitarism following surgical decompression, however, indicate the possibility for mere interruption of the hypothalamic-portal pituitary circulation without true necrosis of glandular tissue.[82,118] Recognition of any potential hypopituitarism preoperatively is imperative, as this may have implications for complication avoidance in the perioperative period (see below).

MEDICAL MANAGEMENT

The success of medical therapy for pituitary tumors is dependent upon the particular type of hormone secreted by the tumor and the reliability of the patient. While no medical therapy will result in cure of a macroadenoma, only a minority of patients with functional macroadenomas will remain free of their disease following surgery alone. The side effects and costs of medical therapy must be weighed against the potential for success of surgery. In cases of nonfunctioning tumors, no pharmacological therapy is available. The following discussion refers to those tumors for which specific medical therapy is available.

Prolactin-Secreting Macroadenomas

The probability of surgery offering chemical cure of prolactin-secreting macroadenomas, the most common functional macroadenomas, especially in large lesions with cavernous sinus invasion, is low. The efficacy of bromocriptine in reducing serum prolactin in addition to reducing tumor size and inhibiting tumor growth is well known. The central considerations related to treating such patients are the ability of the patient to tolerate the medication and the realization that the treatment must continue for the duration of the patient's life. It is our present practice to place *all* patients with large pituitary tumors with endocrinologically documented prolactin secretion on a trial of bromocriptine initially, and monitor clinical status and radiographic appearance accordingly. All solid primary prolactin-secreting tumors should respond to the medication, both clinically by a reduction in tumor size and by a reduction in prolactin level. The tenet of therapy should be absolute normalization of prolactin levels, as a prolonged hyperprolactinemic state may be associated with significant osteoporosis. Surgical resection of these lesions is indicated only in those patients intolerant to the side effects of the medication, unable to afford the cost of the medication for a prolonged period of time, or in whom sustained tumor reduction is not effected. Subsequent to surgery, if hyperprolactinemia is persistent to some extent, the patient may be able to tolerate markedly reduced doses of bromocriptine to effect long-term control, or one would consider the use of postoperative radiotherapy to bring the residual tumor under control.

An uncommon complication related to the reduction of a large invasive tumor by medical means is the development of CSF rhinorrhea. This occurs as a consequence of tumor reduction resulting in fistulous formation in areas of previous tumor invasion. This occurrence requires surgical intervention designed to obliterate the CSF fistula with removal of as much tumor as possible in the recognition that it is likely the individual will still require postoperative bromocriptine for long-term control.

Growth Hormone-Secreting Lesions

Complete surgical removal of pituitary adenomas that secrete growth hormone usually provides rapid control of elevated growth hormone, is capable of producing long-lasting "cure," and is relatively safe.[113] The problem arises in those lesions in which total removal is not possible (large suprasellar extent or cavernous sinus invasion). Also, in those cases in which surgery is not an option, other therapies are limited. The recent introduction of the somatostatin analogue octreotide (Sandostatin, Sandoz Pharmaceuticals, Inc., Hanover, NJ) holds future promise for an approved medical therapy for these patients. In early clinical trials, it reduces tumor size in approximately 60 percent of patients, and one-half of patients normalize their growth hormone (GH) and somatomedin-C levels.[86,111,120] Present therapy, however, demands bid-qid parenteral administration or continuous infusion, which dictates careful selection of reliable patients. Radiotherapy of these lesions,[83,85,89,90,127] as with other pituitary tumors, is moderately effective but not without significant adverse effects (see later).

Cushing's Disease

Fortunately, most patients with Cushing's disease harbor microadenoams, which lend themselves to complete surgical resection; our experience has been gratifying, showing a 91 percent chemical cure rate. On the other hand, patients with Cushing's disease who harbor macroadenomas present a serious problem. These tumors are frequently invasive with respect to adjacent dura and bone and consequently chemical cure by surgical means alone. If elevated adrenocorticotropic hormone (ACTH) levels persist after radical surgical resection, we have recently begun to employ stereotactic radiosurgery and eradicate residual sellar and parasellar invasion while sparing adjacent structures.

SURGICAL CONSIDERATIONS

Preoperative Evaluation

Any lesion proximal to the pituitary or hypothalamus requires adequate endocrine evaluation preoperatively to minimize the potential for an intraoperative or postoperative catastrophe because of inadequate pituitary reserve (Table 14-7). The two most important of these are serum cortisol and thyroxin levels. Because of the universal use of perioperative glucocorticoids in surgery involving this area, the risk of intraoperative hypocortisolemia is generally not a major factor. However, preexistent hypothyroidism may manifest acutely during the early postoperative period, underlining the need for adequate preoperative assessment. In cases with defined hypothyroidism, normalization of thyroid function requires approximately 1 week of therapy prior to any elective surgical procedure. For this reason complete endocrine evaluation is performed on all patients suspected of harboring a pituitary lesion; normalcy preoperatively of course does not guarantee such a state postoperatively, but an understanding of preoperative function may indicate those patients in whom a risk of this occurrence should be considered in the perioperative period. An assessment of electrolyte status is also of importance to define the patient with marginal diabetes insipidus (DI) who may not comment on the long-standing urinary frequency from an historical perspective.

Table 14-7. Preoperative Evaluation and Complication Avoidance

Check for history of diabetes insipidus
Complete endocrine evaluation; especially important to screen for hypothyroidism and hypocortisolemia
Radiographic evaluation
    Coronal MRI; check position of carotid arteries
    Pneumatization of sphenoid
    Sphenoid septum lateralized?

Radiographic evaluation should consist of coronal, sagittal, and axial MRI, with large tumors usually having similar signal intensity to brain on T_1-weighted images. Currently, a T_1-weighted image following the infusion of gadolinium is the method of choice for the delineation of intrasellar pathology. MRI also offers visualization of the major vessels, *specifically the intracavernous carotid, indicating the proximity of these structures to the tumor,* especially important in the rare case of the presence of severely ectatic carotid arteries, which might preclude a transnasal approach for risk of vascular injury. For this reason MRI has rendered a preoperative angiographic exam obsolete in the majority of cases. CT may be performed if MRI is not available, performing direct coronal cuts, or with coronal and sagittal reconstruction of axial sections through the sellar region. On unenhanced CT, the tumor usually has density slightly less than surrounding pituitary or cavernous sinuses. This study may also offer relevant information regarding the bony landmarks by varying the window widths, and reveal sellar enlargement, or sloping, thinning, or erosion of the sellar floor, all indicative of an intrasellar expansile process. Attention to the anatomy of the sphenoid sinus is imperative in planning a surgical attack. The extent of pneumatization of the sphenoid is critical in determining intraoperative strategies, and visualization of the localization of the sphenoid sinus septum or septae enables one to maximize exposure of the sella.

Surgical Approach

Transsphenoidal Approach

The transnasal transsphenoidal approach is currently considered the procedure of choice for surgical access to sellar lesions (Fig. 14-14; Table 14-8). The first successful transnasal approach to a pituitary adenoma was described by Schloffer, an Austrian rhinologist, in 1907.[122] His approach was adopted and modified by other European surgeons, and by Cushing in the United States, who introduced the sublabial incision. Original high morbidity of the proce-

dure, largely from septic complications of CSF leaks encountered, and the unavailability of synthetic glucocorticoids to supplement patients perioperatively with lack of pituitary reserve, led to a waning of interest in its use. The resurgence of Cushing's transsphenoidal approach was popularized by Guiot[103] and Hardy,[104] who further refined it by the introduction of the operating microscope and fluoroscopic monitoring. The increase in popularity of this technique may also be attributed in part to the well-recognized inadequacy of the subfrontal approach to removal of the intrasellar component of the tumor. Accordingly, several reports have demonstrated the inherent benefit of the transsphenoidal approach in the primary surgical management of these lesions.[87,94,96,104,105,129] Moreover, several reports exist of favorable results of the transsphenoidal approach in the management of visual disturbances from macroadenomas using the transsphenoidal route,[93,95,133] establishing this as the approach of choice for the surgical management of most pituitary tumors, regardless of size. Our assessment of over 200 patients who presented with visual loss from among our first 1,000 pituitary patients operated on via the transnasal transsphenoidal route yielded evidence of improved vision in 81 percent, unchanged vision in 16 percent, and worsening of vision in 3 percent. These results are similar to other large series that have reported the efficacy of the transsphenoidal approach to suprasellar tumors and certainly equal or exceed the results of large series of subfrontal explorations for visual loss. In addition, there exists clear documentation of the potential for *improvement in pituitary function* following transsphenoidal adenomectomy with careful preservation of normal gland in cases with preexisting hypopituitarism.[82,118] The efficacy of transsphenoidal surgery in selected patients with microadenomas has been established, with some reports of greater than 90 percent tumor control.[119,126] In series including larger tumors, however, a less optimistic 50 to 85 percent tumor control is expected with surgery alone.[92,93,121]

Transsphenoidal microsurgery for both large and small adenomas done by experienced surgeons has acceptable mortality and morbidity (Table 14-9).[88] Of 2,606 microadenomas and 2,677 macroadenomas reported in the international survey by Zervas,[134] the death rate was 0.27 and 0.86 percent, respectively. Direct injury to the hypothalamus seemed to be the major cause of surgical death, with delayed mortality attributed to CSF leaks and their attendant septic complications, or by vascular injury. Operative morbidity includes persistent or permanent DI, the incidence ranging from 1.8 percent permanent DI in the

Table 14-8.   Hints for Success Using the Transsphenoidal Approach

Make a wide bony opening over sella
Check position of carotid arteries before opening dura, puncture dura with 25-gauge needle before using a No. 11 blade
Avoid "blind" curettage through diaphragma sellae
Use Valsalva maneuver to promote descent of suprasellar tumor into sella, and to check for CSF leaks

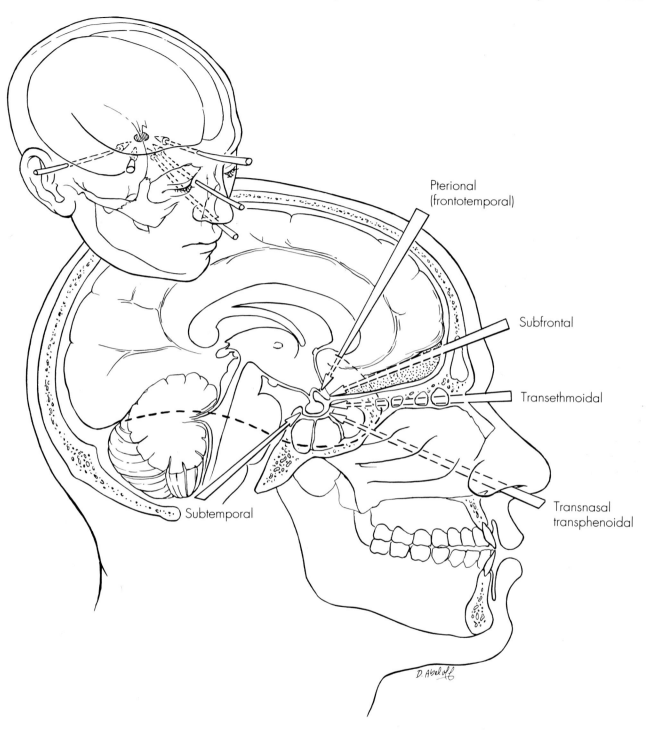

Figure 14-14. Visualization and access to the tumor lying within the sella and suprasellar cisterns. It is important on the preoperative coronal projection on the MRI to note the location of the carotid arteries as well as any septum within the sphenoid sinus so as to allow for wide opening of the sella without compromise to vascular or neural structures surrounding the sella (see Figs. 14-15B and C).

Table 14-9.   Complications of the
Transsphenoidal Approach

Optic nerve/chiasm injury
Intracavernous cranial nerve injury
Carotid artery injury
    Hemorrhage
    Carotid-cavernous fistula
    False aneurysm
CSF rhinorrhea

505 cases reported by Laws and Kern[115] to a 17 percent incidence immediately postoperatively with large adenomas as reported by Cohen.[95] Postoperative CSF fistulas range from 1 to 4.4 percent among different series,[98,132] depending upon the size of the lesion and follow-up time, but occur disproportionately with larger lesions.[88] Of more than 1,500 cases reviewed at the Mayo Clinic by Laws,[112] major morbidity (stroke, visual loss, vascular injury, meningitis, CSF rhinorrhea, cranial nerve palsy) was encountered in 3.5 percent, and minor morbidity [bleeding, nasal or sinus problems, DI, syndrome of inappropriate antidiuretic hormone secretion (SIADH), transient cranial nerve paresis, transient psychosis] occurred in another 3.5 percent of patients. As put forth by all of these authors, complications amount to a relatively small percentage of the overall surgical experience, emphasizing the relative safety of the procedure.

The rare relative contraindications to the transsphenoidal approach would include (1) extensive lateral tumor herniating into the middle fossa with minimal midline mass—these cases *may* require a primary or secondary transcranial procedure to remove tumor inaccessible by a midline approach (see below); (2) ectatic carotid arteries projecting midline, as mentioned above; and (3) acute sinusitis, which may delay the procedure for treatment of the infection. Previous rhinoplasty or submucous resection may increase the difficulty of the dissection planes, but these can invariably be established, and thus this factor should not in itself constitute a contraindication to the transnasal approach.

Apparent lateral extension into the middle fossa requires careful inspection of imaging evidence as to the precise track of such lateral extension. In tumors presenting without previous operative intervention, our experience has been that such lesions gain access to the middle fossa by extension through the cavernous sinus (Fig. 14-15C). For that matter, many of these "middle fossa extension" lesions remain within the confines of the cavernous sinus and extend into the middle fossa by ballooning the lateral wall of the cavernous sinus. Such lesions are optimally approached by the transsphenoidal route, following the extension of the tumor into the cavernous sinus from either the sphenoid or, more commonly, the sella.

A detailed description of the transnasal transsphenoidal procedure performed at our institution has been published previously.[130] The following comments address those aspects of the procedure specifically pertaining to large pituitary tumors. As described above, often cases of nonfunctioning tumors present as large lesions with suprasellar extension or cavernous invasion. As with any surgical endeavor, exposure is critical; this is especially true in intrasellar exposure, due to the long operative corridor and relatively small sellar target. Adequate bony removal is essential to allow complete sellar access. Identification of sphenoid sinus septation is critical in enabling a broad exposure of this structure. There may be numerous cells within the sphenoid sinus defined by these variable septae; failure to recognize this compartmentalization of the sphenoid will result in inadequate exposure of the sella. It is critical to identify the sphenoid ostia at the time of exposure of the rostrum of the sphenoid in order to gain access to the full expanse of the sphenoid upon removal of the rostrum.

The location of the carotid arteries on coronal MRI should be noted, as this information is valuable when opening the dura at the lateral margins of the sella (see below; Figs. 14-15A&B and 14-16B&C). Before opening the dura with a No. 11 blade, we routinely puncture the dura with a 25-gauge needle as further insurance against injury to an ectatic carotid artery in the sella. Characteristically, these tumors are soft and friable, and at surgery may herniate down through the diaphragma sellae after evacuation of the intrasellar component; this may be facilitated by the anesthetist performing a Valsalva maneuver intraoperatively. Other techniques to promote this include the infusion of air or saline through a previously placed cisternal or lumbar catheter.[80,131] A pure suprasellar tumor, or one that requires suprasellar access, may be approached, if necessary, by carrying the bony resection anterior over the tuberculum sellae with exposure of the dura mater lying anterior to the circular sinus. A transverse incision may then be made in the dura rostral and caudal to the circular sinus, with bipolar coagulation and transsection of the circular sinus. This sinus is an intradural structure contained between the leaves of the dura. Transsection of the circular sinus will then allow exposure of the suprasellar cistern itself, and will provide adequate room for surgical resection of tumor in this location.

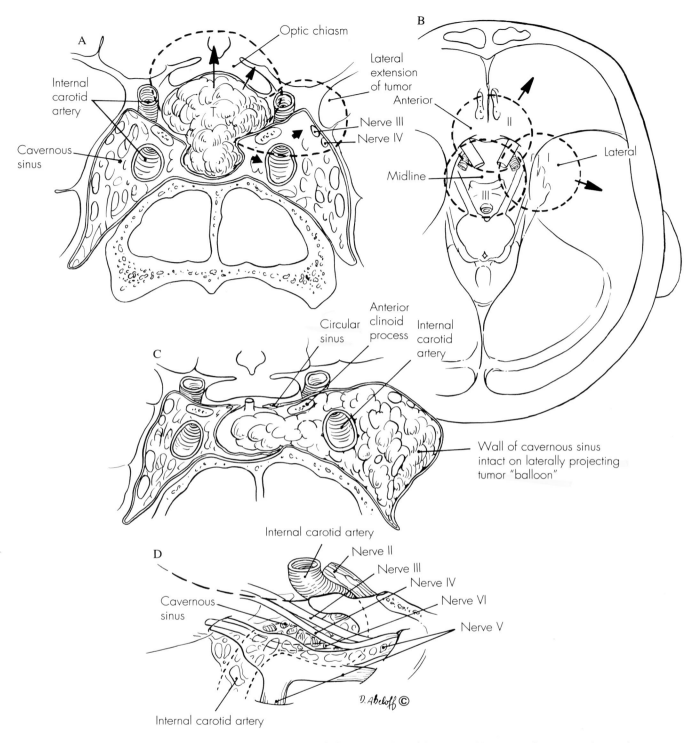

Figure 14-15. (A) Coronal views of tumor (*T*) filling the sella with suprasellar extension; note the optic chiasm stretched over top of tumor, and the relationship of the sellar tumor to the cavernous sinuses containing the carotid arteries. **(B–D)** The usual lateral extension of pituitary adenoma into the cavernous sinus with the "false" appearance of middle fossa extension. This most frequently represents a direct extension through the cavernous sinus with bulging of the cavernous sinus into the middle fossa and is best approached by transsphenoidal dissection, since a subfrontal or subtemporal approach does not allow for resection of as much tumor mass. Tumor extension lateral to the carotid artery frequently defies gross total removal.

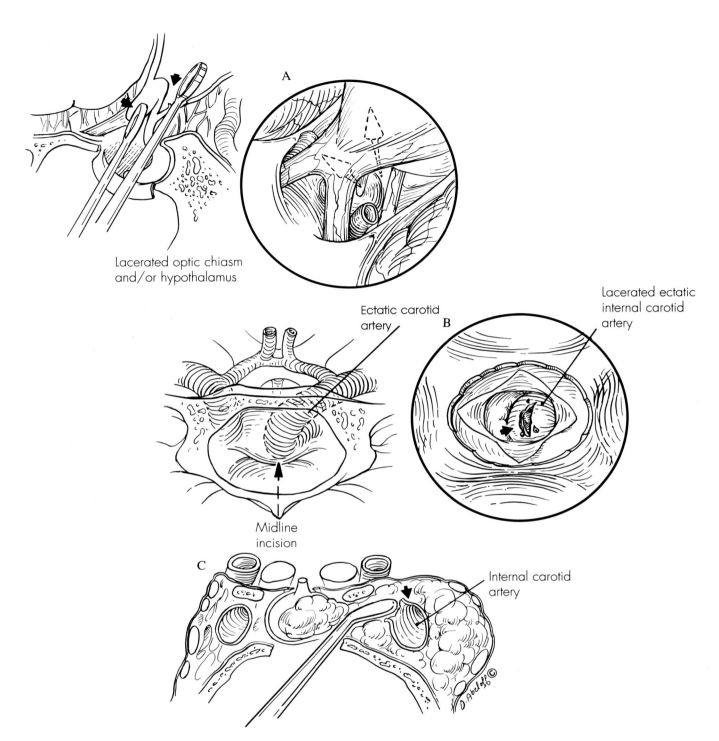

Lacerated optic chiasm and/or hypothalamus

A

Ectatic carotid artery

B

Lacerated ectatic internal carotid artery

Midline incision

C

Internal carotid artery

Figure 14-16. **(A)** A narrow opening in the diaphragma sellae with opportunity for compromise to either optic mechanisms or hypothalamus by "blind" curettage in this recess. The resection should be limited to structures lying below the arachnoid of the suprasellar cistern with the use of instruments that provide direct access to visualized structures. **(B)** An ectatic carotid artery escaping from the cavernous sinus and lying in the midline of the sella. Meticulous attention to preoperative MRIs is essential to define the location of the carotid artery with respect to the pituitary gland. In addition, our practice has been to insert a No. 22 needle through the dura prior to opening it, to reaffirm the absence of any major vascular structure within the sella. Absent such careful analysis, laceration of an ectatic carotid artery is a distinct possibility. **(C)** Dissection into the cavernous sinus in an attempt to resect tumor that has extended laterally into the cavernous sinus. Dissection in and around the carotid artery, which can generally be palpated by appropriately curved dissectors, allows for careful dissection from the carotid artery. However, the use of sharp dissectors may

Profuse intrasellar hemorrhage may be arterial or venous in origin. Extraction of tumor with radiographic extension into the cavernous sinus will entail some obligatory venous bleeding from violation of the cavernous sinus. The venous bleeding in these instances may be abundant but is always controllable with gentle packing with Surgicel. Care should be taken to avoid overzealous application of pressure in this area, as adjacent cranial nerves may be injured. The distinctly rare instance of massive arterial bleeding that may be encountered (most commonly when opening the lateral margins of the dura in the sella) usually signifies a carotid injury (three cases in our series). The immediate management should be a packing of the arteriotomy to stop potentially life-threatening bleeding; the site of the opening is rarely visualized directly, but carefully placed Surgicel with gentle pressure has been sufficient to stop the bleeding initially in our limited experience. Once the bleeding is under control, the sella should be appropriately packed first with fascia and then with muscle to ensure the presence of a nondissolvable material for permanent packing. Immediate postoperative angiography would then be warranted to ascertain the integrity of the vessel and plan any future vascular management. Obviously, careful management of blood pressure and frequent neurological evaluation in this situation is imperative.

Once the tumor mass has been resected, attention must be paid to obliteration of the CSF fistula if the arachnoid has been violated. As early as 1952, Hirsch[106] fully recognized the limitations of any intracranial attempt to control the leak, as he reported the first successful attempt of closing a sphenoidal leak following hypophysectomy using a septal mucoperichondrial flap. During transsphenoidal procedures in which the arachnoid has been breached, we routinely harvest a fascia lata graft of appropriate size to cover the opening; the graft is placed on the intradural side of the opening (within the intrasellar compartment), and a small piece of Marlex mesh is fashioned to reconstruct the sellar floor in order to maintain the apposition of the fascial graft. Placement of the fascial graft is critical, as the intracranial pressure will tamponade the graft to the dura if properly inserted. Prior to closing, the anesthetist is asked to perform a Valsalva maneuver to assess the functional integrity of the graft. The sphenoid behind this graft is then packed with fat obtained at the harvest of the fascial graft to buttress the graft further in position. If there is no CSF leakage around the graft, the retractor is removed, and the posterior nasal pack is placed against the sphenoidal opening. We then perform a routine lumbar puncture (18-gauge needle) in the recovery room and on the first postoperative day to mitigate further against the development of persistent fistula. In the unusual case of a postoperative leak following this protocol, the decision to return to the operating room for a formal repacking is taken early to avoid meningitis; little is to be gained by waiting in these cases, as the relatively avascular graft is less prone to spontaneous closure than in the posttraumatic situation. It has been our routine practice to obtain nasopharyngeal cultures prior to prepping of the nose to guide antibiotic coverage should a postoperative meningitis occur.

The remarkably low morbidity and mortality associated with transsphenoidal resection of even very large tumors has encouraged our group to consider transnasal resection as the preferred primary approach to virtually all macroadenomas. Many of these will herniate into the enlarged sella from the suprasellar cistern, subfrontal space, and cavernous sinus once the sellar component has been evacuated.

The performance of a transcranial approach to even the largest suprasellar tumor has become a rarity on our service since wide opening of the sella turcica, which is usually enlarged with most large tumors, has enabled radical resection superiorly as well as laterally and in an anteroposterior (AP) plane utilizing the integrity of the arachnoid and diaphragma sellae to determine the limits of safe dissection. On the other hand, we have occasionally found that a tumor will extend superiorly from the sella into the suprasellar cistern through a "relatively" competent diaphragma sellae. This anatomical or pathological substrate has proved challenging on two occasions in our present series, numbering 1,321 cases. In these two particular cases, the dissection was carried out above the diaphragma by taking a curved curette and placing it through the opening in the diaphragma sellae that could be visualized once the inferior por-

---

result in laceration of the carotid artery causing a carotid-cavernous fistula or false aneurysm of the carotid artery. The avoidance of sharp curettage around the carotid artery is essential in this circumstance. Bony resection can be carried laterally over the cavernous sinus as tumor extends into the cavernous sinus to follow the tumor into the cavernous sinus. It should be appreciated that tumor extending beyond the lateral aspect of the carotid artery rarely if ever lends itself to gross total resection and is fraught with significant risk with respect to potential neural and vascular compromise.

tion of the tumor was removed and resecting tumor from the suprasellar cistern in a "blind" fashion (Fig. 14-16A). On the two occasions of concern, patients sustained an increase in monocular visual loss presumably because this secondary dissection compromised the integrity of either the vascular supply or a protective arachnoid of the ipsilateral optic nerve. Our present policy calls for dissection of that portion of tumor that is readily accessible through the diaphragma sellae and then utilization of artificially increased intracranial pressure via performance of a Valsalva maneuver. We are reluctant to utilize the exaggerated curved curettes passed anteriorly in the direction of the optic nerve and its entrance into the optic foramen underneath the anterior clinoid (Fig. 14-16A). We feel that the potential for compromise of the integrity of the optic nerve in this very unusual circumstance would not warrant an attempt at radical resection of the anterior portion of the tumor lying under the optic nerves. One can usually obtain a radical resection of tumor lying underneath the chiasm and decompress the chiasm to obtain satisfactory visual decompression utilizing this technique. Resection or penetration through the intact diaphragma sellae may lead to compromise of related vascular structures, which makes such an effort undesirable.

We have, on rare occasions, found tumors that do not enlarge the sella but grow directly into the suprasellar cistern. These may present a particular problem, but, by mobilizing normal gland and opening through the tuberculum sellae as described above, one can frequently gain access to the suprasellar cistern and extract the tumor.

Transcranial Approach

Our experience with pituitary adenomas has enabled us to formulate a plan that essentially obviates the utilization of a transcranial approach for pituitary macroadenomas (Fig. 14-17). On the other hand, there are occasions in which such an approach is desirable. These instances, as outlined above, are when the transsphenoidal approach is hazardous from the presence of ectatic carotid arteries, or when the tumor spills over into the middle fossa or both middle fossae while leaving a small virtually normal-sized sella turcica. Such lesions generally occur because of an incompetent diaphragma sellae, which provides the vehicle for superior and lateral growth of tumor or possibly extensive anterior and/or posterior growth of tumor without the significant or measurable expansion of the sella. Under such circumstances, direct visualization of the tumor by the transcranial approach may be optimal. In addition,

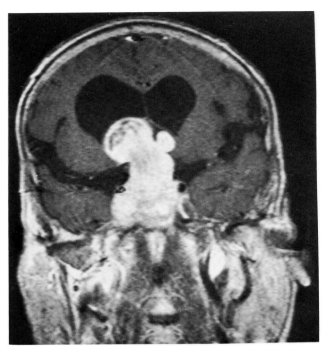

Figure 14-17. Choice of surgical approach: transsphenoidal vs. transcranial? The large invasive nonsecreting adenoma visualized on the gadolinium-enhanced coronal T_1 MRI demonstrates mostly vertical growth with no significant lateral middle fossa extension; for this reason, a primary transsphenoidal approach was chosen with adequate decompression of the visual apparatus. As the likelihood of surgical cure of this tumor is negligible, postoperative radiation therapy is indicated.

there are occasional cases in which the consistency of tumor that is encountered via the transsphenoidal approach is such as to defy an adequate resection of tumor from this approach. This may require a secondary transcranial procedure when inadequate decompression of the optic mechanism has been established. If the optic mechanism has been adequately decompressed, one would generally use postoperative radiation therapy to "mop-up" any residual tumor that may defy resection via the transnasal route.

During the course of transcranial surgery, the significant complicating anatomy presents itself primarily related to the vascular supply to the hypothalamus as well as the optic chiasm in addition to the visual structures themselves. Almost all pituitary tumors should lie below the arachnoid so that one would want to open the arachnoid and then stay below the arachnoid plane so as not to compromise potentially the perforating vasculature to the optic mechanism as well as the hypothalamus. The pterional approach to the suprasellar cistern lends itself best for this procedure (Fig. 14-14), but one must recognize that the ipsilateral optic nerve may prevent adequate visualization of tumor extending beneath it when the tumor undergoes growth in a lateral direction (Fig. 14-15B). The best technique to utilize in these circumstances is to undertake an extensive decompression medial to the optic nerve followed by subsequent mobilization of the tumor from the lateral compartment underneath the optic nerve from lateral to medial so that one can mobilize this final remnant of tumor. Exquisite care must be exercised to attempt to visualize the proximal portion of the carotid artery along with its ophthalmic branch so as to preserve the integrity of these structures while also avoiding any disruption of the perforating vessels coming from the internal carotid artery to the posterior aspect of the optic chiasm as well as optic nerve (Fig. 14-18).

The consistency of the tumor, as from below, is usually that of a soft and friable lesion that is easily debulked by the use of curettes of variable lengths and rotations. The main difficulty encountered with the removal of the lesion is the adherent capsule present, which may preclude total removal without injury to cranial nerves or the midline neuraxis. In such cases it is certainly more prudent to remove the soft interior and leave a densely adherent capsule than to risk cranial and vascular injury for a lesion that is likely not curable by surgery alone. These patients will invariably need radiotherapy for ultimate tumor control. The goals of the operation should primarily be decompression of the optic apparatus and judicious tumor removal without exposing neural or vascular structures to undue risk of injury.

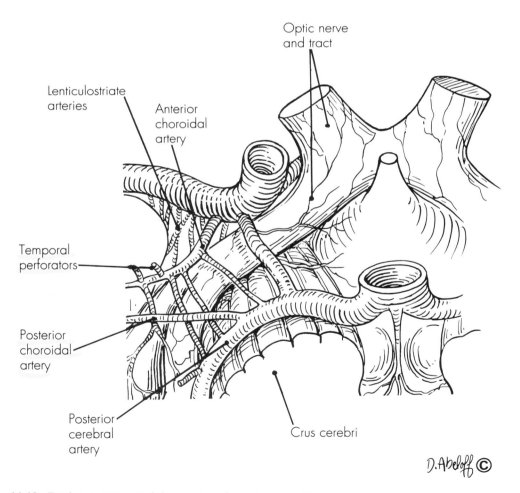

Figure 14-18. During a transcranial exposure for a tumor with suprasellar extension, one must exercise extreme care in the manipulation of low midline neural and vascular structures. The abundant perforating arteries in this region may pose a hazard to manipulation of the adherent capsule of the pituitary tumor.

Perioperative Management of Particular Importance for Avoidance of Complications

Perioperative glucocorticoids should be administered to all patients; this is crucial if preoperative endocrine assessment indicates any hypocortisolemia (Table 14-10). In our institution, we routinely administer methylprednisolone at sizable dosages of 40 mg (or 10 mg dexamethasone) q6h in the immediate perioperative period in those cases with neurological compromise, usually starting the day before surgery and continuing for one to two days postoperatively, then in a tapering dose regimen tailored to the individual patient's projected glucocorticoid needs as anticipated by the preoperative endocrine assessment and intraoperative findings. In those cases without visual compromise, lower dosages of these high-potency glucocorticoids with a more rapid postoperative taper may be employed.

Thyroid function, as mentioned previously, should be assessed preoperatively, and normalized prior to any elective surgical intervention. The stress of surgery may provoke an actual crisis in the patient without sufficient reserve, and should be a consideration in patients with an otherwise unexplained alteration in mental status postoperatively.

We have abandoned the routine use of perioperative antibiotics; the liberal use of bacitracin-impregnated irrigant has been sufficient in our experience to prevent infection; however, it should be emphasized that the transsphenoidal route should be considered only *semisterile*. In the advent of a postoperative meningitis, therapy must include coverage of colonizing organisms identified from the routine preoperative nasopharyngeal culture.

Serial visual field testing is routinely performed in the recovery room and ICU to monitor visual and general neurological condition. In the patient with preoperative visual deficit, careful monitoring in the early postoperative period is essential. Both the

Table 14-10.   Perioperative Tips for Complication Avoidance

Perioperative glucocorticoids
Close intensive care monitoring
  (Frequent vision checks—q1h for the first 12 hours)
  Maintenance of normotension
  Urine-specific gravities and serum sodium levels

---

transfrontal and transsphenoidal routes are successful in improving vision.[93,100,132] Immediate postoperative improvement of vision may occur,[99] with a significant improvement usually within the first 2 weeks, but continued improvement may occur for up to 12 months.[107] More importantly, any *loss* of vision in the postoperative period may indicate an evolving hemorrhagic complication; in this instance emergency CT scanning should be performed to exclude this. Evidence of clot on the postoperative scan with a progressive visual deficit would warrant emergency transsphenoidal reexploration. It should be borne in mind, however, that early postoperative scanning (both CT and MR) may demonstrate false evidence of suprasellar hemorrhage due to postoperative changes that give the false impression of the presence of a suprasellar clot. Consequently, the clinical evidence provided by progressive visual loss remains the primary guide to the need for reexploration supplemented by imaging evidence.

Blood pressure is carefully monitored; hypotensive events are to be avoided, especially in cases with compressive neurological deficit in which tissue perfusion is already marginal. We do not, however, routinely place an intra-arterial line in patients with an uncomplicated medical history.

Urine volumes and specific gravities must be followed in concert with sodium levels in order to understand clearly the dynamics of potential postoperative diabetes insipidus. High doses of corticoids will frequently bring out a subclinical state of DI, so we attempt to taper corticoids as rapidly as possible. In addition, one frequently encounters a secondary stage of water retention (?SIADH) following an initial bout of DI. Once this secondary stage (identified by a low serum sodium) is finished, the patient may transiently excrete a large volume of low specific gravity urine, which simply represents clearance of excess free water and should not be treated since the vast majority of these patients will come into appropriate fluid balance on their own. It is imperative, however, to follow the serum sodium carefully in order to define this process.

Prior to discharge, an AM fasting serum cortisol is obtained to determine the need for cortisol replacement. Intraoperative evidence of residual normal pituitary gland is also a major guide in such considerations. Thyroid evaluation is usually done at 3 to 4 weeks postoperatively since autonomous function of the thyroid may persist for some time postoperatively.

Unless clinically indicated, postoperative imaging is not done for at least 6 weeks postoperatively, or 3 months in most cases. This allows clearance of all operative artefactual changes that might confuse one's decision about the implementation of postoperative adjuvant therapy.

MANAGEMENT OF THE PATIENT WHO PRESENTS A POOR SURGICAL RISK

In the elderly patient or any patient harboring a medical illness that may pose a significant risk to a general anesthesia and surgery, consideration should be given to primary radiation therapy, following an appropriate clinical diagnosis of a nonfunctioning pituitary tumor. The indications for this nonsurgical approach strengthen in cases with hypopituitarism. A dose of 4,000 cGy (rad) by external beam is considered optimal by most radiotherapists.[83,123] In a recently reported series of 12 patients treated with radiation therapy alone, Chun et al.[92] described a 50 percent recurrence rate with a 75 percent local control following salvage treatment. Other authors report a local control rate of 50 to 79 percent, with an adequate salvage in cases of recurrence.[110,127]

Radiation therapy was advocated for the management of pituitary tumors as early as 1907.[101] Radiation therapy *per se*, however, should not be considered a completely benign therapy, or an equivalent alternative to microsurgical resection.[92] Adverse effects from radiation in this region may range from mild to severe. It carries *a significant risk of worsening of preexisting hypopituitarism, with an overt 10 to 15 percent frequency of panhypopituitarism,*[117] may increase the rate of atherogenesis in the major vessels in the field, and may cause visual impairment.[92] These complications increase as a function of total treatment dose.[83] The visual impairment may result from one of several mechanisms, including empty sella syndrome, treatment failure, or direct radiation damage to optic pathways. This latter complication is seen with significant frequency with daily fractionation of greater than 220 cGy.[83] Other minor complications from radiation therapy include epilation, scalp swelling, and otitis.[85]

In the asymptomatic elderly patient with a nonsecreting tumor, intact pituitary function, and no compromise of the visual system, a case can be made for merely monitoring the patient with routine clinical (visual field) and endocrine evaluation, with serial MRI or CT scanning being performed at least yearly; these tumors may exhibit a benign course, without reaching symptomatic dimensions within the remaining life expectancy.

POSTOPERATIVE RADIATION THERAPY

The rationale for the use of postoperative radiation therapy is to reduce the incidence of recurrence, with several studies suggesting improved tumor control with the combination of surgery plus radiation therapy.[89,92,93,102,117] This is especially true in large and invasive lesions, which manifest an increased rate of recurrence. This treatment, however, by no means ensures recurrence-free survival; the time to recurrence may be prolonged, however. Valtonen and Myllymaki[128] have reported a surprisingly high 36 percent recurrence rate in patients with a "total removal" following transfrontal craniotomy and postoperative radiation therapy, with recurrences having occurred up to 18 years following therapy. Thus, published recurrence rates may be misleading in series with short follow-up times. This is an important consideration, as morbidity and mortality both increase with operative intervention in cases of recurrence.[114,128]

With functioning pituitary tumors, evaluation of postoperative endocrine status may give indications as to the effectiveness of the surgical removal; however, in nonfunctioning lesions the judgment of the surgeon supplemented by postoperative imaging are the only parameters to gauge the extent of resection and therefore risk of recurrence. The surgeon's appreciation of the totality of the resection may not be accurate in the face of an invasive tumor. The lack of a chemical marker in a true nonfunctional tumor makes assessment of cure difficult in the postoperative period. Furthermore, in contrast to prolactin and growth-hormone secreting tumors, no adjunctive pharmacotherapy is available.

For these reasons, the criteria for selection of patients for postoperative radiation therapy remains controversial. In general, large tumors, which have a high frequency of invasion of the dura and therefore defy surgical excision, should all be considered candidates for postoperative radiation therapy, especially if the patient has hypopituitarism postoperatively. Similarly, with frank cavernous sinus invasion, postoperative radiation therapy would be advocated. When tumor invasion is not evident, and "total" removal has been achieved, following the patient with routine scanning on a yearly basis may be an appropriate strategy, especially if endocrine function is intact.

THE PROBLEM OF RECURRENCE

The patient with recurrent tumor other than a prolactinoma may present a challenge, especially if young and with a functional pituitary. In these cases, further treatment must be individualized, with options including repeat transsphenoidal surgery, salvage radiation therapy, or merely following patients with serial images if they are functionally intact or stable. Prior radiation therapy may produce thinning of the bone at the skull base, and may predispose to postoperative leaks, but is never a contraindication to transsphenoidal surgery.[113] The situation is quite different following previous frontal craniotomy, which may produce scarring, and distort vascular anatomy, increasing the risk of subsequent procedures.

CONCLUSIONS

It must be remembered that the management of such lesions is predicated upon the nature of the underlying hormonal abnormality. Whereas surgery must be considered the primary mode of therapy for the nonfunctioning adenomas, newer pharmacotherapeutic agents developed for non-prolactin-secreting lesions may constitute a management option in the future.

REFERENCES

General Considerations

1. Adams CBT: The management of pituitary tumors and post-operative visual deterioration. Acta Neurochir (Wien) 94:103, 1988
2. Auer LM, Clarici G: The first 100 transsphenoidally operated pituitary adenomas in a non-specialized centre: surgical results and tumour recurrence. Neurol Res 7:153, 1985
3. Barrow DL, Tindall GT: Loss of vision after transsphenoidal surgery. Neurosurgery 27:60, 1990
4. Bevan JS, Adams CBT, Burke CW et al: Factors in the outcome of transsphenoidal surgery for prolactinomas and non-functioning pituitary tumor, including pre-operative bromocriptine therapy. Clin Endocrinol 26:541, 1987
5. Black PMcL, Zervas NT, Candra GL: Incidence and management of complications of transsphenoidal operation for pituitary adenoma. Neurosurgery 20:920, 1987
6. Candrina R, Galli G, Bollati A: Letter to the editor, Subdural and intraventricular tension premocephalus after transsphenoidal operation. JNNP 51:1005, 1988
7. Ciric I, Mikhael M, Staffors J et al: Transsphenoidal microsurgery of pituitary macroadenomas with long-term results. J Neurosurg 59:395, 1983
8. Cohen AR, Cooper PR, Kupersmith MJ et al: Visual recovery after transsphenoidal removal of pituitary adenomas. Neurosurgery 17:446, 1985
9. Eisele DW, Flint PW, Janas JD et al: The sublabial transseptal transsphenoidal approach to sellar and parasellar lesions. Laryngoscope 98:1301, 1988
10. Fahlbusch R, Buchfelder M: Transsphenoidal surgery of parasellar pituitary adenomas. Acta Neurochir (Wien) 92:93, 1988
11. Fahlbusch R, Buchfelder M, Muller CA: Transsphenoidal surgery for Cushing's disease. J R Soc Med 79:262, 1986
12. Faria MA, Tindall GT: Transsphenoidal microsurgery for prolactin-secreting pituitary adenomas: results in 100 women with the amenorrhea-galactorrhea syndrome. J Neurosurg 56:33, 1982
13. Hashimoto N, Handa H, Yamagami TL: Transsphenoidal extracapsular approach to pituitary tumors. J Neurosurg 64:16, 1986
14. Horwitz NH, Rizzoli HV: Postoperative Complications of Intracranial Neurological Surgery. Williams & Wilkins, Baltimore, 1982
15. Kennedy DW, Cohn ES, Papel IO et al: Transsphenoidal approach to the sella: The Johns Hopkins experience. Laryngoscope 94:1066, 1984
16. Kern EB: Transnasal pituitary surgery. Arch Otolaryngol 107:123, 1981
17. Landolt AM: Transsphenoidal surgery of pituitary tumors: its pitfalls and complications. p. 1. In Villiers JC de (ed): Some Pitfalls and Problems in Neurosurgery. Vol. 13. Progress in Neurological Surgery. Karger, Basel, 1990
18. Laws ER, Jr: Transsphenoidal approach to lesions in and about the sella turcica. p. 309. In Schmidek HH, Sweet WH (eds): Operative Neurosurgical Techniques: Indications, Methods, and Results. Grune & Stratton, Orlando, FL, 1988
19. Laws ER, Jr, Abboud CF, Kern EB: Perioperative management of patients with pituitary microadenoma. Neurosurgery 7:566, 1980
20. Laws ER, Jr, Fode NC, Redmond MJ: Transsphenoidal surgery following unsuccessful prior therapy. J Neurosurg 63:823, 1985
21. Laws ER, Jr, Kern EB: Complications of transsphenoidal surgery. Clin Neurosurg 23:401, 1976
22. Laws ER, Jr, Trautman JC, Hollenhorst RW, Jr: Transsphenoidal decompression of the optic nerve and chiasm: visual results in 62 patients. J Neurosurg 46:717, 1977
23. Lee KS, Kelly DL: Intrasellar persistent trigeminal artery associated with a pituitary adenoma: case report. J Neurosurg 70:271, 1989

24. Maira G, Anile C, de Marinis L, Barbarino A: Prolactin-secreting adenomas: surgical results and long-term follow-up. Neurosurgery 24:736, 1989

25. Mampalam TJ, Tyrrell JB, Wilson CB: Transsphenoidal microsurgery for Cushing's disease: a report of 216 cases. Ann Intern Med 109:487, 1988

26. Martins AN: Pituitary tumors and intrasellar cysts. p. 431. In Vonken PJ, Bruyn GW (eds): Handbook of Clinical Neurology. Vol. 17. North Holland Publishing, Amsterdam, 1974

27. McLanahan CS, Christy JH, Tindall GT: Anterior pituitary function before and after transsphenoidal microsurgical resection of pituitary tumors. Neurosurgery 3:142, 1978

28. Nelson AT, Tucker HS, Jr, Becker DP: Residual anterior pituitary function following transsphenoidal resection of pituitary macroadenomas. J Neurosurg 61:577, 1984

29. Newfield P, Albin MS, Chestnut JS, Maroon J: Air embolism during transsphenoidal pituitary operations. Neurosurgery 2:39, 1978

30. Nichols DA, Laws ER, Jr, Houser OW et al: Comparison of magnetic resonance imaging and computed tomography in the preoperative evaluation of pituitary adenomas. Neurosurgery 22:380, 1985

31. Otenasek FJ, Otenasek RJ, Jr: Dangers of oxidized cellulose in chiasmal surgery: report of two cases. J Neurosurg 29:209, 1962

32. Peer LA: The neglected "free fat graft": its behavior and clinical use. Ann J Surg 92:40, 1956

33. Renn WH, Rhoton AL: Microsurgical anatomy for the sellar region. J Neurosurg 43:288, 1975

34. Ross DA, Wilson CB: Results of transsphenoidal microsurgery for growth hormone-secreting pituitary adenomas in a series of 254 patients. J Neurosurg 68:854, 1988

35. Saitoh Y, Mari S, Nii Y et al: Bilateral epidural hematoma after transsphenoidal operation: report of a case with a rare complication. Neurosurgery 16:658, 1985

36. Sherwin PJ, Patterson WJ, Griesdale DE: Transseptal, transsphenoidal surgery: a subjective and objective analysis of results. J Otolaryngol 15:155, 1986

37. Shields CB, Valdes-Rodriquez AG: Tension premocephalus after transsphenoidal hypophysectomy: case report. Neurosurgery 11:687, 1982

38. Spaziante R, deDivitiis E, Cappabianca P: Reconstruction of the pituitary fossa in transsphenoidal surgery: an experience of 140 cases. Neurosurgery 17:453, 1985

39. Spaziante R, deDivitiis E, Cappabianca P: Techniques of reconstruction of the sella and related structures. p. 321. In Schmidek HH, Sweet WH (eds): Operative Neurosurgical Techniques: Indications, Methods, and Results. Grune & Stratton, Orlando, FL, 1988

40. Staples GS: Transseller intracavernous intercarotid collateral artery associated with agenesis of the internal carotid artery: case report. J Neurosurg 50:393, 1979

41. Tindall GT, Barrow DL: Disorders of the Pituitary. p. 498. CV Mosby, St. Louis, 1986

42. Tindall GT, Barrow DL: Tumors of the sellar and parasellar areas in adults. In Youmans JR (ed): Neurological Surgery, WB Saunders, Philadelphia, 1990

43. Weiss MH: Comment on Black PMcL, Zervas NT, Candra GL: Incidence and management of complications of transsphenoidal operations for pituitary adenomas. Neurosurgery 20:920, 1987

44. Wilson CB, Dempsey LC: Transsphenoidal microsurgical removal of 250 pituitary adenomas. J Neurosurg 48:13, 1978

45. Woodard EJ, Colohan ART: Fibrin glue. Perspect Neurol Surg 1:1990

46. Zervas NT: Surgical results for pituitary adenomas: results of an international survey. p. 377. In Black PMcL, Zervas NT, Ridgeway EC, et al (eds): Secretory Tumors of the Pituitary Gland, Raven Press, New York, 1984

Pituitary Microadenomas

47. Adams CBT: The management of pituitary tumours and post-operative visual deterioration. Acta Neurochir 94:103, 1988

48. Black PMcL, Zervas NT, Candia GL: Incidence and management of complications of transsphenoidal operation for pituitary adenomas. Neurosurgery 20:920, 1987

49. Britt RH, Silverberg GD, Prolo DJ et al: Balloon catheter occlusion for cavernous carotid injury during transsphenoidal hypophysectomy. Case report. J Neurosurg 55:450, 1981

50. Cabezudo JM, Carrillo R, Vaquero J et al: Intracavernous aneurysm of the carotid artery following transsphenoidal surgery. Case report. J Neurosurg 54:118, 1981

51. Cushing H: The Pituitary Body and Its Disorders. JB Lippincott, Philadelphia, 1912

52. Esiri MM, Bevan JS, Burke CW et al: Effect of bromocryptine treatment on the fibrous tissue content of prolactin-secreting and non-functioning macroadenomas of the pituitary gland. J Clin Endocrinol Metab 63:383, 1986

53. Faria MA Jr, Tindall GT: Transsphenoidal microsurgery for prolactin-secreting pituitary adenomas. J Neurosurg 56:33, 1982

54. Griffith HB, Veerapen R: A direct transnasal approach to the sphenoid sinus. Technical note. J Neurosurg 66:140, 1987

55. Gorczyca W, Hardy J: Arterial supply of the human anterior pituitary gland. Neurosurgery 20:369, 1987

56. Hardy J: Transsphenoidal microsurgery of the normal and pathological pituitary. Clin Neurosurg 16:185, 1968

57. Hardy J: Transsphenoidal hypophysectomy: neurosurgical techniques. J Neurosurg 34:582, 1971

58. Hardy J: Transsphenoidal microsurgery of prolactinomas: report of 355 cases. p. 431. In Tolis G (ed):

Prolactin and Prolactinomas. Raven Press, New York, 1983

59. Hardy J, Mohr G: The prolactinoma: surgical aspects. Neurochirurgie 27(suppl 1):41, 1981

60. Hirsch O: Pituitary tumors; a borderland between cranial and trans-sphenoidal surgery. N Engl J Med 254:937, 1956

61. Kishore PRS, Kaufman AB, Melichar FA: Intrasellar carotid anastomosis simulating pituitary microadenoma. Radiology 132:381, 1979

62. Landolt AM: Transsphenoidal surgery of pituitary tumors: its pitfalls and complications. Prog Neurol Surg 13:1, 1990

63. Laws ER, Jr, Kern EB: Complications of transsphenoidal surgery. In Laws ER, Jr, Randall RV, Kern EB et al (eds): Management of Pituitary Adenomas and Related Lesions with Emphasis on Transsphenoidal Microsurgery. Appleton-Century-Crofts, East Norwalk, CT, 1982

64. Nabe-Nielsen J: Nasal complication after transsphenoidal surgery for pituitary pathologies. Acta Neurochir 96:122, 1989

65. Oldfield EH, Chrousos GP, Schulte HM et al: Preoperative localization of pituitary microadenomas by bilateral and simultaneous inferior petrosal venous sinus sampling. N Engl J Med 312:100, 1985

66. Olson DR, Guiot G, Derome P: The symptomatic empty sella: prevention and correction via the transsphenoidal approach. J Neurosurg 37:533, 1972

67. Peele J: Unusual anatomical variations of the sphenoid sinus. Laryngoscope 67:208, 1957

68. Pigott TJD, Holland IM, Punt JAG: Caroticocavernous fistula after transsphenoidal hypophysectomy. Br J Neurosurg 3:613, 1989

69. Renn WH, Rhoton AL, Jr: Microsurgical anatomy of the sellar region. J Neurosurg 43:288,1975

70. Rhoton AL, Jr: Ring curettes for transsphenoidal pituitary operations. Surg Neurol 18:28, 1982

71. Rhoton AL, Jr, Hardy DG, Chambers SM: Microsurgical anatomy and dissection of the sphenoid bone, cavernous sinus and sellar region. Surg Neurol 12:63, 1979

72. Tindall GT, Barrow DL: Disorders of the Pituitary. p. 349. CV Mosby, St. Louis, 1986

73. Tindall GT, Collins WF, Kirchner JA: Unilateral septal technique for transsphenoidal microsurgical approach to the sella turcica. Technical note. J Neurosurg 49:138, 1978

74. Watson SW, Sinn DP, Neuwelt EA: Dental considerations in the sublabial transsphenoidal surgical approach to the pituitary gland. Neurosurgery 10:236, 1982

75. Welch K, Stears JC: Chiasmapexy for the correction of traction on the optic nerves and chiasm associated with their descent into an empty sella turcica. J Neurosurg 35:760, 1971

76. White JC, Ballantine HT Jr: Intrasellar aneurysms simulating hypophyseal tumors. J Neurosurg 18:34, 1961

77. Wilson CB: A decade of pituitary microsurgery. J Neurosurg 61:814, 1984

78. Xuereb GP, Prichard MML, Daniel PM: The arterial supply and venous drainage of the human hypophysis cerebri. Q J Exp Physiol 39:199, 1954

79. Zervas NT: Surgical results in pituitary adenomas: results of an international survey. p. 377. In Black PMcL, Zervas NT, Ridgway EC, Jr, et al (eds): Secretory Tumors of the Pituitary Gland. Raven Press, New York, 1984

Pituitary Macroadenomas

80. Adams CBT: The management of pituitary tumors and post-operative visual deterioration. Acta Neurochir (Wien) 94:103, 1988

81. Antunes JL, Murasko K, Stark R et al: Pituitary portal blood flow in primates: a Doppler study. Neurosurgery 12:492, 1983

82. Arafah B: Reversible hypopituitarism in patients with large nonfunctioning pituitary adenomas. J Clin Endocrinol Metab 62:1173, 1986

83. Aristzabal S, Caldwell WL, Avila J: The relationship of time dos fractionation factors to complications in the treatment of pituitary tumors by irradiation. Int J Radiat Oncol Biol Phys 2:667, 1977

84. Asa SL, Kovacs K: Histological classification of pituitary disease. Clin Endocrinol Metab 12:567, 1983

85. Baglan R, Marks J: Soft-tissue reactions following irradiation of primary brain and pituitary tumors. Int J Radiat Oncol Biol Phys 7:455, 1981

86. Barnard LB, Grantham WG, Lamberton P et al: Treatment of resistant acromegaly with a long-acting somatostatin analogue (SMS 201-995). Ann Intern Med 105:856, 1986

87. Bevin JS, Adams CBT, Burke CW et al: Factors in the outcome of transsphenoidal surgery for prolactinoma and non-functioning pituitary tumor, including pre-operative bromocriptine therapy. Clin Endocrinol 26:541, 1987

88. Black PMcL, Zervas N, Candia GL: Incidence and management of complications of transsphenoidal operation for pituitary adenomas. Neurosurgery 20:920, 1987

89. Bloom HTG: Radiotherapy of pituitary tumors. p. 165. In Jenkins JS (ed): Pituitary Tumors. Butterworth, London, 1973

90. Bloom B, Kramer S: Conventional radiotherapy in the management of acromegaly. p. 179. In Black PMcL, Zervas NT, Ridgeway EC et al (eds): Secretory Tumors of the Pituitary Gland. Raven Press, New York, 1984

91. Christy NP, Warren MP: Other clinical syndromes of the hypothalamus and anterior pituitary, including tumor mass effects. p. 438. In DeGroot LJ (ed): Endocrinology. WB Saunders, Philadelphia, 1989

92. Chun M, Masko GB, Hetelekidis S: Radiotherapy in the treatment of pituitary adenomas. Int J Radiat Oncol Biol Phys 15:305, 1988

93. Ciric I, Mikhael M, Stafford T et al: Transsphenoidal microsurgery of pituitary macroadenomas with long term follow-up results. J Neurosurg 59:395, 1984

94. Ciric IS, Tarkington J: Transsphenoidal microsurgery. Surg Neurol 2:207, 1974

95. Cohen AR, Cooper PR, Kupersmith MJ et al: Visual recovery after transsphenoidal removal of pituitary adenomas. Neurosurgery 17:446, 1985

96. Collins WF: Pituitary tumor management: an overview. p. 179. In Tindall GT, Collins WF (eds): Clinical Management of Pituitary Disorders. Raven Press, New York, 1979

97. Daniel PM, Prichard MML: Studies of the hypothalamus and the pituitary gland with special reference to the effects of transection of the pituitary stalk. Acta Endocrinol 80(suppl. 201):1, 1975

98. Faria MA, Tindall GT: Transsphenoidal microsurgery for prolactin-secreting pituitary adenomas. J Neurosurg 56:33, 1982

99. Feinsod M, Selhosst JB, Hoyt WF, Wilson CB: Monitoring optic nerve functioning during craniotomy. J Neurosurg 44:29, 1976

100. Goldman JA, Hedges TR, Shucart W, Molitch ME: Delayed chiasmal decompression after transsphenoidal operation for a pituitary adenoma. Neurosurgery 17:962, 1985

101. Gramegna A: Un cas d'acromegalie traité par la radiothérapie. Rev Neurol 17:15, 1909

102. Grigsby PW, Simpson JR, Emami BN et al: Prognostic factors and results of surgery and postoperative irradiation in the management of pituitary adenomas. J Radiat Oncol Biol Phys 16:1411, 1989

103. Guiot G: Considerations on the surgical treatment of pituitary adenomas. In Fahlbusch R, Werder KV (eds): Treatment of Pituitary Adenomas. 1st European workshop. p. 202. Thieme, Stuttgart, 1978

104. Hardy J: Transsphenoidal microsurgery of the normal and pathological pituitary. Clin Neurosurg 16:185, 1969

105. Hardy J: Transsphenoidal hypophysectomy. J Neurosurg 34:582, 1971

106. Hirsch O: Successful closure of cerebrospinal rhinorrhea by endonasal surgery. Arch Otolaryngol 56:1, 1952

107. Kayan A, Earl CJ: Compressive lesion of the optic nerves and chiasm: pattern of recovery of vision following surgical treatment. Brain 98:13, 1975

108. Kovacs K, Horvath E: Pathology of pituitary adenomas. In Collu R, Brown G, Van Loon GR (eds): Clinical Neuroendocrinology. Blackwell Scientific Publications, Boston, 1988

109. Kovacs K, Horvath E, Ryan N, Ezrin C: Null cell adenoma of the human pituitary. Virchows Arch [A] 387:165, 1987

110. Kramer S: The value of radiation therapy for pituitary and parapituitary tumors. Can Med Assoc J 99:1120, 1968

111. Lamberts SWJ, Uitterlinden P, del Pozo E: SMS 201-995 induces a continuous decline in circulating growth hormone and somatomedin-C levels during therapy of acromegalic patients for over two years. J Clin Endocrinol Metab 65:703, 1987

112. Laws ER: Editorial comment. Neurosurgery 20:923, 1987

113. Laws ER: Neurosurgical management of acromegaly. p. 53. In Cooper PR (ed): Contemporary Diagnosis and Management of Pituitary Adenomas. AANS Publications Committee, Park Ridge, IL, 1991

114. Laws ER, Fode NC, Redmond MJ: Transsphenoidal surgery following unsuccessful prior therapy. J Neurosurg 63:823, 1985

115. Laws ER, Kern EB: Complications of transsphenoidal surgery. p. 435. In Tindall GT, Collins WF (eds): Clinical Management of Pituitary Disorders. Raven Press, New York, 1979

116. Lees PD, Pickard JD: Hyperprolactinemia, intrasellar pituitary tissue pressure, and the pituitary stalk compression syndrome. J Neurosurg 67:192, 1987

117. Noell KT: Prolactin and other hormone producing pituitary tumors: radiation therapy. Clin Obstet Gynecol 23:441, 1980

118. Ober K, Kelly D: Return of gonadal function with resection of nonfunctioning pituitary adenoma. Neurosurgery 22:386, 1988

119. Post KD, Biller BJ, Adelman LS et al: Selective transsphenoidal adenectomy in women with galactorrhea-amenorrhea. JAMA 242:158, 1979

120. Quabbe H-J, Plöckinger U: Dose-response study and long term effect of the somatostatin analog octreotide in patients with therapy-resistant acromegaly. J Clin Endocrinol Metab 68:873, 1989

121. Randall RV, Laws ER, Abboud CF et al: Transsphenoidal microsurgical treatment of prolactin-producing pituitary adenomas. Mayo Clin Proc 58:108, 1983

122. Schloffer H: Erfulgreiche operation eiwes hypophysewtunions auf nasallam. Weg Wien Klin Wochamschr 20:621, 1907

123. Sheline GF: Treatment of non-functioning chromophobe adenomas of the pituitary. AJR 120:553, 1974

124. Shucart WA: Implications of very high serum prolactin levels associated with pituitary tumors. J Neurosurg 52:226, 1980

125. Smallridge RC, Smith CE: Hyperthyroidism due to thyrotropin-secreting pituitary tumors: diagnostic and therapeutic considerations. Arch Intern Med 143:503, 1983

126. Tyrell JB, Brooks RM, Fitzgerald PA et al: Cushing's disease: selective transsphenoidal resection of pituitary microadenomas. N Engl J Med 298:753, 1978

127. Urdaneta N, Chessin H, Fisher JJ: Pituitary adenomas and craniopharyngiomas. Analysis of 99 cases with radiation therapy. Int J Radiol Oncol Biol Phys 1:895, 1975

128. Valtonen S, Myllymaki K: Outcome of patients after transcranial operation for pituitary adenoma. Ann Clin Res 18(suppl. 47):43, 1986

129. Weiss MH: p. 180. In Horvath K, Kaufman F, Kovacs E, Weiss MH (eds): Pituitary Diseases, CRC Press, Boca Raton, FL, 1980

130. Weiss MH: Transnasal transsphenoidal approach. p. 476. In Apuzzo MLJ (ed): Surgery of the Third Ventricle. Williams & Wilkins, Baltimore, 1987

131. Wilson CB: A decade of pituitary microsurgery. The Herbert Olivecrona Lecture. J Neurosurg 61:814, 1984

132. Wilson CB, Dempsey LC: Transsphenoidal micro-surgical removal of 250 pituitary adenomas. J Neurosurg 48:13, 1978

133. Wray SH: Neuro-ophthalmologic manifestations of pituitary and parasellar lesions. Clin Neurosurg 24:86, 1977

134. Zervas NT: Surgical results in pituitary adenomas: results of an international survey. p. 377. In Black PMcL, Zervas NT, Ridgeway EC, Martin JB (eds): Secretory Tumors of the Pituitary Gland. Raven Press, New York, 1984

15 Craniopharyngioma

General Considerations

N. Scott Litofsky
Michael L. Levy
Michael L.J. Apuzzo

Craniopharyngiomas are epithelial tumors derived from the vanishing hypophyseal duct during the formation of Rathke's pouch.[12] As a group, they have been among the most challenging and difficult tumors for neurosurgeons to treat. Much of the difficulty relates to their pathological characteristics. Since these tumors are often adherent to vital neural and vascular structures, complications may and often do occur with their attempted removal. This chapter discusses the morbidity and mortality of the surgical management of craniopharyngiomas.

Complications of craniopharyngioma surgery relate in part to the anatomical relationships of the tumor to the structures of the brain. The tumors may be intrasellar, suprasellar, intraventricular, or in combinations of these locales. They often extend anteriorly, laterally, superiorly, or posteriorly. Because of their central location within the cranium and frequent extension, they may be anatomically related to many crucial neural and vascular structures. Inferiorly, the pituitary gland and stalk may be in close proximity to the tumor. The suprasellar cistern contains the optic nerves and chiasm, as well as the carotid arteries and their branches. Superiorly, the hypothalamus is present. Posteriorly, the midbrain and cranial nerves III, IV, V, and VI may be encountered, as well as the basilar artery and its branches. Sweet[49] indicated that the most tenacious attachments of the tumor are to the optic chiasm, optic tracts, pituitary stalk, hypothalamus, internal carotid artery, posterior communicating artery, and anterior choroidal artery. Other

authors have likewise warned of dense adhesions in these locations.[20,39,54] Because of these adhesions, complications may ensue with surgical manipulation of the tumor. Additionally, Shillito[44] demonstrated "fingers" of tumor invading the brain, particularly into the hypothalamus. Because the gliotic plane between the tumor and the neural elements referred to by Sweet[49] may not always be present, the removal of the lesion may compromise the structures that have been invaded, leading to difficulties for the patient.

Since the characteristics of craniopharyngiomas are quite variable, and their locations are inconstant, a variety of therapeutic modalities has been developed. Included are total resection, evacuation and marsupialization of the cyst, percutaneous aspiration of the cyst through a previous craniotomy, aspiration of the cyst through a reservoir, ventricular shunting, external radiation therapy, stereotactic radiation therapy, intracystic chemotherapy, systemic chemotherapy, and intracystic radiation therapy.[22] Combinations of these modalities have been employed. Complications of each type of treatment have been reported, related to particular aspects of tumor exposure or manipulation, on either a structural or a molecular level.

A number of surgical routes have been used to reach these tumors, including the subfrontal, transcortical-transventricular, transcallosal, transsphenoidal, subtemporal, pterional, and stereotactic approaches. Which route is used depends on the location and anatomical relationships of the tumor as determined by neuroimagery, as well as on the preference of the individual surgeon. Each of these surgical avenues has its own associated complications, which may or may not also be related to the tumor. The complications of each surgical route are discussed completely in Chapter 17 and will not be addressed here in further detail.

Much of the discussion to follow is based on a review of the literature concerned with craniopharyngiomas and their management. The literature itself limits the complete description of all complications in the surgical management of these tumors. Some studies make no mention of the complications of therapy.[4,12,34,36,38] Other reports do not clearly differentiate between deficits present preoperatively and those present after surgery; most commonly, this lack is seen with endocrine abnormalities.[10,11,13,14,19,32,46] A third group of papers does discuss the complications of craniopharyngioma surgery in some detail, but does not specify which complications result from which surgical route or therapeutic modality.[7,9–11,19–21,23,24,27,37,47,48,55] Many authors report only on patient mortality in considering patient outcome.[1,2,8,9,15,17,21,31,39,40,43,51,52] Finally, some authors do not clearly document the incidence of the complications they discuss.[5,6,53]

In this chapter, the complications that have been discussed are synthesized and compiled to create a comprehensive catalogue of the complications of surgical management of craniopharyngiomas. Patient morbidity (Table 15-1) and mortality (Tables 15-2 and 15-3) from most series are included. The complications include neurological deficits, postoperative infections, cerebrospinal fluid leaks, and patient mortality. Endocrine dysfunction, a major complication of craniopharyngioma surgery, is discussed in great detail in the next section of this chapter. Surgeons aware of these complications and the structural perturbations that lead to them may be more apt to avoid them. The outcome of the management of these difficult lesions can then be improved.

IMPAIRMENT OF NEUROLOGICAL FUNCTION

Craniopharyngiomas are often adherent to or invasive into the hypothalamus. Surgical manipulation of these tumors may result in hypothalamic injury. A wide range of deficits can theoretically result from damage to the various hypothalamic nuclei. *Hypothermia* and *hyperthermia* may result from injury to the posterior and anterior hypothalamus, respectively.[48] In his small series of patients, King[28] noted a 50 percent incidence of *poikilothermia,* a result of damage to the temperature control mechanisms in the hypothalamus. Lipton et al.[35] reported a case of a patient who developed hyperthermia after a transcallosal approach to a craniopharyngioma. Hyperthermia can also occur from indirect effects on the hypothalamus, as in 1 of 14 patients who were given intracystic radioactive yttrium[3]; the stereoopaque medium is thought to have served as a pyrogen in that case. Insult to the preoptic area may diminish its cerebral cortical depression and resulting inhibition of the waking center; the patient may suffer from *hyposomnia.* Alternatively, hypersomnia will occur if the waking center between the mamillary bodies and the third nerve nucleus is harmed.[48] Ten of 108 patients reported by Svolos[48] suffered from hypersomnia. Lateral hypothalamic nuclear injury results in *emaciation,* as in 4 percent of Svolos'[48] patients. Ventromedial damage will lead to obesity.[48] The patient studied by Lipton et al.[35] was hyperphagic, and Svolos[48] reported a 30 percent incidence of *obesity.* Hypogonadism occurs with preoptic injury.[48] This last complication is relatively common, as 74 of 108 patients suffered from *hypogonadism* in one series.[48]

The true incidence of these hypothalamic complications is difficult to determine with the available literature. Either some complications were discussed only as part of a case report[35] or a small series,[28] or the complications did not clearly result from surgical manipulation.[48] Instead, they may have resulted from tumor progression.

While unilateral damage to the hypothalamus should result in relatively few difficulties, some deficits will result from bilateral injury.[55] Neurological or endocrine consequences may occur because the tumor has infiltrated into one side of the hypothalamus, rendering it dysfunctional; the surgeon may manipulate the other side of the hypothalamus, thus creating a bilateral injury. Hypothalamic infarction may occur if the tumor capsule excised was adherent to the hypothalamus[20]; deficits would result.

Visual loss has been frequently reported following craniopharyngioma surgery. After transcranial approaches, the incidence has ranged up to 35 percent of patients, although most series report visual deficits in less than 5 percent[7,19,42] to between 10 and 20 percent.[10,37,46,55] Comparable incidences of visual loss are seen after the transsphenoidal approach to craniopharyngiomas.[32,33] Visual compromise has also been reported after intracystic irradiation in up to 7 percent of cases.[3,29,36,45] Multiple mechanisms of optic apparatus injury have been suggested. Direct surgical manipulation of the optic nerves and chiasm, which may be displaced by the expansile growth of

Table 15-1. Morbidity in Craniopharyngioma Surgery

Complication	Incidence, if Reported (%)	Author(s)
Hypothalamic dysfunction		
Hyperthermia	1/14 (7.1)	Backlund,[3] 1973
	Case report	Lipton et al.,[35] 1981
		Svolos,[48] 1969
Poikilothermia	2/4 (50)	King,[28] 1979
		Svolos,[48] 1969
Hyperphagia	Case report	Lipton et al.,[35] 1980
		Svolos,[48] 1969
Anorexia		Svolos,[48] 1969
Hyposomnia		Svolos,[48] 1969
Hypersomnia		Svolos,[48] 1969
Hypogonadism	74/106 (70)	Svolos,[48] 1969
Coma	2/14 (14)	Fischer et al.,[13] 1985
Visual loss	1/14 (7.1)	Backlund,[3] 1973
	1/74 (1.3)	Baskin and Wilson,[7] 1986
	6/43 (14)	Carmel et al.,[10] 1982
	5/14 (36)	Fischer et al.,[13] 1985
	2/51 (3.9)	Hoff and Patterson,[19] 1972
	1/14 (7.1)	Laws,[32] 1980
	3/20 (15)	Laws,[33] 1986
	4/31 (13)	Matson,[37] 1962
	2/44 (4.5)	Rougerie,[42] 1979
	1/10 (10)	Sturm et al.,[45] 1981
	19/109 (17)	Sung et al.,[46] 1981
Acuity	6/120 (5)	Yasargil et al.,[55] 1990
Fields	18/120 (15)	Yasargil et al.,[55] 1990
Hemiparesis	2/17 (12)	Cavazutti et al.,[11] 1983
		Shillito,[44] 1980
	2/109 (1.8)	Sung et al.,[46] 1981
Cerebral infarction	2/106 (1.9)	Svolos,[48] 1969
		Sweet,[49] 1976
		Sweet,[50] 1980
Intracranial hemorrhage		Kanno et al.,[26] 1989
	1/10 (10)	Sturm et al.,[45] 1981
	2/106 (1.9)	Svolos,[48] 1969
		Sweet,[49] 1976
	1/144 (0.7)	Yasargil et al.,[55] 1990
Neuropsychological deficits		
Confusion	2/4 (50)	King,[28] 1979
Memory loss	1/4 (25)	King,[28] 1979
Korsakoff's syndrome	1/38 (2.6)	Kahn et al.,[24] 1973
Mutism	2/17 (12)	Cavazutti et al.,[11] 1983
Psychiatric disorders	7/17 (41)	Cavazutti et al.,[11] 1983
Seizures	2/17 (12)	Cavazutti et al.,[11] 1983
	3/14 (21)	Fischer et al.,[13] 1985
	1/4 (25)	King,[28] 1979
	3/31 (9.7)	Matson,[37] 1962
		Shapiro et al.,[43] 1979
	2/109 (1.8)	Sung et al.,[46] 1981
Anosmia	12/17 (71)	Cavazutti et al.,[11] 1983
		Shillito,[44] 1980
CSF leak	2/14 (14)	Laws,[32] 1980
	1/31 (3.2)	Matson,[37] 1962
	1/10 (10)	Rougerie,[42] 1979
Meningitis	1/9 (11)	Julow et al.,[22] 1985
	3/31 (9.7)	Matson,[37] 1962
	2/106 (1.9)	Svolos,[48] 1969

Table 15-2.   Mortality with Craniopharyngioma Surgery: Primary Resection

Total (%)	Partial (%)	Unspecified (%)	Author(s)
		31/109 (28)	Arseni and Maretsis,[1] 1972
		2/72 (2.7)	Baskin and Wilson,[7] 1986
		4/45 (8.9)	Cabezudo et al.,[9] 1981
		1/43 (2.3)	Carmel et al.,[10] 1982
1/14 (7.1)			Fischer et al.,[13] 1985
1/8 (12)	2/27 (7.4)		Fischer et al.,[14] 1990
0/18 (0.0)	4/16 (25)		Garcia-Uria,[15] 1978
8/25 (32)	0/26 (0.0)		Gordy et al.,[16] 1949
10/75 (13)			Guidetti and Fraioli,[17] 1979
		4/51 (7.8)	Hoff and Patterson,[19] 1972
5/15 (33)	1/5 (20)		Ivkov et al.,[21] 1979
		2/38 (5.3)	Kahn et al.,[24] 1973
0/34 (0.0)			Katz,[27] 1975
1/14 (7.1)			Laws,[32] 1980
		2/100 (2.0)	Laws,[33] 1986
		5/31 (16)	Matson,[37] 1962
0/57 (0.0)			Matson and Crigler,[38] 1969
		1/25 (4.0)	McClone et al.,[39] 1982
		3/26 (12)	Mori et al.,[40] 1980
1/44 (2.3)			Rougerie,[42] 1979
3/22 (14)	4/22 (18)		Shapiro et al.,[43] 1979
	1/10 (10)		Sturm et al.,[45] 1981
		5/109 (4.6)	Sung et al.,[46] 1981
		3/20 (15)	Svien,[47] 1965
		26/106 (24)	Svolos,[48] 1969
2/30 (6.7)			Sweet,[50] 1980
1/23 (4.3)	1/28 (3.6)		Till,[52] 1982
3/144 (2.1)			Yasargil et al.,[55] 1990

the tumor, can result in visual loss. Alternatively, adherence of the tumor to the optic apparatus may result in damage with attempted total excision as neural elements may be removed with tumor. Compromise of the vascular supply to the optic nerves and chiasm with its origin both superior and inferior to these structures also can contribute to visual impairment.[20] Lastly, visual loss has been ascribed to

Table 15-3.   Mortality with Craniopharyngioma Surgery: Resection for Recurrence

Total (%)	Partial (%)	Author(s)
	5/15 (33)	Cabezudo et al.,[9] 1981
	2/17 (12)	Carmel et al.,[10] 1982
	2/7 (28)	Garcia-Uria,[15] 1978
	6/17 (35)	Gordy et al.,[16] 1949
3/8 (37)		Guidetti and Fraioli,[17] 1979
6/24 (25)		Katz,[27] 1975
	(23)	Laws,[33] 1986
5/?		Matson and Crigler,[38] 1969
2/7 (28)		Sweet,[50] 1980

prolapse of the optic apparatus into the empty sella after surgery.[23]

Occasionally patients develop *hemiparesis*. Since the tumor is usually not anatomically related to the corticospinal tract (except with tumors extending posteriorly toward the cerebral peduncles), direct injury to neural structures is unlikely. Rather, vascular injury with resulting distant cerebral ischemia is much more probable, especially in view of the tenacious attachments to the vascular structures in the suprasellar cistern.[49] Cavazutti et al.[11] reported that 2 of 17 patients suffered from postoperative hemiparesis. In another study, less than 2 percent of patients (2/109) developed hemiparesis after surgery.[46]

Cerebral infarctions have also been reported. Functional effects of the infarctions have not always been discussed.[48,50] Sweet[49] discussed two patients who died from infarction due to spreading thrombosis of the basilar artery. He considered the thrombosis to be related to manipulation of the vessels during tumor removal. Two of 106 patients included by Svolos[48] in his series died after clipping of the anterior cerebral arteries during surgery, with resultant infarction. Retractor pressure, with decreased capillary perfusion, may be a factor in other cases.

Vascular injury can lead to postoperative intracranial *hemorrhage,* as well as cerebral infarction. Svolos,[48] for 2 of 106 patients, and Yasargil et al.,[55] for 1 of 144 patients, noted occurrence of intracranial hemorrhage following craniopharyngioma resection. In a series of 10 patients who were treated by a stereotactic approach for intracystic radiation, one suffered an intracerebral hemorrhage when a vessel was punctured by a probe.[45] Thus hemorrhage may result from direct arterial injury. Ligation of draining veins, followed by retraction, may also be associated with hemorrhage.[25,26] Hemorrhage has also been noted to follow episodes of elevated blood pressure from oozing at the surgical site.[49] *Delayed subarachnoid hemorrhage* has been reported; the hemorrhage source is thought to be the blood vessels in the gliosis surrounding the tumor.[49]

Changes in mental status are not uncommon complications of craniopharyngioma surgery. Fifty percent of King's[28] small series of patients suffered from *confusion* postoperatively, and 25 percent had short-term *memory loss.* Korsakoff's syndrome, a more severe memory deficit, was observed in 1 of 38 patients in another series.[24] Anatomical or physiological explanations for these deficits were not suggested. Cavazutti et al.[11] noted that following extensive surgery, 2 of 17 patients suffered from mutism. Seven of 17 patients in the same series had unnamed psychiatric disorders following surgery. Disturbance of hypothalamic connections to the thalamus, frontal lobes, and other cortical areas was invoked to explain these difficulties. *Coma* was observed in 2 of 14 patients; hypothalamic injury was again the culprit.[14]

Seizures may complicate the postoperative course. Cortical irritability may result from removal of adherent tumor or from retraction during exposure. The incidence of seizures varies greatly from series to series. Less than 2 to 25 percent of patients may have seizures.[11,13,28,37,46] For patients who have had subfrontal exposures of their tumors, *anosmia* is a common complication of surgery. Shillito[44] states that unilateral anosmia should be the minimum morbidity expected after subfrontal surgery, implying that it is almost an expected result. Cavazutti et al.[11] found that 12 of 17 patients had postoperative anosmia. This complication occurs with stretch or disruption of the olfactory tract as the frontal lobe is retracted.

Cerebrospinal fluid leaks have occasionally occurred postoperatively. Most leaks, in 10 to 14 percent of cases, result after transsphenoidal craniectomies.[33,42] Disruption of the arachnoid with tumor removal and subsequent failure to perform an adequate dural graft is responsible for the leak. Transcranial approaches may also be complicated by cerebrospinal fluid leak. Matson[37] had 1 of 31 patients develop a cerebrospinal fluid leak after a subfrontal approach. Inadequate wound closure or the development of hydrocephalus may predispose the patient to the leak. Unrecognized invasion of the tumor into the sphenoid or ethmoid sinuses may also contribute to the egress of cerebrospinal fluid.

With many neurosurgical operations, *meningitis* is a feared complication. Patients who have had surgery for a craniopharyngioma are no different. Svolos[48] reported that 2 of 106 patients had postoperative meningitis. Matson[37] had three cases of meningitis after surgery in 31 patients. These patients all had subfrontal exposures of their tumors. After intracystic radiation therapy, one of nine patients of Julow et al.[22] developed meningitis. The incidence of meningitis for craniopharyngioma patients is comparable to the incidence in other neurosurgical procedures.

MORTALITY

Although many series of craniopharyngioma patients do not adequately address all the complications of therapy, most authors do discuss patient *mortality.* Three major issues need to be considered when examining series of surgical mortality. The first is the historical time period of the series, that is, the years in which the patients were surgically treated. A second issue is whether the surgeon attempted a radical, total excision, or only considered subtotal removal appropriate. The last issue is whether the surgical procedure was the first surgical attack on the tumor, or if the operation was for a recurrent craniopharyngioma.

Mortality has been affected by two major technological advances. In 1950, glucocorticoids became routinely available, and in 1969, the operating microscope became an integral component of surgical procedures. Mortality decreased after each of these advances.[40] Examination of the incidence of surgical mortality reported in various series illustrates this trend. Patients in older series tend to have higher surgical mortality. For instance, Gordy et al.[16] reported on a group of patients treated prior to the availability of glucocorticoids. In their series, mortality was 32 percent for primary attempts at excision, and 35 percent after surgery for recurrent tumors. This mortality was essentially the same as that of Mori et al.[40] in preglucocorticoid, premicroscope–era patients. Several studies include patients treated after the availability of glucocorticoids, but prior to the advent of the microscope. The surgical mortality reported by Mori et al.[40] of this subgroup of patients was 26 percent. Svolos[48] reported a 25 percent mortality. Other authors have reported mortalities of up to 15 percent.[1,47] The best postglucocorticoid, premicroscope incidence of mortality is 0 percent in 57 cases of primary radical excision.[38] Once both glucocorticoids and the microscope became widely used, surgical mortality dropped significantly. Mori et al.[40] reported a 12 percent mortality. Other recent series note a mortality after primary resections ranging from 2 percent[32] to 33 percent,[21] but most series have a mortality less than 10 percent[9,13,14,33,39,50] and several have less than 5 percent.[7,10,42,46,52,55]

Surgical mortality rates are higher after surgery for recurrent craniopharyngiomas than in cases of primary resection. This trend is seen regardless of the historical period of the series. Gordy et al.,[16] in the premicroscope, preglucocorticoid era, noted a 32 percent mortality for primary radical excision, and 35 percent mortality after surgery for recurrent tumors. Before the use of the microscope, but after glucocorticoids became available, Matson and Crigler[38] had a 0 percent mortality for primary radical excision in 57 patients, but had five deaths in a subset of these patients after surgery for recurrence. Following routine use of the microscope and glucocorticoids, surgical mortality continues to be higher when dealing with recurrent tumors. Authors have reported surgical mortalities for primary procedure and recurrent tumors, respectively, as follows:

Cabezudo et al.[9]: 10 and 33 percent

Carmel et al.[10]: 2 and 12 percent

Garcia-Uria[15]: 13 and 28 percent

Guidetti and Fraioli[17]: 15 and 38 percent

Laws[32]: 2 and 23 percent percent

Sweet[50]: 7 and 28 percent

A reason for the increased mortality may be the more tenacious adherence of the recurrent tumor to neural and vascular structures.[50] These increased adhesions may result from previous surgical manipulation with resulting fibroblastic reaction or from progressive tumor invasion. Radiation therapy may also increase scarring and adhesions. The larger size reached by recurrent craniopharyngiomas may make safe removal more difficult as well.[50]

Mortality may also be different when comparing attempts at planned radical excision and subtotal excision. Unfortunately, most recent authors have not reported their data so as to determine such a difference. Fischer et al.[14] reported a 12 percent mortality for radical excision, and a 7 percent mortality for subtotal removal. Ivkov et al.[21] had 33 and 20 percent mortalities for radical and subtotal excision, respectively, in their series. In 1949, Gordy et al.[16] had 32 percent mortality after radical excision, and 0 percent mortality in cases treated by subtotal excision. These studies suggest mortality is lower for subtotal resection, presumably due to less hypothalamic or vascular injury. On the other hand, Till[52] reported a 4 percent mortality in 23 patients treated with radical excision and a 3 percent mortality in 28 patients who had subtotal resection. In two other studies, patients treated with subtotal resection actually had higher surgical mortality than those treated with radical excision. In the series studied by Shapiro et al.,[43] 14 percent of radical surgery patients died, and 18 percent of patients treated with subtotal excision expired. Similarly, Garcia-Uria[15] had no deaths after radical excision, but 25 percent of patients with subtotal resection expired. Thus, mortality differences between radical and subtotal excision remain controversial.

Surgery for a craniopharyngioma is replete with risk for the patient; complications are not uncommon. Patients may suffer severe endocrine deficiencies or neurological consequences. Infection may occur at the time of surgery, or the patient may develop severe delayed infections. Death may occur from surgery as well, in a significant number of cases. Many of these complications are related to the characteristics of the tumor, and to its anatomical relationships with critical neural and vascular structures. Avoidance of these complications is imperative for improved patient outcome.

Hypothalamic Hypophyseal Compromise

Michael L. Levy
N. Scott Litofsky
Michael L.J. Apuzzo

ANATOMIC SUBSTRATES

Anatomy of the Sellar and Parasellar Regions

The adult pituitary gland measures approximately 1.2 to 1.5 cm in its greatest diameter. It is seated in the sella turcica and is attached to the hypothalamus via the pituitary stalk, which occurs through an opening in the diaphragma sellae. The pituitary gland is divided into the anterior lobe, or adenohypophysis, and the posterior lobe, or neurohypophysis. Whereas each lobe has a distinctive embryological origin, the two lobes become intimately related during embryogenesis. The pituitary gland develops from two completely different components, the first of which is an ectodermal outpocketing of the stomodeum, which lies immediately anterior to the buccopharyngeal membrane known as Rathke's pouch. The second is a downward extension of the diencephalon, known as the infundibulum. At approximately 3 weeks, Rathke's pouch appears as an evagination of the stomodeum, and then grows dorsally toward the infundibulum. By the end of 8 weeks it loses its connection with the oral cavity and then becomes closer in contact with the infundibulum. Rarely, a small portion of the pouch may persist in the wall of the pharynx (pharyngeal hypophysis).

With further development, the cells in the anterior wall of Rathke's pouch increase rapidly in number, forming the anterior lobe, or adenohypophysis. A small extension, the pars tuberalis, grows along the stalk of the infundibulum, eventually surrounding it. The posterior wall of Rathke's pouch forms the pars intermedia. The infundibulum gives rise to the stalk and pars nervosa, or neurohypophysis. It is composed of neuroglial cells. In addition, a number of hypothalamically derived nerve fibers are contained within the stalk and neurohypophysis.[150] The pituitary and hypothalamus are connected by a stalk composed of glandular, vascular, and neural components. The glandular portion of the stalk is derived from the pars tuberalis.

The vascular components consist of nutrient arteries, the portal venous system, and a diffuse capillary network. Arterial supply to the pituitary gland, median eminence, and stalk is derived from paired superior hypophyseal arteries originating from the cavernous carotid arteries. The portal vessels are then formed by the confluence of capillary loops of the median eminence into veins lying anteriorly on the pituitary stalk. Portal vessels also anastomose with capillaries of the neurohypophysis, receiving direct arterial supply from the inferior hypophyseal arteries.[73,74] Capillary tufts arise from the arteries, which then come into contact with nerve endings of the hypothalamic peptidergic neurons. These peptidergic neurons synthesize releasing hormones. The transport of hypothalamic hormones to the adenohypophysis depends on the integrity of this vascular component. Specifically, the hypophysis is supplied by the superior and inferior hypophyseal arteries. Arterial branches form sinusoidal capillaries surrounding the infundibulum. Blood from the sinusoids passes to the anterior lobe via the portal vessels, which give rise to a secondary capillary plexus in the anterior lobe. The tuberoinfundibular tract ends in the sinusoids of the infundibular stem, transporting neurosecretory substances called releasing hormones, which enter the sinusoids. The supraoptic hypophyseal tract contains fibers from the supraoptic and paraventricular nuclei, which pass to the neurohypophysis.

Neurosecretory products of these hypothalamic nuclei are conveyed directly toward the neurohypophysis. Cells in the supraoptic and paraventricular nuclei produce both vasopressin and oxytocin.

The neural component of the pituitary stalk is composed of the unmyelinated supraoptic hypophyseal and paraventriculohypophyseal nerve tracts. These tracts originate in the hypothalamic nuclei and terminate in the neurohypophysis. This neural component is essential for transport of the neural hypophyseal hormones, vasopressin and oxytocin, to the posterior lobe. Generally speaking, the hypothalamus and pituitary function as two systems, the first of which is the hypothalamic adenohypophyseal system, and the second, the hypothalamic neurohypophyseal system.[199]

The hypothalamic adenohypophyseal system includes the tuberoinfundibular neurons in the hypothalamus. It is believed that these neurons are the source of the hypophysiotropic hormones. They terminate on the capillary plexus of the hypophyseal portal blood vessels. These vessels serve as a conduit for hypothalamic, hypophysiotropic hormones originating from the tuberoinfundibular neurons. The cell bodies of the tuberoinfundibular neurons are located in the medial basal hypothalamus, the arcuate nucleus, the anterior periventricular area, and the medial preoptic area.[154,203]

The tuber cinereum lies upon the ventral surface of the hypothalamus. The median eminence of the infundibulum arises from the tuber cinereum in the midline. This is a specialized region of the third ventricle that gives rise to the pituitary stalk. The primary plexuses of the hypophysioportal blood vessels are contained within the median eminence. These serve as a connection between the terminals of the tuberoinfundibular neurosecretory neurons and the capillaries of the hypophysioportal circulation. Specialized ependymal cells are situated within the inferior walls of the third ventricle. These cells are referred to as tanycytes. The processes of the tanycytes terminate in the median eminence. Thus, a presumptive link between the cerebrospinal fluid (CSF) and the median eminence is established. The function of the tanycytes remains unknown.

Based upon the complex functions of the hypothalamic-pituitary axis, insult may result in severe dysfunction. In addition to the aforementioned roles in the regulation of anterior and posterior pituitary gland functions, the hypothalamus controls water balance, body temperature, level of consciousness, sleep, emotion, and behavior. Thus, a multitude of neurological dysfunctions, alterations in physiology, endocrinopathies, and changes in behavioral states can result from hypothalamic lesions. Endocrinopathies with dysfunction producing such disorders as diabetes insipidus, hypogonadism, hypothyroidism, growth hormone deficiency, and prolactin deficiency only result from lesions involving the median eminence. These lesions interfere with the ability to synthesize hypophysiotropic hormones, in addition to impairing the transport of these hormones to the pituitary gland. Also, varying degrees of hypopituitarism can result from only minimal compromise of the pituitary stalk or gland. Impairment of the pituitary-adrenal axis can produce nausea, vomiting, postural hypotension, and hyperthermia. Complete loss of adrenal function can result in death.[144]

Injury of the Hypothalamic-Hypophyseal Axis

Injury from Tumor Invasion

Preoperative endocrinopathies in patients presenting with craniopharyngioma most often result from direct tumor invasion and/or compromise of the hypophyseal-pituitary axis. Matson's[161] summary stated that the growth of this lesion is not neoplastic in nature, but results from the desquamation of epithelial debris into a closed space and by simple cellular proliferation of the epithelium.

Numerous studies have concluded that craniopharyngiomas result from metaplastic changes in the anterior pituitary cells with spread into the squamous epithelium. This usually constitutes much of the solid part of the tumor.[170] Additionally, certain investigators have proposed that tumor recurrence can occur from remaining microscopic fragments that remain postoperatively.[184] Despite the relative confines of the suprasellar region in which these tumors usually arise, they can grow in any possible direction.

The appropriate surgical approach is determined by the direction of growth. Craniopharyngiomas are most often suprasellar. In the suprasellar region they can extend anterior to the optic chiasm (pushing it backward), beneath the optic chiasm (pushing it superiorly), or posterior to the optic chiasm (pushing it forward and displacing the hypothalamus laterally to either side). In these latter cases the tumor comes to lie within the third ventricle. Sweet[195] reported that 23 of 40 patients he reviewed had tumors that were suprasellar in nature, lying posterior to the chiasm, pushing it forward and displacing the hypothalamus laterally. Steno,[189] in a review of 30 patients with documented craniopharyngioma at autopsy, noted that four of the tumors were intrasuprasellar. Of the 25 suprasellar tumors, 4 were extraventricular, 14 intraextraventricular, and 8 intraventricular.

Craniopharyngiomas that are exclusively intrasellar are rare. Northfield[167] reported exclusive intrasellar tumors in 3 of 37 patients reviewed. Occasionally intrasellar craniopharyngiomas can have a presentation similar to that of a pituitary adenoma. This is believed to be secondary to neoplastic compression of the hypothalamus or pituitary stalk, which prevents the portal system from delivering prolactin-inhibiting factor.[96,122,172] Petito et al.,[171] in a review of 245 cases of craniopharyngioma, found that 12 percent of the tumors extended into the posterior fossa. It has also been reported that cystic tumors can extend posteriorly and inferiorly the entire length of the posterior fossa to the foramen magnum.[183,193] Though usually originating from cells lying on the outer surface of the infundibulum or thalamus, craniopharyngiomas can arise from above the intact hypothalamic floor and lateral walls, thus involving the third ventricle.[92,142,179]

Craniopharyngiomas often grow superiorly and anteriorly, with displacement of one or both frontoventricular horns.[193] Craniopharyngiomas can also have a "dumbbell" shape, with dilatation of the sella and extension into the anterior part of the interhemispheric fissure. Additionally, craniopharyngiomas may migrate along any of the basal arteries laterally into the sylvian fissure, along the tract of the middle cerebral artery, or posteriorly along the posterior communicating artery, with involvement of the brainstem.

Many authors have reported the presence of a dense gliotic covering to craniopharyngiomas that lies between the epithelial neoplastic cells and normal brain. Histologically this pseudocapsule includes an abundance of Rosenthal fibers.[66,200] This dense gliotic covering is considered by many to make total resection of craniopharyngiomas impossible without severe compromise to surrounding normal brain.[170,183] On the contrary, this dense gliotic covering has been viewed by others as potential plane of cleavage that may allow for complete extirpation, without compromise to surrounding normal brain.[144,149]

Bartlett, in a review of 12 cases of craniopharyngioma, found that the gliotic reaction was a feature of only fast-growing tumors. In the slow growing type of craniopharyngioma he noted that there was little reaction to tumor growth, in addition to minimal tissue invasion.[69] Sweet[195] reports on a series of 43 patients, all of whom had attempted radical tumor removal. He decided against complete removal only in three patients. Only one of these patients showed histological evidence of hypothalamic invasion with normal hypothalamic tissue microscopically. This patient died postoperatively, secondary to wound infection and hypothalamic injury. Given his experience, he concludes that a vast majority of patients do have a natural cleavage plane, either through glia or beyond the capsule, which does not include neuronal nuclei or visual fiber tracts.

Controversy continues to exist with regard to histological differences between childhood and adult tumor types. Kahn et al.[138] report a histological childhood type of tumor in 48 of 60 cases reviewed. This childhood type of tumor differed from an adult type, which was found to have a nonkeratinizing squamous epithelium, in that it was more aggressive, with rapid growth and a high propensity for recurrence. Minaka

et al.,[157] in 1985, reported on enhanced survival for adults with craniopharyngioma as compared with children. This included groups both with and without postoperative irradiation. There was no significant difference in survival in patients with either squamous or adamantinomatous cell types. Cogen and Carmel[95] in a review of 109 patients found no histological differences in tumor type. They reported that children had a much better relapse-free survival time following total removal. Children were found to have a 77 percent relapse-free survival at 5 years, and 47 percent at ten years. Bloom[79] also reported on enhanced survival in children, when compared with adults.

Injury from Radiation

When compared with the pituitary gland, the hypothalamus is more sensitive to the damaging effects of ionizing radiation. Despite this, pituitary insufficiency following radiation of the head and neck for various malignant conditions has been documented.[88,98–100,148] The dose of ionizing radiation that results in pituitary insufficiency is variable. Growth failure in children following radiation is the most frequent manifestation.[126,181] Shalet et al.[181] reported diminished growth hormone secretory reserve in 11 of 16 patients following radiation. Amenorrhea, secondary to gonadotropin failure, has also been reported. The occurrence of growth disturbance is so frequent that routine evaluation of all children receiving radiation therapy should be undertaken. Panhypopituitarism in adults has also been reported following radiation to the head and neck. One study reports that 15 of 1,200 patients had evidence of hypothalamic pituitary dysfunction following whole-brain irradiation.[164] Radiation-induced hypothalamic lesions were believed to result in hypothalamic pituitary dysfunction in these patients.

Peck and McGovern[169] report that repeated courses of radiation to resistant acromegalic patients of 9,775, 8,150, and 10,126 rads resulted in gross necrosis of the hypothalamus. Clinical manifestations of postradiation necrosis include localizing neurological signs, dementia, and papilledema. In addition, postirradiation occurrence of gliomas and sarcomas in the brain have been reported.[114,119] Soni et al.,[188] in a review of 34 children treated prospectively with 2,400 rads of cobalt-60, reported no disturbance in neurological or psychological function at 18 months of follow-up. They do report a significant incidence of growth failure.

There is no treatment for radiation-induced brain damage, only prevention. Numerous authors have elaborated on estimates of the maximum dose that can be tolerated by brain tissue. Boden[81] estimated that the largest dose is 4,500 rads in 17 days for small and medium-sized fields, and 3,500 rads in 17 days for large fields. Arnold et al.[61] reported that the dose should not exceed 4,500 rads in 30 days for centrally located tumors. Peck and McGovern[169] report that "the degree of radiation necrosis is proportional to the total size of the dose and time factors in its administration." They recommend a midplane tissue dose of 4,000 rads through stationary fields over 28 days, using 4 × 4 cm portals at the surface. They also report that the radiosensitivity of the brain varies from region to region. The cortex and subcortical medullary region are more sensitive than the deep-seated white matter.

The value of radiotherapy in the treatment of craniopharyngioma has been demonstrated by multiple authors.[80,145,146,194] This has been documented by combining radiotherapy with the tumor biopsy and cyst aspiration. Unfortunately, it is only rarely that studies indicate the degree of deficit caused by radiation. In addition, endocrinopathies resulting from surgery in patients undergoing adjuvant irradiation have not been indicated. Though it is clear in a number of reports that when surgical removal is short of total resection, the addition of radiotherapy greatly reduces recurrence and improves survival rates, the significance of endocrinopathies that occur following irradiation has not been evaluated.

The quality of survival following radiation has been evaluated by Sung et al.[191] and Baskin and Wilson.[70] Results were based on a number of factors in these studies, none of which included postirradiation endocrinopathies. It is obvious that the true origin of an endocrinopathy occurring postoperatively in a patient receiving adjuvant irradiation will be unclear. Sweet,[195] Fisher et al.,[108] and Cavazzuti et al.[93] have all undertaken complete comparative studies with data regarding the quality of survival following radiation. Evaluation of outcome following irradiation includes IQ, frontal lobe function, learning, memory, manual dexterity, general performance, visual status, and residual tumor recurrence. Postoperative and postirradiative endocrinopathies have not been considered. Fisher et al.[108] and Cavazzuti et al.[93] have reported on two posttreatment complications of delayed coma occurring 1 year following radiation in patients treated with radical surgery plus radiation. One patient at autopsy had severe gliosis and cavitation of the infundibulum and mamillary bodies. It is obvious that the hazards of postoperative radiation cannot be overlooked. Radiation necrosis, endocrine deficiency, optic neuritis, and de-

mentia have all been reported as complications of adjuvant irradiation.[143]

Intracystic irradiation involving the use of the Leksell stereotactic system to inject colloidal β-admitting yttrium-90 into cystic components of the craniopharyngioma has not yielded information on postirradiation endocrinopathies to date.[65]

Complete radiation necrosis of residual craniopharyngioma postoperatively has been described at autopsy by Amacher.[57] Weiss and Raskind[204] have additionally reported the presence of pronounced radiation changes in the meninges, brain, and optic nerves on reexploration in two patients. Fukamachi et al.[111] reported on radiation necrosis following treatment of tumors in the sellar region in 40 adults in a literature review dating to 1951.

It currently is evident that only in a detailed review of patients receiving postoperative irradiation (with regard to the establishment of postirradiation endocrinopathies) can the incidence of hypothalamic and/or pituitary compromise be estimated and preventative measures taken. Given the potential for aggressive management and maintenance of the hypothalamic pituitary axis in patients with postoperative irradiation, issues regarding postoperative intellectual function, visual status, and performance are obviously of more importance. Since the onset of endocrinopathies resultant from postoperative irradiation represents compromise of the hypothalamic-hypophyseal axis, it becomes evident that such compromise also needs to be evaluated.

Injury from Surgical Extirpation

Despite Hoffman's comment[130] "that the very nature of the tumor necessitates sacrifice of the pituitary stalk," the preservation of the pituitary stalk is now technically possible using the operating microscope.[86,141,163] Even with gross violation of the stalk, a remnant reaching from the median eminence may serve as a matrix upon which the pituitary portal system may reform.[59] Sweet[195] reports a patient in which he had presumptively divided the stalk a few millimeters above the pituitary gland, but kept it intact upon the hypothalamus. In 18 years of follow-up the patient rarely required antidiuretic hormone. In addition, he reports noting an excessively thickened stalk intraoperatively in one patient, which upon being sectioned yielded a central core of tumor running through the length of the stalk. This required the subsequent sacrifice of the entire structure.

Rarely, intraventricular tumors that displace the optic chiasm anteriorly against the tuberculum sellae, leaving the anterior wall and floor of the third ventricle intact, can lead to preservation of the stalk. Al-Mefty et al.[56] report preserving the stalk in three of ten cases of radical removal of giant craniopharyngiomas. It is obvious that identification of the pituitary stalk is essential, given any attempt to preserve it. One technique is to identify the stalk as it penetrates the diaphragma sellae. Another identifying feature is the stalk's striated appearance, caused by the long portal veins on the stalk surface, which maintain their parallel arrangement even with severe displacement of the stalk.

A multitude of operative approaches to craniopharyngiomas exist. These are determined by the location and size of the tumor, in addition to the degree of calcification, percentage of cystic portions, and placement within the ventricular cavities. Carmel[89] provides a thorough discussion of the many approaches to craniopharyngiomas. A detailed description of the operative approaches to craniopharyngiomas has also been given early in this chapter, so only a cursory overview with regard to the potential for endocrinological compromise postoperatively will be given here. Carmel reemphasizes certain surgical principles that are inherent to approaches to craniopharyngiomas. Extra-axial approaches are obviously preferred to transaxial approaches, with unilateral approaches being preferable to elevation of both frontal lobes. In addition, resection of functional neural tissue is rarely indicated. Approaches are extra-axial and transaxial in nature.

All approaches have inherent advantages and disadvantages. Subfrontal approaches, while allowing for direct visualization of the optic nerves and chiasm, in addition to visualization of the ipsilateral carotid artery, hinder attempts at visualizing masses within the third ventricle or of the undersurface of the ipsilateral tract and chiasm. Pterional approaches are essentially unilateral, and lead to poor visualization of the contralateral optic nerve. The pterional approach does provide for the shortest distance to the parasellar region, with good visualization of the retrosellar region. Approaches through the lamina terminalis allow for good visualization of the anterior third ventricle, and separation of tumor from choroid plexus, although this approach has the highest associated risk of hypothalamic damage. Transaxial approaches also have a plethora of disadvantages. Transphenoidal approaches, though avoiding craniotomy, can be difficult if the sella and pituitary gland are normal. Transcallosal approaches lead to the risk of bilateral damage of the fornices, in addition to inherent difficulty in identifying operative landmarks and visualization of the anterior corpus callosum.

Transcortical approaches usually result in hydrocephalus and also lead to poor visualization of the walls of the third ventricle. Postoperative seizure disorders following transcortical approaches can be significant.

Aside from surgical approaches, certain intraoperative techniques can allow for successful extirpation of difficult to access tumor and preservation of surrounding normal brain. The preservation of the subarachnoid plane can allow for safe and total tumor removal. Excessive use of electrocautery can disrupt this plane. Although cystic tumors should be aspirated intraoperatively, excessive evacuation of cystic contents may lead to redundancy in the capsule, and make dissection of the planes more difficult, with sacrifice of surrounding normal tissue. Excessive use of electrocautery of the anastomotic ring supplying the undersurface of the chiasm and optic tracts could also lead to visual loss, with inadvertent coagulation.

Following gross initial extirpation, remaining fragments of tumor should be sharply dissected from the undersurface of the optic apparatus and hypothalamus. Carmel[89] and Sweet[195] recommend the use of small-angle dental mirrors. Given the propensity of craniopharyngiomas to distribute themselves in a multitude of directions, intraoperative rotation of the head may be required for a better view of potential invasion. Dislocation of normal structures and unusual directions of tumor growth necessitate frequent checks on one's orientation. Intradural arterial bleeding should be avoided, if possible. Thrombosis spreading from one of these sites into the lumina of a major channel can lead to hypothalamic ischemia. It is obvious that tenacious adhesions of tumor to major arteries can preclude total removal. Although blind manipulation of a craniopharyngioma intraoperatively can lead to compromise of surrounding normal tissue, tenacious attachments tend to be anterior in origin, and thus posterior manipulation can be undertaken with relatively minor risk. Continuous retraction on the tumor capsule is recommended, given its propensity to drop back into the third ventricle, with potential loss of intraoperative visualization. Shunting procedures and cyst aspiration have been discussed previously in this chapter.

Injury from Ischemic Compromise

A comprehensive understanding of the anatomy of the microvascular structures involving the pituitary gland, stalk, and hypothalamus are essential in avoiding intraoperative ischemic compromise of these structures. Vascular injury of the hypothalamic pituitary region can result from a number of distinctive disease processes. White[205] recorded the difficulty in distinguishing between expanding intrasellar aneurysms and hypophyseal tumors radiographically. Hypothalamic damage can obviously result following rupture of a berry aneurysm.

In addition, pituitary ischemia can result from apoplexy, ischemic pituitary necrosis secondary to postpartum hemorrhage, diabetes mellitus, and trauma. It is important for the surgeon to realize that ectasia of the carotid arteries can occur quite often in acromegaly. Hatam and Greitz reported 6 of 13 patients with ectasia of the carotid arteries in acromegaly (in Hodgson et al.[128]) Jordan et al.[135] reported on 11 incidental silent aneurysms found in 183 patients with adenomas and craniopharyngiomas. Intraoperative microhemorrhage consisting of subarachnoid blood forced up the perivascular sheaths of perforating arteries can distend these sheaths, leading to rupture into the cerebral parenchyma through the wall of the sheath, forming small hemorrhages. Such microhemorrhages can often be localized in the periventricular and supraoptic nuclei, with subsequent compromise of the hypothalamus. Confluence of these hemorrhages can result in complete destruction of the paraventricular and supraoptic nuclei. It is evident that uncontrolled intraoperative hemorrhage, in addition to aggressive coagulation of the superior and inferior hypophyseal arteries or branches of these arteries, which form sinusoidal capillaries about the infundibulum, can result in postoperative endocrinopathies.

HYPOTHALAMIC COMPROMISE

Hypothalamic compromise, whether secondary to tumor invasion or to operative manipulation, can result in a multitude of complications. Compromise in temperature regulation, cardiovascular function, neural control of food intake, level of consciousness, and memory have all been well described. Following is a brief discussion of potential aberrancies in hypothalamic function following tumor invasion or operative manipulation.

Hypothalamic evaluation of environmental stimuli, and the transduction of this information to neural signals, has been exhaustively studied.[78,125] The preoptic anterior region of the hypothalamus functions as a thermostat containing mechanisms for regulation of heat loss. The posterior hypothalamus integrates heat production mechanisms. Lesions involving the preoptic anterior hypothalamic region will result in hyperthermia, whereas lesions of the posterior hypothalamus lead to hypo- or poikilothermia.

Physiologically, temperature regulation follows two major sources of input. Central input is via temperature-sensitive neurons in the anterior hypothalamus. Peripheral input is resultant from cold or warm receptors in the skin and internal organs. Although emotional feelings of thermal discomfort and temperature sensation do reach consciousness, these feelings do not reflect the activity of peripheral thermoreceptors alone, but rather the integrated state of the thermoregulatory system. The conscious manifestations of thermoregulation are of major importance. These precede the mobilization of the sympathoadrenal response. Numerous studies support the role of biogenic amines, neurotransmitters, and neuropeptides in temperature regulation.[105] Fever resulting from infection is also mediated at the level of the hypothalamus.

Thermoregulatory neuropeptides include thyrotropin-releasing hormone, neurotensin, opioids, somatostatin, vasopressin, and corticotropin-releasing hormone. Disorders of thermoregulation in humans resulting from tumor invasion are usually central in nature. Central hypothermia may be either chronic or periodic, with craniopharyngioma resulting in chronic hypothermia. The majority of patients will have a structural lesion involving either the posterior aspect of the hypothalamus or the entire hypothalamus. This is compatible with the belief that this region functions to integrate thermoregulatory cold defense mechanisms. Spontaneous periodic hypothermia has also been described, though this is not likely to result from craniopharyngioma.[116]

Hypothalamic disease may also precipitate cardiovascular compromise. The maintenance of arterial blood pressure and heart rate is based upon the delicate interaction by the sympathetic and parasympathetic nervous systems.[139] Changes in volume, blood pressure, FiO_2, and PCO_2 are detected by receptors lying in the heart, lungs, and large resistance vessels. Reflex arcs to the medullary centers travel through the ninth and tenth cranial nerves, with termination in the nucleus tractus solitarius. In patients with acute onset of subarachnoid hemorrhage, cerebral ischemia, central nervous system tumors, or following neurosurgical intervention, a number of cardiac disturbances have been reported. These include ventricular flutter, ventricular fibrillation, paroxysmal ventricular contractions, supraventricular tachycardias, and sinus arrhythmias.[196] Electrocardiographical changes have also been reported. These include prolongation of the ST segment, prolongation of the QT interval, and various manifestations of abnormal T waves and QRS complexes. The pathophysiology of these cardiac disturbances remains unclear. It is likely that arrhythmias may result in central sympathetic nervous system activation. It is unclear whether such control is secondary to sympathetic responses elicited by hypothalamic stimulation or vagal cholinergic mechanisms.[104,110]

The neural control of food intake is related to both pituitary and hypothalamic mechanisms. In 1901 Frohlich[110] described a case of hypogonadism with associated obesity in a 14-year-old boy with a documented pituitary tumor. Although obesity was initially thought to be solely related to pituitary dysfunction, Erdheim[103] later was able to reproduce similar syndromes following induction of hypothalamic lesions. Obesity associated with hypogonadism and hypothalamic dysfunction is currently well recognized. A detailed case by Reeves and Plum[175] documents the association of a dysfunctional affect, characterized by unprovoked rage and overt aggression, in a patient with obesity associated with hypogonadism. The patient had a hypothalamic lesion that produced hyperphagia and obesity. The lesion destroyed the ventral medial nucleus bilaterally, in addition to invading the median eminence. Pathologically the mass was a hamartoma. The patient was a 28-year-old female with excessive appetite, hyperphagia, obesity, diabetes insipidus, amenorrhea, and a dysfunctional affect. Diabetes insipidus is frequently associated, and lesions of the tuberal and medial eminence are also frequently described.[76]

The hypothalamus is noted to have significant involvement in food intake. Noradrenergic fibers from the brainstem project to the lateral hypothalamus and the limbic forebrain. Lesions of the noradrenergic fibers can interfere with normal feeding. α-Stimulation results in enhanced feeding. The ventral medial hypothalamus is connected with the limbic forebrain and the brainstem. Interactions between a feeding center are presumptively present in the lateral hypothalamus, and a ventral medial hypothalamic satiety center may also exist.[159] Certain peptide hormones also regulate food intake. These include cholecystokinin, insulin, opiates, and thyrotropin-releasing hormone. Currently tumor necrosis factor has been identified in multiple tumor types. Tumor necrosis factor has also been noted to induce anorexia and weight loss in experimental animals. It is currently believed that tumor necrosis factor elicited from tumors involving the central nervous system may also lead to anorexia and weight loss in humans.[75,76]

Hypothalamic dysfunction may also result in decreased levels of consciousness. One of the first reports of a decreased level of consciousness resulting from a hypothalamic lesion was by Gayet, in 1875 (cited in Victor et al.[202]). This most likely represents a case of Wernicke's encephalopathy. Hypothalamic dysfunction has also been implicated in alterations of consciousness ranging from mild somnolence to frank coma.[112,186] Anatomic elucidation of the specific hypothalamic origin of these disorders remains unclear.

Lesions range from the bilateral anterior mesial cortical region to the rostral pons.[173] Unilateral dominant lesions or bilateral lesions of the cingulate gyrus have been reported to result in abulia. This syndrome has also been noted to be resultant from injuries of the hypothalamus and midbrain reticular formation.[166] Such lesions may have been implicated in the case documented by Cairns et al.[87] in 1941, reporting on the clinical findings in a 14-year-old girl with craniopharyngioma involving the tuberal region of the hypothalamus. Following craniotomy with cyst drainage under local anesthesia, the patient had a marked increase in her level of consciousness, with complete retrograde amnesia to the preoperative period. This has been referred to as "coma vigil."[91,97]

A similar case was reported by Fulton and Bailey[112] in a 28-year-old woman with polyuria, polydipsia, and amenorrhea, in addition to decreased mental status. Davison and Demuth[101] reported on a lesion in the posterior basal hypothalamus with prolonged somnolence and hypothermia in a patient with hypothalamic involvement of a glioblastoma multiforme. These studies confirm that precise identification of an anatomical substrate with reproducible alterations in level of consciousness following dysfunction remains difficult. Multiple anatomical levels may in fact be involved. It is most likely dysfunction of the midbrain reticular formation and posterior hypothalamus will add the greatest contribution to disturbances in consciousness.

Hypothalamic dysfunction has also been reported to result in difficulty with the acquisition of new memories. Although lesions of the ventromedial nucleus have been reported to result in memory disturbances, anatomical elucidation remains unclear.[175]

ENDOCRINOLOGICAL COMPROMISE AND MANAGEMENT

The assessment of potential compromise of the hypothalamic pituitary axis is necessary to determine the extent of hormonal disturbance in addition to changes in neuroendocrine and behavioral function. A complete history and physical examination must be obtained. A detailed neurological examination and a mental status evaluation, including psychometric testing, is essential. Physical examination is valuable in revealing clinical manifestations of compromise to the hypothalamic-pituitary axis, with documentation of endocrinological dysfunction.

With elucidation of the complex physiology of the hypothalamic-pituitary axis, multiple tests have been developed to assess secretory reserve. Only those tests that are required for diagnosis and management will be discussed. Tests used for investigational evaluation, and the evaluation of function that is not associated with complications in postoperative management, will not be considered here.

In endocrinological compromise there are marked differences between the pediatric and adult populations. This spectrum ranges from mere replacement therapy in adults with postoperative hypopituitarism to the maintenance and promotion of growth, manifestation of secondary sexual characteristics, and prevention of bony disorders in children. The detailed analysis of results in both pediatric and adult populations is discussed elsewhere, and also will not be considered here.

Endocrinological compromise can be differentiated into neurohypophyseal and adenohypophyseal compromise. These will be discussed in turn.

Neurohypophyseal Compromise

Neurohypophyseal compromise is usually manifested by disturbances in fluid and electrolyte balance. Specifically, the disorders of diabetes insipidus and the syndrome of inappropriate antidiuretic hormone secretion (SIADH) will be discussed.

In the postoperative management of patients one must take into account the replacement of abnormal fluid loss. Fluid loss and electrolyte imbalance must be corrected, in addition to meeting maintenance requirements. This requires the calculation of insensible and sensible losses, gastrointestinal losses, urinary losses, and rapid internal shifts of fluid. Volume depletion of extracellular fluid results from loss of sodium and water, in various proportions, depending on the pathological process. Manifestations include anorexia, nausea, vomiting, apathy, weakness, orthostatic dizziness, weight loss, and alterations in level of consciousness. It should be noted that serum sodium concentration is not a guide to volume depletion, but rather a reflection of the relationship between the total amounts of extracellular sodium and water. In volume depletion, the serum sodium may often be normal. In contrast, the blood urea nitrogen (BUN) is usually elevated out of proportion to the serum creatinine, and the specific gravity of the urine is high. Hematocrit and serum protein concentrations will also be elevated. Treatment is aimed at restoring the contracted extracellular fluid volume by administering solutions to replace lost fluid and electrolytes. With severe volume depletion, central venous pressure or pulmonary capillary wedge pressure monitoring may be helpful.

Extracellular fluid volume excess represents an increase in total body salt and water, and can occur in a variety of states. Manifestations most often include edema and evidence of circulatory overload. Treatment is usually directed toward the specific pathological process. The manifestations of neurohypophyseal compromise usually result from attendant electrolyte disturbances. Specifically, alterations in serum sodium need to be carefully followed both in the immediate postoperative period, and in the long-term treatment of patients with neurohypophyseal compromise.

Hyponatremia usually results in reduced serum osmolality, indicating that the amount of sodium present in plasma water is less than normal. Osmolality is determined by electrolyte concentrations, and can be calculated from serum sodium, potassium, urea, and glucose levels. Symptoms resultant from hyponatremia depend on the rate of fall of the serum sodium, as well as the severity of the hyponatremia. Symptoms usually occur when the serum sodium concentration has fallen below 120 to 125 mEq/L.

Hyponatremia without clinical evidence of dehydration or edema, as in SIADH, can result from craniopharyngioma. Diagnostic criteria include hyponatremia with serum hypoosmolality; less than maximally dilute urine; inappropriate amounts of urinary sodium; normal renal, thyroid, and adrenal function; no clinical evidence of volume depletion or overload (in addition, there should be resolution of all manifestations following fluid restriction); and absence of diuretic use or abuse. Treatment includes decreasing water intake to less than that of sensible and insensible losses until the serum sodium has returned to normal. Subsequently, water may be replaced in amounts equal to that of sensible and insensible losses plus urine output. Use of IV furosemide to induce diuresis, followed by hourly replacement of sodium and potassium, can correct severe hyponatremia in 6 to 8 hours.[124] Replacement of urine sodium and potassium loss is with a 0.9 percent saline, with the addition of 20 mEq/L of potassium. This approach is only of temporary benefit, and is reserved for severe symptomatic hyponatremia. Other drugs, including demeclocycline, lithium, dilantin, furosemide, and oral urea, have also been reported to be effective in the treatment of SIADH.[94,124,176,180]

Hypernatremia, although most often occurring in patients unable to obtain water, may occur if hypotonic fluid losses are replaced by inadequate amounts of water or hypertonic solutions. Manifestations most usually include thirst, though this also may be absent in severe hypothalamic dysfunction. Confusion and weakness, in addition to depletion of urine volume and specific gravity, are also evident unless hypernatremia results from polyuria, as in diabetes insipidus. Changes in the hematocrit may not be evident, given proportionate losses of plasma and red cell water. Treatment is based upon the patient's total body sodium stores. In patients with normal sodium stores, such as in diabetes insipidus, water replacement alone is sufficient. If the serum sodium concentration is less than 160 mEq/L, water may be given orally. If hypertonicity is more marked, 5 percent dextrose and water should be given intravenously. Serum sodium concentration should be followed every 6 hours. One-half of the calculated water deficit should be corrected slowly over the first 24 hours, with correction of the remaining deficit over the subsequent 24 to 48 hours. More rapid correction may result in lethargy, seizures, and/or cerebral edema.

The volume of water necessary to restore serum sodium concentration can be calculated by the body water deficit, which is equal to the normal volume minus the current volume. If salt and water deficit are out of proportion, with associated circulatory collapse, isotonic saline should be administered rapidly until the patient is hemodynamically stable. The patient should then be observed closely in an intensive care unit setting for improvement in skin turgor, cardiac output, and urinary output.

Antidiuretic hormone (ADH) is responsible for the maintenance of serum osmolality and volume regulation. Osmolality is controlled within a narrow range, with a mean 280 mOsm/kg. The addition of vasopressin can increase the serum osmolality to greater than 287. Decreases in volume lead to the release of ADH (specifically with a greater than 10 percent decrease in blood volume). Such decreases can result from postural changes. The plasma osmolality is usually the primary determinant. The set point is modulated through the interaction of glucocorticoids. Manipulations in set point secondary to changes in adrenal activity can lead to the release of vasopressin and the fall in serum sodium. Glucocorticoids inhibit ADH release. Volume control receptors are present in the left atrium, in addition to baroreceptors, which are present in the carotid sinus. It is of interest that postoperative nausea may lead to release of vasopressin, secondary to reflex stimulation of the area postrema.

Diagnosis and Management of Diabetes Insipidus

Postoperative occurrence of diabetes insipidus is most often resultant from sectioning of the pituitary stalk. The occurrence of diabetes insipidus is determined by the level of the stalk section. High section of the pituitary stalk results in ADH deficiency, since some axons of the supraoptic hypophyseal tract terminate on blood vessels high in the stalk or in the median eminence. Neurons connecting with the neural lobe converge superficially in the upper stalk and median eminence; they are extremely vulnerable to destruction. ADH deficiency may result from direct intraoperative sectioning of the stalk, aggressive intraoperative manipulation and mobilization of the stalk, tumor invasion by way of the vascular mantle or infundibulum, postoperative basilar meningitis, intraoperative vascular damage of the circle of Willis (specifically that of the anterior infundibulum or supraoptic nuclei) or following intra- or postoperative hemorrhage, with anorexia to the supraoptic neurohypophyseal system, and neuronal death. As previously noted, the diagnosis may not relate to presence of thirst alone, secondary to severe hypothalamic compromise. Hypovolemia, hyperosmolality, hyperpnea, fever, stupor, coma, and progression to death can also become manifest.

In diagnosing a deficiency of antidiuretic hormone, one must initially prove that water restriction is ineffective in decreasing urine output and increasing concentration, in addition to proving that the kidney can respond to direct stimulation by ADH. Subcutaneous vasopressin (Pitressin, 5 units) or d-arginine vasopressin (DDAVP) should be initiated if serum osmolality is increased from 300 to 500 mOsm/L, or if specific gravity becomes more than 1.011. We recommend DDAVP since it has no cardiac pressor activity.

Treatment involves matching oral and intravenous fluids in addition to strict observation of total fluid intake and output. Electrolyte levels must also be closely followed. Although treatment with vasopressin and vasopressin and tannate in oil have been reported, we recommend treatment with DDAVP nasal insufflation. DDAVP is resistant to plasma degradation, and its prolonged action requires only bid dosing. Initial treatment is with 2.5 μg, given each evening, with increases by 2.5-μg increments until the patient can sleep comfortably throughout the night without continued nocturia.[94] Smaller supplemental dosages can be given during the daytime until the dose becomes greater than 1.5 to 2 times the nighttime dose. When this occurs the entire regimen will need to be increased.

Diagnosis and Management of SIADH

In SIADH, the level of ADH is usually only slightly increased. Pathology results from continued ADH secretion despite a hypoosmolar state. Thus, there is a derangement of the osmoreceptor-ADH control. The continued intake of fluids when associated with increases in ADH leads to fluid retention and excessive body water increase. SIADH may result from excessive release of ADH from neurohypophyseal systems, secondary to suprahypothalamic disease. This can result from cerebral contusion, from a tumor, or from neurosurgical intervention. SIADH may also result from hypothalamic disease, which results in a leak of ADH from the supraoptic neurons. SIADH following injury to the hypothalamus most readily apparent postoperatively, following intraoperative vascular compromise, hemorrhage, or pre- or postoperative subarachnoid hemorrhage. Suprahypothalamic compromise is most often resultant from infarct or infection. Certain drugs may lead to secondary SIADH. These include morphine, Tegretol, and barbiturates.

Robertson[17] reported on four types of SIADH, two of which are of interest in the neurosurgical patient. The response of vasopressin to osmotic stimulation of the osmole receptors is linear with a low threshold. Type II disease represents a resetting of these osmole receptors. Type III disease represents a continuous leak of vasopressin, despite normal osmole regulation. Thus, vasopressin can increase in hyponatremic states, but responds only to changes in plasma osmolality at normal thresholds of 280 to 285 mOsm/kg.

Manifestations of disease are usually apparent when the serum sodium is less than 120 to 125 mEq/L. These include anorexia, nausea, vomiting, lethargy, irritability, inattentiveness, forgetfulness, and paranoia. At levels of serum sodium of 100 to 110 mEq/L, stupor, coma, and seizure may result. The critical factor is the total level of brain water.[180]

Treatment includes fluid restriction to 400 to 600 ml/day. In addition to being therapeutic, this can also be diagnostic. Electrolytes should be evaluated every 6 hours. If neurological compromise persists, hypertonic saline, 3 to 5 percent, should be administered.[124] If adrenocortical deficiency accompanies SIADH, glucomineralocorticoids should be administered. Rapid drops in serum sodium to 125 have been associated with a 50 percent mortality.[60] Rapid correction of markedly decreased serum sodium has been reported to result potentially in central pontine myelinolysis. Central pontine myelinolysis is manifested by lesions in the white matter of the centrum semiovale.[107]

We recommend that no immediate correction be undertaken in those patients presenting with serum sodium concentrations of more than 120. With serum sodium ranging from 105 to 120, a level of 125 to 130 should be approached, with changes in serum sodium at approximately 2 mEq/h. With decrease in serum sodium to levels less than 105, a correction of 20 mEq should occur at 2 mEq/h initially.[53,132] Drug management includes lithium, which interferes with vasopressin action on the kidney at serum levels of 0.3 to 0.6 mEq/L and desmocycline, 600 to 1,200 mg each day, which has an onset within 5 days, and acts for 10 days following discontinuation. Side effects include renal damage and photosensitization. Treatment protocols including the use of naloxone and Dilantin have also been reported.

Adenohypophyseal Compromise

Management of Acute Hypopituitarism

Whether secondary to prolonged deficiencies in adrenocorticotropic hormone (ACTH) or occurring in postoperative patients with the acute onset of stressors (i.e., infection) the acute treatment of severe hypopituitarism represents a clinical emergency. Adrenocorticotropic hormone deficiency is best treated with glucocorticoids. Initiation of treatment should be with intravenous hydrocortisone, in doses exceeding 5 to 10 times the current replacement dose for the patient. Intramuscular injection is more erratic, and less dependable. Oral administration is only minimally more efficacious than intramuscular injection, and is not possible in an emergency situation. Rapid replacement with large doses of corticoids may lead to euphoria, and other mental status changes, in patients with long-standing hypopituitarism. Such replacement should be avoided unless clinical emergency exists.

In coma resultant from pituitary insufficiency, both corticoid and thyroid hormone replacement should be initiated. Complications associated with rapid thyroid hormone replacement, including cardiac disturbances, will necessitate close observation during administration. The potential for precipitation of coronary insufficiency or myocardial infarction must be weighed against the occurrence of myxedema coma. It is recommended that IV administration of thyroid hormone, 15 μg/day of T_3 or 150 μg/day of T_4 be administered. This dose can then be decreased after 3 to 4 days of treatment to 50 to 100 μg thyroxine/day, and in 7 to 10 days following initiation of treatment, replacement can be administered in the usual fashion.

Growth Hormone Compromise

Normal growth hormone (GH) secretion ranges from basal levels of less than 1 ng/ml to 5 ng/ml in the early morning. Bursts of secretion can occur throughout the day. These bursts range from 20 to 50 ng/ml and are most pronounced during the early stages of sleep. Elevations peak during adolescence, and wane with increasing age.

GH levels are extremely sensitive to adenohypophyseal compromise and are usually the first to respond to dysfunction. In children GH deficiency results in stunted growth and potential dwarfism. Skeletal maturation is also delayed. Symptoms are not as readily evident following hyposecretion in the adult. Given the sensitivity of GH, evidence of diminished reserve may be the first endocrinological abnormality to be documented following surgery or radiation.[77,118,177]

The loss of the antiinsulin properties of GH may result in hypoglycemia, especially after fasting. This can also occur with concurrent adrenocortical dysfunction. The reserve has also been found to be influenced by steroid administration and obesity.[206] Endocrinological diagnosis of GH insufficiency can be made with the insulin hypoglycemia test (IHT), clonidine test, L-dopa test, and growth hormone-releasing hormone (GRH) test.[159]

With significant hypoglycemia (less than 50 percent of baseline) following the administration of intravenous insulin, stimulation of release of GH (in addition to ACTH and prolactin) will occur in 30 to 60 minutes. Abnormal response of GH is indicative of compromise to the hypothalamic-pituitary axis. The patient is placed NPO at midnight, and an IV dose of 0.1 U/kg of crystalline zinc insulin is administered. Dosage will range from 0.05 U/kg in those patients with likely insufficiency to 0.15 U/kg in resistant patients. Preadministration serum glucose and GH levels, in addition to levels at 30, 60, 90, and 120 minutes, are obtained.

Failure of GH to increase in response to the insulin-induced hypoglycemia is indicative of insufficiency, although 10 to 15 percent of normal patients may fail to have a response. Normal reserve will be evident by rapid increases in serum GH levels to above 10 ng/ml. Response to hypoglycemia may also be suboptimal in patients with gonadotropic insufficiency. This is one of the most useful tests in assessing GH reserve and the integrity of the hypothalamic-pituitary axis.

Following administration of insulin the patient requires close observation. Should neurological signs or symptoms develop, intravenous glucose will need to be given immediately. Patients with the potential for hypopituitarism and/or adrenocortical insufficiency will require aggressive monitoring following induced hypoglycemia. Elderly patients, those with cardiac compromise, and patients with labile seizure disorders should not be tested with hypoglycemia. In these cases, alternative tests are required.

The clonidine and L-dopa tests have fewer potential complications, and can be used instead of induced hypoglycemia. Clonidine is an α-agonist that stimulates release of GRH. The patient is placed NPO at midnight, and 0.025 mg of clonidine is given orally in the morning. Baseline and postadministrative serum GH levels are evaluated at 30, 60, 90, and 120 minutes. Maximal response of a 5 ng/ml increase in GH is evident at approximately 60 minutes in patients without compromise.[165] In children an initial dose of 75 μg/m^2 is given orally. Elevations of GH to greater than 10 ng/ml reflect normal function.[151,152]

Direct stimulation of the pituitary to release GH is also possible. The use of the synthetic peptide GRH as a 100-μg IV bolus with serial determination of serum GH levels at 0, 30, 60, 90, and 120 minutes has been reported following an overnight fast.[159] The potential advantage of this test is the ability to discern between hypothalamic and pituitary dysfunction. Responses of GH to GRH are age and sex dependent (women have a greater response than men).[83,84,120,182]

Treatment in adults following evidence of insufficiency is not recommended. Treatment in children is with recombinant GH. This has replaced the use of cadaver-derived GH, given the potential for transmission of Creutzfeldt-Jakob disease. The suggested treatment is 1 mg orally every other day for 1 week, with an increase to 2 mg orally every other day as needed. Dosage regimens remain to be established.

Adrenocorticotropic Compromise

Adrenal insufficiency, whether acute or chronic, can seriously compromise patient outcome. Secondary insufficiency is usually a component of panhypopituitarism. With diminished ACTH, cortisol secretion is also reduced. With chronic disease, atrophy of the adrenal cortex is evident, with sparing of the medulla. Glucocorticoid deficiency is usually less in these cases than that seen in Addison's disease. With the obvious complications of ACTH deficiency, rapid and accurate diagnosis is essential.

Given the variability of ACTH secretion throughout the day, the use of provocative tests is recommended. Diurnal variations in serum cortisol levels necessitate measurements of serum cortisol in the morning and evening to assess for adrenal failure.

Episodic secretory bursts may occur throughout the day. In addition, postoperative stress or stress resultant from prolonged stay in the intensive care unit may disrupt the normal diurnal variation. Normal AM serum cortisol levels range from 10 to 25 μg/dl, with a trough of less than 10 μg/dl. Morning values of less than 6 μg/dl usually represent either insufficiency or failure. The most accurate indication of basal secretion can be determined in a 24-hour collection of urine unbound cortisol. Levels of less than 15 μg are usually observed in insufficiency. Upon observing diminished AM cortisol levels and 24-hour urine unbound levels, provocative testing should be initiated.[190] Provocative tests include the ACTH stimulation test, the metyrapone test, and the insulin hypoglycemia stress test.

The ACTH test is used to discern between adrenal and pituitary failure. Synthetic ACTH is given as a 250-μg IV dose over 4 to 8 hours, in 500 ml of 5 percent dextrose-normal saline. Pre- and postchallenge serum cortisol levels and 24-hour urine 17-hydroxysteroid levels are measured. The 1-hour cortrosyn test can be used initially to test for ACTH and adrenal failure. Given the population of patients being discussed, tests of pituitary ACTH reserve are more appropriate, and will be discussed here.

Metyrapone inhibits the enzyme 11-β-hydroxylase, which is integral in cortisol synthesis.[127] Both hypothalamic and pituitary compromise may lead to an abnormal response, and thus, metyrapone is ineffectual in distinguishing between the two. Metyrapone, 750 mg IV, is administered every 4 hours for 24 hours.[190] Normal response is a compensatory increase in ACTH and steroid synthesis, and thus, postadministration urinary 17-hydroxycorticosteroid levels should increase by more than 100 percent, when compared with preadministration levels. Failure of this response is indicative of insufficiency. Vasopressin and insulin stress testing also fail to differentiate between hypothalamic and pituitary insufficiency. The insulin stress test has already been described. It must be reiterated that this test is dangerous in the elderly and those patients with cardiac compromise. Patients with suspected insufficiencies should always be pretreated with glucocorticoids prior to initiation of a stress test.

Following documentation of ACTH deficiency, rapid initiation of replacement is essential. Serious compromise may result, secondary to postoperative stressors in these patients.[201] We use prednisone replacement therapy, given its low cost and longer half-life. Attendant aldosterone (mineralocorticoid) deficiency is extremely rare, and only rarely is synthetic mineralocorticoid replacement given (desoxycorticosterone, corticosterone acetate, or fludrocorti-

sone). Maintenance dosage in patients ranges from 2.5 mg orally twice a day to 2.5 mg orally three times a day. These patients must be followed closely as outpatients, with close attendance to serum sodium, weight, appetite, and blood pressure. In the presence of significant stressors, either pre- or postoperatively, dosage regimens should be increased to 5 mg orally twice a day, or 5 mg orally three times a day.

Thyrotropic Compromise

Thyrotropin-releasing hormone (TRH) has traditionally been used to diagnose hypothalamic pituitary dysfunction.[71,72] In the evaluation of abnormality, adjustments need to be made for age and sex.[72,102,106] Usually, 500 μg of TRH is administered as a bolus, given intravenously over 30 seconds. Baseline serum determinations of thyroid-stimulating hormone (TSH) and T_3 are obtained. Serial determinations at 15, 30, 60, and 90 minutes are obtained following administration. Hypothalamic dysfunction will be manifested by delayed peak response. Side effects of these tests include hypertension, hypotension, urinary urgency, and reports of loss of consciousness (in two cases).[58,85] Unfortunately, the TRH test is more effective in the differential diagnosis of hyperthyroidism. It is more difficult to differentiate hypothalamic from pituitary disease, given the variability of response to TRH.[71,102]

GH levels have also been found to have an inverse relationship to TSH response. TRH can be used to assess prolactin reserve. Prolactin responds in similar fashion to a TRH challenge, as does TSH. Other factors that increase TRH-induced TSH release, other than hypothyroidism, include renal failure and sex (greater response in females during luteal phase of cycle).

Secondary hypothyroidism is a failure of pituitary TSH secretion. These patients have minimal to absent TSH levels, and do not respond to TRH.[187] Hypothalamic hypothyroidism (tertiary) may result from hypothalamic neoplastic invasion, trauma, or ischemia to the pituitary stalk. Diagnosis of tertiary hypothyroidism is based upon decreased thyroid function, minimal to absent serum TSH levels, and a normal or increased response to TRH challenge.

TRH is released from the hypothalamus, and stimulates pituitary release of TSH. TSH activates iodine uptake by the thyroid and synthesis and release of T_4 and T_3. Circulating thyroid hormone exerts negative feedback at the level of the pituitary, and possibly hypothalamus. Serum T_4 is measured by protein-binding assay or radioimmunoassay, as is TSH. It should be noted that Dilantin may decrease T_4 and T_3 levels in euthyroid patients.

The objective of treatment of thyroid dysfunction is restore a normal metabolic state. Full replacement of thyroid hormone is accomplished with 100 to 200 $\mu/g.day$ of L-thyroxine. In medically stable patients restoration need not be rapid, and treatment with 100 to 200 μg orally each day of synthetic L-thyroxine will restore normal metabolism. In patients with long-standing pituitary disease, and in the elderly, gradual replacement is indicated. This is based upon the potential of precipitating cardiac arrhythmias and potential for angina following rapid replacement. It is recommended that T_4 be started at 25 μg orally each day for 2 weeks, with increments to 50 μg orally each day for 2 weeks, and increments of 50 μg orally each day at 2-week intervals until replacement is achieved. Measurements of serum T_3 and T_4 levels are an accurate reflection of treatment.

Following surgery, trauma, or infection, rapid treatment of hypothyroidism may be indicated. Correction should be as rapid as possible, allowing for reasonable risk. Treatment with L-iodothyronine (T_3), 50 to 100 $\mu g/day$, in divided doses, should begin immediately. If the parenteral route is required, levothyroxine (100 to 200 μg each day) can be given intravenously.

Myxedema coma is the most severe complication of hypothyroidism. It is usually characterized by myxedema, stupor, hypotension, bradycardia, hyponatremia, hypoventilation, and seizure. Hypothermia is usually also present. The rapid initiation of treatment is essential, given the severity of the disease and its potential sequelae. Treatment is based upon the maintenance of vital functions, thyroid replacement, and treatment of precipitating factors (i.e., infection).

Gonadotropic Compromise

For gonadotropic compromise, treatment in males is effective with testosterone, 12 to 15 mg IM every 2 to 3 weeks.[158] Testosterone enanthate or proprionate can be substituted in a similar regimen. Oral administration of fluoxymesterone is hampered by irregular absorption, and has been reported to cause cholangitis. Management of replacement is based upon preservation of libido, potency, and beard growth. Long-standing deficiency may require prolonged therapy prior to restoration of libido. The full return of function may sometimes never occur.

In women, replacement therapy is accomplished with administration of estrogen (this can be ethinyl estradiol, 10 to 15 μg orally each day for 25 days, followed by induction of menses through administration of oral progestin on days 21 to 25). We prefer medroxyprogesterone, 5 to 10 mg orally each day.

Some regimens substitute oral contraceptives for replacement, with the stipulation that 10 to 20 $\mu g/day$ of estradiol also be administered. Transdermal estrogen preparations are also currently available. These preparations avoid hepatic metabolism, and the stimulation of angiotensinogen (hypertension) and low-density lipoproteins (atherosclerosis). It is currently recommended that women taking estrogenic hormones also take progestin to induce menses, given its ability to reverse endometrial hyperplasia caused by estrogen. This is believed to counter the increased risk of endometrial carcinoma in women undergoing chronic estrogenic replacement. Regular annual gynecological exams are also recommended. Pap smears and breast exams should also be undertaken biannually. Estrogen replacement will maintain secondary sexual characteristics, breast size, and vaginal secretions, in addition to decreasing the risk of osteoporosis.

Long-acting testosterone enanthate or proprionate are required for return of adrenal androgen secretion and return of libido. Dosage is up to 25 mg intramuscularly every 4 to 6 weeks. The optimal dosage regimen (as with estrogen replacement) is the minimal amount required to remain effective. Excessive testosterone replacement can be manifested by hirsutism. The management of infertility is not within the realm of neurosurgical care and will not be discussed here.

Secondary, or hypogonadotrophic, hypogonadism results from compromise of the hypothalamic pituitary axis. Gonadotrophic secretion is low, secondary to gonadal steroidal deficiency. The differentiation of pituitary versus hypothalamic origin can be difficult in the absence of other findings.[67] Hypothalamic deficiency of gonadotropin-releasing hormone (GnRH) causes a reduction in sensitivity of the pituitary to GnRH. Only GH levels are more sensitive to compromise at the hypothalamic pituitary axis. Even mild compromise usually results in amenorrhea and hypogonadism. Laboratory evaluation includes serum testosterone, estradiol levels, luteinizing hormone (LH), and follicle-stimulating hormone (FSH).

HISTORICAL EVALUATION

Pre- and Postoperative Endocrinological Compromise

Given the multitude of studies evaluating patient morbidity and mortality following surgical intervention for craniopharyngioma in both adults and children one would expect an accurate evaluation of endocrinological compromise resulting from surgery and/or irradiation. Unfortunately, this is not necessarily the case. Few studies elucidate on specific pre- and postoperative endocrinological compromise in the patient populations. In those studies that do, the consideration of surgical approach, specific tumor histopathology, and radiographic appearance have not been included.

Despite these shortcomings, an attempt to evaluate pre- and postoperative endocrinological compromise in patients with craniopharyngioma will be attempted. Endocrinological function following total resection, subtotal resection, cyst evacuation and shunting, and irradiation (external beam versus intracystic) will be discussed. In addition, we will attempt to define differences in endocrinological response between adult and pediatric populations.

The extent of hormone replacement therapy, both pre- and postoperatively, has already been discussed. It is obvious that postoperative diabetes insipidus is commonplace in a vast majority of patients in whom an attempt at radical resection was made. It should be noted that the extent of hormonal replacement does not necessarily reflect the complete endocrinological deficit of any particular patient. Hormone replacement is closely correlated with patient age. The administration of hydrocortisone in a number of studies was instituted only in the presence of stressful stimuli. Delay and/or failure of sexual maturation, decreased stature, and obesity are other examples of endocrinological compromise that need to be discussed. The psychological sequelae associated with such disturbances in endocrinological function have, unfortunately, remained unclear, despite the wealth of literature concerning the treatment of craniopharyngioma.

It remains obvious that in the surgical treatment of craniopharyngioma in children, every effort should be made to minimize potential injury to the hypothalamus, in order to maximize performance as an adult. Surgery should be limited to resection of that portion of tumor that is not adherent to the hypothalamis. This poses an additional difficult question. It is obvious that radiation can lead to further endocrinological and psychosocial compromise in children. Thus, the consideration to delay adjuvant radiation for residual tumor needs to be weighed with the clinical and/or radiographical progression of tumor mass. Intracystic radiation has been reported to be beneficial, when indicated. Current experience in treatment of carniopharyngioma with chemotherapeutic regimens remains unclear and will not be discussed.

Compromise following Total Resection

Hoffman et al.[131] report on a series of 48 children (24 girls and 24 boys). They evaluated endocrinological compromise following total resection, subtotal re-

section, and cyst aspiration. They report that greater than 50 percent of children presented with endocrinological compromise. Specifically, 6 had diabetes insipidus, 9 had short stature, 7 were obese, 2 had decreased TSH levels, and 4 had decreased gonadotrophic function. Endocrinological compromise following total tumor excision was most severe. Postoperative diabetes insipidus was evident in 14 patients, hypocortisolemia in 11, hypothyroidism in 13, and hypogonadism in 4. Normal growth was reported in 3.

Among those patients who underwent subtotal resection and/or aspiration, a total of 11 had diabetes insipidus, 10 had hypocortisolemia, 2 had normal growth, 14 had hypothyroidism, and 8 had hypogonadism. In evaluating their results for total excision, they reported only 1 postoperative mortality. There were 15 survivors, ranging from 1 or 12 years. One patient died of endocrinological complications 2 years after surgery. Eighteen patients had tumor recurrence in the groups receiving subtotal resection and aspiration. Hoffman and coworkers concluded that total excision was the treatment of choice. They suggested that irradiation as an adjuvant should be instituted if signs or symptoms recurred.

Yasargil et al.[208] reported on a large series of 144 patients in 1990. Greater than 33 percent of this patient population was reported to have endocrinological compromise preoperatively. Preoperative dysfunction in growth hormone was present in 32 children and 7 adults. Preoperative obesity was present in 22 children and 19 adults. Amenorrhea preoperatively was present in 11 adults, whereas decreased libido was present in 5 adults. Hypogonadism was present in 2 children preoperatively, and diabetes insipidus was present in 24 children and 8 adults preoperatively. Total tumor resection was reported in 90 percent of patients, with a 16 percent morbidity and a 16.7 percent mortality.

Postoperative endocrinological function was assessed in both children and adults with regard to the presence of diabetes insipidus, substitution therapy, and the integrity of the pituitary stalk. As before, preoperative diabetes insipidus was present in 24 children and 8 adults. Postoperative diabetes insipidus was present in 59 children and 23 adults. Whereas postoperative diabetes insipidus was thought to be permanent in 61 children and 50 adults, it was noted to be temporary in 7 children and 20 adults. Whereas there were no children with normal ADH function postoperatively, 3 adults were reported to maintain normal levels; 56 children and 64 adults required postoperative substitution therapy. Substitution therapy was believed to be permanent in 49 children and 46 adults. No postoperative substitution was required in 7 children and 18 adults.

The intraoperative identification of the pituitary stalk was reported in 35 children and 38 adults. Of these patients, only 19 children and 23 adults were able to undergo operative resection without incurring an injury to the pituitary stalk. Yasargil et al.[208] concluded that the larger the tumor, the greater the potential damage, both pre- and postoperatively, to vital intracranial structures. They suggested that early diagnosis, at the stage when the tumor was still small, improved operative results and the chances for complete removal.

Carmel et al.[90] also conclude that total resection should be the goal of operative approaches to craniopharyngioma. In a series of 43 children, including 19 boys and 24 girls, they reported preoperative decreased growth in 33 percent. Diabetes insipidus was present preoperatively in 4 patients, and 80 percent were reported to have less than median height for their age. Diabetes insipidus following total excision was present in 14 patients. Diabetes insipidus following subtotal excision was present in 19 of 29 patients. Twelve of 34 patients had some return of growth, without requiring GH replacement postoperatively. They reported total excision in 14 patients, who received no adjuvant irradiation. Minimal procedures, including shunting and cyst aspiration, were performed in 9 patients. Eight of these patients underwent adjuvant irradiation. Subtotal resection was accomplished in 20 patients, six of whom received adjuvant irradiation. Survival following total resection in 14 patients was 100 percent at both 5- and 10-year intervals. Survival following subtotal resection in 14 patients was reported at 5 years as 71.4 percent, and at 10 years as 52.1 percent. One patient undergoing minimal resection died before follow-up at 5 years.

Garcia-Uria[113] reported on a series of 38 adults (15 men and 23 women). Preoperative dysfunction of gonadotrophin was reported in 5 patients and preoperative diabetes insipidus was reported in 2. Pituitary dysfunction was present in 22 patients (58 percent).

Total resection was achieved in 18 patients, with no mortality and two recurrences. Subtotal resection was achieved in 14 patients with a 28.5 percent mortality and 7 recurrences at 4 years. Following total resection, postoperative endocrinological compromise increased in 3 patients. The 4 patients with preoperative diabetes insipidus continued to have diabetes insipidus postoperatively. Six patients had postoperative onset of diabetes insipidus, which was reported to be permanent in 3 and transient in 3 patients. Endocrinological compromise following subtotal resection was not discussed.

Katz,[140] in a study with 51 children, reported good results following primary radical excision and close endocrinological follow-up. Thirty patients were re-ported to have endocrinological deficit preoperatively. All patients had some endocrinological compromise postoperatively. Twenty-one of 31 patients were reported to have panhypopituitarism. Six of 31 patients had more than three hormonal deficits, for a total of 87 percent.

Total excision was possible in 22 patients. Six patients had residual tumor, and 3 patients had tumor recurrence. There were 3 associated nonoperative deaths. In consideration of the postoperative condition of the patient in relation to their endocrinological deficit, they reported on excellent recovery in 12, good recovery in 9, fair recovery in 9, and poor recovery in 1 patient.

Rougerie[178] reported on a series of 92 children. In 10 patients with intrasellar tumors, postoperative improvement in gonadotropic function was reported in one child and postoperative growth was reported in another. Forty-seven patients were reported to have either intra- or suprasellar tumors. Forty-four patients underwent a subfrontal approach, with 33 considered to have total excisions. In those patients with preoperative diabetes insipidus, no change was found postoperatively. Patients with preoperative obesity were found to improve in four of five cases. Hypothyroidism and hypocortisolemia were frequent postoperatively, and all patients had failure of GH and gonadotrophic function.

Thirty-three patients were reported to have retrochiasmatic lesions, with subfrontal, subtemporal, and transventricular approaches reported. Only two patients were reported to have total excision. Operative mortality was 50 percent, with an 8 percent recurrence rate. Preoperative obesity, polydipsia, and hypernatremia were reported in three patients. Postoperatively all patients were reported to have diabetes insipidus, all were obese, and all had decreased ACTH. One reportedly had normal growth postoperatively, reaching puberty. Three had almost normal growth. They failed to note any improvement following radiation of residual tumor in their series.

Svolos[192] reported on 108 patients (68 males and 40 females). Preoperative GH deficiency was present in 18 patients (15 severe and 3 moderate). Preoperative gonadotrophic dysfunction was present in 74 patients (46 severe, 11 moderate). Twenty-one patients were described as being preadolescent, 18 adolescent, and 35 postadolescent. ACTH deficiency was reported preoperatively in 12 patients, thyroid deficiency in 23, autonomic dysfunction in 2, diabetes insipidus in 27, and obesity in 31.

One hundred and six surgeries were performed. Twenty-five were radical excisions, 53 were subtotal, and 28 were minimal surgeries (aspirations and/or biopsies). They had a 25 percent operative mortality, with 19 endocrinologically related deaths. In addition, he reported 43 recurrences, occurring from 2 months to 23 years. Postoperative endocrinological deficits were present in 50 patients. Twelve patients required postoperative replacement therapy. Only 4 had required preoperative replacement. At the time of the study 30 survivors were reported. Four had diabetes insipidus, 9 had gonadotrophic dysfunction, and 5 had panhypopituitarism.

Hoff and Patterson[129] also concluded that total excision is of greater benefit than subtotal excision and irradiation in a series of 51 patients. Sixteen were children less than 13 years of age, and 35 were adults. Endocrinological compromise was present in 25 percent of children, as was diabetes insipidus and lethargy. Greater than 50 percent of adults were found to be hypogonadotrophic, and 25 percent were additionally found to have diabetes insipidus and lethargy. Pituitary insufficiency was reported in 31 percent of the children and 49 percent of the adults. Postoperative endocrinological deficiencies in ACTH and TSH were present in most patients. Diabetes insipidus was reported to be rare.

Matson[160] also proposed, in 1962, that total excision was warranted in children and subtotal excision was warranted in adults. In a series of 32 patients, 28 of whom were children and 4 of whom were adults, he reported amenorrhea in all adults preoperatively. Diabetes insipidus was present in 2 patients, and short stature in 6. Postoperative deficits were present following total excision in 19 patients and subtotal excision in 10. These included diabetes insipidus in seven, SIADH in 5, and TSH deficiencies in 4 patients. Resumed growth was evident in all but 2 patients.

Follow-up increased the series from 32 to 74 patients.[162] Diabetes insipidus was present in 5 patients preoperatively and short stature was present in 22. Total resection was reported in 44 patients, radical resection in 2, subtotal excision in 11, and other procedures in 18. He reported a postoperative decrease in ACTH in 10 patients, which led to death. Longitudinal measurements of height, weight, bone age, sexual development, ADH levels, fluid intake and output, urine specific gravity, serum electrolytes, and BUN were closely followed in this series. In addition, thyrotropic hormone, ACTH, GH, and gonadotrophic hormone levels were also recorded.

He suggested total excision when possible, reporting numerous problems occurring in association with tumor recurrence after subtotal resection. In addition, he recommended aggressive endocrinological follow-up postoperatively in all patients. Arseni and Maretsis[62] reported on a series of 110 patients, including 56 children. Preoperative GH deficiency was present in 18, and diabetes insipidus in 21 patients.

Primary amenorrhea was present in 4 patients and secondary amenorrhea in 6. Obesity and/or anorexia was present in 6 patients preoperatively. In total, 63 patients had preoperative endocrinological dysfunction. Nineteen patients had total excision, 82 had subtotal excision, and 3 underwent biopsy. There was no benefit following adjuvant irradiation. Preoperative evaluation of anterior pituitary function, posterior pituitary function, and hypothalamic function was accurately detailed. Only vague reports were made as to postoperative endocrinological dysfunction, and suggestions as to mild improvement in the series were made.

Gordy et al.[115] reported on 51 patients including 25 children. In children less than 10 years of age, 11 had decreased height, 7 were obese, and 1 had evidence of precocious puberty. In 12 patients ranging from 10 to 20 years, only 1 had normal growth, 4 were obese, and 5 had decreased GH levels. Twelve patients were reported to have preoperative diabetes insipidus. Total resection in 25 patients was associated with a 30 percent mortality. Subtotal resection in 26 patients was associated with a 52 percent mortality (41 percent believed to be endocrinologically related). Twenty patients were reported to have postoperative diabetes insipidus. This represents a large series reported in 1949, and substantiates the necessity for strict postoperative maintenance of endocrinological homeostasis. Manaka et al.[157] recommends radiation only if total resection is not possible. He reported on 125 patients. Seventy-two were adults and 53 were children. In those patients receiving radiation, 6 had diabetes insipidus and 32 had gonadotrophic dysfunction. In those patients not receiving radiation, 16 were reported to have diabetes insipidus and 53 were reported to have gonadotrophic dysfunction. Twenty-one patients had total resection, 29 had subtotal resection, 42 had partial resection, and 53 underwent aspiration and biopsy.

Sweet[193] has multiple clinical and anecdotal reports throughout the literature. In a series of 99 patients presented in 1980 he reported that endocrinological compromise was evident in 46 children following radiation and surgery. Two of 12 patients died from endocrinological sequelae. An earlier series, in 1976, reviewed 37 patients including 19 children with craniopharyngioma. Thirty patients had total resection and 5 had subtotal resection. There were 5 recurrences and 1 late death secondary to hypothalamic compromise in a child.

A summary of Sweet's and Matson's experience would show that a total of 3 patients suffering from hypothalamic compromise following radical excision were reported. In reoperation a total of 10 patients were reported to have hypothalamic compromise. In

Sweet's report of 43 patients with attempted radical removal operated upon since 1950, behavioral problems were present in 5 of 24 survivors. Five patients were reported to have recurrent behavioral outbursts. He emphasized that multiple late deaths result from failing to follow closely serum cortisol levels and treat associated stressors. In 23 children following total resection, 4 patients (ranging from 3 to 9 years of age) had compromise secondary to suprarenal insufficiency with secondary infection. He recommends doubling or tripling steroid regimens when infection is present.

Kahn[137] reported on a series of 18 patients in 1959. Seventeen had radical procedures. Postoperative diabetes insipidus was permanent in 6 patients, transient in 7 patients, and nonexistent in 5 patients. In further discussion of 5 patients, 3 with deficiency in ACTH levels were reported. Two subsequently died. Three patients were also reported to have global hypopituitarism. Follow-up in 1973 increased the series to 40 patients, including 28 children. Preoperative endocrinological evaluation was not reported, though all patients were found to have hypopituitarism postoperatively. Diabetes insipidus was present in 63 percent of adults.[138] In evaluating survival and outcome, he concluded that adults tended to respond better to surgical excision of craniopharyngioma than did children.

Lipton et al.,[156] in a case report, discusses a transcallosal approach in a 3-year-old boy with craniopharyngioma. The patient had no preoperative deficit but developed diabetes insipidus, hypothyroidism, and hypothermia postoperatively. The patient was still alive at the 1-year follow-up.

Shillito[185] provided another summary of the results of Matson and Sweet in a review of 64 patients. Following initial radical resection, surgical mortality was reported to be nonexistent in Matson's series. Operative mortality occurred in 2 patients in Sweet's series. Mortality following reoperation occurred in 6 of 34 patients in Matson's series, and 5 of 30 patients in Sweet's. Mortality resultant from postoperative hypothalamic compromise was reported in 12 patients in Matson's series following initial radical resection and reoperation. Only 1 patient in Sweet's died from postoperative hypothalamic compromise following reoperation. These results further support the association of severe endocrinological compromise with an aggressive approach to craniopharyngioma.

Till[198] emphasizes that total excision should only be attempted if intraoperative compromise to the hypothalamus can be avoided and is not inevitable. He recommends either staged procedures or initiation of adjuvant irradiation if intraoperative compromise cannot be avoided. In a review of 63 children, 23

patients had total excision, 28 had subtotal excision, and 12 had irradiation. In total, there were 4 deaths related to endocrinological compromise of the pituitary-adrenal axis. In further review of Grant's series, 11 of 116 patients died postoperatively secondary to pituitary-adrenal compromise. Nine were reported to have severe sequelae.

It must be emphasized that the total excision of craniopharyngiomas should be a primary surgical goal. Still, special attention must be centered on the potential for intraoperative hypothalamic compromise. This is even more important in the pediatric population. Subtotal excision in the face of potential hypothalamic compromise is the safest option when considering long-term outcome and devastating endocrinological compromise. Reoperation and/or adjuvant irradiation should be recommended in those patients with obvious subtotal excision and the development of postoperative clinical signs and symptoms resultant from tumor mass. Strict replacement regimens and endocrinological evaluation are essential in all patients in both the immediate and long-term postoperative period following both total and subtotal resection of craniopharyngioma.

Compromise following Subtotal Resection

Gutlin et al.[121] reported on four patients with stereotactic placement of an Omaya reservoir into cystic craniopharyngiomas. An 8-year-old girl with preoperative evidence of diminished stature had a subtotal resection with subsequent cyst aspiration via an Omaya reservoir. She suffered from postoperative hypopituitarism and diabetes insipidus and subsequently died following a third surgical exploration. The second patient was a 33-year-old man who underwent a subtotal resection. He had postoperative diabetes insipidus and hypopituitarism. The third patient reported was a 17-year-old boy with decreased gonadotrophic function preoperatively. No postoperative function was reported following subtotal resection and irradiation.

Hamer[123] also reported on the conservative management of two children. The first was an 8-year-old boy with diminished GH levels preoperatively. Following transphenoidal resection of an intrasellar craniopharyngioma the patient had no change in his GH status. He had no further compromise of endocrinological function. The second patient was a 6-year-old girl with preoperative diabetes insipidus. Following transphenoidal resection of an intrasellar craniopharyngioma, the patient was free from endocrinological compromise postoperatively.

Laws[153] supports the transsphenoidal approach in the presence of an enlarged sella in a report on 26 adults. Preoperative endocrinological abnormalities were represented by the presence of hypopituitarism in 11 patients, GH dysfunction in 10 patients, primary amenorrhea in 4 patients, secondary amenorrhea in 4 patients, galactorrhea in 2 patients, and diabetes insipidus in 1 patient. Operative mortality was 4 percent, representing one intraoperative death and one late death. Postoperative pituitary replacement was required following the first surgery in seven patients. Postoperative diabetes insipidus was reported in two patients. Ivkov et al.[133] also supported the use of a conservative approach. In a review of 38 patients with global intrasellar cystic juvenile-type tumors, 90 percent of patients were noted to have preoperative endocrinological dysfunction. Eight group I patients were noted to have preoperative hypopituitarism. Six group II-A patients were noted to have large tumors and only minimal endocrinological compromise preoperatively. Twenty-four group II-B patients had preoperative hypopituitarism. Seven of 24 patients had diabetes insipidus. Although postoperative endrocrinological compromise was not specifically detailed, they reported that better results were obtained following subtotal excision.

King[142] reported on four patients with subtotal removal through the lamina terminalis. Two of four patients had undergone prior procedures. His series included three males and one female. No preoperative endocrinological evaluation was reported. Three of four patients were reported to have panhypopituitarism postoperatively. One patient was reported to have mild diabetes insipidus while another patient was reported to have permanent diabetes insipidus postoperatively.

Witt et al.[207] reported on subtotal, minimal resection in two elderly women. Both patients had normal preoperative endocrinological examinations. Postoperative ACTH levels were diminished in both patients, and one patient had mild diabetes insipidus. There was no operative mortality or morbidity otherwise reported.

Bartlett,[68] in a series of 85 patients including 30 children, proposed in 1971 that radical resection be attempted if total resection was found to be impossible. Preoperative endocrinological dysfunction was reported in the pediatric group. Diminished GH was present in 40 percent of patients, hypopituitarism in 3 percent, and failure of development of secondary sexual characteristics in 3 percent. In adults, 32 percent of patients had pituitary failure. Six patients had total resection, whereas 112 had subtotal resection. There were 36 cyst aspirations and 22 ventriculostomies placed. Three patients died of late recurrence, anywhere from 17 to 21 years following surgery. Twenty of 73 patients were still alive at a 10-year follow-up.

Grant and Lyer[117] reported a series of 73 children, including 45 boys and 28 girls. Preoperative endocrinological dysfunction was not reported. Fifty-eight patients received subtotal or total excision: 16 of these patients died. Thirteen patients received aspiration with adjuvant irradiation: 5 of these patients died, and 4 had recurrence of tumor. Two patients had no treatment. Postoperative decrease in ADH was present in 46 of 58 patients. Decrease in GH was present in 33 of 42 patients. Decreased ACTH was present in 23 of 35 patients. Decreased TSH levels were present in 14 of 19 patients, and decreased FSH levels were present in 16 of 18 patients. Late deaths were reported in 7 patients. Four patients had hypocortisolemia in addition to diabetes insipidus. Two patients had diabetes insipidus alone and 1 patient had diminished ACTH alone.

Eight patients presented postoperatively for admission secondary to severe hypoglycemia. Six of these patients had diminished ACTH levels in addition to diabetes insipidus. One patient had diminished ACTH alone, while another patient had only diabetes insipidus. Eleven patients required postoperative admission secondary to hypopituitarism. They concluded that the incidence of marked endocrinological deficit with postoperative compromise, and the potential for emergent readmission, was too high with aggressive attempts at surgical excision of craniopharyngioma and recommended subtotal excision.

Jenkins et al.[134] reported the absence of return of gonadotrophic function following prolonged endocrinological dysfunction in their series of 20 patients (6 adults and 14 children). Postoperative endocrinological function was reported in all patients. Postoperative ACTH levels were diminished in 10 patients and diabetes insipidus was present in 5 patients. In addition, all patients but one had diminished GH. Gonadotrophic dysfunction was present in 19 of 20 patients and thyroid dysfunction in 19 of 20. Prolactin levels were present in 15 patients measured.

It is obvious that subtotal excision with sparing of the hypothalamus will preserve a maximum of postoperative endocrinological function. Difficulty in assessing the literature results from the failure of most studies to include accurate pre- and postoperative endocrinological evaluation. Studies also fail to correlate surgical approach and the extent of surgical excision with postoperative endocrinological deficit.

Conservative Management with Adjuvant Irradiation

Thomsett et al.[197] reported that subtotal excision with adjuvant irradiation was associated with less endocrinological dysfunction when compared with attempts at total excision in a series of 42 patients. Accurate pre- and postoperative endocrinological evaluation was completed in all patients. Fourteen total excisions, 11 subtotal excisions, and 17 minor procedures with adjuvant irradiation were reported. Preoperative deficiencies in GH were reported in 13 of 18 patients, deficiencies in ACTH in 4 of 17, deficiencies in TSH in 7 of 29, deficiencies in LH-FSH in 3 of 8, ADH deficiencies in 4 of 24, deficiencies in prolactin levels in 2 of 10, and deficiencies in prolactin-TRF in 1 of 3.

Postoperative deficits in GH were reported in all 39 patients, in ACTH in 30 of 38, in TSH in 35 of 41, and in LH-FSH in 20 of 28. Postoperative deficits in ADH were reported in 29 of 41 patients. Postoperative deficits in prolactin levels were present in 5 of 31 patients and in prolactin TRF in 9 of 14 patients. No patients were reported to be endocrinologically intact postoperatively. Four patients with preoperative endocrinological dysfunction of one hormone were without change. In patients with dysfunction of one to two hormones, 3 had additional compromise postoperatively. Seven patients had additional compromise in three or more hormones postoperatively, and 28 patients had more than four deficiencies postoperatively.

No reversal of endocrinological dysfunction was reported in this series. In 39 patients undergoing total or partial excision, only 3 had normal endocrinological function postoperatively. In those patients with partial resection and adjuvant irradiation, 15 were reported to have normal endocrinological function postoperatively. Thus Thomsett et al.[197] supported conservative partial resection with adjuvant irradiation as opposed to attempts at total excision.

Kramer et al.[146,147] initially reported on a series of 10 patients, including 6 children, in 1960. Preoperative deficits included decreased GH levels in one patient, diabetes insipidus in one patient, decreased gonadotrophic function in one patient, and panhypopituitarism in one patient. In the patient with preoperative decrease in GH, postoperative onset of diabetes insipidus was reported. In the patient with preoperative panhypopituitarism, residual hypopituitarism was evident postoperatively. At a 15-year follow-up, six children and one adult were still alive. The authors reported that they had good results with small procedures and adjuvant irradiation.

The series was increased to 16 patients in 1968, including 10 adults. Preoperative hypopituitarism was present in two patients, with postoperative onset of hypopituitarism in one and a subsequent unrelated death in the second. Twelve patients had subtotal resection, one patient had biopsy, and three patients had cyst aspiration. All received postoperative irradiation. These results further confirm the benefit of

subtotal removal with adjuvant irradiation in preserving endocrinological function.

Sung et al.[191] reported on a series of 109 patients. Preoperative deficiencies in growth hormone levels were present in 30 percent of adults and 9 percent of children. Preoperative panhypopituitarism was present in 47 percent of adults. Diabetes insipidus was present in 8 percent. Postoperatively, all patients were reported to have panhypopituitarism. Diabetes insipidus was reported as being severe in five patients. Fourteen children and 23 adults had total excision, whereas 20 children and 34 adults had subtotal excision. Minor procedures were performed in 9 adults and 9 children. Of those patients undergoing subtotal excision, a total of 6 children and 11 adults had adjuvant irradiation. In those patients with minimal procedures, 8 children and 7 adults had adjuvant irradiation. Tumor recurrence was reported in 22 children and 36 adults.

Baskin and Wilson[70] reported on a series of 74 patients, including 28 children. Preoperative abnormalities in GH levels were present in 93 percent, impotence in 88 percent, amenorrhea in 82 percent, hypopthyroidism in 42 percent, hypoadrenalism in 34 percent, and diabetes insipidus in 23 percent. In this latter group, 12 patients remained untreated preoperatively. Total excision was reported in 7 patients and subtotal resection in 67. Fifteen percent required multiple surgeries. Total excision resulted in one recurrence.

Postoperative deficits in endocrinological function were reported in numerous patients with normal preoperative endocrinological status. Specifically, hypothyroidism was present in 40 percent, hypoadrenalism in 45 percent, and diabetes insipidus in 23 percent of patients postoperatively. Late-onset diabetes insipidus in a subset of patients following irradiation was reported. Remission occurred in 91 percent of patients with seven recurrences to date. There was a 12 percent operative morbidity and 3 percent operative mortality. These data reinforce the use of subtotal resection with adjuvant irradiation.

Leddy and Marshall[155] were among the first to support the benefit of subtotal excision with radiation (1950) in a series of 10 patients, including 3 children. Preoperative mild diabetes insipidus was present in four patients, diminished gonadotropin function was present in three, and diminished GH was present in one. Mild diabetes insipidus was present postoperatively in two patients, while severe diabetes insipidus was present postoperatively in three patients. In addition, two patients had diminished gonadotrophic function, and one patient had diminished TSH. They reported a 20 percent operative mortality, with two additional late deaths. At 3- to 10-year follow-up, six patients were still alive at the time of the series.

Orayama et al.[168] in a series of 30 cases, reported preoperative deficits including hypogonadism in 8 patients, diabetes insipidus in 5, and decreased GH in 1. Total excision was reported in 2 patients, subtotal in 13 patients, and aspiration/biopsy in 17 patients. All patients received postoperative irradiation ranging from 5,500 to 6,000 rads over a 5- to 7-week course. There were no further endocrinological deficits reported in those patients with preoperative endocrinological dysfunction. Five-year mortality was reported at 69 percent, and 10-year mortality at 60 percent.

Fischer et al.[109] reviewed a series of 37 patients attempting to correlate postoperative endocrinological compromise with the extent of surgery. Eight patients were included as group I patients and had total excision. Some patients in this group had adjuvant irradiation, though this group was not further delineated. Group II (six patients) included those patients with subtotal resection and adjuvant irradiation. Group III included 21 patients undergoing radiation or conservative surgery.

Postoperative diabetes insipidus was present in 87.5 percent of those patients in group I, 66 percent of those patients in group II, and 5 percent of those patients in group III. The mean number of hormones requiring replacement was three in those patients in group I, three in those patients in group II, and two in those patients in group III. Long-term mortality was 8 percent, with one patient dying secondary to a hypothalamic crisis. Tumor recurrence was reported to be 14 percent at a 10½-year follow-up. He reported that conservative surgical approaches and irradiation resulted in only minimal hypothalamic compromise.

Cavazzuti et al.[93] reported less frontal lobe dysfunction in patients following irradiation when compared with those undergoing radical surgery. Endocrinological dysfunction was also at a minimum. In a series of 95 patients only postoperative endocrine evaluation was included in 35 patients. Group I patients received conservative management, with associated irradiation, and comprised a total of 18 patients. Group II patients had radical procedures including subfrontal attempts at resection. Eight patients required only one procedure and were designated as group II-A, whereas nine patients who re-

quired more than one procedure and radiation were placed in group II-B.

Postoperative diabetes insipidus was present in one patient in group I, eight patients in group II-A, and seven patients in group II-B. Postoperative complications associated with radiation were present in only one patient in group I. Postoperative endocrinological function was assessed by the number of hormones requiring replacement. Forty-four percent of patients in group I, 0 percent of patients in group II-A, and 22 percent of patients in group II-B required no postoperative hormonal replacement. Hormone replacement was required for one deficiency in 39 percent of patients in group I. All patients in groups II-A and II-B required replacement of at least two modalities. Replacement of two hormones was reported in 11 percent of patients in group I, 37 percent of patients in group II-A, and 34 percent of patients in group II-B. Replacement of three or more was reported in 5 percent of patients in group I, 63 percent of patients in group II-A, and 33 percent of patients in group II-B.

Fischer et al.[108] concluded that subtotal excision with adjuvant irradiation led to less psychosocial impairment in a series of 37 children in 1985. Fourteen patients with total or subtotal resection were placed in group I. Eleven of these patients received adjuvant irradiation. Twenty-three patients with primary irradiation, in addition to cyst aspiration and/or biopsy, were placed in group II. Postoperative endocrinological dysfunction was absent in all patients in group I and four patients in group II. Diabetes insipidus was present postoperatively in 12 patients in group I and two patients in group II. There was one operative death in group I patients. Tumor recurrence was present in two of five patients with presumptive total excision without adjuvant irradiation.

In evaluating postoperative endocrinological dysfunction, it is clear that subtotal excision of tumor with adjuvant irradiation is associated with markedly less postoperative morbidity than attempts at total excision. A number of studies propose the use of intracystic irradiation.[64,136,174] In addition, the use of colloidal gold has been reported.[82] Further experience with these modalities must be reported prior to an accurate estimation of endocrinological compromise following their initiation.

Transcranial Approaches
Peter W. Carmel

The history of craniopharyngiomas has been mired in controversy from early descriptions of this tumor. These unusual epithelial tumors found in the parasellar region intrigued pathologists in the latter part of the nineteenth century.[242] More than one hundred years ago Onanoff[282] felt that these tumors arose from the pituitary gland, and because some of them resembled adamatanomas of the jaw, he coined the term "pituitary adamatanoma." Seven years later, Mott and Barrett[280] postulated that the tumors might arise from the hypophyseal duct or Rathke's pouch. This question appeared to have been resolved in 1904, when Erdheim, in a classical descriptive paper, characterized the histological features of these tumors, and demonstrated that they arose from embryonic squamous cell rests of an incompletely involuted hypophyseal-pharyngeal duct.[242,258,282,284] Examination of squamous cell rests of the pituitary by both light microscopy[229,275] and electron microscopy[268,273,298] seem to support Erdheim's theory. However, Goldberg and Eshbaugh[246] showed that squamous cell rests are found in only 3 percent of neonates, and their presence increases with age, belying a congenital origin. Suggestions that craniopharyngiomas may be tumors analogous to calcifying odontogenic again question their congenital origin.[222,248]

Treatment of these tumors also continues to provoke considerable disagreement.[263] Recent reviews have recommended conservative therapy, such as cyst aspiration followed by radiation,[221,231,243] or reliance on stereotactic techniques such as instillation of intracyst radiation or high-dose radiosurgery,[234,254,260,261] or radical microsurgical excision with the aim of cure.[219,225,226,252,306,311]

Each of these therapeutic approaches will lead to widely differing management decisions. Each approach will have different types of complications that need to be avoided. Those who favor conservative operative treatment have pointed out the complications of endocrine dysfunction, hypothalamic damage, and intellectual deficits suffered by those who undergo radical surgical removal.[231,243,310] Those who advocate radical surgery at initial intervention emphasize the complications of recurrence if the tumor is not totally resected, and point out risks of vascu-litis, development of secondary tumors, and neuropsychological impairment if radiation therapy is relied upon.[209,213,251,269,307,309,311] This chapter examines these controversies and points out the complications inherent in each approach. Knowledge of these complications may lead to steps that will be successful in avoiding many of them.

MICROSCOPIC APPEARANCE

The microscopic appearance of a craniopharyngioma usually shows a well-defined basement membrane separating the tumor from surrounding astroglial tissue. On this basement membrane a band of high columnar cells forms the external tumor layer. Within this layer a second layer of polygonal cells is seen, a central network of epithelial cells that may be of variable depth.[212,293] Regressive changes within these epithelial cells appear to cause liquefaction and deposit of keratin-like material.[336] Matson and Crigler[278] have written that the growth of these lesions is not neoplastic, but rather they grow by desquamation of epithelial debris and simple cellular proliferation of the epithelium. However, these tumors are able to increase in size rapidly by sequestration of cystic fluid.[259] Furthermore, the ability of tumors to regrow rapidly from microscopic fragments left at initial surgery is well documented.[266,289,296,306]

Cyst walls may vary from extremely translucent or even transparent membranes to thick, tough structures that may become hard and rigid because of calcium salt deposition. Calcification is found on microscopic examination in almost half of adult craniopharyngiomas and in the great majority of those in children.[209,217,218,220,286]

CAN CRANIOPHARYNGIOMAS BE TOTALLY REMOVED?

The tendency of these tumors to form villous elongations into the surrounding brain is well documented.[273] However, in most cases these villi do not actually penetrate brain parenchyma but rather are imbedded in the thick glial scar that is promoted at the interface of the tumor and the cerebral pia arachnoid (Fig. 15-1). Sweet[304,306] pointed out that there is a "glial envelope" at the interface between brain and tumor that may provide a plane to dissect the craniopharyngioma safely. Several autopsy reports have shown that the tumor may have minimal attachment to the brain, usually at the region of the tuber cinerium.[251,286]

Most authors who advocate radical removal, including Sweet,[306] Hoffman,[251] Symon and Sprich,[307] and Carmel,[226] have all indicated that the major obstacle to achieving total tumor removal is usually a tenacious adhesion of the tumor to an essential artery on the anterior portion of the circle of Willis. This is in contrast to those who advocate conservative therapy, whose experience indicates that the most complicating factor in attempted aggressive removal of these tumors is damage to the parenchyma.[243,279] Damaged brain includes not only the hypothalamic-pituitary axis but also hypothalamic connections to the thalamus, frontal lobes, and other cortical areas. Complications noted by these authors include not only endocrine deficits, but also uncontrollable anger, aggression, memory deficits, and numerous psychological and social problems.[231]

The author's bias is that radial surgical removal offers the best hope of achieving a lasting, permanent cure. However, the best results concerning tumor remission in a large series of patients with craniopharyngiomas have been reported by Baskin and Wilson.[221] In this series, a less radical surgical approach was taken, and recurrence of tumor was controlled with radiation therapy. There are several large series nearing the reporting stage in which attempted radical removal is combined with extremely low operative mortality and good functional long-term results.[232] Until these series are published, the results of Baskin and Wilson must be regarded as the current standard.

It is apparent that this surgicophilosophical debate will markedly influence the approach taken by the individual surgeon. Management decisions derive from the attitude the surgeon takes toward these tumors, and will alter both the intraoperative and perioperative handling of craniopharyngiomas.

DIRECTION OF GROWTH

Craniopharyngiomas are opportunistic tumors that push along the path of least resistance, spreading along cerebrospinal fluid (CSF) pathways and invaginating the ventricles. The "classic" appearance of these tumors, pushing anterior to the chiasm, while elevating and displacing it backward, and separating the two optic nerves, is found in a minority of cases. It is more usual for these tumors to enlarge behind the optic chiasm, displacing it forward. Those that are directly beneath the chiasm, stretching and distorting it to a thin layer on the surface of the tumor, cause the greatest preoperative visual deficits. In the group that arises posterior to the chiasm, pushing upward into the third ventricle, the invaginated portion is likely to be cystic with a solid calcified portion at or near the basal dura.

Tumors of this configuration pose two particular problems. First, they may be hard to visualize from the subfrontal subarachnoid pathways, as the optic apparatus is pushed forward. Second, the calcified portion is usually within the sella, or immediately suprasellar, underlying the optic chiasm. This calcified portion is very difficult to break up and may pose risk to the optic pathways as the jagged pieces of calcified material are delivered past them.

Craniopharyngiomas especially those that have multiple cysts,[211] may spread in several directions. An analysis of 19 multicystic craniopharyngiomas in our series of 98 operated cases showed that posterior fossa extension was found in 9 of 72 children (13 percent). Petito et al.[281] analyzing a large series of adult and children's craniopharyngiomas in the files of the Armed Forces Institute of Pathology (AFIP), recorded similar percentages.

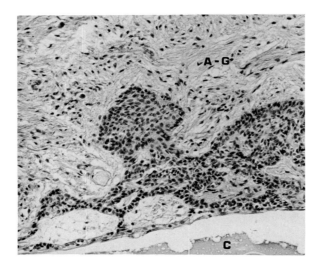

Figure 15-1. Photomicrograph of craniopharyngioma/brain interface. The cystic portion of the tumor is seen at the bottom of the picture (*C*). The tumor epithelium has sent out a "pseudopod" into the surrounding brain tissue. However, it can be seen that this projection of tumor does not penetrate into neural tissue but is largely embedded in an astroglial layer (*A–G*). Sweet[306] has suggested that this layer may provide a natural plane of cleavage between the tumor and the brain parenchyma that will safely permit removal of the tumor.

Neither the size of the cysts, their location, multiple loculations, or CSF pathway obstruction adversely influenced possible total removal of tumor. Those tumors that had calcified walls, particularly when adherent to basal dura or arteries of the anterior circulation, had a lesser chance of total removal. Two children in our series died years after initial surgery, and both deaths were related to recurrent posterior fossa or cerebellar-pontine angle cystic tumors. This unusual subgroup of posterior fossa cystic tumors is a difficult group to treat and the lethal implications of cysts in this location must be kept in mind.

Cystic tumors may have extremely fragile capsules.[296] Sweet[296] has recommended making every effort to preserve the capsule arachnoid so that after intracapsular removal, the sheaths remain even if torn, and the surgeon will avoid leaving behind torn-off bits of thin capsule.[296] Kobayashi et al.[260] have described clinical recurrences when a total removal was thought to have been achieved and have attributed this to fine scraps of tumor left behind at initial surgery.

PREOPERATIVE RADIOLOGICAL EVALUATION

Almost all craniopharyngiomas have their origin from cells in the pituitary stalk. Despite this common origin, the configuration, geometry, and growth patterns vary enormously. In order to select the proper operative approach, initial operative procedure, and evaluation for potential for staging meticulous radio-

logical evaluation of these lesions is necessary. Scans in a single plane are not adequate to evaluate craniopharyngiomas (Fig. 15-2).

The diagnostic procedures currently most employed are computed tomography (CT) and magnetic resonance imaging (MRI). Both are useful in demonstrating the mass of the tumor, its relationship to the ventricular system, major cranial arteries, and general configuration of the tumor. Enhancement with contrast injection often will bring out poorly defined cyst walls, and will allow excellent visualization of the solid portions of the tumor. MRI has the additional facility of varying imaging sequences allowing an estimation of the content of cystic cavities. Tumor cysts may be lucent or signal-intense on CT or MRI, depending on protein content or suspension of calcium salts within the tumor cyst fluid. The sagittal view on MRI is extremely useful, permitting definition of the relationship between the tumor and the optic nerves and chiasm.

It is important on the sagittal and coronal views on both types of scan to discern whether the tumor abuts the CSF pathways in the suprasellar region. Mnay tumors that seem to be wholly within the third ventricle are, in fact, visible in the suprasellar cisterns (Fig. 15-3). These tumors often may safely be removed by a totally extra-axial approach, once the basal portion of the tumor is identified and is exposed in the basal CSF cisterns.

MRI is generally more useful in defining the ramifications of multiple extensions or craniopharyngiomas. However, Kucharczyk and Montanera[166] have pointed out that the solid calcified craniopharyngiomas may be totally overlooked on MRI alone.

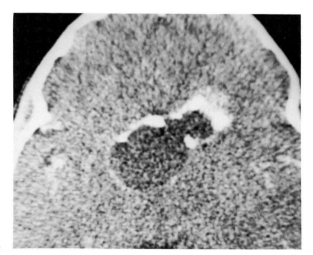
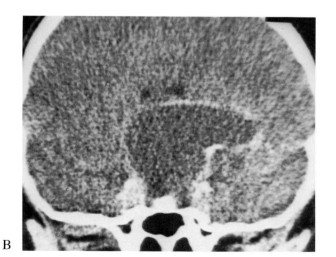

A   B

Figure 15-2. (A) Axial CT scan of craniopharyngioma revealing a large cystic tumor in the suprasellar region. This tumor is partially calcified and penetrates the suprasellar CSF cisterns. **(B)** Coronal CT scan of the same patient. Examination of this scan reveals the complexity and unusual lateral projection of this tumor. This asymmetry changes both the preoperative planning and the operative approach.

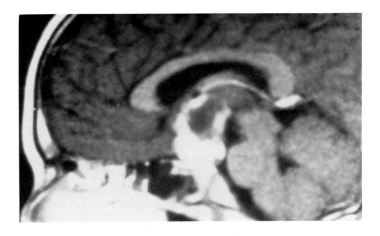

Figure 15-3. Large, partially cystic tumor arising in the suprasellar region and filling the third ventricle. Although the bulk of this tumor is within the third ventricle, it was easily seen in the suprasellar cisternal region using a right subfrontal approach and was removed.

Similarly, small calcified pieces of tumor may not be appreciated on postoperative MRI but may be seen adequately on CT scanning. We generally employ both MRI and CT in both preoperative and postoperative evaluation of craniopharyngiomas.

Some authors feel that preoperative angiography is indispensible in the management of these lesions.[307] The major vessels of the anterior circle of Willis and their relationship to the tumor are well defined on MRI, and this technology has generally obviated the use of preoperative angiographic studies. When a greater definition of the blood vessels is required, MR angiography provides a suitable, noninvasive method of obtaining this information. The vessels that directly supply the craniopharyngioma are quite small and difficult to identify. Angiography does not improve diagnostic accuracy or facilitate operative removal.

MANAGEMENT OF HYDROCEPHALUS

The presence of hydrocephalus complicates the operative management of patients with craniopharyngioma. This difficult factor is found in 15 to 30 percent of patients.[210,221,226] Major complications can arise from inadequate management of hydrocephalus, or failure to appreciate the enormous positional shifts that may occur when treating the tumor and hydrocephalus simultaneously.

Hydrocephalus most often occurs with craniopharyngiomas when the tumor has filled the third ventricle and obstructs the foramina of Monro. When both foramina are obstructed, it may be necessary to shunt both ventricles. The two ventricular catheters are brought together into a single distal shunt, both facing the same outflow resistance. If two separate shunts are used, failure of one not only raises intracranial pressure, but may lead to damaging shifts of midline structures.

When the patient's signs and symptoms are solely related to hydrocephalus, treatment of the hydrocephalus is indicated as a first step. Occasionally decompression of the hydrocephalus will allow the tumor to change position. Thus the tumor that is beneath the optic chiasm may cause greater chiasmatic compression when the hydrocephalus is reduced. In such a case, bitemporal field cuts appeared in a young boy immediately following his shunting procedure (Fig. 15-4).

When a shunt is installed, it is difficult to control the rate of decompression of the hydrocephalus. For this reason some authors have preferred the use of valve-regulated external drainage either immediately before or at the time of definitive operation.[215,216] Major changes in position of intracranial structures may follow the sudden decompression of chronic hydrocephalus. In the case described in Figure 15-5, operation with ventricular drainage was carried out. Numerous complications ensued, related in large part to the rapid decompression of the ventricles, allowing the cortex to fall away from the inner table of the skull. These complications might have been avoided by a slower and more careful management of the patient's chronic hydrocephalus.

OPERATIVE APPROACHES

The choice of operative route will be determined by the shape, size, and direction of growth of the craniopharyngioma. Occasionally characteristics within the tumor such as location of cysts, their size, or location of dense calcification will also effect this choice. The approach may also be dictated by the greatest exposure of the tumor to subarachnoid pathways at the base. Tumors that extend into the lateral

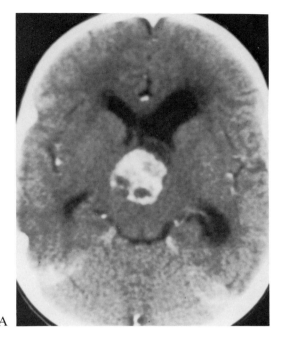
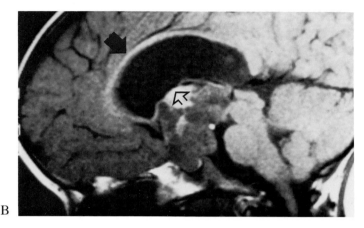

A   B

Figure 15-4. (A) Axial enhanced CT scan of a young boy with a partially cystic craniopharyngioma and hydrocephalus. After completion of this scan the child underwent a left ventriculoperitoneal shunt in another institution. He was admitted as an emergency to the Neurological Institute of New York when his vision rapidly deteriorated. A bitemporal hemianopia had developed within 30 hours following the shunting procedure. **(B)** Sagittal MRI of same boy. There is hydrocephalus, and the tumor fills the third ventricle. At operation the chiasm was severely compressed against the planum sphenoidale. The tumor was removed using a combined subfrontal and transcallosal approach. The factors noted here that are favorable to the transcallosal route include thinning of the corpus callosum (*black arrow*), and wide dilatation of the foramen of Monro (*open arrow*).

ventricles or into the posterior fossa are likely to need staged procedures, and the direction of initial choice will be most affected by the patient's clinical problems and by the area of greatest neural compromise.

Although the choice of approach will be dictated in many ways by the tumor configuration, certain general principles should be followed. In general, approaches that do not sacrifice or divide neural structures are to be preferred to those that do; unilateral approaches are preferable to mobilization of both sides of the brain. Finally, resection of functional neural tissue is rarely indicated in reaching these tumors.

The two approaches in widest general use now are the subfrontal approach,[226,252,296,297] and the pterional route.[307,311] For the right-handed surgeon, the unilateral right-sided flap is preferred, and has the additional advantage of retracting the nondominant hemisphere. Left frontal approaches may be indicated if there is major tumor extension into the left frontal region or into the left middle fossa, or adherence to structures lateral to the left side of the chiasm or left

optic tract. Excellent results have recently been reported utilizing a bifrontal approach.[295]

Both the subfrontal and pterional routes share the advantage of allowing approach below the circle of Willis and excellent visualization of the optic nerves and chiasm. The pterional approach is the shortest, most direct approach to the suprasellar region, and with the removal of the lateral portion of the sphenoid wing places the operator within a few centimeters of the tumor. It offers better direct visualization of the retrochiasmatic area than does the subfrontal approach. The subfrontal approach allows better visualization of the anterior portion of the optic pathways and a more direct approach through the lamina terinalis if that addition to the operative approach is needed. In both approaches the tumor may be approached lateral to the optic nerve and tract or on either side of the carotid artery (Fig. 15-6). The surgeon will evaluate each of these possible routes and should choose the one that allows the greatest exposure of tumor surface. Opening of the lamina terminalis to remove final portions of tumor that extend within the third ventricle is a frequently used

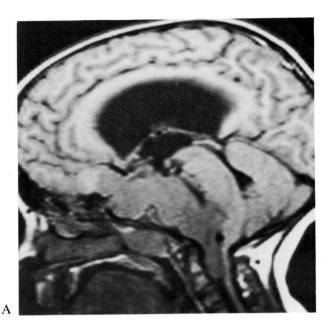

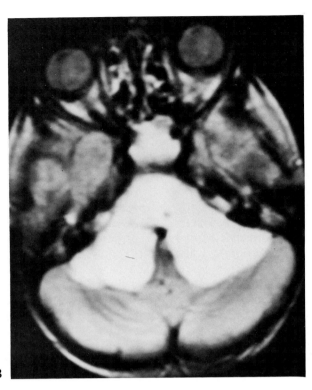

Figure 15-5. (A) Sagittal T₁-weighted MRI in a young boy with a largely cystic craniopharyngioma and hydrocephalus. Despite the rather threatening appearance of the tumor, this little boy was surprisingly intact both visually and endocrinologically. He was operated on without preoperative control of the hydrocephalus and an intraoperative ventriculostomy was employed. Decompression of the massive hydrocephalus and the large volume cystic tumor combined to allow a marked positional shift of brain structures postoperatively. See also Figure 15-15. **(B)** Axial balanced MRI of the same child shown in Figure A. This scan shows the posterior fossa cystic component of the tumor. The brainstem is severely compressed and the cranial nerves are stretched. When the cyst was decompressed at operation there were dramatic changes in the position of these important structures, leading to complications.

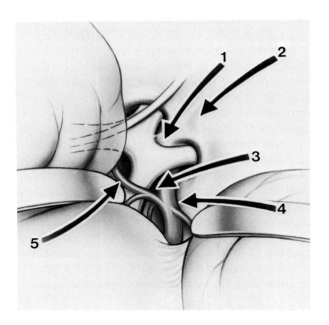

Figure 15-6. Variations available by the subfrontal and pterional approaches. Once the surgical approach has reached the area of the visual apparatus the operator may choose several routes. These will be determined in large part by the area of greatest potential exposure of the tumor surface. (*1*) Traditional approach to suprasellar tumors through the space bounded by the optic nerves and chiasm. (*2*) Transsphenoidal approach by drilling the plenum sphenoidale down to, or even into, the sphenoid sinus. (*3*) Opticocarotid approach, utilizing the space lateral to the optic chiasm and tract and medial to the carotid artery. (*4*) Lateral carotid approach, utilizing the space between the carotid artery and the medial temporal lobe. (*5*) Lamina terminalis approach, opening the lamina terminalis to visualize the tumor directly within the third ventricle.

operative maneuver. Choux[232] recently reported a series of 54 craniopharyngiomas in children and remarked that lamina terminalis opening has been used in nearly all of these cases.

The transsphenoidal approach can be used for those tumors that are wholly within the sella, or in which the suprasellar extension extends directly upward from a widely dilated diaphragm sellae. We do not employ this approach when the sella is of normal size, when pituitary function is intact, or if the suprasellar portion of the tumor extends laterally or anteriorly from a direct line of approach through the sphenoid. Laws[271,272] has described a case in which removal of a densely calcified intrasellar tumor by this approach resulted in damage to both carotid arteries, leading to a fatal outcome.

The transcallosal approach is useful for tumors that have the greatest part of their mass within the third ventricle. It may facilitate removal when the intraventricular portion is solid or calcified, or when the tumor cannot be visualized within the basal subarachnoid pathways. A number of cases of craniopharyngiomas that appear to be entirely within the third ventricle have now been described.[245,247,253,267]

When Long and Chou[274] reported use of the transcallosal approach for craniopharyngiomas in 1973, it was considered an operative tour de force, and a number of severe complications were noted. In the past generation this has become quite a routine operative approach and its techniques have been well described.[311] While the author has employed it only occasionally for craniopharyngiomas, in selected cases it has allowed total removal when other approaches have failed.

Yasargil et al.[311] have noted that a complication of the intrahemispheric retraction is vasospasm of the anterior cerebral arteries as they are dissected and retracted. They recommended topical papavarine to counteract the spasm.

When the corpus callosum is divided, orientation within the lateral ventricles is of prime importance. If the flap is placed anteriorly, the ventricles may be exposed in front of the foramen of Monro. It is necessary to visualize the structures at the foramen for proper orientation (Fig. 15-7A). After orientation is achieved, the septum pellucidum should be widely fenestrated. This will permit easier management of hydrocephalus if the tumor is not removed from the third ventricle.

If the foramen of Monro is not widely dilated, several methods have been described for enlarging access to the roof of the third ventricle. The inset in Figure 15-7A shows the interfornical approach described by Apuzzo et al.[215] This approach permits exposure of the body and caudal portion of the third ventricle. In another approach the choroid plexus may be elevated and the tela choroidea forming the roof of the third ventricle may be entered (Fig. 15-7B).[260] This method may be combined with division of the thalamostriate vein, according to these authors (Fig. 15-7C).

Each of these methods holds the risk of damage to the internal cerebral veins. The last described method, that of sacrificing the fornix (Fig. 15-7D), has the risk of memory loss. While there is some evidence that both fornices must be involved for severe short-term memory loss,[223] the author has not chosen to use this method.

Other approaches to craniopharyngioma will be dictated by the tumor's ability to reach portions of the brain far from the suprasellar site of origin. They have included the subtemporal and transtemporal approaches, suboccipital approaches, and a number of combined approaches. The transcortical approach as described by Dandy[237,238] has now been largely abandoned by most contemporary workers. The disadvantages of requiring hydrocephalus, leaving a transcortical scar, and limited visualization within the third ventricle have largely preempted its role.

AVOIDANCE OF SPECIFIC COMPLICATIONS

Distinguishing the Tumor Capsule from the Arachnoidal Envelope

Craniopharyngiomas are invested with their own layer of pia arachnoid. As they grow toward the basal cisterns they in turn become covered by the cisternal arachnoid nearest their point of origin. As the tumor continues to grow, another layer of cisternal arachnoid will adhere to the surface of the tumor as it escapes from the confines of the suprasellar cistern. Operating in the wrong arachnoidal plane may cause damage to major arteries or cranial nerves. Avoidance of damage to these structures can best be accomplished by a careful search for the arachnoidal plane directly covering the tumor, and it is essential that dissection be carried out between the tumors investing the arachnoid and not in the cisternal plane. As the CSF cisterns are opened, dissection toward the surface of the tumor is carried out. The tumor surface is distinguishable from the overlying arachnoidal planes by its difference in color, texture, and vascular complexity. The surface of the craniopharyngioma will have a much more distinct and often

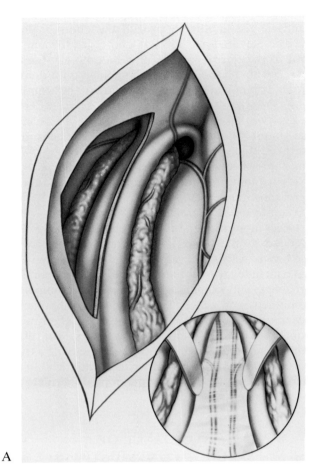

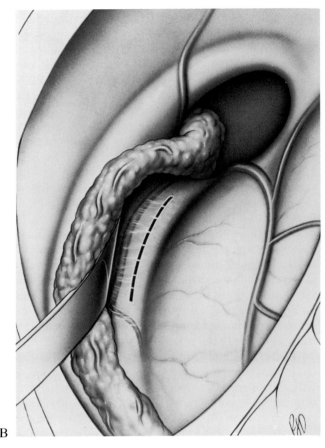

A   B

Figure 15-7. (A) Illustration of intraventricular view in the transcallosal approach. A large fenestration has been made between the ventricles, and the bodies of both ventricles are well seen. The corpus callosum is rarely opened this widely, but adequate visualization of the foramen of Monro is essential for orientation, and for identification of the choroid plexus, fornix, and major veins. **(Insert)** Illustration of the interfornical approach as described by Apuzzo et al.[215] The translucent tela choroidea is stretched, allowing the internal cerebral veins to be identified and thus avoiding their damage. **(B)** Illustration of subchoridal transvelum interpositum approach to the third ventricle. Here again the tela choroidea must be stretched to visualize and avoid damaging the internal cerebral veins. (*Figure continues.*)

more profuse vascular supply than that of the relatively avascular arachnoid.

Because finding the tumor arachnoidal plane is crucial, it is advisable to limit cauterization of the arachnoid until this plane is well seen and at least partially developed. Use of cautery may aneal the arachnoidal planes to each other or may fuse the tumor arachnoid to the tumor capsule itself. Either of these events will make adequate dissection in the tumor-arachnoidal plane more difficult. The number of blood vessels that cross between the arachnoid and the tumor capsule is small and these vessels can be easily identified, cauterized, and divided sharply, as is needed.

Finding the proper plane is most critical in those areas where the tumor forcefully abuts the optic apparatus or the major vessels of the anterior circle of

Wilis. In these regions, dense adhesions can be created between the neural or vascular structures and the tumor arachnoidal. Finding the subarachnoidal plane between the capsule and tumor arachnoid will allow the operator to remove the capsule while preserving the nerve or artery, often allowing small bits of fused arachnoid to remain adherent to these important structures.

In some regions the tumor will have created a significant arachnoidal or glial scar as it impresses itself on neural structures. Sweet[306] has described a cleavage plane that occurs within the layers of the dense glial reaction. His experience has been that ''in the great majority of patients the actual cleavage plane either through glia or beyond a capsule did not include neuronal nucleii or visual fiber tracts.''

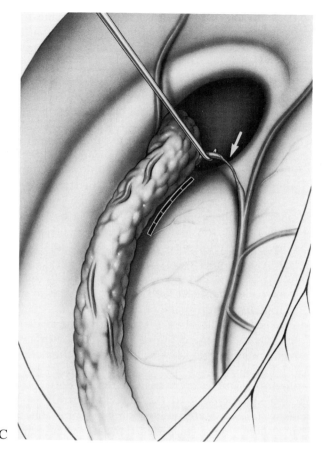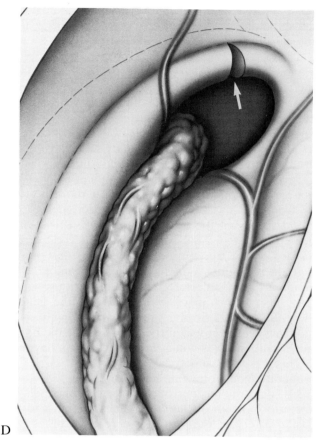

C D

Figure 15-7 *(Continued).* **(C)** Illustration of a variation of the subchoroidal approach, sacrificing the thalamostriate vein. **(D)** Illustration of the method of enlarging the foramen of Monro by dividing the anterior column of the fornix. While several references indicate that unilateral sacrifice of the fornix will not cause memory deficits, the author avoids this method as potentially damaging to learning and memory. (From Carmel,[225] with permission.)

When to Debulk the Tumor

As the tumor grows and stretches, it creates a smooth plane between the tumor arachnoid and tumor capsule. Preservation of this straight, smooth plane is a definite aid in dissection of the tumor capsule. The natural tendency in the operative treatment of craniopharyngiomas is to attempt to reduce the bulk at an early stage of the operation. However, when the tumor is debulked, especially a cystic tumor, both the tumor capsule and the tumor arachnoid become redundant and form folds of capsule and arachnoid that then become much more difficult to separate. Complications may arise from losing the arachnoidal plane; they may be avoided by extensive dissection of the capsule from the arachnoid plane with the tumor either fully intact or with just a small amount of its cystic content removed. This plane is dissected widely around the surface of the tumor until a large area of tumor has been separated from its arachnoidal envelope.

Tumor Adherence to Arteries

The most common obstacle to total removal of craniopharyngioma is a dense adhesion of tumor to a major artery, usually on the anterior circle of Willis. The mesenchymal reaction to the craniopharyngioma capsule appears to be more dense than the glial scar that forms underneath the chiasm or hypothalamus.[226,252,307] Symon and Sprich[307] have pointed out that densely calcified material may adhere to a major artery and preclude development of a plane of cleavage. Both Sweet[305] and Baskin and Wilson[22] report postoperative deaths secondary to removal of such a densely adherent portion of tumor from the wall of the carotid, causing an intraoperative tear.

The arterial blood supply for most craniopharyngiomas is derived principally from the vessels of the anterior circle of Willis. Direct branches from the internal carotid artery, the A-1 portion of the anterior cerebral artery, and the posterior communicating arteries have been described.[286] Within the sella turcica itself, the tumor may be supplied by small perforating arteries directly from the cavernous sinuses.

Pertuiset[286] has stated that craniopharyngiomas do not receive blood from the posterior cerebral arteries or from the basilar artery bifurcation, unless the blood supply of the floor of the third ventricle has been parasitized. This lack of posterior blood supply has led Sweet[308] to note that experience has shown that the tenacious attachments of a craniopharyngioma are only anterior, and that posterior portions may have to be pulled "blindly" into the field of view. Sweet describes a single case in which a craniopharyngioma invaded the arachnoid of the posterior fossa, and was adherent to the vessels beyond.

This vascular supply pattern may be altered in reoperations or following radiation therapy. In such cases, dense adhesions may be formed between the posterior portion of the craniopharyngioma and the basilar artery or the posterior cerebral arteries. Attempts to "slip" these recurrent or irradiated tumors out of their arachnoidal envelope will be unsuccessful and fraught with danger. These adhesions will need to be sharply dissected from neural or vascular structures under direct vision.

Damage to the Optic Nerves

Complications in a series of 99 personally operated craniopharyngiomas include an increase in visual deficits in five patients. Several factors can lead to intraoperative damage to the visual apparatus. The first of these is interruption of the vascular supply to the optic nerves. The nerves and the major portion of the chiasm are supplied from their undersurface by the anastomatic ring of vessels that circles the pituitary stalk fed from the superior hypophyseal arteries. Although most anatomy texts show this anastomotic ring fed only by these two arteries, it has not been unusual to see arterial supply to the ring from the posterior communicating arteries and from the A_1 portion of the anterior cerebral arteries.

The anastomotic ring must be preserved to spare damage to both the visual apparatus and the median eminence region. This may be accomplished by carefully dissecting both the cisternal and tumor arachnoid from the surface of the tumor capsule. The anastomotic vessels travel within the cisternal arachnoidal planes and can be reflected upward as the tumor is being dissected.

Cauterization is to be avoided on the surface of the optic nerves and chiasm. Small arachnoidal vessels over the surface of the visual pathways that may be torn during arachnoidal dissection may be covered with a small cottonoid for a few minutes. This usually results in hemostasis and avoids use of cautery.

There is considerable reference in the literature to the high incidence of prefixed chiasm and congenitally "short" optic nerves associated with craniopharyngioma.[220] In most of these cases the craniopharyngioma lies within the third ventricle and has bowed the chiasm forward, thus creating the impression of "shortening" of the optic nerves. The optic tracts are often pushed laterally by the intraventricular mass as well, cutting off the usually available dissection space between the tracts and the carotid artery (Fig. 15-8). These anatomical distortions may be seen to improve as the tumor is removed and the optic nerves gradually assume a more normal length.

Operating in the small space afforded between the planum sphenoidal and the anterior portion of the chiasm can be extremely difficult. Patterson and Danylevich[285] have suggested removal of the planum sphenoidale in an attempt to achieve more room in this region. These authors advocate drilling through

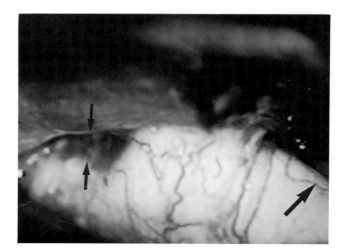

Figure 15-8. Operative view of the right optic nerve, chiasm, and tract in an early-stage removal of a large tumor that had invaginated into the third ventricle. The chiasm is pushed forward toward the planum (*small arrows*), creating the impression of "short" optic nerves. The optic tract is laterally deviated dramatically (*large arrow*). There is only about 1 mm of space in front of the chiasm in this case.

the planum and entering the sphenoid sinus directly. This maneuver affords a large working space anterior and beneath the chiasm. A major disadvantage is the need to repair the sinus opening, usually with a fat graft. It has been our preference to leave the mucosa of the sphenoid sinus intact, simply removing the overlying dura and drilling away several millimeters of bone until the sphenoidal mucosa is barely exposed.[224] This method affords 3 to 6 mm of additional working space and has the advantage of preventing CSF leaks in the postoperative period.

Removal of bone on the edge of the planum sphenoidale can often be supplemented by opening of the lamina terminalis, which allows manipulation of the tumor from both in front and behind the chiasm. The tumor may be debulked via the lamina terminalis as well. Perhaps the best method of dealing with the prefixed chiasm is to debulk the tumor behind it. If the tumor is exposed to the basal subarachnoid cisterns it is possible to enter the basilar portion of the tumor and to manipulate the tumor from the subarachnoid spaces lateral to the optic tract.

The optic nerves and chiasm are extremely sensitive to both retraction and rotation. While it is possible to obtain small amounts of extra room by retraction of the optic nerve, this cannot be done forcefully or carried out for a long period of time. The author has been reluctant to place fixed retractors on the optic nerve or chiasm during the removal of tumor. It must also be remembered that compression over a relatively small area of the nerve by a thin retractor may cause interruption of the anastomotic vessels on the surface and lead to infarction.

Many of the cystic craniopharyngiomas, especially in children, have a dense calcified portion within the base of the cyst. This calcified area of the tumor generally lies on a depressed diaphragm sellae or within the sella itself. It is often necessary to manipulate these calcified fragments past the optic nerve, once they have broken up into small pieces (Fig. 15-9). The breaking up of these calcified lumps may constitute a real chore. Small alligator forceps or micropituitary rongeurs may help to break up these calcifications. It has been occasionally necessary to use a high-speed drill to make the calcified mass small enough to be maneuvered past the visual apparatus. The use of the laser to accomplish reduction of these calcified areas may be dangerous, as the calcified mass will often become extremely hot with use of the laser.

When the calcified lump is small enough to traverse the space available, usually between the optic nerves or between the lateral border of the optic tract and carotid artery, care must be taken with the sharp edges of these fragments. When manipulating a frag-

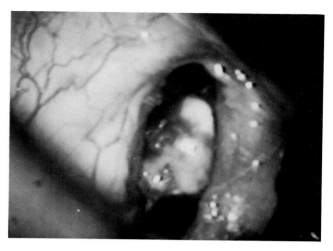

Figure 15-9. Operative view of calcification seen beneath the visual apparatus. The calcified mass is visualized in the space lateral to the right optic nerve and medial to the carotid artery. This dense calcification resisted all efforts to break it up with rongeurs and forceps. Finally, a high-speed drill was used to drill across the waist of the hard mass, breaking it into pieces and allowing its removal.

ment past the optic nerve it is often advisable to place a small retractor as a "bookmark" against the nerve so that the sharp edges will not damage the nerve (Fig. 15-10).

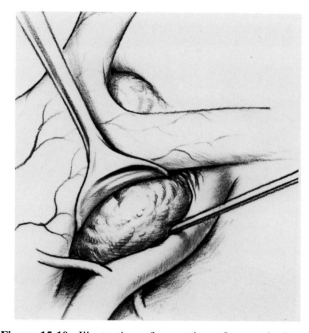

Figure 15-10. Illustration of a portion of a craniopharyngioma being removed past the visual apparatus. The small retractor on the lateral surface of the chiasm serves to protect the nerve in case jagged calcified pieces of the tumor project toward its surface.

Damage to the Pituitary Stalk

Many patients with craniopharyngioma have already functionally disconnected their median eminence from the pituitary gland and are hypopituitary at presentation. Others with normal or almost normal pituitary function at operation have stalks that are paper thin and without any visible pattern of long portal veins on their surface. These stalks do not appear capable of serving normal neural or neurosecretory functions. Many tumors are embedded in the median eminence, and when the tumor is removed the base of the stalk is no longer attached to the brain.

When these cases are excluded, there is a sizable minority of patients in whom the pituitary stalk can be identified and well visualized at operation, and in whom the stalk may be preserved. Preservation of the pituitary stalk is now technically possible using contemporary microscopic visualization and microsurgical techniques.[226,250,311] Although the stalk may be damaged as the tumor is removed, a remnant of stalk reaching from the median eminence to the pituitary gland my serve as a matrix upon which the pituitary portal system may re-form.[228]

The stalk is frequently displaced by the tumor and may be on any of the tumor surfaces. The stalk must be sought early in the dissection and debulking of the tumor to avoid inadvertent damage. Tumor displacement and compression may make the stalk difficult to identify. Its recognition is based on the peculiar striate appearance of the stalk and its known locus of penetration through the diaphragm sellae to the pituitary gland. The striated appearance is caused by the parallel arrangements of the long portal veins on the surface of the stalk (Fig. 15-11). This appearance is unique among suprasellar structures and is extremely distinctive. The parallel striations are maintained even though the stalk is displaced and stretched, disappearing only when the blood flow through the venous channels is obstructed.

The stalk penetrates through the diaphragm sellae to reach the pituitary gland in the center of the diaphragm sellae (Fig. 15-12). From the right subfrontal approach, the stalk lies behind the projection of the right optic nerve. In tumors that are suprasellar in their location, the stalk is best identified by dissecting in the plane beneath the cisternal arachnoid and diaphragm sellae. This plane is usually identified in the anterior portion of the sella or against the lateral walls of the sella. When the diaphragm is visualized dissection toward the fenestration in the diaphragm can be carried out and the stalk identified.

In those tumors that are both intrasellar and suprasellar the stalk may be on any side of the intrasellar extension of the tumor and may even appear to penetrate through its center, as has been recently illustrated by Yasergil et al.[311]

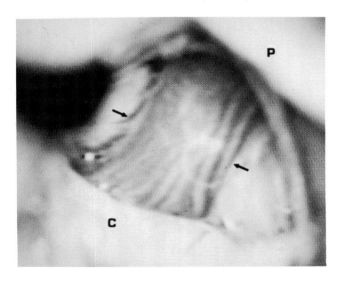

Figure 15-11. Photograph of a pituitary stalk (high microscopic magnification) seen during surgery. In this case the stalk was flattened in a posterior direction along the surface of the diaphragm sellae. The stalk is notable for its distinctive striated appearance, caused by the long portal vessels that run from the hypothalamus to the pituitary sinuses. The stalk is outlined by arrows, and is seen from the chiasm (*C*) to the planum (*P*).

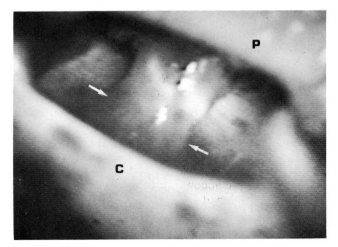

Figure 15-12. Pituitary stalk seen at operation with lower magnification than seen in Figure 15-11. The stalk is visualized in the space between the chiasm (*C*) and the planum (*P*) and is outlined by the arrows. From the right frontal approach the stalk will project in the space behind the right optic nerve. In order to obtain this visualization it was necessary to retract gently on the right optic nerve.

Damage to the Hypothalamus

Many years ago Cushing (cited in Carmel[223]) ointed out that the hypothalamus could function ormally even if severely displaced. This was depen-.ent on the displacement taking place slowly over a eriod of many years. The rapid, traumatic events of craniotomy are more likely to result in hypotha-amic damage. Experimental results have shown that unilateral lesions of the hypothalamus rarely produce clinical symptoms and that most hypothalamic deficiencies require bilateral damage. This same finding is noted clinically as well. Yasergil et al.[311] wrote that "if the hypothalamus was infiltrated by tumor unilaterally there were generally few long-term postoperative problems; whereas, if the hypothalamus was infiltrated bilaterally and the tumor was removed after a good deal of dissection, then the patient needed more careful postoperative neuroendocrine and electrolyte control."

If the patient has a functioning pituitary stalk, cutting of the stalk may cause an almost immediate onset of diabetes insipidus. When the operation is prolonged, this may be noticable before the patient has left the operating room. Frequent analysis of serum electrolytes and osmolarity, as well as urinary electrolytes and osmolarity, is an important feature of adequate postoperative water-balance management.

It is important to remember that in these patients the response to stalk section may be triphasic.[290] In the first phase there is a loss of antidiuretic hormone (ADH) secretion when the stalk is initially cut. However, within 2 to 5 days the posterior lobe of the pituitary gland may begin to involute, especially if its blood supply is interrupted. As these axon terminals begin to die off, stored ADH is released into the systemic circulation, which may cause a temporary normalization of the urinary output and water ingestion. If long-acting agents such as pitressin tanate are given, the patient may go into renal shutdown in this phase. Even shorter acting agents, such as nasal d-arginine vasopressin (DDAVP), can have lengthy response periods extending over 12 or even 24 hours. The period of time of dosage will have to be watched particularly carefully. When all of the stored ADH has been released from the dying axon terminals, the patient once again returns to a state of diabetes insipidus.

In patients in whom the stalk has been left intact, the need for DDAVP may persist, even in those children in whom the need for the nasal spray will only be transient. It appears that there is a period of "shock" of the stalk, which stops the adequate re-lease of ADH. Sweet[306] has reported a patient who found that she worked much more efficiently on DDAVP than while she was on pitressin tanate. Interestingly, while on the pitressin she had incessant hyperphagia and no sense of satiety. After the use of DDAVP she felt satisfied at the end of a normal meal and the fight against weight gain was easier.

Patients are generally kept on large doses of high-potency steroids during the immediate postoperative period for control of postoperative cerebral edema. This substitution is more than adequate to make up for the loss of adrenocorticotropic hormone (ACTH). Too rapid a reduction of steroids may result in a syndrome of a septic meningitis,[241,276] and too slow a reduction increases unwanted side effects of hypercorticoidism.

Management of growth in children has been vastly improved with the availability of synthetic growth hormone. It has been noted that children with radical removal of craniopharyngiomas and with subnormal values of circulating growth hormone when tested can still have accelerated growth following tumor removal.[226,252] Sweet[306] reported normal or accelerated growth in all eight of his patients who underwent radical removal and who were critically studied. In a study of our own patients, postoperative growth without hormone treatment took place in 12 of 34 children, including 5 with radical removal.[235] There had been concern that use of growth hormone replacement might cause an increase in the recurrence rate, or accelerating growth of residual tumor. Recent studies by Clayton et al.[233] seem to dispel this fear.

A common finding following craniopharyngioma removal is abnormal weight gain in many patients. This rapid weight gain starts immediately after surgery. In a series reported by Sorva,[300] two-thirds of the children studied had a weight gain of more than 10 percent during the first 3 postoperative months. Sixty percent of these children were defined as being obese within the following years. These authors noted that the type of operation had no decisive role in the development of obesity, and it was seen as often after partial removal as after total removal. The rapid development of permanent obesity may be due to an alteration in lipid metabolism by a hypothalamic lesion.[223,300]

In addition, there is evidence of abnormal food-seeking behavior after surgery for craniopharyngioma.[299] In such patients the mechanism of obesity seems to be clearly related to an aggressive hyperphagia. In some cases the food-seeking activity becomes bizarre and behavior is abnormal. These patients will engage in many antisocial activities including stealing of money to purchase food to satisfy their need.

Reeves and Plum[291] have reported a woman in whom destruction of the ventral medial nuclei of the hypothalamus bilaterally by a hamartoma resulted in hyperphagia, obesity, and aggressive behavior. Studies of hypothalamic activity have indicated that the ventral medial nucleus forms a "satiety center." Destruction of this nucleus bilaterally experimentally results in abnormal feeding behavior and weight gain.

Another adverse response to bilateral ventral hypothalamic manipulation is an increase in aggressive behavior. In some patients this is signaled by the onset of verbally explosive episodic rage attacks. In children this can lead to disruptions in classrooms and to a need for placement in special education classes.[301,306] In rare cases, the rage may be exhibited as physical abuse of family, friends, or even strangers.

A complication attributed to hypothalamic damage is the onset of fever, cardiovascular collapse, coma, and death at late intervals following craniopharyngioma. Matson and Crigler[278] reported one such case 4 months after operation. Fischer et al.[243] had another child with a similar course 1 year following radical excision. This has been attributed to hypothalamic injury by some authors. However, Till[308] has noted four deaths occurring 3 to 9 years after operation. He attributed each of these to inadequate treatment of the patient's suprarenal insufficiency "at the time of an otherwise straightforward infection." Sweet had a similar case but felt that this might be related to radiation necrosis.[306] Hoffman et al.[251] have reported a similar death that took place during a metapyrone test in another hospital.

Whether all of these deaths are related to some specific hypothalamic problem, or simply reflect inadequate substitution therapy with corticosteroids, remains unclear. In the four autopsied cases studied by Till[308] there was no tumor at the operative site and there is no mention of either necrosis or infarction in the hypothalamic region.

Yasargil et al.[311] have reported two children who died of hypothalamic hemorrhage following incomplete excision by the pterional approach. They also noted that sepsis can be a difficult problem to manage in these cortisone-deficient patients. Pneumonia and shunt infections were found in 4 percent of his patients.

Psychosocial Function

Those who favor conservative therapy with subtotal excision followed by radiation therapy point to the high level of function of their patients in support of this approach. Table 15-4 gives data gleaned from proponents of conservative and radical approaches to craniopharyngioma management.

Table 15-4.   Results in Survivors

	Yasargil et al. (1967–1987)	Sweet (1970–1979)	Cavazzuti, Fischer et al. (1972–1981)	Baskin and Wilson (1969–1985)
General performance				
Number	120	12	21	
Rating (%)				
Excellent	80.8	76	86	
Good		16	14	
Fair	19.2	8	0	
Visual status (acuity) (%)				
Better	37.5	42	33	60
Same	57.5	25		2
Worse	5	33		
Full-scale IQ		97.2	101.4	
Learning and memory				
Wechsler memory scale		101.0	101.6	
Reproduction of figure text (Rey-Osterrich)		26.8	19.3	
Mortality				
(Operation/recurrence) (%)	17.5	16	8	3
Total no. patients in series	141	43	37	74

(Data from Bartlett,[220] Cavazzuti et al.,[231] Sweet,[304] and Yasargil et al.[311])

The group at the Children's Hospital of Boston considers the high number of behavioral problems following attempts at radical excision cited in the literature as a major reason for a conservative attitude.[231,243] This group feels that disturbance of the hypothalamic connections to the thalamus, frontal lobes, and other cortical areas serves to explain some of the psychological and social problems that are seen following radical excision. They also note that children with craniopharyngiomas have other specific problems that are related to their tumor, including visual disturbances, endocrinopathies, and obesity.

Radiation Therapy

The first small group of patients treated with radiation following subtotal removal of suprasellar craniopharyngiomas was reported more than 50 years ago.[230] At that time it was felt that the tumor was not destroyed by x-rays but that cells that produced secretions and formed cysts would be destroyed. Doubts continued for many years as to whether or not craniopharyngioma epithelium would be effectively killed by radiation therapy.[213,251]

A dramatic change in this attitude occurred in 1961 when Kramer and his associates[264,265] reported excellent results with subtotal tumor removal and supravoltage irradiation. Since that time many studies have shown the efficacy of radiation therapy both in increasing the survival rates of patients with operation and radiation therapy, and in even more dramatic improvements in the recurrence-free survival rates.[239,302] A large series of 125 patients was recently reported on by the University of Tokyo.[277] Of this group, 45 patients received postoperative radiation therapy, and the cases with total tumor removal were excluded. The 5- and 10-year survival rates were 88.9 and 76.5 percent for the subtotally removed and irradiated group, whereas the group that underwent similar operations but had no radiation had survival rates of 39.9 and 27.1 percent, respectively.

In 1986 Baskin and Wilson[221] reported a series of 74 patients in whom the operative approach was conservative and was followed by radiation therapy. Although the follow-up period on this group was short, they were able to report that 91 percent of these patients were in remission and that the operative mortality was 3 percent. Unfortunately, this series does not show the overall function or recurrence rate after this conservative management.

A series of patients who were treated conservatively and followed for more than 10 years was re-ported on by Fisher et al.[243] Eight of these patients were treated with radical removal and 29 with subtotal removal and irradiation. Of the conservatively treated group, 2 died (1 of progressive tumor growth and 1 of a radiation-induced brainstem glioma) and 2 of the 27 survivors (7 percent) had tumor recurrence. The authors emphasized the good functional results of this group of patients.

Increasing attention is being given to the effects of high doses of radiation therapy on brains of children. Duffner et al.[240] in 1985 examined the survivors of radiation therapy for posterior fossa tumors. They found that 40 percent of these children had IQs below 70 and only 20 percent had IQs in the normal range. A very detailed and careful study was published by Packer et al. in 1989.[283] In this study, children with malignant brain tumors treated with radiation therapy had a fall in full-scale IQ from 105 at diagnosis to 91 by the end of the second year after radiation therapy. Children who did not receive radiation therapy did not demonstrate a fall in any cognitive parameter over time. The younger the child was at the time of treatment, the greater was the likelihood and severity of damage.

A study of children who had been given brain irradiation under the age of 3 and who had survived for a long period showed that 55 percent required a special education school.[301] Radiation therapy alone was felt to account for the mental sequalae in at least 40 percent of these children. The effects of radiation are likely to worsen over a period of time. In a study of leukemic patients who received only 2,400 cGy, the effects of radiation therapy in general did not begin to appear until 3 years posttherapy and continued to worsen.[240]

A recent report of 21 patients who were subjected to megavoltage external beam irradiation with more than 5-year follow-up showed a marked difference in the complication rate between those patients who had 51.3 to 60 Gy and those that had higher doses in the range of 60 to 70 Gy.[244] In the high-dose group the actuarial risk at 5 years for optic neuropathy was 30.5 percent and for brain necrosis was 12.5 percent. However, there did not seem to be a significant difference in tumor control or recurrence rate in the high- and low-dose groups.

There is increasing enthusiasm for treatment of craniopharyngiomas by stereotactic, focused high-beam radiation.[234] This can be carried out with either proton beam or "gamma knife." It is perhaps premature at this writing to evaluate the efficacy of these modalities. A recent case of delayed cerebral radiation necrosis following proton beam therapy has been reported.[257] One of the long-term hazards of radiation

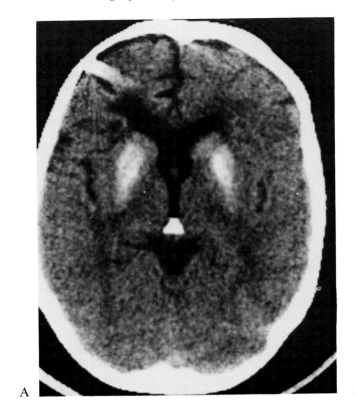

A

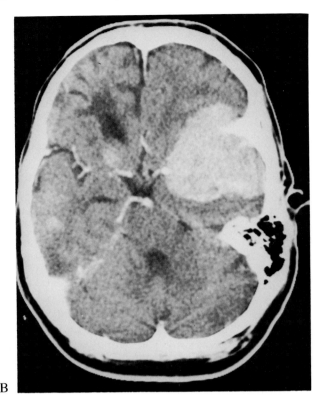

B

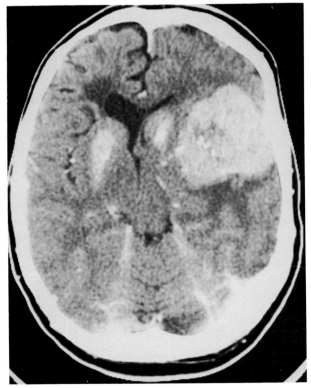

C

Figure 15-13. Tomographic scans of a young man who had been initially treated at age 7. In initial treatment, the tumor was subtotally removed and a course of 5,000 cGy was given. **(A)** Scan taken when the man was 20 years old, suffering from the recent onset of generalized seizures but with no other focal neurological impairment. He was short, obese, and mildly retarded. At that time he was in a state training program. This scan shows the changes that are typical postirradiation. There is calcification in the basal ganglia, and a mild to moderate degree of cerebral atrophy, especially in the frontal regions. **(B&C)** Scans taken 2 years later, 15 years after initial radiation therapy. On these scans a large sphenoid wing meningioma is seen. The tumor had caused a contralateral hemiparesis. This tumor was totally removed and despite its rapid growth was histologically a benign meningioma.

therapy is the induction of a secondary tumor following radiation therapy. Tumors reported following irradiation of craniopharyngiomas include brainstem gliomas, supra- and infratentorial sarcomas, and meningiomas.[226] The case illustrated in Figure 15-13 shows a tumoral complication secondary to radiation therapy, as well as other deleterious changes.

Intracystic irradiation has been used in many locations and several favorable reports, particularly with the use of potassium-32 isotopes, have been published.[260,261] In most of the treatment protocols a precise knowledge of the cyst volume is necessary to determine the amount of radioactive isotope to be injected. Lexell (as quoted by Backlund et al.[216]) has suggested that 100 kilorads delivered to the cyst surface would deliver sufficient dosage to collapse the cyst.

A recent excellent analysis of stereotactic instillation of yttrium-90 has been published by Backlund and coworkers.[216,294] Although these authors have experience with more than 300 craniopharyngiomas treated stereotactically, the published reports describe 44 consecutive patients treated from 1964 to 1976. This study limited those tumors treated stereotactically to those that had the majority of their mass within the cystic component of the tumor. At the end of a long and carefully monitored follow-up period, 31 patients were alive and well and 6 had died of their tumor or related causes. Another two patients died of other causes but were felt to have done so due to failure of therapy. One of the deaths was due to subarachnoid hemorrhage, caused by erosion of a posterior communicating artery. This series of patients has results as good as the operative results that were then published, and we await additional results from the larger series with anticipation.

Vascular Damage following Craniopharyngioma Removal

Two distinct kinds of vasculopathies have been described after craniopharyngioma removal. The first of these is fusiform dilatation of the carotid artery,[303] and the second is related to hemodynamic changes, often at sites distant to the site of operation.

Fusiform Dilatations of the Carotid Artery

Sutton and coworkers[303] at Children's Hospital of Philadelphia have recently reported finding fusiform dilatation of the carotid artery following attempted total removal. This was found in 9 of 31 patients (21 percent) at the time of surgery for recurrence of tumor or on routine surveillance with enhanced CT scanning.

Although their belief was not confirmed by autopsy, these workers felt the abnormalities were unlikely to be either false or dissecting aneurysms. They were not related to visible lacerations of the vessel wall during the surgical procedure. It seemed clear that the dilatation arose as a result of the surgery and was invariably found on the side of the operative approach. This abnormality was attributed to surgical retraction on the carotid artery to gain access to the tumor or was due to weakness of the arterial wall following removal of the tumor capsule from the adventitia. The fact that these were not seen on the immediate postoperative scan, but occurred after only many months or years, suggests that these may be an injury to the vasovasorum that weakens the muscular layer enough to allow the arterial wall to expand.

Although the follow-up on these cases is short, no patient has developed symptoms related to mass effect or hemorrhage. Sutton and coworkers attempted to reduce the size of the carotid artery intraoperatively in one patient, but felt that surgical treatment of the fusiform dilatation was not warranted. Fusiform dilatations may involve only a portion of the supraclinoid internal carotid or may involve the initial portions of the anterior or middle cerebral arteries.

In our own experience with 72 children operated on for craniopharyngioma, 6 cases of carotid dilatation have been noted. In one of these, in whom a total removal had been achieved, a second operation to wrap the supraclinoid carotid artery with muslin was carried out. A second operated case was a child who had been operated on twice at another institution, and had a full course of radiation therapy. The child had recurrent tumor and the artery was dilated (Fig. 15-14). Sutton et al.[303] have recommended operating from the contralateral side if reoperation is indicated with this complication. In the case illustrated in Figure 15-15, we operated from the same side, removed the rest of the tumor, and wrapped the supraclinoid carotid artery with fine muslin.

Vascular Problems at Distant Sites

Konovolov[267] has described two further vascular problems associated with craniopharyngioma surgery. The first of these is the development of ischemic symptoms related to lack of arterial profusion at sites distant from the operative site. In an example cited by Konovolov, a infarct in the distal distribution of the basilar system was found after tumor removal in the suprasellar and lamina terminalis region. The author felt that this might possibly be related to

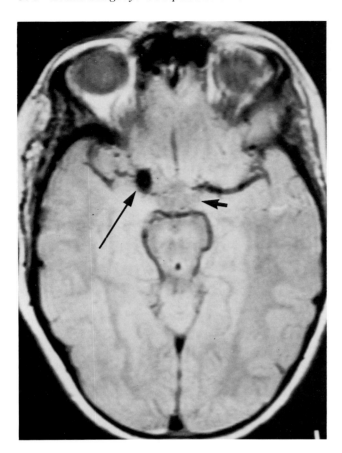

Figure 15-14. Axial MRI showing a fusiform dilatation of the right carotid artery (*long arrow*) in a young girl. This dilatation occurred in the supraclinoid carotid artery up to the bifurcation, without involving the initial portions of either the anterior or middle cerebral arteries. There is tumor recurrence, filling the suprasellar cistern (*short arrow*). This child had undergone two previous operations for her craniopharyngioma at another institution and had received a course of radiation therapy. At reoperation, the tumor was removed and the supraclinoid portion of the carotid artery was wrapped with muslin.

blood in the subarachnoid space and basilar artery spasm associated with intraoperative hypotension.

A second complication was the development of venous stasis or thrombosis secondary to changes in intracranial volume or stretching or bridging veins in the cortex. In a recent case with this complication a child with massive hydrocephalus and a large-volume tumor was operated on with intraoperative ventriculostomy. There was a dramatic colapse of the brain substance and stretching of the veins. This child subsequently went on to develop multiple venous infarcts over the surface of the cortex and other complications (Fig. 15-15). Fortunately, after a stormy period the child has returned to normal function.

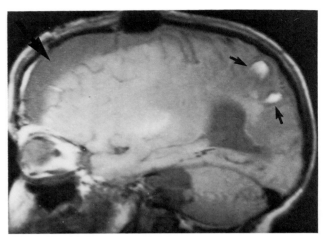

Figure 15-15. Sagittal MRI showing distant complications of cortical collapse. This young boy had massive hydrocephalus and a very large cystic tumor (same case as illustrated in Figure 15-5). The rapid decompression of both the hydrocephalus and the tumor led to stretching of the cerebral veins, causing multiple venous infarcts. In this view the large subdural hygroma is seen in the frontal region (*large arrow*) and two hemorrhagic venous infarcts are seen in the posterior parieto-occipital region (*small arrows*). Despite these complications this child has made a good recovery.

Management of Recurrences

The numerically greatest complication of craniopharyngioma surgery is recurrence. In a study of both adults and children, the recurrence rate of subtotally removed tumor without radiotherapy was almost 90 percent at 5 years, and more than 90 percent at 10 years.[292] Despite the fact that craniopharyngiomas are considered "slow-growing" tumors,[220,249,256,258] they tend to recur early because of the capacity for rapid growth of the cystic portions of the tumor. They are perhaps one of the most rapidly recurring of "benign" tumors. Recurrences from a large series reported by Sung et al.[302] are shown in Figure 15-16. These data reveal that of the 75 recurrences in this series, 52.5 percent (39 patients) recurred in under one year. Seventy-five percent of recurring tumors did so within 3 years, while 85 percent of those that recurred were back within 5 years. While the occasional subtotally removed tumor may appear to be quiescent for long periods without further therapy, this type of anecdotal case must be regarded as an exception.

The decisions made when there is known residual tumor after initial surgery, or when there is recurrence, are very difficult. Megavoltage external beam

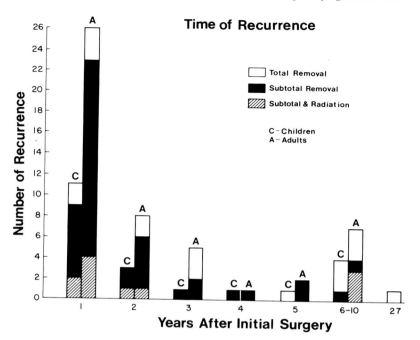

Figure 15-16. Time of recurrences following craniopharyngiomas following initial therapy. Note that in the subtotally removed group, and in the group that had both subtotal removal and irradiation, the majority of the recurrences occurred in the very first years after surgery. Recurrences were noted to be somewhat delayed in the "totally" removed cases.

radiation therapy is fairly effective, but increasingly is thought not to be appropriate in young children. The efficacy and long-term effects of both intracystic radiation and high-beam stereotactic guided radiotherapy remain problematic.

Many surgeons have commented on the increased risks and likelihood of failure upon renewed attempts at tumor removal. Sweet[306] noted that one of eight patients died when an attempt at radical removal was made at a second operation following a less extensive resection at the first procedure. However, he goes on to say, "Death ensued within a maximum of 6 months in every one of the five patients in whom I carried out a second radical removal" following a primary radical resection.

Yasargil et al.[311] also noted greatly increased mortality from a second procedure. In their series of both adults and children, counting all deaths that occurred during the entire follow-up period, the mortality was 9 percent (11 of 125 patients). However, the mortality after secondary microsurgery was 32.5 percent (13 of 40 patients), more than a threefold increase. The direct surgical mortality was 2.1 percent (3 of 144 patients).

On our experience, neither prior surgery nor surgery and radiation precluded a chance at total removal. The operative morbidity and mortality were the same in both groups. However, the chance of radical removal (no observable tumor at operation) was much lower in the secondary procedure group.

Transsphenoidal Surgery

Edward R. Laws, Jr.

The transsphenoidal approach for the management of craniopharyngioma presents a unique set of advantages and complications. For many surgeons the goal of an operation for craniopharyngioma is the gross total removal of most lesions. The transsphenoidal approach permits "total" removal of many lesions, particularly those that are primarily cystic and associated with an enlarged sella turcica. Operations may also be planned with a goal of subtotal removal (often to be followed by radiation therapy), and the transsphenoidal approach may also be suitable in accomplishing this goal. Once again, an enlarged sella and a primarily cystic tumor are features that make the approach feasible. Finally, in cases of recurrent craniopharyngiomas in which the goal is palliation, the transsphenoidal approach may be desirable, effective, and relatively safe. In this instance, enlargement of the sella is less important, but a cystic tumor is more likely to be managed effectively by this approach.

Our experience with surgery for craniopharyngioma now comprises 158 operations in 144 patients. Of these, 126 were primary operations in patients who had no prior therapy. In most of these, the goal was total removal of the lesion. Transsphenoidal surgery was utilized as primary therapy in 76 patients with craniopharyngioma. In 18 patients the transsphenoidal operation was utilized after a prior operation, almost always a craniotomy. The goal in these patients was usually palliation, although the total or radical resection was accomplished in many cases. During the same 16-year time period 61 patients with craniopharyngiomas were treated by craniotomy. The overall results of the transsphenoidal approach for the management of craniopharyngiomas have been excellent. The survival, quality of life, incidence of recurrence after total removal, mortality, and morbidity have been comparable to, and in most instances superior to, results reported in patients treated by craniotomy.

Proper case selection and technical and conceptual knowledge are the keys to success. The importance of the enlarged sella is critical. Enlargement of the sella implies that the tumor took origin below the diaphragma sellae, and therefore, although attached to the pituitary stalk, it is not attached to the hypothalamus or the optic chiasm (Fig. 15-17). This provides the possibility of total removal via the transsphenoidal approach and allows the surgeon to operate successfully.

Most craniopharyngiomas that expand the sella compress the normal anterior pituitary gland so that hypopituitarism is common, and the most likely location for the normal gland is anteriorly within the sella. For this reason, the transsphenoidal approach may be less satisfactory when preservation of the normal gland is essential.

It is obvious that, if complications are to be avoided, judgment must be applied as to the indications for surgery, the route of surgical approach, and the goal of surgery. These judgment decisions will be individualized for each patient, each tumor, and each surgeon. Using a suboptimal approach or setting an unrealistic goal can predispose the patient to complications and a poor outcome. Anatomical features must be studied carefully in planning a surgical approach, and careful surgical technique is also a major factor in avoiding complications.

Complications, including mortality, can be described by considering a number of categories.

HYPOTHALAMIC INJURY

Damage to the hypothalamus may result from direct surgical injury and also from hemorrhage or ischemia provoked by the procedure. Clinical manifestations of hypothalamic damage range from death to diabetes insipidus and may include morbid obesity, uncontrollable hunger or thirst, memory loss, somnolence, and difficulties with body temperature control. Such complications are more frequent in patients with prior surgery or radiation therapy. Hypothalamic injury can be avoided with careful technique and intraoperative video fluoroscopic control when working above the sella.

VISUAL DAMAGE

Damage to the optic nerves and chiasm can also occur from direct surgical trauma, hemorrhage, or ischemia. Fractures of bony structures at the base of the skull can damage optic nerves and can occur from aggressive opening of the retractor or from a misdirected approach. Many patients have preoperative compromise of visual function, making them more susceptible to further damage. Visual complications are also more likely to occur in patients with adhesions from prior surgery and in patients who have received prior radiation therapy. Assessment of the bony anatomy, careful and gentle technique, and confirmation of surgical landmarks are the major methods of avoidance of these complications. Packing of the empty sella can prevent the late complication of visual loss from prolapse of the optic chiasm.

ARTERIAL DAMAGE

Arterial damage is possible, particularly when vessels are adherent to the capsule of the tumor. Arteries may be lacerated, perforated, avulsed, or damaged so that they develop spasm or intraluminal thrombosis. These arterial injuries may result in fatal hemorrhage, intracranial hematoma, or stroke from ischemia or embolization. Laceration of the carotid artery can result in the formation of a false aneurysm or a carotid-cavernous fistula. Arterial complications can also be caused by preexisting aneurysms of the circle of Willis, which may rupture or become symptomatic in the perioperative period. Careful study of

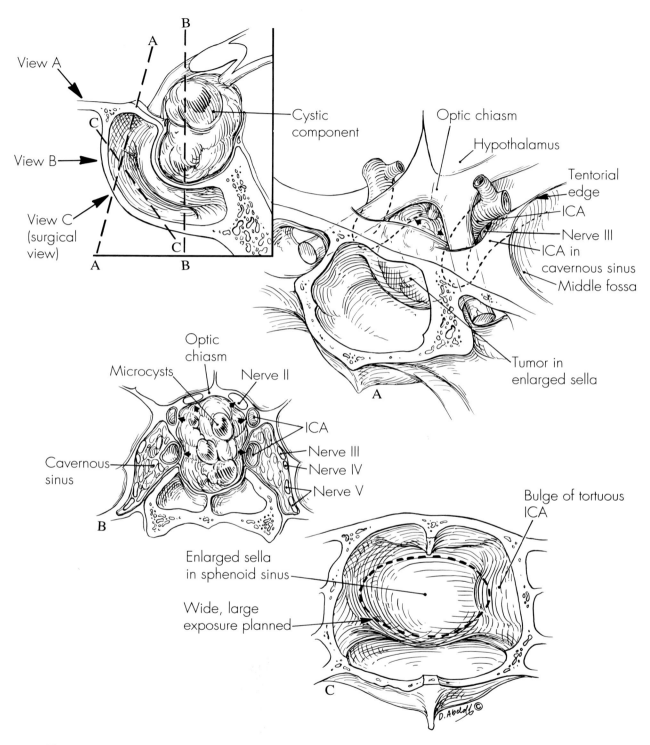

Figure 15-17. Anatomical relationships of a typical sellar/suprasellar craniopharyngioma. Three different planes of pathological anatomy are presented as indicated in the inset. **(A)** View A is a coronal view through the sphenoid sinus, and **(B)** view B is a coronal plane through the tumor—both views show the anatomy as seen by the transsphenoidal surgeon. **(C)** View C is from above, showing relationships of the intracranial structures.

the arterial anatomy on preoperative imaging studies can help avoid these complications.

RHINORRHEA AND MENINGITIS

Cerebrospinal fluid (CSF) rhinorrhea and meningitis are the most common complications of transsphenoidal surgery for craniopharyngioma. Total removal of the tumor usually requires resection of the diaphragma sellae, (Fig. 15-18) and subtotal removal frequently includes violation of the diaphragm. In most cases, therefore, there is a large intraoperative CSF leak that must be sealed as part of the closure. This is usually done with autologous grafts of fascia lata, fat, or muscle. These grafts may be buttressed by the use of fibrin glue, and the sellar floor is reconstructed with cartilage or bone from the nasal septum. Whenever a postoperative CSF leak occurs, the potential for bacterial meningitis exists, and this complication can be fatal. Prophylactic antibiotics are commonly utilized, but when meningitis occurs, prompt and accurate action is necessary to forestall disaster. CSF rhinorrhea can result in pneumocephalus, which may also require prompt corrective action. Violation of the cribriform plate during exposure or surgery can also produce a CSF leak. Ready acknowledgment of an intraoperative or postoperative CSF leak is essential, and careful anatomic reconstruction and sealing of the sella helps in preventing these complications.

CAVERNOUS SINUS DAMAGE

Damage to the cavernous sinus can occur, particularly in the process of stripping the craniopharyngioma capsule away from the dura that forms the wall of the cavernous sinus. In addition to injuring the venous sinus itself, the contents of the cavernous sinus can be damaged. These include the carotid artery, the third, fourth, and sixth cranial nerves and the fifth cranial nerve (Fig. 15-17). Careful technique, good visualization of anatomical structures, and accurate hemostasis with Gelfoam and tamponade help avoid complications.

DAMAGE TO BRAINSTEM, SINUS, NOSE, AND MOUTH

Damage to the brainstem may occur with a misdirected approach that violates the clivus, or when a large tumor erodes this structure, exposing the dura of the clivus. Proper use of anatomical studies should help prevent this complication.

Sphenoid sinus complications include postoperative infection, mucocele formation, and obstruction. The walls of the sinus may be fractured by the speculum, leading to optic nerve damage or hemorrhage. It is our practice to remove all of the sphenoid sinus mucosa and to do the bone work with great precision in an attempt to avoid these complications.

Nasal complications include nasal septal perforation, nasal obstruction, and cosmetic deformities such as caudal tip deformities and septal deviation. Loss of smell can also occur, presumably due to damage to nerve endings in the nasal mucosa. Nondestructive surgical technique and meticulous reconstruction of the nasal structures help to avoid nasal complications.

Complications of the sublabial approach include persistent numbness of the upper lip and teeth or dental problems such as devitalization or discolor-

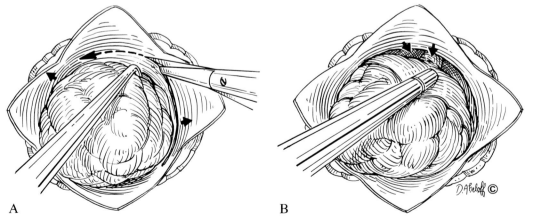

A   B

Figure 15-18. Steps in the total removal of a craniopharyngioma using the transsphenoidal approach. **(A)** Sharp dissection is used to open the diaphragm of the sella, which is fused to the dorsal capsule of the tumor. **(B)** Mobilization of the superior aspect of the tumor. The arrows in Fig. A show reflection of the sellar dura and incision of the diaphragmatic attachment at the tuberculum sellae. The arrows in Fig. B indicate the pituitary stalk where it attaches to the dorsal capsule of the tumor.

ation. The retractor can fracture the hard palate and lead to misalignment of the upper incisors. Once again, care with surgical technique is the key to avoidance of complications.

ENDOCRINE ABNORMALITIES

Postoperative endocrine abnormalities can also be considered to be complications. If a patient has normal anterior pituitary function preoperatively, there is considerable risk of loss of function, particularly if a total removal is attempted. This is a major consideration in the growing child in whom exogenous steroid therapy can result in limitation of growth potential. The implications for fertility should also be considered in appropriate cases; some of our male patients have banked sperm prior to surgery.

DIABETES INSIPIDUS

Diabetes insipidus commonly occurs after removal of a craniopharyngioma, as the tumor is usually attached to the pituitary stalk. Preoperative diabetes

Table 15-5. Complications of Transsphenoidal Surgery in 94 Patients with Craniopharyngioma

Complication	No. Affected
Operative death	2 (hemorrhage, carotid occlusion)
CSF leak	13
Meningitis	7
Stroke	2
Visual loss	1
Subdural empyema	1

insipidus is virtually never reversed by surgery, but postoperative diabetes insipidus may be transient, and at least 50 percent of the patients treated by transsphenoidal surgery recover, usually within 6 to 12 months of surgery. Diabetes insipidus can be avoided by handling the pituitary stalk with great gentleness, avoiding the transmission of force or traction to the hypothalamic nuclei, and using sharp dissection in detaching the tumor from the stalk.

The actual incidence of mortality and complications in our transsphenoidal series is presented in Table 15-5. The incidence of surgical problems is

Table 15-6. Potential Complications of Transsphenoidal Surgery for Craniopharyngioma

Complication	Cause	Avoidance
Hypothalamic damage	Surgical trauma Hemorrhage	Video fluoroscopic control Microsurgical technique
Optic nerve/chiasm damage	Surgical trauma Ischemia Postoperative scarring Postoperative prolapse	Surgical landmarks Microsurgical technique Packing the empty sella
Arterial damage	Surgical trauma Arterial anomalies Arterial pathology (aneurysm, ectasia, etc.) Misdirected approach	Preoperative imaging Microsurgical technique
CSF rhinorrhea/meningitis	Violation of skull/dura Misdirected approach Inadequate closure	Careful technique and anatomic assessment Prophylactic antibiotics
Cavernous sinus/cranial damage	Surgical trauma Misdirected approach	Careful technique and anatomic assessment
Brainstem damage	Misdirected approach Surgical trauma	Careful technique and anatomic assessment
Sphenoid sinus complications	Surgical trauma Retained mucosa	Excision of mucosa Careful technique
Nasal/sublabial complications	Resection of nasal spine Septal mucosal perforation Inadequate reconstruction Devitalization of teeth	Nondestructive technique; reconstruction of nasal structures
Diabetes insipidus	Surgical trauma to or ischemia of stalk/hypothalamus	Microsurgical technique Sharp dissection

acceptable, particularly considering the difficulty in managing some of these tumors. The potential complications, their major causes, and methods of avoidance are given in Table 15-6. The references[312-361] provide a review of the literature with regard to extracranial approaches to craniopharyngioma and include the complications reported by others. Advances in diagnosis, surgical technique, and adjunctive measures should result in continuing improvement in the outcome of therapy for patients with craniopharyngiomas.

Complications and Their Avoidance

Alexander N. Konovalov

Craniopharyngioma surgery is both difficult and risky. Many outstanding neurosurgeons have been interested in the problems inherent in craniopharyngioma surgery.[362,364-372] Although challenged by the difficulties presented by craniopharyngiomas, owing to their proximity to important brain structures, and inspired by the possibility of achieving radical resection of these tumors with the help of microsurgical techniques, early optimism turned to pessimism as the number of complications and the rate of tumor recurrence continued to be high.

CRANIOPHARYNGIOMA DIFFERENTIATION

Surgical complexity, results, and complications are closely related to the location and size of the tumor.

Craniopharyngiomas are usually differentiated in accordance with their position relative to the chiasm. The relation of the tumor to the third ventricle (e.g., beneath the third ventricle, thus compressing and elevating its floor, or penetrating the ventricular floor) is of special importance. In everyday practice the following classification is used[365,366]:

1. *Endosuprasellar craniopharyngiomas.* Pure endosellar craniopharyngiomas are rare and are usually approached transsphenoidally.
2. *Suprasellar craniopharyngiomas.* These start to develop at the level of the pituitary stalk (pituitary stalk craniopharyngiomas). They are most often found in the subarachnoid space beneath the third ventricle, elevating the ventricular floor.
3. *Third ventricle craniopharyngiomas.* These tumors develop from remnants of Rathke's pouch at the level of the infundibulum. They destroy the ventricular floor and occupy its cavity. Part of the tumor usually lies

beneath the third ventricle in the intrapeduncular space or spreads to the para- and retrosellar regions. Tumors of the latter two types correspond roughly to the so-called retrochiasmal craniopharyngiomas.

From a practical point of view we consider it important to differentiate tumors that occupy the third ventricle from those that only elevate its floor (both, as just mentioned, being retrochiasmal craniopharyngiomas), as surgical approaches to each are different. Underestimation of their differences may result in selection of the wrong approach. Our next observation illustrates our point:

A patient was admitted to our institution after computed tomography (CT) and magnetic resonance imaging (MRI) revealed a relatively small retrochiasmal craniopharyngioma (Fig. 15-19). Erroneously, the tumor was thought to be intraventricular, and to reach it a transcallosal approach was chosen. How-

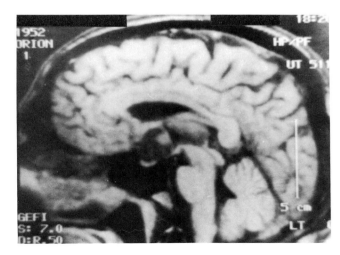

Figure 15-19. Small ''suprasellar-extraventricular'' (retrochiasmal) craniopharyngioma.

ever, no tumor was found in the third ventricle. Instead, the tumor was found to lie beneath the ventricular floor, displacing it upward and compressing the foramen of Monro. Additional frontal trepanation was necessary, and the tumor was successfully removed via the opticocarotid triangle.

This example illustrates that in some cases it is not easy to determine the exact location of the tumor even with the help of CT and MRI. Previously we resorted to ventriculoscopy before opening the skull, as inspection of the foramen of Monro permitted determination of the real location of the tumor.

GIANT CRANIOPHARYNGIOMAS

Craniopharyngiomas can also differ in size, solidity, and cystic content. Giant craniopharyngiomas (those with a diameter of >5 cm) may be met in any of the above-mentioned groups, but are most often pituitary stalk tumors. As a rule, these are cystic tumors. A solid part located in the chiasma-sellar region is usually relatively small and may be intensively calcified. Cysts are more often located in the basal subarachnoid space under the brain in the anterior, middle, and posterior cranial fossae (Figs. 15-20

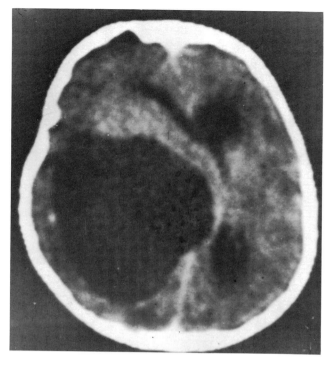

Figure 15-21. Giant cystic craniopharyngioma.

and 15-21). They may protrude into the lateral ventricle through its basal wall (substantia perforata anterior, fissura hypocampi) or into the third ventricle through the intraventricular foramen.

Giant craniopharyngiomas are more common in children. In our practice they constitute about 25 percent of all childhood craniopharyngiomas.

In our experience, in about one-third of all giant cystic craniopharyngiomas, the pituitary stalk and third ventricular floor are not destroyed; rather, they are greatly displaced by the tumor. This is because the tumor has its origin in the subarachnoid space (an explanation of this phenomenon was given by Ciric[363]). Bearing this in mind, the surgeon has to be careful to reveal and preserve the pituitary stalk.

A morphological study by Korshunov[374] revealed that in some cases the tumor does not have its own capsule; rather, the cystic wall is formed by thickened fibrous tunica vasculosa or arachnoidea.

The tumor spreads along cerebral membranes in a thin layer, rounding up cranial nerves (first the optic nerves and chiasm) and basal vessels; in some cases the tumor has no clear border with these structures and a complex of epithelial cells is in close contact with adventitia and perineurium.

In some cases tumor may penetrate the tunica vasculosa and invade the brain.

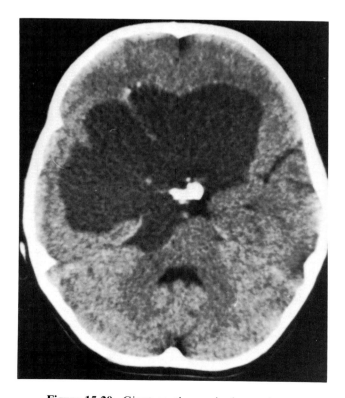

Figure 15-20. Giant cystic craniopharyngioma.

All of the above-mentioned morphological peculiarities make radical removal of these tumors questionable. Surgical complications are strongly related to the anatomical variant of the tumor, its size, and its direction of growth. For example, in a series of third ventricle craniopharyngiomas, mortality was three times that of a series of endosuprasellar craniopharyngiomas. Surgery of giant craniopharyngiomas also results in a high rate of complications and early tumor recurrence.

Only the most important complications of craniopharyngioma surgery and their avoidance will be discussed here.

Direct Damage to the Pituitary Gland, Diencephalon, Optic Pathways, and Other Important Brain Structures

Craniopharyngiomas that develop in the sella may seriously damage the pituitary gland. During surgery it is usually difficult to find and preserve the remnants of the gland. Only in cases of small endosellar tumors in which the gland is not badly damaged can it be preserved after transsphenoidal tumor ablation. In our experience, however, these tumors make up only about 2 to 3 percent of all craniopharyngiomas.

In much more common cases of large endosellar tumors with suprasellar expansion it is usually difficult to find and preserve the remnants of the pituitary gland. Nevertheless, resection of the tumor capsule should always be done with great care, especially in the posterior part of the sella, where tiny strips of light-pink tissue remnants of the gland can be found. In some cases pathologic examination of the tissue for verification of pituitary gland is useful.

Preservation of the pituitary stalk is important to prevent one of the most common complications of craniopharyngioma surgery, namely diabetes insipidus. In some cases in which the stalk is destroyed by the tumor or a previous operation complete compensation for fluid-electrolyte imbalance is possible.

In craniopharyngiomas originating in the sella with suprasellar expansion the pituitary stalk is usually found behind or above the tumor. The stalk can be seriously damaged or destroyed by dislocation and infiltration with the tumor. After evacuation of the cystic contents and removal of the solid part of the tumor the capsule can be displaced downward, which helps to expose the stalk and separate it.

We consider it important to preserve not only the stalk itself but also any vascular connections with the remnants of the pituitary gland. For this reason we leave part of the capsule adherent to the stalk. Once the tumor has been removed we try to suture the remaining part of the capsule to reconstruct the "normal" anatomical relationship and also to prevent dislocation of the optic nerves and the sellar chiasm if it is very large (Fig. 15-22).

As mentioned above, some giant cystic craniopharyngiomas only stretch and displace the stalk. With this in mind the surgeon has to take care to find and preserve this important structure. In cases in which the tumor has infiltrated and destroyed the stalk preservation of its function is highly problematic.

Damage to the Hypothalamus

Damage to the hypothalamus can occur with any type of craniopharyngioma but more often with craniopharyngiomas of the third ventricle. Craniopharyngiomas of this type displace the hypothalamus and often roughly adhere to the walls of the third ventricle—mostly anterior and laterally. Although

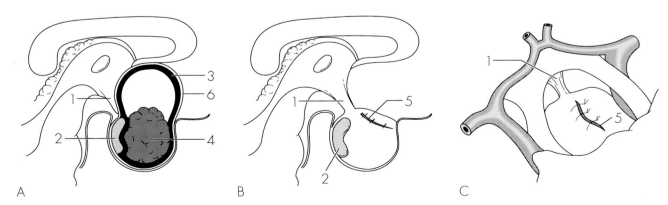

Figure 15-22. (A–C) Stages of removal of endosuprasellar craniopharyngiomas. *(1)* Pituitary stalk. *(2)* Pituitary gland. *(3)* Capsula of craniopharyngioma. *(4)* Solid part of the tumor. *(5)* Sutured diaphragma sellae. *(6)* External layer of craniopharyngioma—distended diaphragma sellae.

there is a layer of glial tissue around the tumor, it may penetrate this capsule and become embedded in the hypothalamus itself; therefore, rough manipulation, especially without good visual control, can be very dangerous. Careful selection of the approach is the best way to avoid this complication. In our experience with direct removal of 200 craniopharyngiomas of the third ventricle a transcallosal approach (alone or in combination with a subfrontal approach) is most appropriate. This approach allows revision of all compartments of the ventricle and separation of the capsule of the tumor under direct visual control. When subchiasmal or transopticocarotid triangle approaches are used, it is difficult at best to expose the tumor penetrating the third ventricle. The lamina terminalis approach provides much better exposure, although only when the tumor is relatively small and localized to the anterior part of the third ventricle. In comparing results of tumor removal with these approaches the percentage of radical tumor removal is found to be much higher and the recurrence rate markedly lower when the transcallosal approach is used.

In our opinion the transcallosal approach also helps to preserve vascularization of the hypothalamus. Vessels supplying the tumor and hypothalamus usually form a rich network on the basal surface of the tumor. Using a basal approach (i.e., subchiasmal, transopticocarotid triangle), I believe that it is more difficult to preserve vessels supplying brain structures than if a transcallosal route is used. In addition, the transcallosal approach allows separation under visual control of the posterior part of the tumor capsule adjacent to the perforating branches arising from the bifurcation of the basilar artery.

Our experience allows us to conclude that a transcallosal (or combined) approach provides better conditions for prevention of hypothalamic damage and for more radical removal of third ventricle craniopharyngiomas.

Damage to the Important Arteries

Damage to the important arteries (carotid, anterior cerebral, posterior communicating arteries, etc.) is rare when microsurgical techniques are used. Damage may occur when the tumor capsule envelops these arteries or when large calcifications, usually localized in the basal part of the craniopharyngioma, have to be removed. Some important arterial branches can be strongly adherent to or even embedded in these calcifications. Lying behind this concretion, they are invisible. Attempts to mobilize and remove such a calcification without breaking it into pieces may result in catastrophic bleeding, which is impossible to control as the damaged artery is not visible. I lost one of my patients with a recurrent highly calcified craniopharyngioma in which one of the posterior communicating arteries was included. An attempt to mobilize this large and very hard calcification resulted in an uncontrollable hemorrhage with tamponade of the third and lateral ventricles. Therefore, with craniopharyngiomas containing large, solid calcifications the surgeon must take care to break them into pieces under visual control with help of rongeurs, scissors, or a special ultrasound knife. Once this is done the peripheral, less hard part of the tumor and its capsule may be displaced and separated from vessels and other important structures.

Disturbances of Brain Circulation

In analyzing causes of death in patients with craniopharyngiomas Vichert and Korshunov of the Burdenko Institute[373,374] found an important fact: in practically all cases of patient mortality after craniopharyngioma removal, spread and in some cases very pronounced disturbances of circulation can be found. These alterations are revealed by obturating arterial thrombosis, exfoliation of an internal elastic membrane or dissecting aneurysm, edema of intima, and multiple necroses of the tunica media (Figs. 15-23 and 15-24). As a result of these alterations there were multiple infarcts in different zones of vascularization (including the diencephalon and brainstem) (Fig. 15-25).

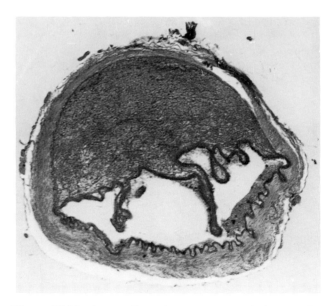

Figure 15-23. Acute dissecting aneurysm of the anterior cerebral artery with occlusion of the arterial lumen after craniopharyngioma removal. (× 40, Weigert's stain.)

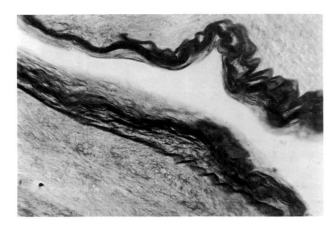

Figure 15-24. Coarse changes in structure of the internal elastic membrane (disorganization, duplication, and distortion) in a branch of middle cerebral artery after craniopharyngioma removal. (× 200, Weigert's stain.)

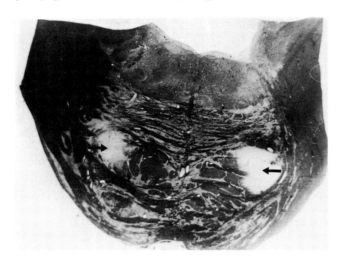

Figure 15-25. Small symmetrical infarction in the pons (*arrows*) after craniopharyngioma removal. (Planar Spielmeyer stain.)

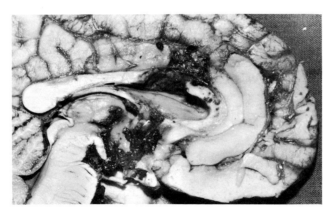

Figure 15-26. Hemorrhage in the diencephalic region after third ventricle craniopharyngioma removal.

It is important to stress that similar changes (usually not very pronounced) can also be observed in patients with craniopharyngiomas who died because of the illness itself and not as a consequence of surgical intervention.

This phenomenon needs special investigation and explanation. Here we can only mention some factors that, in our view, are important:

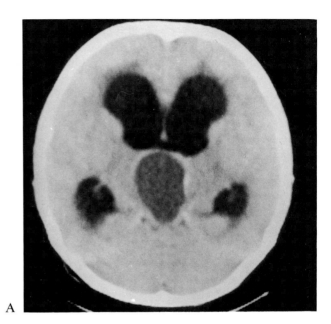

A

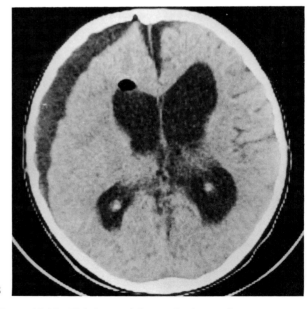

B

Figure 15-27. Third ventricle craniopharyngioma removal. **(A)** Before surgery. **(B)** After tumor removal: brain collapse, with accumulation of air above the right frontal lobe and in anterior horns, and hemorrhagic fluid collection in left frontal region.

1. Acute and chronic changes in vessels as a result of damage to the hypothalamus and pathological secretion of vasoactive peptides and hormones
2. Additional disturbances of microcirculation as a sequela of fluid-electrolyte imbalance and loss of water
3. Spasm of the basal arteries due to postoperative bleeding into the base of the brain (even a small postoperative hemorrhage can be life-threatening, as a spasm of basal arteries can worsen blood circulation that is already seriously compromised)

Control of bleeding during surgery therefore must be extremely thorough. Quite a few patients have been lost as a result of a relatively small hemorrhage in the bed of the removed tumor (Fig. 15-26). As coagulation of bleeding vessels may aggravate ischemic lesions of the hypothalamus, we prefer to control bleeding in this area with small pieces of Gelfoam.

Brain Collapse, Subdural Blood or Fluid Effusion, and Pneumocephalus and Resultant Brain Compression

Brain collapse, subdural effusions, and pneumocephalus may complicate removal of craniopharyngiomas by producing extensive hydrocephalus. Figures 15-27 and 15-28 present some examples of such complications.

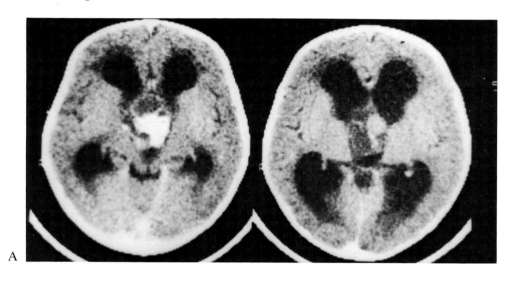

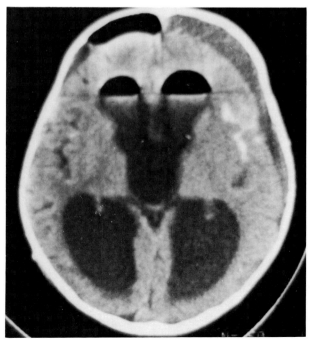

Figure 15-28. Third ventricle craniopharyngioma removal. **(A)** Before surgery. **(B)** After surgery: brain collapse and liquid collection in the right frontal region.

In dealing with giant cystic craniopharyngiomas, we try to anticipate collapse and dislocation by diminishing the volume of cysts with the help of repeated punctures and evacuation of cystic fluid before attempting radical tumor excision. Omaya drainage can also be used for this purpose. In this context the place of shunting procedures in the treatment of craniopharyngiomas needs special discussion.

Our general procedure has been to attempt primary radical removal of the tumor, which usually re-establishes fluid passage while avoiding shunting. If there is a pronounced hydrocephalus, however, radical tumor removal may result in brain collapse, subdural effusions, and brain compression. In such a case we consider it more justified to start with a divergence procedure and to postpone tumor removal until the ventricles became smaller, but not too small, as a hydrocephalus facilitates the approach to the tumor and its removal.

Serial CT imaging is very important in the determination of the most favorable time for radical surgery. We found that in some cases fluid divergence may result not only in diminishing ventricle size, but also in rapid and marked enlargement of cystic tumors, probably owing to intracranial volume-pressure changes. This means that timing of surgery after ventricular shunting is very important in prevention of the above-mentioned serious complications.

CONTRAINDICATIONS TO CRANIOPHARYNGIOMA SURGERY

To prevent some serious complications of craniopharyngioma surgery it is necessary to identify those patients in whom radical tumor removal is too risky. Our experience shows that surgery of recurrent third ventricle craniopharyngiomas engenders many complications. Mortality in this group is more than twice that of primarily operated patients. In adults, and especially in aged patients, results are also markedly worse than in children. In other words, a more conservative strategy in aged patients and in cases of tumor recurrence may greatly lessen the number of complications and mortality.

CONCLUSIONS

It is necessary to emphasize once more that surgery of craniopharyngiomas is still risky and that much must be done to improve results and find ways to prevent the numerous complications that plague patients harboring these tumors.

REFERENCES

General Considerations

1. Arseni C, Maretsis M: Craniopharyngioma. Neurochurgurgia 1:25, 1972
2. Backlund EO: Studies on craniopharyngioma. I. Treatment: past and present. Acta Chir Scand 138:749, 1972
3. Backlund EO: Studies on craniopharyngiomas. III. Stereotaxis treatment with intracystic yttrium-90. Acta Chir Scand 139:237, 1973
4. Backlund EO, Johansson L, Sarby B: Studies on craniopharyngiomas. II. Treatment by stereotaxis and radiosurgery. Acta Chir Scand 138:749, 1972
5. Bartlett JR: Craniopharyngiomas—a summary of 85 cases. J Neurol Neurosurg Psychiatry 34:37, 1971
6. Bartlett JR: Craniopharyngiomas: an analysis of some aspects of symptomatology, radiology, and histology. Brain 94:725, 1971
7. Baskin DS, Wilson CB: Surgical management of craniopharyngiomas: a review of 74 cases. J Neurosurg 65:22, 1986
8. Bond WH, Richards D, Turner E: Experiences with radioactive gold in the treatment of craniopharyngioma. J Neurol Neurosurg Psychiatry 28:30, 1965
9. Cabezudo JM, Vaquero J, Areito E et al: Craniopharyngiomas: a critical approach to treatment. J Neurosurg 55:371, 1981
10. Carmel PW, Antunes JL, Chany CH: Craniopharyngiomas in children. Neurosurgery 11:382, 1982
11. Cavazutti V, Fischer EG, Welch K et al: Neurologic and psychophysiologic sequelae following different treatments of craniopharyngiomas in children. J Neurosurg 59:409, 1983
12. Ciric IS, Cozzens JM: Craniopharyngiomas: transsphenoidal method of approach—for the virtuoso only? Clin Neurosurg 27:169, 1980
13. Fischer EG, Welch K, Bell JA: Treatment of craniopharyngiomas in children. J Neurosurg 62:496, 1985
14. Fischer EG, Welch K, Shillito J et al: Craniopharyngiomas in children. Long-term effects of conservative surgical procedures combined with radiation therapy. J Neurosurg 73:534, 1990
15. Garcia-Uria J: Surgical experience with craniopharyngioma in adults. Surg Neurol 9:11, 1978
16. Gordy PD, Peet MM, Kahn EA: The surgery of the craniopharyngiomas. J Neurosurg 6:503, 1949
17. Guidetti B, Fraioli B: Craniopharyngiomas. Results of surgical treatment. Acta Neurochir Suppl 28:349, 1979
18. Gutin PH, Klemme WM, Lagger RL et al: Management of the unresectable cystic craniopharyngioma by aspiration through Omaya reservoir drainage system. J Neurosurg 52:36, 1980
19. Hoff JT, Patterson RH: Craniopharyngiomas in children and adults. J Neurosurg 36:299, 1972
20. Hoffman HJ, Hendrick EB, Humphreys RP et al:

Management of craniopharyngioma in children. J Neurosurg 47:218, 1977

21. Ivkov M, Ribaric I, Slavik E: Surgical treatment of craniopharyngiomas in adults. Acta Neurochir Suppl 28:352, 1979

22. Julow J, Layni F, Hadja M et al: The radiotherapy of cystic craniopharyngioma with intracystic installation of 90 Y silicate colloid. Acta Neurochir 74:94, 1985

23. Kahn EA: Some physiologic implications of craniopharyngiomas. Neurology 9:82, 1959

24. Kahn EA, Gosch HH, Seeger J et al: Forty-five years experience with the craniopharyngiomas. Surg Neurol 1:5, 1973

25. Kanno T, Kajama A: A pitfall in the interhemispheric translamina terminalis approach for the removal of a craniopharyngioma. Significance of preserving draining veins. Part II. Experimental study. Surg Neurol 32:116, 1989

26. Kanno T, Kajama A, Shoda M et al: A pitfall in the interhemispheric translamina terminalis approach for the removal of a craniopharyngioma. Significance of preserving draining veins. Part I. Clinical study. Surg Neurol 32:111, 1989

27. Katz EL: Late results of radical excision of craniopharyngiomas in children. J Neurosurg 42:86, 1975

28. King TT: Removal of intraventricular craniopharyngiomas through the lamina terminalis. Acta Neurochir 45:277, 1979

29. Kobayashi T, Kageyama N, Ohara K: Internal irradiation for cystic craniopharyngioma. J Neurosurg 55:986, 1981

30. Kramer S, McKissock W, Concannon JP: Craniopharyngiomas. Treatment by combined surgery and radiation therapy. J Neurosurg 17:217, 1961

31. Kramer S, Southard M, Mansfield CM: Radiotherapy in the management of craniopharyngiomas. AJR 103:44, 1968

32. Laws ER: Transsphenoidal microsurgery in the management of craniopharyngioma. J Neurosurg 52:661, 1980

33. Laws ER: Craniopharyngioma. Neurosurgery 19:326, 1986

34. Leksell L, Backlund EO, Johansson L: Treatment of craniopharyngiomas. Acta Chir Scand 133:345, 1967

35. Lipton JM, Rosenstein J, Sklar FH: Thermoregulatory disorders after removal of a craniopharyngioma from the third ventricle. Brain Res Bull 7:369, 1981

36. Manaka S, Teramoto A, Takakura K: The efficacy of radiotherapy for craniopharyngioma. J Neurosurg 62:648, 1985

37. Matson DD: Craniopharyngioma. Clin Neurosurg 10:116, 1962

38. Matson DD, Crigler JF: Management of craniopharyngioma in childhood. J Neurosurg 30:377, 1969

39. McClone DG, Raimondi AJ, Naidich JP: Craniopharyngioma. Childs Brain 9:188, 1982

40. Mori K, Harda H, Murata T et al: Results of treatment for craniopharyngioma. Childs Brain 6:303, 1980

41. Pollack IF, Lunsford LD, Slamovitz TL et al: Stereotaxis intracavitary irradiation for cystic craniopharyngiomas. J Neurosurg 68:227, 1988

42. Rougerie J: What can be expected from the surgical treatment of craniopharyngiomas in children. Childs Brain 5:433, 1979

43. Shapiro K, Till K, Grant DN: Craniopharyngiomas in childhood. A rational approach to treatment. J Neurosurg 50:617, 1979

44. Shillito J: Craniopharyngiomas: the subfrontal approach or none at all? Clin Neurosurg 27:188, 1980

45. Sturm V, Rommel T, Strauss L et al: Preliminary results of intracavitary irradiation of cystic craniopharyngiomas by means of stereotactically applied yttrium-90. Adv Neurosurg 9:401, 1981

46. Sung OI, Chung CH, Harisiadis L et al: Treatment results of craniopharyngiomas. Cancer 47:874, 1981

47. Svien HJ: Surgical experiences with craniopharyngiomas. J Neurosurg 23:148, 1965

48. Svolos DG: Craniopharyngiomas. Acta Chir Scand Suppl 403:4, 1969

49. Sweet WH: Radical surgical treatment of craniopharyngioma. Clin Neurosurg 23:52, 1976

50. Sweet WH: Recurrent craniopharyngiomas: therapeutic alternatives. Clin Neurosurg 27:206, 1980

51. Takahashi H, Nakasawa S, Shimura T: Evaluation of postoperative intratumoral injection of bleomycin in craniopharyngioma in children. J Neurosurg 62:120, 1985

52. Till K: Craniopharyngioma. Childs Brain 9:179, 1982

53. Thomsett MJ, Conte FA, Kaplan SL et al: Endocrine and neurologic outcome in childhood craniopharyngioma: review of effect of treatment in 42 patients. J Pediatr 97:728, 1980

54. Trippi AL, Garner JT, Kassabian JT: A new approach to inoperable craniopharyngiomas. Am J Surg 118:307, 1969

55. Yasargil MG, Curcia M, Kis M et al: Total removal of craniopharyngiomas. Approaches and long-term results in 144 patients. J Neurosurg 73:3, 1990

Hypothalamic Hypophyseal Compromise

56. Al-Mefty O, Hassounah M, Weaver P et al: Microsurgery for giant craniopharyngiomas in children. Neurosurgery 17:585, 1985

57. Amacher AL: Craniopharyngioma: the controversy regarding radiotherapy. Childs Brain 6:57, 1980

58. Amarant TM, Fridkin M, Koch Y: Leutinizing hormone-releasing hormone and thyrotropin-releasing hormone in human and bovine milk. Eur J Biochem 127:647, 1982

59. Arem R, Zoghbi W, Chan L: Amenorrhea-galactorrhea and craniopharyngioma. Surg Neurol 20:109, 1983

60. Arieff AI, Guisado R: Effects on the central nervous system of the hypernatremia and hypernatremic states. Kidney Int 10:104, 1976

61. Arnold A, Bailey P, Harvey RA: Intolerance of the

primate brainstem and hypothalamus to conventional and high energy radiations. Neurology 4:575, 1954

62. Arseni C, Maretsis M: Craniopharyngioma. Neurochirurgica 1:25, 1972

63. Ayus YC, Rhada KK, Arieff AI et al: Changing concepts in treatment of severe symptomatic hyponatremia: rapid correction and possible relation to central pontine myelinolysis. Am J Med 78:897, 1985

64. Backlund EO: Studies on craniopharyngiomas. I. Treatment: past and present. Acta Chir Scand 138:743, 1972

65. Backlund EO: Stereotactic treatment of craniopharyngiomas (1966–1975). Presented at the 6th International Congress of Neurological Surgery, Sao Paulo, June 19–25, 1977

66. Bailey P, Buchanan DN, Bucy PC: Intracranial Tumors of Infancy and Childhood. p. 349. University of Chicago Press, Chicago, 1939

67. Barnea ER, Naftolin F, Tolis G, De Cherney A: Hypothalamic amenorrhea syndromes. In Givens JR (ed): The Hypothalamus. p. 147. Year Book Medical Publishers, Chicago, 1984

68. Bartlett JR: Craniopharyngiomas—a summary of 85 cases. J Neurol Neurosurg Psychiatry 34:37, 1971

69. Bartlett JR: Craniopharyngiomas. An analysis of some aspects of symptomatology, radiology and histology. Brain 94:725, 1971

70. Baskin DS, Wilson CB: Surgical management of craniopharyngiomas: a review of 74 cases. J Neurosurg 65:22, 1986

71. Bennett GW, Sharp T, Brazell M, Marsden GA: TRH and catecholamine neurotransmitter release in the central nervous system. p. 253. In Griffiths EC, Bennett GW (eds): Thyrotropin-Releasing Hormone. Raven Press, New York, 1983

72. Berg GR, Utiger RD, Schalch DS, Reichlin S: Effect of central cooling in man on pituitary-thyroid function and growth hormone secretion. J Appl Physiol 21:1791, 1966

73. Bergland RM, Page RB: Can the pituitary secrete directly to the brain? (affirmative anatomical evidence). Endocrinology 102:1325, 1978

74. Bergland RM, Page RB: Pituitary-brain vascular relations: a new paradigm. Science 204:18, 1979

75. Beutler B, Greenwald D, Hulmes JD et al: Identity of tumor necrosis factor and the macrophage-secreted factor cachectin. Nature 316:552, 1985.

76. Beutler B, Cerami A: Cachectin and tumor necrosis factor as two sides of the same biological coin. Nature 320:584, 1986

77. Blatt J, Bercu BB, Gillin JC et al: Reduced pulsatile growth hormone secretion in children after therapy for acute lymphoblastic leukemia. J Pediatr 104:182, 1984

78. Bligh J: Neuronal models of hypothalamic temperature regulation. p. 315. In Lederis K, Cooper KE (eds): Recent Studies of Hypothalamic Function. S Karger, Basel, 1973

79. Bloom HJG: Recent concepts in the conservative treatment of intracranial tumours in children. Acta Neurochir 50:103, 1979

80. Bloom HJG, Harmer CL: Craniopharyngioma: general aspects and treatment. p. 119. In Bucalossi P, Veronesi V, Emanuelli H et al (eds): I Tumori Infantili. Casa Editrice Ambrosiana, Milano, 1976

81. Boden G: Radiation myelitis of the brain-stem. J Fac Radiol 2:79, 1950

82. Bord WH, Richards D, Turner E: Experiences with radioactive gold in the treatment of craniopharyngioma. J Neurol Neurosurg Psychiatry 28:30, 1965

83. Borges JL, Blizzard RM, Evans WS et al: Stimulation of growth hormone (GH) and somatomedin C in idiopathic GH-deficient subjects by intermittent pulsatile administration of synthetic human pancreatic tumor GH-releasing factor. J Clin Endocrinol Metab 59:1, 1984

84. Borges JL, Blizzard RM, Gelato MC et al: Effects of human pancreatic tumour growth hormone releasing factor on growth hormone and somatomedin C levels in patients with idiopathic growth hormone deficiency. Lancet 2:119, 1983

85. Burger HG, Patel YC: TSH and TRH: their physiological regulation and the clinical applications of TRH. p. 67. In Martin L, Besser GM (eds): Clinical Neuroendocrinology. Academic Press, San Diego, 1977

86. Cabezudo JM, Vaquero J, Areitio E et al: Craniopharyngiomas: a critical approach to treatment. J Neurosurg 55:371, 1981

87. Cairns H, Oldfield RC, Pennybacker JB, Whatteridge D: Akinetic mutism with an epidermoid cyst of the third ventricle (with a report on the associated disturbance of brain potentials). Brain 64:273, 1941

88. Calabrese VP, Selhorst JB, Harbison JW: Cerebrospinal fluid infusion test in pseudotumor cerebri, abstracted. Ann Neurol 4:173, 1978

89. Carmel PW: Craniopharyngiomas. p. 905. In Wilkins RH, Rengachary SS (eds): Neurosurgery. McGraw-Hill, New York, 1985

90. Carmel PW, Antunes JL, Chany CH: Craniopharyngiomas in children. Neurosurgery II:382, 1982

91. Caroff S, Rosenberg H, Gerber JC: Neuroleptic malignant syndrome and malignant hyperthermia. Lancet 1:244, 1983

92. Cashion EL, Young JM: Intraventricular craniopharyngiomas. Report of 2 cases. J Neurosurg 34:84, 1971

93. Cavazutti V, Fischer EG, Welch K et al: Neurologic and psychophysiologic sequelae following different treatments of craniopharyngiomas in children. J Neurosurg 59:409, 1983

94. Cobb WE: Management of neurogenic diabetes insipidus with DAVP and other agents. p. 139. In Reichlin S (ed): The Neurohypophysis. Plenum, New York, 1984

95. Cogen PH, Carmel PW: Craniopharyngioma growth potential: therapy response of children vs. adults, abstracted. Neurosurgery 9:469, 1981

96. Cooper PR, Ransohoff J: Craniopharyngioma originating in the sphenoid bone. Case report. J Neurosurg 36:102, 1972

97. Cravioto H, Silberman J, Feigin I: A clinical and pathologic study of akinetic mutism. Neurology 10:10, 1960

98. Crompton MR: Hypothalamic lesions following the rupture of cerebral berry aneurysms. Brain 86:301, 1963

99. Crompton MR, Layton DD: Delayed radionecrosis of the brain following therapeutic x-radiation of the pituitary. Brain 84:85, 1961

100. Dargeon HW: Considerations in the treatment of reticuloendotheliosis. The Janeway Lecture, 1964. AJR 93:521, 1965

101. Davison C, Demuth EL: Disturbances in sleep mechanism. Clinicopathological study: lesions at diencephalic level (hypothalamus). Arch Neurol Psychiatry 55:111, 1946

102. Dyer RG, Dyball REJ: Evidence for a direct effect of LRF and TRF on single unit activity in nostral hypothalamus. Nature 252:233, 1974

103. Erdheim J: Veber Hypophysengangsgeschwulste und hirn Cholesteatome. Sitzungsb DK Akad Wissensch Math Natur Cl (Wien) 113:537, 1904

104. Evans DE, Gillia RA: Reflux mechanisms involved in cardiac arrhythmias induced by hypothalamic stimulation. Am J Physiol 234:199, 1978

105. Feldberg W, Myers RD: Effects on temperature of amines injected into the cerebral ventricles. A new concept of temperature regulation. J Physiol (Lond) 173:226, 1964

106. Fink G, Koch Y, Aroya NB: Release of thyrotropin releasing hormone into hypophysial portal blood is high relative to other neuropeptides and may be related to prolactin secretion. Brain Res 243:186, 1982

107. Finlayson MH, Snider S, Oliva LA, Gault MH: Cerebral and pontine myelinolysis: two cases with fluid and electrolytic imbalance and hypotension. J Neurol Sci 18:399, 1973

108. Fischer EG, Welch K, Belli JA et al: Treatment of craniopharyngiomas in children: 1972–1981. J Neurosurg 62:496, 1985

109. Fischer EG, Welch K, Shillito J et al: Craniopharyngiomas in children. Long-term effects of conservative surgical procedures combined with radiation therapy. J Neurosurg 73:534, 1990

110. Frohlich A: Ein Fall von Tumor dert Hypophysis cerebri ohne Akromegalie. Wien Klin Runcsch 15:883, 1901

111. Fukamachi A, Wakao T, Akai J: Brain stem necrosis after irradiation of pituitary adenoma. Surg Neurol 18:343, 1982

112. Fulton JF, Bailey P: Tumors in the region of the third ventricle: their diagnosis and relation to pathological sleep. J Nerv Ment Dis 69:1, 1929

113. Garcia-Uria J: Surgical experience with craniopharyngioma in adults. Surg Neurol 9:11, 1978

114. Goldberg MB, Sheline GE, Malamud N: Malignant intracranial neoplasms following radiation therapy for acromegaly. Radiology 80:465, 1963

115. Gordy PD, Peet MM, Kahn EA: The surgery of the craniopharyngiomas. J Neurosurg 6:503, 1949

116. Gowers WR: Epilepsy and Other Chronic Convulsive Diseases: Their Causes, Symptoms and Treatment. Dover Publications, New York, 1885

117. Grant DB, Lyer K: Hypopituitarism after surgery for craniopharyngioma. Childs Brain 8:201, 1982

118. Green WH, Campbell M, David R: Psychosocial dwarfism: a critical review of the evidence. J Am Acad Child Psychiatry 1:39, 1984

119. Greenhouse AH: Pituitary sarcoma: a possible consequence of radiation. JAMA 190:269, 1964

120. Grossman A, Savage MO, Wass JA et al: Growth hormone-releasing factor in growth hormone deficiency: demonstration of a hypothalamic defect in growth hormone release. Lancet 2:137, 1983

121. Gutin PH, Klemme W, Lagger RL et al: Management of the unresectable cystic craniopharyngioma by aspiration through Omaya reservoir drainage system. J Neurosurg 52:36, 1980

122. Hamberger CA, Hammer G, Norlen G et al: Surgical treatment of craniopharyngioma. Radical removal by the transantrosphenoidal approach. Acta Otolaryngol (Stockh) 52:285, 1960

123. Hamer J: Removal of craniopharyngioma by subnasal-transsphenoidal operation. Neuropediatrics 9:312, 1978

124. Hantman D, Rossier B, Zohlman R et al: Rapid correction of hyponatremia in the syndrome of inappropriate secretion of antidiuretic hormone. An alternative treatment to hypertonic saline. Ann Intern Med 78:870, 1973

125. Hardy JD: Control of body temperature. p. 294. In Mogenson GJ, Calaresu FR (eds): Neural Integration of Physiological Mechanisms and Behavior. University of Toronto Press, Toronto, 1975

126. Harrop JS, Davies TJ, Capra LG et al: Pituitary function after treatment of intracranial tumors in children. (Letter to the editor.) Lancet 2:231, 1975

127. Healy DL, Chrousos GP, Schulte HM et al: Increased adrenocorticotropin cortisol and arginine vasopressin secretion in primates after the antiglucocorticoid steroid RU 496: dose response relationships. J Clin Endocrinol Metab 60:1, 1985

128. Hodgson SF, Randall RV, Holman CB et al: Empty sella syndrome: report of 10 cases. Med Clin North Am 56:897, 1972

129. Hoff JT, Patterson RH: Craniopharyngiomas in children and adults. J Neurosurg 36:29, 1972

130. Hoffman HJ: Craniopharyngioma—the continuing controversy on management. Presented at the American Association of Neurological Surgeons, Boston, April 6–9, 1981

131. Hoffman HJ, Hendrick EB, Humphreys RP et al: Management of craniopharyngioma in children. J Neurosurg 47:218, 1977

132. Hou S: Syndrome of inappropriate antidiuretic hormone secretion. p. 165. In Reichlin S (ed): The Neurohypophysis. Plenum, New York, 1984

133. Ivkov M, Ribaric I, Slavik E: Surgical treatment of craniopharyngiomas in adults. Acta Neurochir [Suppl] (Wien) 28:352, 1979

134. Jenkins JS, Gilbert CS, Ang V: Hypothalamic pituitary function in patients with craniopharyngiomas. J Clin Endocrinol Metab 43:394, 1976

135. Jordon RM, Kendall JW, Kerber CW: The primary empty sella syndrome: analysis of the clinical characteristics, radiographic features, pituitary function and cerebrospinal fluid adenohypophysial hormone concentrations. Am J Med 65:569, 1977

136. Julow J, Lanyi F, Hajda M et al: The radiotherapy of cystic craniopharyngioma with intracystic installation of 90Y silicate colloid. Acta Neurochir (Wien) 74:94, 1965

137. Kahn EA: Some physiologic implications of craniopharyngioma. Neurology 9:82, 1959

138. Kahn EA, Gosch HH, Seeger J et al: Forty-five years experience with craniopharyngiomas. Surg Neurol 1:5, 1973

139. Kasting NW, Veale WL, Cooper KE, Lederis K: Effect of hemorrhage on fever: the putative role of vasopressin. Can J Physiol Pharmacol 59:324, 1981

140. Katz EL: Late results of radical excision of craniopharyngiomas in children. J Neurosurg 42:86, 1975

141. Kempe LG: Operative Neurosurgery. Vol. 1: Cranial, Cerebral and Intracranial Vascular Disease. Springer-Verlag, New York, 1968, p. 90

142. King TT: Removal of intraventricular craniopharyngiomas through the lamina terminalis. Acta Neurochir (Wien) 45:277, 1979

143. Kobayashi T, Kageyama N, Ohara K: Internal irradiation for cystic craniopharyngioma. J Neurosurg 55:896, 1981

144. Kobayashi T, Kageyama N, Yoshida J et al: Pathological and clinical basis of the indications for treatment of craniopharyngiomas. Neurol Med Chir (Tokyo) 71:39, 1981

145. Kramer S: Craniopharyngioma: the best treatment is conservative surgery and postoperative radiation therapy. p. 336. In Morley TP (ed): Current Controversies in Neurosurgery. WB Saunders, Philadelphia, 1976

146. Kramer S, McKissack W, Concannon JP: Craniopharyngiomas. Treatment of combined surgery and radiation therapy. J Neurosurg 17:217, 1961

147. Kramer S, Southard M, Mansfield CM: Radiotherapy in the management of craniopharyngiomas. AJR 103:44, 1968

148. Lam KSL, Wang C, Yeung RTT et al: Hypothalamic hypopituitarism following cranial irradiation for nasopharyngeal carcinoma. Clin Endocrinol 24:643, 1986

149. Landolt A: 8. Die Ultrastruktur des Kraniopharyngeoms. Schweiz Arch Neurol Neurochir Psychiatry 111:313, 1972

150. Langman J: Medical Embryology. Williams & Wilkins, Baltimore, 1981

151. Laron Z, Gil-Ad T, Topper E et al: Low oral dose of clonidine: an effective screening test for hormone deficiency. Acta Paediatr Scand 71:847, 1982

152. Laron Z, Topper E, Gil-Ad T: Oral clonidine—a simple, safe and effective test for growth hormone secretion. Evaluation of growth hormone secretion: physiology and clinical application. Pediatr Adolesc Endocrinol 12:103, 1983

153. Laws ER: Transsphenoidal microsurgery in the management of craniopharyngioma. J Neurosurg 52:661, 1980

154. Lechan RM, Nestler JL, Jacobson S, Reichlin S: The hypothalamic "tuberoinfundibular" system of the rate as demonstrated by horseradish peroxidase (HRP) microiontophoresis. Brain Res 195:13, 1980

155. Leddy ET, Marshall TM: Roentgen therapy of pituitary adamantinomas (craniopharyngioma). Radiology 56:384, 1951

156. Lipton JM, Rosenstein J, Sklar FH: Thermoregulatory disorders after removal of a craniopharyngioma from the third ventricle. Brain Res Bull 7:369, 1981

157. Manaka S, Teramoto A, Takakura K: The efficacy of radiotherapy for craniopharyngioma. J Neurosurg 62:648, 1985

158. Martin JB, Copeland PM: Hypothalamic hypopituitarism. p. 71. In Krieger DT, Bardin CW (eds): Current Therapy in Endocrinology and Metabolism. BC Decker, Philadelphia, 1985

159. Martin JB, Reichlin S: Clinical Neuroendocrinology. FA Davis, Philadelphia, 1987

160. Matson DD: Craniopharyngioma. Clin Neurosurg 10:116, 1962

161. Matson DD: Neurosurgery of Infancy and Childhood. Charles C Thomas, Springfield, IL, 1969

162. Matson DD, Crigler JF: Management of craniopharyngioma in childhood. J Neurosurg 30:377, 1969

163. McMurry FG, Hardy RW, Dohn DF et al: Long term results in the management of craniopharyngiomas. Neurosurgery 1:238, 1977

164. Mechanick JI, Hochberg FH, Larocque A: Hypothalamic dysfunction following whole-brain irradiation. J Neurosurg 65:490, 1986

165. Muller E: Growth enhancement by clonidine treatment in children with growth disorders. p. 309. In Muller EE, MacLeod RM (eds): Neuroendocrine Perspectives. Vol. 5. Elsevier, Amsterdam, 1986

166. Nielsen JM, Jacobs LL: Bilateral lesions of the anterior cingulate gyrt. Bull Los Angeles Neurol Soc 16:231, 1951

167. Northfield DWC: Rathke-pouch tumours. Brain 80:293, 1957

168. Orayama Y, Ono K, Yabumoto E et al: Radiation therapy of craniopharyngioma. Radiology 125:799, 1977

169. Peck FC, McGovern ER: Radiation necrosis of the brain in acromegaly. Neurosurgery 25:536, 1966

170. Pertuiset B: Craniopharyngiomas. p. 531. In Vinken PJ, Bruyn GW (eds): Handbook of Clinical Neurology. Vol. 18. Part 3. Tumors of the Brain and Skull. North-Holland, Amsterdam, 1975

171. Petito CK, DeGirolami U, Earle K: Craniopharyngiomas. A clinical and pathological review. Cancer 37:1944, 1976

172. Pheline C, Jamois Y, Engel P et al: One case of atypical craniopharyngioma located in sphenoidal body and operated first by nasal then by maxillary sinus route. Neuro-Chire 27:221, 1981

173. Plum F, Posner J: The Diagnosis of Stupor and Coma. 3rd Ed. FA Davis, Philadelphia, 1980

174. Pollack IF, Lunsford LOP, Slamovitz TL et al: Stereotaxic intracavitary irradiation for cystic craniopharyngiomas. J Neurosurg 68:227, 1988

175. Reeves AG, Plum F: Hyperphagia rage and dementia accompanying a ventromedial hypothalamic neoplasm. Arch Neurol 20:616, 1969

176. Robertson GL: Physiopathology of ADH secretion. p. 274. In Tolis G, Labrie F, Martin JB, Naftolin F (eds): Clinical Neuroendocrinology: A Pathophysiological Approach. Raven Press, New York, 1979

177. Romshe CA, Zipf WB, Miser A et al: Evaluation of growth hormone release and human growth hormone treatment in children with cranial irradiation-associated short stature. J Pediatr 104:177, 1984

178. Rougerie J: What can be expected from the surgical treatment of craniopharyngiomas in children. Childs Brain 5:433, 1979

179. Rush JL, Kusske JA, DeFeo DR et al: Intraventricular craniopharyngioma. Neurology 25:1094, 1975

180. Rymer MM, Fishman FA: Protective adaptation of brain to water intoxication. Arch Neurol 28:49, 1973

181. Shalet SM, Morris-Jones PN, Bearowell CG, Pearson O: Pituitary function after treatment of intracranial tumours in children. Lancet 2:104, 1975

182. Shibasaki T, Sihzume K, Nakahara M et al: Age-related changes in plasma growth hormone response to growth hormone-releasing factor in man. J Clin Endocrinol Metab 58:212, 1984

183. Shillito J: The treatment of cranipharyngiomas of childhood. p. 332. In Morley TP (ed): Current Controversies in Neurosurgery. WB Saunders, Philadelphia, 1976

184. Shillito J: Craniopharyngiomas. Special Lecture. American Association of Neurological Surgeons, New Orleans, April 26, 1978

185. Shillito J: Craniopharyngiomas: the subfrontal approach or none at all? Clin Neurosurg 27:188, 1980

186. Skultety FM: Clinical and experimental aspects of akinetic mutism. Report of a case. Arch Neurol 19:1, 1968

187. Snyder PJ, Jacobs LS, Rasello MM et al: Diagnostic value of thyrotropin-releasing hormone in pituitary and hypothalamic disease. Ann Intern Med 81:751, 1974

188. Soni SS, Marten GW, Pitner SE et al: Effects of central-nervous-system irradiation on neuropsychologic functioning of children with acute lymphocytic leukemia. N Engl J Med 293:113, 1975

189. Steno JG: Microsurgical topography of craniopharyngiomas. Acta Neurochir [Suppl] (Wien) 35:94, 1985

190. Streeten DHP, Anderson GH, Jr, Dalakos TG et al: Normal and abnormal function of the hypothalamic-pituitary-adrenocortical system in man. Endocr Rev 5:371, 1984

191. Sung OI, Ching CH, Harisiadis L et al: Treatment results of craniopharyngiomas. Cancer 47:847, 1981

192. Svolos DG: Craniopharyngiomas. Acta Chir Scand [Suppl] 403:4, 1969

193. Sweet WH: Radical surgical treatment of craniopharyngioma. Clin Neurosurg 23:52, 1976

194. Sweet WH: Recurrent craniopharyngiomas: therapeutic alternatives. Clin Neurosurg 27:206, 1980

195. Sweet WH: Craniopharyngiomas (with a note on Rathke's cleft epithelial cysts and on suprasellar cysts). p. 349. In Schmidek H, Sweet WH (eds): Operative Neurosurgical Techniques: Indications, Methods, and Results. Grune & Stratton, Orlando, FL, 1988

196. Talman WT: Cardiovascular regulation and lesions of the central nervous system. Ann Neurol 18:1, 1985

197. Thomsett MJ, Conte FA, Kaplan SL et al: Endocrine and neurologic outcome in childhood craniopharyngioma: review of effect of treatment in 42 patients. J Pediatr 97:728, 1980

198. Till K: Craniopharyngioma. Childs Brain 9:179, 1982

199. Tindall GE: Tumors of the sellar and parasellar area in adults. p. 3447. In Youmans JR (ed): Neurological Surgery. 3d Ed. WB Saunders, Philadelphia, 1990

200. Van den Bergh R, Brucher JM: L'abord transventriculaire dans les cranio-pharyngiomes du troisième ventricule. Aspects neurochirugicaux et neuropathologiques. Neurochirurgie 16:51, 1970

201. Veldhuis JD: Hypopituitarism. p. 16. In Krieger DT, Bardin CW (eds): Current Therapy in Endocrinology and Metabolism. BC Decker, Philadelphia, 1985

202. Victor M, Adams RD, Collins GH: Wernicke-Korsakoff Syndrome. FA Davis, Philadelphia, 1971

203. Weigand SJ, Price JL: Cells of origin of the afferent fibers to the median eminence in the rat. J Comp Neurol 192:1, 1980

204. Weiss SR, Raskind R: Non-neoplastic intrasellar cysts. Int Surg 51:282, 1969

205. White JC: Aneurysms mistaken for hypophyseal tumors. J Clin Neurosurg 10:224, 1964

206. Williams T, Berelowitz M, Joffe SN et al: Impaired growth hormone response to growth-hormone releasing factor in obesity. N Engl J Med 311:1403, 1984

207. Witt JA, MacCarty CS, Keating FR: Craniopharyngioma (pituitary adamantinoma) in patients more than 60 years of age. J Neurosurg 12:354, 1955

208. Yasargil MG, Curcia M, Kis M et al: Total removal of craniopharyngiomas. Approaches and long-term results in 144 patients. J Neurosurg 73:3, 1990

Transcranial Approaches

209. Adamson TE, Wiestler OD, Kleihues P, Yasargil MG: Correlation of clinical and pathological features in surgically treated craniopharyngiomas. J Neurosurg 73:12, 1990

210. Al-Mefty O, Hassounah M, Weaver P et al: Micro-

surgery for giant craniopharyngiomas in children. Neurosurgery 17:585, 1985

211. Altinors N, Senveli E, Erdogan A et al: Craniopharyngioma of the cerebello-pontine angle. Case report. J Neurosurg 60:842, 1984

212. Alvord EC, Jr: Growth rates of epidermoid tumors. Ann Neurol 2:367, 1977

213. Amacher AL: Craniopharyngioma: the controversy regarding radiotherapy. Childs Brain 6:57, 1980

214. Antunes JL, Muraszko K, Quest DO, Carmel PW: Surgical strategies in the management of tumors of the anterior third ventricle. In Brock M (ed): Modern Neurosurgery. Springer-Verlag, Berlin, 1982

215. Apuzzo MLJ, Chikovani OK, Gott PS et al: Transcallosal interfornicial approaches for lesions affecting the third ventricle: surgical considerations and consequences. Neurosurgery 10:547, 1982

216. Backlund EO, Axelsson B, Bergstrand CG et al: Treatment of craniopharyngiomas—the stereotactic approach in a ten to twenty-three years' perspective. I. Surgical, radiological and ophthalmological aspects. Acta Neurochir (Wien) 99:11, 1989

217. Banna M: Craniopharyngioma in adults. Surg Neurol 1:202, 1973

218. Banna M, Hoare RD, Stanley P, Till K: Craniopharyngioma in children. J Pediatr 83:781, 1973

219. Barrow DL, Spector RH, Takei Y, Tindal GT: Symptomatic Rathke's cleft cysts located entirely in the suprasellar region: review of diagnosis, management and pathogenesis. Neurosurgery 16:766, 1985

220. Bartlett JR: Craniopharyngiomas: an analysis of some aspects of symptomatology, radiology and histology. Brain 94:725, 1971

221. Baskin DS, Wilson CB: Surgical management of craniopharyngiomas: a review of 74 cases. J Neurosurg 65:22, 1986

222. Bernstein ML, Uchino JJ: The histological similarity between craniopharyngioma and odontogenic lesions: a reappraisal. Oral Surg 56:502, 1983

223. Carmel PW: Surgical syndromes of the hypothalamus. Clin Neurosurg 27:133, 1979

224. Carmel PW: Craniopharyngiomas. p. 905. In Wilkins RH (ed): Neurosurgery. Vol. 1. McGraw-Hill, New York, 1985

225. Carmel PW: Tumours of the third ventricle. Acta Neurochir (Wien) 75:136, 1985

226. Carmel PW: Tumors of the disordered embryogenesis. p. 3223. In Youmans JR (ed): Neurological Surgery. 3rd Ed. Vol. 5. WB Saunders, Philadelphia, 1989

227. Carmel PW, Antunes JL, Chang CH: Craniopharyngioma in children. Neurosurgery 11:382, 1982

228. Carmel PW, Antunes JL, Ferin M: Collection of blood from the pituitary stalk and portal veins in monkeys, and from the pituitary sinusoidal system of monkey and man. J Neurosurg 50:75, 1979

229. Carmichael HT: Squamous epithelial rests in hypophysis cerebri. Arch Neurol Psychiatry 26:966, 1931

230. Carpenter RC, Chamberlin GW, Frazier CH: The treatment of hypophyseal stalk tumors by evacuation and irradiation. AJR 38:162, 1937

231. Cavazzuti V, Fischer ED, Welch K et al: Neurological and psychophysiological sequelae following different treatments of craniopharyngiomas in children. J Neurosurg 59:409, 1983

232. Choux M: Craniopharyngioma surgery: techniques, complications and alternatives. Presented at the 59th Annual Meeting of the American Association of Neurological Surgery, New Orleans, April 20–25, 1991

233. Clayton PW, Price DA, Shalet SM, Gattesmaneni HR: Craniopharyngioma recurrence and growth hormone therapy. Lancet: 642, 1988

234. Coffey RJ, Lunsford LD, Bissonette D, Flickinger JC: Stereotactic gamma radiosurgery for intracranial vascular malformations and tumors; report of the initial North American experience in 311 patients. Stereotact Funct Neurosurg 54:535, 1990

235. Cogen PH, Carmel PW: Craniopharyngioma growth potential response of children vs. adults. Neurosurgery 9:469, 1981

236. Critchley M, Ironside RN: The pituitary adamantinomata. Brain 49:437, 1926

237. Dandy WE: Diagnosis, localization, and removal of tumor of the third ventricle. Bull Johns Hopkins Hosp 33:188, 1922

238. Dandy WE: Benign Tumor in the Third Ventricle of the Brain: Diagnosis and Treatment. Charles C Thomas, Springfield, IL, 1933

239. Danoff BF, Cowchock FS, Kramer S: Childhood craniopharyngioma: survival, local control, endocrine and neurological function following radiotherapy. J Radiat Oncol Biol Phys 9:171, 1983

240. Duffner PK, Cohen ME, Thomas PRM, Lansky SB: The long-term effects of cranial irradiation on the central nervous system. Cancer 56:1841, 1985

241. Ellner JJ, Bennett JE: Chronic meningitis. Medicine 55:341, 1976

242. Erdheim J: Ueber Hypophysengangsgeshwulste und Hirncholesteatoma. Sitzungsber Akad Wiss (Wien) 113:537, 1904

243. Fischer EG, Welch K, Shillito J et al: Craniopharyngiomas in children: long-term effects of conservative surgical procedures combined with radiation therapy. J Neurosurg 73:534, 1990

244. Flickinger JC, Lunsford LD, Singer J et al: Megavoltage external beam irradiation of craniopharyngiomas: analysis of tumor control and morbidity. J Radiat Oncol Biol Phys 19:117, 1990

245. Fukushima T, Hirakawa K, Kimura M, Tomonaga M: Intraventricular craniopharyngioma: its characteristics in magnetic resonance imaging and successful total removal. Surg Neurol 33:22, 1990

246. Goldberg GM, Eshbaugh DE: Squamous cell rests of the pituitary gland as related to the origin of craniopharyngiomas: a study of their presence in the

newborn and infants up to age four. Arch Pathol Lab Med 70:293, 1960

247. Goldstein SJ, Wilson DD, Young AB, Guidry GJ: Craniopharyngioma intrinsic to the third ventricle. Surg Neurol 20:249, 1983

248. Gorlin RJ, Pindborg JJ, Redman RS et al: The calcifying odontogenic cyst: a new entity and possible analogue of the cutaneous calcifying epithelioma of Malherbe. Cancer 17:723, 1964

249. Hoff JT, Patterson RH, Jr: Craniopharyngiomas in children and adults. J Neurosurg 36:2922, 1972

250. Hoffman HJ: Comment on paper by Patterson RH, Jr, Danylevitch A. Neurosurgery 7:116, 1980

251. Hoffman HJ: Craniopharyngiomas. Prog Exp Tumor Res 30:325, 1987

252. Hoffman HJ, Hendrick EB, Humphreys RB et al: Management of craniopharyngiomas in children. J Neurosurg 47:218, 1977

253. Ikezaki K, Fujii K, Kishikawa T: Magnetic resonance imaging of an intraventricular craniopharyngioma. Neuroradiology 321:247, 1990

254. Julow J, Lanyi F, HaJda M et al: The radiotherapy of cystic craniopharyngioma with intracystic installation of 90-Y silicate colloid. Acta Neurochir (Wien) 74:94, 1985

255. Kahn EA, Gosch HH, Seeger JF, Hicks SP: Forty-five years experience with the craniopharyngiomas. Surg Neurol 1:5, 1973

256. Katz EL: Late results of radical excision of craniopharyngiomas in children. J Neurosurg 42:86, 1975

257. Kaufman M, Swartz BE, Mandelkern M et al: Diagnosis of delayed cerebral radiation necrosis following proton beam therapy. Arch Neurol 47:474, 1990

258. Kernohan JW: Tumors of congenital origin. p. 1927. In Minckler J (ed): Pathology of the Nervous System. McGraw-Hill, New York, 1971

259. Kjos BO, Brant-Zawadzki M, Kucharczyk W et al: Cystic intracranial lesions: magnetic resonance imaging. Radiology 155:363, 1985

260. Kobayashi T, Kageyama N, Ohara K: Internal irradiation for cystic craniopharyngioma. J Neurosurg 55:896, 1981

261. Kodama T, Matsukado Y, Uemura S: Intracapsular irradiation therapy of craniopharyngiomas with radioactive gold: Indication and followup results. Neurol Med Chir (Tokyo) 21:49, 1981

262. Konovalov A: Craniopharyngioma surgery: techniques, complications and alternatives. Presented at the 59th Annual Meeting of the American Association of Neurological Surgery, New Orleans, April 20–25, 1991

263. Koos WT, Miller MH: Intracranial Tumors of Infants and Children. Thieme, Stuttgart, 1971

264. Kramer S: Craniopharyngiomas: the best treatment is conservative surgery and postoperative radiation therapy. p. 336. In Morley TP (ed): Current Controversies in Neurosurgery. WB Saunders, Philadelphia, 1976

265. Kramer S, McKissock W, Concanon JP: Craniopharyngiomas: treatment by combined surgery and radiation therapy. J Neurosurg 18:217, 1961

266. Kucharczyk W, Montanera WJ: The sella parasellar region. p. 625. In Atlas SW (ed): Magnetic Resonance Imaging of the Brain and Spine. Raven Press, New York, 1991

267. Kunishio K, Yamamoto Y, Sunami N et al: Craniopharyngioma in the third ventricle: necropsy findings and histogenesis. J Neurol Neurosurg Psychiatry 50:1053, 1987

268. Landolt AM: Die Ultrastruktur des Kraniopharyngeoms. Schweiz Arch Neurol Neurochir Psychiatry 111:313, 1972

269. Lapras C, Patet JD, Mottolese C et al: Craniopharyngiomas in childhood: analysis of 42 cases. Prog Exp Tumor Res 30:350, 1987

270. Lavyne MH, Patterson RH, Jr: Subchoroidal transvelum interpositum approach to mid-third ventricular tumors. Neurosurgery 12:86, 1983

271. Laws ER: Craniopharyngiomas in children and young adults. Prog Exp Tumor Res 30:335, 1987

272. Laws ER, Jr, Randall RV, Kern EB, Abboud CF: Management of Pituitary Adenomas and Related Lesions. Appleton-Century-Crofts, E. Norwalk, CT, 1982

273. Liszczak T, Richardson EP, Phillips JP, Jacobson S, Kornblith PL: Morphological, biochemical, ultrastructural, tissue culture and clinical observations of typical and aggressive craniopharyngiomas. Acta Neuropathol (Berl) 43:191, 1978

274. Long DM, Chou SN: Transcallosal removal of craniopharyngiomas within the third ventricle. J Neurosurg 39:563, 1973

275. Luse SA, Hernohan JW: Squamous-cell rests of the pituitary gland. Cancer 8:623, 1955

276. Maier HC: Craniopharyngioma with erosion and drainage into the nasopharynx. An autobiographical case report. J Neurosurg 62:132, 1985

277. Manaka S, Teramoto A, Takakura K: The efficacy of radiotherapy for craniopharyngioma. J Neurosurg 62:648, 1985

278. Matson DD, Crigler JF, Jr: Management of craniopharyngioma in childhood. J Neurosurg 30:377, 1969

279. Mori K, Handa H, Murata T et al: Results of treatment for craniopharyngioma. Childs Brain 6:303, 1980

280. Mott FW, Barrett JOW: Three cases of tumor of the third ventricule. Arch Neurol (Lond) 1:417, 1800

281. Nadich TP, Pinto RS, Kushner MJ et al: Evaluation of sellar and parasellar masses by computed tomography. Radiology 120:91, 1976

282. Onanoff J: Sur un cas d'epithelioma (étude histologique), Paris 1832. Cited in Seemayer TA: Pituitary craniopharyngioma with tooth formation. Cancer 29:423, 1972

283. Packer JR, Sutton LN, Atkins TE et al: A prospective

study of cognitive function in children receiving whole-brain radiotherapy and chemotherapy: 2-year results. J Neurosurg 70:707, 1989

284. Patten BM: Patten's Human Embryology. McGraw-Hill, New York, 1976

285. Patterson RH, Jr, Danylevich A: Surgical removal of craniopharyngiomas by a transcranial approach through the lamina terminalis and sphenoid sinus. Neurosurgery 7:111, 1980

286. Pertuiset B: Craniopharyngiomas. P. 531. In Inken PJ, Bryun GW (eds): Handbook of Clinical Neurology. Vol. 18. Part 3. Tumors of the Brain and Skull. North-Holland, Amsterdam, 1975

287. Petito CK, De Girolami U, Earle KM: Craniopharyngiomas; a clinical and pathological review. Cancer 37:1944, 1976

288. Podoshin L, Rolan L, Altman MM, Payser E: ''Pharyngeal'' craniopharyngioma. J Laryngol Otol 84:93, 1970

289. Ragoowansi AT, Piepgras DG: Postoperative ectopic craniopharyngioma. J Neurosurg 74:653, 1991

290. Ranson SW, Fisher C, Ingram WR: Hypothalamico-hypophyseal mechanism in diabetes insipidus. Assoc Res Nerv Ment Dis 17:410, 1938

291. Reeves AG, Plum F: Hyperphagia, rage and dementia accompanying a ventromedial hypothalamic neoplasm. Arch Neurol 20:616, 1969

292. Rubenstein CL, Varni JW, Katz ER: Cognitive functioning in long-term survivors of childhood leukemia: a prospective analysis. Dev Behav Pediatr 11:301, 1990

293. Russell DS, Rubinstein LJ: Pathology of Tumors of the Nervous System. 4th Ed. Williams & Wilkins, Baltimore, 1977

294. Saaf M, Thoren M, Gerstrand CG et al: Treatment of craniopharyngiomas—the stereotactic approach in a ten to twenty-three years perspective. II. Psychosocial situation and pituitary function. Acta Neurochir (Wien) 99:97, 1989

295. Samii M, Bini W: Surgical treatment of craniopharyngioma. Zentralbl Neurochir 52:17, 1991

296. Shillito J: The treatment of craniopharyngiomas of childhood. p. 332. In Morley TP (ed): Current Controversies in Neurosurgery. WB Saunders, Philadelphia, 1976

297. Shillito J, Matson DD: An Atlas of Pediatric Neurosurgical Operations. p. 497. WB Saunders, Philadelphia, 1982

298. Shuangshoti S, Netsky MG, Nashold BS: Epithelial cysts related to sella turcica: proposed origin from neuroepithelium. Arch Pathol Lab Med 90:444, 1970

299. Skorzewska A, Lal S, Waserman J, Guyda H: Abnormal food-seeking behavior after surgery for craniopharyngioma. Neuropsychobiology 21:17, 1989

300. Sorva R: Children with craniopharyngioma. Early growth failure and rapid postoperative weight gain. Acta Paediatr Scand 77:587, 1988

301. Suc E, Kalifa C, Brauner R et al: Brain tumors under the age of three, the price of survival. Acta Neurochir (Wien) 106:93, 1990

302. Sung DI, Chang CH, Harisiadis L, Carmel PW: Treatment results of craniophangiomas. Cancer 47:847, 1981

303. Sutton LN, Gusnard D, Bruce DA et al: Fusiform dilatations of the carotid artery following radical surgery of childhood craniopharyngiomas. J Neurosurg 74:695, 1991

304. Sweet WH: Radical surgical treatment of craniopharyngioma. Clin Neurosurg 23:52, 1976

305. Sweet WH: Recurrent craniopharyngiomas: therapeutic alternatives. Clin Neurosurg 27:206, 1980

306. Sweet WH: Craniopharyngiomas (with a note on Rathke's cleft cysts). p. 349. In Schmidek HH (ed): Operative Neurosurgical Techniques. Grune & Stratton, Orlando, FL, 1988

307. Symon L, Sprich W: Radical excision of craniopharyngiomas. Results in 20 patients. J Neurosurg 62:174, 1985

308. Till L: Craniopharyngioma. Childs Brain 9:179, 1982

309. Tomita T: Management of craniopharyngiomas in children. Pediatr Neurosci 14:204, 1988

310. Torkildsen A: Should extirpation be attempted in cases of neoplasm in or near the third ventricle of the brain? Experiences with a palliative method. J Neurosurg 5:249, 1948

311. Yasargil MG, Curcic M, Kis M et al: Total removal of craniopharyngiomas: approaches and long-term results in 144 patients. J Neurosurg 73:3, 1990

Transsphenoidal Surgery

312. Bergland RM, Ray BS: The arterial supply of the human optic chiasm. J Neurosurg 31:327, 1969

313. Bergland RM, Ray BS, Torack RM: Anatomical variations in the pituitary gland and adjacent structures in 225 autopsy cases. J Neurosurg 28:93, 1968

314. Bouche J, Rougerie J, Freche C et al: L'abord des craniopharyngiomes par la voie transsphenoidale basse. Ann Otolaryngol (Paris) 84:655, 1967

315. Calcaterra TC: Extracranial surgical repair of cerebrospinal rhinorrhea. Ann Otolaryngol 89:108, 1980

316. Calvert J. Claux J: Les craniopharyngiomes—le traitement par voie basse. Rev Otoneuroophth 27:121, 1955

317. Ciric IS, Cozzens JW: Craniopharyngiomas: transsphenoidal methods of approach—for the virtuoso only? Clin Neurosurg 27:169, 1980

318. Cushing H: The craniopharyngiomas. p. 93. In: Intracranial Tumors. Notes Upon a Series of Two Thousand Verified Cases with Surgical Mortality Percentages Pertaining thereto. Charles C Thomas, Springfield, IL, 1932

319. Fujii K, Chambers SM, Rhoton AL, Jr: Neurovascular relationships of the sphenoid sinus: a microsurgical study. J Neurosurg 50:31, 1979

320. Grant DB, Lyen K: Hypopituitarism after surgery for craniopharyngioma. Childs Brain 9:201, 1982

321. Grisoli F, Vincentelli F, Farnarier P et al: Transsphenoidal microsurgery in the management of non-pituitary tumours of the sella turcia. p. 193. In Brock M (ed): Modern Neurosurgery. Springer-Verlag, Berlin, 1982

322. Guiot G: Par ou faut-il aborder l'hypophyse? Presse Med 78:209, 1970

323. Halstead AE: Remarks on the operative treatment of tumors of the hypophysis. Surg Gynecol Obstet 10:494, 1910

324. Hamberger CA, Hammer G, Norlen G, Sjogren B: Surgical treatment of the transantrosphenoidal approach. Acta Otolaryngol (Stockh) 52:285, 1960

325. Hamlin H: Discussion of Leksell L, Backlund EO: The treatment of craniopharyngiomas (summary of paper.) Acta Neurol Scand 43:249, 1967

326. Hammer J: Removal of craniopharyngiomas by subnasal trans-sphenoidal operation. Neuropediatrie 9:319, 1978

327. Hardy J, LaLonde J: L'éxérèse par voie trans-sphenoidale d'un craniopharyngiome géant. Med Can 92:1142, 1963

328. Harris FS, Rhoton AL, Jr: Anatomy of the cavernous sinus: a microsurgical study. J Neurosurg 45:169, 1967

329. Hirsch O: Successful closure of cerebrospinal fluid rhinorrhea by endonasal surgery. Arch Otolaryngol 56:1, 1952

330. Horwitz NH, Rizzoli HV: Postoperative Complications in Neurosurgical Practice. p. 59. Williams & Wilkins, Baltimore, 1967

331. Horwitz NH, Rizzoli HV: Craniopharyngioma. p. 132. Postoperative Complications of Intracranial Neurological Surgery. Williams & Wilkins, Baltimore, 1982

332. Illum P, Elbrond O, Nehen AM: Surgical treatment of nasopharyngeal craniopharyngioma: radical removal by the transpalatal approach. J Laryngol Otolaryngol 91:227, 1977

333. Johnson NE: Craniopharyngioma—review with a discussion of transpalatal approach. Laryngoscope 72:1731, 1962

334. Landolt AM: Complications and pitfalls of transsphenoidal pituitary surgery. Neurosurgeons 4:398, 1988

335. Laws ER, Jr: Transsphenoidal approach to lesions in and about the sella turcica. p. 327. In Schmidek HH, Sweet WH (eds): Operative Neurosurgical Techniques. Grune & Stratton, Orlando, FL, 1982

336. Laws ER, Jr: Craniopharyngiomas: diagnosis and treatment. p. 321. In Sekhar LN, Schramm VL, Jr (eds): Tumors of the Cranial Base: Diagnosis and Treatment. Futura, Mount Kisco, NY, 1987

337. Laws ER: Craniopharyngiomas in children and young adults. Prog Exp Tumor Res 30:1, 1987

338. Laws ER, Jr: Transsphenoidal microsurgery in the management of craniopharyngioma. J Neurosurg 52:661, 1988

339. Laws ER, Jr, Kern EB: Complications of transsphenoidal surgery. Clin Neurosurg 23:401, 1967

340. Laws ER, Jr, Randall RV, Abboud CF (eds): Management of Pituitary Adenomas and Related Lesions. p. 376. Appleton-Century-Crofts, E. Norwalk, CT, 1982

341. Laws ER, Jr, Randall RV, Abboud CF, Hayles AB: Craniopharyngioma—the transsphenoidal microsurgical approach. p. 335. In Givens JR (ed): The Hypothalamus. Year Book Medical Publishers, Chicago, 1984

342. Laws ER, Jr, Trautmann JC, Hollenhorst RW, Jr: Transsphenoidal decompression of the optic nerve and chiasm. Visual results in 62 patients. J Neurosurg 46:717, 1977

343. Lyen KR, Grant DB: Endocrine function, morbidity, and mortality after surgery for craniopharyngioma. Arch Dis Child 57:837, 1982

344. Majlessi H, Shariat AS, Katirai A: Nasopharyngeal craniopharyngioma. Childs Brain 9:205, 1982

345. Newfield P, Ablin MS, Chestnut JS, Maroon J: Air embolism during transsphenoidal pituitary operations. Neurosurgery 2:39, 1978

346. Patrick BS, Smith RR, Bailey TO: Aseptic meningitis due to spontaneous rupture of craniopharyngioma cyst: case report. J Neurosurg 41:387, 1974

347. Podochin L, Rolan L, Altman MM, Peyser E: 'Pharyngeal' craniopharyngioma. J Laryngol Otol 84:93, 1970

348. Post KD, Kasdon DL: Sellar and parasellar lesions mimicking adenoma. p. 159. In Post KD, Jackson I, Reichlin S (eds): The Pituitary Adenoma. Plenum, New York, 1980

349. Prasad U, Kwi NK: Nasopharyngeal craniopharyngioma. J Laryngol Otolaryngol 89:445, 1975

350. Randall RV, Clark EC, Dodge HW, Jr, Love JG: Polyuria after operation for tumors in the region of the hypophysis and hypothalamus. J Clin Endocrinol 20:1614, 1980

351. Randall RV, Laws ER, Jr, Abboud CF: Clinical presentation of craniopharyngioma: a brief review of 300 cases. p. 335. In Givens JR (ed): The Hypothalamus. Year Book Medical Publishers, Chicago, 1984

352. Renn WH, Rhoton AL, Jr: Microsurgical anatomy of the sellar region. J Neurosurg 43:288, 1975

353. Rhoton AL, Jr, Hardy DG, Chambers SM: Microsurgical anatomy and dissection of the sphenoid bone, cavernous sinus and sellar region. Surg Neurol 12:63, 1979

354. Rhoton AL, Jr, Harris FS, Renn WH: Microsurgical anatomy of the sellar region and cavernous sinus. Clin Neurosurg 24:54, 1977

355. Rhoton AL, Jr, Maniscalco J: Microsurgery of the sellar region. p. 106. In Glaser JS (ed): Neuro-Ophthalmology. Vol. 9. CV Mosby, St. Louis, 1977

356. Rhoton AL, Jr, Yamamoto I, Peace DA: Micro-

surgery of the third ventricle: Part 2. Operative approaches. Neurosurgery 8:357, 1981

357. Riccio A: Su di un caso di craniofaringioma del clivus. Minerva Neurochir 13:13, 1969

358. Schucart WA, Jackson I: Management of diabetes insipidus in neurosurgical patients. J Neurosurg 44:65, 1976

359. Svien HJ: Experiences with craniopharyngiomas. J Neurosurg 23:148, 1965

360. Trautmann JC, Laws ER, Jr: Visual status after transsphenoidal surgery at the Mayo Clinic 1971–1982. Am J Ophthalmol 96:200, 1983

361. Welch K, Stears JC: Chiasmapexy of the correction of traction of the optic nerves and chiasm associated with their descent into an empty sella turcica. Case report J Neurosurg 35:760, 1971

Complications and Their Avoidance

362. Arutynov AI, Rostotskaya VI, Krasnova TS: Principles of treating craniopharyngiomas. p. 114. In Opukholi Golovnogo Mozga. (Tumours of Brain.) Moscow, 1975

363. Ciric IS: Regional embryology. p. 167. In Apuzzo MLJ (ed): Surgery of the Third Ventricle. Williams & Wilkins, Baltimore, 1987

364. Hoffman MT, Hendrick EB, Humphreys RP: Management of craniopharyngioma in children. J Neurosurg 47:218, 1977

365. Konovalov AN: Operative management of craniopharyngiomas: advances and technical standards. Neurosurgery 8:281, 1981

366. Konovalov AN: Technique and strategies of direct surgical management of craniopharyngioma. p. 542. In Apuzzo MLJ (ed): Surgery of the Third Ventricle. Williams & Wilkins, Baltimore, 1987

367. Matson DD, Crigler J: Craniopharyngioma in children. J Neurosurg 30:377, 1969

368. Rougerie J: What can be expected from the surgical treatment of craniopharyngiomas in children. Childs Brain 5:433, 1979

369. Stein BM: Transcallosal approach to III ventricle tumours. p. 247. In Schmidek HH, Sweet WH (eds): Current Techniques in Operative Neurosurgery. Grune & Stratton, Orlando, FL, 1977

370. Suzuki J, Katakura R, Mori T: Interhemispheric approach through the lamina terminalis to the anterior part of the III ventricle. Surg Neurol 22:2, 1984

371. Sweet WH: Craniopharyngiomas (with a note on Rathke's "cleft or epithelial cysts on suprasellar cysts"). p. 349. In Schmidek HH, Sweet WH (eds): Operative Neurosurgical Techniques. 2nd Ed. Grune & Stratton, Orlando, FL, 1988

372. Symon L, Sprich W: Radical excision of craniopharyngioma: results in 20 patients. Neurosurgery 62:174, 1985

373. Vichert TM, Korshunov AG: Cerebral vascular system in craniopharyngiomas. Voprosi Nejrochirurgii (Moscow) 6:9, 1985

374. Vichert TM, Korshunov AG: Pathoanatomical characteristics of acute cerebral circulatory disorders in craniopharyngioma. Voprosi Nejrochirurgii (Moscow) 7:23, 1986

16 Intrinsic Cerebral Neoplasms

Intrinsic Cerebral Glioma

Michael Salcman

Neurological complications in the surgery of intrinsic brain tumors are primarily related to problems in localization and exposure, the extent of resection, and the manner in which tissues are handled. Despite advances in neuroimaging, anesthesia, and surgical instrumentation, difficulties persist, because many of the critical issues remain matters of judgment and experience, skills that are not easily transferred from one surgeon to another. Indeed, many of the principles outlined in this overview are not fully appreciated by neurosurgeons in training until they have either personally witnessed the negative consequences of ignoring them or have participated in the successful extirpation of a particularly difficult lesion, without untoward incident. This pedagogical observation is not unique and is a corollary of the axiom that good judgment is often based on bad experiences, and valued experience is gained from episodes of less than perfect judgment. Of course, morbidity after craniotomy for tumor depends on factors other than technique and surgical experience; these are listed in Table 16-1 and have been discussed elsewhere.[15,18]

LOCALIZATION AND EXPOSURE

Ideally, the lesion should be located in the center of the bone flap with a minimum of normal brain exposed. This requires that the localization of the tumor on computed tomography (CT) or magnetic resonance imaging (MRI) be accurately transposed to the surface markings of the skull. Preoperatively, the relation of the tumor to the ventricle, to the motor strip, to the basal ganglia and thalamus, or to other important structures should be reviewed and the likely position of these structures in the bone flap planned.[12] When the tumor is not centered in the flap, it sometimes forces the surgeon to work under a ledge of bone with less than optimal visibility and control of bleeding. This also means that brain is in the center of the flap and that inadvertent swelling and tightness cannot be easily relieved by rapid resection of the lesion, as opposed to traumatic manipulation of possibly eloquent cortex. In order to select a flap properly, it is first necessary for the surgeon to determine in which lobe, if any, the lesion resides (Fig. 16-1). This is not as simple an exercise as it might first appear, since a proper appreciation of the angle of the CT slice must be made. Confusion is most likely in separating frontal from parietal lesions, and superior temporal from frontal lesions. On the CT scan, it is very useful to note where the pterion is (extreme lateral portion of the sphenoid wing), where the coronal suture is on the bone window scan, and where the pinna of the ear is on a soft tissue slice. The two most useful superficial landmarks of the skull are the external auditory meatus for parietal

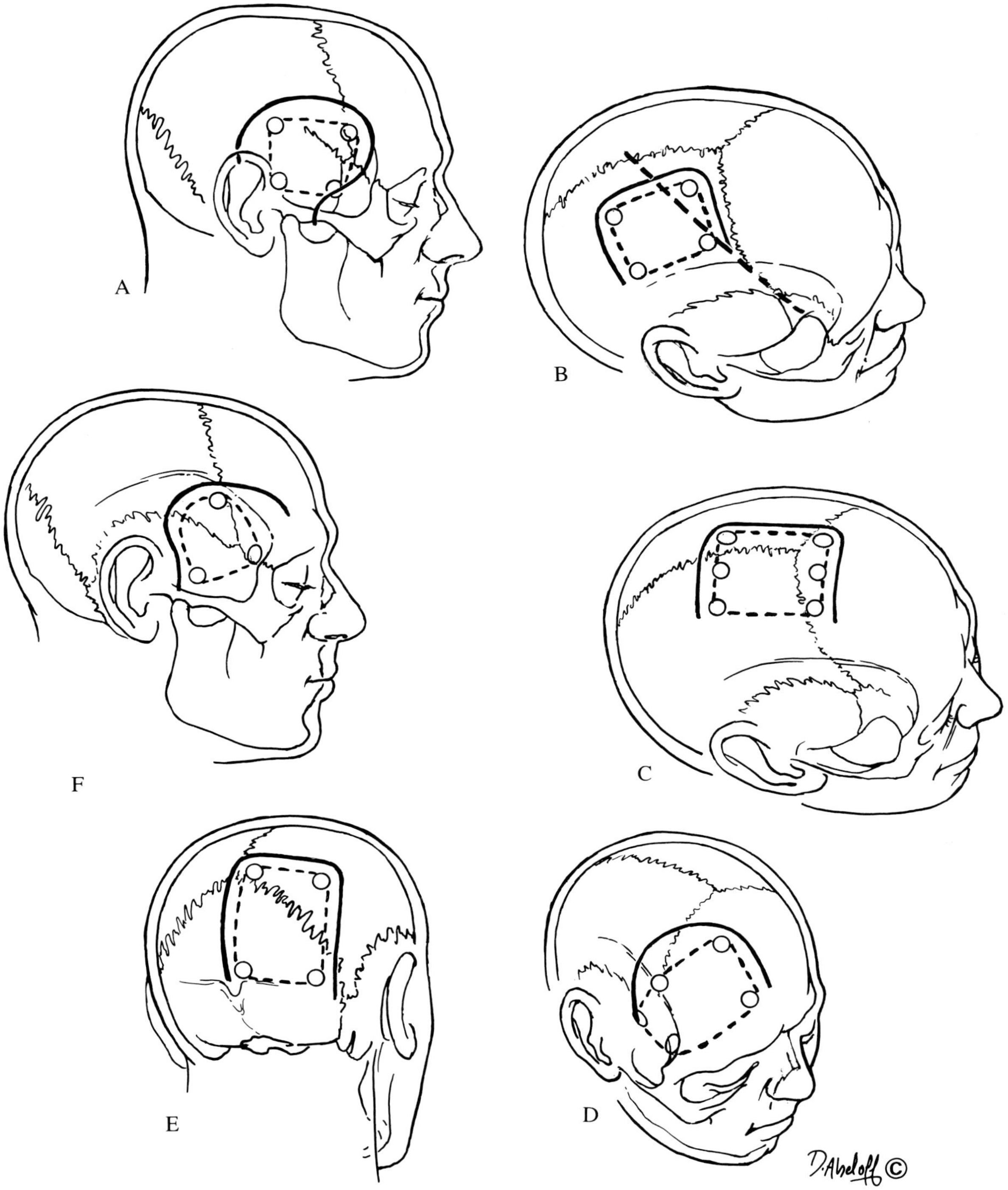

Figure 16-1. Standard flaps for supratentorial tumors. Temporal lobe lesions can be handled through a question mark **(A)** or reverse question mark incision **(F)** with careful exposure of the pterion, the zygoma, and the petrous ridge. Frontal craniotomies usually relate to the midline, the external orbital process (''keyhole''), pterion, and coronal suture **(D).** Craniotomies crossing the sagittal sinus should use burr holes on either side of the midline **(C),** and occipital flaps should reach the midline above the superior nuchal line with control of the lambdoid suture **(E).** Convexity lesions in the frontoparietal region are discussed in Figs. 16-2 and 16-3; the flap is usually situated above the superior temporal line **(B).**

Table 16-1. Factors Influencing Surgical
Outcome

Tumor
    Size
    Location
    Histology
    Vascularity
    Multiplicity
Patient
    Age
    Present disability
    Prior therapy
    General condition
Surgeon
    Ability
    Experience
    Resources

lesions and the coronal suture, as it descends towards the pterion, for frontal lesions.

Throughout the history of neurological surgery, the location of the motor strip has been recognized as the single most important functional consideration in regard to the safe extirpation of space occupying lesions, be they tumors, vascular malformations, or other masses. The first consistently reliable system of superficial measurements were the Taylor-Haughton lines, and they remain a useful method of confirmation when the scalp has not been marked in the CT scanner or by a stereotactic probe (Fig. 16-2). The Rolandic fissure predicted by the Taylor-Haughton method is almost always angled at 45° to the orbitomeatal base line with its origin at the pterion and its termination at the vertex, two inches posterior to the coronal suture. As I have discussed elsewhere, this line is also approximately colinear with the posterior branch of the middle meningeal artery to vertex axis.[12] Except for indicating the relationship of the pterion and coronal suture to a mass, the CT scan did little to improve upon this system. Recently, however, MRI has provided definitive localization of the motor strip.[5] The Rolandic fissure is reliably located posterior to the junction of the superior frontal sulcus and the first sulcus which the latter abuts in the frontoparietal region. For lesions greater than 2 or 3 cm in diameter, the relationship of the mass to the external auditory meatus, the pterion, the motor strip, and the coronal suture should suffice. When in doubt, take the patient back to the CT scanner and place a paper clip or metal-impregnated silastic tube perpendicular to the plane of the CT slice and mark the scalp.

When the lesion is smaller than 2 cm, has indistinct or nonenhancing borders, and is superficially located in the cortex, then hybrid operations, in which craniotomy and stereotaxis are combined, are a recent and almost ideal solution to the localization problem.[10,18] The patient is placed in a CT- or MRI-compatible stereotactic frame and coordinates for the target calculated in the usual fashion. When the patient is returned to the operating room, the stereotactic probe is lowered to the scalp and marks the center of the flap (Fig. 16-3). The probe is elevated and the scalp incision made. The probe is lowered again and the bone flap and the dural incisions are cut around it. When the brain is exposed, the probe can be lowered again to indicate which of several identically appearing gyri should be incised to find the lesion. At this point, the arc of the frame can often be removed and the operating microscope brought into place. Techniques for preoperative localization are summarized in Table 16-2.

Preoperative localization is the essential first step since it allows a bone flap of proper size, location, and orientation to be designed. During the procedure, however, one of the most common mistakes is to make the flap too confining (Fig. 16-4). The saw cuts should be made at the outer edges of the burr holes, otherwise too much exposure in the interior of the bone flap is sacrificed. The bone flap should extend to the edges of the scalp incision; if it does not, either the exposure afforded by the scalp incision has been wasted, the scalp flap was poorly located, or it was designed to be too large. In choosing the size of both the scalp flap and the bone flap, remember that brain tumor exposures need to be considerably larger than aneurysm flaps or other strictly microsurgical approaches, although often smaller than the flaps employed for resection of vascular malformations. The flap needs to be sufficiently large to provide ready access to landmarks in case the localization is in doubt, to provide an opportunity for resection of noneloquent brain or even lobectomy if uncontrollable swelling is encountered and to allow easy access to the tumor without unnecessary (or any!) retraction of the brain against dural or bony margins. All other things being equal, the major portion of the flap and

Table 16-2. Preoperative Localization
Techniques

Superficial landmarks
    Coronal suture, pterion, external auditory
      meatus
Taylor-Haughton lines
Scalp marking by CT
Motor strip by MRI
Image-guided stereotactic craniotomy

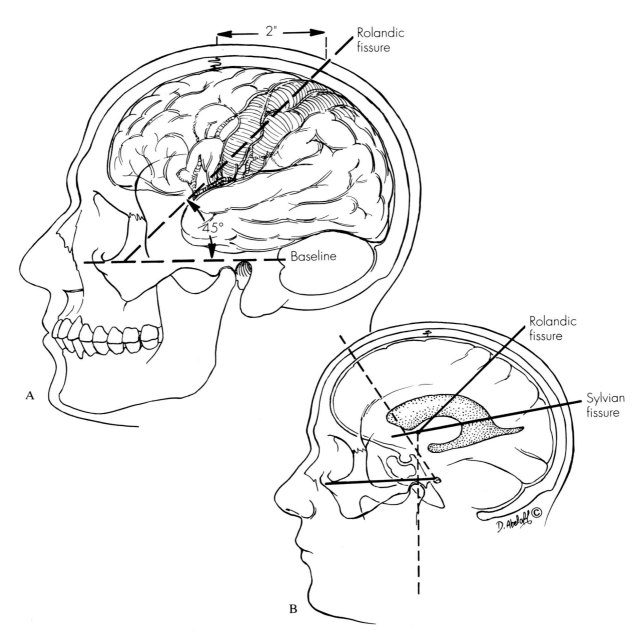

Figure 16-2. Localization methods. **(A)** The rolandic fissure runs along a line angled 45 degrees to the base and ending 2 inches behind the coronal suture. This line is parallel to the origin of the posterior branch of the middle meningeal artery. **(B)** The Taylor-Haughton lines are a more precise estimate of the location of the motor strip from superficial landmarks. (*Figure continues.*)

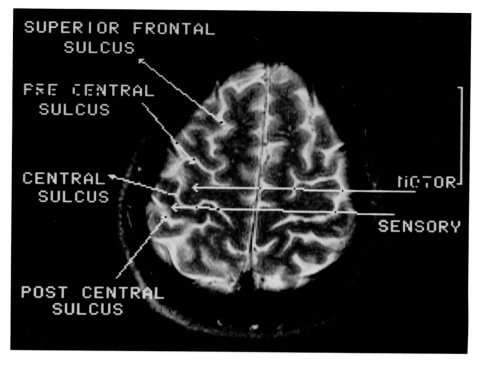

Figure 16-2. (*Continued*). **(C)** The relationship of a mass to the motor strip is best defined on MRI, where the superior frontal sulcus can be seen to join the precentral sulcus and the central sulcus is observed to lie just behind it running perpendicularly to the midline.

the epicenter of the tumor should lie in a plane parallel to the floor of the operating room. This allows the surgeon the greatest degree of free movement over the surface of the exposure and usually provides the most natural gravitational retraction. Some paramedian or midline approaches require that the flap be perpendicular or nearly so to the operating floor so that the hemisphere ipsilateral to the lesion can sag gently downwards.

TISSUE HANDLING

Neurological difficulties are minimized or avoided by keeping the brain moist and avoiding contact with it. Superficial and deep wound infections,[25] postoperative bleeding, and loss of the bone flap are prevented by proper handling of scalp, muscle, bone, and dura. Patients with glial tumors and other intrinsic neoplasms are often subjected to reoperation, for which the principles of gentle and meticulous operative technique are even more critical in the face of the previously irradiated, operated, and otherwise devitalized scalp and bone.[1,8,12,19,27] Remember that most patients undergoing their first craniotomy will soon be subjected to radiation and chemotherapy and that

many of these patients will also become candidates for reoperation and implant procedures.[14,16,22,23]

All craniotomy patients should receive prophylactic antibiotics prior to the scalp incision; a typical regimen consists of 2 g nafcillin every 4 hours and 1.5 mg/kg of gentamicin repeated at 1 mg/kg every 8 hours. The scalp can be injected with a mixture of xylocaine and epinephrine at the initial procedure, but such injections should be avoided at reoperation and after radiation. All scalp incisions should be designed to preserve the blood supply, which enters the scalp from below, and the base of the flap should be at least as broad as its height so as to preserve at least one major feeding artery. Finger pressure should be used to provide temporary hemostasis and the minimum effective number of scalp clips or hemostats should be employed. Clips should not be used at the corners of the incision. Ordinary metal sucker tips should not be applied to soft tissues such as subcutaneous fat, fascia, and muscle since they often stir up as much bleeding as they help stop. Gentle suction through a cottonoid strip or with a two-point suction cautery, frequent irrigation, and meticulous bipolar technique are always preferable at any stage of the operation.

Once the bone flap has been elevated, tack-up su-

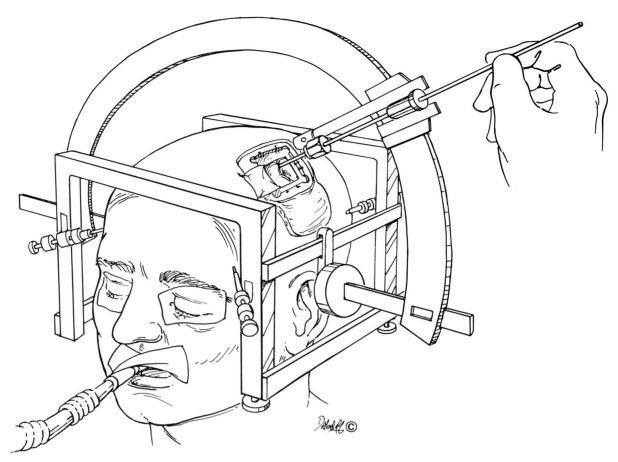

Figure 16-3. Stereotactic guidance of a craniotomy. The stereotactic probe inserted into the electrode holder of the frame guides the placement of the flap and indicates the position of the cortical incision.

tures should be placed in the dura around strips of Gelfoam so as to preclude the formation of postoperative epidural bleeding. Before opening the dura and incising the cortex, it is useful for the surgeon to review a mental checklist of technical points critical to the ease and safety of resection (Table 16-3). A stitch is placed in the dura and a No. 11 blade is used to nick it open with the cutting surface pointed upward so as to avoid lacerating the brain. A microirrigator can be inserted into the incision to float a nar-

row cottonoid strip over the cortical surface. In this way, the brain is gently depressed from beneath the dura and kept out of the way of the small Metzenbaum scissors employed for the dural opening. The dural incision should always be made over normal tissue but as close to the margin of the lesion as possible. The base of the dural flap should always be toward the most eloquent, important, or dangerous structure in the field, that is, the motor strip, the sagittal sinus, Broca's area, or a major artery. In this way, the flap can be opened toward the vital structure and the exposure curtailed when the lesion is uncovered and the minimum amount of cortex has been exposed (Fig. 16-4).

Closure of the dura should begin with the placement of interrupted "cardinal" sutures at the corners of the dural flap with care being taken not to saw into the subjacent cortex; again, cottonoid strips can be used to prevent contact of the sutures with the brain. The limbs of the incision can then be run in the usual fashion. The dura can always be closed if hyperventi-

Table 16-3. Checklist of Technical Points Critical to the Ease and Safety of Resection

Is the lesion centered in the flap?
Is the flap generous enough?
Is the field parallel to the operating room floor?
Is the dural incision based on the critical structure?
Is the brain relaxed?
If not, what is my contingency plan?
Are the tack-up sutures in?

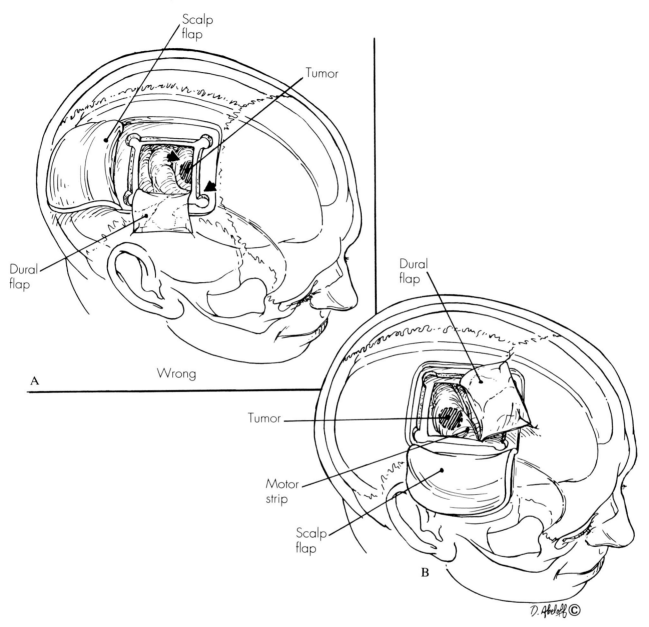

Figure 16-4. A wrong and a right view of a parietal craniotomy. **(A)** The scalp flap has been turned 90 degrees away from its blood supply, which enters inferiorly; the bone flap is centered on the motor strip instead of the tumor and is too confining because the saw cuts are not made at the outer edges of the burr holes; the dura is flapped downward so that unopened dura cannot protect either the motor strip or the sagittal sinus. **(B)** All of those mistakes are corrected.

lation, mannitol, adequate resection, and gentle handling have been properly employed; glioma patients should not be subjected to the risks of cerebral hernia. For similar reasons, the bone flap is sewn in and a central tack-up suture to the dura should be placed to avoid the spread of postoperative epidural bleeding. The scalp is closed in multiple layers and interrupted fine sutures are used in the skin if any suspicion of devitalization is entertained; otherwise skin staples are perfectly adequate and much faster.

EXTENT OF RESECTION

The gentleness with which the brain itself is handled is inextricably linked to the general operative strategy entertained and the extent of the tumor resection actually carried out. Tumors should be approached through the shortest and most direct route possible even if a surface entry needs to be made in the vicinity of eloquent brain (Fig. 16-5). This is because long dark tunnels employed from indirect and "safe" avenues invariably subject the brain to undue retraction or manipulation and subject the surgeon to poor visualization and uncertain hemostasis. In addition, transcortical incisions must result in some white matter loss, and this is kept to a minimum when the pathway is shortened. The safety of cortical incisions in or near eloquent brain is maximized by keeping the incision short (2 to 3 cm in length) and oriented so as to cut or abut the motor strip at a single point along the homunculus, that is to say, the incision should always be at an oblique angle or perpendicular to the motor strip and never run at an acute angle or parallel to it. In hemispheric resections, as in the rest of modern neurosurgery, the smaller the incision or the longer the tunnel, the greater the need for self-retaining retractors and the magnification and illumination provided by the operating microscope. In this way, direct microsurgical approaches can be made through the crown of a gyrus, at the depth of a sulcus, through a major fissure or cistern, or by a standard transcortical tunnel.[11,12]

The cortical incision itself should be made with microinstruments, "painted" on the surface of the brain with a bipolar cautery turned well down, nicked open with a No. 11 blade, and the arachnoid progressively cauterized without char and incised with small scissors. The white matter is spread open with the two-point suction cautery in the long axis of the incision and not sucked out. Retractor blades are always inserted parallel to the long axis of the incision so as to avoid cutting the brain with their edges (Fig. 16-6). Incisions should not be overstretched with retraction; if the corners are fissuring or bleeding or if subpial hemorrhage appears, the incision needs to be lengthened, sometimes just a matter of millimeters. The brain retraction should be released periodically to allow the cortical microcirculation to recover.

A craniotomy should rarely if ever be carried out solely for biopsy, since stereotactic biopsy techniques are safer and easier,[7,18] especially when we consider that a brain tumor disturbed but unresected in a sea of swollen surrounding parenchyma is likely to be more troublesome than not. Brain tumors are like tigers; they are best left undisturbed unless you plan to wound them fatally. Indications for stereotactic surgery as opposed to craniotomy are summarized in Table 16-4 and discussed elsewhere.[15] If a tumor can be safely approached and the major portion of it resected, the patient's neurological status is likely to improve and the subsequent effectiveness of other therapies is likely to increase.[2–4,6,9,16,17,20,24,26] Since there is no precise margin at the interface of an intrinsic tumor and the surrounding brain, it is critical that preoperative estimates be made of the tumor's size and shape. Resection is carried out with the two-point suction cautery, the laser, or the ultrasonic aspirator until intraoperative measurements of the major axes of the resection cavity conform to the preoperative estimates. In addition, one can safely continue the resection until clean white matter is encountered; this tissue will appear bright under the microscope (the tumor will appear dull), especially if peritumoral edema can be seen glistening as it pours out of the brain. A low power setting on the laser can then be used to shave another millimeter or two gently into the apparently "normal" surrounding tissue.[21] This maneuver often succeeds in moving the resection boundary out into or beyond the enhancing rim of the tumor seen on the preoperative scan. The safe surgical boundaries of the tumor are better estimated from the enhanced CT than from the extensive low signal area observed by MRI. The laser is especially useful in the deepest part of the exposure, especially when one wants to minimize the degree of movement or disturbance to the surrounding brain. Most intrinsic tumors are soft enough to be removed with the two-point suction cautery and do not require ultrasonic aspiration. In any case, the latter instrument is sometimes too large and ungainly for safe use in a microsurgical field, especially down long tunnels and through short or narrow cortical incisions.

Absolute hemostasis should be achieved by positive action with the two-point suction cautery, irriga-

Table 16-4.   Indications for Stereotactic Surgery

Tumor
    Is centrally located
    Is poorly demarcated
    Is extremely small
    Has a large cyst
    Has changed character
Patient
    Is too ill for craniotomy
    Is neurologically intact
The next therapy
    Is catheter based
    Requires repeat sampling

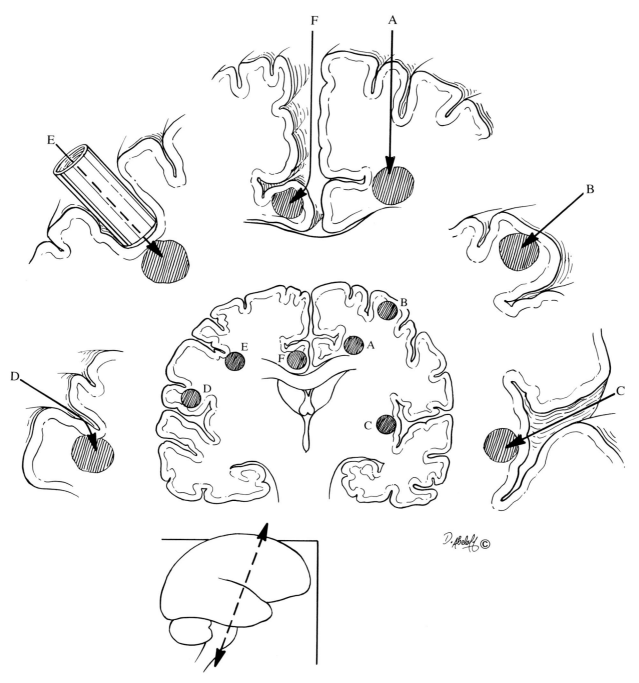

Figure 16-5. General approaches to hemispheric tumors. Many of these approaches are facilitated by the use of the operating microscope. Transcortical approaches can be made through a white matter tunnel **(A)**, at the apex of a gyrus **(B)**, through a fissure **(C)**, through a sulcus along its side **(D)**, or at its deepest portion **(E)**. Paramedian approaches **(F)** are neither subarachnoid nor transcortical but may require a transcortical tunnel at their termination.

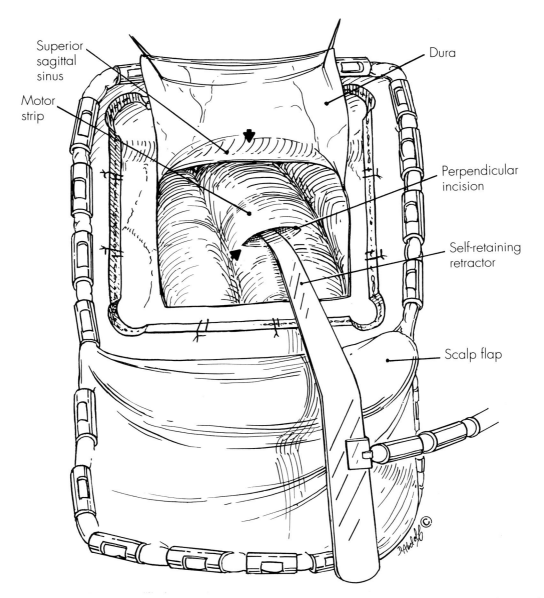

Superior sagittal sinus

Motor strip

Dura

Perpendicular incision

Self-retaining retractor

Scalp flap

Figure 16-6. Transcortical incision. Notice that the dura has been reflected towards the sagittal sinus and that the incision is perpendicular to the long axis of the motor strip. The self-retaining retractor blade is placed flat against the incision edge so as not to cut the brain with the narrow side of the blade nor bruise the cortex by being inserted at a corner.

tion, and laser, and never by packing the wound. Thin wisps of oxidized cotton can be layered into the fissures and cracks of the resection bed, and films of cellulose can be placed on smooth surfaces. Gelfoam should not be left in the resection cavity because it is not as good a hemostatic agent and it tends to swell. At the conclusion of the resection, the irrigating fluid in the tumor bed should be crystal clear, the brain should be relaxed, and the two lips of the cortical incision should just meet without any evidence of puffiness or subpial bruising. Prior to closure of the

dura, mentally review a few critical points (Table 16-5).

In general, the length and quality of survival depend on maximal resection of the tumor and minimal disturbance of the surrounding brain.[2,3,13,16] Lobectomy is a less satisfactory alternative because it substitutes resection of brain for removal of the tumor. Rarely, lobectomy is necessitated by uncontrollable intraoperative swelling, and it is sometimes used to provide a resection margin of normal tissue around a low-grade lesion.[17] There is no evidence that lobec-

Table 16-5. Critical Points to Review After the Resection

Is the resection cavity equal to the preop tumor size?
Is "normal" brain visible on every wall?
Is the cavity dry?
Is the brain relaxed?
If not, what is my contingency plan?
Are the tack-up sutures in?

tomy is superior to tumor resection alone for high-grade tumors. Complications after lobectomy are frequently caused by technical errors and transgression of anatomical landmarks (Fig. 16-7). All lobectomies should be carried out through a subpial approach in which the pia is entered at one point, and circumfer-entially incised in a controlled manner so as to avoid multiple encounters with the pial vessels.

A frontal lobectomy should be carried out in a wedge-like fashion with the resection extended more posteriorly at its superior margin than at the inferior edge. This technique avoids the basal ganglia and thalamus by utilizing a 45-degree plane that begins with its foot at the posterior margin of the planum sphenoidale, grazes the frontal horn of the lateral ventricle at its midportion, and reaches back to the coronal suture superiorly. It is often good judgment to leave a thin margin of brain along the mesial wall of the resection cavity so as to avoid penetrating the arachnoid and damaging the anterior cerebral artery as it winds around the rostrum of the corpus callosum. On the dominant side, frontal lobectomies must spare the posterior third of the inferior gyrus

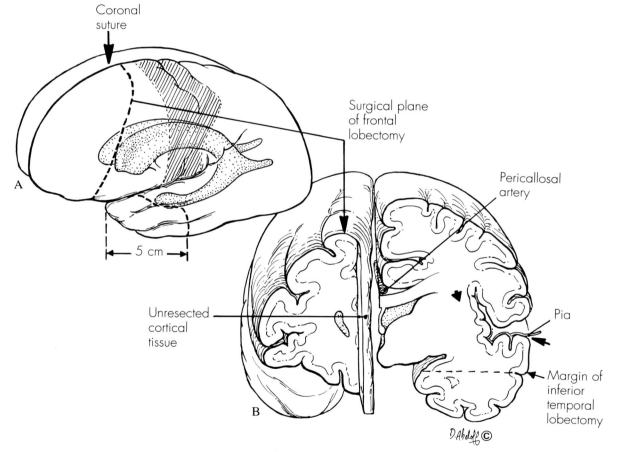

Figure 16-7. Principles of safe lobectomy. **(A)** The safe resection plane for a frontal lobectomy angles backward from inferior to superior so as to avoid the basal ganglia behind the tip of the lateral ventricle's frontal horn and the pericallosal artery. **(B)** The latter can be further protected by leaving a thin strip of subarachnoid tissue unresected on the mesial surface of the frontal lobe. Temporal lobectomies are usually carried out no more than 5 cm from the temporal tip **(A)**, with preservation of the superior gyrus on the dominant side **(B)**.

and temporal lobectomies must end 1 cm anterior to the vein of Labbé or 5 cm from the tip. When possible, avoid resecting the superior temporal gyrus and entering the sylvian fissure, or penetrating the mesial arachnoid and damaging the nerves and vessels running at the tentorial edge in the circummesencephalic cistern.

Temporal lobe resections should not be carried out so far mesially that the surgeon enters the deep hemispheric white matter or the diencephalon and thalamus. Remember that the ''root'' of the temporal lobe follows the ventricle as it curves toward the midline. Conversely, it is possible to extend a temporal lobectomy safely in the posterior direction and remove the temporooccipital junction if only the two inferior gyri need to be resected and the venous drainage is preserved. In this way, 12 or 13 cm of tissue can be removed but not without prior or subsequent embarrassment of the visual field. Intraoperative corticography and microstimulation can be used to increase the safety of both gyrectomy and lobectomy.

The goal of the surgeon in neurooncology should be an increase in the length and the quality of the patient's survival by maximal resection of the tumor and minimal disturbance of the brain. These objectives can be met and complications avoided if diligence is used in tumor localization and exposure, if meticulous technique is employed in handling tissues, and if a thorough plan is developed for the route and extent of the resection.

Stereotactic Surgery for Mass Lesions of the Cranial Vault

M. Peter Heilbrun
Douglas Brockmeyer
Peter Sunderland

Stereotactic localization has become a standard technique for the surgical management of structural lesions in the cranial vault. Starting as an aid to precision point biopsy and gradually expanding as an adjunct for volume resection, stereotactic instruments and techniques have evolved to encompass a wide range of procedures that benefit from precision stereotactic localization.

After a brief review of the literature, this discussion reports a decade's experience in stereotactic localization with the Brown-Roberts-Wells (BRW) system (Radionics, Inc., Burlington, MA) at University of Utah. The report first describes the BRW system and then discusses surgical techniques and protocols for avoiding complications.

LITERATURE REVIEW

Evolution of Image Guided Stereotactic Surgery

Belyaev et al.[31] are credited with the first successful application of computer techniques (as early as 1965) to determine stereotactic target point coordinates in the brain. Since then, computed tomographic (CT) imaging has significantly advanced and broadened computer applications to stereotaxis.

The coupling of CT technology and stereotactic methodology was first reported in 1977 by Maroon et al.,[55] who described three cases in which biopsies and/or aspirations were performed within, and assisted by, the CT scanner. One patient suffered a minor morbidity, and one an unrelated death.

In the late 1970s and early 1980s, many others, including Boethius et al.,[33] Kelly et al.,[48] Mundinger et al.,[58] Gleason et al.,[40] Scarabin et al.,[63] Moran et al.,[57] Shalit et al.,[64] Rushworth,[62] Walsh et al.,[66] and Kelly and Alker,[47] reported success in incorporating CT scan technology into clinical stereotactic surgery. (Table 16-6).

Notable among the early studies was Ostertag et al.'s[60] report of 302 patients who underwent stereotactic localization procedures using the Riechert-Mundinger apparatus. In Ostertag's series a 3 percent minor morbidity rate and a 2.3 percent operative mortality rate was achieved. Other important early studies included 345 patients reported by Edner, and 100 patients reported by Lobato et al.[43] Using the Leksell system, Edner achieved a mortality rate of

Table 16-6. Reported Morbidity and Mortality Rates for
Stereotactic Biopsy and Tumor Resection

Author	Year	No. of Patients	Morbidity Rate (%)	Mortality Rate (%)	System
Ostertag et al.[60]	1980	302	3	2.3	Reichert-Mundinger
Edner[239]	1981	345	2.3	0.9	Leksell
Lobato et al.[53]	1982	100	7	0	Leksell
Heilbrun et al.[143]	1983	75	0	2.6	Brown-Roberts-Wells
Apuzzo et al.[30]	1983	83	4	0	Brown-Roberts-Wells
Lunsford and Martinez[54]	1984	102	5.9	0	Leksell
Apuzzo et al.[29]	1987	500	1	0.2	Brown-Roberts-Wells
Davis et al.[38]	1987	439	<1	<1	Todd-Wells
Kelly[45,46]	1988	226	9.3	0.2	Kelly

0.9 percent and a morbidity rate of 2.3 percent, while Lobato et al.[53] reported no mortality and a 7 percent morbidity rate (Table 16-6).

In the 1980s, further advances and refinements in localization techniques by Brown,[34,35] Perry et al.,[61] Shelden et al.,[65] Boethius et al.,[32] Koslow et al.,[52] and Goerss et al.[41] were described. Advances in computer software as reported by Heilbrun et al.[43] and Kelly et al.[45,49] heralded broader application of stereotactic methods. These enhanced applications include Kelly's computer-guided laser resection of tumors[47,50]; stereotactic craniotomy and traditional resection of intracerebral lesions as reported by Hariz and Fodstad[42] and Moore et al.[56]; as well as stereotactic radiosurgery[67]; brachytherapy[36,56]; and management of brainstem lesions reported by Nauta et al.,[59] Abernathy et al.,[28] and Hood and McKeever.[44] Early case series in this era include those by Heilbrun et al.,[43] Apuzzo and Sabshin,[30] Lunsford and Martinez,[54] Apuzzo et al.,[29] and Davis et al.[38] (Table 16-6).

GENERAL PRINCIPLES OF STEREOTACTIC TRANSFORMATION

Determination of a specific stereotactic target involves the transformation of a two-dimensional position on a reference image such as a CT scan or magnetic resonance image (MRI) to a three-dimensional position in space. To accomplish this transformation, an external reference for three-dimensional stereotactic space must be defined that can be geometrically related to intracranial structures. This external reference must be fixed to the head and have a specific relation to external fiducial markers so that there

is no change in the position of the reference system throughout the stereotactic operative procedure.

Practical Considerations in the Brown-Roberts-Wells Design

What Is Being Calculated

The stereotactic system determines the three-dimensional stereotactic coordinate by defining the position of a CT image point in reference to the plane of the top of the BRW head ring. By referencing the CT scan to rods that are fixed to the patient's head, the BRW system provided a more uniform calibration for vertical accuracy than had been achieved by stereotactic reference systems that attached to a CT scanner table or gantry (Fig. 16-8).

The BRW system includes a preprogrammed laptop computer for the mathematical transformation. Once the two-dimensional scan coordinates of the rods' fixed reference points and the selected cranial target points are entered, the computer transforms the selected points into three-dimensional space. The position established by this calculation is termed the BRW "target." The trajectory to the BRW target is determined by an "approach menu," which calculates precise angle settings and distance between a chosen entry point and the target. The computed angles and distance to the target are then manually set on the mechanical device.

The Mechanical Device

The BRW head ring was designed for versatile attachment to multiple skull position points by pins attached to carbon posts, which are attached to driv-

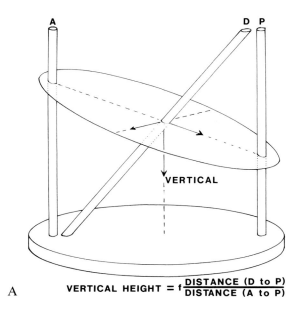

A

$$\text{VERTICAL HEIGHT} = f\frac{\text{DISTANCE (D to P)}}{\text{DISTANCE (A to P)}}$$

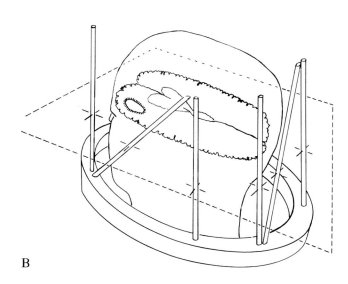

B

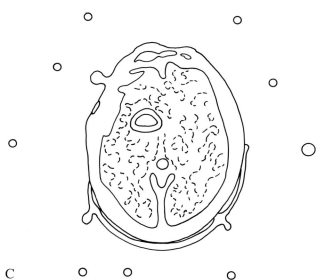

C

Figure 16-8. **(A)** A single set of vertical and diagonal rods (picket fence) mounted on a platform, which serves as the stereotactic coordinate system reference plane. This picket fence is intersected by a plane representing a CT scan or MRI. The intersecting three-dimensional position on the plane can be calculated by measuring the ratio of the distance of the diagonal rod to the vertical rods. **(B)** The localizer with two of the three sets of vertical and diagonal rods (picket fence) required to fix the intersecting image plane in space related to the reference head ring. The two-dimensional position of the rods on the intersected plane is used to calculate the three-dimensional stereotactic coordinate. **(C)** A drawing of a CT scan image showing an axial image of the brain containing a ring-enhancing lesion. The brain is surrounded by the nine vertical and diagonal rods making up the three picket fences. The two-dimensional position of the rods seen on the image is used to calculate the three-dimensional stereotactic coordinate.

ers. In practice, the carbon posts provide an offset distance that ensures that the aluminum head ring does not create CT image artifact (Fig. 16-9).

When the head ring is fixed to the patient's skull, it also serves as a platform to hold localization and guidance devices. To reduce error in conceptualizing right and left and anterior and posterior positions, the attachment feet and receptors are designed with a slight distance offset so that the attached components maintain a specific orientation on the head ring. Attached to the basic head ring is a vertical arc seated on a horizontal arc. Located on the vertical arc is a slide for holding stereotactic probes (Figs. 16-10 and 16-11).

A phantom simulator provides a physical check that the target values have been calculated correctly. By first setting the calculated guidance angles and distances on a phantom, the surgeon can simulate the operative procedure before sterilizing and attaching the arc to the patient's head ring (Fig. 16-12).

To accommodate the move from point biopsy to stereotactically guided volume resection, several modifications have evolved over the decade of BRW use. The head ring has been modified to attach to a plate that connects to the standard operating room (OR) table Mayfield type head-holder, thereby allowing the patient's head to be adjusted for approaches to intracranial lesions and structures from multiple

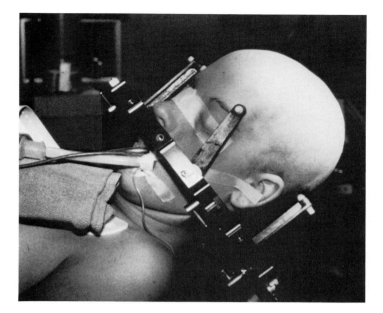

Figure 16-9. The head ring attached to the skull and fixed to the OR table demonstrating that its design and position of fixation allows both artifact-free localization and unimpeded access to the cranial vault for operative procedures.

directions. In addition, threaded openings around the circumference of the ring hold a variety of retractor systems.

There have also been multiple adaptations to the BRW arc to provide more working distance from the arc to the central trajectory. The National Institutes of Health (NIH) arc enables the use of grids for parallel placement of catheters. Initially used for brachytherapy, such grids may also be used to define tumor margins after a central trajectory to the middle of a lesion has been calculated. For open craniotomy and volumetric resection, standard ventricular catheters can be guided to targets and cut off at the surface of the cortex to serve as markers from the surface of the cortex to the lesion target points. A plastic sleeve fitted into the slide located on the vertical arc has simplified this type of catheter placement.

The difficulty of intubating around the head ring has been solved with a swivel head ring, which has a hoop-shaped piece in the front that can be swiveled up out of the way for intubation and then back down for attaching the arcs (Fig. 16-13).

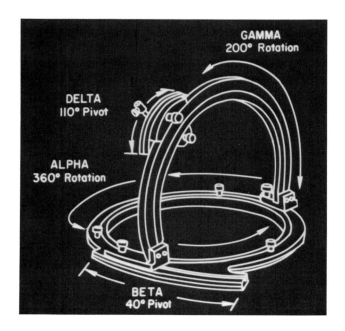

Figure 16-10. The classic Brown-Roberts-Wells guidance arc that allows the definition of a wide range of trajectories to an intracranial target.

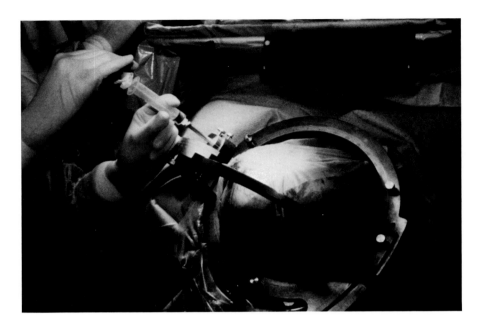

Figure 16-11. Fully draped stereotactic system ensuring both sterility and full access to the cranial vault during a point biopsy through a perforator skull opening.

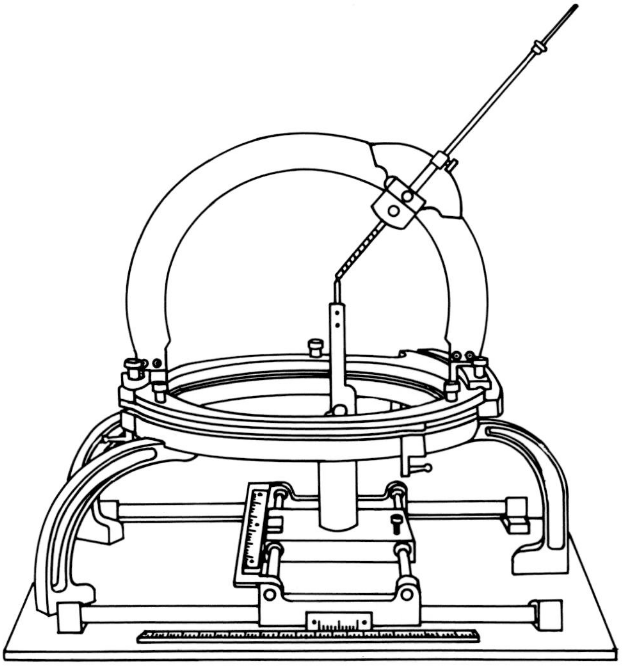

Figure 16-12. The phantom simulator used for simulating the stereotactic operative procedure and verifying the accuracy of the computed frame settings and distances from the arc to the target.

Software Advances—Graphics Workstation as an Aid to Planning Stereotactic Surgery

A surgeon utilizes images of brain structures from many different perspectives and intuitively translates those images into his planned operative approach to lesions within the brain. By using computer graphic reformatting techniques to create a view of brain structures along as well as orthogonal to the probe track, a surgeon can change targets and positions of probe entry points on the scalp or the surface of the brain, and then recalculate probe trajectories until the most appropriate trajectory is visualized and accepted. The new probe paths can be reviewed and accepted or rejected depending on the surgeon's visual analysis of the position of the probe path to critical brain structures (Fig. 16-14). Such computer graphics techniques are useful in increasing options available to the neurosurgeon in the OR for planning safer operations.

LOCALIZATION TECHNIQUES: ATTACHING BRW HEAD RING TO THE SKULL

Attachment Under Local Anesthesia

For the majority of head ring fixations, localizing scans, lidocaine local anesthesia supplemented with intravenous midazolam (Versed) IV is sufficient.

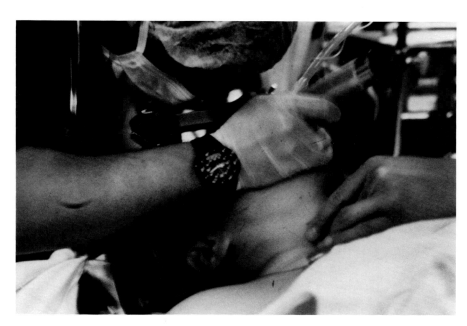

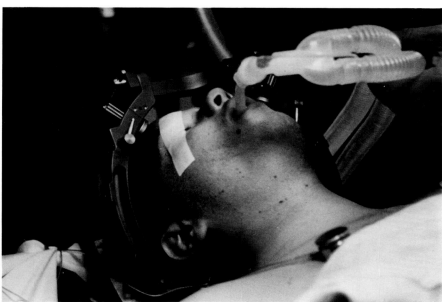

Figure 16-13. The swivel head ring, which allows easier postlocalization intubation for the anesthesiologist.

This eliminates the risks of general anesthesia in the CT scanner area and of transporting an anesthetized patient from the scanner to the operating room. Once the Versed is given, the head ring is strapped in the appropriate position in front of the nose parallel to the orbitomeatal line laterally, and parallel to the intercanthal line anteriorly (Fig. 16-15).

The scalp is cleaned and the post positions are adjusted to appropriate positions a few millimeters from the scalp. Five to 7 ml of 1 percent lidocaine with epinephrine is injected through the pin opening in the post to raise a wheal, which pushes the scalp out

firmly to the post. If the patient is to wear the head ring throughout the day while awake, 2 to 3 ml of a long-acting local anesthetic such as 0.25 percent bupvacaine (Marcaine) is added.

Waiting 5 to 10 minutes ensures good local anesthesia for screwing the pins through the scalp into the bone. Once the pins are screwed in, the straps are removed. The head is moved by holding the head ring to various positions to ensure that the ring is rigidly secured. Neither the pins nor the posts need to be tightened with excessive force. No torque wrench is needed. Following application of the head ring, the

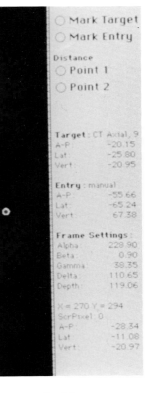

Figure 16-14. The OR workstation computer console image of CT scan annotated with target, entry, and frame setting data used for the stereotactic procedure.

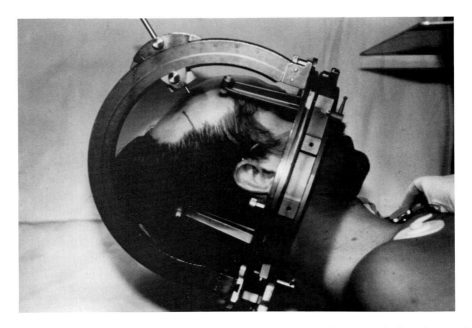

Figure 16-15. The normal fixation position of head ring and arc for the majority of procedures.

patient is taken into the scanner room in the wheelchair and is properly assisted in transfer to the scanner table.

Strategies for Placing the Head Ring

The normal position of the head ring at the level of the nose parallel to the orbitomeatal and intercanthal lines should be shifted depending on the location of the target.

To approach *temporal lobe lesions,* the head ring can be angled so that the guidance arc can be set with a low trajectory. In this situation, the anterior post on the side of the lesion should be rotated about 15° so that the pin is fixed to the skull in the frontal bone approximately at the pupillary line. This allows a trajectory with an anterior temporal entry to a anteromesial temporal position and ensures that the guidance arc clears the anterior pin (Fig. 16-16). *Caution:* Using the BRW guidance arc in some circumstances, it is not possible to compute a low enough trajectory to get a temporal target that avoids the vasculature in the sylvian fissure.

To reach *posterior fossa* lesions by a transcerebellar approach, the head ring is fixed to the skull with the anterior marker reversed 180 degrees and below the occiput. This reversal allows the head ring to be attached to the Mayfield table adapter so that the patient can be fixed to the OR table in either the sitting or the prone position. The head ring is also fixed higher frontally and lower occipitally so that a trajectory can be designed that is paramedian over the cerebellar hemisphere and that will avoid the

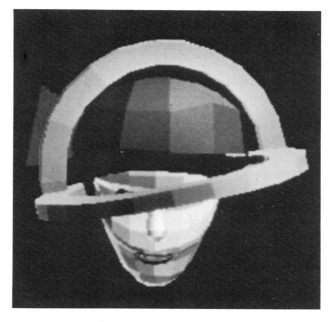

Figure 16-16. The tilted position of head ring to improve access to middle fossa.

transverse and sigmoid sinus and the midline (Fig. 16-17). *Caution:* In older patients with cervical spondylosis and with kyphosis limiting flexion, it may not be possible to accomplish posterior fossa approaches with the BRW ring. With posterior fossa approaches, the guidance arc may not clear the vertex of the skull, so that an oblique lateral approach must be designed for anterior and medial cerebellar and brainstem lesions.

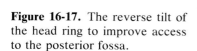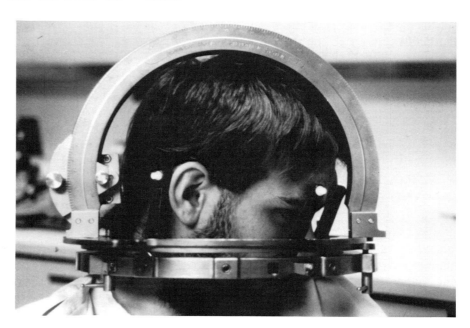

Figure 16-17. The reverse tilt of the head ring to improve access to the posterior fossa.

IMAGE ACQUISITION

Although the BRW concept does not require that the head ring be fixed to the CT scanner table, doing so is comfortable for the patient and provides images with scalp contours with no movement from slice to slice.

Once the patient is lying comfortably on the scanner table, the table is moved superiorly and rostrally until the horizontal laser arming light of the gantry projects on the large No. 1 rod of the BRW localizer and the vertical laser arming beam projects on the top of the head ring. Scan parameters including field of view (FOV), scan slice thickness, and contiguous or overlap images need to be planned. The FOV that will give the largest screen image of the head yet will still include the nine fiduciary rod images should be chosen.

For lesions larger than 2 cm, 3-mm-thick contiguous slices are appropriate. Lesions smaller than 2 cm require smaller, 1.5-mm-thick contiguous slices.

The study begins when the technician records a scanogram, which consists of a lateral or anterior-posterior (AP) image of the skull. The lateral scanogram can then be marked with the line cursor to delineate the range of scan slices so that the lesion and potential entry points are encompassed by the series of scans.

If an entry point from a superior image is planned, the images should be obtained approaching the top of the skull. Obtaining images through the entire head adds only an extra 5 minutes to the total scan time.

For record keeping, the technician files two sets of images; one set for the radiology file, and a second set for the surgeon to take to the operating room for hard copy reference. The study can also be saved on a standard 9-inch magnetic data tape for use in an operating room computer graphics workstation. For stereotactic localization utilizing multiple trajectories for open craniotomy, this type of computer use becomes essential.

IMAGE SELECTION FOR TARGET AND ENTRY POINT CALCULATION

When image acquisition is completed, the surgeon quickly reviews all of the images on the console. If the set is satisfactory, the patient is removed from the scanner table and transported by wheelchair or stretcher to the operating room.

Orienting Console Display

Standard CT consoles display images in the body mode, that is, from the feet up. To place the image in the appropriate orientation for actual surgery, that is, looking from the top of the head down, the image must be flipped right to left on its AP axis.

The surgeon then selects the specific images to be used for target calculation and any other images that might be used for entry point calculation.

Choice of Image and Targets

Center Target

For *lesions smaller than 2 cm* in diameter, an image that represents the center of the lesion and a target in the center of the lesion will yield the least false-negative biopsies. A target in the center of the lesion is also appropriate if the lesion is larger than 2 cm, but shows homogeneous low density on the scan with the presumptive diagnosis of a lower grade astrocytoma, or if the presumptive diagnosis is an abscess rather than a malignant astrocytoma (Fig. 16-18).

Enhancing Border

For *large lesions that are heterogeneous,* a central biopsy might only yield tissue that is 100 percent necrotic and nondiagnostic. In the case of large lesions

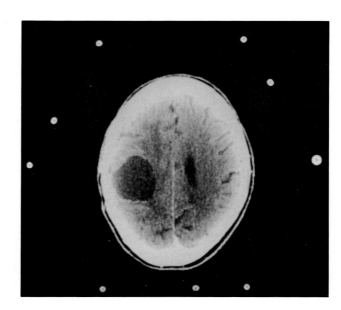

Figure 16-18. The biopsy position in the center of a low-density homogeneous lesion.

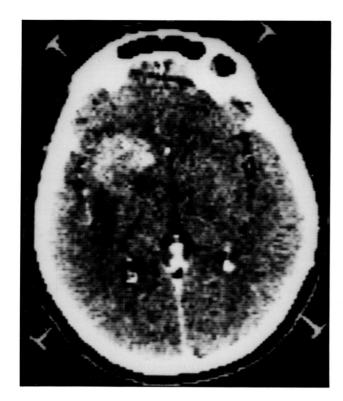

Figure 16-19. The biopsy position at the enhancing border of a hyperdense heterogeneous lesion.

with a ring-enhancing border with the presumptive diagnosis of a malignant astrocytoma, a target in the enhancing border tissue results in the highest diagnostic yield (Fig. 16-19). Biopsying a target on an image that shows the superior border of the lesion will produce a biopsy sample that starts at the outside edge of the enhancing border and passes to the center of the lesion.

When stereotactic localization is combined with open craniotomy for lesion excision, choosing multiple targets allows catheters to be passed to the superior surface and to the borders of the lesion. Selecting an image in the center of the lesion and marking its anterior, posterior, lateral, and medial target positions will produce an outline of the lesion. By using a point on a superior slice image as an entry point and a position on a lower slice as a target, the surgeon can define a trajectory that back-projects an entry point at the scalp. If that position is not satisfactory, the entry point determined at the superior surface of the lesion can be moved to a new position and a new trajectory calculated. In a similar fashion, an inferior lesion slice is chosen to determine the inferior aspect of the lesion (Fig. 16-20). *Caution:* When parallel catheter trajectories are being used to define tumor borders, if the lesion is large, it is possible that a parallel catheter would pass outside the craniotomy margin. In this situation, additional entry points can be used to pass catheters to the lesion margins.

Figure 16-20. Multiple trajectories outline the center and borders of a lesion.

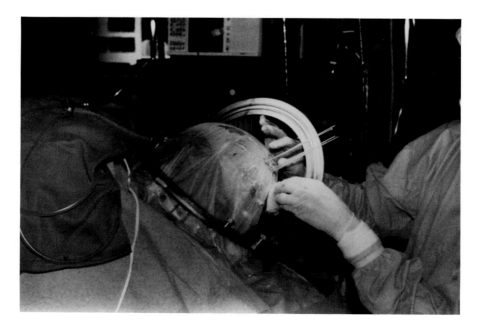

Procedure for Marking Targets

A trackball cursor is used to register the *x* and *y* coordinate of any point on the console. Beginning with rod No. 1, the surgeon registers and records points for each of the nine picket fence rods. Once all the rod positions are recorded in the proper order, the cursor is moved to a target and the *x* and *y* position of one or multiple targets are recorded. Multiple target positions can be recorded from a single image without remarking the rods. However, if alternate targets are chosen on different images, the rod positions must be rerecorded. The BRW data sheet is set up to record rod positions on three different images. If more images are used, multiple data sheets can be used.

Calculation of more than one target with the standard BRW computer becomes cumbersome. The use of an operating room graphics workstation becomes valuable in this situation because trajectories can be adjusted instantaneously to view the simulated probe tracts as they pass to target points within and around the lesion.

TRAJECTORY SELECTION

Once the target has been determined, the surgeon plans a trajectory by one of two methods: (1) by selecting a specific entry point on the surface of the scalp or skull, or (2) by the azimuth-declination method in which the appropriate quadrant of the head is selected. An optimal trajectory will pass the shortest distance, avoid critical neural and vascular structures, and require only a single initial entrance from the arachnoid space into the brain parenchyma.

Target Location

To design a trajectory, the target position is categorized as supratentorial or infratentorial, surface and subcortical, frontal, parietal, temporal, occipital, or cerebellar, central white matter, paraventricular, intraventricular, or midline. Extra-axial lesions are rarely approached stereotactically, although occasional small meningiomas and suprasellar lesions are approached using stereotactic guidance.

Using this classification, entry points are determined in the following fashion. For *surface or subcortical lesions,* an entry point is chosen that is directly over the lesion. *Caution:* In approaching surface or subcortical lesions in the region of the sylvian fissure and insula, it is prudent to combine stereotactic localization with a small trephine or craniot-omy for direct visualization of the probe track to the lesion. The distance is short, the cortical incision is almost as small as using a biopsy instrument, and the direct visualization will help avoid the large middle cerebral artery opercular branches.

For all other *supratentorial lesions,* except mesial temporal lobe, standard classical paramedian entry positions that traverse silent watershed areas of the brain can be used. For example, for posterior frontal or anterior thalamic lesions, an appropriate entry point is at, or anterior to the coronal suture, 2 to 3 cm from the midline. For a lesion that is subependymal or on the caudate, the entry point might be more lateral and anterior to avoid the frontal horn. For deep parietooccipital, posterior corpus callosum, or pineal region lesions, a watershed entry point posterior to the parietal boss, 2 to 3 cm from the midline, is appropriate. For pineal region lesions, it is essential to review the position of the internal cerebral veins on coronal MRI, adjusting the entry point laterally to avoid the veins. If the internal cerebral veins are irregular, for example in pineal lesions, a standard open supratentorial or infratentorial approach may be prudent.

Defining a Trajectory by Azimuth-Declination Technique or Entry Point Technique

Azimuth-Declination Technique

The BRW computer is used to define a trajectory by the azimuth-declination technique. Depending on the quadrant containing the lesion, an azimuth value from 0 to 360 degrees is selected. For example, a right frontal lesion is in the quadrant from 0 to 90 degrees so a reasonable azimuth would be 25 degrees. For a left parietooccipital lesion, a reasonable azimuth is 210 degrees. The declination is the number of degrees above horizontal zero. A declination of 55 to 80 degrees will yield a trajectory generally perpendicular to the curve of the skull. The computer will output a set of four arc angle settings and a distance to the target. When the procedure is simulated on the phantom, of the trajectory is not satisfactory, a new azimuth and/or declination can be entered. Thus if the declination of 70 degrees provides too oblique a trajectory, a new declination of 80 degrees can be entered, and the phantom trajectory reset accordingly. Alternatively, for minor adjustments, a revised trajectory may be set up manually without using the computer—by adjusting all four angles on the arc, directing a pointer through a sleeve to the phantom target, and reading the four settings and depth directly off of the arc. This method is useful, although it may not save much time over recomputation using the computer.

Entry Point Techniques

Physical Placement

The most common method of choosing the entry point is by placing the arc on the head ring fixed to the patient's head and moving the arc randomly until the end of a sleeve is positioned on the patient's scalp. All fittings of the arc are tightened, the arc is moved to the phantom, the phantom pointer is moved to the sleeve, and the coordinates are recorded. *Caution:* To account for the thickness of the scalp and skull, we generally add 10 mm to the distance of the entry point coordinate. This additional distance moves the fulcrum of the trajectory closer to the inner table or surface of the brain so that an instrument will adequately clear the bony edge of a perforator opening in the skull.

CT Scan Point on Bone

An entry point can also be determined from the CT scan by picking a point on the bone, calculating it as a target, and then using those values as the entry point. In this method, the cursor is placed on the target and moved to a position laterally and anteriorly that will provide a satisfactory angle to the target. The scan window is then changed from the brain tissue to the bone window and scrolled upwards through the images until the cursor hits the inner table. This cursor position is recorded along with the rod positions on this image and the target entry point. Alternatively, an entry point target can be determined from the image slice with the coronal or lambdoid suture, by measuring an appropriate paramedian distance from the midline.

VERIFICATION

Although phantom verification is not an essential component of the BRW system, it does provide an additional safety feature. The capability of simulating the operative procedure provides an extra assurance that the computation procedure is correct. Not only does the simulator verify the actual numbers, it allows the surgeon to conceptualize the actual operative procedure in three-dimensional stereotactic space.

The phantom simulator consists of a head ring mounted on a platform containing a pointer that can be moved to any point in calculated stereotactic space. The guidance arc can be placed on the phantom and the precision of the trajectory can be checked by ensuring the phantom pointer meets a pointer or sleeve on the arc. In addition, manual adjustment to the arc and entry points can be made easily with the phantom.

However, for sophisticated parallel approaches to plan placement of catheters for interstitial brachytherapy and hyperthermia, an operating room graphics workstation is more efficient than the phantom.

BIOPSY AND OPEN CRANIOTOMY FOR TUMOR RESECTION

Although the ideal goal of all surgical procedures is complete removal of the lesion without precipitating any morbidity, the essential surgical judgment is: Which lesions can be removed completely and which lesions should only be biopsied or only partially resected?

The natural history of the presumed disease process together with the lesion's size, shape, and location, and a determination of whether it is focal, multicentric, or crosses the midline, and whether it appears to be encapsulated or infiltrating, all enter into the surgical judgment.

Biopsy

If the lesion is homogeneous and of low density, a lower grade astrocytoma is likely. In such cases, a biopsy specimen should be obtained from the center of the lesion with the Nashold-Seddon-type side cutting forceps, and the target coordinate is the center of the opening in the forceps (Fig. 16-21). However, if the lesion is heterogeneous and has an enhancing border, the finding is generally a higher grade astrocytoma with a partially necrotic center. In such cases, the most reliable site of biopsy is the edge of the enhancing lesion toward the center. A target coordinate at the proximal portion of the opening in the forceps will provide a 10-mm-long piece of tissue within the lesion.

Once the biopsy is completed, a ventricular catheter can be passed along the central trajectory to the inferior border of the lesion. A standard corticotomy is made and dissection is carried down to the superior border of the lesion, following which various blade retractors are used to explore the lesion for resec-

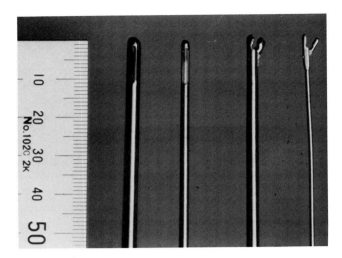

Figure 16-21. Nashold-Seddon-type side cutting forceps and 2-mm cup forceps used for biopsy.

tion. Depending on the nature of the tissue and the vascularity, the tissue dissection can be carried out as either an internal debulking or an extracapsular dissection using the ultrasonic aspirator or classic suction and coagulation. Previously placed ventricular catheters guide the dissection limits. The guidance arc can be kept in place, pivoting it out of the way on its fulcrum, or the vertical arc can be removed, and the horizontal arc left in place in order not to break the sterile field (Fig. 16-22).

Complete Resection

For lesions anticipated to be astrocytomas, if the lesion is in a polar position, such as the frontal or temporal lobe, and MRI T$_2$-weighted studies show that it does not cross the corpus callosum or involve presylvian structures, then complete resection can be considered.

If complete resection is the goal, choosing a central trajectory provides certain advantages: a central position for a craniotomy flap, a position in the superior portion of the lesion, a position for biopsy in the center of the lesion, and a position in the inferior aspect of the lesion. Choosing a target on the lowest slice and an entry point on the highest slice defines a trajectory from the top to the bottom of the lesion. From this slice, parallel trajectories to the anterior, posterior, medial, and lateral limits of the lesion can be determined. The position at which the border trajectories meet the bone can be used to determine the size and limits of the bone opening. Or, the size of the bone flap may be reduced by designing trajectories from the intersection of the central trajectories with the surface of the brain (which serves as a fulcrum) to the selected borders (Fig. 16-23).

Once the craniotomy is accomplished and the dura has been opened, straight ventricular catheters are passed to the tumor borders. The central trajectory is used to obtain a biopsy specimen.

Recently we have explored the technique made possible with MRI imaging of designing a trajectory starting at the surface of the sulcus, microsurgically opening the sulcus to its depth, and then traversing deep gray matter at the depth of its sulcul fold into the white matter, and then to the lesion. To date, we do not have evidence that this procedure is associated with less morbidity than transgyral dissections. In the past, we developed a set of cylindrical retractors similar to those described and used by Kelly.[46,48]

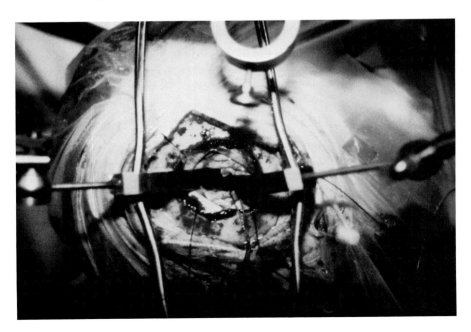

Figure 16-22. Small open craniotomy with the guidance pivoted to the side.

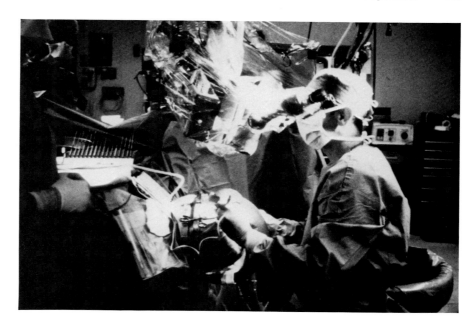

Figure 16-23. Surgeon comfortably performing microsurgical removal of an arteriovenous malformation (AVM) through a craniotomy combined with adjunct stereotactic guidance.

To utilize those retractors with a diameter greater than 10 mm, we gradually dilated the tract through the brain to the target with malleable gallbladder duct dilators. Nevertheless, we found that cylindrical retractors greater than 10 mm in diameter caused unacceptable distortion of the brain, and we returned to the use of standard-blade-type retractors.

Once a lesion is reached, several surgical resection instruments can be used depending on the surgeon's preference. The most useful is the classical combination of suction and bipolar coagulation. The improvement of the bipolar coagulation by the addition of nonstick features and combined irrigation capabilities is useful. Although CO_2 laser vaporization is available, the loss of tactile feedback when using the laser may decrease the surgeon's ability to define dissection planes. Ultrasonic aspiration is also utilized, although the size of the standard instruments requires enlarged openings.

COMPLICATIONS

A review of the complications in our series of 357 stereotactic cases performed from December 1979 through June 1990 reflects a learning curve in the techniques of stereotactic localization for the management by biopsy and resection of intracranial lesions.

In our evaluation of complications, we compared four groups of 100 cases from late 1979 to June 1984, July 1984 to June 1986, July 1986 to June 1988, and July 1988 to June 1990 (Table 16-7).

In the first 100 cases from 1979 to June 1984, there was an operative mortality rate of 3 percent (deaths within 30 days of the procedure), a major morbidity rate of 2 percent secondary to hemorrhage, and a minor morbidity rate of 3 percent. Two of the three deaths were associated with postbiopsy exacerbation of brain edema and occurred within 24 hours of the biopsy. The third death was a complication of a craniotomy 13 days following a stereotactic biopsy of a large oligodendroglioma.

The first death mentioned above involved a neurologically intact patient with a large frontal lesion. Stereotactic biopsy under local anesthesia showed an anaplastic astrocytoma. The patient was found dead in her hospital bed at night many hours after the biopsy. No hemorrhage was found at autopsy. It was postulated she had an unrecognized seizure. Our protocol now requires patients to be in an intensive care environment for at least 24 hours following the procedure.

The second death involved a patient who had an open stereotactic biopsy of the border of a ring-enhancing heterogeneous glioblastoma. Several hours after biopsy, he deteriorated and was taken immediately to the operating room, where craniotomy revealed only swelling and no hemorrhage. Swelling was confirmed by CT and the patient died several hours later.

In the second 100 cases, from July 1984 to July 1986, two perioperative deaths occurred. One death occurred several days after a stereotactic biopsy of a malignant lymphoma. A postoperative bleeding disorder resulted in a large intracranial hemorrhage, which was not treated pursuant to the family's

Table 16-7.   Complications

	Years (case nos.)				
	1979–1984 (1–100)	1984–1986 (101–200)	1986–1988 (201–300)	1988–1990 (300–357)	Total
Death within 30 days	3	2	0	1	6
Major morbidity					
Hemorrhage with deficit	2	1	2	2	7
Major deficit without hemorrhage	0	0	0	1	1
Minor morbidity					
Transient deficit	1	1	5	3	10
Brachytherapy catheter misplacement	0	2	0	0	2
Sinus pin puncture	1	0	0	0	1
Wound infection	1	0	0	1	2
Other					
Failed procedure	0	1	0	0	1
Head ring removal for intubation	0	0	1	0	1

wishes. Another death unrelated to the stereotactic procedure occurred in a patient with acute myelogenous leukemia.

No deaths occurred in the third 100 cases from July 1986 to June 1988. From July 1988 to June 1990, one death occurred when it was elected not to treat a dominant hemisphere hemorrhage into a glioblastoma 2 days after stereotactic biopsy.

In the first 100 cases from 1979 to June 1984, two major morbidities occurred following hemorrhage at the biopsy site in two patients with malignant astrocytomas. In the second 100 cases, from July 1984 to July 1986, one major morbidity occurred. A neurologically intact young female had presented with a persisting mild deficit secondary to a hematoma. High-quality angiography did not show an arteriovenous malformation (AVM). After stereotactic aspiration of the hematoma, the collapsed wall was biopsied with the cup forceps to rule out tumor. A 3-mm length of a 1-mm-diameter blood vessel was present in the biopsy tissue, and there was brisk arterial bleeding from the cannula through which the aspiration and the biopsy had been performed. A craniotomy was quickly accomplished, and the probe was followed down to the hematoma cavity. Hemorrhage was eventually controlled with difficulty after dissection through deep gray and white matter structures. The patient was left with a permanent hemiparesis. We no longer biopsy collapsed walls of lesions containing fluid. In the two cases since then, fluid was sent for cytology, which suggested metastatic tumor cells. One case was treated with subsequent open resection of the wall of the lesion; the second was treated with radiation.

There was a period during July 1988 to June 1990 (cases 201 through 357) in which our major morbidity increased. Influenced by Kelly's description of volume resection of deep-seated intracranial lesions, we became more aggressive in our attempts to resect lesions completely. In spite of stereotactic definition of tumor borders, in one case hemiplegia occurred when a calcified portion of the lesion extended into the genu of the internal capsule. We have subsequently returned to a more conservative approach of biopsy and subtotal resection. This determination is consistent with Kelly's later description of the Dumas-Duport classification of infiltrating lesions, and his report that there was no significant increase in survival in patients with malignant astrocytomas following complete stereotactic volume resection.[45,46] Less aggressive resection followed Coffey et al.'s retrospective report[37] that prolonged survival following stereotactic biopsy of malignant astrocytomas depends more on completion of radiation therapy than either the time or extent of resection. In addition, during these latter years, two postbiopsy hemorrhages occurred that resulted in increased motor deficits. The first was a small thalamic hemorrhage into the internal capsule. The deficit did not clear. A second hemorrhage occurred when a frontal approach was misdirected laterally to the enhancing border of the lesion and a sylvian vessel bled, requiring an open procedure. A third hemorrhage occurred during open guided resection of a suspected encapsulated cavernous angioma in the internal capsule. The lesion was an occult AVM with intermixed normal brain tissue, which bled actively at the time of resection.

Table 16-8. False-Positive/False-Negative Diagnoses*a*

	Years (case nos.)				
	1979–1984 (1–100)	1984–1986 (101–200)	1986–1988 (201–300)	1988–1990 (300–357)	Total
False positive	7	3	0	0	10
False negative	6	2	2	1	11

a False positive defined as original pathological diagnosis later disproven. False negative defined as nondiagnostic tissue obtained from biopsy position confirmed on postop image study.

In the entire series, minor complications occurred in ten patients with transient deficits, two patients requiring brachytherapy catheter adjustment, one patient with a frontal sinus puncture by a pin that required minor repair, one patient with a pin site infection that was easily treated with antibiotics, and one patient with a bone flap infection that required removal and subsequent cranioplasty. One patient had a procedure terminated when she developed severe facial pain as the biopsy instrument contacted either the tentorial edge or the fifth nerve root entry zone. This problem has been solved by utilizing multiplanar MRI, particularly oblique coronals, for viewing the planned trajectory path into the brainstem.

A significant problem in the first 200 cases was the percentage of false-positive and false-negative diagnoses (Table 16-8). We defined false-positive diagnoses as those in which the original diagnosis at the time of the stereotactic procedure was later disproved. False-negative diagnoses were defined as nondiagnostic tissue obtained from an image-confirmed biopsy site. Such diagnoses often occurred when firm lesions were displaced by the biopsy instrument, resulting in biopsy of perilesion tissue. Often the diagnosis was normal brain or gliosis. In the first 100 cases from 1979 to June 1984, we had 14 percent false-positive and false-negative diagnoses, 7 percent in each category. In the second 100 cases, from July 1984 to July 1986, we had 5 percent false-positive and false-negative diagnoses. Only one further false-negative case occurred in the subsequent 157 cases. This improvement resulted from better neuropathological support in conjunction with a protocol for taking more samples or converting from a closed procedure to an open stereotactic procedure if the microscopic diagnosis on frozen section or smear did not fit the expected diagnosis from the clinical course and imaging studies. Conversion to an open procedure provides both direct guidance and visualization at the time of biopsy and resection. The recognition of the problems of false-positive and false-negative diagnoses directly resulted in our moving to stereotactically guided craniotomy for biopsy coupled with resection.

SUMMARY

This chapter part describes the evolution of the BRW system in using image-guided stereotactic localization for biopsy and volume resection. Like the operating microscope, stereotactic localization and guidance is now considered a standard for approaching intra-axial cerebral lesions and structures. The University of Utah experience is documented along with the description of the methods that have been developed to avoid complications. An analysis of the actual complication rate and a discussion of strategies and techniques to avoid complications when utilizing stereotactic methods is presented.

Techniques and Refinements of Anesthesia for Stereotaxy

Stephen N. Steen
Vladimir Zelman
Peter Gruen
Abdolmajid Bayat
Michael L.J. Apuzzo

Don't shout at the crocodile until after you have crossed the river.

South African proverb

HISTORY OF STEREOTACTIC INSTRUMENTATION

''Neolithic skulls nearly twelve thousand years old appear not only to have been carefully cut by a skilled hand but also to have healed following the operation"[102]—all presumably without the use of antiseptics, antibiotics, or anesthesia. Perhaps even then they had the use of coca or some similar leaf to chew in order to allay anxiety, produce sedation, and reduce pain.

In recent years, improvements for entering the skull to locate specific areas for sampling, ablation, stimulation, and recording have been developed.

David Zernov of Moscow University demonstrated the first stereotactic apparatus, an "encephalotome," in 1889 to the Society of Mathematical Physics, reported in French the following year in the Revue Générale des Clinique et Thérapeutique.[95] That same year, the encephalotome was used in humans with epilepsy.

In 1906, Horsely and Clark[91] developed stereotactic equipment with "the idea of applying geometry to the study of the brain to ascertain the functions of various cerebellar structures in the cat."

Forty years later, Speigel et al.[103] reported their stereotactic operation, a dorsomedian thalamotomy, in the human. Initially "the stereotactic apparatus was applied and stabilized by a plaster bandage cast of the shaved skull and a brace containing a mold of the patient's teeth. This tooth mold contained a large circular hole for the anesthesiologist's access." Arnold St. J. Lee, a technician in the Physiology and Experimental Neurology Department of Temple University, reiterated the need for three points screwed into the skull—a proposal that was rejected out of hand by Spiegel in that he felt any additional surgery would be immoral. (A.S.J. Lee, personal communication, 1991).

Subsequently Lee devised a system for exact repositioning of the stereotactic apparatus after x-ray analysis.[70] In his application of physical science to medical research and patient care, Lee conceived of, designed, and developed many different types of human stereotactic instruments for brain surgery including a freezing probe. This original cryosurgery system for brain operations, which allows the surgeon to "turn off" a specific area of the brain reversibly before destroying it, is on permanent exhibit at the Smithsonian Institution.[82] (For a brief history of different forms of stereotactic apparatus, the reader is referred to Chapter 12 by Perkins et al. in *Clinical Neuroanesthesia* by Cucchiara and Michenfelder.[83])

In 1957, a neurosurgical operation suite was constructed that included anesthesia induction and electronic rooms with unique x-ray and monitoring facilities. A specially modified operating room (OR) table with head and x-ray cassette holders, instant Trendenlenburg, and vacuum bottles was designed as well as a facility panel for the anesthesiologist's use.[105] This appears to have been the forerunner of the modern stereotactic OR but without some of the present-day built-in anesthetic improvements in monitoring and recording of the patient's condition.

Anesthesia

Originally, local anesthesia was employed for stereotactic surgery. This may be a trying experience for a conscious patient whose cooperation is needed for evaluating the responses to the surgical intervention. To improve the situation, many drugs and combinations thereof were tried.

In 1959, Ingvar et al.[92] administered either thiopental or ether with succinyl choline and placed a flexible oroendotracheal tube that had an extra cuff with perforations so that lidocaine could be administered intratracheally during the procedure. Maintenance was with nitrous oxide and meperidine. During the testing and recording, the drugs were discontinued to permit the patient to respond to some commands, though obviously verbalization was not possible. This technique was used to decrease the risk of administration of light pentothal anesthesia without endotracheal intubation and to avoid any barbiturate influence on the electrocorticogram.[92] In the same year, Hall et al.[89] used general endotracheal anesthesia with nitrous oxide, halothane, and a continuous intravenous drip of succinyl choline. Patients were difficult to manage with these techniques and were placed at risk. In 1960, Deligne et al.[84] reported on their use of a mixture of 2028 M.D (dextromoramide) 10 mg and Palfium 5 mg following premedication in 139 neurological procedures (predominantly stereotactic neurosurgery) and noted wide variations in subject doses.

In 1960, Steen reported the use of thiamylal, a barbiturate, with local analgesia in over 1,000 patients with Parkinson's syndrome who underwent basal ganglia surgery. The barbiturate was the sole agent used intravenously in addition to a local analgesic, and the anesthetic management was described in detail with the proviso that "verbal contact with the patient should be maintained at all times." Steen stated that "perhaps the management of these patients may be termed pharmacologic hypnosis with the emphasis varying from the adjective to the noun, depending on the suggestibility of the patient and the ability of the anesthesiologist."

For the 5-year period ending in 1961, Steen[106] also described "the anesthetic management of 128 patients suffering from movement disorders other than Parkinsonism." The seven categories of movement disorders fell into two groups with regard to anesthetic management: an intravenous analgesic technique with local anesthesia was used 57 times in 41 patients, and for the rest general anesthesia was administered.

For basal ganglia surgery 216 anesthesias were administered, of which 133 were successful with "an ultra-short-acting barbiturate and intermittent small doses of intravenous narcotic, sufficient to maintain a level no deeper than that of amnesia-analgesia." General anesthesia was administered to 83 patients, including 17 for whom the analgesic technique was unsuccessful. This 20 percent failure rate is comparable to that reported elsewhere.[107]

In 1961, Nilsson and Janssen[98] used neuroleptanalgesia (i.e., a combination of phenoperidine [a major tranquilizer] and haloperidol [a potent analgesic] to produce a state of analgesia, immobility, and indifference on the part of the patient) with endotracheal intubation and a muscle relaxant. Until 1961, halothane or trichloroethylene was added to a mixture of nitrous oxide and oxygen by Brown et al.[76]

In 1964, Coleman and DeVilliers[80] published their anesthesia technique of intermittent, intravenous doses of methohexitone for 29 cases of movement disorders and 64 patients with parkinsonism. Subsequently, the relaxant gallamine triethoiodide was added (to reduce muscle movement without the need for increasing the dose of methohexitone) in the remaining 253 parkinsonism patients.

In the 1960s various anesthetic agents were used: no one technique was universally adopted. Microelectrode techniques were also developed to target "tremor cells" in the nucleus ventralis intermedius of the thalamus for the treatment of Parkinson's disease. Anesthesia was listed by Tasker et al.[108] as general anesthesia (for the radiological localization) with local anesthesia for the placement of lesions, whereas Ohye[99] stated that the surgery is "usually performed under local anesthesia" and that "in cases with severe abnormal movements some sedation is given, and in patients under ten years of age a general anesthesia is preferred."

In 1964, Brown[75] reported on a neuroleptanalgesic technique using phenoperidine with droperidol in 90 operations for Parkinson's disease and over 150 other procedures such as lumbar air encephalography, craniotomy, and electrocorticography, stating in his conclusion that complete satisfaction for the patient, surgeon, and anesthesiologist occurred for those with parkinsonism. Previously, he had tried haloperidol (instead of droperidol) and substituted dextromoramide or fentanyl for phenoperidine.

In 1965, Tasker and Marshall[107] reported on 53 consecutive stereotactic procedures performed chiefly for dyskinesia with their "modified neuroleptanalgesia technique, whereby the use of a moderate degree of the analgesic phenoperidine, secured useful, though not total, anesthesia" with a "sufficiently small degree of respiratory depression to avoid endotracheal intubation." With their technique, 80 percent of patients showed striking analgesia, while fewer than 10 percent developed sedation severe enough to interfere with the operation.

From 1967 to 1976 one of us (V.Z.) administered various anesthetic techniques to approximately 2,500 patients with parkinsonism and other movement disorders upon whom stereotactic procedures were performed by Kandel. In the beginning, local infiltration with sedation, and general anesthesia were used. Later, neuroleptanalgesia with the patient awakened for testing was employed; some patients were endotracheally intubated.[95]

In 1980, 7,469 craniocerebral operations from November 1965 to November 1978 were reported to have been successfully performed under acupuncture anesthesia.[79] This study involved 21 units of neurosurgery in China and does not appear to have been randomized or blinded. The results are not clear in that while the success rate is claimed to be about 90 percent, the analgesic effects of acupuncture were satisfactory in 76.6 percent of these cases. Moreover, drugs such as sodium phenobarbital, meperidine, and haloperidol were administered preoperatively as well as intraoperatively, and scalp infiltration of up to 15 ml 0.1 percent procaine was used when indicated. These findings question the efficacy of acupuncture except perhaps in selected cases.

In 1983, Zukic and Kelly[119] described a neuroleptic analgesia technique in 51 patients aged 6 to 80 years who underwent various stereotactic procedures lasting 2.5 to 4.0 hours. Fentanyl and droperidol, with supplemental local anesthesia at the pin sites, were used. They "did not follow any dosage schedule or miligram per kilogram curves but titrated these agents to patient response, until an optimum level of sedation and analgesia was achieved, while preserving the ability of the patient to communicate verbally in a qualitative manner.'' They considered this technique to ''give consistent results and [to be] a very safe and reliable alternative to general anesthesia or other techniques of intravenous sedation''—if administered and monitored properly!

Between July 1984 and July 1988, 46 stereotactic ventrolateral thalamotomies were performed under sedation at the Mayo Clinic and 8 adrenal medullary transplants under general anesthesia.[96,100]

Between July 1987 and June 1988, 10 patients with Parkinson's disease underwent stereotactic placement of autologous adrenal medulla in the basal ganglia at our Medical Center.[118] The anesthetic management consisted ''of three separate phases: 1) local standby for the CT determination of targets, 2) general anesthesia for adrenal harvesting, and 3) repositioning and 'lighter' general anesthesia for the stereotactic grafting.''

In the classic book, *Modern Stereotactic Neurosurgery,* edited by L. Dade Lunsford, which was published in 1988,[77] Bullard and Nashold reported on a study involving 14 patients with posttraumatic movement disorders. They preferred local anesthesia and, when sedation was absolutely right, used a short-acting narcotic sedative compound such as fentanyl before the head was shaved, marked, and anesthetized (with 1 percent lidocaine infiltration).

Apuzzo and Fredricks[69] performed more than 600 procedures up to 1981 using the Brown-Roberts-Wells system to evaluate and manage mass lesions and used local infiltration with sedation as indicated.

In 1989, a report appeared on the use of alfentanil in lieu of fentanyl or sufentanil with droperidol and 50 percent nitrous oxide in oxygen for resection of epileptogenic foci for awake craniotomy in four cases.[115]

In 1990, Janczur and Stewart[93] described their technique, ''a continuous infusion of alfentanil supplemented by 1.26–2.50 mg droperidol and 1–2 mg midazolam for approximately 20 patients undergoing stereotactic brain biopsy.''

That same year, Allan et al.[68] published their findings in which they compared two sedation techniques for neuroradiology; one group of 25 patients received fentanyl and midazolam while the other group of 25 patients was given fentanyl and a two-stage infusion of propofol in a subanesthetic dose. They reported ''little difference in quality of sedation with either technique, but there is a surprising degree of hypoxia if supplementary oxygen is not used.'' Their means of PaO_2 were lower (70 mmHg without oxygen) in contrast to those reported by Varassi and Panella[110] (95.3 mmHg, with patients breathing spontaneously on room air and who received only IV propofol). Of 48 patients, only ''two patients made involuntary

movements and showed muscular hypertonus at induction,'' and they felt that ''the doses used were just sufficient to keep the patients asleep and permit the test to be performed in a technically perfect manner and without any risk to the patient.''

Although the mean doses of propofol and the mean times for awakening in these two reported studies are about the same, all the patients appear to have been heavily sedated; in fact, ''bidirectional verbal contact was not usually maintained'' in the study of Allan et al.[68]

In 1991, Bone and Bristow[73] reported their ''total intravenous anesthetic'' technique on 16 patients undergoing stereotactic surgery for biopsies, implants, and excision. Preoperative medication consisted of oral diazepam 0.2 mg/kg 90 minutes before lidocaine 1 mg/kg and fentanyl 2 μg/kg IV, and then an induction dose of propofol over 30 seconds. Failure to respond to verbal communication was accepted as loss of consciousness, at which time vecuronium 0.1 mg/kg IV was administered. Endotracheal intubation was performed and maintenance of anesthesia was with propofol via an infusion pump. The three-step infusion of Roberts et al.[101] was used initially (but without nitrous oxide), which was later adjusted to clinical depth of anesthesia. ''Muscle relaxation was achieved with an infusion of vecuronium,'' being adjusted so that ''only the first twitch from a train-of-four stimulus was noted.''[73] Regardless of the fact that these patients were intubated (a possible necessity) and that the initial anesthetic technique appears to be somewhat by rote (this chapter's authors' sentiments), they felt that ''this technique was associated with stable hemodynamic conditions'' and that it provided ''good operative conditions for stereotactic surgery.''

That same year, a randomized, double-blind study (the first to our knowledge) was conducted by Gignac et al.[87] on 30 patients presenting for awake craniotomy for seizures. ''The effectiveness of sufentanil (S) and alfentanil (A) to fentanyl (F) in providing analgesia with minimal side effects'' was compared. The authors found that drugs ''S, F, and A given as a bolus followed by an infusion are equally effective in providing patient comfort and good surgical conditions without any difference in the incidence of side effects.''

PROCEDURAL GUIDELINES

The anesthetic requirements for stereotactic neurosurgical procedures are different from those normally encountered in the general practice of anesthesia. They are even more restrictive than the maintenance of "a perfect airway, adequate ventilation, low venous pressure, a slack brain, minimal bleeding, the absence of coughing or straining and a rapid return to consciousness,"[81] as summarized by Bozza Marrubini.[74] The requirements of the operation and the characteristics (physical, physiopathological, and psychological) of the patient subjected to it oftimes determine the anesthetic technique.[74]

Stereotactic procedures afford the neurosurgeon the opportunity to reach previously inaccessible brain regions with relative safety and great precision. As the indications proliferate, patient characteristics become more diverse and the technique of conscious sedation more complex. Current stereotactic procedures include biopsy, aspiration, implantation, radiosurgery, and functional neurosurgery.

Logistic Considerations

Stereotactic procedures entail certain logistical considerations that impact on anesthetic delivery and maintenance. The stereotactic base ring is affixed to the skull in a position above or in front of the nose, where it obstructs access to the mouth with a laryngoscope. Extending the head for visualization of the vocal cords is difficult with the base ring in place and impossible once the head is fixed to the modified Mayfield head rest apparatus used in our institution. Accordingly, if possible, the base ring of the frame should be applied so as not to impede rapid access to the airway in the event of an emergency.

Positioning the Patient

Application of the base ring is done with the patient in the sitting position. This permits access to the head from all sides and enables multiple observers to verify simultaneously the accurate placement and angulation of the ring. The sedated patient may have decreased head control and neck muscle tone—it is thus essential that at least one assistant hold and steady the head in an erect position. This assistant's touch also reassures the patient during the injection and infiltration of local anaesthetics prior to the application of the base ring pins.

Protecting the Neck

The vertebral column is vulnerable in patients with decreased control and tone. With a bulky base ring the unsupported neck is liable to twist or acutely flex, especially on moving between the OR table and transport gurney or in going from a supine to an erect position or vice versa. Minimization of such movements is an obvious means of avoiding such injuries. The guiding and controlling hand of an ever-present assistant on the base ring cannot be overemphasized. In the event that a stereotactic procedure is performed under general anesthesia, attention to neck control is even more vital. Any untoward or suspicious movement of the head with respect to the body can result in a spinal injury in an essentially "unexaminable" patient. A high index of suspicion is imperative. The C-spine should be promptly evaluated either by plain film or by computed tomography (CT) "scout" at the time that this study is obtained in the course of a stereotactic procedure. If possible, it is desirable for a fully conscious sedated patient to participate in all transfers. OR and CT capabilities are variable, but most institutions where stereotactic procedures are performed still require at least one transport for the patient.

Transportation

Transportation requires placing the patient in a supine position. In patients with underlying respiratory compromise this position in the context of sedation may result in hypoventilation. Portable electroencephalographic (ECG) and oximetry monitors should, under optimal conditions, accompany the patient during transport; their accurate functioning should be reverified before moving the patient from the OR.

All drugs and equipment necessary for cardiopulmonary resuscitation should be transported with the patient. This includes laryngoscope, endotracheal tube, and an anesthesia reservoir breathing bag (e.g., Ambu-type). Both the anesthesiologist and the surgeon need to be vigilant for any indication of respiratory decompensation or mental status deterioration during transport.

Pharmacologic Agents

The drugs used by the anesthesiologist may result in adverse effects, the more common ones being respiratory depression, nausea, vomiting, oversedation, and hypermotility.

Pharmacologic agents for conscious sedation anesthesia in stereotactic procedures are generally diluted to enable more precise titration to desired effect, and the use of tuberculin syringes is recommended. Narcotics, benzodiazepines, and butyrophenones are most frequently used, although no dose combinations can be categorically prescribed. The anesthesiologist must use drugs with which he/she is familiar to achieve the above-stated desired effects in the patient with a given personality profile. Edelman et al.[85] believe nitrous oxide can be safe to use for the majority of neurosurgical procedures. They stated that it should not, however, be used in the following situations:

> 1) patients with increased ICP [intracranial pressure], unless there is concurrent administration of cerebral vasoconstrictors or hyperventilation; 2) patients who will be exposed to periods or regions of cerebral ischemia; 3) immediately before dural closure and for the remainder of intracranial procedures in the head-up position; and 4) during and immediately following episodes of VAE [venous air embolism].

Use of Monitors

Routine monitoring for stereotactic procedures includes "pulse oximetry, ECG, blood pressure cuff, precordial or esophageal stethoscope and temperature probe."[100] Equipment to monitor these parameters should also accompany the patient during any transport and while imaging is being undertaken.

In the CT or magnetic resonance (MR) scanner anesthesiologists find themselves in the suboptimal position of being separated from the patient during the time required for image acquisition. Distances from console room to scanner gantry vary, but usually are greater than 20 feet. A further hazard is that the patient's head is inaccessible once within the CT or MR scanner ring. Several seconds are required to move the gantry mechanically or to slide the patient manually. The monitors must, therefore, be continuously and carefully scrutinized for any sign of change from baseline. At this most vulnerable stage, verbal encouragement to remain still is preferable to further doses of sedative medication since "verbal contact with the patient remains the experienced anesthesiologist's best and most precise form of surveillance."[109]

In the scanner metallic and electronic components may interfere with monitoring devices. This consideration may be decisive in the determination of a particular patient's eligibility for stereotactic surgery or may preclude MRI, which may force recourse to CT imaging. In fact, a recent report from the Mayo Clinic indicated the need for the careful selection and testing of monitoring equipment when 1.5-tesla scanners are used.[94] A significant measurement error in the accuracy of pressure transducers when inside an MRI magnet has been described, with the means to overcome such errors "by placing the transducer away from the center of the magnet and/or by re-zeroing the transducer in its final scan position."[90] A pneumatic pulse monitor for use during MRI that is noninvasive, battery-operated, and without detectable effect on MRI quality has been developed for remote 7.5 m (25 feet) electronic monitoring of the pulse.[112]

Quiet in the Operating Room

New alarm standards in comparing "Patterson sounds" for use on medical equipment in Europe have been proposed, but Weinger[114] believes that establishment "of strict alarm standards . . . may be undesirable at this time because to do so may stifle innovation in alarm technology," and that "the use of Patterson alarms in individual (non-integrated) devices will certainly worsen existing problems of noise and stress in the OR environment."

Trop,[109] who employed exclusively conscious-sedation analgesia (CSA) in approximately 1,400 patients who underwent operations for seizures at the Montreal Neurological Hospital since 1963, emphasized that "quiet in the operating room is a prerequisite for all well-conducted CSA techniques" but that it did "not imply absolute silence but referred to the character and amplitude of the background noise level." He further stated that "controversial or disquieting conversation among [operating personnel] can severely distress the patient, resulting in such an intense anxiety reaction that additional anesthesia may seem to be the only method for control." He also remarked, however, that "additional anesthesia may result in apnea, loss of reflexes and all the attendant problems." Over 120 years ago, William Ferguson, Water's predecessor at King's College Hospital in London, "embarrassed onlookers at operations by observing total silence. This practice bears emulation today."[113]

The present authors concur with the above and believe that "canned, environmental, globally penetrating noise fills no human need" in the OR, especially when broadcasts of news and advertisements are intermingled with music that may not cater to every taste simultaneously and may constitute a dangerous distraction for the team.[97]

Postoperative Care

Postoperative care is required not only for postanesthesia recovery but also for patients who (1) may have received heavy sedation, (2) had neurological compromise preoperatively, or (3) have lesions in dangerous locations associated with mass effect and/ or increased intracranial pressure. Such patients are best observed in a monitored intensive care setting.

Stereotactic procedures involve different degrees of stimulation, discomfort, and need for patient cooperation; the anesthesiologist must know the timing of each surgical step with its attendant demands and stresses on the patient so that sedation can be adjusted accordingly.

COMPLICATIONS

Complications and their management are summarized in Table 16-9.

Respiratory Problems

A first case of respiratory distress associated with stereotactic irrigation of a craniopharyngioma cyst has been recently published,[111] although pulmonary edema has been previously reported following rupture of an intracranial aneurysm.[117] There are several other potential complications in whose management the anesthesiologist should have an important, if not primary, role. These would include hiccups, which

can also interfere with diagnostic studies and therapeutic interventions.

Of interest is the report by Bannon[72] in which "smelling salts" under the nose of a 2-year-old child undergoing radiation treatment for cerebellar neuroblastoma was successful within one respiratory cycle. Subsequently he "used this technique on several other patients, either awake or sedated with 100% success and no adverse effects."

Allergy

Allergy to latex may result in anaphylactic shock during dental work, barium enema, or surgery, and the incidence may be expected to increase with the more frequent use of gloves because of concern with AIDS. Natural latex products are widely used and include not only surgical gloves, but also breathing bags, compressive bandages, catheters, condoms, balloons, etc.[88] If the history of rubber allergy is in doubt, it has been recommended that specific skin tests be performed.[78]

Allergy to contrast dye manifesting by a cutaneous reaction and itching is another complication, which may be managed with nothing more than timely antihistamine administration. More fulminant reactions

Table 16-9. Complications and Management

Complication	Clinical Picture	Management	Avoidance
Dye allergy	Mild 　Cutaneous rash 　Itch Severe 　Respiratory distress 　Hypotension 　Shock	Mild 　Antihistamine 　Reassurance Severe 　Intubation 　CPR	Obtain history of past allergic 　reactions Antihistamine ⎫ 　　　　　　⎬ preoperative Steroid　　 ⎭
Seizure	Spectrum from focal motor to tonic 　clonic	Medical 　Check anticonvulsant/ 　　electrolyte levels 　Bolus anticonvulsant 　Benzodiazepine for immediate control Procedural 　Reschedule procedure 　Remove ring 　Remove intracranial instruments	Check preoperative anticonvulsants and electrolytes
Respiratory arrest	Hypoxia Absence of spontaneous respirations	Remove base ring Intubate (hyperventilate, mechanical ventilation as necessary)	Avoid oversedation 　Vigilant observation of pulse 　oximeter and CO_2 monitor
Oversedation	Decreased responsiveness Shallow respirations	Reversal narcotics Postoperative ICU Intubation/mechanical ventilation if necessary	Maintain verbal interaction with 　patient Dilution and careful titration to 　effect

with respiratory distress, hypotension, or shock may require intubation and full cardiopulmonary resuscitation (CPR). While exceedingly rare, such a complication occurring with a base ring and localizer frame in place on a patient whose head is deep in an MR scanner can be potentially catastrophic and requires continuous attention to monitors on the part of an ever-vigilant anesthesiologist.

Seizures

Seizures occur in patients undergoing stereotactic procedures intra- or postoperatively as a consequence of their intracranial pathology, due to metabolic disturbances or subtherapeutic anticonvulsant levels and, infrequently, as a result of the surgical manipulation itself. The well-prepared anesthesiologist safeguards the patient against this complication by review of blood chemistry and anticonvulsant levels preoperatively. In the event of an intraoperative seizure, immediate airway control must be secured; any intracranial instruments and the base ring must be rapidly removed in anticipation of possible endotracheal intubation and mechanical ventilation. Medication to abort ongoing epileptic activity should be administered.

"Stat" electrolytes and anticonvulsant levels should be sent before administration of a bolus of anticonvulsant medication. Once seizure activity has stopped, the patient's mental status must be assessed and if intubation has not been performed, it may be deferred if the patient is fully awake and alert with only a localized Todd's paralysis. In general, the procedure should be terminated and rescheduled for another day for any but the mildest focal seizure unless failure to perform such procedure at the current time would jeopardize the patient's life or eventual neurological recovery.

Oversedation

Oversedation is a sometimes unavoidable anesthetic complication. Its avoidance requires good knowledge of the patient's personality and expectations. Dilution of administered agents and careful monitoring of effect help prevent oversedation.

Not infrequently oversedation in a patient with marginally elevated intracranial pressure and depressed alertness results in hypoventilation with consequent hypercarbia, cerebrospinal fluid (CSF) acidosis, vasodilatation, and further increased intracranial pressure. Over several hours, postoperatively initially awake patients may progress to drowsiness,

obtundation, lethargy, stupor, and coma. If elevated intracranial pressure is associated with herniation or compromise of cerebral perfusion, oversedation may result in irreversible cerebral damage. Thus, whenever oversedation is suspected in patients with increased ICP, postoperative observation is prudent if not mandatory. Reversal of the opiate component of sedating medications is accelerated by naloxone; the other classes of medications cannot be readily reversed. Intubation with mechanical ventilation may be necessary if sedation results in airway obstruction or ventilatory compromise.

"Difficult" Patients

Problems presented by "difficult" patients are presented in Table 16-10.

Agitated Patients

Special anesthetic consideration must be given to certain patients. Among these "difficult" patients are those who for psychological or neurological reasons are agitated. Agitation can be anticipated following the preoperative visit. Sedation can usually overcome anxiety and agitation, but resort to general anesthesia may be required in the event that the patient is moving about too unpredictably to ensure safety, especially during potentially dangerous interventions such as insertion of the base ring pins, drilling through the calvarium, and passage of an intracranial cannula.

Obesity and Other Anatomical Variants

Obesity and certain other variations of thoracic anatomy predispose to respiratory decompensation, which can be exacerbated by sedation. These particularities of body habitus in addition to any other medical problems should be fully queried, investigated, documented, and addressed with appropriate diagnostic and therapeutic action at the time of the preoperative visit.

Increased Intracranial Pressure

Patients with increased intracranial pressure present another anesthetic problem. Intraoperative reduction of pressure in a nonintubated patient may require diuresis; thus consideration should be given to placement of a Foley catheter at the outset before administration of mannitol and/or furosemide. Patients with significant increased intracranial pressure are candidates for stereotaxis under general anesthe-

Table 16-10. Difficult Patients

Patient Type	Associated Complication	Management	Avoidance
Obese	Ventilatory and respiratory compromise	Reverse sedation Airway control Possible intubation	Preoperative examination Pulmonary function test ⎤ Arterial blood gas ⎬ preoperative Pulmonary consult ⎦
Increased intracranial pressure Mass lesion	Obtundation Herniation	Intubation/hyperventilation Diuresis	Intubate preoperatively General endotracheal anesthesia Foley catheter Diuresis early in procedure
Agitated	Displacement of ring Movement of target Compromise of safety	Increase sedation Possible intubation and general anesthesia	Quiet in OR Reassurance Intubate preoperatively (general anesthesia)
Children	Overdosage	Reversal (if possible) Airway control (possible intubation)	Titrate medication according to body weight
	Excess movement	Increase sedation Possible intubation	General endotracheal anesthesia

sia, especially if they are obtunded or stuporous prior to arrival at the OR. An appreciation for the patient's intracranial pathology is essential for delivery of appropriate anesthesia. The location of a mass lesion may mitigate against sedation in favor of general anesthesia. In processes associated with increased intracranial pressure, oversedation and hypoventilation must be scrupulously avoided. Although an embolism is rare in stereotactic surgery, the use of a Doppler precordial monitor and an atrial catheter should be considered.

Children

Children who undergo stereotactic procedures require special attention to dosing. Accurate body weight must be obtained preoperatively, although dosage adjustment is not limited to body weight alone. Most children under 16 cannot (whether through fear or inadequate comprehension) cooperate sufficiently to ensure their safety during a stereotactic procedure. General anesthesia will obviate much of the risk of a procedural misadventure in the pediatric age group.

Badgwell and Lerman,[71] reporting on the Annual Scientific Session of the American Academy of Pediatrics Section on Anesthesiology in 1990, mentioned "an extensive review of the anesthetic implications of stereotactic radiosurgery in children" by Baesik et al. from Harvard; Ferrari et al. from Cornell "presented data to indicate that ketamine maintains cardiac contractility during induction and maintenance of anesthesia in Adriamycin-exposed patients, whereas thiopental does not."

Remote anesthesia and monitoring of 12 children aged 1 to 5 years who underwent over 100 radiotherapeutic procedures under general anesthesia was reported in 1970 without any anesthetic complications. Visual observation was maintained either through leaded glass or via closed circuit TV, and the monitoring system "provided both visual and auditory contact with the patient, his respirations, and his pulse."[86]

An oxygen analyzer was not attached at induction of anesthesia in a healthy 4-year old boy in order to gain the child's confidence. Cyanosis resulted in 2 minutes, with improvement with 100 percent oxygen. Examination later revealed a loose oxygen flow tube with gas escaping from the top and hence selective delivery of nitrous oxide.[116]

CONCLUSIONS

Anesthetic objectives in stereotactic surgery are that the patient be comfortable (but not oversedated), with adequate pain control while retaining the conscious ability to communicate and cooperate, and with adequate motor strength and control to move from table to gurney and maintain a sitting position.

Attainment of these anesthetic goals requires, in addition to careful administration and titration of pharmacologic agents, an accurate appraisal and appreciation of the individual patient's personality profile and expectations. The preoperative visit is of paramount importance in gaining insight into the patient's psychology. Cognizant of the patient's emotional, cultural, educational, and socioeconomic background, the anesthesiologist can more effectively titrate medications to effect.

Despite remarkable advances in both basic and applied neuroscience over the past 30 years, the conclusion reached in 1965, that "there is no one ideal method for the administration of anesthesia to patients with movement disorder" and that "each case required individualization with regard to surgical requirements and the skill and judgement of the anesthesiologist" remains unchanged today with respect to anesthesia for stereotactic neurosurgery.[106]

Special Considerations in Point Stereotactic Procedures

Lawrence S. Chin
Chi-Shing Zee
Michael L.J. Apuzzo

Point access imaging-directed stereotaxy has entered as a primary component of the general neurological surgery armamentarium during the past decade. This methodology has been fueled by the need for tissue assay based on abnormal imaging disclosure and safe, reliable conduit entry and placement in fluid collections at a multitude of basal and intracerebral sites.

A number of mechanical systems have evolved that offer components capable of stereotactic intracranial point access based on imaging. Principles described later in this section are specifically related to the Brown-Roberts-Wells (Radionics, Inc., Burlington, MA) and Cosman-Roberts-Wells systems (Radionics, Inc.) but are relevant to all imaging stereotactic procedures for which point access is required. Comments are based on over 3,500 stereotactic procedures performed at our hospitals over the past decade. During this period, techniques for complication, avoidance, and management were based upon the rudimentary principles that follow.[120,121,125]

COMPLICATION LITERATURE REVIEW (BIOPSY)

With proper consideration and experience, modern image-directed stereotactic biopsy is one of the safest procedures performed by neurosurgeons today. The greatest risk to the patient lies at the site of biopsy, with hemorrhage being the most hazardous complication. The most common scenario in which this occurs is during the biopsy of an unexpected vascular lesion such as a cavernous angioma or a highly vascular tumor. This danger is further compounded by the closed nature of the procedure, preventing direct visual inspection of the bleeding area. Adequate preoperative evaluation to exclude a vascular lesion is the best method to avoid this complication. A magnetic resonance image (MRI) is critical in assessing the potential for a vascular component to the lesion.

Cavernous angiomas have a mixture of high- and low-intensity regions on T_1-weighted images and are often surrounded by a rim of low intensity corresponding to hemosiderin-filled macrophages. A suspected cavernous angioma should not be biopsied. Arteriovenous malformations and aneurysms will present as low intensity on T_1 and T_2, corresponding to a "flow-void" signal. Certain metastatic tumors can be highly vascular: melanoma, choriocarcinoma, and renal cell carcinoma. A thorough metastatic workup in patients with risk factors for neoplasms elsewhere and patients with multiple enhancing lesions at the gray-white interface is mandated.

Other potential complications include a worsening of neurological deficit from edema at the point of biopsy. The pathogenesis may be obscure but is usually related to lesion manipulation from insertion of the cannula and extraction of tissue. This is a potential problem in firm lesions where pressure to surrounding brain may be transferred during lesion penetration or other biopsy manipulations. Alternatively, injury to cortical draining veins during insertion of the biopsy cannula may result in local edema. Multiple passes of the probe to obtain specimens should be avoided in order to minimize iatrogenic trauma to the lesion or surrounding target area. Intraoperative or postoperative seizures are likely due to cortical injury at the site of cannula entry, transit, or focal manipulations. Hemorrhage and edema may also exacerbate an underlying seizure disorder. Therapeutic levels of an appropriate anticonvulsant should be ensured prior to the biopsy, and cortical suppressants should be delivered intravenously during surgery. Infections may arise anywhere along the transit line of the biopsy but are quite rare. We do not routinely use antibiotic prophylaxis in our biopsy procedures.

Table 16-11 lists 12 large published series of stereotactic biopsy using computed tomography (CT) or MRI[122–124,126,127,133–140] A variety of stereotactic systems and biopsy techniques are represented. A total of 2,941 cases were reported. In addition, an unpublished series of biopsies from our institution will be presented in a later section.

Table 16-11. Complications and Mortality Rates Reported in Stereotactic Biopsy Series

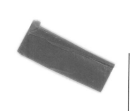

Author	No. of Cases	Hemorrhage Symptomatic	Hemorrhage Asymptomatic	Deficit without Hemorrhage	Seizures	Infection	Misc.	Morbidity	Mortality
Kelly, 1991[133]	547	5 (0.9%)	—	5 (0.9%)	6 (1.1%)	—	—	16 (2.9%)	2 (0.3%)
Blauuw and Braakman, 1988[123]	243	3 (1.2%)	—	1 (0.4%)	6 (2.5%)	—	—	10 (4.1%)	1 (0.4%)
Lunsford, 1988[136]	240	5 (2%)	3 (1.3%)	—	—	2 (0.8%)	1 (0.4%)	11 (4.6%)	0
Niizuma et al., 1988[137]	121	—	5 (4.1%)	3 (2.5%)	—	—	1 (0.8%)	8 (6.6%)	0
Apuzzo et al., 1987[122]	500	2 (0.4%)	—	1 (0.2%)	1 (0.2%)	1 (0.2%)	—	5 (1%)	1 (0.2%)
Levin, 1985[134]	88	1 (1.1%)	3 (3.4%)	—	—	—	—	4 (4.5%)	0
Scerrati and Rossi, 1984[139]	68	2 (2.9%)	—	—	—	—	—	2 (2.9%)	1 (1.5%)
Sedan et al., 1984[140]	318	11 (3.5%)	—	—	—	2 (0.6%)	2 (0.6%)	15 (4.7%)	2 (0.6%)
Lobato et al., 1982[135]	109	1 (0.9%)	—	—	—	—	—	1 (0.9%)	0
Edner, 1981[126]	345	5 (1.4%)	—	5 (1.4%)	—	—	—	10 (2.9%)	3 (0.9%)
Bosch, 1980[124]	60	—	—	—	—	—	—	0	2 (3.3%)
Ostertag et al., 1980	302	9 (2.9%)	—	1 (0.3%)	—	—	—	10 (3.3%)	7 (2.3%)
Total	2941	44 (1.5%)	11 (0.4%)	16 (0.5%)	13 (0.4%)	5 (0.2%)	4 (0.1%)	92 (3.1%)	19 (0.6%)

The most common complication was symptomatic hemorrhage as characterized by a hematoma seen on CT scan and a new or exacerbation of an existing deficit. This was seen in 1.5 percent of total cases (range, 0 to 3.5 percent). The hematoma generally was found intracerebral, but (rarely) subdural or epidural hematomas have resulted. The most common deficit was hemiparesis or hemiplegia. Asymptomatic hemorrhages were much less commonly reported and occurred in only 0.4 percent (range, 0 to 4.1 percent) of the total cases. Neurological deficit without hemorrhage usually correlated with increased edema near the site of the lesion, causing mass effect. This complication was seen in 0.5 percent (range, 0 to 2.5 percent). Seizures were a complication in 0.4 percent and infection was reported in only 0.2 percent. The cases involving infection consisted of two superficial wound infections, one infected bone flap, and two bouts of meningitis. The four miscellaneous complications (0.1 percent) included a case of wound seroma and one report of tumor tracking along the biopsy track. The other two complications were not specified. The total morbidity was 3.1 percent.

Mortality following stereotactic biopsy was a rare occurrence. Of 2,941 cases, only 19 deaths were reported, for an incidence of 0.6 percent (range, 0 to 3.3 percent). Overwhelmingly, the most common cause was hemorrhage.

Most of the world's literature concerning stereotactic biopsy is focused on the supratentorial space. Posterior fossa stereotaxis, however, has achieved greater popularity with the advent of modern imaging. Table 16-12 summarizes data from 6 series of posterior fossa stereotactic biopsy of lesions primarily in the brainstem.[127–132] A total of 143 cases are represented. Forty-one were performed from the suboccipital approach, either transtentorial or infratentorial, and 102 were performed from the coronal region. This technique requires passing the probe down the long axis of the brainstem. The total morbidity was 10.5 percent (range, 0 to 21 percent). A difference in morbidity between the coronal approach versus the suboccipital approach was not discernible. Deficits manifested as cranial nerve palsies and motor weakness. There were five cases of hydrocephalus reported by Frank et al.,[127] which were presumably due to obstruction of cerebrospinal fluid (CSF) outlet flow by small hemorrhages in the fourth ventricle. There was one mortality involving the biopsy of a pontine telangiectasia. The overall mortality rate was 0.7 percent. Biopsy in the infratentorial space appears to be slightly more risky than in the supratentorial region, as evidenced by the morbidity rates (3.1 vs. 10.5 percent). The close proximity of cranial nerve nuclei and long tracts to other critical areas such as the respiratory centers make the posterior fossa less forgiving to postbiopsy hemorrhage or edema. Approach to lesions in the posterior fossa must be undertaken very carefully.

SURGEON PREPARATION

To ensure avoidance of either a complication or an unsatisfactory result, surgeons must ensure that they, along with members of the stereotactic team, are prepared for the procedure and informed related to the specifics of the individual undertaking. Imaging, nursing, and pathology personnel should understand all elements of their role in relation to the procedure in both a general and specific sense. For biopsy procedures, an *experienced pathologist* who is confident in appraisal of small tissue specimens and skilled in neuropathology is essential and a primary component of the team in *real time,* not on a later consultation basis. Biopsy procedures are dynamic events that require interplay between surgeon and pathologist for optimization of outcome. At times a specialized neuropathologist becomes an essential part of the equation.

The surgeon should have *complete contemporary* imaging appraisal of the case in question with magnetic resonance detail in three planes with and without contrast. A recent CT scan is important if images for targeting are based on CT technology. These should be reviewed with a competent radiologist and concepts of entry, target, and transit established.

The complexity of the *instrumentation* applicable for the procedure should be reviewed and checked for operation prior to the procedure.

Table 16-12. Complications in Posterior Fossa Biopsy

Author	No. of Cases	Morbidity	Mortality
Guthrie et al., 1989[131]	4	0	0
Giunta et al., 1989[130]	35	4 (8.6%)	0
Frank et al., 1988[127]	33	7 (21%)	1 (3%)
Franzini et al., 1988[127]	45	2 (4.4%)	0
Hood et al., 1986[132]	14	1 (7%)	0
Galanda et al., 1984[129]	12	0	0
Total	143	15 (10.5%)	1 (0.7%)

THE PROCEDURE

In approaching the procedure, an attitude of *attention to detail* and *moderation of pace* is essential for optimization of outcome with minimization of complete avoidance of complication. Events in each setting are controlled and directed with *concentration*. Compromise and distraction will set the stage for problems.

Applications of the Base Ring

The base ring application is optimally undertaken in the operating room with a full head shave, which affords a complete view of the cranium for pin placement and relation of pin and platform site to images. If required, intravenous contrast is administered prior to operating room entry with a second unit administered with base ring application if necessary.

Anesthesia and sedation is administered by the attendant *neuroanesthesiologist*. In our experience, general anesthesia is rarely required in any point stereotactic procedure performed on an adult.

The ring, posts, and pins are checked for proper operation, and the skull is prepared with the patient on the operating room table in a sitting position. Two nurses assist in this stage with the anesthesiologist maintaining proper head and ring alignment. The ring and pins are brought into proper alignment with the cranium, and placement sites are marked with a pen. Three milliliters of local anesthetic (0.5 percent lidocaine with 1 : 200,000 epinephrine) are injected at each site with care taken to ensure pericraneal and soft tissue infiltrations. The pins are then fixed at the site and hand tightened to ensure fixation. Care should be taken that rostral migration of the ring does not occur. An error of the neophyte is to apply the ring too close to the vertex, a placement that allows

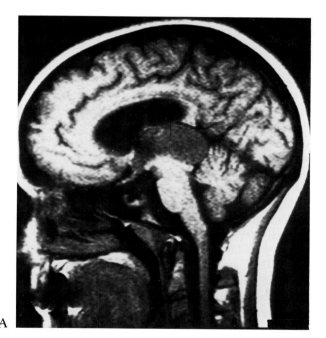

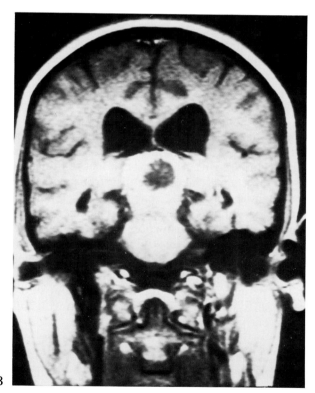

A   B

Figure 16-24. Pineal lesion. **(A)** T_1 sagittal unenhanced MRI shows a mass in the pineal region with extension into the third ventricle and compression of the tectum. **(B)** T_1 MRI with gadolinium in coronal view showing enhancement of lesion. Ring placement should be relatively high or needs to be very low to avoid artifact from the pins. Entry can be a standard twist drill craniostomy in the right parietal area, and the target should be the lateral enhancing portion with a secondary target planned in the center of the lesion. The tentorium and great vein must be avoided.

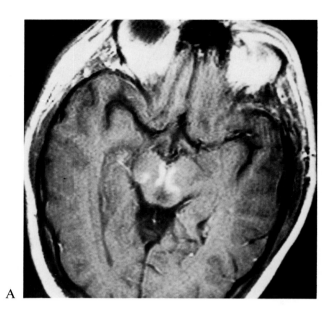
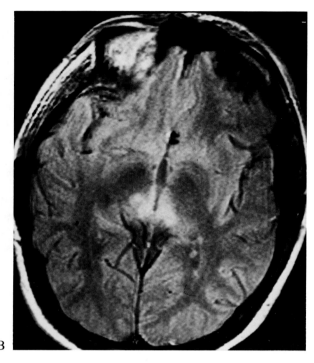

A   B

Figure 16-25. Midbrain-pulvinar lesion. **(A)** T_1 with contrast MRI in axial cut showing irregular enhancement of midbrain. **(B)** T_1 MRI in same sequence; one cut cephalad reveals extension of the lesion into posterior thalamus. This lesion should not be planned as a brainstem biopsy via pericoronal approach. Instead, a posterior pass to the pulvinar region is the safest and most direct method. The lateral enhancing edge should be targeted and care taken to avoid the ventricular surface.

migration of pins or torsion distortion of the base with fixation of the ring in the final position prior to drilling and transit. This creates offset of transit lines to the target, which could be disastrous as the target is shifted in stereotactic space.

Care is required to avoid ring placement that will provide artifactual distortion on targeting images. This may be avoided by studying MR images in multiple planes (especially sagittal) and then relating calvarial contour, target, and pin position.

The patient is transferred to the imaging suite for target selection and transit determination with appropriate entry.

Entry Point, Target, and Transit Determinations

In the imaging suite, the localizer system is fixed to the base ring with care taken to ensure proper fixation. After transfer to the couch, image acquisition is facilitated by fixation of the ring to the couch. A scalp mark or two may be placed for approximate entry markers. In general, the anterior two-thirds of the cerebrum, centrum, and brainstem may be acquired

through pericoronal entry. Posterior third cerebral, pineal region, and temporal targets are approached via superior parietal-occipital entry (Fig. 16-24). Slice optimization is individualized, but 5-mm slices taken through the entry marker and parallel to the base ring are usually optimal. Softwear included in the scanner console assists with finalization of entry, target, and transit line to the target as the three are optimized according to neurosurgical principles.

For optimization of outcome and biopsy, the process of *target selection* is key. It is our practice to attempt to target enhancing areas well within a lesion. This at times requires double-dose contrast with a delay of 30 to 60 minutes after administration. Obviously, critical and subcortical targeting carries increased risk because of vascularity and should be avoided if possible. Biopsy from ventricular or cyst walls adjacent to a fluid volume increases the risk of hemorrhage as tamponade and chemical factors are not operant protectors (Fig. 16-25). Biopsy adjacent to poles, particularly frontally and temporally, pose increased risk and should be avoided. *Sylvian and peri-insular regions are dangerous* (Fig. 16-26).

Entry points then determine the line of transit to

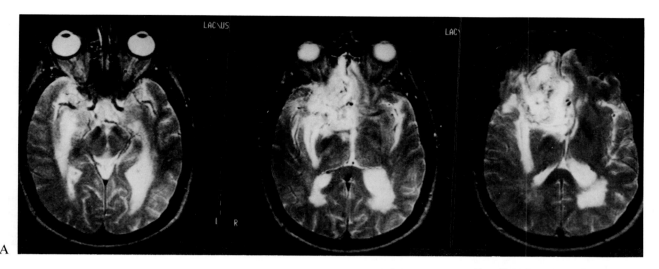

Figure 16-26. Right frontotemporal lesion. **(A)** Axial T_2 MRIs reveal a large lesion in the frontal pole and temporal tip with uncinate fasciculus tracking through the sylvian region and insula. **(B)** Sagittal T_1 MRI with gadolinium demonstrates frontal extent of lesion. Ring placement must not be too low for this lesion as pin artifact will interfere with targeting. The sylvian and insular regions are areas of hazard for passage or biopsy. A precoronal entry is planned with the target being midanterior and medial. The medial aspect of the frontal pole is preferable because tethering by the corpus callosum affords less motion, thus minimizing the chances of brain torsion and disruption of bridging veins.

the target point, and are best selected in a physiological "silent" area (Fig. 16-27). Transits should avoid ependymal penetration if possible, as risk is increased. In general, transit to target is an inocuous event if a 13-gauge blunt cannula is employed. Regions of concern include the cortical surface and brain-lesion interface (Fig. 16-28). Alternate entry and transit lines should be designated with console software to achieve optimum tailoring of the procedure to the individual needs.

The method of cranial perforation is as important as selection of the site of entry. If possible, a transit perpendicular to the dural surface should be achieved. Drilling on a curved or angulated surface is potentially problematical. We prefer to use a quarter-inch *twist drill* for entry. This requires a tight or minimal subdural-subarachnoid compartment. With atrophy this is often generous. With all factors considered, it is at times important to select a *burr hole*

methodology to avert the potential subdural hematoma that may evolve secondary to a lack of tamponade effect (in minor venous injury during transit) (Fig. 16-29). This is assessed on preprocedure coronal and sagittal images as well as the targeting images.

Data Process and Instrumentation Check

Following standard data process with target determination in stereotactic space, all instrumentation, function, length, and settings are checked meticulously on the extracranial phantom base target representation of the individual case. Each setting is checked by the surgeon and the cosurgeon in repetitive order.

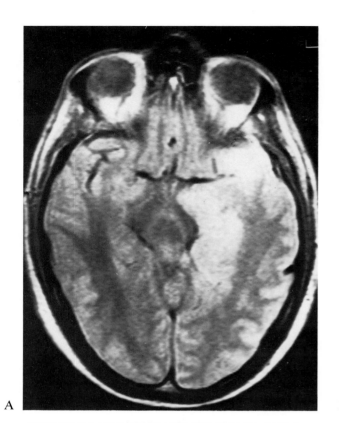

A

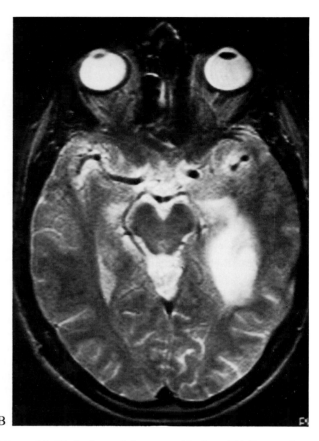

B

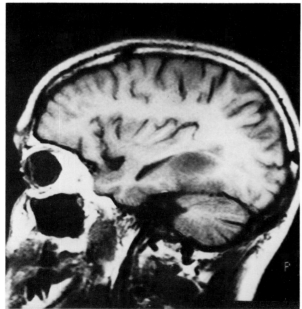

C

Figure 16-27. Left mesial temporal lesion. **(A)** Proton density axial MRI showing increased signal intensity in left uncus and parahippocampal gyrus. There is slight mass effect on the midbrain and swelling of the left temporal lobe. **(B)** T_2 axial MRI confirms the abnormality in the uncus and also white matter edema in the left temporal lobe. **(C)** Sagittal T_1 MRI illustrates low signal intensity in the left posterior temporal lobe with elevation of the temporal horn. The lateral orthogonal approach to a temporal lobe mass is problematic for several reasons. It requires traversing the temporalis muscle, which can result in bleeding and can deflect the transit of the probe. Placement of the base ring may need to be altered for a true lateral entry. Insertion of the biopsy probe into a hard lesion may cause displacement of the mesial temporal lobe, resulting in direct pressure on the brainstem and incisura. Finally, the risk of injury to the temporal lobe cortex in the dominant hemisphere is potentially devastating. A posterior approach via a twist drill is the recommended course. The planned passage is down the long axis of the temporal lobe with the entry into the cortex occurring in a relatively silent area of the occipital lobe.

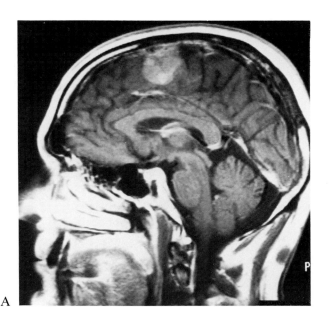

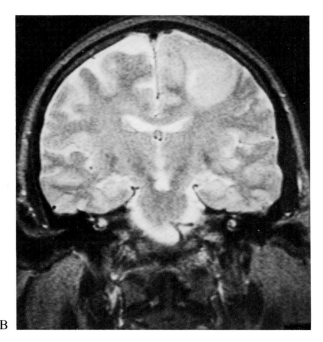

A   B

Figure 16-28. Large left frontal cortical and subcortical lesion. **(A)** T_1-enhanced sagittal MRI shows a uniformly enhancing 2.5 × 3.0 cm lesion in the posterior frontal lobe. **(B)** T_2 coronal MRI showing lesion extending up to the cortical surface with fullness of surrounding gyri and decreased subarachnoid space compared with the contralateral side. A burr hole is not necessary in this circumstance because the mass of the lesion is enough to tamponade a small amount of bleeding at the biopsy site. Also, the relative lack of subarachnoid space makes development of a subdural hematoma less likely. A twist drill placed over the lesion and a target planned in the center of the lesion are recommended.

Transcranial Access and Acquisition of Procedural End Points

The base ring is fixed to the table by a Mayfield adaptor unit. It is important to set table flexion and back elevation prior to final fixation of the ring-table interface as distortion may occur with alteration of body position after the head is fixed. It has been our practice to determine the head and nose positions visually in relation to the ring from a vertex view in the scanner and to ensure that such relation is absolutely maintained as the final preoperative position is fixed.

After local infiltration of the entry region, the arc system is brought into the field and securely fixed. In the event that a twist drill entry is utilized, a 7-mm incision is made and squared at each limit with pericranial transection completed. *Guide tubes* in line of transit are employed. *Stops* are essential and are used once the tip is set at the pericranial level to approximate calvarial thickness, which is estimated

for images. An effort is made to achieve a clean and precise intercalvarial table perforation with minimal dural peripheral pocketing. The difficulty of this is increased in the event that drilling is done on a cranial slope. In elderly patients, dural perforation may occur with drilling. A precise dural perforation is then accomplished with a sharp probe that has a 1-cm stop applied. These maneuvers make the occurrence of epidural hematoma rare. The 13-gauge cannula is passed to the target without delay and the scalp entry sealed with a cottonoid.

Cortical or dural venous hemorrhage may occasionally be present as the sharp probe is removed. The tamponade of the cannula placement controls this problem satisfactorily. Should unusual bleeding be encountered, a burr hole may be placed for greater superficial exposure to attain hemostasis. This is a rare evolution; however, burr instrumentation bipolar forceps and headlights are available and are part of our setup on each case. For biopsy, we prefer long, flexible broncoscopy cup forceps with the as-

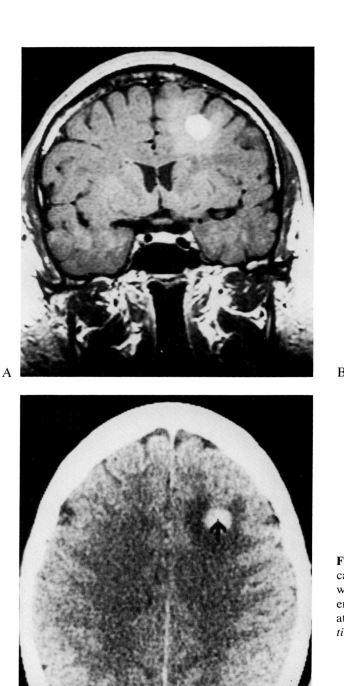

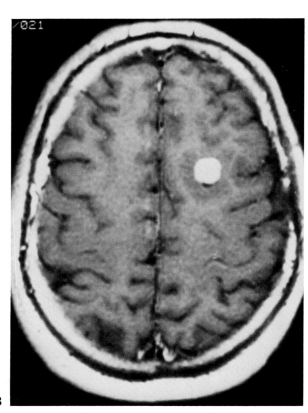

A

B

C

Figure 16-29. Mid- and posterior frontal cortical-subcortical lesion. **(A)** Round, uniformly enhancing lesion at gray-white junction in coronal view on T$_1$ MRI. **(B)** Axial T$_1$-enhanced MRI. **(C)** CT scan with contrast showing lesion at gray-white junction near the centrum. (*Figure continues.*)

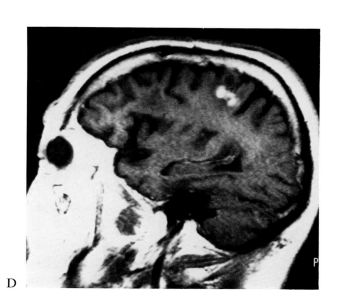

D

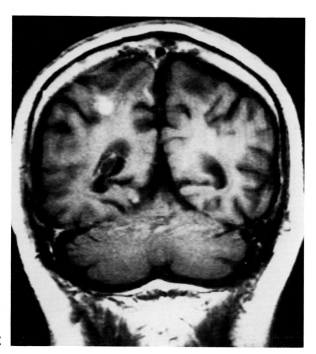

E

Figure 16-29 (*Continued*). **(D)** T$_1$ image with enhancement in sagittal cut shows a similar lesion further posterior in the motor strip. **(E)** Coronal T$_1$ MRI with enhancement. **(F)** Axial CT scan with contrast shows edema surrounding the lesion. Both lesions are located superficially in the frontal subcortical region with one well anterior to the motor strip and the second in the motor cortex. Entry for biopsy should be accomplished via a burr hole, as the superficial location carries a higher risk of significant hemorrhage from injury to a draining vein and also lacks tamponade effect should a small bleed occur within the lesion. The burr hole is planned directly over the lesion.

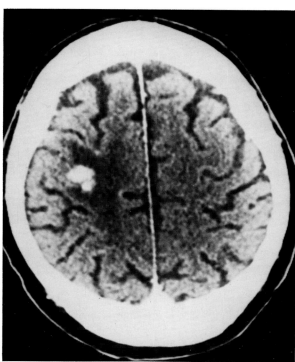

F

Table 16-13. Complications and Avoidance Measures

Complication	Avoidance
Hemorrhage	
Epidural	Ensure stop is secured on drill
	Avoid obliquely angled entry
	Perform dural penetration briskly with a 1-cm stop on a sharp probe
Subdural	Avoid cortical biopsy if possible
	Use burr hole if cortex is biopsied
	Use burr hole if subarachnoid space is generous
	Place burr hole directly over lesion for cortical biopsy
	Avoid polar targets
Intraparenchymal	Check bleeding parameters preop
	Avoid long transit lengths
	Avoid multiple passes
	Avoid sylvian and insular regions
Intraventricular or Intracavitary	Avoid biopsy of ependymal surfaces
	Avoid passage through ventricles
	Avoid cyst wall biopsy
Intralesional	Perform careful preoperative evaluation to avoid biopsy of a vascular lesion or hemorrhagic met.
	Avoid excessive biopsy manipulation or number of samples
	Avoid multiple passes
	Reinsert cannula to tamponade bleeding
Perilesional	Avoid biopsy of potentially vascular capsule or brain-lesion interface
	Biopsy center of lesion if solid
Deficit without hemorrhage	Use preoperative corticosteroids
	Ensure stability of hardware
	Employ guide tubes for all stages
	Phantom check all instrumentation
	Avoid excessive manipulation of lesion with passes or biopsy
Seizures	Check levels of preoperative seizure medications
	Avoid rolandic or perirolandic entry
Failed biopsy	Acquire preoperative laboratory data scrupulously
	Assess preoperative imaging carefully
	Use double-dose delayed contrast for faintly enhancing lesions
	Target enhancing regions
	Target multiple areas if necessary
	Avoid unenhancing, low-intensity, potentially necrotic center of lesion as sole biopsy target
	Phantom check all instrumentation
	Review all studies and suspected diagnoses with pathologist
	Do not stop procedure until pathologist feels comfortable with preliminary result
	Repeat biopsy if clinical or radiological course is atypical for pathological diagnosis on appropriate treatment
	Avoid ring migration
	Avoid ring torsion due to body position on operating table
Infection	Maintain sterile technique
	Irrigate thoroughly
	Avoid piercing air cells or sinuses with pins or twist drill
Pin artifact	Study preoperative three-view MRI to decide pin placement
	Shave entire head to study contour in relation to images
Ring movement	Shave entire head for precise pin penetration
	Avoid seating pins too close to vertex
	Avoid body or head readjustment once base ring is anchored to Mayfield adapter-table amalgam

sistant opening and closing the tip while palpation is undertaken by the operator. Side-cutting aspiration instrumentation is simply not a uniformly satisfactory mode of tissue retrieval when the spectra of lesion type and texture are considered. Forceps are fully opened at the cannula tip, slightly advanced, and then closed with palpation by the operator as the flexible barrel of the instrument is removed by the operator. Two specimens are satisfactory for information maximization in experienced hands. Hemorrhage may be apparent as the second specimen is retrieved; significant hemorrhage is rare. The cannula should be replaced and left at the site while tissue is reviewed with the pathologist. Our practice is to review all specimens with the pathologist during the procedure and to access third and fourth specimens if required. However, this is an unusual event.

Upon tissue review, the cannula is carefully withdrawn, the wound copiously irrigated with bacitracin solution, and a single monofilament suture placed.

An immediate postoperative scan is part of every procedure (Table 16-13).

MORTALITY AND COMPLICATIONS (USC)

In consideration of more than 3,500 point image-directed stereotactic procedures, *one death* occurred very early in the series. This was following biopsy of a thalamic cavernous angioma (1981) and was prior to availability of MRI. In addition, *seven hemorrhages* have occurred, which have required surgical evacuation with no adverse sequelae. These included three at the target site (two melanoma, one glioma), three acute subdural hematoma (twist drill), and one epidural hematoma (drill stop not employed). Three transient *focal seizures* have been observed with transit. Two *generalized convulsions* occurred. In all of these instances, rapid control was achieved by intravenous medications immediately administered by the neuroanesthesiologist. No adverse sequelae were noted.

Two *infections* have been observed, one case manifesting as a superficial scalp infection following a burr hole biopsy, and one as a subgaleal abscess after multiple catheter placement. In consideration of the numbers involved, the safety of these procedures (provided proper attention to detail is followed and judgment for application is used) is remarkable.

Problems Relating to Pathological Interpretation in Stereotactic Biopsy Procedures
Parakrama T. Chandrasoma

Stereotactic brain biopsy represents the ultimate in terms of efficiency in pathological diagnosis. While the initial response of the pathologist to the small size of the specimen obtained at stereotactic biopsy is one of dismay, there is a rapid realization that it is adequate for diagnosis in most cases. Specimen quality is the key rather than specimen quantity. If the pathologist is given a good specimen, there is little difficulty with histological diagnosis. This is true even when the pathologist has not had specialized training in neuropathology, an important fact if stereotactic biopsy is to be done by general neurosurgeons in community hospitals.

At the heart of this somewhat euphoric assessment of stereotactic brain biopsy and its feasibility in terms of providing tissue for pathological diagnosis is the ability of the neurosurgeon to obtain a high-quality specimen. This is the limiting step that determines the success or failure of stereotactic brain biopsy. It behooves us, therefore, to consider what represents a "good" specimen.

Modern radiological imaging techniques such as computerized tomography (CT) and magnetic resonance imaging (MRI) produce superb images of lesions of the brain. It is less certain that we understand clearly what these images really mean. Since these modalities have developed in an era when brain neoplasms are treated with surgery, radiation, and chemotherapy, we have had very little opportunity to compare the radiological images with the removed lesion in a truly meaningful way. While one does not wish for the old days when one could study at autopsy a lesion untouched by treatment, one must realize that this kind of invaluable correlative information is no longer available. Thus we compare the radiological images to small samples from the lesions and attempt to extrapolate this information to the entire image. Lesions that are studied at surgical resection are commonly piecemeal fragments that cannot be oriented in relation to the radiological images, and autopsies are limited to studying lesions that have been altered dramatically by treatment.

From the standpoint of stereotactic biopsy interpretation, a neoplastic brain lesion can be classified

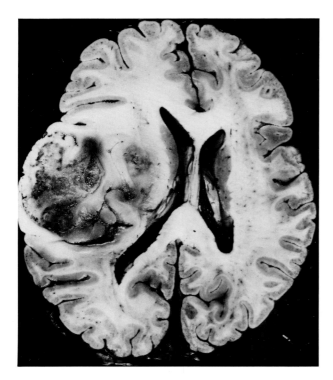

Figure 16-30. Fairly well circumscribed example of a glioblastoma multiforme. Note the presence of less involved brain elements within the confines of the mass lesion.

into the following groups: (1) encapsulated and very well-circumscribed neoplasms (Figs. 16-30 and 16-31), and (2) infiltrative neoplasms of varying degrees of malignancy (Fig. 16-32). Nonneoplastic lesions such as infarcts, demyelinating plaques, and a variety of infections may produce either localized or diffuse lesions.

In neoplastic lesions, the pathological changes involved are neoplastic cellular proliferation and the host response to the presence of the neoplasm. The following areas can be recognized within a neoplastic lesion (Fig. 16-30): (1) areas where the brain tissue has been completely replaced by neoplastic cells; (2) areas where the neoplastic cells infiltrate brain tissue; (3) areas where there are no neoplastic cells, but where there are host-reactive phenomena such as neovascularity, inflammation, reactive astrogliosis, and edema; and (4) areas of necrosis, usually in the central region of highly malignant neoplasms. These areas vary in their extent and pattern in different neoplasms. In encapsulated and well-circumscribed neoplasms, the central region is composed entirely of neoplastic cells, and the periphery composed entirely of reactive tissue without infiltrating neoplastic cells. In an infiltrative neoplasm, the lesion frequently contains areas where the neoplastic cells are admixed with reactive brain tissue. In such cases, it is important to realize that the different areas are not neatly

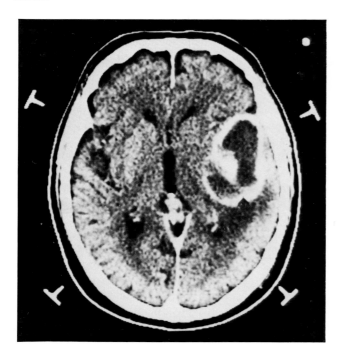

Figure 16-31. CT scan of a glioblastoma multiform comparable in appearance to the tumor shown in Fig. 16-30. Note that the radiologic image does not permit fine definition of different areas within the tumor mass.

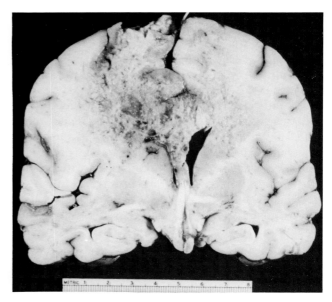

Figure 16-32. Highly infiltrative glioblastoma multiforme. The center of the mass will be composed entirely of tumor with necrosis. The peripheral infiltrative component will be an intimate mixture of neoplastic cells and reactive brain tissue.

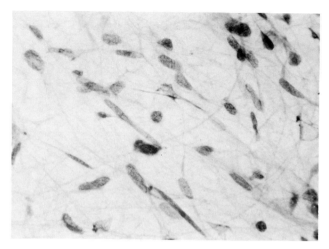

Figure 16-33. Anaplastic astrocytoma, smear. The smear is composed entirely of neoplastic astrocytes of moderately high cellularity and moderate cytologic atypia. The neuropil of normal brain is absent, the background of the smear consisting entirely of cytoplasmic processes of the neoplastic astrocytes. (Hematoxylin & eosin [H&E], × 100.)

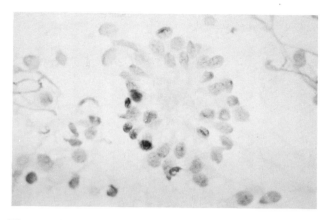

Figure 16-35. Smear of ependymoma showing the small, round ependymal cells arranged in a rosette. (H&E, × 100.)

stratified, but may be admixed with each other throughout the lesion that appears on the radiological image. In nonneoplastic lesions, the variations are even greater, and the pathognomonic changes frequently less easy to identify than neoplastic cells.

Translation of these pathological elements to the radiological image is difficult, if not impossible (Fig. 16-31). There is very little data that permits accurate correlation of radiological images with these different pathological components within a lesion. It is a mistake to look at a CT or MRI abnormality and equate all of it to neoplastic cellular proliferation. Very clearly, areas of reactive change in and around the neoplastic cells can produce abnormalities on CT and MRI.

Selection of the target for biopsy within the CT or MRI lesion is all important in providing an adequate sample.[143,161] The instrumentation for stereotactic biopsy is so accurate that the tissue is removed from, or very close to, the selected target point. The neurosurgeon must have an excellent understanding of the nature of pathological lesions when selecting the target point, if the biopsy is to have the highest likelihood of providing diagnostic tissue.

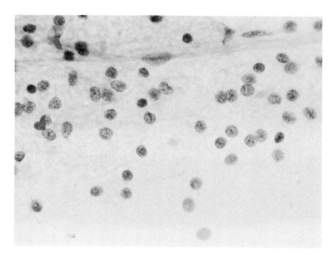

Figure 16-34. Smear of oligodendroglioma showing the uniform, round, naked nuclei in the clean background. (H&E, × 100.)

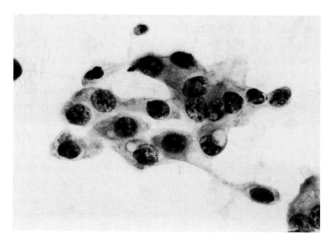

Figure 16-36. Smear of metastatic carcinoma, showing cohesive group of epithelial cells in a clean background. Note the presence of cytoplasmic vacuolation due to mucin, indicating this is an adenocarcinoma. (H&E, × 100.)

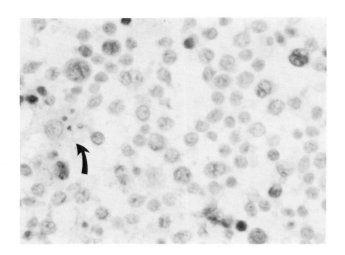

Figure 16-37. Smear of malignant lymphoma, showing dyscohesive round cells resembling transformed lymphocytes. Note the presence of the tingible body macrophage (*arrow*). (H&E, × 100.)

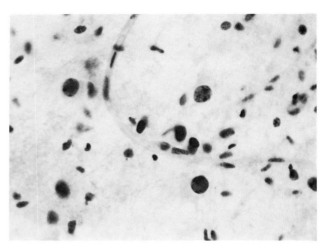

Figure 16-38. Smear of progressive multifocal leukoencephalopathy, showing enlarged glial cells with ground glass inclusions. (H&E, × 100.)

From a pathological standpoint, the ideal diagnostic tissue in a neoplastic lesion is defined as nonnecrotic cellular material from an area of the lesion where the neoplastic cells have completely replaced the brain tissue. When such tissue is examined, either by smear or frozen section, the pathologist sees only neoplastic cells, and can make an accurate diagnosis without difficulty. It is a relatively simple matter with such a specimen to differentiate between astrocytoma (Fig. 16-33), oligodendroglioma (Fig. 16-34), ependymoma (Fig. 16-35), metastatic carcinoma (Fig. 16-36), malignant lymphoma (Fig. 16-37), and virtually any other neoplasm that may be encountered. The cytological and histological features of these different neoplastic cells have been extensively described in the literature.[141,144,147,150,153,155,158]

When the specimen is from a suboptimal target point, the pathological diagnosis can be very difficult and will be associated with a significant error rate. For example, when a biopsy shows an astrocytic proliferation admixed with lymphoid cells, it is often difficult to identify which component is neoplastic and which is reactive based on the smear or frozen section. A malignant lymphoma may be associated with a florid, highly atypical astrocytic proliferation, and this may be difficult to differentiate from an anaplastic astrocytoma with a reactive lymphocytic infiltrate. Special studies such as immunological lymphoid marker studies and gene rearrangement studies can differentiate reactive from malignant lymphoid proliferation, but these are difficult to use in the setting of the small specimen size obtained at stereotac-

tic biopsy.[156] The answer in such cases is not to depend on special techniques, but to obtain a better specimen that is composed only of neoplastic cells without admixed reactive material.

In a nonneoplastic lesion, the situation is even more complex.[145] These lesions are not known to be nonneoplastic before biopsy, and exclusion of a neoplasm is frequently the major point of the biopsy. Nonneoplastic lesions are absolutely diagnostic only when an infectious agent is identified (Figs. 16-38 and 16-39). When an infectious agent is not found, all that

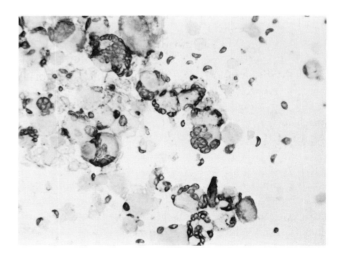

Figure 16-39. Smear stained by immunoperoxidase technique using antibody directed against *Toxoplasma gondii*. Note the presence of numerous crescent-shaped trophozoites, both in and outside cells. (H&E, × 160.)

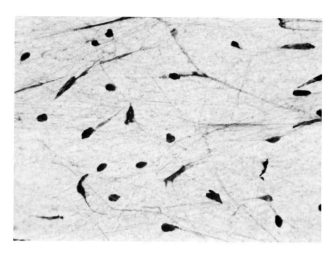

Figure 16-40. Smear of well-differentiated astrocytoma of cerebral hemisphere, showing neoplastic astrocytes of low cellularity and mild cytological atypia. The background shows the processes of the neoplastic astrocytes. Differentiation of this smear from reactive gliosis requires clinical and radiologic correlation. (H&E, × 100.)

is present in the biopsy is reactive tissue. It is difficult in such cases to make specific diagnoses, or even decide whether the host reaction is against an infectious agent or a neoplasm that is not represented in the biopsy. These biopsies provide the greatest degree of difficulty in terms of pathological diagnosis.

While target point selection is the step that limits the accuracy of the stereotactic brain biopsy, it is also the step for which there is least guidance for the neurosurgeons. The absence of correlative information between radiological images and pathological elements in the lesion makes target point selection an inherently inaccurate process. It has been my experience that pathological interpretation is easy when the neurosurgeon is experienced, somewhat compulsive about details, and understands the pathology of brain lesions. However, even with care and experience, the biopsy does not always produce diagnostic tissue, and both neurosurgeon and pathologist must be aware of this if error is to be avoided.

Let us examine critically the broad principles that govern target point selection by the neurosurgeon. In a large, low-density, homogeneous, nonenhancing CT lesion that has a high likelihood of being a well-differentiated astrocytoma, the target is in the central part of the lesion. A biopsy from such a target is likely to be from an area composed of well-differentiated neoplastic astrocytic cells that have replaced the normal brain tissue. Smear and frozen section of such a specimen show neoplastic astrocytes that show low cellularity, mild nuclear abnormalities, and

prominent cytoplasmic processes. The finely granular eosinophilic background that characterizes normal brain is lost, and the background contains only the cytoplasmic fibers of the neoplastic astrocytes (Fig. 16-40). The smear is superior to frozen section in this neoplasm because it permits more accurate evaluation of the background. The peripheral area of well-differentiated astrocytoma consists of normal brain infiltrated by the neoplastic cells. Biopsies from this infiltrative zone of a well-differentiated astrocytoma are very difficult to differentiate from reactive gliosis. Open biopsies of these lesions commonly provide tissue from the peripheral infiltrating edge, and are much more difficult for the pathologist than stereotactic biopsies.

In anaplastic astrocytomas, the CT appearance is usually more circumscribed with contrast enhancement due to the neovascularity that is common in these neoplasms. The lesion may also be heterogeneous on imaging, with areas of low density within the enhancing zone. Areas of low density may represent necrotic tissue, poorly vascularized neoplasm, or areas of less involved brain. CT scans and MRIs cannot reliably differentiate anaplastic astrocytoma from glioblastoma multiforme, other malignant neoplasms, and even some nonneoplastic lesions.[161] It is the general rule in these lesions to target an enhancing area within the CT lesion. It is our experience also that this area provides the highest frequency of diagnostic tissue. The danger of finding only necrotic tissue in the central nonenhancing zone makes this area less desirable for biopsy. When the tissue is composed of neoplastic cells alone, or when an infectious agent is identified, the diagnosis is easy. When an admixture of pathological processes is present, there may be great difficulty and significant danger of error. In such cases, diagnosis may be easy when the neoplastic cells are easily recognizable such as in metastatic carcinoma, melanoma, and highly anaplastic astrocytoma. On the other hand, in lower grade gliomas and lymphomas, differentiating neoplastic and reactive glial and lymphoid cells can be very difficult. Additional material is crucial in these difficult cases. Since the problem here is not so much with accurate tissue procurement from the target, but with inherent variability of the pathology at the target point, it is usually adequate to obtain a second sample by slightly (0.5 to 1 cm) adjusting the biopsy site. Retargeting for a second biopsy is rarely necessary in our experience.

The mortality in our series of over 3,000 stereotactic biopsies has been limited to one death. This occurred early in our series and was due to a massive hemorrhage from a lesion that at autopsy was found to be a cryptic vascular malformation.[142] The morbidity has been similarly very low (seven clinically significant hemorrhages). With this background, it is reasonable to suggest that our technique provides results that will be difficult to improve in terms of safety. We use one target point and obtain tissue using a biopsy forceps that has either a 1 or 2 mm cup. The average specimen consists of two to three tissue fragments. A second sample obtained by slightly adjusting the needle is required in about 10 percent of cases. It is extremely rare that a second target point be biopsied. The level of accuracy that we have achieved with this protocol has been in the 95 percent range recorded in the literature for neoplastic lesions.[151,152,154,157,160] We have had a lower rate of success with identifying a specific etiology in nonneoplastic lesions.

Different centers have different protocols for stereotactic biopsy in terms of type of biopsy apparatus, number of specimens taken, and number of target point biopsied.[151,152,154,157] Most authorities that use a side-cutting needle (providing a 1- to 2-cm core of tissue) believe this is safer than a biopsy forceps because the latter requires a pulling action that theoretically increases the risk of vascular injury. We have found this not to be true. However, we have no strong reasons not to use the side-cutting needle as long as an equivalent safety record can be demonstrated in the long term. Certainly the amount of tissue is greater, and while this is probably not essential for diagnostic accuracy, it provides tissue for research and special studies that may be beneficial. Having demonstrated that two to three pieces of tissue from one target point achieves the objective of accurate pathological diagnosis at a rate equivalent to any other, we find it difficult to justify biopsy of multiple target points, because of a theoretical risk of increasing morbidity and mortality. Again, it is impossible to argue against this practice without data proving there is an increased risk associated with multiple biopsies. It may be true that multiple biopsies are indicated in those lesions in which a pathological diagnosis is not readily apparent on smear or frozen section of the first sample.

Stereotactic biopsy has obvious limitations of sampling that must be addressed if its use is to be justified in clinical diagnosis of neoplasms. For this consideration, neoplasms can be divided into two types: (1) regionally homogeneous neoplasms such as metastatic carcinoma, craniopharyngioma, malignant lymphoma, meningioma, oligodendroglioma, primitive neuroectodermal tumor etc., and (2) regionally heterogeneous neoplasms such as astrocytomas[146,149] and pineal germ cell tumors.[159] In regionally homogeneous neoplasms, the identification of the neoplastic type in a biopsy provides a diagnosis that can be accurately extrapolated to the entire neoplasm. In regionally heterogeneous neoplasms, one area of the neoplasm may be significantly different from another, so that extrapolation is not justified.

Pineal germ cell neoplasms may have mixed elements that include teratoma, germinoma, embryonal carcinoma, yolk sac carcinoma, and choriocarcinoma.[159] A biopsy may show only one of these elements and therefore be inadequate. There are two ways to overcome this problem: (1) to take multiple biopsies with its potential risks in these neoplasms, which may be highly vascular; and (2) to use a combination of radiology, histopathology, and tumor markers for diagnosis. We utilize the second option. If a pineal neoplasm is solid, negative for α-fetoprotein and chorionic gonadotropin, and the smear shows germinoma, a diagnosis of pure germinoma is rendered. If it has cystic areas, is marker negative, and has histological features of teratoma, we diagnose it as a pure teratoma. If serum or cerebrospinal fluid α-fetoprotein or chorionic gonadotropin levels are elevated, we diagnose a yolk sac or choriocarcinoma element in it. If the histology shows a different component, a diagnosis of mixed germ cell tumor is made. In this way, we reach clinically relevant accuracy with a single biopsy.

Astrocytomas are regionally heterogeneous in that different areas within a given malignant astrocytoma will show different histological grades. If biopsy of an astrocytoma results in significant undergrading, this may impact significantly on management and prognosis. To evaluate the risk of undergrading, we compared stereotactic biopsies with the resected specimens of astrocytic neoplasms.[148] This showed that there was a tendency to undergrade glioblastoma multiforme at stereotactic biopsy. This was due to the fact that target selection actively attempted to avoid necrotic areas, and necrosis was a prerequisite in our system of classifying an astrocytoma as a glioblastoma multiforme. The only other discrepancy that we found was an oligodendroglial admixture in two cases of well-differentiated astrocytomas. We consider these two errors small enough that they did not adversely affect clinical management. As such, we concluded that stereotactic biopsy using a single target point provided valid pathological diagnoses in astrocytic neoplasms. Again, the question of increasing risk by obtaining multiple biopsy samples must be balanced against the value of more accurate histological grading. The individual neurosurgeon and pathologist can develop their technique in a manner that best suits their needs.

In conclusion, stereotaxy has provided the neurosurgeon with a superb tool to obtain tissue samples from lesions virtually anywhere in the brain. The instrumentation is so good that a biopsy can be taken almost exactly from a predetermined target point in a lesion imaged by CT or MRI. Unfortunately, the selection of the target point that will provide the most diagnostic tissue is still an art rather than a decision based on scientific fact. The general rules for target selection are accurate in most cases, but when the pathologist experiences diagnostic difficulty, the neurosurgeon-pathologist team must recognize that the most common reason for this is that the selected target, although in the lesion, is from an area that does not provide a diagnostic specimen. How the team handles these difficult cases will determine their overall accuracy and satisfaction with the procedure.

Craniotomy

Internal Decompression of Intra-axial Supratentorial Tumors (Malignant Supratentorial Gliomas and Metastatic Tumors)

Ivan S. Ciric
David Weinsweig

The surgical treatment of malignant supratentorial gliomas is still somewhat controversial. The preponderance of literature on the subject over the past 25 years, however, favors radical resection of malignant supratentorial gliomas. There is abundant evidence in the literature[163,167–169,171,173,174,177,179–182,186,187] that the length and quality of survival are directly proportional to the extent of the resection. Even more importantly, the literature shows clearly that the residual postoperative tumor burden adversely influences the long-term outcome.[164,178,179,188] Naturally, the enthusiasm of some authors who claim that "cerebral glioblastomas can be cured"[166] should be tempered with the reality that malignant supratentorial gliomas must be considered incurable regardless of the treatment modality used. To be sure, long-term high-quality survivals after radical resection of malignant supratentorial gliomas including glioblastoma multiforme are possible and have been reported in the literature.[163] Indeed, radical resection has also been advocated in a select group of patients with recurrent malignant supratentorial gliomas as being associated with longer and better quality survivals.[162,172,184] In contrast, only a few reports in the literature refute that the extent of surgery is a positive prognostic factor for the length and quality of survival, claiming that biopsy alone and radiation therapy are associated with equally good results.[170] While we firmly believe that there is a definite positive relationship between the extent of the surgical resection and the outcome in terms of length and quality of survival, a randomized prospective study would be necessary to make this conviction an unequivocal certainty.[183]

GENERAL CONCEPTS

Serial stereotactic biopsies of malignant supratentorial gliomas have shown that there are three zones of tumor that can be correlated with computed tomography (CT) and magnetic resonance imaging (MRI). The CT scan-enhanced area (solid or ring enhancement) and the T_1-weighted images of the tumor on the infused MRI represent the central core of the tumor comprised of pure tumor cell population.[176] The low attenuation area surrounding the CT scan-enhanced area and the high-intensity signal abnormality on the T_2-weighted MRI images, which surround the central core of the tumor, represent infiltrating tumor in the surrounding edematous brain. Indeed, tumor cells have been found even beyond the abnormality demonstrated by the T_2-weighted images of MRI. This anatomical constellation of malignant supratentorial gliomas has been confirmed by us during microsurgical operations for removal of these tumors.

A malignant supratentorial glioma can present on the cortical surface or it can be totally submerged

Table 16-14. Correlation of CT and MRI Characteristics of Malignant Supratentorial Gliomas with Histology and Surgical Indications

Imaging Diagnosis	Surgical Anatomy/Histology	Surgical Correlate
CT scan, enhanced area MRI T_1 with gadolinium	Macroscopic tumor Pure tumor cell population (and necrosis)	Resectable
CT scan, low density MRI T_2	Edematous brain-infiltrating tumor	Not resectable Biopsy recommended
"Normal" CT (beyond "edema") and MRI	Normal-appearing brain, ± infiltrating tumor	No surgical considerations

below the cortex. It has been our experience that gliomas presenting on the cortical surface have often involved a single gyrus, resulting in a marked gyrus distension and thus giving the impression of a more extensive involvement. The confinement of a glioma to a distended gyrus also continues along the banks of the gyrus, with a clear cleavage plane between it and the adjacent sulcus. At the bottom of the sulcus, the glioma merges with and expands into the subcortical white matter. Within the white matter itself, however, most of the gliomas continue to have a macroscopic boundary except in the depth, where they may blend imperceptibly with the subependymal white matter. Thus, most malignant supratentorial gliomas have a macroscopic boundary easily recognizable at the time of surgery along a fairly distinct cleavage plane between the tumor on one hand and the surrounding sulcal cortex and edematous white matter on the other. The discreet and well-definable tumor within the macroscopic boundary of a glioma corresponds to the CT scan-enhanced abnormality (solid or ring enhanced) and to the enhanced lesion on the gadolinium-infused T_1-weighted MRI images and is histologically represented by a pure tumor cell population (with or without necrosis). This is more true for high-grade than low-grade gliomas since the latter may not enhance. Our experience shows that a gross total removal of the CT scan-enhanced abnormality or of the enhanced lesion on the gadolinium-infused T_1-weighted MRI images, representing the macroscopic part of a malignant supratentorial glioma, is associated with low morbidity of less than 5 percent and longer and better quality survivals.[163,167] In contrast, a mere debulking of the macroscopic part of the tumor (subtotal removal) is associated with a 10-fold increase in morbidity.[167] A gross total removal indicates absence of any demonstrable postoperative enhancement on the CT scan or on the MRI, attributable to residual tumor tissue. Thus, the goal of an operative procedure designed to remove a malignant supratentorial glioma is to perform a gross

total removal of the macroscopic part of the tumor as represented by the CT scan-enhanced area or gadolinium-infused T_1-weighted MRI images. The lower attenuation area on the CT scan and the high-intensity signal abnormality seen on the T_2-weighted MRI images represent areas of tumor infiltration into the surrounding brain in conjunction with edema. This area must not be resected in eloquent regions of the brain while it can be incorporated into a greater resection in terms of a lobectomy in noneloquent regions. Table 16-14 correlates the CT and MRI imaging characteristics of malignant supratentorial gliomas with histology and surgical indications.

INSTRUMENTATION

Vision magnification facilitates removal of a supratentorial glioma. In our practice, the operating microscope is used routinely in all glioma surgery. In contrast to the loupes, the operating microscope provides a much needed stereoscopic perception of the tumor at all depths of the operative site; it facilitates the recognition of the cleavage plane between the tumor and the often distended, thinned-out cortex of the neighboring gyrus, as well as the interface between the tumor and the underlying edematous white matter. The operating microscope will also facilitate detection of small, but critically important arterial blood vessels, thereby preventing their injury in areas such as the medial temporal lobe, the banks of the sylvian fissure, the central and precentral sulcus, the calcarine fissure, etc. Finally, the operating microscope provides for a more precise, targeted hemostasis at both the arterial and venous level.

Self-retaining retractors, microsurgical instruments, an appropriate selection of microsuction tips, and bipolar coagulation are an essential part of the armamentarium necessary to remove a supratentorial glioma. Bipolar coagulating units and forceps with

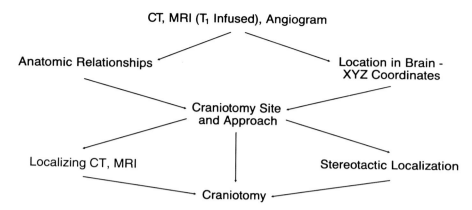

Figure 16-41. Preoperative strategy algorithm for supratentorial craniotomy for intra-axial lesions.

nonadhering tips and of different lengths and sizes are necessary.

Stereotactic approach to deep-seated malignant supratentorial gliomas, be it for purposes of biopsy,[165,170,185] or as an integral part of the surgical technique of their resection,[175,177] has been well established and is presently frequently used in a variety of ways by a number of neurosurgeons. We use CT- and MRI-assisted stereotactic guidance to all deep-seated tumors routinely. Thus, the majority of these patients are operated upon in the stereotactic frame.

SURGICAL TECHNIQUE

Patient position, selection and planning of the scalp-skull flap, localizing techniques, and general principles of a supratentorial craniotomy including complications and their management were described in detail in Chapter 4 (Fig. 16-41).

If the dura is tight due to raised intracranial tension, the head of the operating table should be raised in relationship to the feet (reversed Trendelenburg position), hyperventilation should be instituted so as to lower the PCO_2 into the 20 to 22 mmHg range (occasionally lower), and a rapid infusion of an osmotic diuretic can also be given. These measures usually suffice to lower the intracranial tension within a matter of minutes. The dura can then be opened safely. If an intra-axial cyst formation is present in conjunction with the tumor, the cyst can be cannulated via a very short dural incision. The cyst contents should be aspirated only partially, just enough to achieve relaxation of the brain, but not to empty the entire cyst, since the presence of the cyst will facilitate detection of a deep-seated tumor and make the resection easier and safer. Generally, it is preferable to reflect the dural flaps toward major venous sinuses in order not to injure bridging veins. It is

critical to preserve as many bridging cortical veins as possible. In this respect, it is imperative to preserve the bridging veins in the posterior two-thirds of the cerebral convexity and by all means the vein of Labbé draining into the lateral sinus.

TECHNIQUE OF GROSS TOTAL TUMOR REMOVAL

The first step in the removal of a supratentorial glioma presenting on the surface (Fig. 16-42) is to divide the arachnoid, which spans from the surrounding normal cortex over the tumor (Fig. 16-43). This is accomplished with the use of a nonadherent bipolar coagulating forceps and microscissors (Fig. 16-44). This maneuver brings the surgeon to the interface between the tumor and the banks of the neighboring sulcus. Utilizing brain retractors, the plane of cleavage between the tumor and the surrounding sulcus is then developed with the use of bipolar coagulating forceps and a microsuction tip (Fig. 16-45). Arterial vessels not part of the tumor surface must be preserved. Venous channels spanning the two structures should be coagulated and divided. We prefer to keep this cleavage plane open with sterile strips made of Vaseline-impregnated burn dressing (Adaptic), which does not adhere at all to the cortical surface (Fig. 16-46). Once the cortical part of the tumor has been clearly demonstrated, it may be necessary to decompress the tumor before tracing it into the subcortical white matter in order to prevent undue traction on the surrounding structures. The choice of instrument at this stage of the operation will depend on the tumor structure, consistency, and vascularity. A tumor with a necrotic, soft, relatively avascular center is ideally suited for decompression with an ultrasonic cavitating aspirator (Figs. 16-46 and 16-47). On the other hand, a tenacious, highly septate and rather

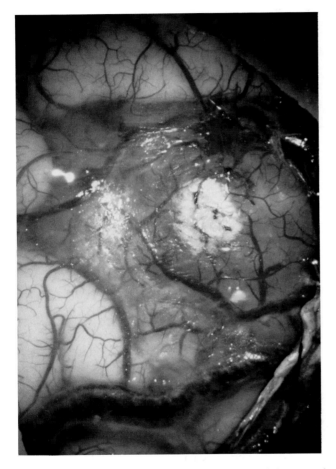

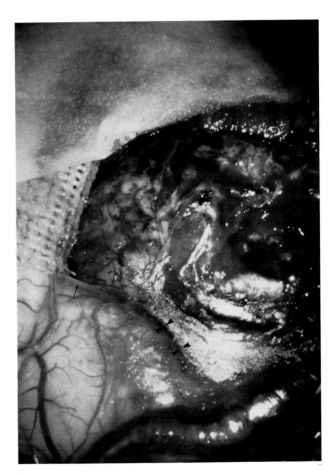

Figure 16-42. Glioblastoma multiforme in the right central region.

Figure 16-43. Arachnoid spanning between the cortex and the tumor (*arrowheads*) and partially divided (*arrow*).

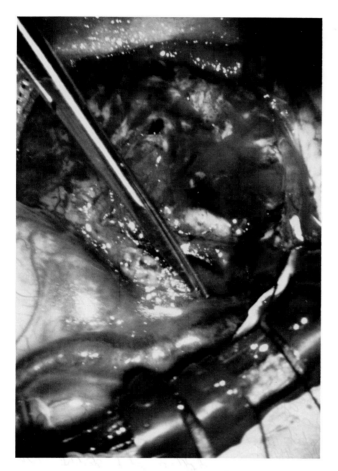

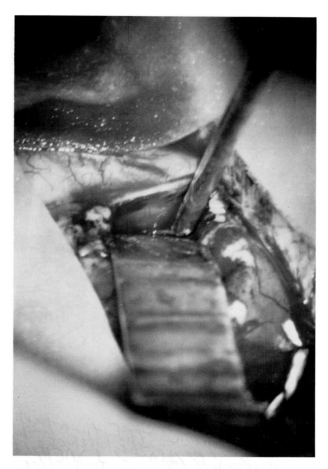

Figure 16-44. Further division of arachnoid in order to establish a plane of cleavage between the tumor and the surrounding cortex circumferentially and mobilization of a cortical vein.

Figure 16-45. Tumor-neighboring sulcal cortex interface.

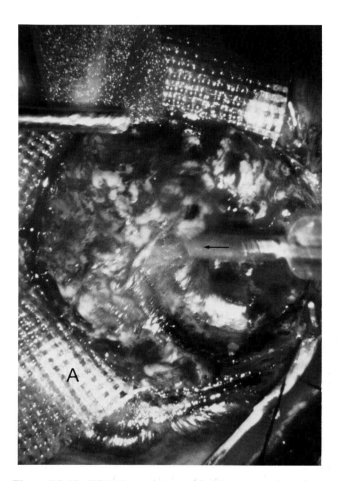

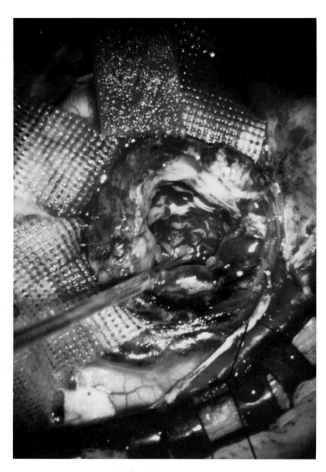

Figure 16-46. With the tumor-surrounding cortex interface circumferentially established, the tumor is decompressed utilizing either the CO_2 laser or an ultrasonic cavitating aspirator (*arrow*). Plane of cleavage between tumor and neighboring sulcal cortex kept open with strips of Adaptic (**A**).

Figure 16-47. Tumor decompression completed. This will permit further dissection along the macroscopic tumor margins without undue retraction.

vascular tumor is better decompressed using the CO_2 laser set at a defocused modality. Bipolar coagulation can also be used to segregate the tumor into segments, which can then be removed with sharp dissection. The presence of a cystic component can facilitate tumor decompression after it is aspirated. With a portion of the tumor decompressed, the surgeon will now be able to trace the macroscopic tumor along its margins in the subcortical white matter with greater ease and with less need for retraction on the surrounding structures.

At the depth of the sulcus the cortex of the gyrus will be found distended and blending imperceptibly with the underlying tumor (Fig. 16-48). This is a critical stage in the operative procedure since from this point on the surgeon will lose the relatively distinct boundaries, comfort, and protection of the neighboring sulcus and gyrus with its distinct pial surface. Before the tumor is traced into the subcortical white matter, it should be completely freed from its cortical confinements (Fig. 16-49). Exceptions to this rule would be a tumor that abuts the sylvian fissure or a tumor adjacent to eloquent areas of the brain, where it might be preferable to leave that portion of the tumor undisturbed and deal with it after the tumor has been decompressed and rolled out from its bed in less critical areas.

Magnification will allow the surgeon to find the nearly always existent plane between the macroscopic tumor boundary and the surrounding edematous white matter, which is not easily discernible to the naked eye or even to loupe magnification. The tumor surface, while at times pale and avascular, will nevertheless appear different from the surrounding stark white and avascular edematous white matter (Fig. 16-50). Presence of bleeding usually indicates that the surgeon is within the tumor. In contrast, an avascular, bloodless field indicates a proper cleavage

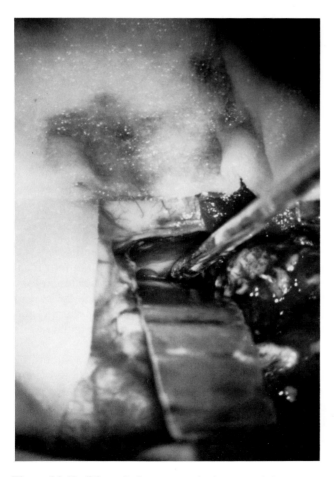

Figure 16-48. Distended cortex at the bottom of the sulcus.

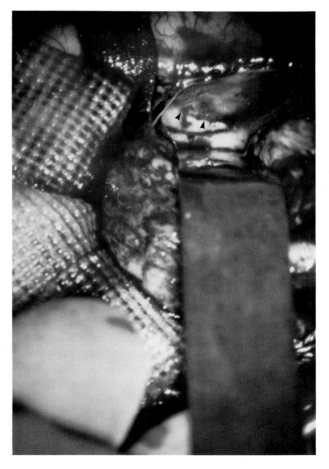

Figure 16-49. Interface between tumor (retracted) and the bottom of the sulcus-white matter junction (*arrowheads*).

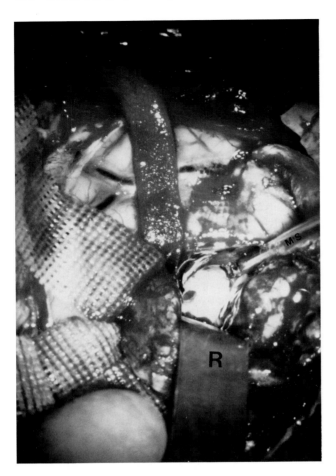

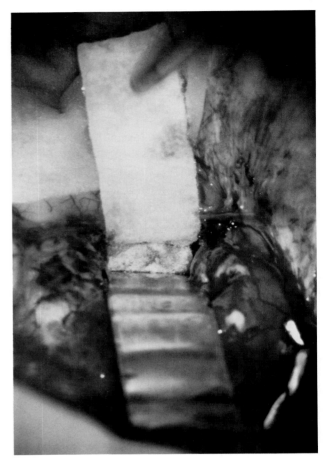

Figure 16-50. Tumor (macroscopic boundary)–white matter interface. Note that retraction is only against the decompressed tumor. Retractor (*R*) can be used as a dissector and the microsuction tip (*MS*) can be used as a retractor.

Figure 16-51. Plane of cleavage between tumor and the white matter in the depth can be kept open with moist cotton patties, which also elevate the tumor from its bed.

plane between the tumor and the edematous white matter. A tenacious cleavage plane can mean that a surgeon has wandered away from the tumor-white matter interface into the more normal white matter. More often than not, it will be necessary to alternate internal tumor decompression with dissection around the tumor surface before the entire macroscopic part of the tumor can be separated from its bed. When retraction is necessary during surgery, it should be applied principally against the tumor rather than against the surrounding brain. A retractor on the cortical and white matter surface can keep the tumor-brain interface open and should serve as a protector of the underlying brain rather than as a retractor. The established planes of separation between the tumor and the surrounding brain are kept open with strips of

Adaptic, moist Telfa cotton paddings, and moist cotton gauze (Fig. 16-51). Separation of the tumor from the surrounding white matter should be done along the opposing tumor poles, leaving for last the part of the tumor adjacent to critical areas of the brain, major vascular structures, and the ventricular walls (Figs. 16-52 and 16-53).

With the tumor resected the tumor bed should be inspected for soft clots, all of which must be meticulously removed lest there be a small artery or venule underneath that could result in a postoperative tumor bed hematoma. All such vessels must be thoroughly coagulated under vision magnification. The use of high-power magnification at this stage of the operation is very useful since it allows for precise, targeted vessel search and coagulation. The tumor bed is then

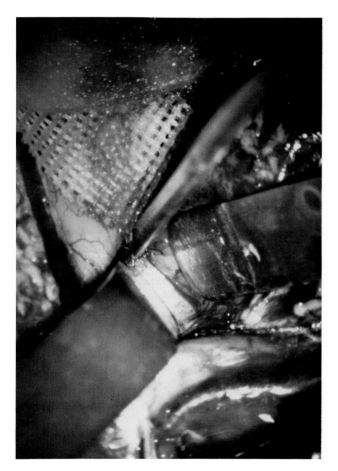

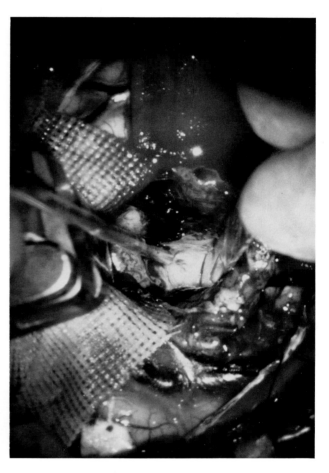

Figure 16-52. The process of tumor dissection along its macroscopic boundaries is repeated along the opposing poles of the tumor. Tumor-depth of sulcus–white matter interface.

Figure 16-53. Opposing pole, tumor depth–white matter interface.

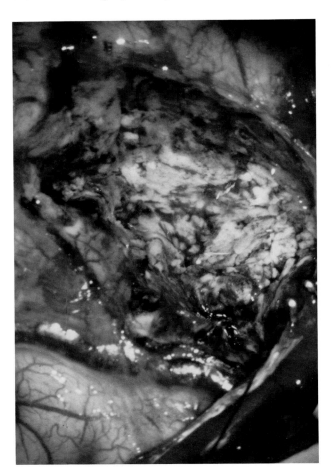

Figure 16-54. Postresection tumor bed filled with normal saline. All soft clots must be meticulously cleaned out and secure hemostasis achieved.

inspected for residual tumor tissue, again under vision magnification with the microscope, and all such residual tissue meticulously removed. Thorough, repeated irrigation of the tumor bed with normal saline at body temperature should yield a field completely free of any blood contamination even under conditions of raised intrathoracic pressure provided by the anesthesiologist (Fig. 16-54). Failure to do so can prove unforgiving in the postoperative period because of a possible tumor bed hematoma.

The technique of approach and removal of malignant supratentorial gliomas not presenting on the cortical surface will depend on their location relative to the surrounding neovascular structures (eloquent areas of the brain, arterial and venous structures, proximity to the midline or major fissures, etc.) and their depth (Figs. 16-55 to 16-57). Subcortical tumors in noneloquent areas of the brain are approached and removed in essentially the same way as are tumors presenting on the brain surface. Their exact location is easily established based on cortical landmarks and with the use of ultrasound. In eloquent areas of the brain subcortical tumors should be approached along the sulcus of the most distended gyrus, preferably farthest away (and yet as close to the tumor as possible) from the eloquent cortex. Deep-seated tumors are best localized and approached using stereotactic craniotomy techniques as described in Chapter 4 via a sulcus in the noneloquent cortex and along a white matter corridor away from important neurovascular structures. Precise localization, a sparing yet sufficient cortical incision at the depth of the sulcus, minimum retraction with self-retaining retractors, use of

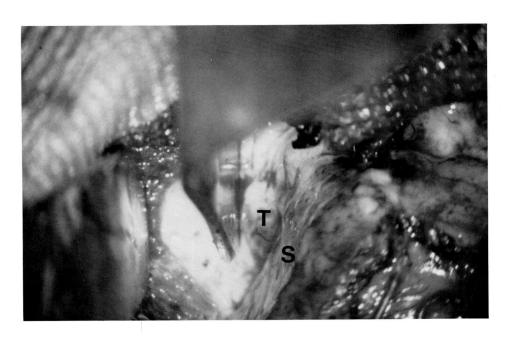

Figure 16-55. Sulcal incision in the central sulcus exposing the subcortical tumor (*T*). *S*, sulcal cortex.

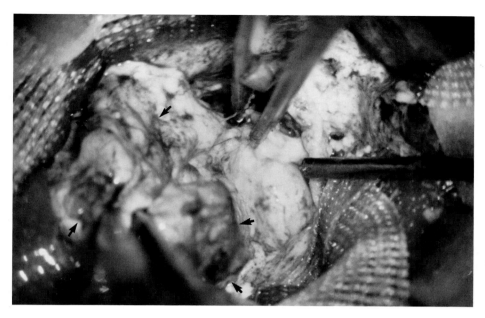

Figure 16-56. Tumor (between *short arrows*) freed from its bed utilizing bipolar coagulation.

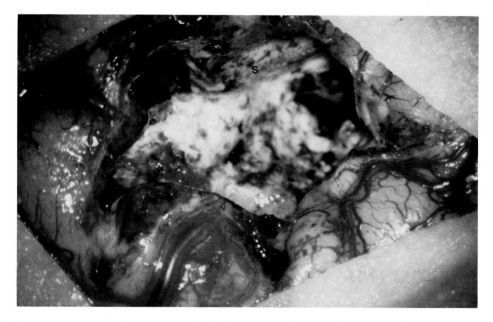

Figure 16-57. Postresection view of tumor bed. Please note intact sulcal cortex circumferentially (*S*). No cortex was resected in this case.

the operating microscope, internal decompression with the CO_2 laser, or use of an ultrasonic cavitating aspirator and meticulous hemostasis throughout the procedure are cornerstones of the surgical technique for removal of deep-seated malignant supratentorial gliomas.

CONCLUSIONS

There is ample evidence in the literature to support the contention that resection of the macroscopically definable tumor mass during operations for malignant supratentorial gliomas (gross total removal) is associated with excellent immediate postoperative results and longer and better quality survivals. The macroscopically definable tumor is represented on imaging studies by the CT scan-enhanced area and the enhancement seen on the gadolinium-infused T_1-weighted MRI images. In contrast, a mere "debulking" of the macroscopically definable tumor is associated with an unacceptable immediate postoperative morbidity that precludes any quality survival. Greater degrees of resection also encompassing the infiltrating tumor into the surrounding edematous but otherwise structurally intact brain (partial lobectomy) is acceptable and at times advisable in noneloquent areas of the brain only. Stereotactic biopsies of malignant supratentorial gliomas cannot be considered as a surgical therapy, and consequently they do not alter the dismal natural course of these lesions. The cornerstones of the surgical therapy described in this chapter consist of a precise preoperative tumor localization, meticulous surgical planning, a cortical and white matter corridor approach that does not interfere with the eloquent cortex and important vascular structures, and internal tumor decompression in large tumors, and, finally, separation of the tumor along its macroscopic borders from the neighboring cortex (in surface tumors) and the surrounding deep white matter. Stereotactic approach to deep-seated tumors, the use of the operating microscope and microsurgical techniques, and attention to detail during all phases of surgery are also essential technical standards in the surgical treatment of malignant supratentorial gliomas.

Cerebral Lobectomies
Robert E. Maxwell

Cerebral gliomas encompass a spectrum of pathology; prognostic implications are clouded by vagaries in tissue biology, the changing sensitivity of detection methodologies, and the absence of adequate data from scientifically valid, well-controlled, randomized treatment. The cornerstone of diagnosis and optimal management of cerebral gliomas rests on early tissue diagnosis by either needle aspiration or excisional biopsy. The primary goal of glioma management (having defined the size, location, and precise pathology of the neoplasm) is to perform as complete an extirpation of the lesion as possible without compromising the patient's capacity to function at a level

understood and acceptable to the patient and family. Compromises are unfortunately often necessary when the size, configuration, or location of a cerebral glioma make the goal of complete excision of the tumor with maximum tumor resection margins unattainable. The subject of this chapter is the assessment of risk and avoidance of complications in the most favorable situations, those in which tumor characteristics suggest that prolonged survival, significant palliation, alleviation of symptoms, and preservation of function can be expected and hopefully achieved by lobectomy.

PREOPERATIVE RISK MANAGEMENT

A lobectomy, when feasible, offers definite advantages over an excisional biopsy or internal decompression by tumor excision. The lower grade neoplasms favorably located in the frontal and temporal lobes are particularly amenable to this approach. Failure of the neurosurgeon to excise totally a cerebral neoplasm for which the location and characteristics of the lesion are consistent with the goal of achieving a surgical cure is a risk not to be underestimated and represents a serious complication and lost opportunity for the patient to experience a completely successful outcome. The preoperative evaluation is designed to avoid or lessen the risks of suboptimum outcome because of inadequate excision of the pathological tissue or unnecessary trauma to brain, cranial nerve, or vascular tissues important for neurological function.

Neuropsychological Testing

Pre- and postoperative neuropsychological testing is often indicated for patients undergoing lobectomy. The tests guide the surgeon in assessing and documenting cerebral dominance, preexisting deficits, and the potential for deficits resulting from the procedure. The patients and their families can be better counseled when this information is available before surgery.

The avoidance of unacceptable neurological deficits requires the surgeon to be aware of the location of the lesion and its relationship to motor, sensory, language, and memory cortex and the respective projection pathways. The cerebral hemisphere dominant for speech and memory must always be documented when a temporal lobectomy or an aggressive frontal or occipital lobectomy is being considered. There is obviously more surgical leeway in the nondominant hemisphere.

The Wada (intracarotid amobarbital injection) test is used to lateralize speech and verbal and nonverbal memory function. The medial temporal structures posterior to the amygdala should not be excised without confirming that the contralateral temporal lobe can support near term memory needs. A number of neuropsychological test batteries are available for lateralizing deficits and suggesting the location of subtle structural lesions such as mesial temporal sclerosis not always readily apparent on computed tomography (CT) scans or magnetic resonance imaging (MRI).

Visual Field Testing

Preoperative ophthalmologic assessment includes formal visual field testing on patients considered for temporal or parietooccipital lobectomy. The ventral fibers representing the ipsilateral inferior retina (contralateral superior visual field) loop forward over the inferior horn of the lateral ventricle before reaching the striate cortex beneath the calcarine fissure (Figure 16-58).

The posterior extent of temporal lobectomy determines the size of the contralateral superior quadrantic field deficit. The deficit is considered a side effect rather than a complication of temporal lobectomy, but nevertheless needs to be carefully explained to the patient and family in advance of surgery. The expected "pie in the sky" deficit resulting from a 4½ to 5-cm anterior temporal lobectomy is usually not noticable to the patient. It is prudent, however, to warn the patient and family before surgery that significant contralateral visual field loss can result from vascular injury or direct trauma to the optic tract or retrolenticular fibers of the geniculocalcarine radiation. Avoidance of this complication presents important technical consideration during temporal lobectomy. Occipital lobectomy, of course, commits the surgeon and patient to expect and accept a contralateral, congruous, homonymous hemianopsia.

Electrodiagnostic Testing

Scalp electroencephalography (EEG) is an adjunct to lateralizing and localizing hemispheral lesions. The distance of scalp electrodes from the cortex and artifacts resulting from muscle activity may result in inconclusive recordings. Interictal discharges

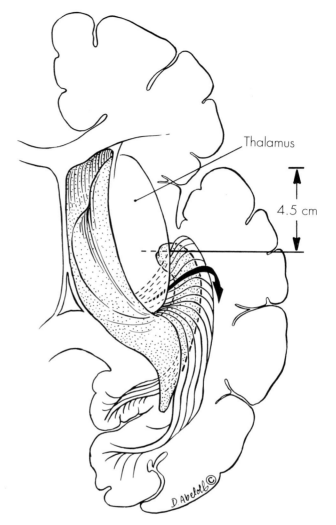

Thalamus

4.5 cm

Figure 16-58. Temporal lobectomy extending posterior to the tip of the inferior horn of the lateral ventricle interrupts the ventral loop of the geniculocalcarine radiation resulting in a contralateral superior quadrantic visual field deficit. Vascular or traumatic injury to the densely packed retrolentricular portion of the geniculocalcarine pathway causes a dense hemianopsia.

(spikes) are not as reliable as ictal discharges in defining the site of seizure origin and require converging lines of evidence derived from clinical features of the disorder, neuropsychological studies, and structural abnormalities on radiographic studies.

Invasive electrodiagnostic monitoring is usually not necessary in patients with obvious structural lesions. There are circumstances, however, in which a structural lesion is either not apparent, is located adjacent or subjacent to cerebral tissue suspected of

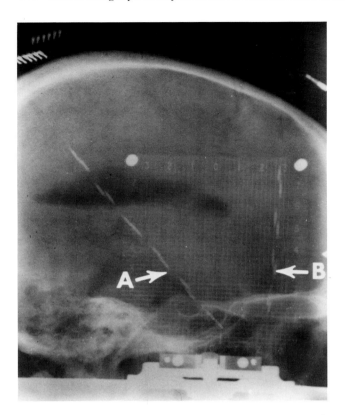

Figure 16-59. Lateral skull radiograph showing the position of depth electrodes placed stereotactically to provide electrophysiological monitoring of the basifrontal regions and the amygdala and hippocampus of both hemispheres.

serving eloquent neurological functions, or is associated with an epileptic focus that needs to be better defined or mapped before proceeding with resection. A neoplasm associated with a seizure disorder may require more than excision of the tumor if seizure control is a concomitant goal of surgical treatment.[201]

Sphenoidal electrodes are a minimally invasive technique of particular value when a temporal lobe lesion is suspected. Electrodes placed in the trigeminal cistern by means of a percutaneous transforamen ovale approach[208] or depth electrodes inserted stereotactically into the medial temporal lobe or other cerebral areas[206] may assist the surgeon in lateralizing seizure onset in difficult cases. The stereotactic placement of depth electrodes carries the immediate risk of hemorrhage and the delayed risk of infection. The risk of hemorrhage can be reduced by using a semiflexible electrode with a removable style.[197] Bilateral frontal and temporoparietal chains of electrodes with contacts equidistant at 1-cm intervals provide adequate sampling of the basifrontal regions and the amygdala and hippocampus of the temporal lobes (Fig. 16-59). The risk of infection is reduced by meticulous sterile surgical technique, by the administration of an appropriate prophylactic antibiotic while the electrodes are in place, and by limiting the duration of monitoring. Subdural strips of four to six electrodes can also be slid over the cortical surface by means of strategically placed burr holes.

When the side of cerebral involvement is known, but the precise site of the lesion or extent of the planned resection or lobectomy needs refinement,

Figure 16-60. Photograph of 8 × 8 cm subdural grid electrode array with 64 platinum alloy contact points positioned over the cortical area of interest. Precise mapping of motor, speech, and language cortex can be achieved by electrical stimulation and the recording of cortical evoked sensory responses. Spontaneous cortical ictal and interictal activity can also be captured and localized by this technique. Cables from strip electrodes placed beneath the left temporal lobe are also seen.

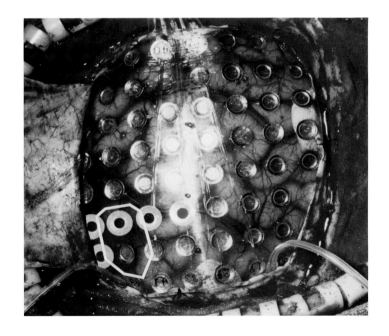

placement of a larger grid electrode array in the subdural space permits detailed mapping of ictal and interictal discharges and mapping of cortical function by electrical stimulation and elicitation of cortical evoked responses.[195] These techniques give the surgeon confidence to pursue the goal of achieving the maximum resection of neoplastic and epileptogenic tissue consistent with the preservation of important cortical functions.

Sensory, motor, and language cortex can be mapped by electrical stimulation intraoperatively under local anesthesia or by implantation of electrodes over the surface of the cerebrum for chronic monitoring and recording (Fig. 16-60). If excision of epileptogenic tissue is an important consideration, the implantation of subdural electrodes permits the capture and localization of ictal events by video EEG. Chronically implanted electrodes also provide the patient and clinicians an opportunity to carry out both cortical electrical stimulation and the recording of cortical evoked sensory responses in an unhurried and less stressful setting. Findings can also be confirmed and documented by different examiners, further reducing the risk of false localization. Platinum alloy contacts on the depth and subdural electrodes provide artifact-free MRI-compatible images useful not only to confirm electrode placement, but also to correlate electrodiagnostic findings with topographic anatomy or with any lesions seen on the MRI scan.

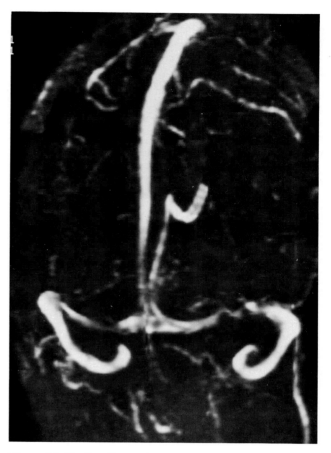

Figure 16-61. Gradient echo reconstruction of venous flow by MRI provides an effective means for assessing asymmetry of the sagittal and transverse sinuses without the risks and complications of angiography. The location of bridging cortical veins entering the sinuses can also be assessed by this technique.

Neuroradiography

MRI, particularly with gadolinium enhancement, may demonstrate lesions such as ganglioglioma, pleomorphic xanthochromic astrocytomas, hamartomas, glial ectopia, and mesial temporal sclerosis that are not readily apparent on CT scans.[198] MRI is also helpful in assessing the size of the temporal lobe and the distance of a lesion from the temporal pole. MRI spectroscopy may also be of value for assessing focal areas of altered cerebral metabolism. The risks and complications of angiography may be avoided and improved three-dimensional views of venous anatomy achieved by means of gradient echo reconstructions of venous flow on MRI (Fig. 16-61).

Positron emission tomography (PET) with the administration of metabolic tracers such as 18F-fluorodeoxyglucose, which measures cerebral glucose utilization, can demonstrate an area of hypometabolism interictally in patients in whom no lesion is apparent on CT or MRI. The same area may become hypermetabolic during seizures.[191]

Medical Management

The dose and timing of steroid administration depends on the underlying condition for which lobectomy is indicated. Conventional dosage started the night before surgery is appropriate for seizure surgery. High-dose steroid therapy may be indicated to control elevated intracranial pressure (ICP) associated with malignant edema. Dexamethasone is a potent synthetic glucocorticoid with the advantages of no sodium retention and a biological half-life up to 4 days. Symptomatic improvement and relief of elevated ICP associated with reduction in cerebral edema occurs in 3 to 6 hours. It is recommended and conventional practice to administer antacids or H-receptor antagonists to patients on steroids. Cimetidine has been associated with altered mentation in the elderly, however, and can interfere with the metabolism of anticonvulsant medication.[204]

Patients with intractable epilepsy are maintained on their optimum anticonvulsant regimen as much as possible through the perioperative period. Pre- and postoperative blood levels are monitored and dosage adjusted as indicated. Valproate therapy may be associated with low fibrinogen levels and prolonged bleeding time. Coagulopathy is usually corrected within 3 weeks of stopping the medication.

Drug interactions must always be kept in mind. Carbamazepine may lower hydantoin levels. Isoniazid, chloromycetin, dicumarol, and disulfiram can interfere with hydantoin inactivation, resulting in elevated plasma levels and toxicity. Patients on carbamazepine can have severe and prolonged nausea and vomiting following administration of anesthetic agents. Tissue and serum epoxide levels may become elevated and result in severe drug toxicity. During the perioperative period, changes can occur in the administration, absorption, and liver metabolism of anticonvulsant drugs. Anticonvulsant levels must be closely monitored and adjustments in dosages made promptly to avoid inadequate drug levels or tissue toxicity.

There is a temptation to taper anticonvulsant medication rapidly in order to expedite invasive seizure monitoring and thereby lessen the risk of infectious complications. Unless anticonvulsant drugs are withdrawn slowly in small increments, however, there is the risk of precipitating severe status epilepticus or provoking atypical epileptic events. The former is risky for the patient and the latter misleading for the surgeon.

The use of prophylactic antibiotics at the time of craniotomy is controversial. It is the policy of the author to administer a single intravenous dose of the currently most appropriate antibiotic at the time of induction of anesthesia for craniotomy. If a foreign body exiting through the scalp such as a ventricular drain or subdural electrodes is left in place, then antibiotics are continued until the foreign body is removed. This approach has been associated with a 2 percent infection rate with subdural electrode arrays left in place for 1 to 3 weeks and a 1.3 percent infection rate following craniotomy and temporal lobectomy.

INTRAOPERATIVE RISK MANAGEMENT

Frontal Lobectomy

Consideration for adequate exposure is paramount, but attention to the location of previous incisions and the potential need for other procedures in the future are also important when planning the scalp incision. A transcoronal scalp incision starting at the zygoma just in front of the ear ipsilateral to the lobectomy and extending across the midline to the inferior temporal line provides adequate exposure. The temporal branch of the facial nerve to the frontalis muscle is spared, and the incision is entirely behind the hairline, thereby avoiding the risk of facial disfigurement (Fig. 16-62).

The medial burr holes are placed 1.5 cm lateral to the midline, avoiding the sagittal sinus. Craniotomy near the midline dictates that burr holes be carefully positioned neither too close nor too far from the midline so that adequate control of the sagittal sinus and bridging cortical veins can be achieved without undue risk of air emboli or uncontrolled bleeding. Preoperative assessment of bridging cortical veins by angiography or MRI guides the placement of burr holes near the vertex so as to avoid unplanned or uncontrolled disruption of the veins if the dura is

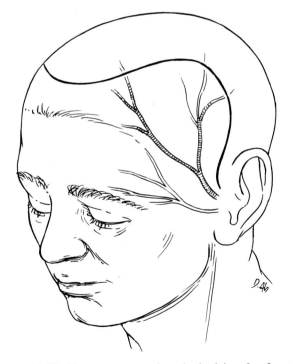

Figure 16-62. The transcoronal scalp incision for frontal lobectomy spares the temporal branch of the facial nerve supplying the frontalis muscle and is entirely behind the hairline.

prematurely fenestrated (Fig. 16-61). The frontal craniotomy edges are beveled using a Gigli saw and the burr holes filled with bone dust or chips before closing the scalp in order to give a more cosmetically acceptable result. The size and location of the frontal sinus is studied before placing the frontal burr hole, thereby avoiding the risk of cerebrospinal fluid (CSF) leakage and postoperative infection. The anterior margin of a frontal craniotomy is carefully inspected for evidence of frontal sinus exposure. Exposure of the frontal sinus at the time of frontal craniotomy increases the risk of early or delayed scalp infection, mucopyocele, osteomyelitis of the skull or bone flap, epidural or subdural empyema, or brain abscess. The incidence of these complications following frontal craniotomy is not well documented.[192]

Complications have in general not been frequent following craniofacial surgery in which the frontal sinus was entered.[189,194] The risk of such complications is present, however, and is increased in patients with a history of sinusitis and nasal allergies who undergo frontal craniotomy.[205] Frontal lobectomy does not necessitate a particularly low frontal craniotomy, and the frontal sinus can be avoided with careful preoperative planning. When the CT scan suggests an unusually large or asymmetrical frontal sinus, the Caldwell view on the plain skull radiograph may assist with the preoperative assessment so that the craniotomy can be planned to avoid the sinus.

If the frontal sinus is entered during frontal craniotomy, experience has shown that the surgeon can preserve the residual mucosa except that attached to the bone flap, which is completely removed. The bony window to the sinus is covered with fascia. The sinus is not obliterated and the frontonasal ducts are preserved. Bone wax is not used in or around an opened sinus, and care is taken to not pass sutures through the sinus mucosa.

A prefrontal lobectomy designed so as not to fenestrate the anterior horn of the lateral ventricle is best achieved by separating the frontal cortex from the falx cerebri in the longitudinal fissure and thereby identifying the genu of the corpus callosum. If the plane of cortical incision at the medial margin of the resection is anterior to the corpus callosum, the ventricle will not be opened and the anterior cerebral and pericallosal arteries are also avoided. The frontopolar branch of the anterior cerebral artery will have to be coagulated and divided but only after taking care either to identify the frontopolar branch to the opposite hemisphere or absolutely assuring oneself that the ipsilateral frontopolar artery is an end artery supplying only the tissue to be excised. The frontopolar arteries both course within the interhemispheric fissure and may crisscross one another. To disrupt the frontopolar artery contralateral to a prefrontal lobectomy mistakenly or inadvertently may result in a "frontal lobe syndrome" with apathy, changes of personality, and alterations in judgment and ability to plan. Prefrontal lobectomy is not expected to result in postoperative deficit in the absence of complications or damage to the contralateral frontal lobe, but occasionally evidence for recent memory impairment, apathy, or reduced control of voluntary micturition or other complicated motor acts is noted.[199]

Intraoperative ultrasonography is often useful for locating and determining the boundaries of intracerebral tumors. Glioblastomas arising in the hemisphere above the level of the corpus callosum tend to infiltrate the corpus callosum and extend into the contralateral hemisphere. Tumors arising below the level of the corpus callosum are more likely to involve the basal ganglia.[196] Lobectomy is rarely indicated when ultrasonography or radiography indicates that the neoplasm infiltrates the opposite hemisphere or the basal ganglia.

Temporal Lobectomy

A temporal lobectomy is usually performed with the head in full lateral position. In order to avoid twisting of the neck and compromise in venous drainage, the shoulder is supported with a rolled blanket, bringing the body into a three-quarter supine position.

The question mark-shaped skin incision is started just anterior to the pinna at the level of the zygomatic arch. The incision is carried above the ear and then is brought posterior a distance appropriate for the anticipated resection. This incision spares the temporalis branch of the facial nerve to the frontalis muscle. It is usually not necessary to bring the frontal limb of the incision anterior to the hair line, thereby avoiding facial disfigurement (Fig. 16-63).

An osteoplastic bone flap can be used, but adequate exposure is more easily achieved by turning a free bone flap. The temporalis fascia and muscle is incised 0.5 to 1 cm from its line of incision and reflected with the scalp flap. More adequate exposure is achieved if the reflection of the temporalis muscle is carried 2 to 3 cm forward along the zygomatic arch. The temporalis muscle and scalp are retracted with fish hooks.

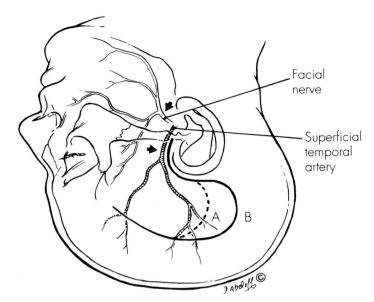

Figure 16-63. The curvilinear incision for an anterior temporal lobectomy need extend no further than back of ear **(A)**, although a particularly large intrinsic temporal lobe glioma may dictate a more posterior flap **(B)**. The temporal branch of the facial nerve is spared by limiting the inferior extent of the incision to the level of the zygoma and keeping the incision close to the pinna.

Trephination of the skull is performed at sufficiently close intervals that the dura mater can be separated from the inner table of the skull before turning the bone flap with a craniotome. Extra attention to this detail can lessen the risk of tearing the dura mater and lacerating the cortex and cortical vessels prematurely. The skull and bone flap are best prepared for closure at this time by drilling well-spaced suture holes in the bone flap and skull before opening the dura mater. Thorough hemostasis is also achieved at this stage of the procedure by waxing the diploe and stoping epidural venous ooze if necessary.

The middle meningeal artery is coagulated and the dura mater is opened at least 0.5 cm from the skull margin. The dura mater is usually reflected anteriorly over the sphenoid wing and temporalis muscle. The dura mater is protected by moist cotton pledgets in order to avoid shrinkage and the need for duraplasty at the time of closure. If duraplasty is necessary to accomplish a tight dural closure, autologous grafts with fascia or other suitable tissue from the patient are preferable to cadaver dura or synthetic dural substitutes.

It is important to inspect the temporal bone carefully for fenestration of the mastoid air sinus. Such an opening must be carefully sealed or packed off and extra attention given at the time of dural closure to a watertight suture line. The middle fossa will be in direct communication with the inferior horn of the lateral ventricle and the basilar cisterns after temporal lobectomy. Failure to exercise due precaution in these details enhances the risk of a CSF fistula and meningitis or ventriculitis.

Conventional wisdom contends that the anterior 4.5 cm of the dominant temporal lobe and anterior 6 cm of the nondominant temporal lobe can usually be resected without significant compromise of neurological function. A small "pie in the sky" contralateral superior quadrantic visual field deficit is accepted as the price of doing business in the anterior temporal lobe because of interruption of fibers in the geniculocalcarine loop of Meyer and Rochambeau (Fig. 16-58).

It is recognized, however, that there is considerable variability in temporal lobe size and functional localization, particularly in brains damaged early in development. Crossed brain dominance for speech and handedness is more common as determined by neuropsychometry and the Wada amytal test. Cortical brain mapping and functional localization by electrical stimulation and cortical sensory evoked responses suggest considerable variability in patients with chronic lesions and cortical dysfunction.

The relevance of speech arrest with electrical stimulation is still a subject open to interpretation. Speech arrest has been elicited by electrical stimulation within 2.5 cm of the temporal tip.[200] Electrical stimulation has also failed to elicit speech arrest in

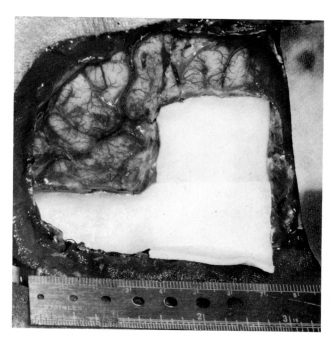

Figure 16-64. Photograph taken immediately after extensive resection of the left temporal lobe including a large parietal topectomy. The patient suffered from intractable seizures associated with a large intraparenchymal schwannoma in the temporal and parietal lobes. The Wada amobarbital test lateralized language to the left hemisphere, but cortical mapping, by electrical stimulation through a subdural grid electrode array, elicited speech arrest only in areas above the line of resection. The schwannoma and epileptogenic cortex were excised with preserved speech.

the temporal lobe of the dominant hemisphere in patients with chronic lesions and a long history of epilepsy. Subsequent temporal lobectomy and temporoparietal corticectomy produced only transient partial dysnomia (Fig. 16-64). Similar wide variation in the size, configuration, and location of the motor and sensory cortex is elicited by electrical stimulation. Confirmation of the sensory cortex is obtained by cortical sensory evoked responses.

Intraoperative ultrasonography is also a useful tool during temporal lobectomy to complement careful preoperative assessment of CT and MRI. The size, configuration, and posterior extent of the neoplasm can be determined and the posterior extent of the lobectomy tailored accordingly.

There is some evidence that tumors arising in the temporal lobes are less likely to spread to contiguous areas of brain and are, therefore, more amenable to complete resection by means of lobectomy. Encapsulated glioblastomas with a tendency to occur in the temporal lobes have been described.[190,193] The prog-

nosis of cystic pilocystic astrocytomas is particularly weighted by the willingness and ability of the surgeon to attempt total excision of the tumor.[202]

The temporal lobe dissection is initiated by bipolar coagulation of the pia mater and pial vessels along the superior temporal gyrus and across the middle and inferior temporal gyri at the posterior limit of the resection. The pia mater is sectioned and subpial dissection of the cortex and underlying white matter is carried out by aspiration. The middle cerebral veins (superficial sylvian veins) are often not precisely located over the sylvian fissure (Fig. 16-65). It is important to identify the margins of the sylvian fissure before commencing with the pial dissection over the superior temporal gyrus.

The first pia-arachnoid plane to be sought and respected during temporal lobectomy is that separating the superior temporal gyrus from the frontal lobe and insula (Fig. 16-66). Failure to appreciate and protect this plane may result in injury to the candelabra branches of the middle cerebral artery and a postoperative hemiparesis (Fig. 16-66B).[203] Electrocorticography following resection of the temporal lobe may show residual interictal spikes emanating from the insular cortex. Corticectomy of the insula is contraindicated, however, because of the risk of damage or spasm of the middle cerebral vessels over the insula.[203] It is, therefore, generally prudent to limit resection to the temporal lobe when a glioma is found to be crossing the sylvian fissure and infiltrating the insula. An expeditious and safe approach to temporal lobectomy is to carry the primary line of dissection down through the inferior horn of the lateral ventricle and the parahippocampal commissure, sectioning the pia-arachnoid along the floor of the middle fossa (Fig. 16-66A). The choroid plexus is identified and protected by cotton pledgets as soon as the inferior cornu of the lateral ventricle is entered. It is safe to electrocoagulate the choroid, but aspiration or traction on the choroid may result in hemiparesis and hemianopsia caused by stretch injury to branches of the anterior choroidal artery supplying the internal capsule, optic tract, and cerebral peduncle (Fig. 16-67).

The bridging cortical veins draining the anterior, inferior, and lateral temporal lobe are coagulated and divided close to the brain as the final step before evacuating the lateral anterior temporal lobe from the middle fossa. Venous drainage is thereby adequate and venous stasis with secondary edema and hemorrhage avoided as the dissection proceeds.

The operating microscope facilitates the dissection of the uncus and hippocampus and delivery of the mesial temporal structures from the incisura. This

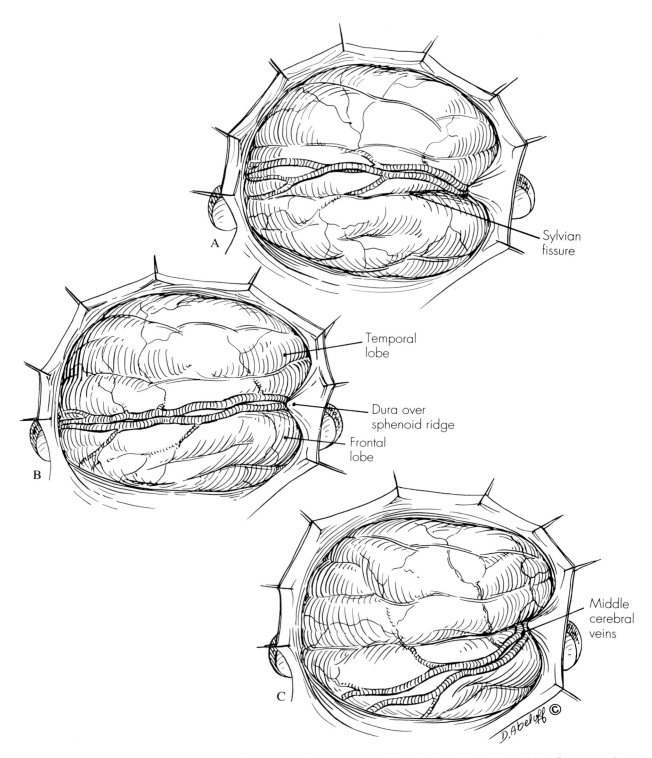

Figure 16-65. The middle cerebral veins are not always a true guide to the location of the sylvian fissure, and the temporal lobe can vary in size and gyral configuration. The veins may lie **(A)** inferior to the fissure over the temporal lobe **(B)**, within the sylvian fissure, or **(C)** superior to the fissure over the frontal lobe.

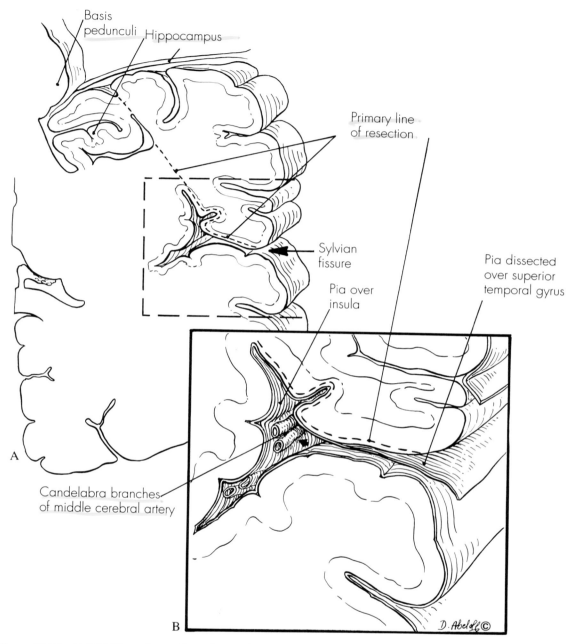

Basis pedunculi

Hippocampus

Primary line of resection

Sylvian fissure

Pia over insula

Pia dissected over superior temporal gyrus

Candelabra branches of middle cerebral artery

A

B

D. Abeloff ©

Figure 16-66. (A&B) The primary line of resection through the superior temporal gyrus respects the integrity of the pia arachnoid plane over the candelabra branches of the middle cerebral artery. The line of resection extends through the inferior horn of the lateral ventricle, care being taken to protect terminal branches of the choroidal vessels. Complete en bloc excision of the mesial temporal structures with preservation of the arachnoid membrane at the incisura is facilitated by use of the operating microscope.

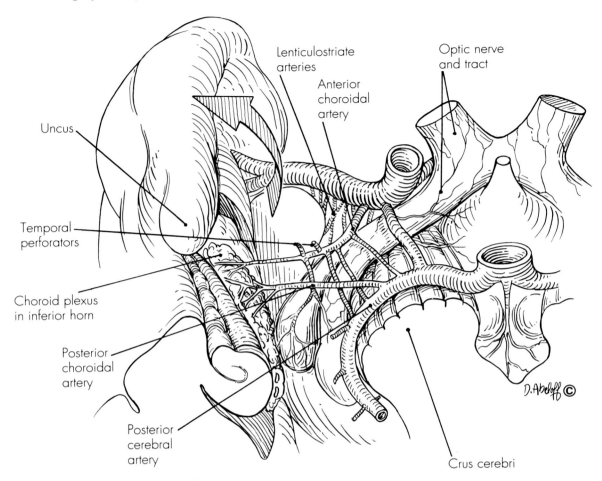

Figure 16-67. During a transcranial exposure for a tumor with suprasellar extension, one must exercise extreme care in the manipulation of low midline neural and vascular structures. The abundant perforating arteries in this region may pose a hazard to manipulation of the adherent capsule of the pituitary tumor.

phase of the temporal lobectomy can vary in degree of difficulty depending upon the consistency of the mesial temporal tissues and contiguous pathology, tissue herniation through the incisura, and adhesive arachnoiditis along the inferomedial surface of the uncus and hippocampus.

The pia-arachnoid plane separating the uncus and hippocampus from the interpeduncular and ambient cisterns is not encroached (Fig. 16-66A). Observance of this anatomical principle lessens the risk of damage to the oculomotor and trochlear nerves, posterior communicating, anterior choroidal, and posterior cerebral arteries, optic tract, and cerebral peduncle. This precaution also prevents surgical tissue debris and blood products from gaining ready access to the basilar cisterns, lessening the risk of postoperative

aseptic meningitis and meningismus. Premature or brusque delivery of the uncus from the incisura can transmit traction to the oculomotor or trochlear nerves when the nerve is adhered to the pia-arachnoid overlying the uncus causing a stretch injury to the nerves and a postoperative diplopia (Fig. 16-68).

The anterior choroidal artery is a very important vessel supplying the optic tract, internal capsule, and basis pedunculi before terminating in the tela choroidea. Traction or injury to this vessel can cause infarction injury to any of these structures resulting in a contralateral hemianopsia and hemiparesis (Fig. 16-69). Temporopolar branches of the anterior choroidal artery can be safely electrocoagulated and divided where they enter the uncus without stretching

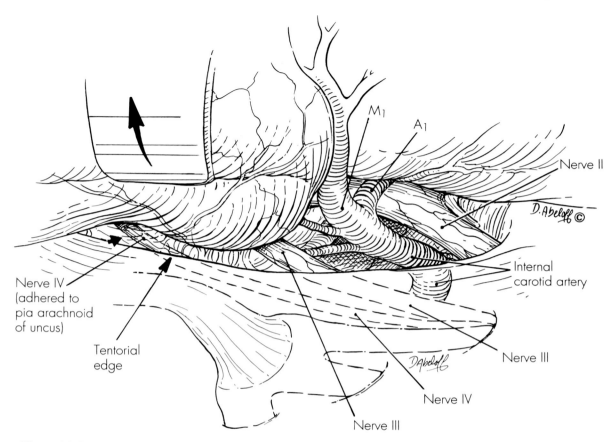

Figure 16-68. The uncus, amygdalar complex, and hippocampus are not infrequently packed into the incisura when temporal lobe pathology is evident. Gentle handling of the mesial temporal tissues and preservation of the arachnoid planes over the oculomotor and trochlear nerves, posterior communicating and anterior choroidal arteries, and cerebral peduncle lessens the risk of transient or permanent neurological dysfunction.

the main trunk (Fig. 16-67). The anterior choroidal branches to the optic tract and internal capsule are also subject to stretch injury if the tela choroidea and terminal branch of the artery are subjected to traction. The tela choroidea and anterior choroidal artery can be safely electrocoagulated, but traction transmitted to the more proximal branches of the artery can result in several neurological deficit. Great care is exercised to protect the tela choroidea from traction injury once the inferior cornu of the lateral ventricle is exposed (Fig. 16-67). A lateral branch of the posterior choroidal artery can also supply the anterior choroid plexus of the temporal horn.

The inferior horn of the lateral ventricle is more lateral in the posterior temporal lobe and slants towards the midline in the more anterior temporal lobe before dipping and terminating just behind the amygdala approximately 4 cm from the temporal pole. The choroid plexus and anterior choroidal artery vary in size and length, sometimes extending almost to the tip of the inferior cornu, but more often tapering off 1 to 2 cm from the anterior tip of the inferior horn. The anterior choroidal artery is accordingly at greater risk of aspiration and traction injury when the plane of resection is more posterior in the medial temporal lobe.

It is possible to damage the optic tract and interrupt fibers passing from the internal capsule into the basis pedunculi by direct trauma, but this is less likely than vascular injury under conditions of normal anatomy as this complication requires surgical transgression of two pia-arachnoid planes and their contained CSF space (Fig. 16-66). Maldevelopment of the brain and tissue planes, neoplasms or adhesive arachnoiditis from previous trauma, or meningoencephalitis may distort this anatomy, however, suggesting the value of careful preoperative assessment of this region on MRI.

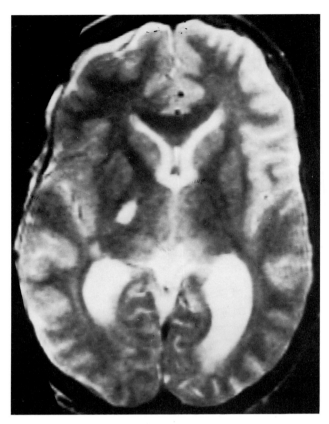

Figure 16-69. MRI showing small infract in posterior limb of right internal capsule. Patient awoke from anesthesia with left hemiparesis after extensive right temporal lobectomy extending 8 cm back from temporal tip. The infarct was presumably caused by either stretch injury or occlusion of a capsular branch of the anterior choroidal artery.

Occipital Lobectomy

Asymmetry of the occipital region is frequent, but may or may not be apparent from the appearance of the skull. Asymmetry of the sagittal and transverse sinuses is important. This anatomy can be assessed on the venous phase of the anteroposterior (AP) angiogram or on gradient echo reconstructions of venous flow on MRI (Fig. 16-61).

It is prudent, particularly in the elderly, to avoid trephination near the large venous sinuses in this region. Dural adhesions to the inner table of the skull increase the risk of injury to these structures. Prompt control of vigorous bleeding from the torcular herophili, superior sagittal sinus, or transverse sinus may be difficult to achieve at an early stage of the craniotomy, air embolus is a significant risk, and sacrifice of these venous structures is often not compatible with survival of the patient.

Asymmetry of the skull, superior sagittal sinus, and confluence of the sinuses is common near the occipital pole, but may not be apparent from the external appearance of the skull at craniotomy (Figs. 16-70 and 16-71). Careful inspection of the dura mater for location of the sagittal and transverse venous sinuses will lessen the risk of disorientation. If the surgeon does become disoriented in the occipital region and occipital lobe because of asymmetry, injury to the corona radiata could result in hemihypesthesia or hemiparesis. Orientation can always be achieved by observing the location of the falx cerebri and tentorium cerebelli, however.

Whereas the width of the falx cerebri is variable in the frontal region, the occipital falx extends to the corpus callosum and consistently measures approximately 60 mm from the occipital pole to the splenium. In the nondominant hemisphere the cortical

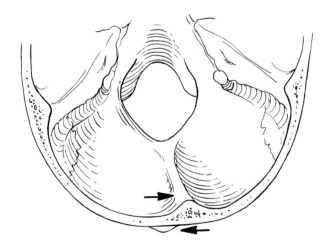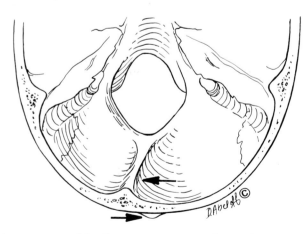

Figure 16-70. Asymmetry of the skull at the occipital pole is common and is often not apparent on inspection of the external surface.

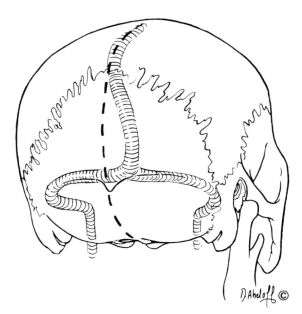

Figure 16-71. The location of the superior sagittal sinus and confluence of the sinuses is variable and may be well off the midline.

small rent occur in one of the sinuses, a piece of Avitene sponge placed on the rent and tamponade for a few minutes with a cotton pledget is almost always adequate to accomplish hemostasis. The cavity is filled with sterile saline before closing the dura mater. A final precautionary measure is to ask the anesthesiologist to increase the intracranial venous pressure transiently by increasing the end-expiratory respiratory pressure; the neurosurgeon then observes if this physiological maneuver elicits bleeding from a venous dural sinus.

One advantage of placing the patient in the prone or three-quarter prone position rather than the semi-sitting position for occipital lobectomy is the reduced risk of air emboli if a sinus or bridging vein is opened. Particularly dangerous is a fenestrated venous sinus or diploic channel not noticeably bleeding, but sucking air because the venous pressure is less than atmospheric pressure. Transesophageal Doppler ultrasonography, transesophageal echocardiography, end-tidal/CO_2 monitoring, and a central venous catheter for aspirating air from the right atrium are important adjuncts to intracranial surgery when the head is elevated.

incision can be safely placed 6 cm anterior to the occipital pole. In the dominant hemisphere, however, the anterior extent of the resection is more conservative unless cortical mapping with electrical stimulation has clearly shown the functional angular gyrus to be located more anteriorly (Fig. 16-72). Speech arrest has been elicited by electrical stimulation of the angular gyri, which in cadavers has been measured 3.5 cm from the occipital pole.[207]

Surgical injury to posterior parietal cortex in this region of the dominant hemisphere may result in receptive dysphasia, dyslexia, dysgraphia, and dyscalculia in addition to deficits in visuospatial and body imagery. Injury to the fibers of the splenium of the corpus callosum combined with occipital lobectomy in the dominant hemisphere isolates the language cortex from the residual visual cortex in the nondominant hemisphere and results in the syndrome of alexia without agraphia.

The occipital horns are variable in size and location and may or may not be entered as the subpial dissection proceeds towards the midline. The fenestrated ventricle is covered to prevent soilage of the ventricular system and rapid and excessive egress of cerebrospinal fluid. The vessels in the calcarine fissure are coagulated and divided as the falx cerebri is approached. Draining veins entering the sagittal and transverse sinuses and torcular herophili are coagulated and divided close to the brain before lifting the occipital lobe away from the occipital pole, thereby sparing injury to the large venous sinuses. Should a

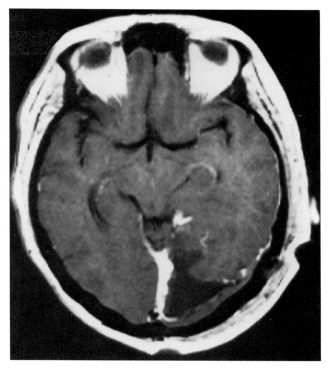

Figure 16-72. MRI showing occipital lobectomy for neoplasm in dominant hemisphere. The anterolateral extent of the lobectomy is quite conservative, in order to avoid injury to the parietal language association cortex. It is also important in such cases not to injure the splenium of the corpus callosum in order to avoid the complication of alexia.

REFERENCES

Intrinsic Cerebral Glioma

1. Ammirati M, Galicich JH, Arbit E et al: Reoperation in the treatment of recurrent intracranial malignant gliomas. Neurosurgery 21:601, 1987
2. Ammirati M, Vick N, Liao Y et al: Effect of the extent of surgical resection on survival and quality of life in patients with supratentorial glioblastomas and anaplastic astrocytomas. Neurosurgery 21:201, 1987
3. Andreou J, George AE, Wise A et al: CT prognostic criteria of survival after malignant gliomas surgery. Am J Neuroradiol 4:488, 1983
4. Beaney RP, Brooks DJ, Leenders KL et al: Blood flow and oxygen utilization in the contralateral cerebral cortex of patients with untreated intracranial tumors as studied by positron emission tomography, with observations on the effect of decompressive surgery. J Neurol Neurosurg Psychiatry 48:310, 1985
5. Berger MS, Cohen WA, Ojemann GA: Correlation of motor cortex brain mapping data with magnetic resonance imaging. J Neurosurg 72:383, 1990
6. Ciric I, Ammirati M, Vick N et al: Supratentorial gliomas: surgical considerations and immediate postoperative results. Gross total resection versus partial resection. Neurosurgery 21:21, 1987
7. Coffey RJ, Lunsford LD, Taylor FH: Survival after stereotactic biopsy of malignant gliomas. Neurosurgery 22:465, 1988
8. Harsh FR, IV, Levin VA, Gutin PH et al: Reoperation for recurrent glioblastoma and anaplastic astrocytoma. Neurosurgery 21:615, 1987
9. Jelsma R, Bucy PC: The treatment of glioblastoma multiforme of the brain. J Neurosurg 27:388, 1967
10. Kelly PJ, Kall BA, Goerss S et al: Computer-assisted stereotaxic laser resection of intra-axial brain neoplasms. J Neurosurg 64:427, 1986
11. Pia HW: Microsurgery of gliomas. Acta Neurochir (Wien) 80:1, 1986
12. Salcman M: Supratentorial gliomas: clinical features and surgical therapy. p. 573. In Wilkins RH, Rengachary SS (eds): Neurosurgery. McGraw-Hill, New York, 1985
13. Salcman M: The morbidity and mortality of brain tumors. A perspective on recent advances in therapy. Neurol Clin 3:229, 1985
14. Salcman M: Resection and reoperation in neuro-oncology: rationale and approach. Neurol Clin 3:831, 1985
15. Salcman M: Surgical decision making for malignant brain tumors. Clin Neurosurg 35:285, 1988
16. Salcman M: The role of surgical resection in the treatment of malignant brain tumors: who benefits? Oncology 2:47, 1988
17. Salcman M: Radical surgery for low grade glioma. Clin Neurosurg 36:353, 1989
18. Salcman M: Malignant glioma management. Neurosurg Clin 1:49, 1990
19. Salcman M, Kaplan RS, Ducker TB et al: Effect of age and reoperation on survival in the combined modality treatment of malignant astrocytoma. Neurosurgery 10:454, 1982
20. Salcman M, Kaplan RS, Samaras GM et al: Aggressive multimodality therapy based on a multicompartmental model of glioblastoma. Surgery 92:250, 1982
21. Salcman M, Robinson WL, Montgomery E: Laser microsurgery: a review of 105 intracranial tumor. J Neurooncol 3:363, 1986
22. Salcman M, Samaras GM: Interstitial microwave hyperthermia for brain tumors. J Neurooncol 1:225, 1983
23. Salcman M, Sewchand W, Amin PP, Bellis EW: Technique and preliminary results of interstitial irradiation for primary brain tumors. J Neurooncol 4:141, 1986
24. Shapiro WR: Treatment of neuroectodermal brain tumors. Ann Neurol 12:231, 1982
25. Tenney M, Vlahov T, Salcman M, Ducker TB: Wide variation in risk of wound infection following clean neurosurgery—implications or perioperative antibiotic prophylaxis. J Neurosurg 62:243, 1985
26. Wood JR, Greene SB, Shapiro WR: The prognostic importance of tumor size in malignant gliomas: a computed tomographic scan study by the brain tumor cooperative group. J Clin Oncol 6:338, 1988
27. Young B, Oldfield EH, Markesbery WR et al: Reoperation for glioblastoma. J Neurosurg 55:917, 1981

Stereotactic Surgery for Mass Lesions of the Cranial Vault

28. Abernathey CD, Camacho A, Kelly PJ: Stereotaxic suboccipital transcerebellar biopsy of pontine mass lesions. J Neurosurg 70:195, 1989
29. Apuzzo MLJ, Chandrosoma PT, Cohen D et al: Computed imaging stereotaxy: experience and perspective related to 500 procedures applied to brain masses. Neurosurgery 20:930, 1987
30. Apuzzo MLJ, Sabshin JK: Computed tomographic guidance stereotaxis in the management of intracranial mass lesion. Neurosurgery 12:277, 1983
31. Belyaev VV, Ivannikov YG, Usov VV: A method for calculating stereotactic coordinates in an arbitrary system by converting coordinates on computer. Vopr Neirokhir 4:58, 1965 (in Russian)
32. Boethius J, Bergstrom M, Greitz T: Stereotaxic computerized tomography with a GE 8800 scanner. J Neurosurg 52:794, 1980
33. Boethius J, Collins VP, Edner G et al: Stereotactic biopsies and computer tomography in gliomas. Acta Neurochir (Wien) 40:223, 1978
34. Brown RA: A computerized tomography-computer graphics approach to stereotactic localization. J Neurosurg 50:715, 1979

35. Brown R: A stereotactic head frame for use with CT body scanners. Invest Radiol 14:300, 1979

36. Coffey RJ, Friedman WA: Interstitial brachytherapy of malignant brain tumors using computed tomography-guided stereotaxis and available imaging software: technical report. Neurosurgery 20:4, 1978

37. Coffey RJ, Lunsford LD, Taylor FH: Survival after stereotactic biopsy of malignant gliomas. Neurosurgery 22:465, 1988

38. Davis DH, Kelly PJ, Marsh R et al: Computer-assisted stereotactic biopsy of intracranial lesions. Appl Neurophysiol 50:172, 1987

39. Edner G: Stereotactic biopsy of intracranial space occupying lesions. Acta Neurochir (Wien) 57:213, 1981

40. Gleason CA, Wise BL, Feinstein B: Stereotactic localization (with computerized tomographic scanning), biopsy and radiofrequency treatment of deep brain lesions. Neurosurgery 2:217, 1978

41. Goerss S, Kelly PJ, Kall B, Alker GJ: A computed tomographic stereotactic adaptation system. Neurosurgery 10:375, 1982

42. Hariz MI, Fodstad H: Stereotactic localization of small subcortical brain tumors for open surgery. Surg Neurol 28:345, 1987

43. Heilbrun MP, Roberts TS, Apuzzo MLJ et al: Preliminary experience with Brown-Roberts-Wells (BRW) computerized tomography stereotaxic guidance system. J Neurosurg 59:217, 1983

44. Hood TW, McKeever PE: Stereotactic management of cystic gliomas of the brain stem. Neurosurgery 24:373, 1989

45. Kelly PJ: Volumetric stereotactic resection of intra-axial brain mass lesions. Mayo Clin Proc 63:1186, 1988

46. Kelly PJ: Stereotactic biopsy and resection of thalamic astrocytomas. Neurosurgery 25:185, 1989

47. Kelly PJ, Alker GJ: A stereotactic approach to deep-seated central nervous system neoplasms using the carbon dioxide laser. Surg Neurol 15:331, 1981

48. Kelly PJ, Alker GJ, Goerss S: Computer-assisted stereotactic laser microsurgery for the treatment of intracranial neoplasms. Neurosurgery 10:324, 1982

49. Kelly PJ, Kall B, Goerss S: Transposition of volumetric information derived from computed tomography scanning into stereotactic space. Surg Neurol 21:465, 1984

50. Kelly P, Kall B, Goerss S, Earnest FI: Computer assisted stereotaxic laser resection of intra-axial brain neoplasms. J Neurosurg 64:427, 1986

51. Kelly PJ, Olson MH, Wright AE: Stereotactic implantation of iridium 192 into CNS neoplasms. Surg Neurol 10:349, 1978

52. Koslow M, Abele MG, Griffith RC et al: Stereotactic surgical system controlled by computed tomography. Neurosurgery 8:72, 1981

53. Lobato RD, Rivas JJ, Cabello A, Roger R: Stereotactic biopsy of brain lesions visualized with computed tomography. Appl Neurophysiol 45:426, 1982

54. Lunsford LD, Martinez AJ: Stereotactic exploration of the brain in the era of computed tomography. Surg Neurol 22:222, 1984

55. Maroon JC, Bank WO, Drayer BP, Rosenbaum AE: Intracranial biopsy assisted by computerized tomography. J Neurosurg 46:740, 1977

56. Moore MR, Black PM, Ellenbogen R et al: Stereotactic craniotomy: methods and results using the Brown-Roberts-Wells stereotactic frame. Neurosurgery 25:572, 1989

57. Moran CJ, Naidich TP, Gado MH, Marchosky JA: Central nervous system lesions biopsied or treated by CT-guided needle placement. Radiology 131:681, 1979

58. Mundinger F, Birg W, Ostertag CB: Treatment of small cerebral gliomas with CT-aided stereotaxic curietherapy. Neuroradiology 16:564, 1978

59. Nauta HJW, Contreras FL, Weiner RL, Crofford MJ: Brain stem abscess managed with computed tomography-guided stereotactic aspiration. Neurosurgery 20:476, 1987

60. Ostertag CB, Mennel HD, Kiessling M: Stereotactic biopsy of brain tumors. Surg Neurol 14:275, 1980

61. Perry JH, Rosenbaum AE, Lunsford LD et al: Computed tomography-guided stereotactic surgery: conception and development of a new stereotactic methodology. Neurosurgery 7:376, 1980

62. Rushworth RG: Stereotactic guided biopsy in the computerized tomographic scanner. Surg Neurol 14:451, 1980

63. Scarabin JM, Pecker J, Brucher JM et al: Stereotactic exploration in 200 supratentorial brain tumors. Neuroradiology 16:591, 1978

64. Shalit MN, Israeli Y, Matz S, Cohen ML: Intra-operative computerized axial tomography. Surg Neurol 11:382, 1979

65. Shelden CH, McCann G, Jacques S et al: Development of a computerized microstereotactic method for localization and removal of minute CNS lesions under direct 3-D vision. J Neurosurg 52:21, 1980

66. Walsh PR, Larson SJ, Rytel MW, Maiman DJ: Stereotactic aspiration of deep cerebral abscesses after CT-directed labeling. Appl Neurophysiol 43:205, 1980

67. Winston KR, Lutz W: Linear accelerator as a neurosurgical tool for stereotactic radiosurgery. Neurosurgery 22:454, 1988

Techniques and Refinements of Anesthesia

68. Allan MWB, Laurence AS, Gunawardena WJ: A comparison of two sedation techniques for neuroradiology. Eur J Anaesth 6:379, 1989

69. Apuzzo MLJ, Fredericks CA: The Brown-Roberts-Wells system. In Lunsford LD (ed): Modern Stereotactic Neurosurgery. Martinus Nijhoff Publishing, Boston, 1988

70. Austin G, Lee ASJ: A plastic ball-and-socket type of stereotaxic director. J Neurosurg 15:264, 1958

71. Badgwell IM, Lerman T: Reports of scientific meetings. Anesthesiology 74:801, 1991

72. Bannon MG: Termination of hiccups occurring during anesthesia. Anesthesiology 74:385, 1991

73. Bone ME, Bristowe A: Total intravenous anesthesia in stereotactic surgery—one year's clinical experience. Eur J Anesth 8:47, 1991

74. Bozza Marrubini M: General anaesthesia for intracranial surgery. Br J Anaesth 37:268, 1965

75. Brown AS: Neuroleptanalgesia for the surgical treatment of Parkinsonism. Anaesthesia 19:70, 1964

76. Brown AS, Horton JM, Macrae WR: Anesthesia for neurosurgery. Anaesthesia 18:143, 1963

77. Bullard DE, Nashold BS: Posttraumatic movement disorders. p. 341. In Lunsford LD (ed): Modern Stereotactic Neurosurgery. Martinus Nijhoff Publishing, Boston, 1988

78. Calenda E, Durand JP, Petit J et al: Anaphylactic shock produced by latex. Anesth Analg 72:845, 1991

79. Chen G: Acupuncture anaesthesia in neurosurgery. Am J Med 8:271, 1980

80. Coleman DJ, De Villiers JC: Anaesthesia and stereotactic surgery. Anaesthesia 19:60, 1964

81. Conway CM: Neurological anesthesia. p. 765. In Churchill-Davidson HC (ed): A Practice of Anaesthesia. Year Book Medical Publishers, Chicago, 1984

82. Cooper IS, Lee ASJ: Cryothalamectomy—hypothermic congelation. J Am Geriatr Soc 9:714, 1961

83. Cucchiara RF, Michenfelder JD (eds): Clinical Neuroanesthesia. Churchill Livingstone, New York, 1990

84. Deligne P, Talairach J, David M: Essais de'anesthésie en neuro-chirurgie avec l'association 2028 M.D-dextromoramide. Neurochirurgie 8:356, 1960

85. Edelman GL, Baughman VL, Albrecht RF: Nitrous oxide and neuroanesthesia. Surv Anesthesiol 33:117, 1991

86. Feingold A, Lowe HJ, Holaday DA, Griem ML: Inhalation anesthesia and remote monitoring in children. Anesth Analg 49:656, 1970

87. Gignac EA, Manninen PH, Gelb AW et al: The comparison of the use of three narcotics during awake craniotomy. Anesth Analg 72:S91, 1991

88. Gold M, Swartz JS, Braude BM et al: Intraoperative anaphylaxis: an association with latex sensitivity. J Allergy Clin Immunol 87:662, 1991

89. Hall K, Baldwin M, Norris F: Succinylcholine drip during craniotomy. Anesthesiology 20:65, 1959

90. Hillier SC, CB MB, Presson RG et al: Pressure transducer performance inside a magnetic resonance imaging scanner. Anesth Analg 72:S109, 1991

91. Horsley V, Clark RH: The structure and functions of the cerebellum examined by a new method. Brain 31:45, 1908

92. Ingvar DH, Jeppsson ST, Nordstrom L: A new form of anaesthesia in surgical treatment of focal epilepsy. Acta Anaesthesiol Scand 13:111, 1959

93. Janczur EA, Stewart FC: Continuous alfentanil infusion for stereotactic brain biopsy. Anesth Analg 71:312, 1990

94. Jorgensen NA, Messick JM, Nugent M et al: Patient monitoring during MRI. Anesth Analg 72:S130, 1991

95. Kandel EI: Functional and Stereotactic Neurosurgery. Publishing House Meditsina, Moscow, 1981

96. Kelly PJ, Ahlskog JE, vanHeerden JA et al: Adrenal medullary autograft transplantation into the striatum of patients with Parkinson's disease. Mayo Clin Proc 64:282, 1989

97. Morrow L: In one ear, in the other. Time, January 7, 1991, p 84

98. Nilsson E, Janssen P: Neurolept-analgesia—an alternative to general anesthesia. Acta Anaesthesiol Scand 5:73, 1961

99. Ohye C: Selective thalamotomy for movement disorders: Microrecording stimulation techniques and results. p. 315. In Lunsford LD (ed): Modern Stereotactic Neurosurgery. Martinus Nijhoff Publishing, Boston, 1988

100. Perkins WJ, Kelly PJ, Faust RJ: Stereotactic surgery. p. 379. In Cucchiara RF, Michenfelder ID (eds): Clinical Neuroanesthesia. Churchill Livingstone, New York, 1990

101. Roberts FL, Dixon J, Lewis GTR et al: Induction and maintenance of propofol anaesthesia. Anaesthesia 43(suppl.):14, 1988

102. Root-Bernstein RS: Ends & Means: Physic Forgotten and True. Sciences 31:10, 1991

103. Spiegel EA, Wycis HT, Marks M, Lee AJ: Stereotaxic apparatus for operations on the human brain. Science 106:349, 1947

104. Steen SN: Anesthetic management for basal ganglia survey in patients with Parkinson's syndrome. NY State J Med 60:3230, 1960

105. Steen SN: Patient monitoring in the operating room. Ann NY Acad Sci 118:408, 1964

106. Steen SN: Anesthetic management for basal ganglia surgery patients with movement disorders. Anesth Analg 44:66, 1965

107. Tasker RR, Marshall BM: Analgesia for surgical procedures performed on conscious patients. Can Anaesth Soc J 12:29, 1965

108. Tasker RR, Yamashiro K, Lenz F, Dostrovsky JO: Thalamotomy for Parkinson's disease: microelectrode technique. p. 297. In Lunsford LD (ed): Modern Stereotactic Neurosurgery. Martinus Nijhoff Publishing, Boston, 1988

109. Trop D: Conscious-sedation analgesia during the neurosurgical treatment of epilepsies—practice at the Montreal Neurological Institute. Int Anesthesiol Clin 24:175, 1986

110. Varrassi G, Panella L: Propofol infusion for magnetic resonance imaging. Eur J Anaesth 7:247, 1990

111. Vitkun SA, Madder BL, Zipkin M, Poppear PJ: Respiratory distress associated with stereotactic irrigation of a brain cyst. J Clin Anesth 3:53, 1991

112. Volgyesi GA, Doyle DJ, Kucharczyk W, Hele MJ: Design and evaluation of a pneumatic pulse monitor for use during magnetic resonance imaging. J Clin Monit 7:186, 1991

113. Wangensteen OH, Wangensteen SD (eds): The Rise of Surgery: from Empiric Craft to Scientific Discipline. p. 9. University of Minnesota Press, Minneapolis, 1978

114. Weinger MB: Proposed new alarm standards may make a bad situation worse. Anesthesiology 74:791, 1991

115. Welling EC, Donegan J: Neuroleptanalgesia using alfentanil for awake craniotomy. Anesth Analg 68:57, 1989

116. Wishaw K: Hypoxic gas mixture with Quantiflex Dual Mixer and induction room safety. Anesth Intens Care 19:127, 1991

117. Yabumoto M, Kuriyama T, Iwamoto M et al: Neurogenic pulmonary edema associated with ruptured intracranial aneurysm: Case report. Neurosurgery 19:300, 1986

118. Zelman V, Apuzzo MJ, Henle A et al: Anesthetic management during stereotactic placement of autologous adrenal medulla in the basal ganglia. p. 41. In Matsuki A, Hironori I, Oyama T (eds): Endocrine Response to Anesthesia and Intensive Care. Proceedings of the 46th International Symposium on Endocrinology in Anesthesia and Surgery, Osaka, Sept. 14–15, 1989. Excerpta Medica, Amsterdam, 1990

119. Zukic A, Kelly PJ: Neuroleptic analgesia for stereotactic surgery. Appl Neurophysiol 46:167, 1983

Special Considerations in Point Stereotactic Procedures

120. Apuzzo M, Chandrasoma P, Breeze R et al: Applications of image-directed stereotactic surgery in the management of intracranial neoplasms. p. 73. In Heilbrun MP (ed): Stereotactic Neurosurgery. Williams & Wilkins, Baltimore, 1988

121. Apuzzo MLJ, Chandrasoma P, Zelman V et al: Applications of computerized tomographic guidance stereotaxis. p. 751. In Apuzzo MLJ (ed): Surgery of the Third Ventricle. Williams & Wilkins, Baltimore, 1987

122. Apuzzo MLJ, Chandrasoma P, Cohen D et al: Computed imaging stereotaxy: experience and perspective related to 500 procedures applied to brain masses. Neurosurgery 20:930, 1987

123. Blaauw G, Braakman R: Pitfalls in diagnostic stereotactic brain surgery. Acta Neurochir (Wien) Suppl. 42:161, 1988

124. Bosch DA: Indications for stereotactic biopsy in brain tumors. Acta Neurochir (Wien) 54:167, 1980

125. Chandrasoma P, Apuzzo MLJ: Stereotactic Brain Biopsy. Igaku-Shoin, New York, 1989

126. Edner G: Stereotactic biopsy of intracranial space occupying lesions. Acta Neurochir (Wien) 57:213, 1981

127. Frank F, Fabriziz AP, Frank-Ricci R et al: Stereotactic biopsy and treatment of brain stem lesions: combined study of 33 cases (Bologna-Marseille). Acta Neurochir (Wien) Suppl. 42:177, 1988

128. Franzini A, Allegranza A, Melcarne A et al: Serial stereotactic biopsy of brainstem expanding lesions. Considerations on 45 consecutive cases. Acta Neurochir (Wien) Suppl. 42:170, 1988

129. Galanda M, Nadvornik P, Sramka M et al: Stereotactic biopsy of brainstem tumors. Acta Neurochir (Wien) Suppl. 33:213, 1984

130. Giunta F, Grasso G, Marini G et al: Brainstem expanding lesions: stereotactic diagnosis and therapeutic approach. Acta Neurochir (Wien) Suppl. 46:86, 1989

131. Guthrie B, Steinberg G, Adler J: Posterior fossa stereotaxic biopsy using the Brown-Roberts-Wells stereotaxic system. J Neurosurg 70:649, 1989

132. Hood T, Gerbarski S, McKeever P et al: Stereotaxic biopsy of intrinsic lesions of the brain stem. J Neurosurg 65:172, 1986

133. Kelly P: Tumor Stereotaxis. WB Saunders, Philadelphia, 1991

134. Levin A: Experience in the first 100 patients undergoing computerized tomography-guided stereotactic procedures utilizing the Brown-Roberts-Wells guidance system. Appl Neurophysiol 48:45, 1985

135. Lobato R, Rivas J, Cabello A et al: Stereotactic biopsy of brain lesions visualized with computed tomography. Appl Neurophysiol 45:426, 1982

136. Lunsford L: Diagnosis and treatment of mass lesions using the Leksell stereotactic system. p. 145. In Lunsford L (ed): Modern Stereotactic Neurosurgery. Martinus Nijhoff Publishing, Boston, 1988

137. Niizuma H, Otsuki T, Yonemitsu Y et al: Experiences with CT-guided stereotaxic biopsies in 121 cases. Acta Neurochir (Wien) Suppl. 42:157, 1988

138. Ostertag C, Mennel H, Kiessling M: Stereotactic biopsy of brain tumors. Surg Neurol 14:275, 1980

139. Scerrati M, Rossi G: The reliability of stereotactic biopsy. Acta Neurochir (Wien) Suppl. 33:201, 1984

140. Sedan R, Peragut J, Farnarier P: Intra-encephalic stereotactic biopsies. Arch Neurochir (Wien) Suppl. 33:207, 1984

Problems Relating to Pathological Interpretation in Stereotactic Biopsy Procedures

141. Adams JH, Graham D, Doyle D: Brain Biopsy: The Smear Technique for Neurosurgical Biopsies. p. 1. JB Lippincott, Philadelphia, 1981

142. Apuzzo MLJ, Chandrosoma PT, Cohen D, et al: Computed imaging stereotaxy: experience and perspective related to 500 procedures applied to brain masses. Neurosurgery 20:930, 1987
143. Apuzzo MLJ, Hinton DR: Clinically relevant issues attendant to pathology. p. 19. In Apuzzo MLJ (ed): Malignant Cerebral Glioma. American Association of Neurological Surgeons, Park Ridge, IL, 1990
144. Burger PC: Use of cytological preparations in the frozen section diagnosis of central nervous system neoplasia. Am J Surg Pathol 9:344, 1985
145. Burger PC: Surgical pathological considerations in inflammatory and transmissible diseases of the central nervous system. Am J Surg Pathol 11(S1):38, 1987
146. Burger PC: Classification, grading and patterns of spread of malignant gliomas. p. 3. In Apuzzo MLJ (ed): Malignant Cerebral Glioma. American Association of Neurological Surgeons, Park Ridge, IL, 1990
147. Chandrasoma PT, Apuzzo MLJ: Stereotactic Brain Biopsy. p. 65. Igaku-Shoin, New York, 1989
148. Chandrasoma PT, Smith MM, Apuzzo MLJ: Stereotactic brain biopsy in brain masses: comparison of results at biopsy versus resected surgical specimen. Neurosurgery 24:160, 1989
149. Daumas-Duport C, Scheithauer BW, Kelly PJ: A histologic and cytologic method for the spatial definition of gliomas. Mayo Clin Proc 62:435, 1987
150. Eisenhardt L, Cushing H: Diagnosis of intracranial tumors by supravital technique. Am J Pathol 6:541, 1930
151. Heilbrun MP: Computed tomography-guided stereotactic systems. Clin Neurosurg 31:564, 1983
152. Kelly PJ, Kall BA, Goerss SG: Computer-assisted stereotactic biopsies utilizing CT and digitized arteriographic control. Acta Neurochir (Wien) 33(suppl.):233, 1984
153. Liwnicz BH, Henderson KS, Masukawa T, Smith RD: Needle aspiration cytology of intracranial lesions. Acta Cytol 26:779, 1982
154. Lunsford LD: Diagnosis and treatment of mass lesions using the Leksell stereotactic system. In Lunsford LD (ed): Modern Stereotactic Neurosurgery. Martinus Nijhoff Publishing, Boston, 1988
155. Mouriquand C, Benabid AL, Breyton M: Stereotaxic cytology of brain tumors. Review of an eight year experience. Acta Cytol 31:756, 1987
156. Namiki TS, Nichols P, Young T et al: Stereotaxic biopsy diagnosis of central nervous system lymphoma. Am J Clin Pathol 90:40, 1988
157. Ostertag CB: Reliability of stereotactic brain tumor biopsy. In Lunsford LD. Modern Stereotactic Neurosurgery. Martinus Nijhoff Publishing, Boston, 1988
158. Russell DS, Krayenbuhl A, Cairns H: The wet film technique in the histological diagnosis of intracranial tumors: a rapid method. J Pathol 45:501, 1937
159. Scheithauer BW: Neuropathology of pineal region tumors. Clin Neurosurg 32:351, 1984
160. Willems JGMS, Alva-Willems JM: Accuracy of cytologic diagnosis of central nervous system neoplasms in stereotactic biopsies. Acta Cytol 28:243, 1984
161. Zee C-S, Apuzzo MLJ, Clark C et al: Neuroradiology for imaging-directed stereotactic biopsy. p. 45. In Chandrasoma P, Apuzzo MLJ (eds): Stereotactic Brain Biopsy. Igaku-Shoin, New York, 1989

Internal Decompression of Intra-axial Supratentorial Tumors

162. Ammirati M, Galicich JH, Arbit JH et al: Reoperation in the treatment of recurrent intracranial malignant gliomas. Neurosurgery 21:607, 1987
163. Ammirati M, Vick N, Liao YL et al: Effect of the extent of surgical resection on survival and quality of life in patients with supratentorial glioblstoma and anaplastic astrocytomas. Neurosurgery 21:201, 1987
164. Andreou J, George AE, Wise A et al: CT prognostic criteria of survival after malignant glioma surgery. AJNR 4:488, 1983
165. Apuzzo ML, Sabshin JK: Computed tomographic guidance stereotaxis in the management of intracranial mass lesions. Neurosurgery 12:277, 1983
166. Bucy PC, Oberhill HR, Siqueira EB et al: Cerebral glioblastomas can be cured! Neurosurgery 16:714, 1985
167. Ciric I, Ammirati MA, Vick N et al: Supratentorial extraganglionic gliomas. Surgical considerations and immediate postoperative results. Gross total resection versus debulking. Neurosurgery 21:21, 1987
168. Ciric I, Rovin R, Cozzens J et al: Role of surgery in the treatment of malignant cerebral gliomas. p. 141. In Apuzzo MLJ (ed): Malignant Cerebral Glioma. American Association of Neurological Surgeons, Park Ridge, IL, 1990
169. Ciric I, Vick NA, Mikhael MA et al: Aggressive surgery for malignant supratentorial gliomas. Clin Neurosurg 36:375, 1990
170. Coffey RJ, Lunsford LD, Taylor FH: Survival after stereotactic biopsys of malignant gliomas. Neurosurgery 22:465, 1988
171. Fadul C, Wood J, Thaler H et al: Morbidity and mortality of craniotomy for excision of supratentorial gliomas. Neurology 38:1374, 1988
172. Harsh GR, Levin VA, Gutin PH et al: Reoperation for recurrent glioblastoma and anaplastic astrocytoma. Neurosurgery 21:615, 1987
173. Jelsma R, Bucy PC: The treatment of glioblastoma multiforme of the brain. J Neurosurg 27:388, 1967
174. Kelly PJ: Stereotactic biopsy and resection of thalamic astrocytomas. Neurosurgery 25:185, 1989
175. Kelly PJ: Stereotactic imaging, surgical planning and computer-assisted resection of intracranial lesions: methods and results. Adv Tech Stand Neurosurg 17:77, 1990
176. Kelly PJ, Daumas-Duport C, Kispert DB et al: Imaging-based stereotaxic serial biopsies in untreated intracranial glial neoplasms. J Neurosurg 66:865, 1987

177. Kelly PJ, Kall BA, Goerss S et al: Computer-assisted stereotaxic laser resection of intra-axial brain neoplasms. J Neurosurg 64:427, 1986

178. Levin VA, Hoffman WF, Heilbron DC: Prognostic significance of the pretreatment CT scan on time to progression for patients with malignant gliomas. J Neurosurg 52:642, 1980

179. Levin VA, Wara WM, David RL et al: Northern California Oncology Group Protocol 6G91: response to treatment with radiation therapy and seven-drug chemotherapy in patients with glioblastoma multiforme. Cancer Treat Rep 70:739, 1986

180. Salcman M: Resection and reoperation in neuro-oncology. Rationale and approach. Neurol Clin 3:831, 1985

181. Shapiro WR, Green SB, Burger PC et al: Randomized trial of three chemotherapy regimens and two radiotherapy regiments in postoperative treatment of malignant glioma. Brain Tumor Cooperative Group Trial 8001. J Neurosurg 71:1, 1989

182. Vecht CJ, Avezaat CJ, van Putten WL et al: The influence of the extent of surgery on the neurological function and survival in malignant glioma. A retrospective analysis in 243 patients. J Neurol Neurosurg Psychiatry 53:466, 1990

183. Vick NA: Removal of malignant astrocytomas. Correspondence reply. Neurosurgery 22:440, 1988

184. Vick NA, Ciric IS, Eller TW et al: Reoperation for malignant astrocytoma. Neurology 39:430, 1989

185. Wild AM, Xuereb JH, Marks PV et al: Computerized tomographic stereotaxy in the management of 200 consecutive intracranial mass lesions. Analysis of indications, benefits and outcome. Br J Neurosurg 4:407, 1990

186. Wilson CB: Glioblastoma: the past, the present and the future. Presented at the Congress of Neurological Surgeons Annual Meeting, Los Angeles, California, October 25, 1990

187. Winger MJ, Macdonald DR, Cairncross JG: Supratentorial anaplastic gliomas in adults. The prognostic importance of extent of resection and prior low-grade gliomas. J Neurosurg 71:487, 1989

188. Wood JR, Green SB, Shapiro WB: The prognostic importance of tumor size in malignant gliomas: a computed tomographic scan study by the Brain Tumor Cooperative Group. J Clin Oncol 6:338, 1988

Cerebral Lobectomies

189. Bridger GP: Radical surgery for ethmoid cancer. Arch Otolaryngol 106:630, 1980

190. Davidoff LM, Feiring EH: Circumscribed glioblastoma multiforme. J Neuropathol Clin Neurol 1:161, 1951

191. Engel J, Jr, Kuhl DE, Phelps ME: Patterns of human local cerebral glucose metabolism during epileptic seizures. Science 218:64, 1982

192. Farmer JC, Jr: The paranasal sinuses: neurosurgical considerations. p. 177. In Wilkins RH, Renegachary SS (eds): Neurosurgery Update I. Diagnosis. Operative Technique and Neuro-oncology. McGraw-Hill, New York, 1990

193. Jelsma R, Bucy P: Glioblastoma multiforme—its treatment and some factors effecting survival. Arch Neurol 20:161, 1969

194. Ketcham AS, Wilkins RH, Van Buren JM et al: A combined intracranial facial approach to the paranasal sinuses. Am J Surg 106:698, 1963

195. Lesser RP, Luders H, Klem G et al: Extraoperative cortical functional localization in patients with epilepsy. J Clin Neurophysiol 4:27, 1987

196. Maxwell HP: The incidence of interhemispheric extension of glioblastoma multiforme through the corpus callosum. J Neurosurg 3:54, 1946

197. Maxwell RE, Gates JR, Fiol ME et al: Clinical evaluation of a depth electroencephalography electrode. Neurosurgery 12:561, 1983

198. Maxwell R, Gates J, McGeachie R: Magnetic resonance imaging in the assessment and surgical management of epilepsy and functional neurological disorders. Appl Neurophysiol 50:369, 1987

199. Needham CWL: Neurosurgical Syndromes of the Brain—Frontopolar Syndromes. p. 11. Charles C Thomas, Springfield, IL, 1973

200. Ojemann GA: Individual variability in cortical localization of language. J Neurosurg 50:164, 1979

201. Ojemann GA: Surgical treatment of epilepsy. p. 2517. In Wilkens RH, Rengachary SS (eds): Neurosurgery. McGraw-Hill, New York, 1985

202. Palma L, Guidette B: Cystic pilocystic astrocytomas of the cerebral hemispheres. J Neurosurg 62:811, 1985

203. Penfield W, Lende RA, Rasmussen T: Manipulation hemiplegia: an untoward complication in the surgery of epilepsy. J Neurosurg 18:760, 1961

204. Priebe HJ, Skillman JJ, Bushnell LS et al: Antacid versus cimetidine in preventing acute gastrointestinal bleeding. N Engl J Med 302:426, 1980

205. Schramm VL Jr, Maroon JC: Sinus complication of frontal craniotomy. Laryngoscope 89:1436, 1979

206. Talairach J, Bancaud J: Stereotaxic approach to epilepsy. Prog Neurol Surg 5:297, 1973

207. Van Buren JM, Fedio P, Frederick GC: Mechanisms and localization of speech in the parietotemporal cortex. Neurosurgery 2:233, 1978

208. Wieser HG, Elger CE, Stodieck SR: The 'foramen ovale electrode.' A new recording method for the preoperative evaluation of patients suffering from mesiobasal temporal lobe epilepsy. Electroencephalogr Clin Neurophysiol 61:314, 1985

17 Pineal Region Masses

General Considerations

Keiji Sano

Since the pineal body is located in the center of the cranial cavity, René Descartes (1596–1650), the greatest philosopher of 17th century France, thought that the pineal body might be the seat of the soul. This concept is, of course, wrong. The pineal body, however, is certainly the seat of various kinds of tumors. Because of the central location of the pineal body, the distance between it and the surface of any portion of the scalp is almost the same, whatever surgical approach to the pineal region a surgeon will take (Fig. 17-1). Therefore, one should choose the surgical approach to this region according to the size and extension of the tumor so that removal of the tumor will be most extensive or complete and damage to the normal brain will be minimal. In the following commentary, falcotentorial meningiomas and gliomas of the mesencephalodiencephalon are not mentioned, and only the so-called germ cell tumors are discussed as to their surgery and management. Here, germ cell tumors include germinoma, embryonal carcinoma, endodermal sinus tumor, choriocarcinoma, mature teratoma, immature (malignant) teratoma, and so-called mixed germ cell tumors, although I believe that only germinoma derives from primordial germ cells and, hence, the true germ cell tumor.[11]

THERAPEUTIC PRINCIPLES

Diagnosis of a medium-sized or large tumor arising in the pineal region and the posterior third ventricle is not difficult because of the presence of increased in-

tracranial pressure, paralysis of the conjugate upward gaze (Parinaud's sign), pseudo-Argyll Robertson pupil, and so forth. Cerebral angiography is useful to detect the extent and vascularization of the tumor. Calcification in plain craniograms may sometimes be pathognomonic, especially in patients under 10 years of age. The most powerful and noninvasive diagnostic tool, however, is computed tomography (CT) or magnetic resonance imaging (MRI). Examination of levels of α-fetoprotein (AFP), human chorionic gonadotrophins (HCG), and carcinoembryonic antigen (CEA) in the serum or in the cerebrospinal fluid should be done in all cases. The first two tumor markers (AFP and HCG) are especially informative as to the nature of tumors in this region.

If HCG is positive, the tumor must be choriocarcinoma or a mixed germ cell tumor with choriocarcinomatous elements or a mixed germ cell tumor with syncytiotrophoblastic giant cells. If AFP is positive, the tumor must be endodermal sinus tumor or a mixed germ cell tumor with endodermal sinus tumor elements. Prognosis of choriocarcinoma or endodermal sinus tumor is rather poor even after surgical removal of the tumor and postoperative radiation therapy of the whole neuraxis. Recently, chemotherapeutic agents such as actinomycin D, cis-platinum, vinblastine, and bleomycin, or their combinations are reported to be worthy of use.

If AFP and HCG are negative, the tumor may be either germinoma, embryonal carcinoma, mature teratoma, immature teratoma, mixed germ cell tumors with combination of these tumor elements, or pineal parenchymal tumors (pineocytoma, pineoblas-

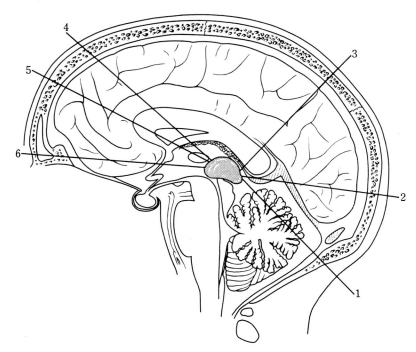

Figure 17-1. Various approaches to tumors in the posterior third ventricle, *1*, infratentorial supracerebellar; *2*, occipital transtentorial; *3*, posterior transcallosal or posterior transventricular; *4*, anterior transcallosal transvelum interpositum; *5*, transcallosal interfornicial; *6*, translamina terminalis.

toma, or pineocytoma with lymphocytic infiltration[11]). If 2,000 rads of local radiation effectively abolishes the tumor on CT or MRI scan, it may be germinoma or two-cell-pattern-type tumor of pineal parenchymal origin that I call pineocytoma with lymphocytic infiltration (or used to call pinealoma in honor of Krabbe).[3] However, if the size of the tumor is more than 2 cm (or sometimes more than 1.5 cm) in diameter, direct surgery and removal of the tumor followed by radiation (for germinoma and pineocytoma with lymphocytic infiltration, local radiation is usually sufficient) should be recommended. Mature teratoma can be cured only by removal of the tumor, and its prognosis is good. Embryonal carcinoma and immature teratoma with malignant transformation usually show poor prognosis even after surgical removal and postoperative radiation therapy of the whole neuraxis. The above-mentioned chemotherapeutic agents are also recommended.

Stereotactic biopsy of tumors of this region has recently been gaining in popularity. However, I am not particularly enthusiastic about this procedure, because different parts of the same tumor of this region may show different histology so that biopsy of a small piece of the tumor may be misleading as to the true nature of the tumor. Therefore, I prefer exploration and debulking (unless removal is possible) of the tumor. Cytological examination of the cerebrospinal fluid is important for diagnosis. If malignant neoplastic cells are identified at cytology, the case may develop dissemination metastases in the cerebrospinal fluid (CSF) space. For diagnostic purposes, I recommend millipore filter-cell culture[12] of the CSF. This method is more sensitive than conventional cytological studies. Therefore, positive culture does not necessarily mean that the probability of dissemination metastases is high. After treatment is finished, during follow-up, repeated examinations of the tumor markers are useful to detect recurrence of the tumor producing these markers at the earliest possible stage.

IMPORTANT ARTERIES AND VEINS IN THE PINEAL REGION

The artery that supplies the pineal body is the medial posterior choroidal artery (ramus chorioideus posterior medialis). This artery arises from the posterior cerebral artery lateral to its junction with the posterior communicating artery (pars postcommunicalis), runs in the ambient cistern, parallel to the posterior cerebral artery, supplies the pineal body, superior and inferior colliculi, and then runs forward in the tela chorioidea of the third ventricle, turns backward at the foramen of Monro, runs in the choroid plexus of the lateral ventricle, and anastomoses with the lateral posterior choroidal arteries, sending branches to the anterior thalamic nucleus, the medial geniculate body, and the pulvinar. This artery is usually single (69 percent), or sometimes double (23.9 percent), or triple (6.2 percent), or quadruple (0.9 percent).[5]

The lateral posterior choroidal arteries (rami chorioidei posteriores laterales) are usually two in number (but range from one to four),[5] arise from the posterior cerebral artery (pars postcommunicalis), run in the ambient cistern, go through the choroidal fissure, run into the choroid plexus of the lateral ventricle, and anastomose with the medial posterior choroidal artery and the anterior choroidal artery, sending branches to the lateral geniculate body and the parts of the thalamus. The arteria laminae tecti (arteria quadrigemina) arises from the posterior cerebral artery medial to its junction with the posterior communicating artery (pars precommunicalis), runs in the ambient cistern, and supplies the superior coliculus. A branch of the superior cerebellar artery supplies the inferior colliculus. From the peripheral trunk of the posterior cerebral artery, the arteria occipitalis medialis arises and sends the calcarine artery (ramus calcarinus) to the calcarine sulcus and the parietooccipital artery (ramus parietooccipitalis) to the parietooccipital sulcus and its neighborhood. These are listed in Table 17-1 and diagramed in Figure 17-2. The arteries supplying various portions of the brainstem should always be preserved at surgery.

The draining veins from the pineal body and the habenular trigone are named the superior and inferior pineal veins by Tamaki[14] and flow into the vein of Galen or the internal cerebral veins. The veins from the superior and inferior colliculi, the superior and inferior quadrigeminal veins (Tamaki) or the tectal veins (Matsushima[6]), flow into the vein of Galen or the superior vermian vein. The basal veins of Rosenthal flow directly into the vein of Galen (28 percent[5]), or into the internal cerebral veins (34 percent), or the confluence of the bilateral internal cerebral veins (28 percent). Many veins draining the frontal base, the lateral ventricle, and the hippocampus flow into the basal veins.

The anterior septal vein, the anterior caudate vein, the choroidal vein of the choroid plexus, and the thalamostriate (terminal) vein flow into the internal cerebral vein at the posterior rim of the foramen of Monro. In addition, the internal cerebral vein receives the posterior septal vein, the medial atrial vein (trigonal vein), and the direct lateral veins. The internal cerebral veins flow into the vein of Galen, which is 0.5 to 1.5 cm in length and flows into the straight sinus (sinus rectus). The precentral cerebellar vein (one in 46 percent, two in 54 percent[5]) and the superior vermian vein (one in 70 percent, two in 30 percent) flow into the vein of Galen or directly into the straight sinus.

These are listed in Table 17-2 and diagramed in Figure 17-3. The veins draining portions of the brainstem should always be preserved at surgery.

Table 17-1. Arteries Supplying the Pineal Region and its Neighborhood

From the posterior cerebral artery (arteria cerebri posterior)
    From the pars precommunicalis
        Arteria laminae tecti (arteria quadrigemina)
            Colliculus superior
    From the pars postcommunicalis
        Medial posterior choroidal artery (ramus chorioideus posterior medialis)
            Pineal body
            Corpora quadrigemina
            Tela chorioidea ventriculi tertii
            Thalamus
        Lateral posterior choroidal arteries (rami chorioidei posteriores laterales)
            Choroid plexus of the lateral ventricle
            Lateral geniculate body
            Thalamus
    From the peripheral trunk
        Arteria occipitalis medialis
            ⎧ Calcarine artery (ramus calcarinus)
            ⎨   Sulcus calcarinus
            ⎩ Parietooccipital artery (ramus parietooccipitalis)
               Sulcus parietooccipitalis and its neighborhood
        Posterior pericallosal artery
From the superior cerebellar artery (arteria cerebelli superior)
        Colliculus inferior

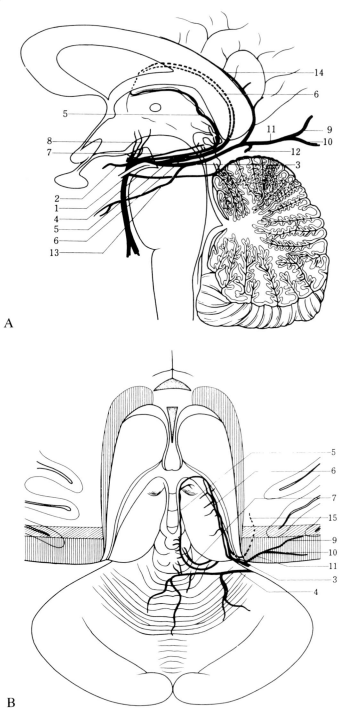

Figure 17-2. (A) Lateral view. **(B)** View from above. Arteries supplying the pineal region and its neighborhood. *1*, a. basilaris (basilar artery); *2*, a. communicans posterior (posterior communicating artery); *3*, a. cerebri posterior (posterior cerebral artery); *4*, a. cerebelli superior (superior cerebellar artery); *5*, ramus chorioideus posterior medialis (medial posterior choroidal artery); *6*, rami chorioidei posteriores laterales (lateral posterior choroidal arteries); *7*, a. laminae tecti, sive a. quadrigemina (quadrigeminal artery); *8*, thalamoperforating arteries; *9*, ramus parietooccipitalis (parietooccipital artery); *10*, ramus calcarinus (calcarine artery); *11*, a. occipitalis medialis; *12*, a. temporalis posterior (posterior temporal artery); *13*, a. temporalis anterior (anterior temporal artery); *14*, a. pericallosa posterior (posterior pericallosal artery); *15*, a. chorioidea anterior.

Table 17-2. Veins Draining the Pineal Region and its Neighborhood

Great cerebral vein of Galen (vena cerebri magna)
   Pineal veins (superior and inferior)
     Pineal body
     Trigonum habenulae
   Quadrigeminal veins (superior and inferior) (tectal veins)
     Corpora quadrigemina
   Superior vermian vein
     Superior vermis
   Precentral cerebellar vein
     Cerebellum, superior cerebellar peduncle
   Posterior pericallosal vein
   Internal occipital vein

Internal cerebral veins (venae cerebri internae)
   Septal veins (anterior and posterior)
     Septum pellucidum
   Anterior caudate vein
     Caput nuclei caudati
   Thalamostriate vein (vena thalamostriata, terminal vein)
   Choroidal vein (vena chorioidea)
     Choroid plexus of the lateral ventricle
   Medial atrial vein (trigonal vein)
     Trigonum of the lateral ventricle
   Direct lateral veins

Basal veins of Rosenthal (venae basales)
   Vena cerebri media profunda
   Venae centrales (striatae) inferiores
   Vena cerebri anterior
   Vena apicis cornus temporalis (hippocampal vein)
   Vena atrii lateralis (lateral atrial vein)
   Vena cornus temporalis (atriotemporal vein)

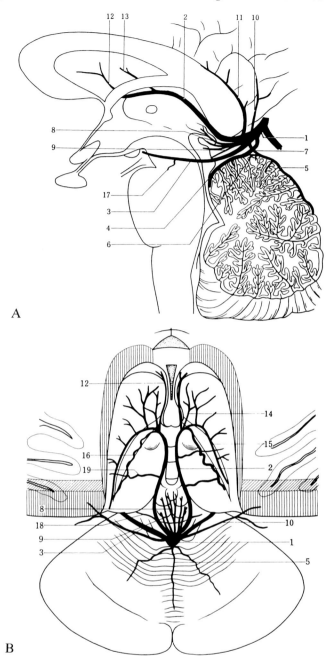

COMPARISON OF VARIOUS APPROACHES

Among various operative approaches to tumors in this region, I prefer (1) the *occipital transtentorial approach* (Poppen and Marino,[8] Jamieson,[2] and others) or (2) the *infratentorial supracerebellar approach* (Krause,[4,7] Zapletal,[15] Stein[13]) if the tumor is medium-sized or small; if, however, the tumor is large enough to reach anterior to the adhesio interthalamica, then (3) the *anterior transcallosal transventricular transvelum interpositum approach* (originally described as the frontal transcallosal approach by Sano[9,10]) may be recommended.

Occipital Transtentorial Approach

For the occipital transtentorial approach to a pineal tumor, I prefer the incision (usually on the nondominant side) illustrated in Figure 17-4. The midline portion of the incision can be elongated to the suboccipital region if it is necessary to open the posterior fossa.

Figure 17-3. (A) Lateral view. **(B)** View from above. Veins draining from the pineal region and its neighborhood. *1*, v. cerebri magna (great cerebral vein of Galen); *2*, v. cerebri interna (internal cerebral vein); *3*, v. basalis (basal vein of Rosenthal); *4*, precentral cerebellar vein; *5*, supraculminate vein; *6*, pre- and intraculminate veins; *7*, superior vermian vein; *8*, superior and inferior pineal veins (Tamaki et al.)[14]; *9*, superior and inferior quadrigeminal (tectal) veins; *10*, internal occipital vein; *11*, posterior pericallosal vein; *12*, anterior septal vein; *13*, posterior septal vein; *14*, anterior caudate vein; *15*, v. thalamostriata (thalamostriate vein, terminal vein); *16*, choroidal vein (v. chor(i)oidea); *17*, lateral mesencephalic vein; *18*, medial atrial vein (trigonal vein); *19*, direct lateral vein.

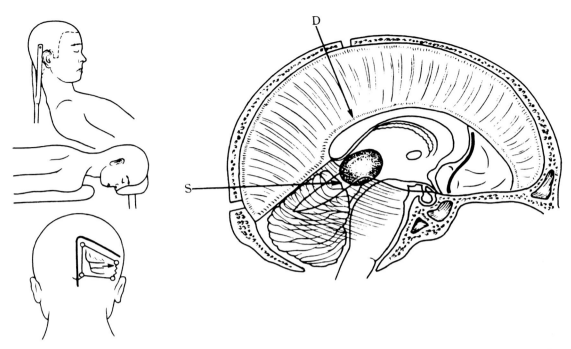

Figure 17-4. Occipital transtentorial approach (*S*) and parietal transcallosal approach (*D*) (From Sano,[9] with permission.)

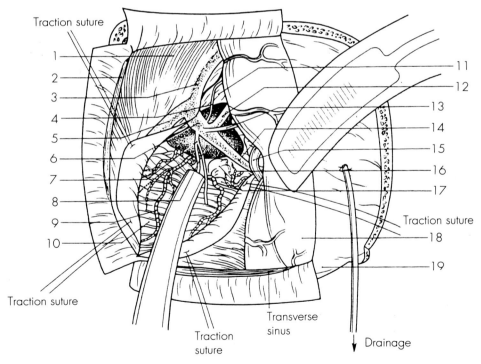

Figure 17-5. Occipital transtentorial approach. Detailed view. *1*, Falx; *2*, superior sagittal sinus; *3*, inferior sagittal sinus; *4*, splenial vein or posterior pericallosal vein; *5*, sinus rectus; *6*, vein of Galen; *7*, precentral cerebellar vein; *8*, pineal tumor; *9*, superior cerebellar artery; *10*, cerebellum; *11*, splenium; *12*, internal cerebral vein; *13*, internal occipital vein; *14*, basal vein; *15*, posterior cerebral artery; *16*, medial posterior choroidal artery; *17*, colliculi; *18*, occipital lobe; *19*, dura.

Craniotomy is close to the superior sagittal sinus and the transverse sinus. The patient is either in the prone position (the operating table had better be slightly tilted to the side of craniotomy, namely the right side, so that the right occipital lobe sinks laterally) or the lounging position, as seen in Figure 17-4. The occipital lobe is punctured through the dura mater, and a silicone rubber tube is inserted into the posterior portion of the lateral ventricle and secured to the dura (Fig. 17-5). The tube drains the CSF during the operation and makes lateral retraction of the occipital lobe easier. The operating microscope is used from this stage. The tentorium is split close to the straight sinus, and the superior surface of the cerebellum is exposed. A pineal tumor is often visible rostral to the vermis, underneath the vein of Galen. If the tumor is located further rostrally, the splenium of the corpus callosum is split by suction to expose the tela choroidea of the third ventricle. If the tumor is large, it is often already breaking through the tela choroidea; if not, the tela is incised along the midline or close to the nondominant occipital lobe after cauterization with a bipolar coagulator.

Therefore, this approach enables the operator to use the lower (parieto-) occipital approach (as proposed by Poppen and Marino[8] and Jamieson[2]) and, if necessary, the high parietooccipital approach (as proposed by Dandy[1]) as well.

If the tumor is a pineocytoma with lymphocytic infiltration or a germinoma (germinoma is usually slightly tougher), the tumor is removed piecemeal. If the tumor is a teratoma, removal en bloc will often be feasible. After removal of the tumor, the other end of the silicone rubber tube (which has been inserted into the lateral ventricle) is brought into the lateral cistern or the pontine cistern to secure the cerebrospinal fluid pathway. This is done because the rostral portion of the aqueduct is often compressed by the tumor, and even after removal of the tumor the effect of the compression may remain for a certain period.

Table 17-3. Occipital Transtentorial Approach

Advantages
  Providing an excellent view both above and below the tentorial notch
Disadvantages
  May damage the occipital lobe
  May damage the splenium of the corpus callosum
  May be difficult to reach parts of lesions extending to the opposite side
Indication
  Tumors that straddle the tentorial notch or those located above the notch

This approach provides an excellent view both above and below the tentorial notch. It may, however, be difficult to reach the part of a large tumor extending to the opposite side. There may be a danger of damaging the occipital lobe and also damaging the splenium of the corpus callosum, resulting in the split-brain syndrome. The approach is indicated in surgery of tumors that straddle the tentorial notch or those located above the notch. The advantages and disadvantages of this approach are listed in Table 17-3.

Infratentorial Supracerebellar Approach

The infratentorial supracerebellar approach is utilized when the pineal tumor is not too large. The superior surface of the cerebellum is pressed down after electrocauterizing and severing the bridging veins between the cerebellum and the tentorium (Fig. 17-6). The tumor can be seen beneath the vein of Galen and between the basal veins of Rosenthal. The precentral cerebellar vein and the superior vermian vein are identified and severed. The tumor is usually removed piecemeal.

I previously performed the infratentorial supracerebellar approach with the patient in a sitting position as advocated by Stein.[13] However, because of the fear of air embolism I am now using this approach with the patient in an oblique prone position. The operator stands to the left of the patient and looks down on the pineal region through the operating microscope.

Another point that should be mentioned and has hitherto never been described is that in rare cases the tectal veins or the superior and inferior quadrigeminal veins are so well developed that the tumor cannot be reached directly from behind. In that case the tumor should be approached slightly obliquely between these veins and the basal vein of Rosenthal. Another alternative for such cases is the occipital transtentorial approach.

In this approach, there is only minimal damage to neural tissues. The approach allows the surgeon to avoid crossing the deep veins. Disadvantages of this approach are narrow operative field, sacrificing the precentral cerebellar vein and the superior vermian vein, and difficulty in reaching paramedian tumors, portions of a tumor extending to the inferoposterior part of the third ventricle, and tumors above the tentorial notch. The approach is indicated in cases of small tumors in the pineal and quadrigeminal region. These are listed in Table 17-4.

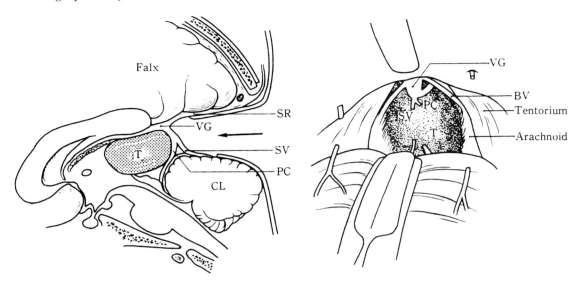

Figure 17-6. Infratentorial supracerebellar approach. *BV,* basal vein; *SV,* superior vermian vein; *CL,* cerebellum; *SR,* sinus rectus; *PC,* precentral cerebellar vein; *T,* tumor; *VG,* vein of Galen. (From Sano,[9] with permission.)

Anterior Transcallosal Transventricular Transvelum Interpositum Approach

The patient is positioned supine. A coronal or horseshoe-shaped skin incision is made on the right (nondominant) side, in the frontal region. A quadrangular bone flap extending to the midline and anterior to the coronal suture is elevated (Fig. 17-7). The dura is hinged toward the midline. The right frontal lobe is retracted away from the falx to expose the corpus callosum and the anterior cerebral arteries. The anterior part of the corpus callosum is split between these arteries, 3 to 4 cm in length, proceeding posteriorly to open the pars centralis of the right lateral ventricle

Table 17-4.   Infratentorial Supracerebellar Approach

Advantages
  Minimal damage to neural tissues; allowing the surgeon to
    avoid crossing the deep venous system
Disadvantages
  Narrow space (small distance between the colliculi and the
    tentorial hiatus)
  Sacrificing the precentral and superior vermian veins
  Difficult to reach paramedian lesions in the third ventricle
  Difficult to reach portions of tumor extending to the infero-
    posterior part of the third ventricle
  Difficult to reach lesions above the tentorial notch
Indications
  Small tumors in the pineal region and the quadrigeminal
    area
  Biopsy

(Fig. 17-8). The velum interpositum is cut just lateral to the tenia fornicis and medial to the choroid plexus (Fig. 17-9) under the microscope. The bilateral fornices and the internal cerebral veins are retracted to the medial side to explore the tumor between these structures and the right thalamus (Fig. 17-10). Section of the choroid plexus or the thalamostriate vein is not necessary. Thus the tumor and the surrounding structures are viewed from above and below. Microsurgical manipulation of the tumor is easy because of the ample space. This approach provides an excellent view of tumors in the third ventricle and allows the surgeon to manage parts of tumors extending to the lateral ventricle. There is, however, damage to the anterior portion of the corpus callosum and there may be possible damage to the fornix. This approach is indicated in cases of huge tumors in the pineal region or in the posterior third ventricle extending anterior to the adhesio interthalamica. These are listed in Table 17-5.

In all patients submitted to surgery, steroids are administered before, during, and after the operation. Postoperative irradiation is indicated in cases of germinoma or pineocytoma with lymphocytic infiltration, usually using Co-60 or LINAC, the total dose being 5,000 to 6,000 rads (daily dose 100 to 200 rads). The field of irradiation is 6 × 6 cm to 8 × 8 cm, centering on the pineal region. In cases of malignant tumors, whole-brain irradiation and spinal cord irradiation are added, but even in these cases the total dose does not exceed 5,000 to 6,000 rads.

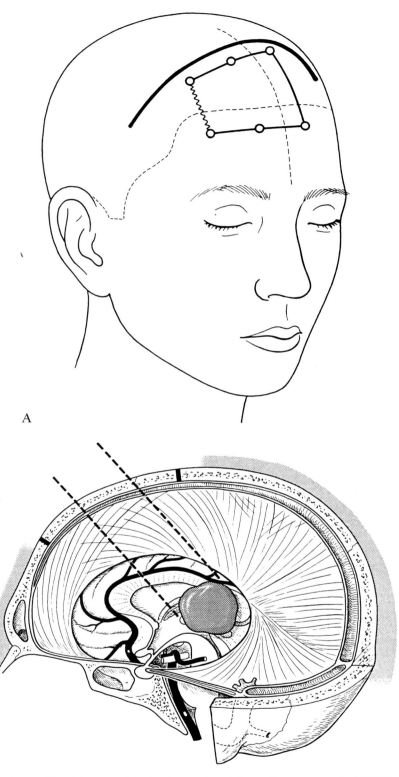

A

B

Figure 17-7. Anterior transcallosal transventricular transvelum interpositum approach. **(A)** Skin incision and craniotomy. **(B)** Approach to a tumor. (From Sano,[9] with permission.)

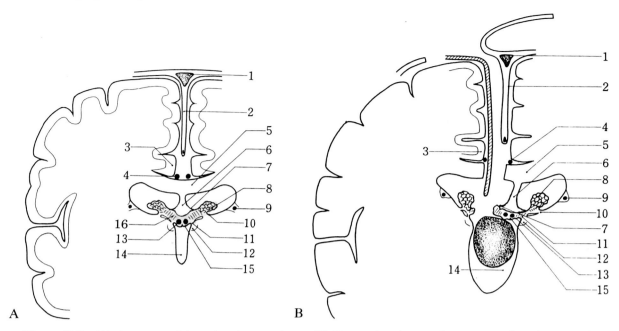

Figure 17-8. **(A)** Anatomy of the velum interpositum. **(B)** Transvelum interpositum approach and a tumor in the third ventricle. *1,* sinus sagittalis superior; *2,* falx; *3,* gyrus cinguli; *4,* a. cerebri anterior; *5,* corpus callosum; *6,* fornix; *7,* tenia fornicis; *8,* plexus chorioideus ventriculi lateralis; *9,* v. thalamostriata, stria terminalis, lamina affixa; *10,* tenia chorioidea; *11,* tenia thalami; *12,* stria medullaris thalami; *13,* v. cerebri interna; *14,* ventriculus tertius; *15,* plexus chorioideus ventriculi tertii; *16,* tela chorioidea ventriculi tertii; 8+16+15, velum interpositum.

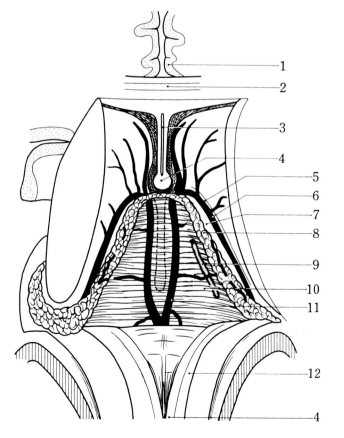

Figure 17-9. Incision of the velum interpositum on the right side (schematic). *1,* gyrus cinguli; *2,* corpus callosum; *3,* septum pellucidum; *4,* fornix; *5,* stria terminalis; *6,* v. thalamostriata; *7,* lamina affixa; *8,* plexus chorioideus ventriculi lateralis; *9,* section of the velum interpositum; *10,* velum interpositum; *11,* v. cerebri interna; *12,* tenia fornicis.

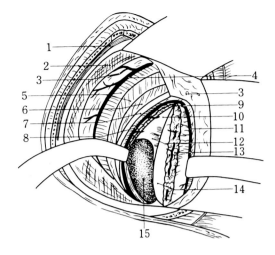

Figure 17-10. Anterior transcallosal transvelum interpositum approach. Actual operative view. *1*, sinus sagittalis superior; *2*, falx; *3*, gyrus cinguli; *4*, a. cerebri anterior sinistra; *5*, corpus callosum; *6*, septum pellucidum; *7*, fornix; *8*, v. cerebri interna dextra; *9*, foramen interventriculare; *10*, ventriculus tertius; *11*, v. thalamostriata dextra, lamina affixa; *12*, adhesio interthalamica; *13*, plexus chorioideus ventriculi lateralis dexter; *14*, thalamus dexter; *15*, tumor.

Table 17-5. Anterior Transcallosal Transventricular Transvelum Interpositum Approach

Advantages
    Providing an excellent view of lesions in the (posterior) third ventricle
    Allowing the surgeon to manage parts of lesions extending to the lateral ventricle
Disadvantages
    Damage to the anterior portion of the corpus callosum
    Possible damage to the fornix
Indication
    Huge tumors in the pineal region or in the posterior third ventricle
    Tumors extending anterior to the level of the adhesio interthalamica

Selection of an Operative Approach

Kintomo Takakura
Masao Matsutani

Although a variety of tumors develop in the pineal region, the pattern of the tumor growth is different according to tumor type. Germ cell tumors grow mainly into the third ventricle, but most gliomas or malignant lymphomas grow generally into the brain parenchymal tissue and not into the third ventricle. Teratomas and meningiomas are well demarcated and clearly separated from brain tissue, but anaplastic gliomas or other malignant tumors invade diffusely into the normal brain parenchymal tissue. The surgical approach is, therefore, selected by the location, size, and biological characteristics of each tumor.

According to the recent Japanese Brain Tumor Registry,[16] germ cell tumors accounted for 76.1 percent of all verified pineal region tumors (504 cases, Table 17-6). Germ cell tumors are classified into three major histological types: germinoma, teratoma, and malignant (immature) germ cell tumors. The malignant germ cell tumors include choriocarcinoma, endodermal sinus tumor (yolk sac tumor), embryonal carcinoma, or malignant teratoma. Such purely malignant tumors are extremely rare, and those tumors are generally found as a mixed histological type with germinoma or teratoma. The current registered germ cell tumors include 301 germinomas, 49 teratomas,

Table 17-6.   Tumors in Pineal Region
(Japanese Brain Tumor Registry, 1990)

Diagnosis	No. of Cases		
	Total No. (%)	Male	Female
Germ cell tumor	384 (76.1)	346	38
Germinoma	301 (59.7)	268	33
Teratoma	49 (9.7)	45	4
Malignant germ cell tumor	34 (6.7)	33	1
Epidermoid and dermoid	10 (2.0)	7	3
Pineocytoma	9 (1.8)	8	1
Pineoblastoma	15 (3.0)	12	3
Glioma	43 (8.5)	25	18
Other tumors	43 (8.5)	33	10
Total	504 (100.0)	431	73

(Data from Brain Tumor Registry of Japan.[16])

and 34 malignant germ cell tumors. Pineal parenchymal tumors (9 pineocytomas and 15 pineoblastomas) accounted for about 5 percent of all pineal region tumors. Gliomas (43 cases) accounted for 8.5 percent. Other tumors are meningioma, malignant lymphoma, metastatic, and others. The incidence of tumors in the third ventricle is shown in Table 17-7. Gliomas accounted for 41.4 percent, while germ cell tumors accounted for 22.7 percent of all 390 cases. Since the cases in Table 17-6 and 17-7 did not overlap, the overall incidence of germ cell tumors in the

Table 17-7.   Tumors in the Third Ventricle[a]
(Japanese Brain Tumor Registry, 1990)

Diagnosis	No. of Cases (%)
Astocytoma	77 (19.7)
Anaplastic astrocytoma	16 (4.1)
Glioblastoma	18 (4.6)
Ependymoma	38 (9.7)
Oligodendroglioma[b]	13 (3.3)
Craniopharyngioma	54 (13.8)
Pituitary adenoma	7 (1.8)
Germinoma	59 (15.5)
Teratoma	28 (7.2)
Malignant lymphoma	2 (0.5)
Meningioma	12 (3.0)
Other tumors	62 (15.9)
Total	390 (100.0)

[a] The cases in Table 17-7 do not include cases in Table 17-6.
[b] Some cases of oligodendroglioma are central neurocytoma.
(Data from Brain Tumor Registry of Japan.[16])

Table 17-8.   Pineal Region Tumors
(University of Tokyo, 1990)

Diagnosis	No. of Cases
Germinoma	78
Teratoma	21
Malignant germ cell tumor	18
Glioma	21
Pineocytoma and pineoblastoma	4
Meningioma	3
Metastatic tumor	2
Malignant lymphoma	3
Total	150

pineal region and the third ventricle was about 52.7 percent (471 germ cell tumors in all 894 cases) in Japan. This incidence might be the highest in the world. In my own experience of 150 pineal region tumors, 117 cases (78.0 percent) were the germ cell type (Table 17-8).

Germinoma is extremely sensitive to radiation and is cured by radiation therapy. The statistics demonstrate that the 5-year survival rate of germinoma treated from 1979 to 1981 in all of Japan was 79 percent.[16] Our Brain Tumor Study Group (consisting of six university clinics) has accumulated 83 cases of germinoma treated recently. The 5-year survival rates were 100 percent for female and 93 percent for male patients. On the other hand, teratoma is resistant to radiation, and surgical removal is the only choice of treatment. In cases of malignant germ cell tumors, combined treatment with surgery, radiation therapy, and chemotherapy is inevitable. For malignant gliomas, when radical surgical removal of the tumor is feasible, the effectiveness of postsurgical adjuvant therapy with radiation and chemotherapy improves.

Recent diagnoses by CT scan and MRI as well as tumor marker studies have made it possible to differentiate fairly well the histological types or the biological characteristics of the pineal region tumors before surgical removal. Therefore the surgical approach to the pineal region tumors is selected by location, size, and biological characteristics.

AFP, HCG PLAP .

SELECTION OF SURGICAL APPROACH BY IMAGING DIAGNOSIS

As noted above, selection of surgical approaches to the pineal region tumors depends on the location, the size, the extension and the biological characteristics of the tumor diagnosed by MRI or CT scan. Various approaches from every conceivable angle have well been reported.[19,21,23,25] The most popular approaches are the interhemispheric transcallosal (anterior or posterior), the transventricular (anterior or posterior), the occipital transtentorial, and the infratentorial supracerebellar approaches. Since the pineal region tumors are not as common, the surgeon's experience and preference are another factor.

I mostly use the suboccipital transtentorial approach for small or middle-sized pineal region tumors. This approach was initially introduced by Foerster in 1928.[27] Tumors such as those shown in Figure 17-11 could be removed easily by this approach. The patient is placed in the prone position with the head rotated slightly (10 to 20 degrees) toward the contralateral side of the craniotomy.

The suboccipital supracerebellar approach is also useful for midline vascular tumor-like meningioma. This approach was initially reported by Krause in 1926[18] and later developed by Stein[25] using a microsurgical technique. For meningiomas such as that shown in Figure 17-12, I used the suboccipital supracerebellar approach with minimum bleeding from the tumor tissue during the operation. The tumor was totally removed piece by piece without any damage of deep venous system. This is a midline approach and does not call for retraction of the occipital lobe; thus the risk of hemianopia after the operation is avoided.

For tumors growing into the anterior part of the third ventricle, the interhemispheric transcallosal approach is preferable. Since most of the tumor inside the third ventricle can be seen directly under the microscope, we can remove the tumor by a well-oriented view during the operation. For tumors growing into the lateral ventricle, as shown in Figure 17-13, the transcortical-transventricular approach from the silent cortical area might be the best, to avoid the postoperative risk of neurological deficit. On the other hand, most of the malignant gliomas developed near the pineal body grow into the parenchymal glial tissue rather than into the third ventricle. Furthermore, the tumor generally grows unevenly into one side of the brain, as shown in Figures 17-14 and 17-15. In such cases, a two-step operation using the transcortical and the suboccipital transtentorial approaches (described later) might be the best approach.

FRONTAL TRANSCORTICAL-TRANSVENTRICULAR APPROACH TO THE LARGE GERM CELL TUMOR

The interhemispheric transcallosal approach is widely used and might be standard for tumors located inside the third ventricle. This is probably the most reliable approach to the small or middle-sized tumor located inside the third ventricle, preventing disconnection syndrome after the surgery, when a small callosal incision of 2.5 cm or less is properly performed. The anterior callosal section is safer than the posterior callosal section to prevent postoperative disconnection syndrome. However, if the tumor is extremely large and extends from the anterior part of the third or lateral ventricle to the fourth ventricle, as shown in Figure 17-16, the frontal transcortical-transventricular approach is preferable. By using this approach, we can access the tumor without strong retraction of the brain.

Large germ cell tumors located in the third ventricle are generally teratoma or malignant germ cell tumors containing some teratomatous component in the tumor tissue. For the transcortical-transventricular approach, a small corticotomy less than 3 cm on the frontal silent area is enough to visualize the tumor located in the lateral and third ventricles. Even tumors inside the fourth ventricle can be seen in the straight operative view under the microscope.

Patients are placed in a supine position with the head flexed 10 degrees laterally. The frontal skin incision is made as shown in Figure 17-17. Two skull burr holes are placed parallel to the sagittal sinus. The rectangular bone flap, 6 × 4 cm, is enough for this approach. After the dural opening, a 2 to 3 cm corti-

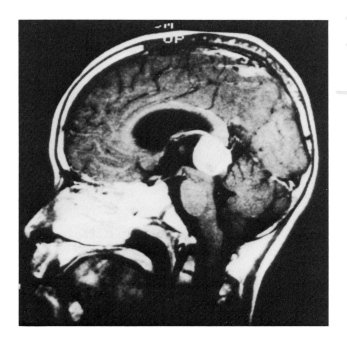

Figure 17-11. Germinoma (MRI, T_1-weighted).

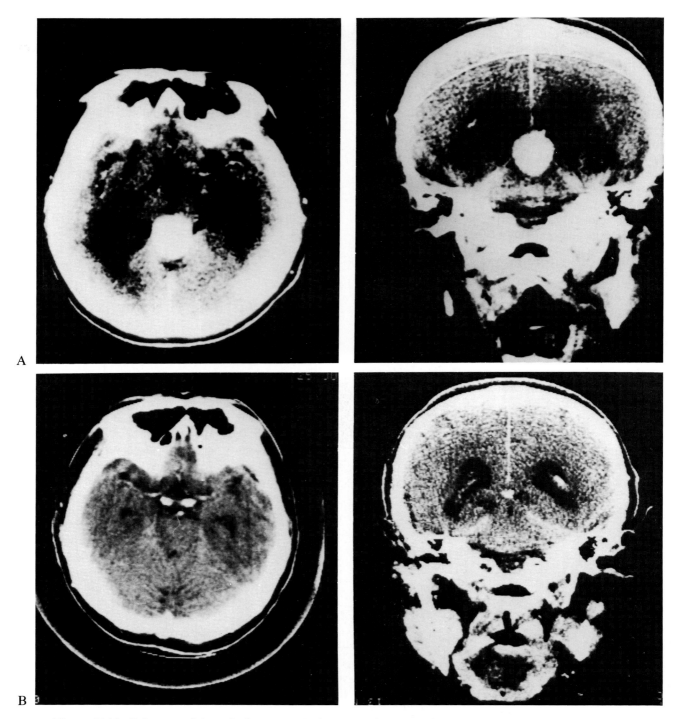

Figure 17-12. Falcotentorial meningioma. **(A)** Before operation. **(B)** After total removal of the tumor by the infratentorial supracerebellar approach.

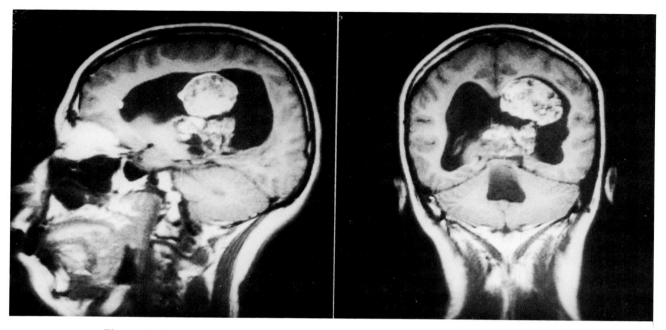

Figure 17-13. Teratoma in the third, lateral, and fourth ventricle (MRI, T₁-weighted).

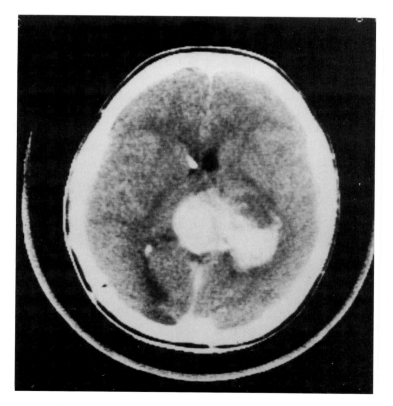

Figure 17-14. Glioblastoma near the pineal region.

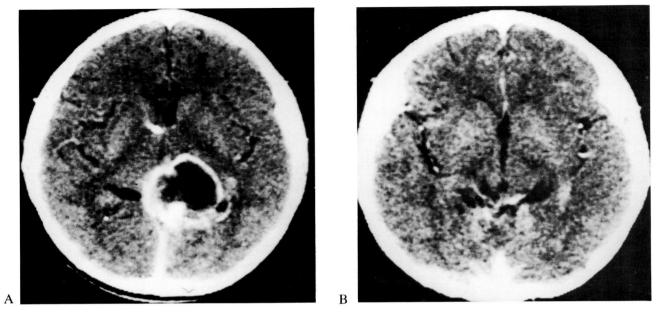

Figure 17-15. Glioblastoma near the pineal region in a 10-year-old girl, **(A)** before and **(B)** after surgery.

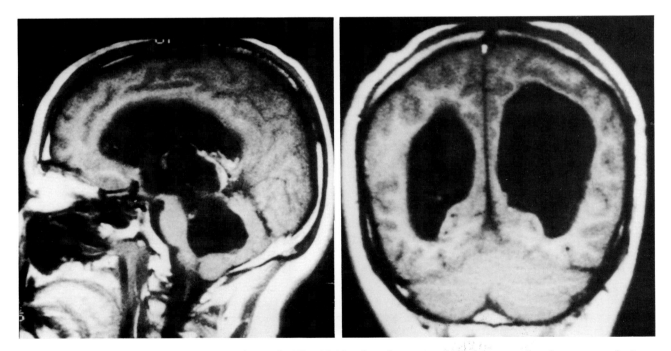

Figure 17-16. The same case as shown in Fig. 17-13, after the removal of the tumor by the transcortical transventricular approach.

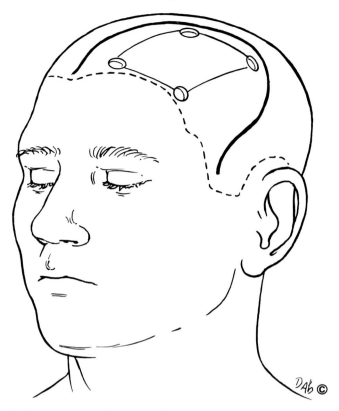

Figure 17-17. Transcortical-transventricular approach for the teratoma shown in Fig. 17-13. Skin incision and the craniotomy.

cotomy is made parallel to the superior sagittal sinus. By mild retraction using the spatula, the surface of the enlarged lateral ventricular wall is easily accessed. After a straight incision on the ventricular wall, the tumor can be visualized inside the lateral ventricle (Fig. 17-18). Teratoma tissue is usually heterogeneous. Soft tissue (fat or epidermoid tissue) can be easily aspirated by suction. The hard osseous or cartilaginous tissue is removed piece by piece using pituitary or other forceps. Ultrasound suction is useful to remove the tumor.

The merits of this approach are avoidance of unnecessary strong retraction of brain tissue, prevention of the disconnection syndrome, possibly engendered by the interhemispheric transcallosal approach and a wide surgical view. Figures 17-13 and 17-16 demonstrate a large teratoma before and after surgical removal. This 19-year-old boy with epileptic seizures, cerebellar ataxia, and disturbance of ocular movement has shown an excellent recovery after removal of the tumor by this approach. The tumor con- tained a variety of tissues including bone, cartilage, hair, waxy fatty tissue, and epidermoid-like tissue.

TWO-STEP SURGERY BY OCCIPITAL TRANSCORTICAL AND THE SUBOCCIPITAL TRANSTENTORIAL APPROACHES TO THE LATERALLY EXTENDED PINEAL REGION TUMOR

The suboccipital transtentorial is probably the most frequently used approach to large pineal region tumors. Although the germ cell tumor generally grows into the third ventricle, the glioma grows expansively into the glial parenchymal tissue laterally from the pineal region, as shown in Figures 17-14 and 17-15. When the glioma expands laterally, strong retraction of the occipital lobe by a spatula is needed, if we apply the occipital transtentorial or transcallosal approach. Furthermore, brain edema surrounding the glioma increases the danger of damage to the

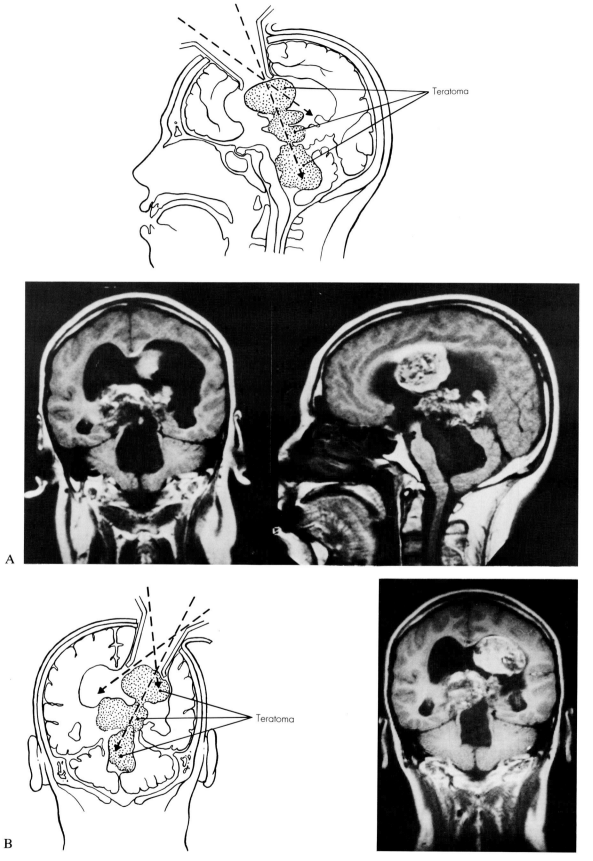

Figure 17-18. Transcortical-transventricular approach to a teratoma in the whole ventricular system. **(A)** Sagittal view. **(B)** Coronal view.

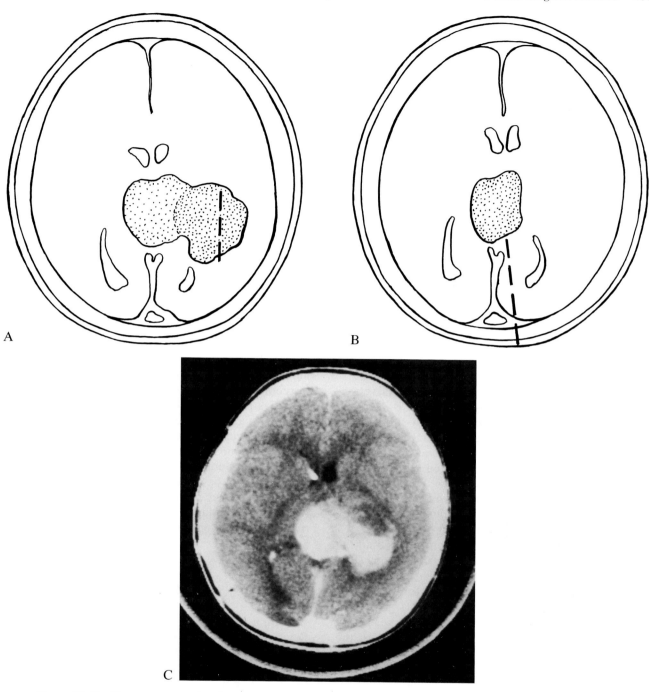

Figure 17-19. Two-step operation for the pineal region glioma shown in Figure 17-15. **(A)** First step. Removal of the right lateral side of the tumor by the transcortical approach (*dashed line*). **(B)** Second step. Removal of the tumor remnant by the suboccipital transtentorial approach (*dashed line*). **(C)** CT scan showing tumor.

parenchymal brain tissue by retraction. In such later-ally extended gliomas, I therefore use the following two-step operation. In the first step, the laterally ex-tended tumor is removed as much as possible by the occipital transcortical approach. The small cortico-tomy is enough for this maneuver, and a large bulk of

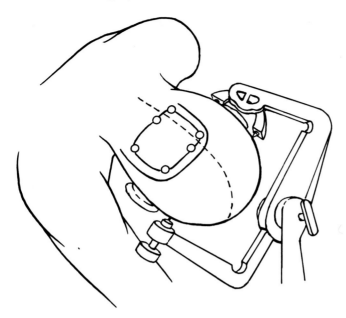

Figure 17-20. The position, skin incision, and craniotomy for the two-step operation shown in Fig. 17-19.

the tumor can be safely removed with minimal retraction of the occipital lobe (Fig. 17-19A & B).

In the second step, the conventional suboccipital transtentorial approach is applied for removing the remnant of tumor in the central pineal region. After the removal of the laterally extended tumor, the occipital lobe can always be retracted easily by the spatula with minimal pressure, which prevents unnecessary damage to the parenchymal brain tissue, and postsurgical complications can be avoided.

I prefer an oblique-prone position rather than the sitting position in order to avoid air embolisms (Fig. 17-20). The skin incision is made slightly larger than usual laterally, to make enough space for removal of the laterally extended tumor (Fig. 17-21). Two burr holes are made in the contralateral side of the sagittal sinus in order to open the dura mater close to the sagittal sinus. Other burr holes are made in proper position to the torcular herophili, the transverse sinus, and the lateral occipitoparietal region. After the dural opening, the place of the corticotomy is selected above the laterally extended tumor. Special care must be taken to avoid the postsurgical visual field and other neurological deficits. A 2- to 3-cm corticotomy is enough for the removal of the tumor, which is performed by ultrasound suction. Minor bleeding from the tumor tissue can easily be controlled by using hemostatic materials such as Surgicel, Oxycel, or fibrous collagen with gentle pressing using a cotton pledglet. After removal of the bulk of

the tumor, the retractors are taken out. In the second step, the remnant tumor is removed by the usual suboccipital transtentorial approach (Fig. 17-21C). The occipital lobe is retracted laterally and superiorly if necessary. In this step, retraction by a spatula is quite easily done without tight swelling of the brain. The preservation of the bridging vein is necessary. The tumor can be seen easily and the tentorial incision is made more than 1 cm lateral to the midline forward of the tumor surface. At this stage of the operation, vascular structures such as the vein of Galen, the basal vein of Rosenthal, and the internal cerebral vein are generally identified. The tumor is removed using ultrasound suction, carefully avoiding any damage to the arteries and the vein of Galen and the basal vein of Rosenthal. Since the operative viewing field for this surgical maneuver is quite broad, it is not difficult to see and preserve those vessels. The border of the glioma is clear in some place, but obscure in other regions where the glioma may be diffusely growing into the normal brain tissue. Since total removal of the malignant glioma is essentially not possible, extension of the tumor removal is up to each surgeon's decision. I would like to recommend, however, removal of as much of the tumor as possible, in order to decrease the mass effect and to achieve maximal tumor suppressive effect by postsurgical adjuvant therapy. After removal, complete hemostasis is necessary, before closing the dura mater. Sometimes covering the surface of the resected brain or tumor tissue with a sheet of Surgicel and fibrin glue prevents postsurgical hemorrhage. In cases of anaplastic glioma or glioblastoma, radiotherapy with chemotherapy is inevitable after surgery.

COMPLICATIONS

Complications are different for each approach. Several risks are well summarized by Sawaya et al.[23] The suboccipital transtentorial approach is quite safe if great care is taken not to damage bridging veins and the deep venous system. If retraction of the occipital lobe is too tight, the bridging veins or medial occipital veins are damaged causing a hemianopia. In my series, a large pineoblastoma in a 1-year-old boy was almost totally removed by this approach (Fig. 17-22). Although the patient's condition was good after the surgery, extensive subdural effusion was noted by MRI (Fig. 17-22B). The pineoblastoma recurred later, even though the boy was treated by radiochemotherapy following the surgical removal. The controversial problems of whether such huge malignant

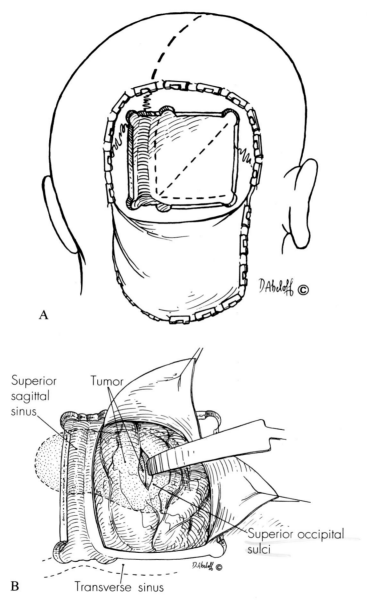

A

Superior
sagittal
sinus

Tumor

Superior occipital
sulci

B   Transverse sinus

Figure 17-21. The two-step operation shown in Figs. 17-19 and 17-20. **(A)** Skin incision, craniotomy, and the dural incision. **(B)** The first step. Transcortical approach. (*Figure continues.*)

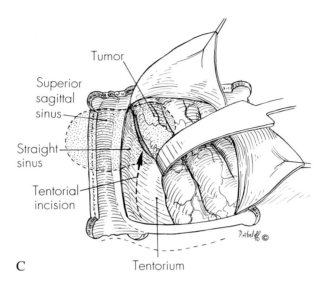

C

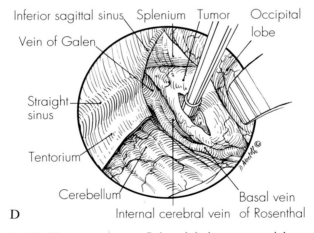

D

Figure 17-21. (*Continued*). **(C)** The second step. Suboccipital transtentorial approach. **(D)** The remaining tumor near the pineal region invading to the splenium.

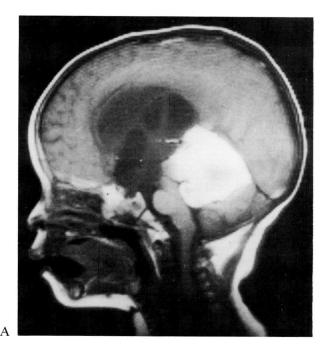 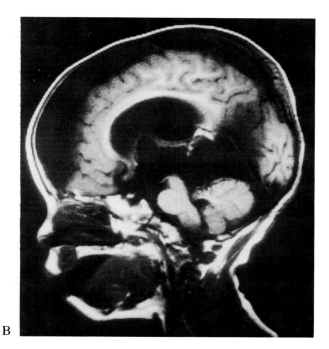

Figure 17-22. Pineoblastoma (MRI). **(A)** Before treatment. **(B)** After surgical removal.

tumors should be radically removed, or treated by chemotherapy alone after the biopsy remain.

The subtentorial supracerebellar approach is also safe, if care is taken not to damage the internal cerebral veins and other deep veins.[22,24] The major problem in this approach is inevitably a risk of air embolism in a sitting position. Every possible monitoring device must be set up before the operation. No hazardous complications have, however, been encountered in my series. The transcortical transventricular approach to tumors located mainly inside the third ventricle is safely performed under the microscope, since the small corticotomy (less than 3 cm in the silent area of the cortex) and gentle manipulation of the spatula with minimum pressure can prevent unexpected damage to the cerebral cortex. This approach provides good visualization inside the ventricle, which is often widely dilated at the time of operation. The risk of memory impairment is always present, however, if the contralateral fornix is damaged during the operation, after the widening the foramen of Monro by sectioning the ipsilateral fornix superiorly or anteriorly. To prevent damage to the fornix, it has been reported that the subchoroidal approach (dividing the thalamostriate vein) could prevent major complications.[17,20,26] Regarding the transcallosal approach disconnection syndrome is a major complication. The anterior transcallosal approach is safer than the posterior sectioning and a callosal incision less than 2.5 cm was not associated with detect-able disconnection syndrome.[23] In any case of operation for pineal region tumors, the risk of epileptic seizure after the surgery must be prevented by the appropriate administration of antiepileptic drugs. Phenytoin and phenobarbital should be administered starting from the preoperative period. Glucocorticoid is also administered at the time of surgery and in the postoperative period.

CONCLUSIONS

There are a variety of tumors in the pineal region, in terms of histological or biological characteristics as well as shape, size, and extension of the tumor. Several standard approaches each have their merits and demerits. Since MRI or CT scans can give us accurate morphological information, we can select the most reliable surgical approach for each tumor. Benign tumors such as teratoma, meningioma, or pineocytoma should be removed as completely as possible. Even in cases of malignant tumors such as malignant germ cell tumor, glioma, or pineoblastoma, radical surgical removal of the tumor can improve the effectiveness of adjuvant treatment with radiation and chemotherapy, as well as with biological response modifiers like interferon. The modifications for the standard approaches or the two-step operation as described here might improve the surgical result of pineal region tumors with minimal postoperative complications in certain cases.

Supratentorial Approaches to the Pineal Region

Michael L.J. Apuzzo
Howard Tung

Pineal region tumors are uncommon lesions comprising about 1 percent of intracranial neoplasms. A wide variety of histologically distinct tumor types may occur. Germ cell tumors, gliomas, and pineal cell tumors comprise the majority of neoplasms encountered in this region. The anatomical substrate of the pineal region and posterior part of the third ventricle, with its surrounding vital nervous and vascular structures draining delicate cerebral areas, have made surgical approaches to this region historically both difficult and dangerous. Harvey Cushing once stated that he "never succeeded in exposing a pineal tumor sufficiently well to justify an attempt to remove it."[40] Despite Cushing's lack of enthusiasm, various surgical approaches have been proposed for access to the pineal region since the early part of the century. These primary surgical corridors are separated into the infratentorial supracerebellar approach and the supratentorial approaches, which include the posterior transcallosal, the posterior transventricular, and the occipital transtentorial approaches. (Figs. 17-23 and 17-24).

The initial early experience with direct surgical access to the pineal region was extremely discouraging, creating high mortality and morbidity.[43,62,63,83,87,88,106] In an initial 10-year period Dandy[43] experienced seven consecutive deaths. In three other patients, one died 3 months after operation; one was well 4 months after operation; and one developed recurrence 2½ years after surgery.[43] In 1950, Horrax[62] reported 50 percent mortality within 3 months in 10 patients in which a radical removal of tumor was performed by a modified Dandy technique. Rand and Lemmen[83] reported a 70 percent mortality among 17 patients undergoing direct surgical approach for tumors located in the posterior portion of the third ventricle, and in 1954 Ringertz et al.[87] reported a 58.8 percent operative mortality in 51 patients who had either gross total or partial removal of their tumor.

Since these early attempts at surgery resulted in such poor outcome, the treatment bias at the time advocated ventricular shunting followed by radiation therapy.[28,36,39,62,67,81,83,87,102] However, subsequent reports began to document improved results with direct surgical approaches. In 1960 Kunicki[69] reported two operative deaths in eight patients with pineal tumors over 10 years utilizing the posterior interhemispheric transcallosal approach. In 1965, in one of the first reports supporting surgical intervention, Suzuki[101] optimistically reported on 19 patients with neoplasms of the posterior third ventricle. In all but two cases he obtained total or almost total extirpation with an operative mortality of 10 percent. In 1968, Poppen and Marino[81] described 45 cases of posterior third ventricular tumors. They reported that their early results by either the posterior transcallosal or the posterior intraventricular routes had met with disastrous results. However, the authors noted that more recently, after utilization of the occipital transtentorial route, better results were obtained in their series. In 1971, Jamieson[65] presented successful excision of eight pineal tumors without an operative death using a modification of the Poppen technique. In 1978, Reid and Clark[84] reported their experience with 15 patients undergoing excision of masses in the pineal region with only one postoperative death, presumably from brainstem edema.

With improvements in imaging, anatomical comprehension, neuroanesthesia, postoperative intensive care, microneurosurgical techniques, and recognition of CSF diversion for hydrocephalus, direct surgical approaches to the pineal region no longer carry the poor surgical prognosis of past years and may now be undertaken with acceptable risk.[39,45,49,59,65,71,72,79,89,98] In recent years, surgical mortality has been reported from 0 to 5 percent, with a minimal amount of long-term morbidity.[48,60,73,95,105] (Table 17-9). Moreover, since approximately 25 percent of pineal region tumors are marginated, surgery in this area affords an opportunity for an excellent outcome in cases in which gross total surgical excision is possible.[77,95,96] Furthermore, modern stereotactic techniques have provided a safe and accurate method for achieving direct tissue sampling for diagnosis and thus have avoided treating patients with "blind" radiotherapy or unnecessary or poor yield surgery[29,78] (Fig. 17-25).

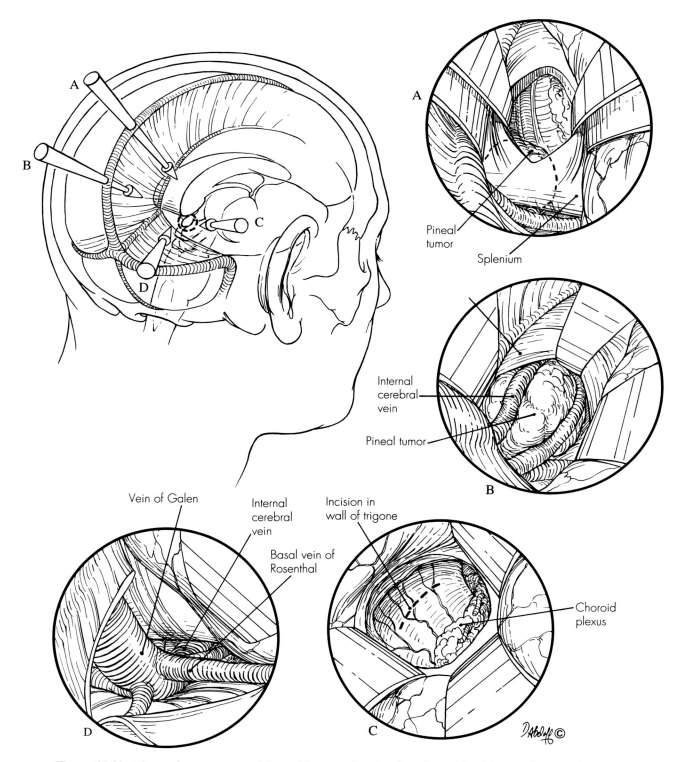

Figure 17-23. The major supratentorial corridors to the pineal region with ultimate view at pineal and parapineal site. **(A&B)** Posterior interhemispheric (transcallosal, retrocallosal.) **(C)** Posterior transventricular. **(D)** Occipital transtentorial.

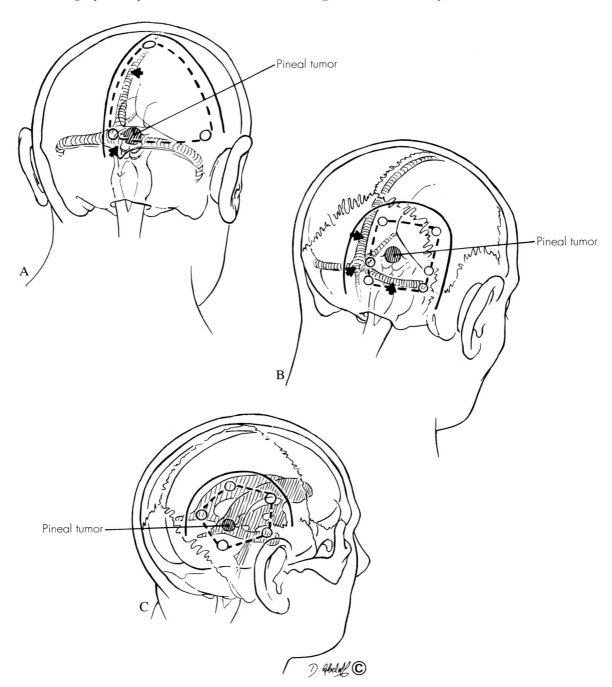

Figure 17-24. The basic scalp and bone flap positioning for entry in major supratentorial corridors. **(A)** Posterior interhemispheric (transcallosal, retrocallosal). **(B)** Occipital transtentorial. **(C)** Posterior transventricular.

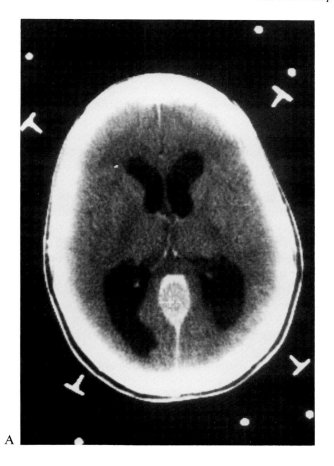

A

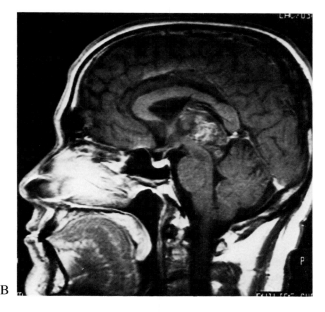

B

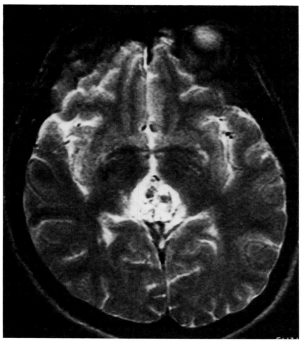

C

Figure 17-25. **(A)** Retropineal region mass in falcine leaflets. Histology debatable prior to stereotactic biopsy, which disclosed atypical teratoma. This rapidly resolved with radiation. **(B)** Sagittal T_1-weighted and **(C)** axial T_2-weighted MRI images of glioblastoma multiforme (stereotactic biopsy-proven) arising from left thalamic mass to occupy midline fluid void. Lesion managed with stereotactic biopsy verification, field and focused radiosurgical boost radiation without direct exploration with 26-month survival in a 42-year-old man.

Table 17-9.   Mortality Rates of Supratentorial
Approaches to the Pineal Region

Author	Year	Mortality (%)	No. of Cases
Dandy[43]	1936	70	10
Horrax[62]	1950	50	10
Rand and Lemmen[83]	1953	70	17
Ringertz et al.[87]	1954	59	51
Kunicki[69]	1960	25	8
Suzuki and Iwabuchi[101]	1965	10	17
Poppen and Marino[81]	1968	44	9[a]
Jamieson[65]	1971	0	8
Neuwelt et al.[76]	1979	5	16
Ventureyra[105]	1980	10	10[b]
Hoffman et al.[60]	1983	5	22
Lapras et al.[70,71]	1987	1	86
Edwards et al.[48]	1988	0	30
Luo[73]	1989	3	64

[a] Occipital transtentorial approach only.
[b] Single death was giant vein of Galen arteriovenous malformation.

Despite improved microsurgical technique and results over the years, direct surgical approaches to the pineal region and the avoidance of complications remain one of the most challenging ventures for the contemporary neurosurgeon. The various supratentorial approaches to the posterior third ventricle may require manipulation, incision, or excision of various neural or vascular structures.[86] This may include transcallosal or transcortical incisions; manipulation or division of the columns of the fornix, the walls of the third ventricle, and the deep venous system; and dissection and separation of a tumor from the quadrigeminal area. Reported complications and potential complications are related to the regional neural and vascular structures encountered, manipulated, or sacrificed during surgery. Injury to these neural and vascular structures in approaches to the third ventricle can produce well-defined deficits with anatomical-pathological correlation corresponding to the area injured and at other times can produce variable and inconstant deficits (Table 17-10).

THE DEEP CEREBRAL VENOUS SYSTEM

The components of the deep cerebral venous system, where the internal cerebral and basal veins converge to form the great vein (Galen's vein), provide an important potential threat for satisfactory outcome in all surgical approaches to the pineal region.

In addition, tributaries of the deep cerebral venous system are intimately related to the walls of the third ventricle. The paired internal cerebral veins originate behind the foramen of Monro and course posteriorly within the velum interpositum, where they exit above the pineal body to enter the quadrigeminal cistern and join Galen's vein. The terminal segment of the medial posterior choroidal artery courses anteriorly in the tela choroidea of the third ventricle close to the midline and inferior and medial to the internal cerebral veins. The velum interpositum is the space between the two layers of the tela choroidea in the roof of the third ventricle. The basal vein originates in the anterior incisural space and courses posteriorly between the midbrain and temporal lobe, exiting the ambient cistern to join the great vein of Galen. The great vein, formed by the union of the internal cerebral veins and basal veins, courses posteriorly and superiorly around the splenium to join the straight sinus at the anterior aspect of the falcotentorial junction. The straight sinus then courses posteroinferiorly along the falcotentorial junction to join the torcula. Along its course, the great vein receives many tributaries, accounting for a high density of veins in this area.[85,86]

Thrombosis of the deep venous system is rare and has been infrequently reported. Thrombosis of the internal cerebral venous channels has been associated with serious neurological defects. Majerszki and Majteni[74] described a clinical syndrome of headaches, altered mental status, nausea, dizziness, and rigidity of the neck muscles from thrombosis of the internal cerebral veins. Similarly, Ehlers and Courville[49] reported that thrombosis of the internal cerebral venous channels in infancy and childhood resulted in a variety of clinical symptoms including seizure, drowsiness, or coma, raised intracranial pressure, and elevated temperature. On the other hand, Johnson et al.[66] reported two cases of internal cerebral vein thrombosis of which both patients survived without serious neurological deficit, although one patient developed hydrocephalus and required a ventriculoperitoneal shunt.

Unfortunately, it is almost impossible to extrapolate information obtained from thrombosis of the deep cerebral venous system to possible neurological consequences after surgical occlusion of the deep cerebral venous system. Thrombosis of the galenic system is often related to trauma or infection and invariably involves branches of the superficial venous system or anastomotic channels with the deep venous system.

There is a paucity of information related to surgical occlusion of the deep venous system. Surgical sacri-

Table 17-10. Complications of Supratentorial Approaches to the Pineal Region

Author	Year	Approach	Complications
Dandy[43]	1936	Posterior transcallosal	Acutely raised intracranial pressure Transient blindness Homonymous hemianopsia Extraocular palsies Decreased upgaze
Horrax[62]	1950	Posterior transcallosal	Lethargy Parinaud syndrome Hemiparesis Homonymous hemianopsia Diabetes insipidus
Ringertz et al.[87]	1954	Posterior transcallosal	Hyperthermia (30%) Progressive coma Respiratory disturbances
Kunicki[69]	1960	Posterior transcallosal	Indifference and somnolence (100%) Hemiplegia (50%) Paralysis of upward gaze (83%)
Suzuki and Iwabuchi[101]	1965	Posterior transcallosal	Convulsions (57%) Hemiplegia (50%) Indifference and somnolence (36%) Decubitus (36%)
		Posterior transventricular	Indifference and somnolence (100%) Hemiplegia (100%) Decubitus (100%)

Jamieson[65]	1971	Occipital transtentorial	Homonymous hemianopsia
			    Transient (25%)
			    Permanent (12%)
			Intracerebral hemorrhage (12%)

Neuwelt et al.[76]	1979	Occipital transtentorial	Homonymous hemianopsia (17%) Transient hemiparesis (5%) Posterior fossa epidural clot (5%)
Ventureyra[105]	1980	Occipital transtentorial	Temporarily worsened Parinaud syndrome (28%) Temporary homonymous hemianopsia (14%) Temporary ataxia (14%) Seizure (14%)

Edwards et al.[48]	1988	Not specified	Immediate morbidity (27%)
			Persistent morbidity (10%)
			    Seizures
			    Hemiparesis
			    Homonymous hemianopsia
			    Meningitis

Luo[73]	1989	Occipital transtentorial	Morbidity (9%) Not specified

fice of branches of the superficial and deep cerebral venous system has produced inconsistent deficits. In a survey of neurosurgical program directors, of the 28 that replied, Smith and Sanford[93,94] reported that 35 percent believed cerebral infarction would ensue after surgical ligation of the internal cerebral vein while 47 percent believed cerebral infarction would follow surgical ligation of the great vein of Galen.

Experimentally, Bedford[32] reported on five monkeys who remained in good health and established collateral circulation after occlusion of the great vein of Galen.[32] In addition, Hammock et al.[56] selectively occluded the vein of Galen in rhesus monkeys without untoward clinical effects. They showed angiographic evidence of dilated major draining veins and sinuses, and microscopic dilatation of the smaller diencephalic and choroidal veins with occlusion of the great vein. Examination of the brains after vein of Galen occlusion revealed no evidence of vascular infarction or encephalomalacia.

Clinically, Dandy[43] noted that not infrequently sacrificing one internal cerebral vein could be accomplished without effect, and on a few occasions ligation of both internal cerebral veins and even the great vein could be carried out without serious neurological sequelae. Caron et al.[37] reported two cases in which there were no ill effects attributable to the obstruction of both internal cerebral veins during the resection of a pinealoma. Postoperatively, there was thrombosis of internal cerebral veins and of the basal vein of Rosenthal. Futhermore, Sakaki et al.[90] reported a case of a large pineal meningioma in which the vein of Galen was sacrificed without clinical sequelae. They suggested that obstruction of the great vein of Galen may be well tolerated in some cases, especially if the obstruction is gradual, allowing collaterals of the deep venous system to develop.

Nevertheless, every effort should be made to preserve the deep venous system because obliteration of the major vessels have been known to cause major deficits. Many complications have been reported with injury to this complicated venous network including diencephalic edema, mental symptoms, somnolence, coma, mutism, hyperpyrexia, tachypnea, tachycardia, rigidity of limbs, and exaggeration of deep tendon reflexes.[31,69,97,101,110]

SUPRATENTORIAL SURGICAL APPROACHES

As noted earlier, three major supratentorial corridors to the pineal region have been employed (Figs. 17-23 and 17-24).

Posterior Transcallosal Approach

In 1921, Dandy[42] reported a supratentorial parasagittal posterior parietal approach to the pineal region that apparently had as its basis an earlier report by Brunner in 1913.[34] This approach required an intraoperative ventricular puncture for egress of CSF, retracting the right hemisphere laterally, splitting the corpus callosum, and occasionally sacrificing the internal cerebral veins and several superior cerebral veins to obtain adequate exposure of the posterior third ventricle and pineal region. If required, an occipital lobectomy was also performed. This approach is best suited for posterior third ventricular masses arising in the corpus callosum above the great vein of Galen and extending to the posterior portion of the third ventricle or for masses in the third ventricle with the majority of the mass extending superiorly to the posterior part of the corpus callosum.

Although primary consideration must be given to parasagittal venous tributaries during anterior callosal approaches, this is a less important issue in posterior callosal approaches involving the posterior third of the nondominant cerebral hemisphere, which rarely gives significant tributaries to the posterior one-third of the sagittal sinus.[30,85,100] However, sacrificing the veins coursing between the cerebrum and the superior sagittal sinus anterior or posterior to the rolandic vein, although usually not causing a deficit, may be accompanied by hemiplegia.[69,92]

The posterior parietal lobe is retracted from the falx, exposing the corpus callosum. The cerebral retraction for the posterior interhemispheric approach has been associated with convulsions, hemiplegia, mutism, indifferent affect, somnolence, and visual field loss.[48,61,68,69,101]

The posterior portion of the corpus callosum is incised in the midline to enter the third ventricle and has been associated with a disconnection syndrome.[54] This incision may also divide the hippocampal commissure and open the lateral ventricle. Posterior callosal or splenial incision commonly results in left hemialexia and color anomia.[33,41,53,64,99,103,107] If accompanied by a left occipital lesion or any lesion causing a right hemianopsia, the syndrome *alexia without agraphia* becomes apparent, as first described by Dejerine.[44,52,53] When the splenial incision required is small, as in the case of a small vascular malformation, transverse sectioning of the splenium along the direction of its fiber tracts may reduce the complication rate for this procedure.[91,111] Midcallosal trunk section has produced inconsistent and minimum physiological sequelae including temporary mutism, generally inconsequential auditory effects, and possible tactile interactive deficits.[33] Dimond et al.[46] reported that surgical section of the posterior portion of the body of the corpus callosum can produce some memory defect. However, in this case, the corpus callosum was approached by a right-handed surgeon by retraction of the left cerebral hemisphere. More anteriorly, other deficits reported with callosal incisions include disorders of interhemispheric transfer of information, visuospatial transfer, the learning of bimanual motor tasks, and memory.[33,41,46,51,53,82,91,104] Memory loss has also been reported with extensive commissurotomy in which the hippocampal commissure was sectioned.[112] Heilman and Sypert[58] reported a patient with amnesia and a glioma in the region of the hippocampal commissure; after subtotal excision, the patient manifested a profound and persistent amnestic deficit.

The medial posterior choroidal arteries and their branches are intermingled with the internal cerebral veins and are frequently exposed in approaches through the corpus callosum. Although a potential source for infarction, usually at this point they have given off the majority of their neural branches.[85,109,110]

Below pineal tumors lies the area of the quadrigeminal plate including the superior and inferior colliculi, superior cerebellar arteries, and trochlear nerve. Often the most dangerous dissection is in this area as tumors may be tightly adherent to or embedded in this area. Dissection of the area of the quadrigeminal plate may cause disorders of eye movement, extraocular palsies due to edema of the nuclei of the nerves or central pathways in the brainstem, blindness from edema in the colliculi or geniculate bodies, or acute hydrocephalus from edematous closure of the aqueduct of Sylvius.[43] In particular, dissection in this sensitive area may exacerbate or create a complete or partial Parinaud syndrome.[43,61,62,69,72,165] Injury to the superior cerebellar artery in approaches to the posterior third ventricle and pineal region may cause a cerebellar deficit.

Posterior Transventricular Approach

The posterior transventricular approach for the excision of pineal tumors was first suggested by Van Wagenen in 1931[104] (Fig. 17-26). This represents a feasible but infrequently applied corridor.[104] He utilized a parietooccipital bone flap and a cortical incision extending from the posterior end of the superior temporal gyrus into the inferior part of the parietal lobe to enter a dilated right lateral ventricle. In his original case, the patient had initial postoperative complications including Biot-type respirations, left hemiplegia, left hemianopsia, and sensory deficits of hypoaesthesia with astereognosis on the patient's left side. Since its introduction, the temporal approach has been rarely used because of the likelihood of postoperative neurologic deficits such as hemianopsia and hemiparesis.[61,81,101] Horrax[61] reported successful extirpation of a large pineal tumor utilizing the transventricular approach, but the patient experienced hemiplegia, homonymous hemianopsia, lateral gaze palsy, and lethargy postoperatively.

A more preferable approach has been through a high parietal bone flap using a cortical incision in the superior parietal lobule.[55] This avoids the visual pathways traversing the parietal lobe and the speech areas at the junction of the parietal and temporal lobes in the dominant hemisphere. This approach provides adequate exposure of the atrium and posterior portion of the body of the lateral ventricle. It is best suited for posterior thalamic and parathalamic tumors involving the third ventricle, for third ventricular tumors extending from the third ventricle to the

posterior portion of the lateral ventricle, or for lesions involving predominantly the atrium or glomus of the choroid plexus.

Through a medial parietal bone flap, the dura is opened medially with sparing of the bridging veins to the sagittal sinus. The cortical incision is made with the long axis of the superior parietal lobule behind the postcentral gyrus. If the cortical incision is carried too far anteriorly, a potential for sensory deficits exists. The cortical incision and cereberal retraction used in the posterior transventricular approach has resulted in postoperative complications including convulsions, hemiplegia, hemianopsia, sensory disturbances, somnolence, and impaired consciousness.[62,81,102] In three cases utilizing this approach for pineal region tumors Suzuki's[101] patients experienced uniform postoperative mental clouding, indifferent attitude and hemiplegia; two conditions were temporary. Approaches through the dominant hemisphere have the theoretical potential of causing the Gerstmann syndrome as a postoperative complication.

Upon entering the lateral ventricle, the choroid plexus along the choroidal fissure provides an orienting landmark. To expose the third ventricle, an incision through the body and crus of the fornix in the direction of the fibers of the fornix is carried out, sparing the contralateral half of the fornix. An amnestic syndrome may potentially accompany manipulation and excision of the fornices bilaterally, although this is usually associated with more anterior approaches. There is no agreement in the literature on whether fornix integrity is required for normal memory. Bilateral fornical sectioning has been implicated in causing memory deficit,[58,96] while other reports have shown absence of memory disturbance with bilateral fornical sectioning.[35,47,50,108] It seems probable that an additional abnormality must accompany bilateral fornical damage for a flagrant amnestic syndrome to appear.

The internal cerebral veins, great vein, and medial posterior choroidal artery often are distorted and may obstruct direct exposure of a pineal tumor. As with the posterior transcallosal approach, sacrifice and manipulation of the deep venous system may result in neurological deficit, as well as dissection in the sensitive region of the quadrigeminal area.

Occipital Transtentorial Approach

The occipital transtentorial approach was initially described by Poppen in 1966.[80] In his description, Poppen utilized the sitting position and a small right occipital craniectomy in approaching the pineal region (Fig. 17-27). Because of limited exposure, this

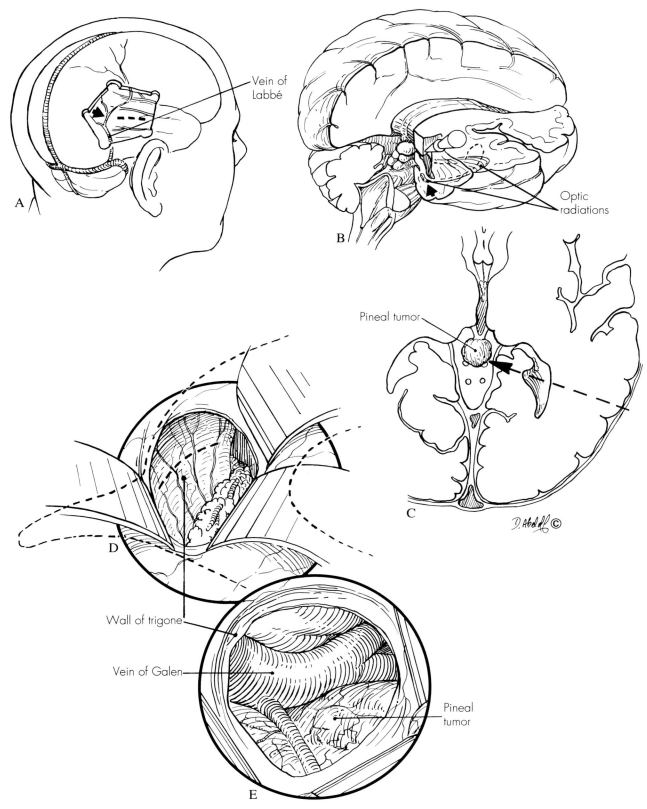

Figure 17-26. The posterior transventricular approach to the pineal region (Van Wagenen[104]) with **(A&B)** original transtemporal entry depicted to gain access to **(C)** dilated ventricular system at trigone. **(D&E)** Subsequent exposure yields visualization of lateral view of pineal and retropineal mass. This approach requires retraction, and a neural sacrifice that is not a risk with other supratentorial corridors and *is not recommended.*

494

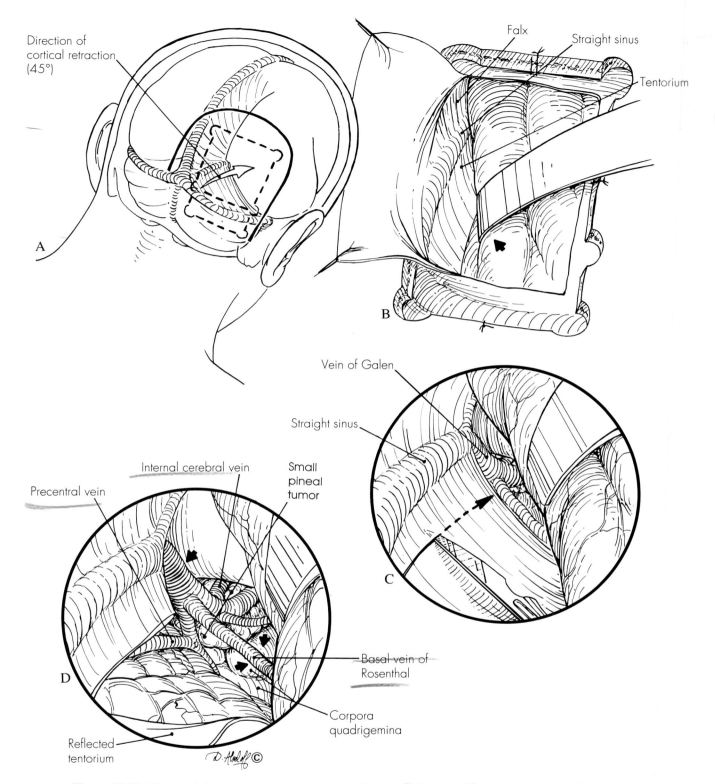

Figure 17-27. The occipital transtentorial approach (Poppen,[80] Jamieson[65]). **(A)** An occipital craniotomy placed at the peritorcular region allows **(B)** retraction of the medial and basal occipital parietal axis with **(C)** tentorium and subsequent incisural exposure. **(D)** A para-straight sinus tentorial incision provides pineal region exposure. Exposure requires midline and tentorial access for minimization of retraction and reduction of potential for calcarine injury.

technique was later modified by Jamieson in 1971.[65] In his series of eight patients, Jamieson did not experience a single operative mortality, but two patients had immediate morbidity of temporary homonymous hemianopsia from cerebral retraction, while a third patient suffered a permanent homonymous hemianopsia from a postoperative hemorrhage in the occipital lobe. Jamieson concluded that the pineal region could be approached safely surgically with low mortality and morbidity and also underscored the importance of obtaining a histological diagnosis for masses in the pineal region. This approach is suitable for those tumors in the pineal region centered at or above the tentorial edge without major extension into the posterior fossa.

In Jamieson's technique, a right occipital craniotomy is performed and the dura is opened. The occipital pole is retracted superiorly and laterally. Retraction of the occipital lobe has been related to postoperative visual complications of transient or permanent homonymous hemianopsia as well as transient hemiplegia.[65,76,81,84] In a series of 17 patients, Clark[38,76] experienced three instances of hemianopsia; however, with subsequent utilization of the park bench position and gravity-assisted retraction of the occipital lobe, postoperative visual field deficits have been reduced significantly. There are usually no bridging veins between the medial occipital pole and transverse sinuses such that the occipital lobe may be retracted without sacrificing bridging veins.

However, sacrifice of bridging veins to the transverse sagittal sinus may potentially cause venous infarction with subsequent visual deficit.[110] The internal occipital vein may be seen usually originating from the inferior medial surface of the occipital lobe and running anteromedially toward the pineal region ending in the vein of Galen. Sacrifice of the internal occipital vein, although usually occurring without deficit, has been associated with hemianopsia.[57,109]

The tentorium is incised approximately 1 to 1.5 cm parallel to the straight sinus, and injury to the straight sinus may result in cerebral edema or coma. The arachnoid is next opened and often the vein of Galen and its tributaries obstruct the approach to a tumor. As with the other supratentorial approaches, injury to the deep venous system may cause significant neurological deficit or no deficit at all. The precentral cerebellar veins are sagittally arranged in the midline and join the great vein inferiorly. These are usually sacrificed without neurological consequence.[70,95] Lapras[70,71] has operated on 58 patients; none (with late follow-up) have had cerebellar sequelae following sacrifice of these veins. The splenium is usually ele-

vated by a pineal tumor and may be spared, but the lower portion may be encountered and divided if necessary with the possible ensuing complication of a disconnection syndrome. Finally, as with the other supratentorial approaches, meticulous attention is directed toward dissection in the quadrigeminal area, especially in the contralateral half, which may be inadequately visualized. Damage to the quadrigeminal area may cause a worsening Parinaud syndrome, palsies of the extraocular muscles, or acute hydrocephalus from closure of the sylvian aqueduct.

OPERATIVE CONSIDERATIONS

As with anterior and mid-third ventricular masses, primary objectives in the management of pineal region masses include:

1. Defining histology of the process
2. Normalizing cerebral spinal fluid dynamics
3. Achieving maximum lesion excision
4. Decompressing focal pressure effects

As always, these objectives must be achieved with minimization of patient risk. Direct supratentorial approaches to the region are attended by risks of cortical, midhemispheric, thalamic, rostral brainstem, and cerebellar injury. In addition, major hypothalamic injury and central hemispheric injury may be initiated by venous damage to the vein of Galen and internal cerebral and basilar veins of Rosenthal. In our opinion, anterior transcallosal and lateral transcortical approaches carry either excessive tissue sacrifice or excessive corridor lengths for strictly "pineal region" (posterior third ventricular-quadrigeminal cistern) masses and therefore are not generally employed or advised. In the event that a supratentorial corridor to the pineal region is indicated, posterior interhemispheric approaches have proved superior from standpoints of view line, flexibility, and safety of application and therefore will be dealt with extensively in this section of avoidance and management of problems (Figs. 17-28 to 17-30).

SELECTION

The posterior interhemispheric approach is an appropriate operative corridor for:

1. Lesions that occupy the posterior third ventricle and quadrigeminal cisterns or straddle the same (Fig. 17-31)
2. Lesions with dural involvement or attachment in the region of the vein of Galen and straight sinus regions (Fig. 17-32)

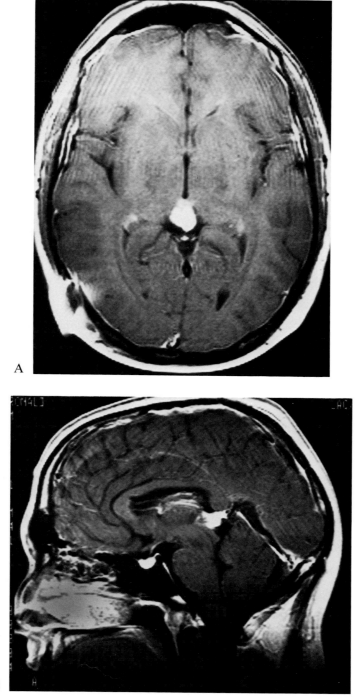

Figure 17-28. **(A)** Axial and **(B)** sagittal contrast-enhanced T$_1$-weighted MRIs of subsplenial pineal region mass with distortion of the superior quadrageminal plate (pineocytoma). Intrahemispheric transtentorial corridor affords good visual access.

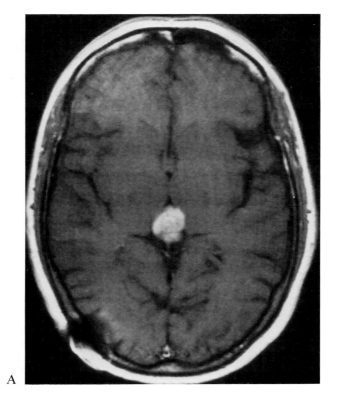

A

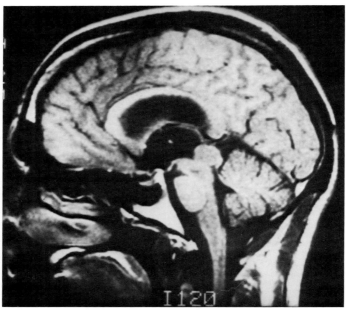

B

Figure 17-29. **(A)** Axial and **(B)** sagittal T_1-weighted MRIs of astrocytoma straddling posterior third-ventricular-quadrageminal cisternal space. Retrocallosal corridor with transtentorial exposure affords good access.

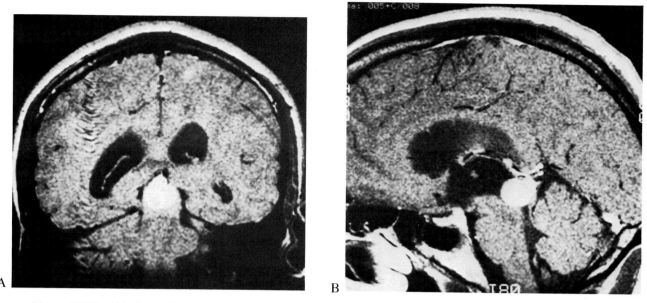

Figure 17-30. **(A)** Coronal and **(B)** sagittal contrast-enhanced T₁-weighted MRIs of pineocytoma distorting iter entry with posterior displacement of quadrageminal plate. Interhemispheric line of sight 5 cm above torcular provides short and accessible corridor for excision by retrosplenial transtentorial route.

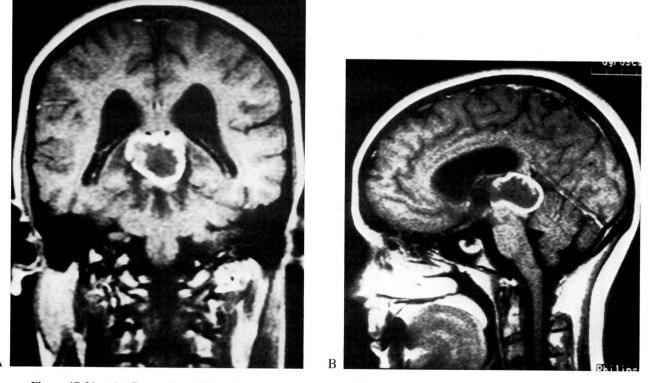

Figure 17-31. **(A)** Coronal and **(B)** sagittal contrast-enhanced T₁-weighted MRIs of 3.5 × 3.0 cm apparently cystic lesion straddling subspleneal space. Note line of sight 5 cm superior to torcula in interhemispheric corridor. Glioblastoma multiforme in a 20-year-old woman.

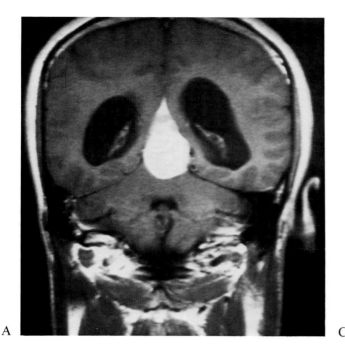

A

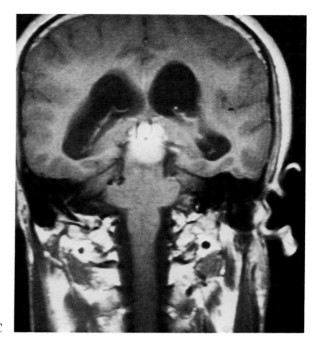

C

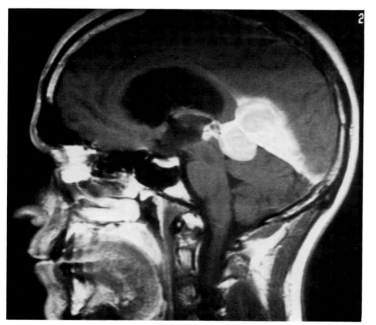

B

Figure 17-32. Contrast-enhanced **(A)** posterior coronal, **(B)** sagittal, and **(C)** anterior coronal T$_1$-weighted MRIs in a 26-year-old man. This complex structural lesion is ideally approached employing the options attendant to the interhemispheric corridor. Tentorial meningioma.

Its major advantages with respect to the infratentorial supracerebellar approach are:

1. Ability to perform surgery comfortably with the patient in a semiprone position, thus reducing the danger of air emboli
2. A shorter corridor to the operative target site
3. Wide and comfortable access to the entire region of the straight sinus, posterior falcine, tentorial junction

Its major disadvantages with respect to infratentorial supracerebellar approaches include:

1. A more difficult anatomical orientation
2. Superior transvenous access to mass lesions required
3. Anatomy less constant to the region of pathology
4. Ventriculomegaly required for optimization of safety. Although not an absolute requirement for its undertaking, ventriculomegaly facilitates the approach and re-

duces the incidence of cortical complications in most hands

TECHNIQUE OF POSTERIOR INTERHEMISPHERIC CORRIDOR IN PINEAL REGION EXPOSURE

The exploration of the pineal region by any corridor presents a complex anatomical and physiological undertaking. Avoidance of complications relates to an obsessive attention to detail from all aspects of patient evaluation and therapeutic action during preoperative, intraoperative, and postoperative settings. An *adagio di molto* attitude is essential.

Preoperative Assessment

Imaging

Contemporary imaging is imperative in defining lesion position, size, contour, extent, vascularity, and variabilities in content; all of these are determinants of intraoperative action during corridor selection, modification, and lesion excision. These images govern three-dimensional comprehension of the surgeon during the surgical event. In this complex approach, safety of excision and avoidance of unsatisfactory results cannot be maximized without full exploitation of magnetic resonance imaging in multiple planes of perspective. Concurrently, absolute definition of distortion of normal anatomy are displayed that are critical for orientation at the falcine tentorial junction, where critical neural and vascular structures are to be recognized and preserved.

Presurgical Preparation

Instrumentation

Proper availability of microinsturmentation peculiar to "long-reach" midline exposures are necessary. Comfortable working lengths of instrumentation should attain 10 cm. Self-retaining retractor systems in proper working order with availability of multiple tapered blades are key to the safety of the procedures. Operators should be familiar with all nuances of the systems operation. We have employed a Buddie system with multiple blade modifications.

Zeiss Contraves microinstrumentation with a 275 objective or a variable focal length system provides the basis for ease of access and maximum flexibility of view line and instrument accessability.

Intracranial Pressure

There is no doubt that improper or suboptimal control of mass intracranial content will create a substrate for multiple complications and possibly premature termination of the operative procedure. High-potency glucocorticoids should be employed. If ventriculomegaly is apparent, ventriculostomy should be employed and noted to be in working order before field draping is undertaken at the time of the procedure.

In the event that ventriculostomy is not required before the operative event, care should be taken not to "overdrain," thus losing the advantages of temporal reduction of the enlarged ventricular system at the time of the procedure. A right-sided placement of the pericoronal catheter is utilized for this approach. As always, preoperative or intraoperative drainage should be undertaken carefully with slow decompression and consideration of remote subdural bridging venous injury.

Obviously, from the purely technical sense, ventriculostomy is preferrable to preoperative shunting, especially with this corridor or in cases in which a high probability for restoration of CSF pathways exists within the direct surgical undertaking.

Surgical Procedure

Stage I: Positioning

We employed the three-quarter prone body position with the head in the oblique 45-degree angle and the right hemispheric dependent (i.e., three-quarter prone dependent oblique). This position has the advantage of reduction of possibility of air embolism during the opening, gravity enhancement of the interhemispheric slot, and absolute surgeon comfort for extended periods. Its major disadvantages are the complexity of the positioning and the oblique head position, which at times may be a source of disorientation to the surgeon. To avoid problems during positioning, the Mayfield head-holder is applied in proper orientation prior to turning the patient to the initial prone position. The left thorax is then elevated on a roll, two pillows are placed to elevate the interior legs and flex the feet, and an axillary roll is placed under the right axilla as the right arm is allowed to fall flexed over the head end of the table partially supported by the head-holder connection.

The head is fixed in the dependent 45-degree oblique position and the foot of the operating table dropped, elevating the head to a supracardiac position. All pressure surfaces are afforded soft foam padding, and the pelvis is fixed with a stationary belt. Finally, all potential intraoperative modifications of table position are accessed to ensure patient stability and pressure point protection (Fig. 17-33).

It should be stressed that during this evolution, three personnel are required in addition to the operating room surgeon and anesthesiologist to ensure the safety and optimization of positioning.

Stage II: Establishing the Corridor to the Pineal Region

Scalp and Bone Flap

To avoid problems and lack of access, overretraction, and obscuration of view lines, absolute midline access from 1 cm superior to the torcula to 9 cm from the torcula is essential. Scalp and bone flaps are de-

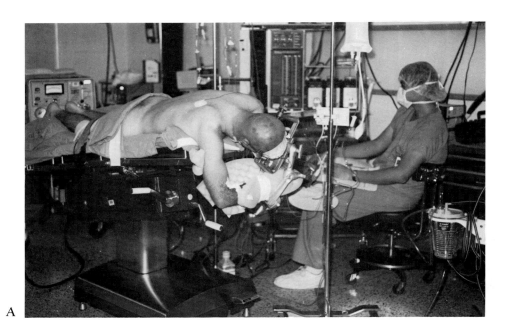

A

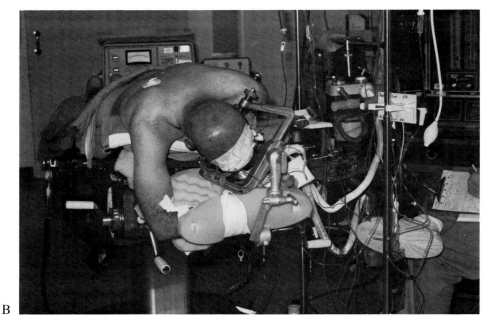

B

Figure 17-33. Demonstration of the 45-degree oblique patient position (semiprone/semilateral) with head in dependent oblique position. Note **(A)** angulation of table and securing of pelvis and **(B)** axillary roll, forearm padding adjacent to table, and Mayfield adaptor system. (*Figure continues.*)

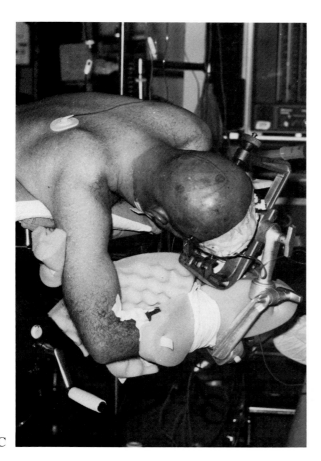

C

Figure 17-33 (*Continued*). Note **(C)** angle of head with dependent fixation, ventriculostomy tube, and scalp marking. Three individuals other than the surgeon are required for rapid and safe evolution of positioning.

signed to achieve this end. In contrast to the anterior hemispheric approaches, the posterior interhemispheric corridor does not usually present, difficulties of management of parasagittal venous drainage. However, injury to the sagittal sinus in its posterior third is particularly hazardous (Figs. 17-24, 17-33C, and 17-34).

A 10-cm incision is marked 2 cm lateral to the midline on the left, extending from the inion to the vertex; at its apex the second limb of the mitre is extended laterally 8 cm. This incision gives midline orientation by identification of the sagittal suture. Care is taken to orient properly before draping because of the oblique head position. We generally employ a three-hole bone flap with burr holes placed adjacent to the midline with secondary blunt dissection over the sagittal sinus. A third hole is placed over the right lateral extent of the exposed cranium with the intent of fashioning a mitre with its base on the lateral sinus line. In the event that epidural dis-

section is difficult or unsatisfactory, it is imperative that further midline burr holes be placed to avoid venous sinus injury. An alternative method is right paramedian craniectomy with rongeur craniectomy to the midline, a more cumbersome and less satisfactory technique.

Prior to turning the bone flap, all hemostatic materials and sutures should be ready in the event that sinus injury is apparent. Rapid action is required to minimize blood loss at the time the bone flap is turned. For orientation, a strip of Surgicel is placed over the sagittal sinus. Tenting sutures are placed immediately at the craniotomy edge with care taken to avoid excessive remote epidural dissection, which could be a source of hemorrhage once the ventriculostomy is opened for volume reduction. The Buddie retractor system is brought in to the field.

Midline Exposure and Parafalcine Dissection

The dura is opened laterally (inferiorly) and reflected medially, as opposed to the anterior paramedian approach; parasagittal venous tributaries and granulations are not usually problematical; the ventriculostomy is opened for hemispheric decompression with care being taken not to overdrain to the point of creating an excessive decompression, setting the stage for a subdural or epidural hemorrhage. As the sagittal sinus is approached, care is taken not to lacerate the structure, and as the dura is reflected across the midline, excessive retraction is not employed, which could occlude the outflow. The occipital pole is identified and a direct parafalcine midline view is established. The operating room microscope and a 19-mm tapered (to 5-mm) retractor blade is brought into the field, and very gentle retraction is employed to initiate and develop the midline slot. The calacrine region is adjacent to the medial wall and should be protected by awareness, gentle retraction, and the barrier protection of Biocol or soft cottonoids as the exposure is developed. The combination of osmotic agents, CSF drainage, and gravity generally makes deep midline access a simple and nonthreatening surgical exposure. However, problems may occur related to deep orientation due to the lack of definition and of the falx tentorial junction, which commonly blends without either angulation or visual cues of color change provided by the straight sinus (Fig. 17-35). There may be a tendency to over-retract at this point. It is important to be aware of the fact that the midline slot should not exceed 2 cm from medial to lateral extent, with no more than 7 cm of deformation from the occipital pole. The dissection

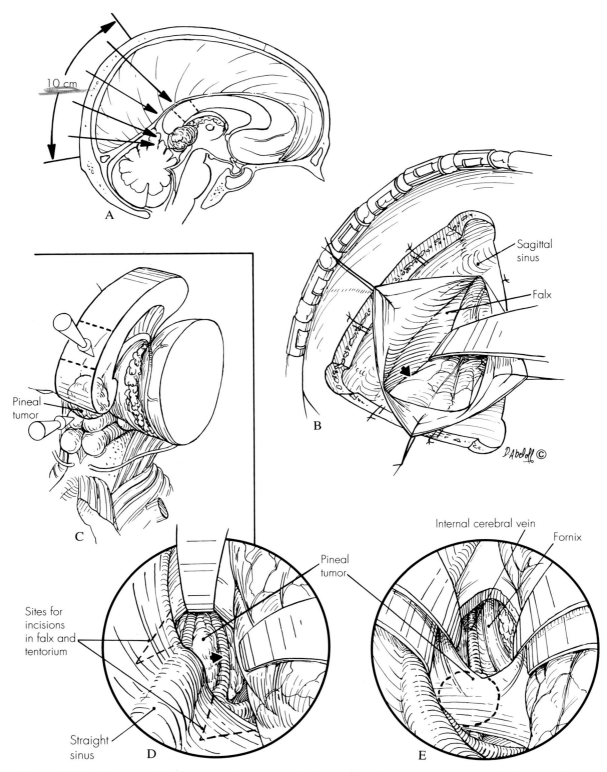

Figure 17-34. The essential elements of interhemispheric exposure by posterior access. **(A)** Ten-centimeter midline exposure for its flexibility of view line and access. **(B)** Visualization of sagittal sinus with excellent midline exposure and dependent position minimizes retraction requirements. **(C)** Access to region may be directed through transcallosal or retrocallosal routes. **(D)** Retrocallosal exposure to pineal region may be enhanced by retraction maneuvers or tentorial section adjacent to straight sinus. **(E)** Transcallosal exposure should avoid splenial or venous injury during transit.

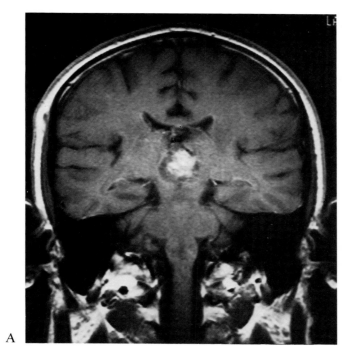

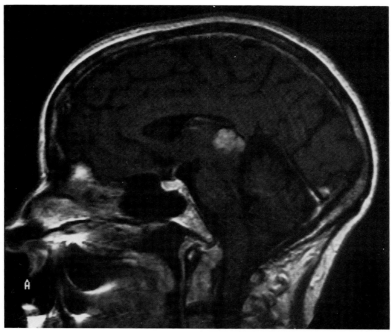

Figure 17-35. **(A)** Coronal and **(B)** sagittal contrast-enhanced T₁-weighted MRIs of dermoid in posterior third ventricle **(C–H)** demonstrate relation of tentorium and falx to cisterns, neural elements, and tumor in the posterior anterior progression. Note tentorial curvature and slope of falx junction and slope to falx junction and incisura. The straight sinus, an anticipated landmark for orientation, is frequently not easily identifiable, and disorientation occurs along the slope of the tentorium unless the incisura is identified. (*Figure continues.*)

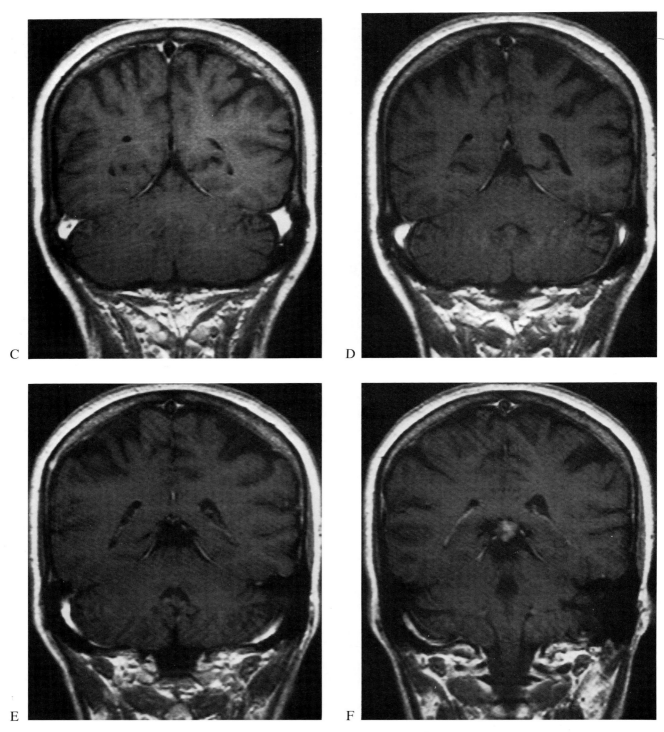

Figure 17-35 (*Continued*).

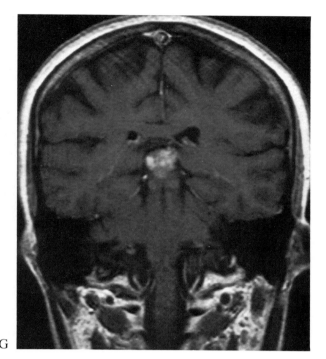

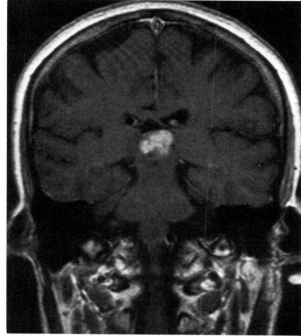

G

H

Figure 17-35 (*Continued*).

plane should proceed anteriorly along the falx with orientation provided by appreciation of head position, falx alignment, and measurements attained from images. The inferior falcine border, corpus callosum, and posterior incisura may be readily appreciated. The white splenium frequently provides a visually striking landmark for orientation.

Stage III: Lesion Identification and Excision

Keys to maximizing excision and minimizing problems and outcome include:

1. Recognizing anatomical distortion as defined by images
2. Identification and preservation of the vein of Galen, internal cerebral veins, and basal veins of Rosenthal
3. Maximizing exposure of the region by fenestration of dural leaflets (falx and tentorium)
4. Preservation of neural surfaces in the quadrigeminal cistern (tectal plate) and third ventricle (thalamic and hypothalamic walls)
5. Variations of microscopic view lines in corridors to gain visual access secondarily
6. Preservation of continuity of the splenium of the corpus callosum if possible to avoid transferred deficits

Exposure Options

Following identification of the target regions exposure may be enhanced to maximum dimensions by a combination of retraction and sacrifice of dural leaf-

lets in the region. In addition, (rarely) neural sacrifice is required to maximize exposure corridors by lesion excision or emergent exposure access. Maximization and visualization at the onset of lesion excision will minimize potential complications (Fig. 17-34). Technical maneuvers for access in direct lines of sight include:

1. Incision of the tentorium
2. Incision of the falx
3. Retraction of the splenium
4. Incision of the splenium
5. Incision of the posterior trunk
6. Alteration of microscope angulation for line of sight
7. Utilization of angulated mirror systems
8. Retraction of anterior vermian components
9. Incision and resection of cerebellar vermian components

In affecting each of these exposure options, care must be taken to make every effort to preserve the major venous elements in the region. Once achieved, the maximized exposure will afford not only increased view of mass surface and contour, but also better appreciation of all major components of venous anatomy. In the event that venous laceration occurs, every effort must be made to avoid complete venous tributary sacrifice or occlusion. Temporary Gelfoam, Surgicel, and cottonoid tamponade is preferred to coagulation. Temporary changes in head position may be required to attain desired control and

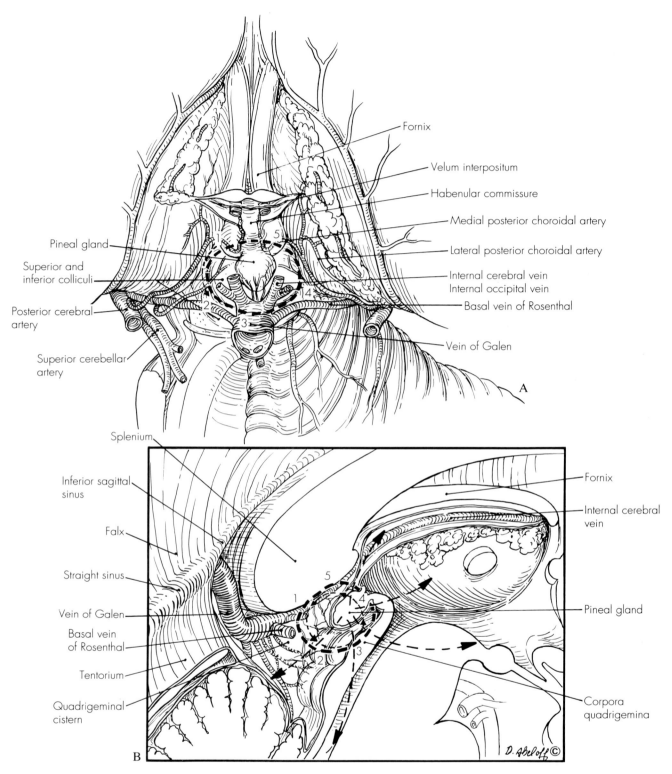

Fornix

Velum interpositum

Habenular commissure

Medial posterior choroidal artery

Lateral posterior choroidal artery

Internal cerebral vein
Internal occipital vein

Basal vein of Rosenthal

Vein of Galen

Pineal gland

Superior and inferior colliculi

Posterior cerebral artery

Superior cerebellar artery

A

Splenium

Inferior sagittal sinus

Falx

Straight sinus

Vein of Galen

Basal vein of Rosenthal

Tentorium

Quadrigeminal cistern

B

Fornix

Internal cerebral vein

Pineal gland

Corpora quadrigemina

D. Abeloff©

Figure 17-36. (A&B) Demonstration of regional anatomy at pineal region target area with growth dispersal pattern **(B).** The pattern for stepwise lesion excision is noted numerically on the illustrations. Internal decompression is followed by capsular dissection with care taken to avoid pressure transmission to adjacent neural structures. Capsular dissection from neurovascular structures is continued only in the event that planes are identifiable and easily achieved. Preservation of major venous tributaries is essential. Variation of microscope view lines and applying maneuvers for enhancement of exposure are key principles for successful excision.

hemostasis. In achieving exposure, tentorial incision is the most commonly used maneuver with a No. 11 blade knife used for initial incision 2 to 3 cm posterior to the incisural margin and 1.5 cm lateral to the straight sinus. The free edge may then be retracted or a wedge removed, giving free visual access to the posterior third ventricle and quadrigeminal cystern region. A secondary tapered retractor blade may then be introduced to displace the cerebellum or splenium to enhance exposure further caudally or rostrally. Occasionally the splenium is displaced or thinned by the mass. In these circumstances, some limited resection is feasible.

Lesion Dissection and Excision

With exposure maximized, distortion of venous anatomy with identification of the vein of Galen, proximal internal cerebral veins, and right basal vein

of Rosenthal should be apparent. The mass may be obscured by a veil of arachnoid, and this is opened. In general, it is our practice to obtain histological verification of a lesion before progressing with aggressive excision. Our approach is modified by the nature of the lesion. In most cases, internal decompression is initiated with biopsy followed by standard microscopic peripheral dissection with piecemeal excision of walls in the following stepwise fashion (Fig. 17-36):

1. Superior and left lateral mass component
2. Inferior left lateral mass component
3. Inferior mass component
4. Inferior and right lateral mass component

Ranging and angulation changes with the operating microscope are essential during these stages to maximize view lines and minimize line dissection and excessive tugging on capsular surfaces, which may

Table 17-11. Intraoperative Complications

Problem	Avoidance
Intracranial mass/brain swelling	Proper bone flap placement Minimization of retraction High potency glucocorticoids Diuresis Hyperventilation Proper head positioning Ventriculostomy Surface brain protection
Intracranial pressure control/ hydrocephalus	Ventriculostomy functioning well Temporal reduction of ventricular system Microdissection, irrigation
Deep venous system injury	Identification and preservation of venous anatomy Tamponade rather than coagulation if possible Optimization of exposure
Sagittal sinus injury	Care in placement of burr holes and bone flap Proper hemostatic materials and sutures Careful retraction of falx/sagittal sinus when necessary
Local neural injury	Recognition of normal and pertinent anatomy Preservation of neural surfaces (tectal plate, thalamic and hypothalamic walls) Microdissection, judgement to stop, irrigation
Inadequate intraoperative exposure	Selection of appropriate operative corridor Adequate definition of lesion by neuroradiological imaging Development of local exposure Maneuver to enhance access
Disorientation during initial corridor development	Relation of images to observed anatomy and anatomical landmarks that are observable Reorientation of retractor angle Identification of tentorial or falcine edge Identification of (white) splenium
Suboptimal lesion excision	Optimization of corridor Optimization of local exposure Understanding specific anatomy Changing view lines Availability of all proper microinstrumentation

result in remote injury or hemorrhage. Constant use of microirrigation to the field and particularly to lateral margins of interface enhances dissection planes. It cannot be overemphasized that *all* planes of dissection and peripheral attachment in these lesions are key. In the event that dissection planes are resistant, prudence demands *retreat*.

Exophytic components of intrinsic tumors are excised, but intra-axial components of dorsal brainstem and thalamic neoplasms, particularly if malignant, are not aggressively pursued.

Tenuous attachments are often encountered in the region of the Iter outlet and superior quadrigeminal plate; these attachments resist excision and are generally not the subject of aggressive surgical action.

Soft lesions that are readily aspiratable are simple matters of technical excision in the event that adequate exposure has been established. At completion of excision, visualization of the complete third ventricle with both foramina of Monro is achieved. A satisfactory excision yields healthy thalamic, hypothalamic, and quadrageminal surfaces for inspection.

Stage IV: Closure

Copeous irrigation with bacitracin and Ringer's lactate solution sets the stage for a complete hemo-

Table 17-12. Postoperative Complications

Complication	Avoidance
Intracranial hemorrhage	Patience (intraoperative) Meticulous hemostasis (with proper hemostatic materials) Irrigation SABP control
Pneumocephalis/remote subdural hematoma	Slow ventricular drainage intraoperatively, no overdrainage of ventricular system, refill ventricles with irrigation at termination of procedure, subdural drain
Brain swelling	Minimization of retraction intraoperatively, continued high-potency glucocorticoids; fluid management as regulated Venous preservation
Intracranial pressure control/ hydrocephalus	Ventriculostomy with drainage as necessary
Seizures	Prophylactic anticonvulsants (level adequate)
Infection, meningitis	Intraoperative antibiotics Preoperative antibiotics Postoperative antibiotics Copious irrigation
Infarction	Recognition and preservation of deep venous and arterial anatomy, surface protection Hydration SABP control
Parinaud syndrome	Maximization of local exposure Gentle dissection, preservation of neural surfaces Avoidance of sinus retraction or injury
Hemiparesis	Minimization of cerebral retraction intraoperatively Preservation of neural surfaces
Brain transfer deficits	Preservation of continuity of splenium of corpus callosum
Homonymous hemianopsia	Avoidance of minimization of calcarine retraction Proper positioning of patient intraoperatively Proper brain relaxation intraoperatively
Coma, death	Preservation of important neural surfaces Avoidance of brainstem injury Avoidance of deep vascular injury Maximization of local exposure Avoidance of sagittal sinus and peritorcular sinus injury Meticulous deep hemostasis

Abbreviation: SABP, systemic arterial blood pressure.

stasis with bipolar forceps. Good general relaxation and pulsation of brain surfaces should be observed. The field should be completely filled with body temperature solutions before dural closure is initiated; all air should be displaced. Retractors are removed and intrahemispheric surfaces inspected (particularly exposed and remote areas) with either the microscope or the headlight. After a watertight dural closure has been established, the bone flap is replaced with middle dural tenting sutures in place. We employ no drains in the subgaleal space on this procedure (Table 17-11).

Postoperative Period

Major complications in the early postoperative period will relate to hemorrhage and uncontrolled CSF obstruction. Monitoring of interventricular pressure is essential during the first 48 hours whether or not shunting was undertaken. This vigilance applies to "total" excision of benign lesions as well. Neurological defects of the regional nature will manifest early in the postoperative course, and imaging is required to rule out a surgically remediable cause (Table 17-12).

Supracerebellar Approaches in the Pineal Region

Jeffrey N. Bruce
Bennett M. Stein

Advances in neuroanesthesia, microsurgical technique, and neuroradiological imaging have combined to lower the mortality and morbidity associated with pineal region surgery. Increased experience and sophistication have led to a better recognition of potential complications of this surgery, enabling neurosurgeons to avoid them or to manage successfully those that are inevitable. Optimal management strategies for pineal region tumors require an aggressive surgical approach for diagnostic and therapeutic purposes.

COMPLICATIONS OF PINEAL REGION SURGERY

Complications of pineal region surgery can be conveniently classified into three categories: complications related to the operative approach and exposure, complications from intraoperative tumor resection, and postoperative complications.

Complications of Operative Approach

Open Procedures

The pineal region can be accessed infratentorially through a supracerebellar approach or supratentorially through either a transcallosal-interhemi- spheric or occipital transtentorial approach (Fig. 17-37).[119,120,127,138,160,165,166] The specific risks inherent in each approach stem from the structures that must be retracted and the patient positioning that must be utilized to facilitate tumor exposure. Although this chapter focuses on the infratentorial approach, a knowledge of all approaches is helpful to enable the surgeon to balance the specific risks with the selective anatomical advantages a given approach may offer for each tumor. The choice of approaches is also influenced by the degree of confidence and familiarity that a surgeon has with each technique.

The infratentorial-supracerebellar approach involves a corridor under the tentorium and over the cerebellum, providing a central midline trajectory to the tumor.[143,169] The advantages of this approach include (1) a direct trajectory to what are usually midline tumors, (2) minimal interference during tumor resection from the deep venous structures lying dorsal to the tumor, (3) lowered venous pressure and pineal region congestion as gravity enables the cerebellum to drop downward in the sitting position, and (4) facilitated microsurgical dissection around the deep veins as gravity assists the tumor in dropping away from these structures.[119,167,169] For tumors with a large supratentorial component or lateral extension to the atrium of the lateral ventricle, this exposure is sufficient, and a supratentorial approach is recommended. The major risks of the infratentorial approach are mainly related to the use of the sitting

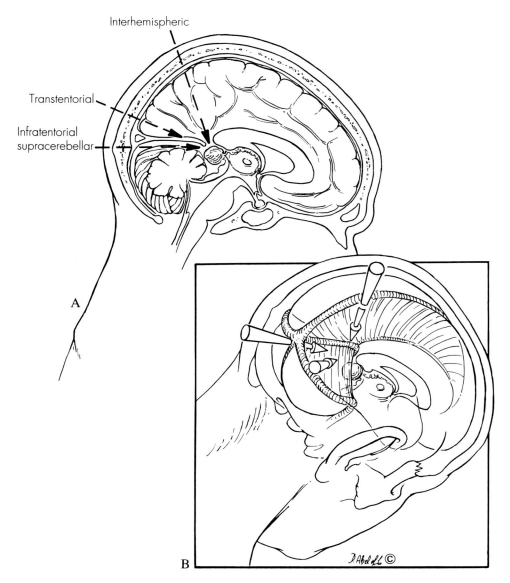

Figure 17-37. Head position and trajectory for the three basic approaches to the pineal region: transcallosal interhemispheric, occipital transtentorial, and infratentorial supracerebellar.

position where the potential for air embolism or ventricular collapse with subdural hematoma exist.

The risks of the sitting position can be minimized by utilizing the prone or "Concorde" position.[140] This position, however, negates the advantages of gravity assistance, making tumor removal and exposure more difficult.

Stereotactic Biopsy

Stereotactic biopsy of pineal tumors has been proposed as an alternative to open procedures.[125,146,147,153] Because of the high propensity for

sampling error due to limited amounts of biopsy material, stereotactic biopsy should be reserved for those patients with extensive medical problems or evidence of widespread tumor dissemination.[119,123,131] Mixed tumors may contain small malignant portions surrounded by benign tumor tissue that can be easily overlooked in a small sample (Fig. 17-38). Similarly, granulomatous inflammation often accompanies germinomas and can obscure the diagnosis.[142] An incorrect diagnosis can lead to unnecessary or insufficient postoperative adjuvant treatment.

Although the technical difficulties of stereotactic

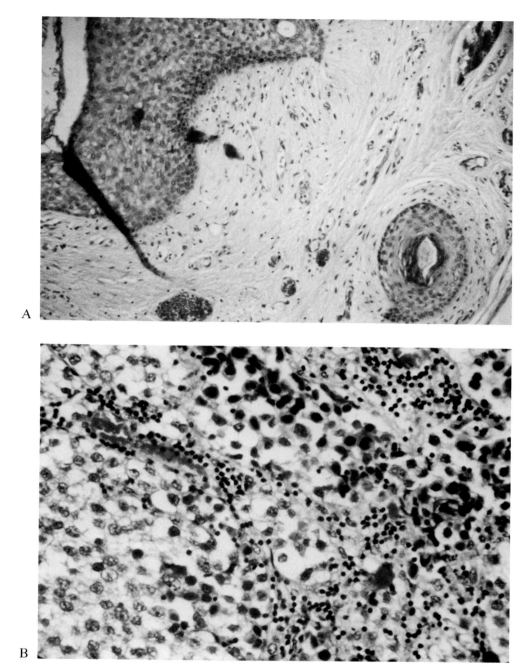

Figure 17-38. Histology of a mixed dermoid-germinoma in an 18-year-old man. **(A)** The benign dermoid portion of the tumor is seen. **(B)** The malignant germinomatous elements are seen. Adequate sampling is necessary to avoid erroneous diagnosis.

biopsy are less compared with open procedures, the potential gains from debulking or possible total resection cannot be ignored.[144,164,169] Furthermore, stereotactic biopsies result in operative duplicity for the one-third of pineal tumors that are benign and will subsequently require a craniotomy for surgical removal. Other risks of stereotactic biopsy include implantation metastases and hemorrhage, both intratumoral or from damage to the deep venous system.[153,155,161] While open operations certainly carry a risk of hemorrhage as well, bleeding can be controlled more definitively under direct vision.

Complications from Intraoperative Tumor Removal

Complications from Manipulation of Neural Structures

Neurological deficits stemming from manipulation of surrounding anatomical structures account for the most common complications of pineal region surgery. Most tumors are situated below the tentorium and expand into the posterior third ventricle or over the dorsal surface of the quadrigeminal plate and cerebellum. The vessels of the deep venous system are displaced dorsally or laterally. Growth of the tumor can involve the quadrigeminal portion of the midbrain, thalamus, or superior portion of the cerebellum. Postoperative deficits are usually related to manipulation of these structures during retraction or tumor removal. The most common neurological deficits include extraocular movement dysfunction, altered mental status, and ataxia. Most deficits are transient and resolve spontaneously. When tumor growth has caused deficits preoperatively, they are nearly always worse following surgery. The incidence and severity of these deficits are increased with large, invasive tumors and prior radiation therapy.[144,168] Radiation causes decreased vascularity and resiliency of the neural tissue while increasing fibrosis and obscuring tissue planes.

Alterations of extraocular movements and other variations of Parinaud syndrome account for the most common neurological deficits seen following pineal region surgery. Impaired upgaze or convergence occur in nearly all patients postoperatively for a brief period, but are rarely permanent. These deficits are of little consequence except for infrequent instances in which impairment of conjugate eye movements results in diplopia.

Postoperative cognitive disturbances can range from mild lethargy to a unique syndrome of akinetic mutism. These disturbances most likely reflect alterations in the reticular activating system; however, thalamic and third-ventricular disruption may be contributory. The development of alterations in mental status seems to be particularly sensitive to prior radiation therapy.

Ataxia is a frequent complication and is probably associated with cerebellar retraction and manipulation interfering with the cerebellar efferent pathways. When ataxia does occur, there is often simultaneous impairment of cognitive function and extraocular movements.

Complications from Damage to Vascular Structures

Several deep venous systems converge in the pineal region, including internal cerebral veins, vein of Galen, and veins of Rosenthal. Bleeding from damage to these structures intraoperatively can be difficult to control. Occlusion can result in venous infarcts of the thalamus or midbrain.

Branches of the choroidal arteries coming off the posterior cerebral arteries supply critical structures in the midbrain. Profound neurological deficits can result from disruption of these vessels.

Damage to major vessels includes the possibility of aneurysm formation. An example of this was a patient of ours who was referred following what was thought to be a recurrence of a previously resected sarcoma (Fig. 17-39). Upon reexploration he was found to have an enlarging posterior cerebral artery aneurysm probably caused by laser damage to the vessel during the initial surgery. The aneurysm was subsequently clipped through a subtemporal approach.

Postoperative Complications

Hemorrhage

The most serious complication associated with pineal region surgery is hemorrhage into a partially resected tumor bed.[119] Hemorrhage into pineal region tumors is a well-described phenomenon and can occur even in nonoperated tumors (Fig. 17-40).[114,135,171] Postoperative hemorrhages can occur up to several days following surgery and are most common in tumors of pineal cell origin (pineocytoma, pineoblastoma) (Fig. 17-41, Table 17-13). This may be a reflection of both the prominent vascularity and invasive nature of these tumors, which make complete resection and adequate hemostasis difficult to achieve.[114,134,155,171]

In certain instances, hemorrhages can occur in the cerebellum and may be secondary to venous infarcts from dividing bridging veins between the cerebellum and tentorium or excessive cerebellar retraction. Cerebellar hemorrhages are rarely symptomatic, are usually discovered on routine postoperative scans, and are well tolerated with conservative management.

The hemorrhagic complications associated with pineal cell tumors make optimal management difficult to define. Although the future holds some promise for the isolation of new tumor markers to identify tumors

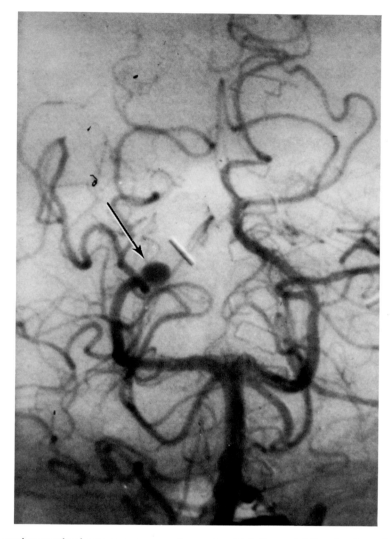

Figure 17-39. Posterior cerebral artery aneurysm (*arrow*), which formed following laser injury to the vessel during removal of a pineal region sarcoma.

with hemorrhagic potential by nonsurgical methods, currently there is no substitute for a tissue diagnosis.[141] Biopsies obtained stereotactically have not proved satisfactory for avoiding this complication.[155,170] Additionally, up to 25 percent of these tumors are fully resectable with surgery and are not radiosensitive, making surgical indications more compelling.[163]

Hydrocephalus

Hydrocephalus is present in approximately 90 percent of patients with pineal region tumors and can be an additional source of complications (Fig. 17-42). In general, a preoperative shunt is preferred for controlling hydrocephalus prior to tumor resection to allow a gradual reduction in ventricular size. Although tumor seeding has been reported following shunt placement, in reality this occurs rarely and is usually associated with an end-stage intracranial recurrence.[136,165] Although filters can reduce the risk of tumor dispersion, the rare incidence of seeding does not justify the increased risk of shunt obstruction associated with filters. Overall, shunt malfunction rates tend to be high and are probably related to inflammatory debris or tumor cells within the CSF.

Infectious and Inflammatory Complications

Infectious complications do not appear to be any more common with pineal region surgery than other types of intracranial surgery despite the sometimes

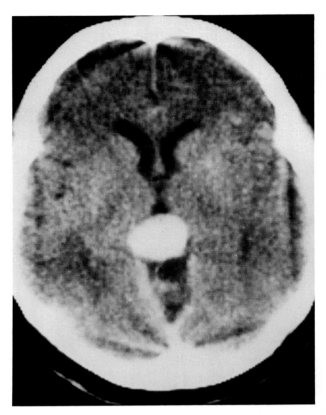

Figure 17-40. CT scan demonstrating preoperative hemorrhage into a pineocytoma. This 38-year-old woman presented with headache and hydrocephalus.

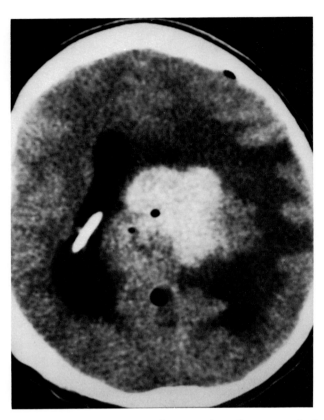

Figure 17-41. Hemorrhage into a subtotally resected pineoblastoma on postoperative day 2. Patient eventually made a full recovery with conservative management.

lengthy operations. Inflammatory symptoms can occur from aseptic meningitis or "posterior fossa syndrome" consisting of fever, headache, lethargy, and stiff neck.[121] These symptoms respond well to dexamethasone and are rarely problematical, although they often mimic a bacterial infection. This phenomenon is related to steroid withdrawal and possibly to the inflammatory effects of CSF bathing the wound space and ebbing back into the surrounding brain. The incidence of this complication can be reduced by

Table 17-13.   Summary of Operative-Related Deaths in 146 Operations for Pineal Region Tumors

Tumor	Cause of Death
Pineocytoma	Hemorrhage into subtotally resected tumor; remained comatose and died postoperative day 2
	Hemorrhage into subtotally resected tumor; died postoperative day 4
Ependymoma	Hemorrhage into subtotally resected tumor; while making gradual recovery; died of sudden pulmonary embolus on postoperative day 16
	Initially made excellent recovery following gross total resection on tumor; on postoperative day 6 had hemorrhage in cerebellum that filled third ventricle resulting in acute hydrocephalus and herniation; had urgent surgical removal of clot; died 3 days later after recurrent hemorrhage and failure of ventricular drainage
Astrocytoma	Initially made excellent recovery following subtotal tumor resection; hemorrhage into tumor bed on postoperative day 10 and became comatose; died 17 days later
Teratoma	Presented in vegetative state due to massive diencephalic tumor recurrence 17 years after previous subtotal resection of tumor and radiation therapy; had gross total resection of tumor at second operation; postoperative course complicated by shunt malfunction, pneumonia, gastrointestinal bleeding, and coagulopathy; died on postoperative day 10 from multiple medical problems associated with compromised preoperative clinical state

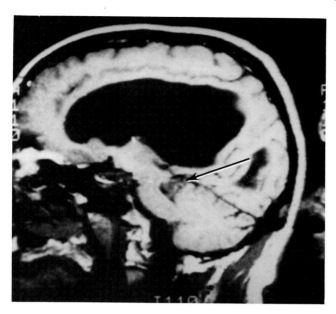

Figure 17-42. Hydrocephalus in a 41-year-old man with a pineocytoma (*arrow*) presenting with mild ataxia.

routinely performing a craniotomy with rewiring of the bone flap following a thorough dural closure.

Medical and Iatrogenic Complications

Medical and iatrogenic complications may be somewhat less frequent, since most patients are relatively young and in otherwise good health. Side ef-

fects from steroids are occasionally a problem due to the high dosage used for lengthy intervals.

HISTORICAL PERSPECTIVE

Dandy's[127] pioneering efforts with pineal region surgery began 70 years ago with his initial interhemispheric approach to these deep-seated tumors. Despite his innovative attempts, the lack of suitable anesthesia and microsurgical technique resulted in poor outcomes.[128] Other early approaches, developed by such individuals as Van Wagenen[173] and Poppen,[157,158] were abandoned following high mortality and morbidity rates. Krauss[143] was one of the forerunners of the currently used supracerebellar approach, which he used to explore the pineal region in three individuals. The infratentorial approach currently used, improved by the addition of microsurgical techniques, has evolved from his initial efforts.

Following the initially poor results with pineal region surgery, conservative management became the accepted form of treatment, combining a shunting procedure and radiation therapy without histological confirmation of tumor type.[113,126,129,130,159] As improvements were made in microsurgical technique and neuroanesthesia, complications rates became more acceptable and newer approaches were developed or modified (Table 17-14).[119,124,131,137,139,148,150,156]

Interest in surgical approaches to the pineal region in the era of microsurgery were rekindled with

Table 17-14. Results following Microsurgery in the Pineal Region

Author	Year	No. of Patients	Approach	Mortality (%)	Permanent Morbidity (%)
Stein[167]	1971	6	IT	0	0
Page[152]	1977	9	IT	11	0
Reid and Clark[160]	1978	15	ST,IT	7	7
Chapman and Linggood[124]	1980	8	ST,IT	0	0
Ventureyra[174]	1981	11	ST,IT	9	0
Wood et al.[176]	1981	21	ST,IT	0	<10
Jooma and Kendall[139]	1983	20	ST,IT	0	0
Kobayashi et al.[140]	1983	14	IT	0	0
Sano[165]	1985	32	ST,IT	0	—[a]
Boyd and Steinbok[116]	1985	18	ST,IT	0	0
Neuwelt[149]	1985	29	ST,IT	3	3
Lapras and Petit[144]	1985	85	ST,IT	0	—[a]
Pendl[154]	1985	25	ST,IT	8	12
Nagao et al.[148]	1988	16	ST,IT	0	6
Edwards et al.[131]	1988	30	ST,IT	0	10
Pluchino et al.[156]	1989	25	IT	8	—[a]
Bruce and Stein[120]	1992	141	ST,IT	4	3

Abbreviations: ST, supratentorial; IT, infratentorial.
[a] Insufficient data.

Stein's[167] description of six patients operated on through the infratentorial supracerebellar approach without mortality or significant morbidity. This was followed by Page's[152] report of nine patients who underwent pineal region surgery through a similar approach. One patient with a subtotally resected glioblastoma died from tumor swelling and hydrocephalus on the second postoperative day.

Ventureyra[174] approached eight pineal tumors through several supratentorial approaches, achieving a total resection in half without mortality or significant morbidity. The series included a vein of Galen aneurysm that was successfully thrombosed in situ through a supracerebellar infratentorial approach.

Reid and Clark[160] compared the infratentorial and transtentorial approaches in 15 patients. There were no complications among the four patients approached infratentorially. Of the 11 patients approached transtentorially, 1 died from brainstem edema, 1 had a small inconsequential superior temporal field defect, and 1 had a permanent homonymous hemianopsia.

Eight patients were approached mostly through the infratentorial route by Chapman and Linggood[124] without mortality or permanent morbidity. Total removal was achieved in one case, with extensive subtotal resection in three, and biopsy in four.

Wood et al.[176] were successful in obtaining histological diagnosis in 21 patients without mortality and less than 10 percent morbidity. The transcallosal approach was preferred more often than the infratentorial, although details on approaches and complications were not provided.

There were no operative deaths in a series of 20 patients undergoing pineal region surgery by Jooma and Kendall,[139] which included one patient approached infratentorially. Of the remaining 19 explored through the occipital transtentorial approach, there was 1 patient who had persistent ocular signs and hemiparesis.

Kobayashi et al.[140] introduced the Concorde position for the infratentorial approach in 1983. Gross total removal without complications was possible among 14 operations for three pineal tumors, three arachnoid cysts, one superior cerebellar tumor, three meningiomas, and four arteriovenous malformations.

Sano[165] used both the infratentorial and occipital transtentorial approach in 32 patients with no deaths.[165] A prone position was generally preferred. Aggressive surgical resection was felt to increase the effectiveness of radiotherapy even when radiosensitive tumors were involved.

Pendl[154] had two deaths in a series of 25 patients, using mostly the infratentorial approach. One patient died with edema secondary to intracerebral hemor-

rhage and the other from complications following an unexplained extensive abdominal hemorrhage. Permanent morbidity occurred in three patients including two debilitated patients who died several months following surgery for malignant astrocytoma and medulloblastoma. Two patients had some minor persistent extraocular motility problems, one of whom also had persistent ataxia.

With the use of the operating microscope, 18 patients underwent successful surgery without mortality or morbidity, as reported by Boyd and Steinbok.[116] The infratentorial approach was used for all but one patient, and gross total resection of eight tumors was possible. Of eight patients undergoing surgery prior to the use of the operating microscope, one patient improved, five were unchanged, and two deteriorated including one death.

Using the occipital tentorial or infratentorial approach Neuwelt[149] achieved a gross total excision in 9 of 13 patients with malignant primary pineal tumors. Operative complications included three patients with persistent hemianopsia, one with mild transient hemiparesis, one with epidural hematoma of the posterior fossa, and one with epidural hygroma. Many complications including worsening Parinaud syndrome and visual field defects proved to be transient. Overall, there was one operative death among 29 patients with both malignant and benign lesions.

In one of the larger pineal series, Lapras and Patet[144] operated on 85 patients without mortality. The occipital transtentorial approach in the sitting position was preferred in the majority of patients.

Nagao et al.[148] had no complications among several patients approached infratentorially.[148] In the one patient approached through the occipital transtentorial approach, truncal ataxia and slurred speech developed postoperatively. The transcallosal approach was utilized in eight cases resulting in four patients with disconnection syndromes. Six patients developed transient sensorimotor disturbances and homonymous hemianopsia.

In a series by Edwards et al.[131] on 30 pediatric patients with pineal region tumors, the infratentorial approach was utilized in 19 patients, occipital transtentorial in six, transcallosal in 3, and stereotactic biopsy in 2. There were no operative deaths although eight children had some degree of postoperative deficits. Morbidity was permanent in three, including two patients with mild, nondisabling hemiparesis, and one with severe neurological dysfunction secondary to meningitis and seizures. Curiously, histologic evaluation was erroneous in both patients undergoing stereotactic biopsy.

The infratentorial approach was used in 25 patients reported by Pluchino et al.,[156] including 9 who underwent surgery based on the results of an initial ste-reotactic biopsy. One patient died from complications related to hemorrhage and another from acute hydrocephalus. Morbidity was low and mostly related to extraocular motor and gaze disturbances.

SURGICAL TECHNIQUE

Surgical Considerations and Patient Selection

A wide spectrum of pathological entities can occur in the pineal region, including tumors, nonneoplastic cysts, vascular malformations, and inflammatory lesions.[119,166] The most common tumors are of germ cell, glial cell, or pineal parenchymal cell origin (Table 17-15). Within each category of tumor type, subtypes can range from benign and even nonneoplastic to highly invasive and malignant. Certain tumor types, notably of germ cell or pineal cell origin can be of a mixed-cell variety.

Surgical intervention is essential for obtaining adequate tissue samples to establish a histological diagnosis. Optimal clinical management depends on ac-curate histological diagnosis to guide adjuvant radiation or chemotherapy.[118,119,124,131,139,146,156] Management strategies incorporating radiation without histological confirmation as an alternative to surgery are obsolete. As the number of long-term postradiation survivors has increased, it is evident that radiation therapy, particularly if administered unnecessarily, is not without complications. Among the more extreme delayed complications of radiation are cerebral necrosis, progressive cognitive deficits, endocrine dysfunction, and de novo tumor formation (Fig. 17-43).[151]

The benefits of surgery extend beyond its role in providing tissue for definitive histological tumor identification. Notably, up to one-third of pineal region tumors are histologically benign and curable by surgery alone (Table 17-16).[119,162] Although the role of tumor debulking for invasive tumors is inconclusive, there is anecdotal evidence for improved survival following aggressive surgical removal.[144,164,169] Additionally, a significant percentage of malignant tumors are resectable (Table 17-16).[119] The benefits of aggressive surgical removal for malignant tumors will be better appraised with long-term follow-up in these patients.

Table 17-15. Summary of Pathology and Approaches in 146 Operations for Pineal Region Tumors at the New York Neurological Institute

Tumor	Total No.	Supracerebellar/ Infratentorial	Supratentorial
Germ cell	53	44	9
Germinoma	24	22	2
Teratoma	9	5	4
Other benign germ cell	3	3	0
Mixed malignant germ cell	12	11	1
Immature teratoma	3	1	2
Embryonal cell carcinoma	2	2	0
Pineal cell	31	26	5
Pineocytoma	17	14	3
Pineoblastoma	7	5	2
Mixed pineal cell	8	8	0
Glial cell	43	42	1
Astrocytoma	23	22	1
Anaplastic astrocytoma	3	3	0
Glioblastoma	4	4	0
Ependymoma	10	10	0
Oligodendroglioma	2	2	0
Choroid plexus papilloma	1	1	0
Miscellaneous	19	15	4
Pineal cysts	4	4	0
Meningioma	9	6	3
Other malignant	3	2	1
Other benign	3	3	0
Total	146	127	19

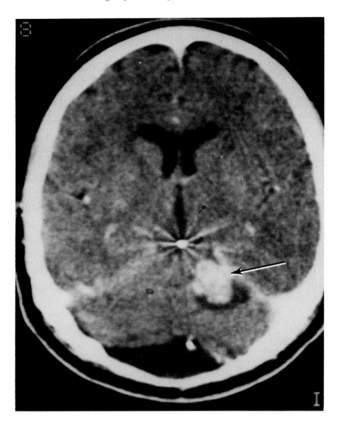

Figure 17-43. Radiation-induced meningioma (*arrow*) occurring 21 years after treatment. This patient had been needlessly radiated at the age of 8 before subsequently undergoing resection of his pineal teratoma.

Given the wide variety of pathology that occurs in the pineal region, open exploration is recommended for all patients with symptomatic pineal region tumors. Stereotactic biopsy is reserved for patients in poor medical condition or those who have disseminated tumors. Special consideration should be given to patients with suspected pineal cysts.[132] Benign cysts of the pineal gland are being diagnosed more frequently as CT and MRI usage increases for routine neurological complaints (Fig. 17-44). They are usually seen as incidental findings on radiographical studies. Histologically, they are normal variants of the pineal gland consisting of a cyst surrounded by a flattened pineal gland. They are generally 1 to 2 cm in diameter and do not cause distortion of the surrounding structures or aqueduct. An associated hydrocephalus or other localizing symptoms are sufficient grounds for doubting this diagnosis and suspecting a cystic tumor. Several patients have had operations for this condition before the full extent of their nature was recognized. It is now apparent that these are anatomical variants that should be followed and not treated surgically.

Preoperative Workup

CT and MRI, with and without contrast, are a necessity in all patients, and should include axial, coronal, and sagittal views to optimize surgical management strategies (Fig. 17-45). These images can provide valuable information concerning the size of the tumor and the surrounding anatomical relationships with the third ventricle, corpus callosum, quadrigeminal plate, aqueduct of Sylvius, anterior cerebellar vermis, and anterior medullary velum. A tumor that extends far above the tentorium or far laterally toward the atrium of the lateral ventricle is often better managed through a supratentorial approach. MRI is particularly useful for identifying the tumor's relationship to the surrounding blood vessels including the vein of Galen, internal cerebral veins, veins of Rosenthal, and precentral cerebellar vein. The location of the internal cerebral veins may have some diagnostic value since they are nearly always located dorsal to the tumor, except with some meningiomas. Other important radiographical features include irregular tumor borders, which are suggestive of tumor invasiveness. Additionally, contrast can provide information on the vascularity of the lesion and the degree of intratumoral heterogeneity. Scans are also important for identifying the hydrocephalus that often occurs with these patients. Despite significant advances in recent years with diagnostic imaging, it continues to be ineffective in reliably predicting tumor histology.[133,177]

Table 17-16. Surgical Results in 146 Operations (141 Patients) for Pineal Region Tumors

Histology	Biopsy	Subtotal Resection	Total Resection	Transient/ Minor/No Morbidity	Permanent Major Morbidity	Death	Total
Benign	0	6	43	48	0	1	49
Malignant	6	67	24	88	4	5	97
Total	6	73	67	136	4	6	146

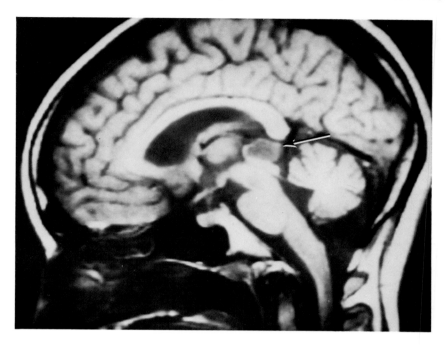

Figure 17-44. Benign pineal cysts (*arrow*) are anatomical variants and rarely become symptomatic. They should be followed without surgery with serial MRIs.

Angiography is reserved for patients whose CT scan or MRI suggest the presence of a vascular lesion such as an arteriovenous malformation or a vein of Galen aneurysm (Fig. 17-46). Although certain pineal region tumors such as pineocytomas and pineoblastomas can be very vascular, arteriography is of little benefit. The vascularities of these tumors will be readily apparent at the time of operation, and angiography is unlikely to change the operative approach.

The preoperative workup should include CSF analysis for tumor markers and cytology. Tumor markers are useful for follow-up purposes and predicting histology in certain instances. α-Fetoprotein and β-human chorionic gonadotropin (HCG) are the two most commonly associated markers and correspond to certain malignant germ cell tumors.[115] When elevated, they are measurable in the CSF with slightly lower levels in the serum.

When hydrocephalus is present, it is best controlled prior to undergoing surgical resection of the tumor. Placement of a ventriculoperitoneal shunt at least several days prior to surgical resection permits a gradual reduction in the ventricular size, avoiding ventricular collapse and potential subdural hemorrhage (Fig. 17-47). Although abdominal seeding for certain types of tumors has been reported following shunt placement, we have not found this to be a problem.[136,175] For this reason, we do not recommend placement of a shunt filter as it merely increases the risk of shunt malfunction. When tumor resection is likely to unblock the aqueduct of Sylvius, a ventricular drain may be placed at the time of surgery. The ventricular drain can then be removed within several days following surgery, avoiding the necessity for a permanent shunt. Externalized drains carry a risk of infection; however, this is not problematic if they are removed in a timely fashion.

Operative Technique

Set-up and Position

The infratentorial-supracerebellar approach may be performed using the sitting slouch position or prone in the Concorde position (Fig. 17-48).[120,140,169] The sitting position is most commonly used, but, unlike the prone position, it carries the risk of air embolism and cortical collapse. The main advantage is that gravity minimizes venous pressure while assisting in retraction of the cerebellum and the dissection of the tumor off the surrounding structures. Bleeding is more easily controlled and the operative field less obscured from pooling. The Concorde position places the patient prone with the surgeon sitting at the patient's left shoulder. This reduces the risks of the sitting position but negates the advantages of gravity-assisted retraction and hemostasis.

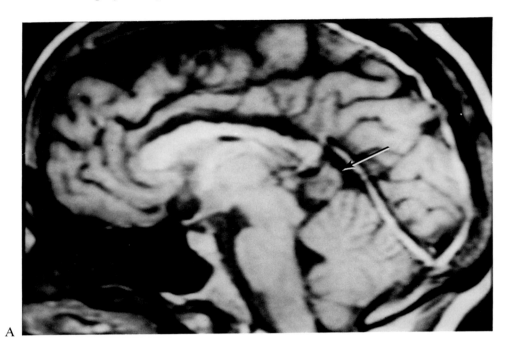

A

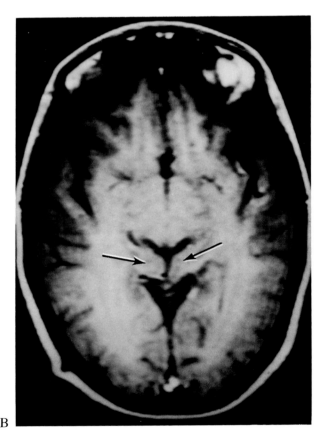

B

Figure 17-45. (A) Sagittal MRI from a man who was referred for a second opinion when histology revealed normal brain tissue following a suboccipital craniectomy for a biopsy of his "pineal region mass" (*arrow*). **(B)** Careful review of the axial MRI shows posterior temporal lobes (*arrows*) projecting into the quadrigeminal cistern. This is a normal variant, which, when viewed sagittally, gives the erroneous impression of a pineal region mass.

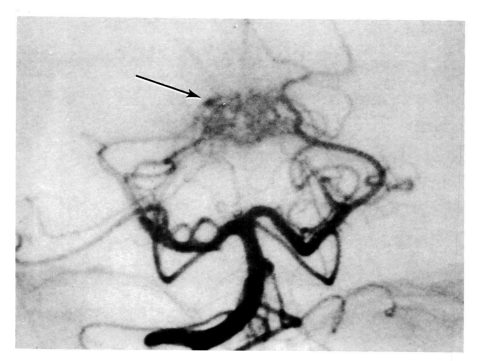

Figure 17-46. Angiography for pineal region masses is reserved for suspected vascular anomalies such as this arteriovenous malformation (AVM) involving the pineal gland (*arrow*). This patient underwent successful resection of her AVM through a supracerebellar infratentorial approach.

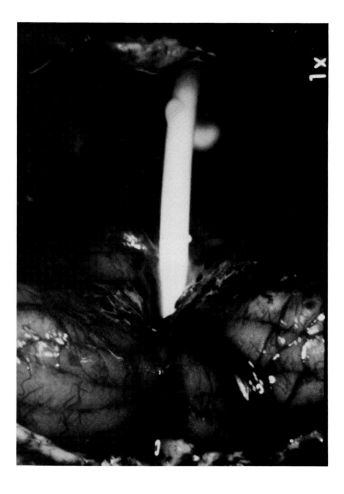

Figure 17-47. Catheter left in place to permit CSF flow between the third ventricle and cisterna magna following resection of a germinoma. The cerebellum is at the bottom of the photo with the tentorium above.

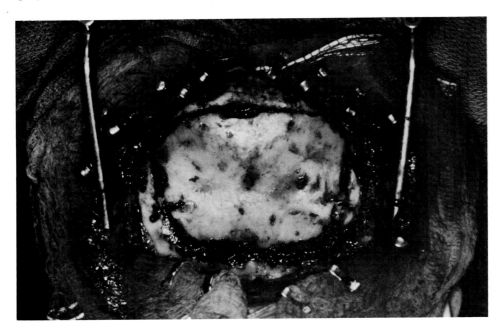

Figure 17-48. Bone flap rewired into place following a suboccipital craniotomy for a germinoma.

When the sitting position is used, precordial Doppler monitoring and monitoring of end-tidal carbon dioxide should be utilized for early detection of air emboli. Air embolism risks can be minimized by elevating the lower extremities. Most air emboli occur during the opening of bone or from tearing of emissary veins adjacent to the dural sinuses. Measures can be taken to seal the sinuses and veins with bipolar cautery and hemostatic agents while meticulously waxing all bone edges. Although small amounts of air are frequently encountered during surgery, they rarely result in serious complications since the source is usually easily identified and controlled.

The potential for ventricular collapse and subdural hematoma in the sitting position is heightened by the ventricular enlargement that often accompanies pineal tumors. Subdural collections of air are common following surgery and, if sizable, can lead to headaches and prolonged lethargy until the air is spontaneously absorbed.

Optimal patient positioning is important for minimizing surgeon fatigue. Generally the patient is placed in the sitting slouch position so that the body forms a C configuration on the operating room table (Fig. 17-49A). A pillow is placed under the lumbar lordosis for support, and the buttocks should rest on an oscillating air mattress to avoid pressure ischemia. The patient should be well down on the operating room table to ensure that the sitting height is not uncomfortably high. The head is flexed so that the tentorium is approximately horizontal to the floor.

Since this requires a significant amount of flexion, overflexion can be prevented by ensuring that a distance of at least two fingerbreadths is maintained between the patient's chin and sternum. A three-point pin-vise type of head-holder such as the Mayfield is necessary to keep the head rigid. Flexing the patient's head preoperatively while he or she is still awake will ensure that it will be suitably tolerated. The operating room table should be adjusted so that the final positioning is not too high to prevent the surgeon from sitting during the operation. An operating microscope is essential for proper magnification and illumination of the operating room field. To shorten the distance between the surgeon and the operative field, a 275-mm lens objective is used along with reversed angled eyepieces (Fig. 17-49A). A freestanding, adjustable arm rest maximizes comfort. A Greenberg self-retaining retractor, with the holder attached to the operating table, optimizes retraction capabilities.

For the Concorde position, the patient is placed prone and brought to the far left side of the table (Fig. 17-49B$_1$ & B$_2$). The head is flexed, tilted to the right, and elevated higher than the heart. The final position should allow the surgeon to be seated on the patient's left side.

Regardless of the position used, the surgery proceeds in a similar fashion. All patients should wear pneumatic compression stockings to prevent lower extremity deep venous thrombosis. Preoperative medications include 10 mg of dexamethasone and a

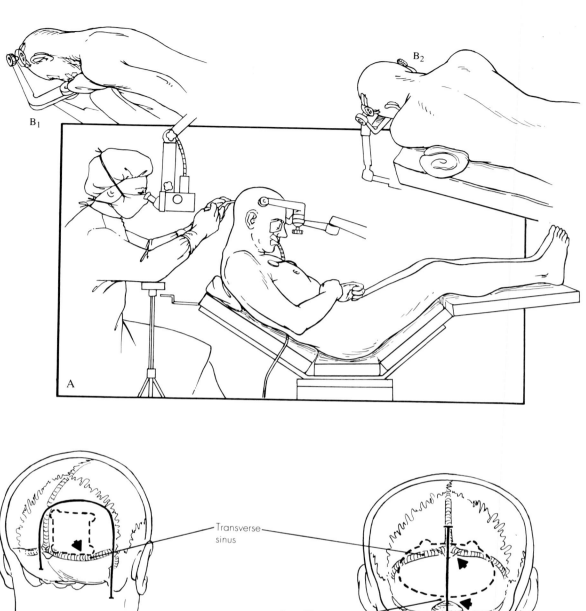

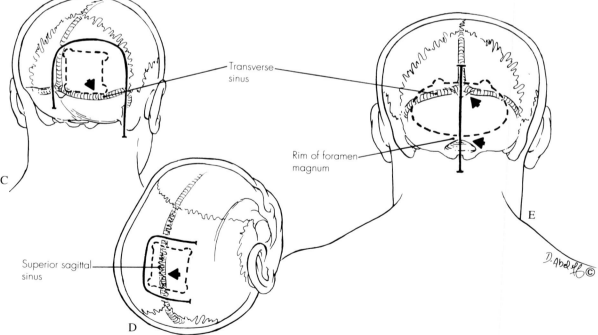

Figure 17-49. **(A)** Sitting-slouch position for the infratentorial supracerebellar approach. The body assumes a C-shaped configuration, and the head should be flexed so that the tentorium is horizontal. An angled eyepiece with a 275-mm lens objective minimizes the distance between the surgeon and the operative site. **(B₁&B₂)** The Concorde position has the patient prone with the head flexed and tilted to the right. **(C)** Incision and exposure for occipital transtentorial approach. **(D)** Incision and exposure for transcallosal interhemispheric approach. **(E)** Infratentorial approach showing suboccipital incision and extent of bony removal to expose the torcula and lateral sinus while leaving the foramen magnum intact.

broad spectrum antibiotic. If intracranial pressure is increased, mannitol can be given. When hydrocephalus is uncontrolled, a ventricular drain is placed through a right occipital burr hole before beginning the craniotomy.

Opening

The suboccipital area is exposed using a midline incision and preserving muscle and fascia for a watertight closure (Fig. 17-49C & D). The incision should extend from approximately 1 cm or so above the external occipital protuberance down to the C4 spinous process (Fig. 49-17E). A longer incision length makes reapproximation of the muscle and fascia easier at the conclusion of the operation. The craniectomy should extend from just above the transverse sinus and torcula but need not include the foramen magnum. Since the foramen magnum remains intact, a subperiosteal dissection of the C1 spinous process is not necessary. Although the majority of our operations were craniectomies, all recent patients have had craniotomies using a high-speed craniotome with replacement of the bone flap at the conclusion of the operation. When a craniotomy is performed, however, it is essential that the sinuses be exposed before traversing them with the craniotome. It is also helpful to drill down the midline keel separately or to thin it down and break it. A self-retaining retractor to retract the muscle and fascia is brought up from above to minimize interference with the surgical opening. Since the operative route is below the torcula and along the tentorium inferiorly, the lateral sinus and torcula must be exposed. Any bleeding from the sinus is easily controlled with a combination of cautery and hemostatic agents.

Following bone removal, the posterior fossa dura should be palpated, and, if overly tense, additional mannitol may be given or further ventricular fluid may be removed. The Greenberg retractors are assembled to frame the operative exposure with a retractor arm positioned superiorly and another inferiorly (Fig. 17-50A). A tray for cottonoids is attached and another arm is directed toward the opening to hold an irrigation system consisting of an 18-gauge spinal needle connected to a length of tubing and a 60-cc syringe filled with irrigating solution. The needle can be positioned to allow the assistant to irrigate easily when the cautery is in use.

Exposure

The dura is opened in a manner that will provide optimal exposure over the superior surface of the cerebellum. A curved dural opening is made extending from the most lateral exposure of the transverse sinus bilaterally (Fig. 17-50B). Secondary dural cuts are made toward the central portion of the lateral sinus on each side to facilitate exposure in the midline. The result is a three-flap configuration, which is then tented upward with a suture and a rubber band attached to the Greenberg retractor. By keeping some tension on this dural flap, shrinkage of the dura is prevented, facilitating closure later on. Once the dura is opened, the bridging veins and arachnoidal adhesions between the surface of the cerebellum and the tentorium can be visualized, enabling them to be cauterized and sharply divided. This causes the cerebellum to drop downward, exposing the supracerebellar-infratentorial corridor. The exposure to this point is more easily accomplished without the microscope. Telfa is placed over the exposed superior surface of the cerebellum to protect it during retraction. An L-shaped retractor may be helpful to retract the tentorium upward, taking care to avoid excessive compression of the sinus. An S-shaped retractor is molded to provide downward retraction on the cerebellum (Figs. 17-50A and 17-51A). The tip of the retractor should be at the most anterior aspect of the cerebellum to expose the arachnoidal adhesions between the quadrigeminal area and the anterior vermis. By this point, any bridging veins out laterally that might be stretched and torn during the cerebellar retraction should be cauterized and divided.

The operating microscope is brought in and the pineal region with its overlying, thickened arachnoid can be visualized. Using a small arachnoid knife or bayonet microscissors, the arachnoid overlying the incisura and the pineal mass should be opened bloodlessly to avoid obscuring tissue planes. The few arachnoidal vessels can be cauterized if necessary. As the arachnoid is sharply dissected, the precentral cerebellar vein that comes into view extending from the anterior vermis toward the vein of Galen should be cauterized and divided (Fig. 17-50C). Arachnoidal dissection should be continued laterally on each side, taking care to avoid the vein of Rosenthal on the medial aspect of the temporal lobe. The tumor is invariably fed by branches of the choroidal and superior cerebellar arteries, which overlie the tumor in the thickened arachnoid. These can be cauterized and divided as long as they are not supplying the quadrigeminal plate.

During this initial phase of the pineal region exposure, the trajectory of the microscope has been aimed up toward the vein of Galen (Fig. 17-51A). The trajectory should then be angled downward 15 to 20 degrees, changing the trajectory from dorsal to the tumor in line with the vein of Galen to a more caudal

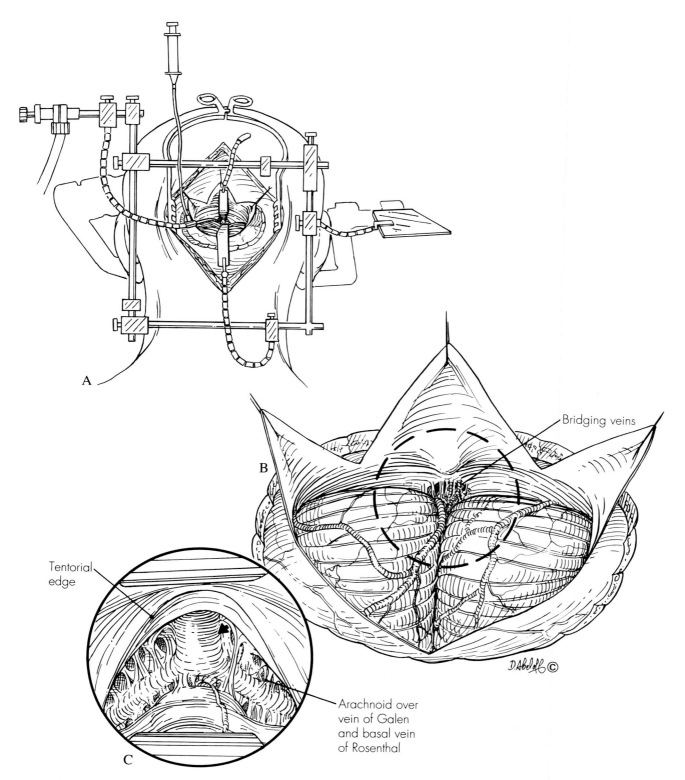

Figure 17-50. **(A)** Operative set-up for the infratentorial approach. A retractor is placed superiorly to pull up on the tentorium while a second retractor is placed on the cerebellum with the retraction directed posteriorly and inferiorly to avoid pressure on the brainstem. A tray for cottonoids is attached on the right, and a irrigation apparatus consisting of a 60-ml syringe and plastic tubing is attached on the left. **(B)** The dural opening is completed to optimize the rostral exposure in the midline and the lateral exposure on each side. Bridging veins extending from the surface of the cerebellum to the tentorium should be cauterized and divided. **(C)** As the arachnoid over the quadrigeminal cistern and pineal region is dissected, the tumor and the precentral cerebellar vein are visualized.

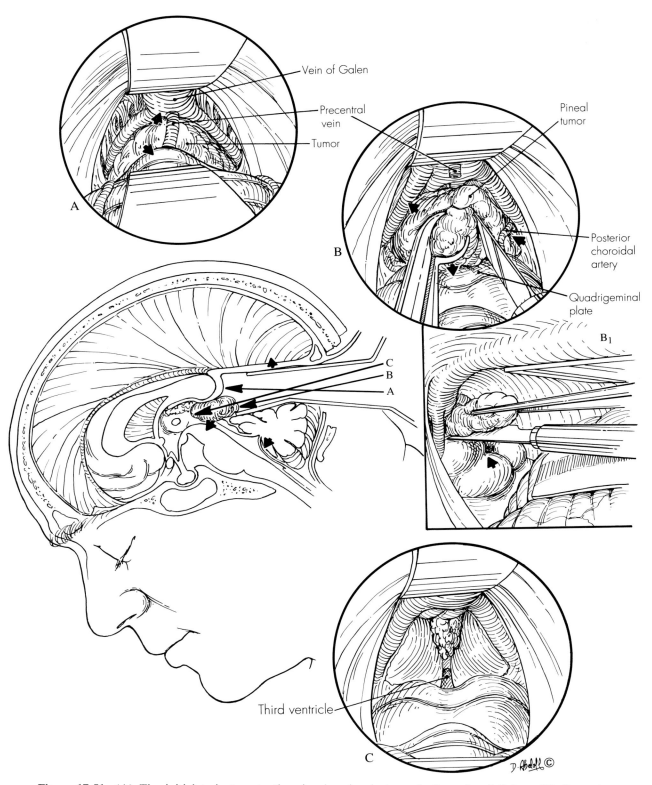

Figure 17-51. (A) The initial trajectory to the pineal region is towards the vein of Galen. **(B)** Once the arachnoid overlying the tumor has been dissected, the microscope should be angled several degrees caudally towards the maximal diameter of the tumor, to avoid injury to the deep venous system. Instruments of extra long length are necessary to facilitate tumor removal. The inferior portion of the tumor is the most difficult to remove since the interface between the tumor and brainstem must be carefully preserved. **(C)** Following removal of the tumor, the roof of the third ventricle can be visualized.

direction, more consistent with tumor exposure and removal (Fig. 17-51B). This avoids any injury to the vein of Galen. As the cerebellum is further freed from its arachnoidal adhesion between the quadrigeminal plate and the pineal region, the cerebellum can be retracted further caudally to expose the inferior aspect of the tumor. The retractor should be placed on the cerebellum and pulled downward and posteriorly to avoid any compression of the quadrigeminal plate.

Tumor Removal

Once the surface of the tumor has been adequately exposed superiorly and laterally, the surface is cauterized and opened with a knife or bayonet scissors. From this point on, specialized instruments of extra length are needed (Fig. 17-51B). Portions of the tumor can be removed with a tumor forceps, pituitary forceps, or other suitable instrument and sent for a frozen tissue diagnosis. Cautery should be used judiciously to preserve specimens for optimal histopathological inspection. The diagnosis on the frozen tissue section can be helpful in guiding operative decisions, although limitations in the degree of accuracy should be kept in mind. More crucial to the operative decision making is whether the tumor is encapsulated or not; this should take precedence over the tentative frozen tissue diagnosis. Depending on the consistency and vascularity of the tumor, as much of the interior should be decompressed as possible. A variety of instruments can be used to accomplish this, including the laser, cavitron aspirator, or combination of sharp and blunt instruments. The choice of instruments is limited by the degree of operative exposure. In view of the wide variety of tumor possibilities, the high incidence of mixed tumor varieties, and the sometimes heterogenous tumor composition, an adequate amount of tissue should be sent for permanent fixation and neuropathological examination. Once the interior of the tumor has been debulked, the degree of tumor encapsulation will become much more evident. After internal decompression, the superior and lateral margins of the tumor can be dissected from the surrounding velum interpositum, pulvinar, and walls of the third ventricle. In tumors that are obviously infiltrating, radical resections are usually not warranted as these tumors often extend well into the surrounding structures where extensive resection can result in significant neurological deficits.

The superior portion of the tumor can be dissected off the vein of Galen and internal cerebral veins by retracting slightly down on the tumor and sharply dissecting between the plane of the tumor and the venous structure. This is a potentially hazardous portion of the resection since the tumor is often very adherent, and injury to the deep venous system is difficult to control. When the vein has been violated, cautery can sometimes be helpful in sealing a pinhole; however, this can cause enlargement of the opening or occlusion of the deep venous system. Usually some combination of hemostatic agent and compression or packing will control this low-pressure bleeding. If the dissection of this portion of the tumor is not possible, a small amount of tumor may be cauterized and left attached to the vein.

The lateral dissection proceeds along the walls of the third ventricle and the thalamus. Encapsulated tumors are usually freed up easily from the thalamus, but as the dissection advances anteriorly the tumor often melds with the ependymal lining of the third ventricle, temporarily obscuring the tissue planes until the intraventricular surface of the tumor is encountered. When tumor margins are hard to discern, it is sometimes helpful to bisect the tumor until an opening is made into the third ventricle providing some reference point as to the depth of the tumor. Removal of the inferior portion of the tumor is the most difficult since it is often adherent to the midbrain where manipulation is poorly tolerated and the interface between the tumor and the quadrigeminal plate is obscured. It is usually possible to lift the tumor upward with a tumor forceps and then continue a microdissection along the inferior margin using a sharp microdissecting instrument and avoiding cautery. With experience, it is possible to determine which tumors may be totally resected and which ones would benefit most from either a limited biopsy or subtotal resection. Nearly all benign and encapsulated tumors can be removed in their entirety. Certain tumors of an invasive nature, such as ependymomas, germinomas, and pineal cell tumors can often be minimally invasive and fairly discrete, particularly when they are small in size. It is sometimes possible to resect these tumors totally as well. Most malignant tumors, however, are invasive and are best treated with a subtotal resection.

Closure

Following resection of the tumor, hemostasis is important. It is important to be judicious with the use of cautery, particularly along the brainstem. If the tumor bed is still oozing, then pieces of Surgicel can be placed along the tumor bed and brought out over the cerebellar surface. It is important not to let small pieces of Surgicel float into the third ventricle, where they can block the aqueduct or the shunt. In certain cases, particularly following a subtotal resection or when shunting is problematic, hydrocephalus can be controlled by a catheter left in the third ventricle, brought out over the surface of the cerebellum, and diverted to the cisterna magna as a modified Torkildsen's procedure (Fig. 17-47).

After the retractors are removed, an attempt is made to close the dura as completely as possible. A small piece of cervical fascia can be sewn in to improve the closure and avoid extradural CSF collection and pseudomeningocele. Performing a craniotomy and wiring the bone flap back in upon completion improves the completeness of the closure (Fig. 17-48). Closure of the muscles and fascia should be sufficient to prevent CSF leak. Subcutaneous drain placement is usually unnecessary if hemostasis is adequate.

The patient should be extubated in the operating room, and manipulation of the head should be minimized to avoid tearing the bridging veins, which have been stretched to some degree by the loss of CSF and ventricular collapse. Postoperatively, patients should remain on a high dose of dexamethasone, which is slowly tapered. Antibiotics are continued for 36 hours and then stopped. If a ventricular drain has been placed at the time of surgery, this should remain in for 1 or 2 days and then removed or converted to a shunt as needed. Leaving the drain externalized for longer periods of time invites infection.

Postoperative Management

Patients should be evaluated periodically with MRI or CT scan to detect early recurrences. The timing of these intervals will depend on the anticipated growth rates of the tumor as determined by histological examinations and the degree of residual tumor. Patients with positive tumor markers can undergo periodic measurement of these as well, for they can be sensitive indicators of further recurrence.

Recurrences may be treated with radiosurgery, chemotherapy if appropriate, or conventional external beam radiation therapy if not previously given to its maximum dose. Decisions regarding reoperation are made on an individual basis. In general, reoperation is limited to patients with benign, slow-growing tumors who are in otherwise stable clinical condition with reasonable expectations for longevity and favorable outcome from previous operation. Reoperation is often complicated by prior radiation, making the surgery more difficult. In our series, five patients have undergone reoperation and all but one had a significant benefit from the procedure. In four of the

five, a gross total removal was accomplished at the second operation. The only patient without significant benefit was a 27-year-old man who had been well for 16 years following an initial tumor resection of a teratoma. He returned with a 1-year history of progressive and profound deterioration with a diencephalic syndrome secondary to tumor recurrence and an ill-advised course of radiation therapy. Reoperation was a desperate attempt to reverse his decline. Although his tumor was completely removed at the second operation, he died from medical complications 10 days postoperatively brought on by his compromised preoperative medical condition.

Several tumors including malignant term cell tumors, ependymomas, and pineal cell tumors have a propensity to seed along the CSF pathways. Patients with these tumors should be evaluated in the postoperative period with a CT scan, myelogram, spinal MRI, and spinal fluid cytology as part of a postoperative stage and workup (Fig. 17-52).[119,170] In our experience spinal MRI is the most sensitive test for diagnosing spinal seeding.

Radiation therapy is given for all malignant pineal tumors including those that have been totally resected.[17] In certain cases in which a particularly low-grade pineal cell tumor or ependymoma has been resected with good margins, the radiation therapy is sometimes delayed indefinitely to follow the progress of recurrences with serial scans. Some of these tumors seem to have a particularly benign clinical behavior and, besides having a better prognosis, are

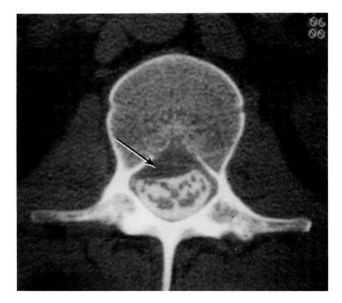

Figure 17-52. CT scan showing an asymptomatic lumbar drop metastases (*arrow*) found during routine postoperative staging in a 33-year-old man with a pineocytoma.

unlikely to be radiosensitive. Identification of these more benign tumors is based on operative findings and corroborated by histological analysis.

Spinal radiation is not given prophylactically but is reserved for those patients who have documented spinal seeding on radiographic examination.[117,119,131,145] The role of radiosurgery appears promising but it has not been fully defined.[122] Chemotherapy is limited to certain nongerminomatous malignant germ cell tumors.[170] The results, however, have been variable.

SURGICAL OUTCOME AND COMPLICATIONS

Surgical results in our series of 141 patients undergoing 146 operations for pineal region tumors have been very encouraging (Table 17-16). A histological diagnosis was made in each patient. The overall incidence of death or permanent major morbidity was 7 percent. Fifteen patients experienced significant postoperative complications; however, nine of them fully recovered to at least their preoperative status, and two others have had only a short follow-up period but are expected to recover fully (Table 17-17). The most common postoperative deficits included extraocular movement disorders and mental status changes, although few remained permanently (Table 17-18). Hemorrhage was the most significant factor in postoperative deaths (Table 17-13). Patients with benign, encapsulated tumors fared much better, with no cases of permanent major morbidity and only one death out of 49 operations performed (Table 17-16). The sole death was in the previously described man who underwent reoperation for a radiated recurrent teratoma.

Surgery for malignant tumors generally resulted in a higher incidence of complications for a variety of reasons. The invasive nature of these tumors often led to more surgical manipulation of critical structures surrounding the tumor as tissue planes and boundaries between tumors and the abnormal tissue were obscured. Additionally, patients preoperatively tended to have more profound and frequent symptomatology than their benign counterparts. Major complications occurred in 18 patients out of 97 operations performed, including five deaths. Of the 13 patients with major postoperative morbidity, 7 have recovered to at least their postoperative status, and 2 others are expected to make a full recovery in the near future (Table 17-17). In the five patients who died, postoperative hemorrhage was a common factor.

Surgical Complications

Ocular motility deficits were the most common complications, although they were present in nearly all patients immediately following surgery, significant or prolonged deficits occurred about 33 percent of the time. Of these 48 patients with prolonged deficits, all but 16 cleared within 1 month. The patients with prolonged extraocular movement problems are hindered mostly by intermittent diplopia. The degree of diplopia in all cases, however, is compensated by the patient and does not cause undue hardship. This group of patients also includes several who have had less than a 1-year follow-up and, based on past experience, many of these patients should improve with more time.

Cognitive deficits developed in 27 patients but usually cleared after several days and have remained permanent to some degree in only 4 patients. Cognitive impairment was present to some degree in all of these four patients preoperatively, including two who were markedly impaired. Prior radiation therapy was a contributory factor in two of the four. Postoperative hemorrhage played a role in one patient with a permanent deficit.

Ataxia was a problem in 26 patients, with only 2 patients significantly affected on a permanent basis, both of whom had symptoms prior to surgery. Ataxia was presumably from cerebellar or efferent cerebellar pathway manipulation.

Complications Related to Operative Positioning

Cervical Spine Compromise

Two patients developed significant weakness related to the sitting-slouch position. One patient awoke with a weakness of the right upper extremity and both lower extremities that resolved spontaneously within 48 hours. This was thought to be related to central spinal cord ischemia since radiographical evaluation failed to reveal any structural abnormalities.

The other patient with weakness is notable for his tragic result and unusual circumstances. This 17-year-old boy's pineal tumor was diagnosed on a routine CT scan following an automobile accident. His complaint was simply headaches without cervical pain or discomfort. Using the sitting-slouch position he underwent an elective subtotal resection of a malignant astrocytoma, and awoke quadriplegic. Cervical spine films, myelogram, and flexion-extension films showed no evidence of cervical pathology. A

Table 17-17. Summary of Patients with Significant Postoperative Morbidity in 146 Operations for Pineal Region Tumors

Tumor	Preoperative Status	Preoperative Radiation Therapy	Postoperative Complications	Follow-up
Germinoma[a]	Good	No	Pleural empyema; steroid psychosis	Made full recovery; died of disease 2 years postoperative
Teratoma/choriocarcinoma[b]	Good	Yes	Seizures; mute; hemiparesis; lethargy	Made full recovery; died of metastatic disease 2 years postoperative
Teratoma/germinoma[a]	Good	No	Obtunded; CSF leak from head pins; pulmonary embolism; subdural hygroma	Made full recovery; alive and well 10 years postoperative
Meningioma[b]	Fair	No	Hemorrhage → hemianopsia, hemiplegia, altered mental status, respiratory insufficiency; ruptured ulcer	Made full recovery; alive and well 4 years postoperative
Pineoblastoma[b]	Good	No	Hemorrhage → lethargy, seizures, hydrocephalus	Made full recovery; alive and well 1.5 years postoperative
Pineocytoma[a]	Fair	Yes	Akinetic mutism and somnolence	Returned to preoperative baseline status 2 months postoperative
Oligodendroglioma[a]	Poor	No	Vegetative state—slightly worse than preoperative	Persistent vegetative state 4 months postoperative
Malignant astrocytoma[a]	Good	No	Quadriparetic from unrecognized, asymptomatic neck fracture from preoperative motor vehicle accident	Died of recurrent tumor 9 years postoperative after minimal improvement in quadriparesis
Pineocytoma[a]	Good	No	Hemorrhage → obtunded	Made full recovery
Pineocytoma[a]	Fair	Yes	Akinetic mutism	Made minimal improvement; died of disease 10 months postoperative
Adenocarcinoma[b]	Fair	Yes	Obtunded	Died of disease 4 months postoperative without recovery
Mixed pineal cell[a]	Fair	No	Akinetic mutism	Made full recovery
Germinoma[a]	Good	No	Akinetic mutism; deranged eye movements	Making progress 2 months postoperative; full recovery expected
Pineocytoma[b]	Fair	No	Confused; deranged eye movements; ataxia; extrapyramidal syndrome	Making progress 2 months postoperative; full recovery expected
Teratoma[b]	Fair	No	Seizures; tracheostomy; preoperative cognitive deficits worse	Made full recovery to preoperative status

[a] Supracerebellar infratentorial approach.
[b] Transcallosal interhemispheric approach.

CT scan showed fractures of the C5 and C6 lamina and pedicles that evidently dated back to his recent automobile accident. Although the fractures were nondisplaced in a neutral position, the spinal distortion associated with the sitting-slouch position was probably sufficient to compromise his spinal canal and compress the cord. This is a unique example of the possible complications of the sitting-slouch position on a compromised cervical spine but nevertheless underscores the necessity of investigating any

Table 17-18. Number of Patients with Significant Complications
following Pineal Region Surgery (146 Operations Performed)

	Transient Morbidity	Permanent Morbidity
Surgical complications		
Extraocular movement dysfunction	48	16
Altered mental status	27	4
Ataxia	26	2
Aseptic meningitis	8	
Symptomatic hemorrhage	4	6
Extrapyramidal syndrome	5	
Hemiparesis	5	
Seizures	4	
Hemianopsia	2	1
Bacterial meningitis	1	
Facial weakness	1	
CSF collection in wound	1	
Complications related to operative positioning		
Subdural hematoma/hygroma	1	
Paraparesis/quadriparesis	1	1
Pin site fracture with CSF leak	1	
Sciatic nerve palsy	1	
Shunt complications		
Shunt malfunction	29	
Shunt infection	1	
Medical and iatrogenic complications		
Respiratory infection/insufficiency	4	
Steroid psychosis	3	
Erythema multiforme	1	
Pulmonary embolus	2	1
Deep vein thrombosis	2	
Pleural empyema	1	
Hepatitis	1	
Ruptured gastric ulcer	1	
Multisystem failure	0	1

question of cervical abnormality. Any questions should be resolved preoperatively and the operative approach adjusted accordingly.

Ventricular Collapse and Subdural Collections

Ventricular collapse and subdural air leading to lethargy is a frequent postoperative finding, yet such collapse resolves spontaneously without significant morbidity (Fig. 17-53). There was only one instance of a significant subdural hygroma, which occurred in a 16-year-old boy following removal of a mixed teratoma-germinoma. A CSF leak had resulted from a fracture of the temporal bone at one of the pin sites from the Mayfield three-point head holder. He ultimately had a satisfactory outcome following an operation on postoperative day 7 for repair of the fracture

and dural tear with a subdural hygroma to peritoneal shunt.

Complications of Supratentorial Approaches

Although 90 percent of operations were performed using the supracerebellar-infratentorial approach, several complications occurred using the transcallosal or occipital-transtentorial approach and are included for the sake of completeness. Six of the 15 patients with significant postoperative morbidity underwent a transcallosal approach (Table 17-17). Additionally, five patients had postoperative seizures following an interhemispheric transcallosal approach. These seizures were easily controlled following therapeutic doses of anticonvulsants. Five patients developed hemiparesis that resolved sponta-

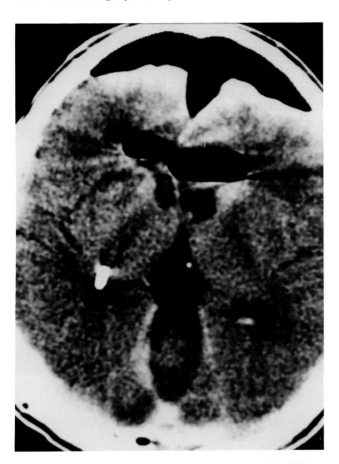

Figure 17-53. Ventricular collapse and subdural air following removal of a mixed germ cell tumor operated on in the sitting position. Patient made a full recovery as air resolved spontaneously over several days.

neously within several days postoperatively following the interhemispheric approach. Two patients had postoperative field deficits that disappeared spontaneously without significant impairment in one patient. All of these patients had undergone an interhemispheric approach except for one with an occipital-transtentorial approach. There were no instances of seizures, hemiparesis, or visual field deficits following the supracerebellar-infratentorial approach.

Postoperative Complications

Hemorrhage

Postoperative hemorrhage proved to be the most devastating complication, leading to five deaths; one patient had significant morbidity (Table 17-19). Hemorrhages were most commonly associated with sub-

totally resected pineal cell tumors and usually resulted from bleeding into the tumor bed. In several instances, this occurred several days into the postoperative period, even after the patient was making a full recovery. The decision to remove the clot is made on an individual basis, but in general we have not found aggressive management to improve the outcome necessarily. Often hemorrhages occurred into a large tumor bed and responded to conservative management with careful attention to sufficient CSF diversion. Hydrocephalus played a prominent role in the fatality of at least one patient following hemorrhage.

Three patients had hemorrhages in the cerebellum, which in two cases were seen only on routine follow-up scans. Presumably this was related to cerebellar retraction. Whenever the infratentorial approach is used, the precentral cerebellar vein is sacrificed, but we do not have any evidence that this contributes to cerebellar hemorrhage.[144,169]

Inflammatory and Infectious Complications

Eight patients developed aseptic meningitis, which in all cases responded to dexamethasone. The incidence of this complication has been reduced by the use of craniotomies rather than craniectomies and by meticulous wound closure. Bacterial meningitis occurred in only one patient, who responded readily to appropriate antibiotics. There were no instances of wound infection or CSF leak.

Hydrocephalus and Shunt Complications

Shunt malfunction occurs in over 20 percent of patients postoperatively. As a result, we often leave a separate ventricular drain in during surgery and allow it to remain for several days. It is removed only when there is clear evidence of a functioning shunt or reopened normal CSF pathways. Hydrocephalus played a significant role in one patient's death.

Medical and Iatrogenic Complications

Patients with pineal tumors are generally young and otherwise healthy; hence the incidence of medical and iatrogenic complications is relatively low. Five patients developed pulmonary compromise or infection. Pulmonary embolus accounted for one death in a patient with an ependymoma who had been making a gradual recovery following a postoperative hemorrhage. Steroid usage was associated with psychosis in three patients and probably contributed to a ruptured gastric ulcer in another patient. Erythema

Table 17-19. Summary of Patients with Hemorrhage in 146 Operations for Pineal Region Tumors

Tumor	Extent of Tumor Resection	Timing of Hemorrhage	Location of Hemorrhage	Outcome
Cystic astrocytoma	Total	Postoperative day 0–2?	Cerebellum	Asymptomatic
Pineocytoma	Subtotal	Postoperative day 3	Tumor bed	Made full recovery
Germinoma	Subtotal	Intraoperative	Cerebellum	Made full recovery
Meningioma	Total	Postoperative day 0	Tumor bed	Made full recovery
Pineoblastoma	Subtotal	Postoperative day 2	Tumor bed/3rd ventricle	Required ventricular drain; made full recovery
Pineocytoma	Subtotal	Postoperative day 3	Tumor bed	Made full recovery
Pineocytoma	Biopsy	Immediately postoperative	Tumor bed/3rd ventricle	Hemorrhage followed uncontrollable high blood pressure; died postoperative day 2
Pineocytoma	Subtotal	Several hours postoperative	Tumor bed/3rd ventricle	Died postoperative day 4
Astrocytoma	Subtotal	Postoperative day 10	Tumor bed	Initially had made full recovery until hemorrhage; died postoperative day 27
Ependymoma	Subtotal	Several hours postoperative	Tumor bed	Died from pulmonary embolus on postoperative day 16 after making gradual improvement
Ependymoma	Total	Postoperative day 6	Cerebellum/3rd ventricle	Developed acute hydrocephalus and herniation → clot removed, ventricular drain placed; died postoperative day 9

multiforme due to a phenytoin reaction occurred in one patient with prophylactic anticonvulsants for the interhemispheric approach. The most significant medical complication occurred in the patient described earlier who died of multisystem failure following reoperation for his recurrent teratoma.

CONCLUSIONS

Successful pineal region surgery requires a thorough understanding of the surrounding anatomy and operative approaches with an appreciation of the possible complications. Avoiding excessive manipulation of neural structures requires experienced intraoperative judgement for guiding the extent of tumor resection. Meticulous attention to hemostasis can minimize the incidence of postoperative hemorrhage with its own devastating sequelae, although this may not always be preventable. Strict attention to detail in the operative setup is necessary to avoid intraoperative fatigue, which can increase the rate of errors. As with any surgery, experience is invaluable for avoiding complications when possible and for managing those that are inevitable.

With the recent improvements in microsurgical technique and neuroanesthesia, a favorable surgical outcome is possible more than 90 percent of the time. The one-third of tumors that are benign and encapsulated have the most favorable results, with a cure rate approaching 100 percent. Although malignant tumors are only occasionally resectable, an aggressive approach is necessary to provide an accurate histological diagnosis and tumor debulking when possible to improve the response to adjuvant therapy. Further progress will follow the development of refinement of adjuvant therapy strategies.

REFERENCES

General Considerations

1. Dandy W: An operation for the removal of pineal tumors. Surg Gynecol Obstet 33:113, 1921
2. Jamieson KG: Excision of pineal tumors. J Neurosurg 35:550, 1971
3. Krabbe KH: The pineal gland, especially in relation to the problem of its supposed significance in sexual development. Endocrinology 7:379, 1923
4. Krause F: Operative Freilegung der Vierhügel nebst Beobachtungen über Hirndruck und Dekompression. Zentralbl Chir 53:2812, 1926
5. Lang J: Praktische Anatomie. Kopf Teil B Gehirn- und Augenschädel, Springer, Berlin, 1979

6. Matsushima T, Rhoton AL Jr, de Oliveira E, Peace D: Microsurgical anatomy of the veins of the posterior fossa. J Neurosurg 59:63, 1983

7. Oppenheim H, Krause F: Operative Erfolge bei Geschwülsten der Sehhügel-und Vierhügelgegend. Berl Klin Wochenschr 50:2316, 1913

8. Poppen JL, Marino R Jr: Pinealomas and tumors of the posterior portion of the third ventricle. J Neurosurg 28:357, 1968

9. Sano K: Pineal region tumors: problems in pathology and treatment. Clin Neurosurg 30:59, 1983

10. Sano K: Treatment of tumors in the pineal and posterior third ventricular region. p. 309. In Samii M (ed): Surgery in and around the Brain Stem and the Third Ventricle. Springer, Berlin, 1986

11. Sano K, Matsutani M, Seto T: So-called intracranial germ cell tumours: personal experiences and a theory of their pathogenesis. Neurol Res 11:118, 1989

12. Sano K, Nagai M, Tsuchida T, Hoshina T: New diagnostic method of brain tumors by cell culture of the cerebrospinal fluid-millipore filter-cell culture method. Neurol Med Chir 8:17, 1966

13. Stein BM: The infratentorial supracerebellar approach to pineal lesions. J Neurosurg 35:197, 1971

14. Tamaki N, Fujiwara K, Matsumoto S, Takeda H: Veins draining the pineal body: an anatomical and neuroradiological study of "pineal veins." J Neurosurg 39:448, 1973

15. Zapletal B: Ein neuer operativer Zugang zum Gebiet der Incisura Tentorii. Zentralbl Neurochir 16:64, 1956

Selection of an Operative Approach

16. Committee of Brain Tumor Registry of Japan: Brain Tumor Registry of Japan. Vol. 7. National Cancer Institute, Tokyo, 1990

17. Cossu M, Labinu MD, Orunesu MD et al: Subchoroidal approach to the third ventricle: microsurgical anatomy. Surg Neurol 21:325, 1984

18. Krause F: Operative Freilegung der Vierhugel, mebst Beobachtungen über Hirndruck und Dekompression. Zentralbl Chir 53:2812, 1926

19. Lapras C: Surgical therapy of pineal region tumors. p. 289. In Neuwelt EA (ed): Diagnosis and Treatment of Pineal Region Tumors. Williams & Wilkins, Baltimore, 1984

20. Lavayne MH, Patterson RH: Subchoroidal transvelum interposition approach to mid-third ventricular tumors. Neurosurgery 12:86, 1983

21. Neuwelt EA (ed): Diagnosis and Treatment of Pineal Region Tumors. Williams & Wilkins, Baltimore, 1984

22. Reid WS, Clark WK: Comparison of the infratentorial and transtentorial approaches to the pineal region. Neurosurgery 3:1, 1978

23. Sawaya R, Hawley DK, Tobler WD et al: Pineal and third ventricle tumors. p. 3171. In Youmans JR (ed): Neurological Surgery. 3rd Ed. Vol. 5. WB Saunders, Philadelphia, 1990

24. Stein MB: The infratentorial supracerebellar approach to pineal lesions. J Neurosurg 35:197, 1971

25. Stein BM: The suboccipital, supracerebellar approach to the pineal region. p. 213. In Neuwelt EA (ed): Diagnosis and Treatment of Pineal Region Tumors. Williams & Wilkins, Baltimore, 1984

26. Viale GL, Turtas S: The subchoroidal approach to the third ventricle. Surg Neurol 14:71, 1980

27. Zülch KJ: Reflection on the surgery of the pineal gland (a glimpse into the past). Neurosurg Rev 4:159, 1981

Supratentorial Approaches to the Pineal Region

28. Abay E, Laws ER, Grado GL et al: Pineal tumors in children and adolescents. Treatment by CSF shunting and radiotherapy. J Neurosurg 55:889, 1981

29. Apuzzo MLJ, Chandrasoma PT, Zelman V et al: Computed tomographic guidance stereotaxis in the management of lesions of the third ventricle. Neurosurgery 15:502, 1984

30. Apuzzo MLJ, Giannotta SL: Transcallosal interforniceal approach. In Apuzzo MLJ (ed): Surgery of the Third Ventricle. Williams & Wilkins, Baltimore, 1987

31. Bailey P: Peculiarities of the intracranial venous system and their clinical significance. Arch Neurol Psychiatry 32:1105, 1934

32. Bedford THB: The nervous system of the velum interpositum of the rhesus monkey and the effect of the experimental occlusion of the great vein of Galen. Brain 57:255, 1934

33. Bogen JE: Physiological consequences of complete or partial commissural section. In Apuzzo MLJ (ed): Surgery of the Third Ventricle. Williams & Wilkins, Baltimore, 1987

34. Brunner C, quoted by Rorschach H: Zur Pathologie und Operabilitat der Tumoren der Zirbeldruse. Beitr Z Klin Chir 83:451, 1913

35. Cairns H, Mosherg WH: Colloid cyst of the third ventricle. Surg Gynecol Obstet 92:545, 1981

36. Camins MB, Schlesinger EB: Treatment of tumours of the posterior part of the third ventricle and the pineal region: a long term follow-up. Acta Neurochir (Wien) 40:131, 1978

37. Caron JP, Debrun G, Sichez JP, Comoy J: Ligature des veines cérébrales internes et survie: à propos de deux pineal anatomies. Neurochirurgie 20:81, 1974

38. Clark WK: Occipital transtentorial approach. In Apuzzo MLJ (ed): Surgery of the Third Ventricle. Williams & Wilkins, Baltimore, 1987

39. Cummins FM, Taveras JM, Schlesinger EB: Treatment of gliomas of the third ventricle and pinealomas. Neurology 10:1031, 1960

40. Cushing H: Intracranial Tumors: Notes upon a Series of Two Thousand Verified Cases with Surgical Mortality Pertaining Thereto. p. 64. Charles C Thomas, Springfield, IL, 1933

41. Damasio AR, Chui HC, Corbett J, Kassel N: Posterior callosal section in a non-epileptic patient. J Neurol Neurosurg Psychiatry 43:351, 1980

42. Dandy WE: An operation for the removal of pineal tumors. Surg Gynecol Obstet 33:113, 1921

43. Dandy WE: Operative experience in cases of pineal tumor. Arch Surg 33:19, 1936

44. Dejerine J: Contribution à l'étude anatomo-pathologique et clinique des differentes variétés de cecite verbale. CR Seances Memoires Soc Biol 44 (second section—Memoires) 4:61, 1892

45. Demakas JJ, Sonntag VKH, Kaplan AM et al: Surgical management of pineal area tumors in early childhood. Surg Neurol 17:435, 1982

46. Dimond SJ, Scammell RE, Brouwers EYM, Weeks R: Functions of the centre section (trunk) of the corpus callosum in man. Brain 100:543, 1977

47. Dott NM: Surgical aspects of the hypothalamus. In Clarke WEL, Beattie J, Riddoch GG, et al (eds): The Hypothalamus: Morphological, Functional, Clinical and Surgical Aspects. Oliver and Boyd, London, 1938

48. Edwards MSB, Hudgins RJ, Wilson CB et al: Pineal region tumors in children. J Neurosurg 68:689, 1988

49. Ehlers H, Courville CB: Thrombosis of the internal cerebral veins in infancy and childhood. J Pediatr 8:600, 1936

50. Garcia-Bengochea F, de la Torre O, Esquivel O, et al: The section of the fornix in the surgical treatment of certain epilepsies. Trans Am Neurol Assoc 79:176, 1954

51. Gazzaniga MS, Risse GL, Springer SP et al: Psychologic and neurologic consequences of partial and complete cerebral commissurotomy. Neurology (NY) 25:10, 1975

52. Geschwind N: Disconnexion syndromes in animals and man. Brain 88:237, 584, 1965

53. Geschwind N, Fusillo M: Color naming defects in association with alexia. Arch Neurol 15:137, 1966

54. Glasauer FE: An operative approach to pineal tumors. Acta Neurochir (Wien) 22:177, 1970

55. Fujji K, Lenkey C, Rhoton AL, Jr: Microsurgical anatomy of the choroidal arteries: lateral and third ventricles. J Neurosurg 52:165, 1980

56. Hammock MK, Milhorat TH, Earle K, et al: Vein of Galen ligation in the primate: angiographic, gross, and light microscopic evaluation. J Neurosurg 34:77, 1971

57. Harris W, Cairns H, Adelaide B: Diagnosis and treatment of pineal tumors with report of a case. Lancet 1:3, 1932

58. Heilman KM, Sypert GW: Korsakoff's syndrome resulting from bilateral fornix lesions. Neurology (NY) 27:490, 1977

59. Hirsch JF, Zouaoui A, Renier D, Pierre-Kahn A: A new surgical approach to the third ventricle with interruption of the striothalamic vein. Acta Neurochir (Wien) 47:135, 1979

60. Hoffman HJ, Yoshida M, Becker LE et al: Pineal region tumors in childhood. Experience at the Hospital for Sick Children. p. 360. In Humphreys RP (ed): Concepts in Pediatric Neurosurgery 4. S Karger AG, Basel, 1983

61. Horrax G: Extirpation of a huge pinealoma from a patient with pubertas praecox: a new operative approach. Arch Neurol Psychiatry 37:385, 1937

62. Horrax G: Treatment of tumors of the pineal body. Arch Neurol Psychiatry 69:227, 1950

63. Horsley V: Discussion. Proc R Soc Med 3(Pt 2):77, 1910

64. Iwata M, Sugishita M, Toyokura YY et al: Etude dans le syndrome de disconnexion visuo-linguale apres la transection du splenium du corps calleux. J Neurol Sci 23:421, 1974

65. Jamieson KG: Excision of pineal tumors. J Neurosurg 35:550, 1971

66. Johnson S, Greenwood R, Fishman MA: Internal cerebral vein thrombosis. Arch Neurol 28:205, 1973

67. Jooma R, Kendall BE: Diagnosis and management of pineal tumors. J Neurosurg 58:654, 1983

68. Kahn EA: Surgical treatment of pineal tumor. Arch Neurol Psychiatry 38:833, 1937

69. Kunicki A: Operative experiences in eight cases of pineal tumor. J Neurosurg 17:815, 1960

70. Lapras C, Patet JD: Controversies, techniques, and strategies for pineal tumor surgery. In Apuzzo MLJ (ed): Surgery of the Third Ventricle. Williams & Wilkins, Baltimore, 1987

71. Lapras C, Patet JD, Mottolese C, Lapras C, Jr: Direct surgery for pineal tumors: occipital-transtentorial approach. Prog Exp Tumor Res 30:268, 1987

72. Lazar ML, Clark K: Direct surgical management of masses in the region of the vein of Galen. Surg Neurol 2:17, 1974

73. Luo SQ, Li DZ, Zhang MZ et al: Occipital transtentorial approach for removal of pineal region tumors: report of 64 consecutive cases. Surg Neurol 32:36, 1989

74. Majerszki C, Majtenyi C: Thrombosis of the internal cerebral veins. p. 641. In: Proceedings of the 7th International Congress of Neuropathology. Excerpta Medica, Amsterdam, 1975

75. McComb JG, Apuzzo MLJ: Posterior intrahemispheric retrocallosal and transcallosal approaches. In Apuzzo MLJ (ed): Surgery of the Third Ventricles. Williams & Wilkins, Baltimore, 1987

76. Neuwelt EA, Glasbery M, Frenkel E, Clark WK: Malignant pineal region rumors. J Neurosurg 51:597, 1979

77. Obrador S, Soto M, Gutierrez-Diaz JA: Surgical management of tumors of the pineal region. Acta Neurochir (Wien) 34:159, 1976

78. Pecker J, Scarabin JM, Vallee B et al: Treatment of tumours in the pineal region: value of stereotaxic biopsy. Surg Neurol 12:341, 1979

79. Popo I, Salvolini U: Meningiomas of the free margin

of the tentorium developing in the pineal region. Neuroradiology 7:237, 1974

80. Poppen JL: The right occipital approach to a pinealoma. J Neurosurg 25:706, 1966

81. Poppen JL, Marino R: Pinealomas and tumors of the posterior portion of the third ventricle. J Neurosurg 28:357, 1968

82. Preilowski BFB: Possible contribution of the anterior forebrain commissures to bilateral motor coordination. Neuropsychologie 10:267, 1972

83. Rand RW, Lemmen LJ: Tumors of the posterior portion of the third ventricle. J Neurosurg 10:1, 1953

84. Reid WS, Clark WK: Comparison of the infratentorial and transtentorial approaches for the pineal region. Neurosurgery 3:1, 1978

85. Rhoton AL, Jr: Microsurgical anatomy of the third ventricular region. In Apuzzo MLJ (ed): Surgery of the Third Ventricle. Williams & Wilkins, Baltimore, 1987

86. Rhoton AL, Jr, Yamamoto I, Peace DA: Microsurgery of the third ventricle: Part 2. Operative approaches. Neurosurgery 8:357, 1981

87. Ringertz N, Nordenstam H, Flyger G: Tumors of the pineal region. Exp Neurol 13:540, 1954

88. Russel WO, Sachs E: Pinealoma: a clinicopathologic study of 7 cases with a review of the literature. Arch Pathol 35:869, 1943

89. Sachs E, Jr, Avman N, Fischer RG: Meningiomas of the pineal region and posterior part of the third ventricle. J Neurosurg 19:325, 1962

90. Sakaki S, Shiraishi T, Takeda S et al: Occlusion of great vein of Galen associated with a huge meningioma in the pineal region. J Neurosurg 61:1136, 1984

91. Schijman E: Microsurgical anatomy of the transcallosal approach to the ventricular system, pineal region and basal ganglia. Childs Nerv Syst 5:212, 1989

92. Shucart WA, Stein BM: Transcallosal approach to the anterior ventricular system. Neurosurgery 3:339, 1978

93. Smith RR, Sanford RA: Disorders of the deep cerebral veins. In Rapp JP and Schmidek HH (eds): The Cerebral Venous Systems and its Disorders. Grune & Stratton, Orlando, 1984

94. Smith RR, Sanford RA, Schmidek HH: Deep veins. In Apuzzo MLJ (ed): Surgery of the Third Ventricle. Williams & Wilkins, Baltimore, 1987

95. Stein BM: The suboccipital, supracerebellar approach to the pineal region. p. 213. In Neuwelt EA (ed): Diagnosis and Treatment of Pineal Region Tumors. Williams & Wilkins, Baltimore, 1984

96. Stein BM: Infratentorial supracerebellar approach. In Apuzzo MLJ (ed): Surgery of the Third Ventricle. Williams & Wilkins, Baltimore, 1987

97. Stern WE, Batzdorf U, Rich JR: Challenges of surgical excision of tumors in the pineal region. Bull Los Angeles Neurol Soc 36:105, 1971

98. Stone JL, Cybulski GR, Rhee HL, Bailey OT: Excision of a large pineal hemangio-pericytoma (angioblastic meningioma hemangiopericytoma type). Surg Neurol 19:181, 1983

99. Sugishita M, Shirohara A, Shimoji T: Does posterior lesion of the corpus callosum cause hemialexia? In Reeves A (ed): Epilepsy and Corpus Callosum. Plenum, New York, 1985

100. Sugita K, Hongo K: Posterior transcortical approach. In Apuzzo MLJ (ed): Surgery of the Third Ventricle. Williams & Wilkins, Baltimore, 1987

101. Suzuki J, Iwabuchi T: Surgical removal of pineal tumors (pinealomas and teratomas): experience in a series of 19 cases. J Neurosurg 23:565, 1965

102. Sweet WH, Talland GQ, Ervin FR: Loss of recent memory following section of the fornix. Trans Am Neurol Assoc 84:76, 1959

103. Trescher HH, Ford FR: Colloid cyst of the third ventricle: report of a case. Operative removal with section of posterior half of the corpus callosum. Arch Neurol Psychiatry 37:959, 1937

104. Van Wagenen WP: A surgical approach for the removal of certain pineal tumors. Report of a case. Surg Gynecol Obstet 53:216, 1931

105. Ventureyra ECG: Pineal region: surgical management of tumours and vascular malformations. Surg Neurol 16:77, 1981

106. Ward A, Spurling RG: The conservative treatment of third ventricle tumors. J Neurosurg 5:124, 1949

107. Wechsler AF: Transient left hemialexia. Neurology (NY) 22:628, 1972

108. Woolsley RM, Nelson JS: Asymptomatic destruction of the fornix in man. Arch Neurol 32:566, 1975

109. Yamamoto I, Kageyama N: Microsurgical anatomy of the pineal region. J Neurosurg 53:205, 1980

110. Yamamoto I, Rhoton AL, Jr, Peace DA: Microsurgery of the third ventricle: Part 1. Microsurgical anatomy. Neurosurgery 8:334, 1981

111. Yasargil MG, Jain KK, Antic J, Laciga J: Arteriovenous malformations of the splenium of the corpus callosum: microsurgical treatment. Surg Neurol 5:5, 1976

112. Zaidel D, Sperry KW: Memory impairment after commissurotomy in man. Brain 97:263, 1974

Supracerebellar Approaches to the Pineal Region

113. Abay EO, Laws ER, Grado GL et al: Pineal tumors in children and adolescents. Treatment by CSF shunting and radiotherapy. J Neurosurg 55:889, 1981

114. Burres KP, Hamilton RD: Pineal apoplexy. Neurosurgery 4:264, 1979

115. Bjornsson J, Scheithauer BW, Okazaki H et al: Intracranial germ cell tumors: pathobiological and immunohistological aspects of 70 cases. J Neuropathol Exp Neurol 44:32, 1985

116. Boyd MC, Steinbok P: Pineal region tumors. Can J Neurol Sci 12:35, 1985

117. Bruce JN, Fetell MR, Stein BM: Incidence of spinal metastases in patients with malignant pineal region

tumors: avoidance of prophylactic spinal irradiation. J Neurosurg 72:354A, 1990

118. Bruce JN, Stein BM: Pineal region tumor. p. 73. In Long DM (ed): Current Therapy in Neurological Surgery. 2nd Ed. BC Decker, Toronto, 1989

119. Bruce JN, Stein BM: Pineal tumors. Neurosurg Clin North Am 1:123, 1990

120. Bruce JN, Stein BM: Subtentorial approach to pineal tumors. p. 63. In Wilson CB (ed): Neurosurgical Procedures: Personal Approaches to Classic Operations. Williams & Wilkins, Baltimore, 1992

121. Carmel PW, Frazer RAR, Stein BM: Aseptic meningitis following posterior fossa surgery in children. J Neurosurg 41:44, 1974

122. Casentini L, Colombo F, Pozza F et al: Combined radiosurgery and external radiotherapy of intracranial germinomas. Surg Neurol 34:79, 1990

123. Chandrasoma PT, Smith MM, Apuzzo MLJ: Stereotactic biopsy in the diagnosis of brain masses: comparison of results of biopsy and resected surgical specimen. Neurosurgery 24:160, 1989

124. Chapman PH, Linggood RM: The management of pineal area tumors: a recent reappraisal. Cancer 46:1253, 1980

125. Conway LW: Stereotaxic diagnosis and treatment of intracranial tumors including an initial experience with cryosurgery for pinealomas. J Neurosurg 38:453, 1973

126. Cummins FM, Taveras JM, Schlesinger EB: Treatment of gliomas of the third ventricle and pinealomas. With special reference to the value of radiotherapy. Neurology 10:1031, 1960

127. Dandy WE: An operation for the removal of pineal tumors. Surg Gynecol Obstet 33:113, 1921

128. Dandy WE: Operative experience of cases of pineal tumor. Arch Surg 33:19, 1936

129. DeGirolami U, Schmidek H: Clinicopathological study of 53 tumors of the pineal region. J Neurosurg 39:455, 1973

130. Donat JF, Okazaki H, Gomez MR et al: Pineal tumors. A 53-year experience. Arch Neurol 35:736, 1978

131. Edwards MSB, Hudgins RJ, Wilson CB et al: Pineal region tumors in children. J Neurosurg 68:689, 1988

132. Fetell MR, Bruce JN, Burke AM et al: Non-neoplastic pineal cysts. Neurology 41:1034, 1991

133. Ganti SR, Hilal SK, Stein BM et al: CT of pineal region tumors. AJNR 7:97, 1986

134. Herrick MK, Rubinstein LJ: The cytological differentiating potential of pineal parenchymal neoplasms (true pinealomas). Brain 102:289, 1979

135. Higashi K, Katayama S, Orita T: Pineal apoplexy. J Neurol Neurosurg Psychiatry 42:1050, 1979

136. Hoffman HJ, Yoshida M, Becker LE et al: Pineal region tumors in childhood. Experience at the Hospital for Sick Children. p. 360. In Humphreys RP (ed): Concepts in Pediatric Neurosurgery 4. S Karger AG, Basel, 1983

137. Hoffman HJ, Yoshida M, Becker LE et al: Experience with pineal region tumours in childhood. Neurosurg Res 6:107, 1984

138. Horrax G, Daniels JT: The conservative treatment of pineal tumors. Surg Clin North Am 22:649, 1942

139. Jooma R, Kendall BE: Diagnosis and management of pineal tumors. J Neurosurg 58:654, 1983

140. Kobayashi S, Sugita K, Tanaka Y et al: Infratentorial approach to the pineal region in the prone position. Concorde position. J Neurosurg 58:141, 1983

141. Korf HW, Bruce JN, Vistica B et al: Immunoreactive S-antigen in cerebrospinal fluid: a marker of pineal parenchymal tumors? J Neurosurg 70:682, 1989

142. Kraichoke S, Cosgrove M, Chandrasoma PT: Granulomatous inflammation in pineal germinoma. Am J Surg Pathol 12:655, 1988

143. Krause F: Operative Frielegung der Vierhugel, nebst Beobachtungen uber Hirndruck unk Dekompression. Zentralbl Chir 53:2812, 1926

144. Lapras C, Patet JD: Controversies, techniques, and strategies for pineal tumor surgery. p. 649. In Apuzzo MLJ (ed): Surgery of the Third Ventricle. Williams & Wilkins, Baltimore, 1987

145. Linstadt D, Wara WM, Edwards MS et al: Radiotherapy of primary intracranial germinomas: the case against routine craniospinal irradiation. Int J Radiat Oncol Biol Phys 15:291, 1988

146. Lunsford LD: Pineal region masses in adults. Neurosurg Consultations 1:1, 1990

147. Moser RP, Backlund EO: Stereotactic techniques in the diagnosis and treatment of pineal region tumors. p. 236. In Neuwalt EA (ed): Diagnosis and Treatment of Pineal Region Tumors. Williams & Wilkins, Baltimore, 1984

148. Nagao S, Kuyama H, Murota T et al: Surgical approaches to pineal tumors: Complications and outcome. Neurol Med Chir (Tokyo) 28:779, 1988

149. Neuwelt EA: An update on the surgical treatment of malignant pineal region tumors. Clin Neurosurg 32:397, 1985

150. Neuwelt EA, Glasberg M, Frenkel E et al: Malignant pineal region tumors. A clinico-pathological study. J Neurosurg 51:597, 1979

151. Noell KT, Herskovic AM: Principles of radiotherapy of CNS tumors. p. 1084. In Wilkins RH, Rengachary SS (eds): Neurosurgery. Vol. 1. McGraw-Hill, New York, 1985

152. Page LK: The infratentorial-supracerebellar exposure of tumors in the pineal area. Neurosurgery 1:36, 1977

153. Pecker J, Scarabin JM, Vallee B et al: Treatment in tumours of the pineal region: value of stereotaxic biopsy. Surg Neurol 12:341, 1979

154. Pendl G: Case material. p. 128. In Pendl G (ed): Pineal and Midbrain Lesions. Springer-Verlag, Wien, 1985

155. Peragut JC, Dupard T, Graciani N et al: De la prevention des risques de la biopsie stereotaxique de cer-

taines tumeurs de la region pineale. Neurochirugie 33:23, 1987

156. Pluchino F, Broggi G, Fornari M et al: Surgical approach to pineal tumours. Acta Neurochir 96:26, 1989

157. Poppen JL: The right occipital approach to a pinealoma. J Neurosurg 25:706, 1966

158. Poppen JL, Marino R: Pinealomas and tumors of the posterior portion of the third ventricle. J Neurosurg 28:357, 1968

159. Rand RW, Lemmen LJ: Tumors of the posterior portion of the third ventricle. J Neurosurg 10:1, 1953

160. Reid WS, Clark K: Comparison of the infratentorial and transtentorial approaches to the pineal region. Neurosurgery 3:1, 1978

161. Rosenfield JV, Murphy MA, Chow CW: Implantation metastasis of pineoblastoma after stereotactic biopsy. J Neurosurg 73:287, 1990

162. Rout D, Sharma A, Radhakrishnan VV et al: Exploration of the pineal region: observation and results. Surg Neurol 21:135, 1984

163. Rubinstein LJ: Cytogenesis and differentiation of pineal neoplasms. Hum Pathol 12:441, 1980

164. Sano K: Diagnosis and treatment of tumors in the pineal region. Acta Neurochir (Wien) 34:153, 1976

165. Sano K: Pineal region and posterior third ventricular tumors: a surgical overview. p. 663. In Apuzzo MLJ (ed): Surgery of the Third Ventricle. Williams & Wilkins, Baltimore, 1987

166. Sawaya R, Hawley DK, Tobler WD et al: Pineal and third ventricle tumors. p. 3171. In Youmans JR (ed): Neurological Surgery. WB Saunders, Philadelphia, 1990

167. Stein BM: The infratentorial supracerebellar approach to pineal lesions. J Neurosurg 35:197, 1971

168. Stein BM: Surgical treatment of pineal tumors. Clin Neurosurg 26:490, 1979

169. Stein BM: Supracerebellar approach for pineal region neoplasms. p. 401. In Schmidek HH, Sweet WH (eds): Operative Neurosurgical Techniques. Vol. 1. Grune & Stratton, Orlando, 1988

170. Stein BM, Fetell MR: Therapeutic modalities for pineal region tumors. Clin Neurosurg 32:445, 1985

171. Steinbock P, Dolmen CL, Kaan K: Pineocytomas presenting as subarachnoid hemorrhage. Report of 2 cases. J Neurosurg 47:776, 1977

172. Sung D, Harisiadis L, Chang CH: Midline pineal tumors and suprasellar germinomas: Highly curable by irradiation. Radiology 128:745, 1978

173. Van Wagenen WP: A surgical approach for the removal of certain pineal tumors: report of a case. Surg Gynecol Obstet 53:216, 1931

174. Ventureyra ECG: Pineal region: surgical management of tumours and vascular malformations. Surg Neurol 16:77, 1981

175. Wilson ER, Takei Y, Bikoff WT et al: Abdominal metastases of primary intracranial yolk sac tumors through ventriculoperitoneal shunts: report of three cases. Neurosurg 5:356, 1979

176. Wood JH, Zimmerman RA, Bruce DA et al: Assessment and management of pineal-region and related tumors. Surg Neurol 16:192, 1981

177. Zimmerman RA: Pineal region masses: radiology. p. 680. In Wilkins RH, Rengachary SS (eds): Neurosurgery. Vol. 1. McGraw-Hill, New York, 1985

18 Surgery in and around the Anterior Third Ventricle

Michael L. J. Apuzzo
N. Scott Litofsky

The region in and around the anterior third ventricle is an area of the brain dense with vital anatomical structures. Lesions of this area may be solely within the anterior portion of the chamber or may invade or compress various walls.

The anterior portion of the third ventricle is bounded anteriorly by the columns of the fornix, the foramina of Monro, the anterior commissure, the lamina terminalis, the optic recess, and the optic chiasm. The lateral margins include the thalamus superiorly and the hypothalamus inferiorly. The roof consists of the body of the fornix medially, choroid fissure with the tela choroidea, and thalamus laterally. Inferiorly, the floor is composed of the optic chiasm, infundibulum of the hypothalamus, tuber cinerium, and mamillary bodies.

Arteries of note in the area include the internal carotid, posterior communicating, anterior choroidal, anterior cerebral, anterior communicating, pericallosal, recurrent artery of Heubner, and branches of these arteries. The major draining veins are the septal, caudate, choroidal, and thalamic groups of veins, and the thalamostriate and internal cerebral veins.[89] These structures are all at risk of injury from lesions in the area or surgery upon these lesions.

While lesions of the anterior third ventricle are relatively uncommon, they encompass a wide spectrum of pathological entities. Some lesions are primarily intraventricular in location but may have attachments to the walls of the chamber. Such lesions include colloid (neuroepithelial) cysts, choroid plexus papillomas or carcinomas, ependymomas, giant cell astrocytomas (of tuberous sclerosis), craniopharyngiomas, meningiomas, xanthogranulomas, cysticercosis cysts, and hemorrhages from vascular lesions, such as aneurysms, cavernous angiomas, or arteriovenous malformations. Other lesions are found primarily in the walls of the ventricle, but may have intraventricular extension. Astrocytomas, including those of the hypothalamus and optic nerves, lymphomas, subependymomas, craniopharyngiomas, abscesses, metastatic carcinomas, cavernous angiomas, arteriovenous malformations, and inflammatory reactions such as sarcoidosis and histocytosis are among these lesions. Lastly, lesions that are primarily extra-axial in basal locations may compress or invade the walls of the anterior third ventricle. Lesions to consider here are diaphragma sellae or planum sphenoidale meningiomas, pituitary adenomas, craniopharyngiomas, epidermoids, dermoids, suprasellar germinomas, arachnoid cysts, and giant aneurysms of the circle of Willis.[6,16,43]

This multitude of lesions can be accessed by a variety of operative approaches. The most appropriate approach for a given lesion depends on the exact location of the lesion as determined by neuroimaging studies, the size of the lesion, the differential diagnosis being considered, and the clinical status of the patient. The transcortical and transcallosal approaches will allow the surgeon to reach the lateral ventricle. From there, the surgeon must gain access to the third ventricle via an approach through the foramen of Monro, with or without enlargement, an interfornical pathway, or a subchoroidal transvelum interpositum approach. Alternative corridors into the third ventricle include a subfrontal or a bifrontal anterior interhemispheric approach, both through the lamina terminalis. Extra-axial basal lesions can be reached via subfrontal, pterional, subtemporal, or transnasal transsphenoidal operations. Some lesions, especially those with cystic components, lend themselves to the use of stereotactic techniques for diagnosis and treatment.[5]

The interior of the anterior third ventricle can only be reached through an incision of a neural structure.[65] Complications may result from the anatomical disruption necessary for access in this location. Other complications result because of the proximity of anterior third ventricular lesions to the vital delicate neural and vascular structures of the area, and the need to manipulate these structures, however gently, to treat these lesions successfully. This chapter reviews and discusses the complications associated with the surgical approaches to the mass lesions of the anterior third ventricle.

It is important to consider complications associated with a surgery in relation to (1) the corridor, (2) the pathology, and (3) the manipulation at the target end point.

LITERATURE REVIEW

Transcortical–Transventricular Approach

The transcortical-transventricular approach, as the name implies, requires incision or a topectomy to reach the lateral ventricle. Once in the lateral ventricle, a secondary maneuver, such as the transforaminal approach or the subchoroidal transvelum interpositum approach, is necessary to reach the third ventricle. This approach is best for lesions with a substantial component within the third ventricle and with enlarged lateral ventricles.

The most frequently discussed complication (Table 18-1) of the transcortical transventricular approach is postoperative seizures.[1,6,10,33,44,48,57,61,71] The frequency of seizures has been reported to be as high as 27 percent.[10] This complication appears to result from the cortical incision, which creates an epileptogenic focus.

Neurological deficits have been reported following transcortical-transventricular approaches to the anterior third ventricle. In more recent series, hemiparesis occurred in up to 20 percent of patients,[1,10,33,48] though Poppen et al.[61] reported a 42 percent incidence in an early series. They felt that hemiparesis resulted from the retraction of the cortex and centrum necessary to visualize the ventricle through the cortical incision. Memory loss has also been reported. Fornix section has been undertaken, presumably with resulting memory loss.[1,23,57] Other patients may have memory deficits from retraction of the caudate nucleus, which was necessary in 27 percent of patients in Cairns and Mosberg's[10] series due to small ventricles. Confusion[10,57,61] and mutism were also reported. If the lateral ventricles are large, drainage of the ventricles through the cortical incision can lead to cortical collapse[20,61] and subdural fluid collections[29] with resulting neurological deficits. Cranial nerve VI paresis can occur.[61] This complication can result from postoperative elevated intracranial pressure. Acute hydrocephalus also may result, its etiology being either hemorrhage into the third ventricle with the clot obstructing the foramen of Monro[61] or obstruction secondary to debris and local edema.

Meningitis and ventriculitis are potential difficulties that may arise after the transcortical-transventricular operation. Shucart[71] stated that 15 percent of patients with intraventricular surgery develop aseptic meningitis from blood or other substances released into the cerebrospinal fluid spaces. One of 23 cases (4.3 percent) of Antunes et al.[1] became ill postoperatively from bacterial ventriculitis. Bacterial meningitis occurred in approximately 9 percent of patients of Cairns and Mosberg[10] and Little and MacCarty.[48] Elevated body temperative without infection was reported by others.[57,61]

Mortality of up to 28 percent has been reported.[61] More recently, death rates approximate 14[48] to 17[1] percent, although Kahn et al.[39] reported a 5 percent mortality. Unmanageable elevated intracranial pressure has been a precipitating cause of death.[1] Meningitis has also been a significant factor in patient mortality.[48] One of the two deaths reported by Poppen[61] occurred in a patient with hyperthermia without infection. This sign may reflect severe hypothalamic injury.

Attempted excision of invasive hypothalamic and thalamic gliomas infiltrating into the third ventricle was responsible for the deaths of two patients of Kahn et al.[39] Finally, pulmonary embolism, though not a complication unique to neurosurgical patients, has been a factor in patient mortality after transcortical-transventricular surgery.[39,61]

Table 18-1. Transcortical-Transventricular Approach

Complication	Incidence (if reported)[a]	Author
Seizure	2/23 (8.6)	Antunes et al., 1980
	3/11 (27)	Cairns & Mosberg, 1971
	—	Hirsch et al., 1979
	—	Lavyne & Patterson, 1987
	2/21 (9.5)	Little & MacCarty, 1974
	Case report	Patterson & Leslie, 1935
	2/7 (28)	Poppen et al., 1953
	—	Shucart, 1987
Hemiparesis	1/23 (4.3)	Antunes et al. 1980
Transient	—	Cairns & Mosberg, 1971
Transient	2/10 (20)	Hirsch et al., 1979
Transient	2/21 (9.5)	Little & MacCarty, 1974
	3/7 (42)	Poppen et al., 1953
Memory loss	1/23 (4.3)	Antunes et al., 1980
	Case report	Geffen et al., 1980
	Case report	Patterson & Leslie, 1935
	3/11 (27)	Cairns & Mosberg, 1971
Confusion	—	Cairns & Mosberg, 1971
	Case report	Patterson & Leslie, 1935
	—	Poppen et al., 1953
Mutism	—	Cairns & Mosberg, 1971
	1/7 (14)	Poppen et al., 1953
Subdural fluid collections	1/5 (20)	Hall & Lundsford, 1987
Cranial nerve VI paresis	1/7 (14)	Poppen et al., 1953
Acute hydrocephalus	1/7 (14)	Poppen et al., 1953
Meningitis	1/11 (9)	Cairns & Mosberg, 1971
Bacterial	2/21 (9.5)	Little & MacCarty, 1974
Aseptic	(15)	Ehni & Ehni, 1987
Ventriculitis	1/23 (4.3)	Antunes et al., 1980
Elevated body temperature	Case report	Patterson & Leslie, 1935
	1/7 (14)	Poppen et al., 1953
Death	4/23 (17)	Antunes et al., 1980
	2/40 (5)	Kahn et al., 1973
	3/21 (17)	Little & MacCarthy, 1979
	3/7 (42)	Poppen et al., 1953

[a] Percent in parentheses.

Transcallosal Approach

The transcallosal corridor permits the surgeon to enter the lateral ventricle and subsequently the third ventricle without a cortical incision. Ventriculomegaly is not a necessary prerequisite for this approach.[1,6,12] A wide variety of complications (Table 18-2) have been noted with transcallosal operations for anterior third ventricular lesions. Some of these complications are obvious and easily observable; others require specialized testing to be elicited.

Hemiparesis has been reported by several authors.[5,19,20,29,50,71,72,89] Shucart and Stein[72] reported a 16 percent incidence of hemiparesis in a series of 25 patients who had a transcallosal operation, and Hall and Lundsford[29] noted a 25 percent incidence. This neurological deficit may be caused by one of several different mechanisms of injury. During the exposure of the corpus callosum the frontal midline of the hemisphere is usually retracted laterally to facilitate visualization. Bridging cortical veins draining into the sagittal sinus are stretched or coagulated and sec-

Table 18-2. Transcallosal Approach

Complication	Incidence (if reported)[a]	Author
Hemiparesis	—	Apuzzo & Giannotta, 1987
	—	Ehni, 1984
	—	Ehni & Ehni, 1987
	—	Shucart, 1987
	4/25 (16)	Shucart & Stein, 1978
	—	Yamamoto et al., 1981
	2/8 (2.5)	Hall & Lundsford, 1987
	—	Long & Leibrock, 1980
	3/34 (8.8)	Harper & Ehni, 1979
Memory loss, transient	10/30 (33)	Apuzzo, 1986
	4/11 (36)	Apuzzo et al., 1982
	—	Ehni, 1984
	1/3 (33)	Jeeves et al., 1979
	—	Reigal, 1978
	3/4 (75)	Winston et al., 1974
	—	Yamamoto et al., 1981
	Case report	Trescher & Ford, 1932
Confabulation *(compensatory)*	—	Long & Leibrock, 1980
	2/5 (40)	Petrucci et al., 1987
Akinetic mutism, transient	—	Apuzzo, 1986
	—	Ehni, 1984
	—	Shucart, 1987
	1/12 (8.3)	Shucart & Stein, 1978
	Case report	Dimond et al., 1977
Aphasia	2/52 (3.8)	Enhi, 1984
Worsening stupor or obtundation	5/52 (9.5)	Ehni, 1984
Tactile transfer deficits	3/3 (100)	Jeeves et al., 1979
	1/52 (1.9)	Ehni, 1984
	—	Reigal, 1978
	—	Long & Leibrock, 1980
	—	Yamamoto et al., 1981
Auditory transfer deficit	—	Apuzzo, 1986
	Case report	Dimond et al., 1977
	—	Reigal, 1978
Astereognosis	1/5 (20)	Petrucci et al., 1987
	Case report	Trescher & Ford, 1932
Cranial nerve VI and VII paresis	—	Ehni, 1984
Cranial nerve VII paresis	—	Ehni, 1984
Meningitis		
Bacterial	1/8 (12)	Hall & Lundsford, 1987
Aseptic	(15)	Shucart, 1987
	3/25 (12)	Shucart & Stein, 1978
Bone flap infection	1/8 (12)	Hall & Lundsford, 1987
	1/52 (1.9)	Ehni, 1984
Hyperthermia	Case report	Lipton et al., 1981
Gastrointestinal hemorrhage	4/16 (67)	Long & Chou, 1973
Death	2/34 (5.8)	Harper & Ehni, 1979

[a] Percent in parentheses.

tioned to enhance exposure. Apuzzo and Giannotta[5] showed that 42 of 100 patients had significant cortical veins within 2 cm of the coronal suture. Compromise of these draining veins can lead to venous infarction with resulting hemiparesis, or a variety of cortical deficits, depending on the pattern of venous drainage in a given patient.[29,50,71] Retraction of the hemisphere laterally can also cause transient cerebral edema, which may result in hemiparesis, as in 8 percent of Harper and Ehni's patients.[31] Hemiparesis has occurred after occlusion of the superior sagittal sinus by retractor pressure.[72] Injury to a pericallosal artery[19,71] from retractor placement or dissection is another cause.

Mental status changes have been noted by many investigators following transcallosal surgery. The cause is debatable but probably relates to paraventricular midline injury. Memory disturbances have been a frequent topic of concern.[2,4,19,36,63,88,89] This loss usually involves short-term memory, and it is generally transient.[88] Winston et al.[88] reported that three of four children had transient diffuse memory loss, and Apuzzo[2] reported a 33 percent incidence. One of three patients of Jeeves et al.[36] had postoperative recent memory loss that resolved over time. After using a posterior transcallosal approach for a colloid cyst in the anterior third ventricle, Trescher and Ford[85] described a patient with transient memory loss with compensatory confabulation. Ehni[19] also noted that confabulation occurred in a patient. Confusion occurs postoperatively[50] as well in up to 40 percent of patients.[59] Some patients will develop a disparity of intelligence testing, with high verbal I.Q. and low performance I.Q.[36] On the other hand, in the acute postoperative period, some patients have been noted to have transient mutism.[2,10,71,72] This complication is felt to result from retraction of the cingulate gyri bilaterally to expose the superior corpus callosum or from thalamic injury.[2] Diamond et al.[17] reported a patient with postoperative mutism who subsequently improved, but still had significant verbal deficits, including difficulty naming, loss of ability to verbally express emotion, loss of technical vocabulary, and verbal memory loss. Aphasia has occurred in 4 percent of patients in one series.[19] Worsening stupor or obtundation occurs occasionally, in as many as 10 percent of patients.[19] Behavioral charges have also been noted.[19]

Much issue has been made in the literature regarding the transfer of information between the cerebral hemispheres after section of the corpus callosum. Complete section of the corpus callosum leads to profound deficits in the interhemispheric transfer of sensory information. Partial section is thought to result in specific sensory modality transfer disruption.[22] Others[24] feel that deficits should be minimal if the splenium is preserved. The transcallosal approach to the anterior third ventricle requires section of approximately 3 cm of the anterior to midcallosum, sparing the splenium. Despite many reported series of patients who have had transcallosal surgery and have no apparent signs of disconnection deficits,[1,4,88] others have described sometimes subtle interhemispheric transfer deficits. Jeeves et al.[36] noted that three of three patients had tactic transfer deficits. Ehni[19] had 1 patient of 52 (2 percent) with a tactile deficit. Reigel,[63] Long and Leibrock,[50] and Yamamoto[89] comment that tactile transfer deficits are common complications of transcallosal surgery. Petrucci et al.[59] also acknowledge tactile transfer difficulties, but in their three patients (of five), the deficits were present preoperatively. Perhaps these deficits reflect the nature of the pathological lesion rather than the surgical approach.

Auditory transfer deficits have also been noted,[63] but special dichotic testing is required to elicit the deficit.[2] The patient of Diamond et al.[17] showed a switch from right to left ear superiority. Astereognesis can be a complication after anterior[59] or posterior callosal section.[85] Visual transfer deficits can also result[63] but usually require splenium section,[22] which should not be necessary in approaching the anterior third ventricle.

Ehni[19] noted transient paresis of the sixth and seventh cranial nerves in several patients. He also noted transient visual loss in another patient. He provided no explanations for these complications. It is doubtful that these observations directly related to the corridor.

As with all surgical procedures, infectious complications also occur with transcallosal approaches. Meningitis and bone flap infections each occurred in as high as 12.5 percent of patients.[29] Ehni[19] noted a 2 percent incidence of bone flap infections in his series. Shucart[71,72] remarked that 15 percent of patients will suffer from aseptic meningitis, as with other patients in whom a ventricle is entered.

Hyperthermia without infection may complicate the postoperative course, as with the transcortical-transventricular approach.[47] This change probably reflects hypothalamic injury from tumor removal or the release of endogenous pyrogen from cellular material in the ventricles.

Long and Chou[49] reported one rather odd complication following transcallosal surgery for anterior third ventricular lesions. Four of six patients (all adults) with intraventricular craniopharyngiomas suffered massive gastrointestinal hemorrhages 1 week after surgery. Three of these four died from their hemorrhages. Since other authors did not experience such a complication with transcallosal approaches, Long and Leibrock[50] subsequently indicated that they felt such hemorrhages were a complication of the tumor type, and not a complication of the approach. It is of note that in describing the bifrontal interhemispheric approach through the lamina terminalis, Suzuki[75] also warned of the complication of gastrointestinal hemorrhage.

Transcallosal approaches to the anterior third ventricle can be attended by patient mortality. This event is not related directly to the corridor. Harper and Ehni[31] had eight deaths in 34 patients, but their discussion indicates that only two patients clearly suffered perioperative deaths, a 6 percent incidence. One of these patients, a neonate, succumbed to fluid mismanagement, and the other suffered bilateral occlusion of the anterior cerebral arteries.

Chamber Entry

Transforaminal Approaches

The most frequently employed route of third ventricular access is directly through the foramen of Monro. If the foramen is enlarged by hydrocephalus or by the mass, removal of a third ventricular lesion can be accomplished through the foramen with relative safety. Colloid cysts, in particular, lend themselves to this operative approach.

Often, the lesion will present through the foramen of Monro into the lateral ventricle. Puncture and drainage of a cyst will reduce its volume and make removal easier. The major complication (Table 18-3) of such a maneuver occurs if the lesion that was felt to be a colloid cyst in reality is an anterior communicating artery or basilar tip aneurysm within the third ventricle.[20] The hemorrhage that might occur with puncture could be devastating. Attempts to dissect a cyst from its superior attachments can yield hemorrhage from disruption of the lesion's vascular supply.[20]

Very commonly, the foramen of Monro is not large enough to effect treatment of anterior third ventricular lesions. Transforaminal removal of these lesions requires enlargement of the foramen. One method of such enlargement is to remove neural tissue from the posterior-inferior aspect of the foramen—a portion of the anterior nucleus of the thalamus.[18,25,31] Complications with this technique have not been clearly reported. Greenwood[25] used posterior enlargement of the foramen of Monro in some of his five patients who had colloid cysts, but he did not specify whether such an approach was used in the one patient who died, the one patient with verbal deficits, or the one patient who developed a pyschoneurosis. Regardless, exposure is less optimal than with the subchoroidal tranvelum interpositum approach.[20] Furthermore, Little and MacCarty[48] suggested that removal of posterior foraminal tissue has the risk of uncontrollable venous bleeding from the internal cerebral vein.

Alternatively, the fornix can be sectioned inferiorly to enlarge the foramen.[25,36,48,57,72] While many authors feel that section of a single fornix should not be associated with memory loss,[11,15,21,35] as previously discussed, others have noted that patients have had transient short-term memory loss after fornix section. Patterson and Leslie[57] reported one patient with memory loss following transcortical surgery for a colloid cyst including section of the fornix. This may be secondary to diffuse midline manipulation and not specifically to isolated unilateral fornical sacrifice. The one patient with fornix section in the series of Antunes et al.[1] had marked memory loss. On the other hand, none of six patients of Little and MacCarty[48] had memory loss after fornix section; one patient did remain comatose following surgery, but the authors felt that the complication was not a result of fornix section. Other authors[25,72] report no memory loss after fornix section in their patients. Therefore, fornical section itself may not be associated with memory loss. The point of this discussion, however, is that memory loss does occur as a complication in some patients who have had surgical section of a fornix. The fornical section may just be one com-

Table 18-3. Transforaminal Approaches

Complication	Incidence (if reported)[a]	Author
Hemorrhage	—	Ehni & Ehni, 1987
	—	Little & MacCarty, 1974
Memory loss	Case report 1/23 (4.3)	Patterson & Leslie, 1935 Antunes et al., 1980

[a] Percent in parentheses.

Table 18-4. Interfornical Approach

Complication	Incidence (if reported)[a]	Author
Memory loss transient	10/30 (33)	Apuzzo, 1986
	—	Ehni & Ehni, 1987
	4/11 (36)	Apuzzo et al., 1982
Paresis, transient	(10)	Apuzzo & Giannotta, 1987

[a] Percent in parentheses.

ponent of a multifocal injury to the structures involved with memory. Other injury may occur from effects of the lesion itself, or manipulation of the lesion and adjacent neural and vascular structures during surgery.

Interfornical Approach

In the event that foraminal exposure is inadequate, dissection may be required for third ventricular exposure.

The major problem (Table 18-4) associated with the interfornical component of this surgical approach is transient memory loss. Apuzzo and Giannotta[5] had a 33 percent incidence of transient memory loss in their series of patients using the interfornical approach. Seventy percent of patients had resolution of their deficit within 1 week, and all patients had normal memory after 3 months. Patients with softer lesions such as cysticercosis cysts had a lower incidence of memory loss, about 20 percent, while those with firmer lesions requiring more extensive manipulation had a much higher incidence (57 percent). The etiology of this memory loss is uncertain. Bilateral fornical injury may be responsible for memory loss.[20] Heilman and Sypert[32] reported a case of Korsakoff's syndrome in a patient with a tumor which destroyed both fornices. *Alternative viewpoints indicate that*

memory loss results from more diffuse, multifocal midline injury.[2,15,21,35,50] Injury to the fornix may alter cholinergic input to the hippocampus from the basal nucleus of Meynert, which can compound basal nuclear injury from the lesion or surgery and could alter cortical cholinergic function. Projections from the nuclei reuniens and paraventricular nuclei of the thalamus to the hippocampus may also be injured with fornical damage.[2,56] These two mechanisms, however, require some fornical injury for the memory deficit. A last possible explanation involves the inferior thalamic peduncle projecting from the amygdala to the dorsal medial nucleus of the thalamus. Each of these structures is vital to the memory process. Injury to a component of this pathway can result in memory loss complications.[2,35] The dosal medial nucleus of the thalamus is closely related to the body of the fornix, and is probably the most susceptible structure of this pathway during the interfornical approach.

A transient paresis has also been noted in 10 percent of patients following transcallosal interfornical approaches to anterior third ventricular lesions.[5]

Subchoroidal Transvelum Interpositum Approach

Entry to the third ventricular chamber may also be obtained by the subchoroidal transvelum interpositum route. Because of the concern of memory disturbances that might occur after fornix section to gain access to the third ventricle, especially if the contralateral fornix is comprised by the lesion,[33,34] exposure via elevation of the choroid plexus division of the thalamostriate vein and incision of the velum interpositum has been developed.[33,44,86] The fornix is left undisturbed in this approach.

The major potential complications (Table 18-5) occurring from this approach theoretically result from

Table 18-5. Subchoroidal Transvelum Interpostum Approach

Complication	Incidence (if reported)[a]	Author
Hemorrhage infarction of basal ganglia	—	McKissock, 1951
	—	Ono et al., 1984
	—	Viale & Turtus, 1980
Hemiplegia, transient	2/10 (20)	Hirsh et al., 1929
	—	Ono et al., 1984
Mutism	1/10 (10)	Hirsh et al., 1929
	—	Ono et al., 1984
Drowsiness, transient	3/10 (30)	Hirsh et al., 1929
	—	Ono et al., 1984

[a] Percent in parentheses.

the occlusion of the thalamostriate vein and other veins at the foramen of Monro. McKissock[53] stated that occlusion of these veins will lead to hemorrhagic infaction of the basal ganglia. This opinion was echoed by others.[55,86] Neurological deficits that are thought to occur after occlusion of the thalamostriate vein include hemiplegia, mutism, and drowsiness. Ono et al.[55] based their opinion on the work of Hirsch et al.,[33] who reported a series of 10 patients with ligation of the thalamostriate vein in which 3 developed temporary hemiparesis, 3 had temporary drowsiness, and 1 patient became mute. Hirsch et al.[33] stated, however, that ligation of the thalamostriate vein is harmless "due to anastomotic connections." They did not consider these deficits as complications of the transvelum interpositum approach per se. Lavyne and Patterson[44] also indicated that complications are few and are mostly related to the transcortical access to the lateral ventricle usually used. Indeed, all of the complications reported by Hirsch et al.[33] have also been seen in patients operated upon with a transcortical transventricular approach not involving a transvelum interpositum component to the surgery. However, even if these complications are not a result of section of the thalamostriate vein, they are potential complications of the procedure taken in whole. *Sacrifice of a unilateral thalamostriate vein is not considered to place the patient at risk.*

Subfrontal Approach

The structures in and around the anterior third ventricle can be compressed or invaded by lesions near the base of the skull anterior and inferior to the third ventricle. The more common of these lesions include pituitary adenomas, craniopharyngiomas, meningiomas, and gliomas. These lesions can be approached by a frontal craniotomy with a unilateral or bilateral subfrontal dissection. Some complications (Table 18-6) are the result of the operative approach and are not dependent on the pathology of the lesion. Other complications reflect the nature of the lesion, either by its compression or its invasion of neural and vascular structures.

As with other procedures requiring cortical manipulation, seizures are not uncommon after a subfrontal exposure. Incidence has ranged from 2[73] to 25 percent.[42] Symon and Rosenstein[82] divided their patients into a group with early seizures and a group with late seizures with incidences of 11 and 7 percent, respectively. A possible mechanism may be cortical injury and irritation from retractor pressure. Not all patients who have postoperative seizures have them as a complication of surgery. In one series of patients with anterior parasellar meningiomas, 9 of the 51 patients had a seizure disorder preoperatively; 7 patients (and it is not clear if any of these were the same patients) had postoperative seizures.[81]

Table 18-6.   Subfrontal Approach

Complication	Incidence (if reported)[a]	Author
Seizure	1/55 (1.8)	Solero et al., 1983
	1/4 (25)	King, 1979
	7/51 (14)	Symon & Jakubaush, 1929b
	18/101 (18)	Symon & Rosenstein, 1984
Anosmia	(30-50)	Patterson, 1987
	15/108 (15)	Symon & Rosenstein, 1984
	—	Shillito, 1980
Visual loss	1/23 fields (4.3)	Gregorius et al., 1975
	5/23 acuity (21)	Gregorius et al., 1975
	24/101 (24)	Rosenstein & Symon, 1984
	7/19 (37)	Jefferson & Aassam, 1979
	4/55 (7.2)	Solero et al., 1983
	2/51 (3.9)	Symon & Jakubouski, 1979a
	—	Hoffman et al., 1978
	—	Sweet, 1976
	2/47 (4.3)	Rougerie, 1979
Cranial nerve III paresis	3/101 (3.0)	Symon & Rosenstein, 1984
Confusion	8/101 (7.9)	Symon & Rosenstein, 1984
Hemiparesis	—	Shillito, 1980
	4/101 (3.9)	Symon & Rosenstein, 1984

(Continued)

Table 18-6. Subfrontal Approach (*Continued*)

Complication	Incidence (if reported)[a]	Author
Intracranial hemorrhage	3/101 (2.9)	Symon & Rosenstein, 1984
	—	Shillito, 1980
Cerebral swelling	—	Solero et al., 1983
Coma/cerebral infarction	1/48 (2.1)	Hoffman et al., 1978
Diabetes insipidus	—	Clar, 1979
	(49)	Symon & Jakubowski, 1979a
Transient/permanent	10/101 (10); 5/101 (4.9)	Symon & Rosenstein, 1984
		Solero et al., 1983
	4/47 (8.7)	Rougerie, 1979
	21/28 (75)	Hoffman et al., 1978
Transient	—	Shillito, 1980
Hypopituitarism	1/55 (1.8)	Solero et al., 1983
	11/51 (22)	Symon & Jakubowski, 1979a
	4/101 (3.9)	Symon & Rosenstein, 1984
	5/51 (9.8)	Matson & Crigler, 1969
	—	Hoffman et al., 1978
	5/42 (11)	Rougerie, 1979
	—	Sweet, 1976
SIADH	4/101 (3.9)	Symon & Rosenstein, 1984
Obesity	1/42 (2.2)	Rougerie, 1979
	—	Sweet, 1980
Meningitis	1/55 (1.8)	Solero et al., 1983
	1/101 (.99)	Symon & Jakubowski, 1979b
Wound infections	3/101 (2.9)	Symon & Rosenstein, 1984
CSF leak	3/101 (2.9)	Symon & Jakubowski, 1979b
	4/101 (3.9)	Symon & Rosenstein, 1984
Systemic infection	20/116 (17)	Till, 1982
	4/25 (16)	McClone et al., 1982
	2/23 (8.6)	Gregorius et al., 1975
Death	1/48 (2.1)	Hoffman et al., 1978
	1/19 (5.3)	Jefferson & Aassam, 1979
	1/25 (4.0)	McClone et al., 1982
	1/47 (2.2)	Rougerie, 1979
	13/55 (23.6)	Solero et al., 1983
	3/20 (15)	Svien, 1965
	2/30 (6.7)	Sweet, 1976
	1/101 (.99)	Symon & Jakubowski, 1979a
	6/101 (5.9)	Symon & Rosenstein, 1984

[a] Percent in parentheses.

Neurological deficits can complicate subfrontal approaches to anterior third ventricular lesions. Both cranial nerve and hemispheric injuries can occur. Anosmia is the most common deficit that occurs, due to olfactory nerve injury by contusion, retraction, or section. Patterson[58] reported a 30 percent incidence with unilateral approaches and a 50 percent incidence with bilateral approaches. Using a subfrontal approach with occasional olfactory nerve section, Symon and Rosenstein[82] noted that 15 of 101 patients had anosmia postoperatively. Shillito[70] indicated that the minimal morbidity of the approach would be unilateral anosmia.

Visual loss from injury to the optic nerves or chiasm is also relatively common, although highly variable in incidence. Many patients have preoperative visual deficits from lesions in the area; following surgery, they have additional deficits, which may or may not be transient. Both visual fields and visual acuity can be affected.[27,57] The incidence of postoperative visual worsening appears to be related in part to the pathology of the lesion. As little as 4 percent of patients with suprasellar pituitary adenomas approached subfrontally have had some visual loss following surgery. Slightly more[2,47] have visual deterioration after subfrontal approaches to craniopharyngiomas.[68] In patients with suprasellar meningiomas, however, the incidence of visual deterioration can be much higher. Although Solero et al.[73] reported a 7 percent incidence, Rosenstein and Symon[67] noted that 24 of 101 patients experienced postoperative visual loss, and Jefferson and Azzam[37] reported a 37 percent incidence of deterioration in 19 patients. Such changes in visual function may be related to manipulation of structures necessary because of tumor attachments. Sweet[78] indicated that in craniopharyngiomas, at least, attachments to the optic chiasm and optic tracts are among the most tenacious. Hoffman et al.[34] felt that although the capsule of the craniopharyngioma is often attached to vessels inferior to the optic chiasm, usually it can be separated from these vessels with the use of the microscope. On rare occasions when the capsule is firmly adherent, the capsule can be detached from the vascular supply, but the risk of visual loss is much higher. Rosenstein and Symon[67] showed that visual worsening following surgery in patients with suprasellar meningiomas occurred more commonly in those patients who had had preoperative visual symptoms for longer than 2 years and in those with monocular rather than binocular involvement. Tumor size and optic disc status were not clearly correlated to postoperative decrease in visual function, but their study was designed to look at visual recovery, not worsening function. Solero et al.[73] suggested that visual worsening with subfrontal approaches to suprasellar meningiomas results because of direct surgical injury to the optic nerves or chiasm or, alternatively, impairment of their blood supply by surgical maneuvers.

Another cranial nerve that may be compromised with subfrontal approaches is the oculomotor nerve. In one series, a 3 percent incidence of transient third nerve palsy was reported.[82] The mechanism of injury was not addressed by these authors. Most likely, manipulation in the area of the cavernous sinus resulted in such injury. Conceivably, the fourth, fifth, and sixth cranial nerves could also be subject to similar injury.

Neurological deficits from cerebral injury are varied. Confusion occurs in approximately 8 percent of patients.[82] Onset is generally delayed. Half of these patients have only transient confusion, with the remainder having permanent deficits. Hemiparesis also occurs,[70,82] though not commonly. Symon and Rosenstein[82] had a 1 percent incidence of permanent motor weakness, with a 3 percent incidence of transient weakness. Patient weakness can result from intracranial hemorrhage (3/101)[82] or vascular injury from dissection of tumor from around the carotid artery.[70] Cerebral swelling may occur[73] and may contribute to a transient hemiparesis. Postoperative coma due to massive cerebral infarction has also been observed. Hoffman et al.[34] had one such case in a series of 48 patients; they did not have use of the microscope in this particular case.

Endocrine and metabolic dysfunction is a relatively common complication of subfrontal approaches to lesions of the anterior third ventricle, regardless of the pathological nature of the lesion. Transfrontal approaches to pituitary adenomas result in diabetes insipidus[14] in up to 49 percent of cases. In three-fourths of these patients, the diabetes insipidus improved, but all patients required hormonal replacement. Patients with suprasellar meningiomas also have postoperative endocrinopathies. Diabetes insipidus is the most common endocrinopathy in these patients. Ten percent of Symon and Rosenstein's[82] patients had transient diabetes insipidus, and 5 percent had permanent diabetes insipidus. Solero et al.[73] also noted postoperative diabetes insipidus in suprasellar meningioma patients. Other complicating endocrinopathies include hypopituitarism and syndrome of inappropriate antidiuretic hormone secretion,[73,80,82] ranging in incidence from 2 to 20 percent of patients with craniopharyngiomas. Diabetes insipidus is usually present postoperatively,[14] although it is usually transient.[70] Rougerie[68] reported an incidence of 8.7 percent and Hoffman et al.,[34] in a series of children, reported 21 of 28 with postoperative diabetes insipidus. Hypopituitarism occurs in approximately 10 percent of patients.[51,68] Sweet[78] stated that he was required to cut the pituitary stalk in 31 of 37 cases, but he did not discuss resulting endocrinopathy. One would expect at least transient diabetes insipidus. Obesity following surgery has also been noted.[68,79] No doubt this results from hypothalamic dysfunction. Temperature dysregulation occurs as well.[14]

Meningitis is infrequent, reported in 1 percent[81] and 2 percent[73] of cases. Wound infections also occur, with an incidence of up to 3 percent.[82] A complication that is closely related to meningitis and wound infections—cerebrospinal fluid (CSF) leaks—has been observed slightly more commonly, with a 3 to 4 percent incidence.[81,82] Of more concern than these local infections are systemic infections that have occurred in craniopharyngioma patients postoperatively with particularly severe consequences. Till[83] reported that 11 of 116 patients (9.5 percent) died from systemic infections and another 9 patients required strenuous resuscitative efforts. In another series, 16 percent of patients died from a flu-like illness.[52] These infections are thought to have such devastating consequences because the patients were suffering from previously undiagnosed or undertreated pituitary insufficiency. Such systemic infections have not been reported with subfrontal approaches to suprasellar meningiomas, pituitary adenomas, or other lesions. Therefore, this particular complication probably reflects injury from removal of the lesion and not from the subfrontal approach per se.

Patient mortality may occur in the immediate postoperative period.[27,34,37,52,68,73,77,78,79,81] While most series have a 2 to 5 percent operative mortality, Solero et al.[73] reported 23.6 percent. Often, death results from hypothalamic dysfunction. Svien[77] reported a perioperative death after a longitudinal sinus thrombosis. The major contributing factor to the high mortality of Solero et al.[73] appears to be clipping of the internal carotid, anterior cerebral, or anterior communicating arteries, which was necessary during surgery to prevent catastrophic hemorrhage if the vessel was torn during surgery or as a planned maneuver during surgery to ensure complete removal of the surrounding tumor. Operative mortality is higher for repeat surgery for craniopharyngioma than for the initial procedure. Sweet's[78] mortality was 6.6 percent for the primary operation and 28 percent for recurrent tumors. Matson's operative mortality increased from 0 percent for his initial exposure to 25 percent in the reoperation group.[40] This increased mortality may reflect more radical attempts at tumor removal during surgery for recurrent tumor with more hypothalamic injury resulting. Alternatively, recurrent tumors may have more hypothalamic invasion, and the patient cannot tolerate the manipulation necessary during removal attempts.[69]

Subfrontal Translamina Terminalis Approach

The lamina terminalis constitutes the anterior wall of the third ventricle. Lesions within the anterior third ventricle can be reached via a subfrontal approach with incision of the lamina terminalis (Table 18-7). Although the exposure into the ventricle is limited, some lesions can be effectively treated with this approach.

Mental status changes can occur with the subfrontal translamina terminalis approach. This observation is related to multiple factors. The patient may have transient confusion, as did 50 percent of King's[42] four patients. One of his patients also had short-term memory loss, which was initially profound, but improved slightly with time. Another patient had "mental slowness." Memory dysfunction may result from injury to the pillars of the fornix,[56] which form the lateral borders of the lamina terminalis. Alteration in consciousness can occur from injury to the descending pathways from the medial frontal lobe entering

Table 18-7. Subfrontal Translamina Terminalis Approach

Complication	Incidence (if reported)[a]	Author
Confusion, transient	2/4 (50)	King, 1979
Memory loss	1/4 (25)	King, 1979
	—	Page, 1987
Decreased level of consciousness	—	Garretson, 1987
	—	Page, 1987
Hypothalamic injury	—	Ehni & Ehni, 1987
Hyperphagia	Case report	Greenwood, 1950
Diabetes insipidus	—	Patterson, 1987
	—	Page, 1987
Gonadotropic dysfunctions	—	Page, 1987
Hypopituitarism	2/4 (50)	King, 1979
Temperature dysregulations	1/4 (25)	King, 1979

[a] Percent in parentheses.

the medial forebrain bundle to the mesencephalon and tegmentum. This injury can result from retraction or vascular injury.[21,56] Injury to the nucleus basalis of Meynert, which is located laterally, can result in higher cortical dysfunction due to alteration in its cholinergic output.[56]

Metabolic and endocrine abnormalities may complicate the approach through the lamina terminalis. The hypothalamus is closely related to the lamina terminalis laterally. Injury to the hypothalamus due to its sensitivity to pressure and manipulation can cause severe hypothalamic injury.[20] Carmel[11] stated that unilateral injury to the hypothalamus rarely causes symptoms. Lesions in the anterior third ventricle may cause preoperative hypothalamic dysfunction on one side, and surgery can injure the other side, thereby causing manifestation of the injury. Hyperphagia and polydipsia can be seen.[26] Gonadotropic dysfunction can occur if the preoptic area of the hypothalamus is injured.[56] Salt and water metabolic abnormalities result from injury to the organosum vasculosum, the subfornical organ, or the supraoptic nuclei.[56] Diabetes insipidus commonly occurs.[58] King[42] noted hypopituitarism in 50 percent of his four patients. Lastly, temperature dysregulation, with tendencies to poikilothermia, may also be present.[42]

Bifrontal Anterior Interhemispheric Approach

An alternative to the subfrontal translamina terminalis is the bifrontal anterior interhemispheric approach, which is designed to minimize injury to neural and vascular elements in the anterior third ventricular region.[75,76] This approach is particularly helpful for suprasellar lesions that displace the third ventricle inferioposteriorly and lesions within the third ventricle.

Neurological deficits (Table 18-8) can occur if intraoperative or postoperative hemorrhages occur. Clips may fail at cut ends of the anterior communicating artery, or ligatures may loosen at the sectioned superior sagittal sinus. Hemorrhage may also occur if a perforating branch becomes separated from its parent trunk artery. Blood in the CSF recesses may cause vasospasm with subsequent ischemia and neurological deficits. Bitemporal hemianopia will result if the chiasm is sectioned for adequate exposure.

Gastrointestinal hemorrhage may uncommonly occur. Endocrinopathy, specifically diabetes insipidus and Addison's syndrome is possible.[75] In fact, diabetes insipidus occurred in 76 percent of patients in one series, although it was usually transient.[76] Acute hydrocephalus occurring postoperatively is also a concern. Infection may result from the frontal sinus exposure necessary during the opening of the procedure. CSF leak may complicate the procedure, especially in older patients in whom the dura is firmly adherent to the skull and is damaged by the craniotome. This leak may also lead to infection. Lastly, bone wax placed in the frontal sinus to obliterate dead space can lead to a sterile epidural abscess.[75]

Pterional Approach

Many lesions in the basilar anterior third ventricular area can be reached by drilling down the sphenoid ridge in the pterional approach. Many lesions are accessible by this approach, but aneurysms of the

Table 18-8. Bifrontal Anterior Interhemispheric Approach

Complication	Incidence (if reported)[a]	Author
Hemorrhage	—	Suzuki, 1987
Vasospasm	—	Suzuki, 1987
Diabetes insipidus	—	Suzuki, 1987
Transient	12/17 (76)	Suzuki et al., 1984
Hypopituitarism	—	Suzuki, 1987
Gastrointestinal hemorrhage	1/17 (5.9)	Suzuki et al., 1984
	—	Suzuki, 1987
Acute hydrocephalus	—	Suzuki, 1987
Infection	—	Suzuki, 1987
CSF leak	—	Suzuki, 1987
Sterile epidural abscess	—	Suzuki, 1982
Temperature dysregulation	1/17 (5.9)	Suzuki et al., 1984

[a] Percent in parentheses.

Table 18-9. Pterional
Approach Complications[a]

Frontalis paresis
Cerebral swelling
Hemorrhage
Hypothalamic injury
Diabetes insipidus
Hypopituitarism
SIADH
Infection

[a] All complications reported by Tindall & Tindall, 1987.

circle of Willis are most commonly dealt with in this manner.

One complication (Table 18-9) unique to this approach is injury to the frontalis branch of the facial nerve during the development of the skin/fascia/muscle flap. The nerve can be damaged by traction, dissection, or division, and can lend to unilateral forehead paralysis. Intracerebral swelling or hemorrhage can occur from retraction of the frontal and temporal lobes; hemiparesis, aphasia, or drowsiness can result. Excessive retraction can also harm bridging veins, leading to hemorrhage. Injury to neurological structures around the lesion may complicate surgery. As in all dissections in the region, hypothalamic injury may lead to coma. Endocrinopathy, such as diabetes insipidus and hypopituitarism can result from pituitary stalk injury. The syndrome of inappropriate antidiuretic hormone secretion (SIADH) can occur as well. Visual loss may complicate the procedure. Most of these complications are nonspecific.[84]

Subtemporal Approach

Another, less commonly used, approach to basilar lesions around the anterior third ventricle is the subtemporal approach. This approach is usually not used as a primary procedure for lesions in this area, except

Table 18-10. Subtemporal Approach

Complication	Incidence (if reported)[a]
Diabetes insipidus	33/33 (100)
Obesity	33/33 (100)
Abnormal growth	29/33 (88)
Visual worsening	2/33 (6.0)
Hemianopsia	1/33 (3.0)
Memory loss	3/33 (9.0)
Cranial nerve III paresis	1/33 (3.0)

[a] Percent in parentheses. All cases reported by Rougerie, 1979.

for lesions with lateral extension.[6] Rather, the access is used for second-stage operations to treat lesions from the anterior third ventricular area that have retrochiasmatic or posterior hypothalamic extension.[68]

In a subset of 33 patients, Rougerie[68] used a subtemporal approach as a second stage. All patients developed diabetes insipidus and obesity. Almost all had abnormal growth. Visual worsening, hemianopia, third nerve paresis (transient and permanent), and memory loss (transient and permanent) also occurred as complications[68] (Table 18-10).

Transnasal Transsphenoid Approach

Midline lesions of the base of the skull may affect the structures of the anterior third ventricle, either by compression or invasion. The transnasal transsphenoidal route can be used to reach these lesions. The lesions that most readily lend themselves to this approach are those located in the sella turcica or the suprasellar area, and that extend superiorly. Lesions with an enlarged sella are particularly accessible.[45] Those lesions that have a narrow base and lateral or anterior extension are not as well treated by this surgical technique. Craniopharyngiomas that are entirely intra-arachnoid and do not enlarge the sella should not be approached in this manner.[13] Accessible lesions include pituitary tumors, craniopharyngiomas and suprasellar germinomas.[30,87]

Complications (Table 18-11) can occur throughout the initial exposure. Disruption of the mucosa within the basal cavity can lead to drainage and unusual noises. Nasoseptal perforation can also occur; Laws and Kern[46] reported a 3.1 percent incidence. Diastasis of the palate may result from placement of retractors.[46] Disruption of the arachnoid will cause CSF rhinorrhea if the tissue graft is inadequately positioned.[87] A 3.1 percent incidence was noted in one series of patients with a variety of lesions.[46] In patients with craniopharyngiomas, Rougerie[68] had a 10 percent incidence of CSF leak, and Laws[45] had a 14 percent incidence. The increased incidence in craniopharyngioma patients may occur because these lesions are more often intra-arachnoid than pituitary lesions. Epistaxis, nasal deformity, and mucocoeles may occur too.[46]

Neurological deficits may complicate transnasal transsphenoidal approaches to anterior third ventricular lesions. These deficits may result from vascular injury or direct surgical trauma. Due to anatomic variation carotid artery injuries may occur.[65,87] Laws and Kern[46] noted a 1.5 percent incidence of carotid artery injury, including two patients (of 193) who suffered cerebral infarction. Hemorrhage may follow cavernous sinus injury as well.[46] The postoperative

Table 18-11.   Transnasal Transsphenoidal Approach

Complication	Incidence (if reported)[a]	Author
Nasal drainage	—	Weiss, 1987
Airway noises	—	Weiss, 1987
Nasoseptal perforation	6/193 (3.1)	Laws & Kern, 1976
Palatial diastasis	2/193 (1.0)	Laws & Kern, 1976
CSF leak	6/193 (3.1)	Laws & Kern, 1976
	—	Weiss, 1987
	2/14 (14)	Laws, 1980
	1/10 (10)	Rougerie, 1979
Epitaxis	—	Laws & Kern, 1976
Nasal deformity	—	Laws & Kern, 1976
Mucocoele	—	Laws & Kern, 1976
Hemorrhage	—	Rhoton et al., 1981
	—	Weiss, 1987
Cerebral infarction	2/193 (1.0)	Laws & Kern, 1976
Visual loss	—	Weiss, 1982
	2/50 (4.0)	Laws & Kern, 1976
	—	Rhoton et al., 1981
Anosmia	—	Rhoton et al., 1981
Cranial nerve paresis	—	Rhoton et al., 1981
Transient	4/193 (2.0)	Laws & Kern, 1976
Hypothalamic injury	—	Rhoton et al., 1981
	—	Weiss, 1987
	1/193 (.5)	Laws & Kern, 1976
Diabetes insipidus	7/177 (4.0)	Laws & Kern, 1976
	2/14 (14)	Laws, 1980
Transient/permanent	2/10 (20)	Rougerie, 1979
	1/10 (10)	
Hypopituitarism	9/14 (64)	Laws, 1980
	6/137 (4.4.)	Laws & Kern, 1976
Meningitis	3/193 (1.5)	Laws & Kern, 1976
Sinusitis	—	Laws & Kern, 1976
Death	4/193 (2.0)	Laws & Kern, 1976
	1/14 (7.1)	Laws, 1980

[a] Percent in parentheses.

course may be marred by visual loss.[87] Laws and Kern[46] had a 4 percent incidence of visual field worsening following transnasal transsphenoidal surgery. Mechanisms of injury include direct damage to the optic nerve (by surgical manipulation), injury to the vascular supply of the nerves or chiasm, compression of the optic apparatus from the tissue graft, and prolapse of the optic nerves into the empty sella.[46] The optic nerves can also be injured if the sphenoid bone is eroded and the speculum clips are placed too deep, or if the optic foramen is fractured by forcefully opening the speculum.[65] The olfactory nerves can be injured if the intranasal dissection is directed too superiorly. Speculum tips placed in the cavernous sinus can damage the oculomotor, trochlear, trigeminal, and abducers nerves.[65] A 2 percent incidence of transient cranial nerve injury is reported.[46] Hypothalamic injury with resulting coma or death may follow direct trauma or vascular injury.[46,65,87]

Surgeons using a transnasal transsphenoidal approach to an anterior third ventricular lesion should be alerted to possible endocrinopathy complicating the postoperative course.[45,46,56,68,87] Diabetes insipidus occurred in 4 percent of cases in one series.[46] In patients with craniopharyngiomas, the incidence is higher, reported as 14 percent by the same author. Rougerie[68] reported an incidence of 20 percent transient diabetes insipidus and 10 percent permanent diabetes insipidus in children. Other endocrinopathies from postoperative pituitary dysfunction occurred in 4.4 percent of patients with a variety of lesions[46] and in 64 percent of patients with craniopharyngiomas.[45]

Infection is always a concern with any surgical approach. Transnasal transsphenoidal approaches are no different. Meningitis has been reported to occur in 1.5 percent of cases. Sinusitis may also result.[46]

Death is an occasional complication. Laws and Kern[46] reported a 2 percent incidence for patients with a variety of lesions and a 7 percent incidence for patients with craniopharyngioma.[45] Etiological factors leading to mortality include meningitis, hypothalamic injury, and vascular occlusion.[46]

Free-Hand Needle Approach

Lesions of the anterior third ventricle have been treated by free-hand needle passage to the lesion (Table 18-12). A burr hole is made at the coronal suture and a needle is directed toward the foramen of Monro where the lesion is located. This technique has been used both for cyst drainage[28] and lesion biopsy.[64]

In five patients, Gutierrez-Lara et al.[28] reported no complications. Rekate et al.[64] reported 1 patient of 14 who had a transient worsening of an unspecified preoperative neurological deficit and a 12 percent incidence of inability to make a diagnosis by this technique. Ehni and Ehni,[20] however, felt that more severe complications could occur. Injuries to the internal cerebral vein, choroid plexus, fornix, hypothalamus, and thalamus are all possible, with resulting neurological or endocrine deficits, or devastating hemorrhage. Spillage of cyst fluid into the ventricle could also be troublesome. *In our opinion, this technique is no longer appropriate or justifiable in view of the availability of stereotactic methods.*

Sterotactic Approach

A last approach to anterior third ventricular lesions is through stereotaxy. Currently, most stereotactic procedures utilize computed tomography (CT) or magnetic resonance imaging (MRI). Lesions can be biopsied, drained, or removed depending on their consistency. A ventriculoscope can be directed stereotactically to enhance removal efforts. On occasion, radioactive substances can be stereotactically directed into cysts to provide radiation therapy.[2,3] The method is remarkably safe.

While a large number of patients have been operated upon without problems,[3] some authors have noted complications (Table 18-13). Vascular injury is potentially the most severe complication. Backlund[7] reported that 1 patient of 16 (approximately 6 percent) died after puncture of an anterior cerebral artery with resulting occlusion of the artery and diffuse vasospasm; hypothalamic insufficiency resulted. Sturm et al.[74] discussed a patient with an intracranial frontal hematoma after a stereotactic procedure, fortunately without neurological deficit. Intraventricular hemorrhage can occur as well, as in 9 percent of the cases of Powell et al.[62]

Seizures are a possible postoperative complication.[9,41] Passage of the probe through the cortical surface can create a small irritative focus.

Blindness occurred in 11 percent of patients in one series, but the patient had a preoperative visual deficit.[60] The etiology was felt to be multifactorial. Sturm et al.[74] reported a 10 percent incidence of postoperative visual loss after the introduction of radioactive yttrium into craniopharyngioma cysts. Osmotherapy resolved the deficits. They hypothesized that visual loss occurs from radiation-induced local edema, or alternatively, minute displacement of previously injured optic nerves from cyst shrinkage.

Infection can occur to complicate stereotactic procedures. Meningitis and ventriculitis, resulting in death, have been observed in 11 percent of patients who had stereotactic aspiration and placement of ra-

Table 18-12.   Free-Hand Needle Approach

Complication	Incidence (if reported)[a]	Author
Worsening of preoperative neurological deficit	1/14 (7.1)	Rekate et al., 1981
Hemorrhage	—	Ehni & Ehni, 1987
Hypothalamic injury	—	Ehni & Ehni, 1987
Thalamic injury	—	Ehni & Ehni, 1987
Spillage of cyst fluid	—	Ehni & Ehni, 1987

[a] Percent in parentheses.

Table 18-13. Stereotactic Approach

Complication	Incidence (if reported)	Author
Hemorrhage	1/11 (9.1)	Powell et al., 1981
	1/10 (10)	Sturm et al., 1981
Vascular occlusion	1/16 (6.5)	Backlund, 1973[a]
Seizure	—	Bosch et al., 1978[a]
	—	Kelly, 1983
Visual loss	1/11 (9.1)	Powell et al., 1981
	1/10 (10)	Sturm et al., 1981
Meningitis	1/9 (11)	Julow et al., 1985
Ventriculitis	1/9 (11)	Julow et al., 1985
Abscess	1/12 (8.5)	Mohadjer et al., 1987
Inability to locate cyst	1/11 (9.1)	Powell et al., 1981
Inability to puncture cyst	1/7 (14)	Hall & Lundsford, 1987
	1/11 (9.1)	Powell et al., 1981
	1/7 (14)	Hall & Lundsford, 1987
Inability to drain cyst	—	Rivas & Loberto, 1985
	—	Ehni & Ehni, 1987
Spillage of cyst fluid	—	Backlund, 1973[a]
	—	Apuzzo, 1986
Death	1/9 (11)	Julow et al., 1985
	1/16 (6.5)	Backlund et al., 1972[a]

[a] Preimaging directed data.

dioactive isotope into cystic craniopharyngiomas.[38] Abscess formation occurred in eight percent of patients in another series.[54]

Inability to accomplish the goal of surgery may also complicate the procedure. Occasionally, the cyst cannot be located.[60] If the cyst is located, it may not be able to be punctured,[29] and, if it is punctured, the fluid may be so viscous that drainage is difficult or impossible.[29,60,66]

Spillage of cyst fluid into the ventricle may cause some difficulties[20] by eliciting an inflammatory reaction. Likewise, when radioactive material or certain radioopaque materials have been placed into a cystic lesion, spillage has occurred into the CSF spaces. Meningeal irritation and elevated body temperature can result from such spillage.[8]

Death has complicated stereotactic procedures uncommonly. In 150 cases, Apuzzo[2] reported 1 death. Cause of death is usually hemorrhage[7] or infection.[38]

Summary

A large variety of lesions occur in the region of the anterior third ventricle. A wide variety of surgical approaches are available for application, depending on multiple factors. Complications can occur with each approach. Hemorrhage, infection, and death, which can occur with any procedure, neurosurgical or otherwise, are possible with approaches to anterior third ventricular lesions. Other complications may result from injury to the neural and vascular structures closely related to the anterior third ventricle. These complications include visual loss, memory loss, alteration in consciousness, and endocrinopathy, as well as many others. Some complications occur as a result of the dissection necessary in approaching the lesion. Others follow surgery because lesions in this area are attached to, compress, or invade vital neural and vascular structures. The manipulation of the lesion or its attachments may cause subsequent dysfunction and postoperative complications.

OPERATIVE CONSIDERATIONS

Primary objectives in management of masses affecting the third ventricular chamber include:

1. Defining histology of the process
2. Normalizing CSF dynamics

3. Achieving maximum lesion excision
4. Decompressing focal pressure effects

These objectives must be achieved in the frame of minimal neural injury and alteration of the patient's physiological status.

Major problems associated with operative approaches to the region are failure to achieve primary objectives as well as associated cortical injury, midhemispheric injury, and thalamic and hypothalamic injury. As noted in the literature review, multiple approaches are feasible, depending on lesion presentation; however, this section will deal with complication avoidance and management related to superior transventricular approaches to the third

ventricular chamber. Because of its ease and versatility the interhemispheric transcallosal corridor will be stressed.

Selection

In our opinion the superior interhemispheric approach is an appropriate operative corridor under the following structural and clinical situations:

1. A lesion clearly contained in third ventricular region and appearing structurally extra-axial with or without minor intra-axial components i.e., colloid cyst, craniopharyngioma, ependymoma (Figs. 18-1 to 18-3)

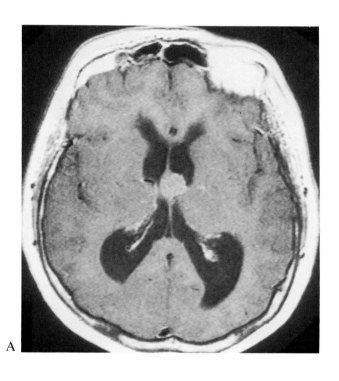

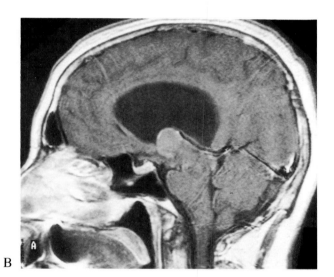

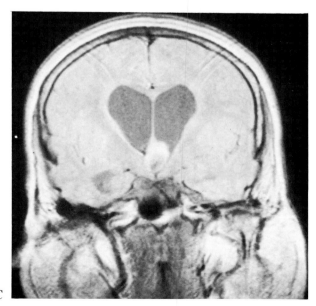

Figure 18-1. T_1-weighted MRIs in **(A)** axial, **(B)** sagittal, and **(C)** coronal views of classic third ventricular colloid cyst. In this case, presentation is predominantly in the left foramen of Monro. Note small right foramen. Visualization at the right foramen would be difficult and would require subchoroidal or interfornical exposure.

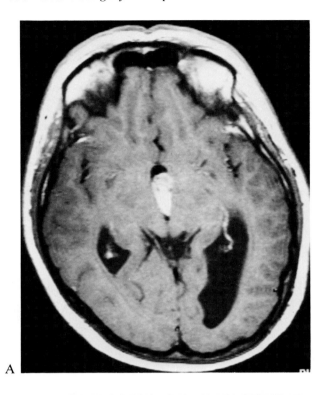

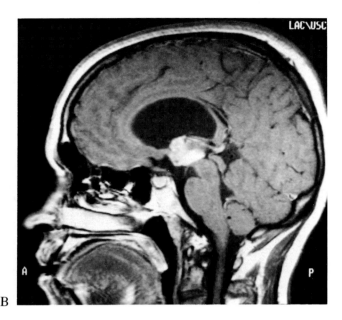

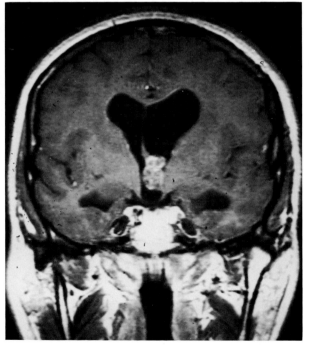

Figure 18-2. (A–C) MRIs in three planes of third ventricular mass presenting at the left foramen of Monro (contrast enhanced, T_1). This ganglioglioma was approached by a left interhemispheric corridor with subchoroidal third ventricular exposure. Note small right foramen of Monro with asymetrical ventriculomegaly.

2. A lesion with major components in the third ventricular region with a small (2 cm) or questionable basal origin, i.e., craniopharyngioma (Fig. 18-4)
3. A lesion with a major third ventricular component for which subfrontal, temporal, or combined basal approaches have been unsuccessful in dealing with the

superior component, i.e., craniopharyngioma meningioma

Although the interhemispheric approach is feasible in the absence of ventriculomegaly, it should be stressed that retractor pressure gradient and view

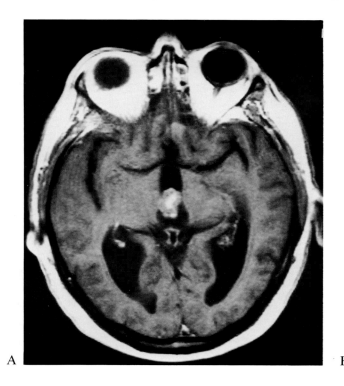

A

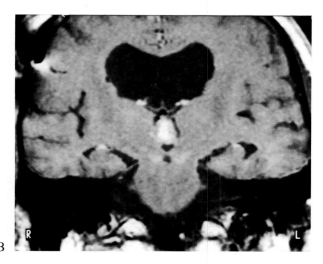

B

Figure 18-3. **(A & B)** MRIs and **(C)** CT scan (unenhanced) of mid-third ventricular mass (ependymoma) with attendant ventriculomegaly. Note right thalamic origin on coronal view. Right-sided interhemispheric approach with interfornical corridor provided excellent exposure. No visualization was apparent through the moderately enlarged foramen of Monro.

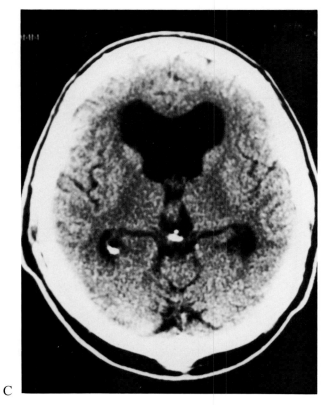

C

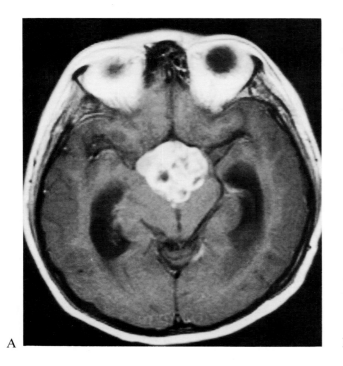

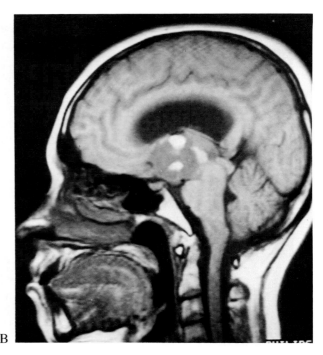

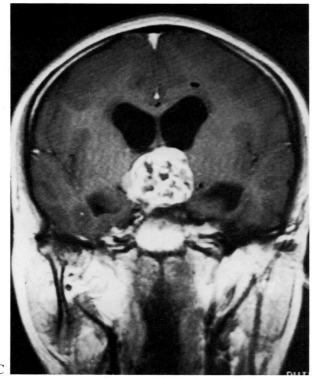

Figure 18-4. T_1-weighted MRIs of moderate-sized basal and third ventricular mass. **(A)** enhanced; **(B)** unenhanced; **(C)** enhanced. This craniopharyngioma was totally excised through a right interhemispheric corridor with simultaneous dissection apertures through the foramen of Monro and the fornical raphe.

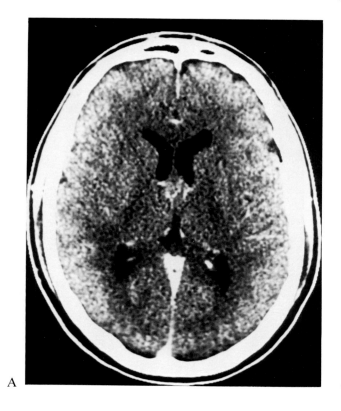

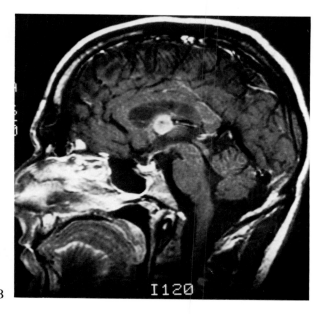

Figure 18-5. (A) CT scan (enhanced), **(B)** enhanced T_1-weighted MRI, and **(C)** unenhanced T_2-weighted MRI of colloid cyst. The ventricles are slightly enlarged and provide an excellent corridor for excision.

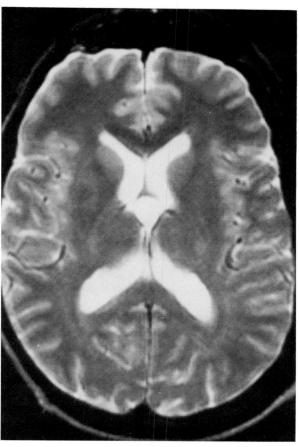

A

B

C

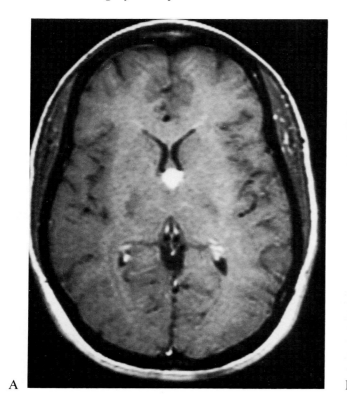

A

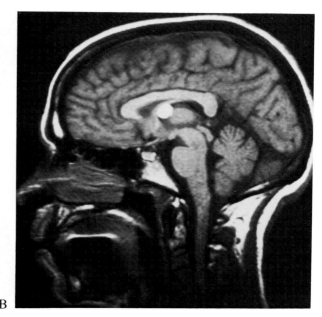

B

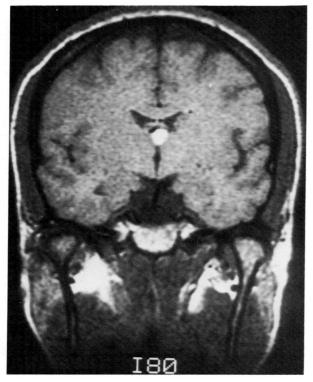

C

Figure 18-6. (A–C) Three planes of view and T$_1$-weighted enhanced MRIs of an 8-mm colloid cyst. Ventricular reservoirs are small and foramenal access is limited **(A)**; the case presents high risk because of overall attendant anatomical factors independent of approach used.

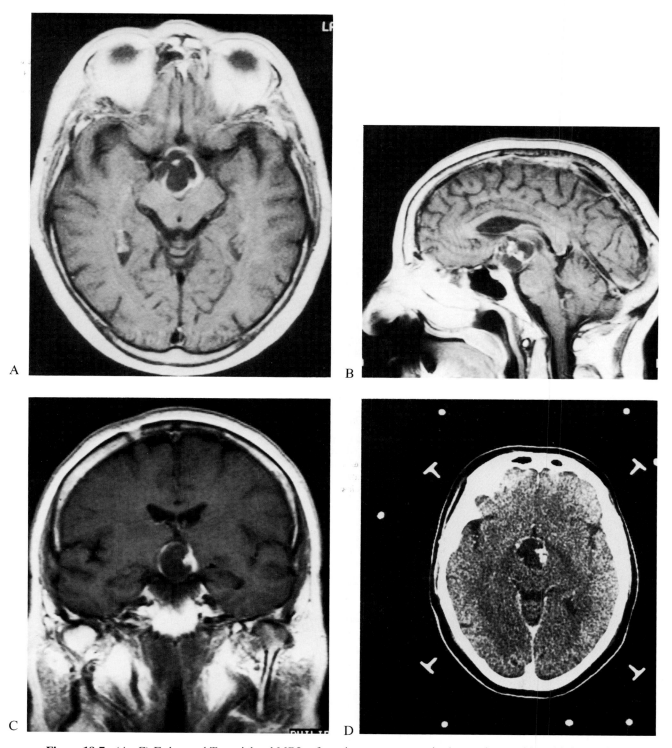

Figure 18-7. **(A–C)** Enhanced T_1-weighted MRIs of cystic recurrent craniopharyngioma with a third ventricular component. Although the basal approach would be an option or consideration, stereotactic aspiration (with CT targeting) **(D)** offers a satisfactory visual system decompression by a procedure of considerably less magnitude. Transcerebral corridors by microsurgery would not be advisable.

line corridors are enhanced by its presence, thus increasing the margin for error of such exposures (Figs. 18-5 and 18-6).

It should be noted that recurrent cystic lesions in this location may be satisfactorily managed by stereotactic aspiration (Fig. 18-7).

TECHNIQUE OF THE MIDLINE CORRIDOR IN THIRD VENTRICULAR EXPOSURE

The interhemispheric approach to the diencephalic roof and third ventricular chamber offers a direct corridor with view line advantages and flexibility at the target region, but with many potential sites for the genesis of intraoperative complications and postoperative problems (Fig. 18-7). From the standpoint of practicality this discussion will progress through the stages of preoperative assessment, intraoperative events, and postoperative periods, and focus upon issues of complication, avoidance, and management. Table 18-14 summarizes the major points of discussion.

Preoperative Assessment by Imaging

Contemporary imaging is imperative in defining lesion position, size, contour, extent, vascularity, and variabilities in content; all of these are determinants of approach and intraoperative action during exci-

Table 18-14. Superior Approaches to Anterior Third Ventricular Lesions

Complication	Avoidance	Management
Intraoperative		
Sinus laceration	Identify sagittal suture Place medial burr hole lateral to suture Carefully dissect dura free of bone; multiple burr holes in event of difficult dissection	Oversew laceration Apply Gelfoam to laceration Then elevate head
Air embolism	Avoid sinus injury Wax bone Use rapid tamponade of sinus laceration Control venous injury	Use Trendelenberg position Rotate patient to right-side up position Aspirate atrial catheter
Cerebral edema or mass in corridor	Do not overretract sagittal sinus Preserve venous tributaries Use gentle and minimal retraction Use osmotic agents Use hyperventilation	Reduce retraction Use Osmotic agents Use Ventriculostomy
Arterial injury	Concentrate precise microsurgical technique Have anatomical awareness	Maintain SAP[a] Maintain blood volume Use tamponade (no biopolar)
Dissection into cingulate gyrus	Have anatomical awareness Follow falx as plumbline Diagnose herniation on preoperative imaging Microdissect	Recognize microdissection of corticopial dissection plane
Intraventricular hemorrhage	Meticulously coagulate ependymal layer Control blood pressure	Use gentle catheter gravity irrigation Identify point of hemorrhage
Inability to locate foramen	Properly position bone flap Do midline callosal opening for appropriate view line to foramen of Monro Identify choroid plexus Properly angulate retractor Have septal herniation into field	Reevaluate images and external landmarks Identify choroid plexus Identify venous landmarks Fenestrate septum
Posterior view line and inadequate access	Properly position bone flap Have callosotomy in proper line of sight Have absolute anatomical orientation for staged development of view line	Extend callosotomy forward Develop subchoroidal or interfornical corridor
Inability to identify forniceal raphe	Have knowledge of specific patient anatomy Identify septum	Coagulate septum to fornical base and open along line of attachment

(Continued)

Table 18-14. Superior Approaches to Anterior Third Ventricular Lesions (*Continued*)

Complication	Avoidance	Management
Suboptimal lesion exposure (excision)	Optimize view lines Consider maneuver to enhance exposure	Employ exposure options at site Alter microscopic line of sight Use microretraction
Postoperative		
Hemorrhage		
Epidural	Control blood pressure Tent dura	Exploration and evacuation
Subdural	Do not overdrain Control blood pressure Have adequate coagulation of sectioned draining veins Apply protection to retracted surfaces of brain Replace CSF	Exploration and evacuation
Intraparenchymal	Control blood pressure Minimize retractor pressure Minimize section of draining veins Protect surfaces	Exploration and evacuation Fluid restriction
Intraventricular	Control blood pressure Have adequate coagulation of ependymal lining Irrigate ventricles until fluid is clear Minimize choroid plexus manipulation	Exploration and evacuation Ventriculostomy (single or double with irrigation)
Hemiparesis	Avoid hemorrhage Minimize retraction Minimize section of draining veins Avoid sinus retraction	Image Glucocorticoids Fluid balance
Memory loss	Identify and preserve hippocampal commissure Minimize fornical manipulation Minimize manipulation of dorsal medial nucleus of thalamus Do not section fornix; use subchoroidal or interfornical approach Avoid transmitted pressure	Image Glucocorticoids Fluid balance
Mutism	Do not perform bilateral cingulate retraction	Image Observe
Hydrocephalus	Make large septal window Visualize patent foramen; bilaterally pass catheter Visualize open iter Use copious ventricular irrigation until clear	Use ventriculostomy
Obtundation	Avoid hemorrhage Minimize hypothalamic manipulation Internally decompress lesion	Image Observe
Pneumocephalus	Irrigate ventricles Use anterior drain	Use catheter decompression
Transfer deficits	Use anterior callosotomy	Take no action
Meningitis, bacterial	Have strict asepsis Use prophylactic parenteral antibiotics Use antibiotic irrigation	Use parenteral antibiotics
Meningitis, aseptic	Use copious irrigation of ventricles	Use glucocorticoids
Seizure	Use anticonvulsants (level) Use meticulous cortical handling and protection	Use anticonvulsants
Aphasia	Perform nondominant craniotomy	Image to rule out contralateral event

[a] SAP, systemic arterial pressure.

sion, and govern operative three-dimensional comprehension during lesion excision. Safety of excision and avoidance of unsatisfactory results cannot be maximized without full exploitation of MRI in multiple planes of perspective. Concurrently, absolute definition of the distortion of normal anatomy is displayed as guidance in corridor development. With the midline exposure, comprehension of the parame-

dian venous tributaries and flow patterns are important informational elements in determining flap placement for entry corridors and should receive the utmost scrutiny by magnetic resonance venography. Corridor angles, entry, and stepwise strategy for each operative stage should be laboriously detailed with the imaging definition of all neural and vascular elements (Fig. 18-8).

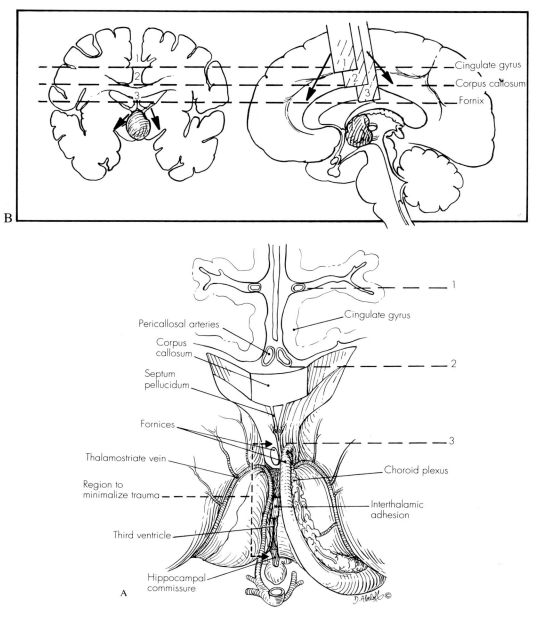

Figure 18-8. (A) The interhemispheric corridor offers multiple options for visualization of the diencephalic roof and exercise of exposure corridors to the third ventricular chamber in vertical and lateral planes. Posterior-coronal view of anatomical elements in region for comprehension of corridors, landmarks, and structures at risk. The procedure may be considered in three stages: (*1*) setting orientation for accessing the lateral ventricle; (*2*) ventricular entry and orientation, strategy development; (*3*) surgery within the third ventricular chamber. **(B)** Progressive stages in lateral ventricular entry: (*1*) dissection to cingulate, (*2*) cingulate to callosum, (*3*) callosum transit.

Presurgical Preparation

Instrumentation

Proper availability of microinstrumentation peculiar to the ''long reach'' of this type of midline exposure is essential. The key selection factor relates to instrument working length (9 to 12 cm from the scalp barrier). Self-retaining retractor systems in proper working order with a wide selection of blade widths and thicknesses are key to the safety of this procedure and the operator's familiarity with the use of the system is imperative. The Budde system provides the basic rudiments and is the ''ideal'' system; however, blade modification in taper and thickness has been found necessary in the event that fornical retraction is required.

Zeiss Contravess microinstrumentation with a 300-mm objective or variable focal length system provides maximum flexibility of view line and instrumentation accessibility.

Intracranial Pressure

Problems of midline access are possible in the event that proper preparation of brain mass and CSF dynamics are inadequate. High-potency glucorticoids, and possibly placement of a ventriculostomy, should be considered. In general, mid- and anterior third ventricular masses present as semielective procedures with subacute or chronic ventriculomegaly and do not require preoperative ventriculostomy. In the event that ventriculostomy is employed, care must be taken not to overdrain, creating a surgically ''unfavorable'' structural setting with either normal size or silt ventricles. We have encountered such a setting frequently in patients referred after unilateral shunting procedures with unilateral slit ventricles and midline shift secondary to contralateral (usually left-sided) ventriculomegaly.

Surgical Procedure

Stage I. Accessing the Lateral Ventricle

Position and Preparation

The head is firmly fixed in a slightly flexed position (10°), with straight alignment to the ceiling in a Mayfield pin fixation head rest (Figure 18-9). Anatomical cues are maximized for operator orientation if *careful* head positioning is accomplished and fixed. There is a tendency to place the Mayfield head rest too high on the calvarium with this position, thus making self-retaining retractor mechanism placement excessively high and cumbersome as later stages of the procedure evolve.

Intravenous high-potency glucocorticoids, anticonvulsants, and antibiotics are administered following induction. We use prophylactic antibiotics for the first 48 hours following surgery if no ventriculostomy is positioned. In the event that a ventriculostomy is used intravenously, antibiotics are used 24 hours following its removal or a shunting procedure.

Scalp and Bone Flap

A two-limbed scalp flap is optimal for bone flap development in this paramedian exposure (Fig. 18-9). This scalp flap should afford visual access to the coronal suture and at least 1 cm of the sagittal suture for orientation.

It should afford 2 cm of exposure to the contralateral parietal frontal surface. A nondominant free bone flap is preferred because it presents less physiological threat and offers the right-handed surgeon better access. Problems of view lines to the lesion and potential complications are minimized by careful consideration of bone flap placement in relation to the coronal suture and a knowledge of venous anatomy in the region. As a general rule, a 7-cm bone flap will afford generous midline access. It is placed one-third posterior to the coronal suture and two-thirds anterior to this structure. However, venous structures should be considered in placement, with flap disposition modeled accordingly. Placement of this flap more than 2 cm posterior to the coronal suture significantly increases the possibility of hemiparesis and should be avoided if possible. Three centimeters of exposure is required to the right of the midline. Midline exposure is optimized in our experience by contralateral exposure of 1 to 2 cm. *Absolute midline exposure is imperative to reduce midline slot retraction and optimize deep view lines.* This flap is accomplished generally with two burr holes, one on each side of the midline. More holes are occasionally required if the dura is adherent, especially adjacent to the sagittal sinus.

Midline Exposure

Cortical and subcortical injury is the major problem to be avoided during this step of the exposure. The dural flap is opened to the lateral component of the bone flap and is reflected medially to the sagittal sinus. Venous structures and Pacchionian granulations should be carefully dissected and preserved. Maintaining venous drainage and cortical pial integrity is critical. Frequently, careful microdissection is required for this stage of the procedure. As the dura is turned to the sagittal sinus and reflected over that structure, *care must be taken not to "overturn" the sinus,* focally occluding it and creating venous compromise, which may be evident bilaterally (Fig. 18-9).

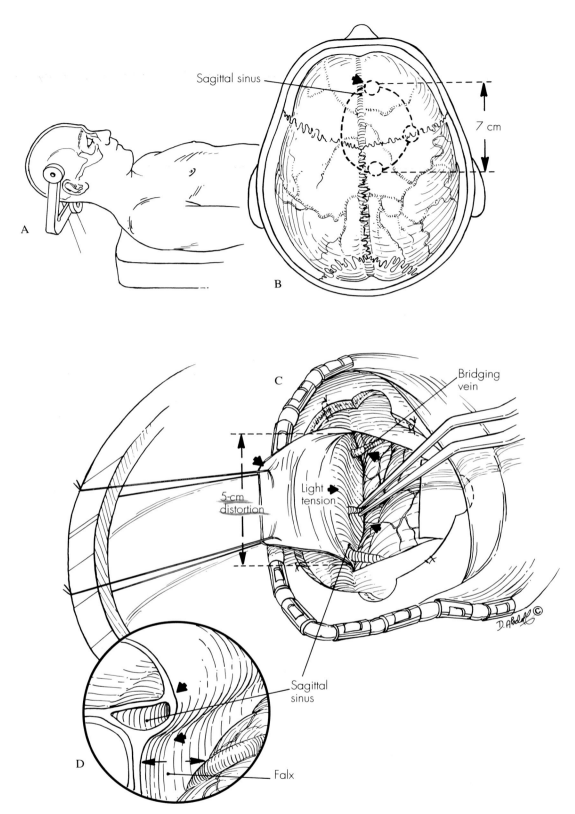

Sagittal sinus

7 cm

A

B

C

Bridging vein

5-cm distortion

Light tension

D.Abdell©

Sagittal sinus

D

Falx

Figure 18-9. Illustration of key elements in early stages of ventricular access. **(A)** Head position. **(B)** Bone flap positioning in consideration of sagittal sinus. Corridor angulation and venous sacrifice must be considered. **(C)** Careful midline exposure and dissection to develop initial stages of corridor. Cortical preservation and protection are key. **(D)** Excessive rotation of sinus will cause occlusion and venous infarction. Entry slot should not exceed 1.5 cm from falx to medial hemispheric margin.

568

With initiation of midline retraction, two considerations are key: (1) cortical protection and (2) retraction minimization.

This stage should not be undertaken until proper brain relaxation is achieved.

The end point of this step in the corridor is a *callosal carpet of 1 × 3 cm, with a 5-cm surface slot* that is *less than 2 cm maximally retracted from the midline* (Fig. 18-10). This is carefully attained with the aid of the microscope and self-retaining retractor systems as well as cortical protection materials such as Biocol or soft 100 percent cotton paddies. A 19-mm flat-based blade is optimal. Problems may evolve secondary to subfalcine herniation, which obscures the dis-

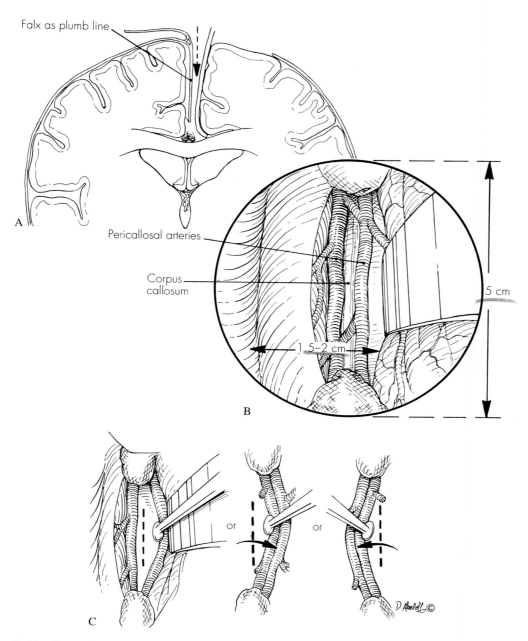

Figure 18-10. Illustrations of interhemispheric entry corridors with selection of callosotomy site. **(A)** Falx provides orientation to midline. Corridor is minimized without overretraction. **(B)** Basal exposure at callosum measures 1.5 × 3 cm. Cotton balls maintain anterior and posterior shape of aperture. **(C)** Pericallosal arteries are visualized and manipulated with microsurgical technique to optimize midline corridor.

section planes, particularly at the cingulum level. Dissection along the falx is essentially clean. Anteriorly, adhesions are often encountered even at parafalcine levels. Careful attention should be taken to identify the callosal marginal artery and pericallosal arteries if they present in the dissection field. At times this is not the case and excessive dissection should not be undertaken to identify them.

Callosal trunk identification is obvious by its white hue as opposed to the cream-tan cingular cortex. Retraction of this slot and maintenance of exposure is facilitated by placement of elongated cotton balls saturated with saline solution prior to placement at both ends of the exposure. This technique reduces blade compression in the central slot (Fig. 18-10).

Callosotomy

For entry orientation, the falx should be used as a plumbline, to avoid disorientation by improper angulation (Fig. 18-11). At the same time, the coronal suture landmarks should be considered along with head angulation as related to sagittal MRI, midline cuts to orient for angulation to the foramen of Monro. An *oval callosotomy* is then performed in stepwise fashion. The aperture is 2.5 × 2 cm in size and developed in careful stepwise fashion employing bipolar coagulation and a 5 French suction. *Great care is necessary at the ependymal level to coagulate vascular tributaries, especially at the posterior margin.* These are potential problems during the intraoperative or

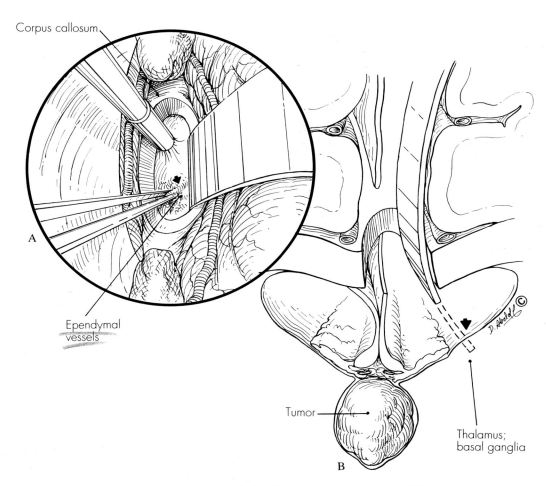

Figure 18-11. (A) Callosotomy (2.5 cm) is performed with bipolar forceps and 5 French aspirator in oval pattern. Care is taken to coagulate all ependymal vessels especially posteriorly. **(B)** Retractors advanced to incorporate callosal trunk to enhance exposure. Care is taken *not* to overadvance blade to basal ganglia. Bilateral cingula retraction risks mutism.

postoperative periods. Visualization of the lateral ventricular system is obvious, with initial graying of the callosum followed by black viewing of CSF. The retractor is carefully advanced for retraction of the right lateral callosal margin with care taken *not to overretract* into the medial hemisphere or the lateral ventricular floor.

Stage II. Lateral Ventricular Entry, Visualization, Orientation, and Development of Strategy for Third Ventricular Entry

Orientation is provided by the choroid plexus. Confusion may be created by left ventricular entry during a right-sided approach. This is easily recognized by a general lateral to medial course of the choroid ribbon. Right-sided entry may then be achieved by retractor removal, lateral resection of the corpus trunk, or identification of the septum pellucidum with subsequent penetration and resection of that structure.

Occasionally with right-sided entry the *septum pellucidum will bellow into the field, obscuring the midline and paramedian ventricular contents.* This is to be expected with bilateral foramen of Monro obstruction and right lateral ventricular decompression. It is easily managed by fenestration of the septum. In all cases, it is easily managed by fenestration of the septum. In all cases, it is important to perform a generous septum fenestration to visualize the contralateral ventricle and to create a single ventricular chamber should postoperative drainage be required. Rapid identification of anatomy and immediate determination of actual entry angulation can then be determined. *Problems may develop if entry is posterior to the foramen and visualization is difficult.* This is managed by anterior development of the callosotomy. In experienced hands this is seldom necessary (Fig. 18-12).

The size of the foramen is evaluated in consideration of the attendant pathology (vascularity and texture are determinants of the degree of access required). To reduce occurrence, longevity, and severity of memory loss consideration must be given to factors of lesion histology, vascularity, and texture; midline manipulation required; and personal skills and experience with microsurgical expertise in this region. A balance is required for ultimate outcome. The softer-textured avascular lesion requires less exposure, and midline structures are subjected to less surgical trauma than when lesions are firm and

vascular lesions are encountered. In any event, *the foramen is the primary corridor of entry* to the third ventricular chamber, and before any other maneuvers are indicated to manipulate the fornix and associated components of the diencephalic roof, the lesion should be evaluated through the foramen of Monro. If the lesion character, foramen size, and view lines combine to a suboptimal operative summation, consideration should be given to (1) developing the fornical raphe or (2) developing the subcoroidal plane with or without sacrifice of the thalamostriate vein.

All strategy should be directed toward avoiding or reducing midline alteration, manipulation, or transmitting pressure gradients to paraventricular structures.

Since both the interfornical and subchoroidal approaches require microsurgical handling and manipulations of the fornix and roof structures, they should be undertaken only after strict consideration of optimization of the approach. At surgery, presenting anatomy or surgical view lines will dictate the optimum choice.

Interfornical Exposure

Problems arise from failure to identify the interfornical raphe, a natural plane between the fornical bodies (Fig. 18-13). The key to its identification depends on the anatomy of the septum pellucidum in the individual case. At times this can be appreciated on MRI (Fig. 18-14). In optimal circumstances, the septum has a fully developed cavum; under these circumstances, the lesion will present with cavum entry. More frequently, the two septal leaves are opened to identify the raphe, which is secondarily opened with a sharp microdissector. Sometimes the septal leaves are fused. In this case, bipolar forceps are used to reduce the septum to the fornix level. This will then be the mark for the raphe, which may be developed with a sharp microinstrument. Frequently, the mass present will form an internal pressure, which will establish a natural presentation into the field of fornical division once the raphe has been surgically developed. *To reduce potential deleterious effects on memory, the raphe should be opened from the foramen of Monro level to 1.5 cm to 2 cm posteriorly with care taken to identify the hippocampal commissure and preserve this structure.* This entry provides the ability to perform simultaneous manipulation of masses through both foramina as well as raphe entry, which allows visualization of the entire chamber.

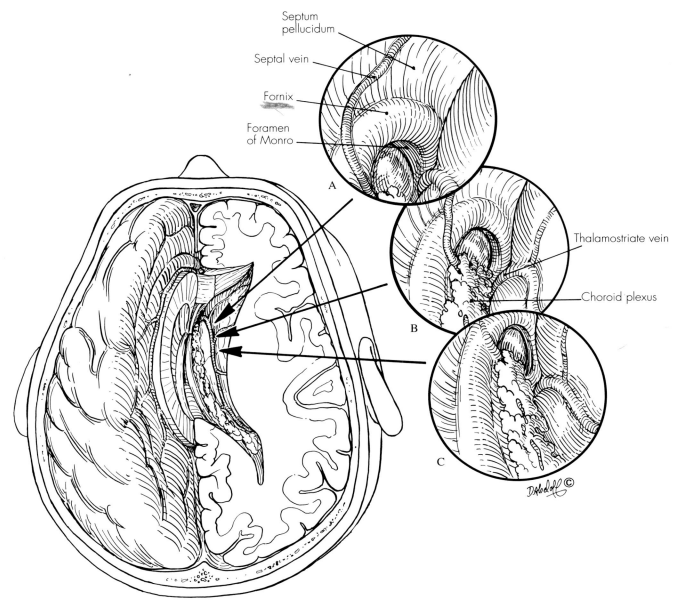

Figure 18-12. Illustration of view lines to foramen of Monro with visualization at end point dependent on angle of entry: **(A)** anterior, **(B)** middle (coronal line), and **(C)** posterior. The entry in Fig. C is suboptimal and should be avoided in general.

Subchoroidal Plane

The subchoroidal plane provides a natural space for entry into the velum interpositum with a tether posterior to the foramen of Monro created by the thalamostriate vein. This vein may be sacrificed to enhance exposure without apparent unwanted physiological effects.

As in the interfornical approach, the mass occasionally balloons into the field as the space is opened by placement of a sharp microdissector.

With small lesions that do not deform the superior thalmus, this structure may obscure visualization of the lesion. In addition, the paramedian rather than the midline approach provides certain view line problems with the interhemispheric exposure and is more optimally employed with a transcortical view line.

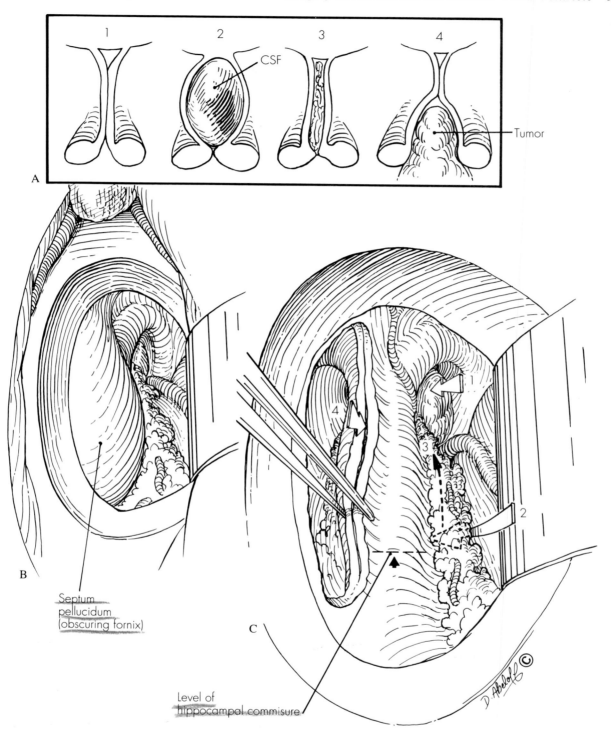

Figure 18-13. Considerations in an orientation within the lateral ventricle and options for third ventricular entry and exposure. **(A)** Variance of anatomy at fornix-septum pellucidum complex: (*1*) septum and two distinct leaflets; (*2*) cavum septum pellucidum; (*3*) fused septum; (*4*) fornical body separated and leaflets space developed by mass. This presentation will impact upon the ease of identification of the forniceal raphe. **(B)** Septum may bellow toward the decompressed side of obscuring foramen and anatomy for orientation. **(C)** Entry options to third ventricular chamber: (*1*) foramen; (*2*) subchoroidal; (*3*) subchoroidal with striothalamic vein sacrifice; (*4*) interfornical.

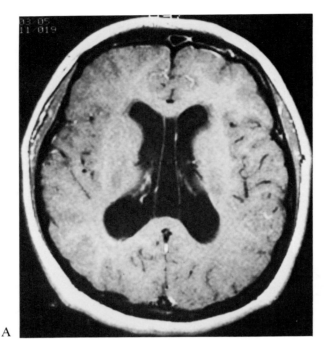

A

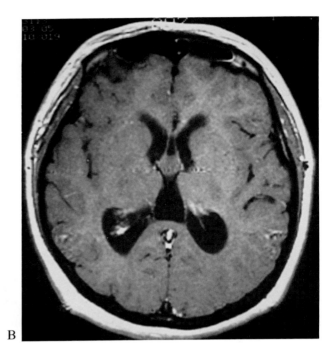

B

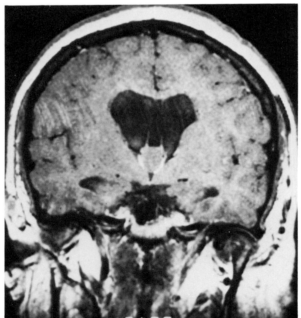

C

Figure 18-14. T$_1$-weighted MRIs of a colloid cyst with cavum septum pellucidum. **(A)** Axial, **(B)** axial, and **(C)** coronal views. This anatomical presentation allowed entry in midline through cavum space and direct visualization of cyst.

Stage III. Surgery within the Third Ventricular Chamber

The keys to safe and optimal excision of third ventricular masses include:

1. Adequacy of view line
2. Adequacy of exposure
3. Development of opportunity for simultaneous lesion manipulation from variable perspectives (if necessary)
4. Minimization of transmitted trauma via the mass to peripheral neural elements
5. Minimization of dissection to obtain excision corridors
6. Protection and maintenance of all entry corridors

Employing transforaminal, subchoroidal, and interfornical options this is often possible with satisfactory results and optimization of outcome with respect to the entire clinical situation (Fig. 18-15). Simplisti-

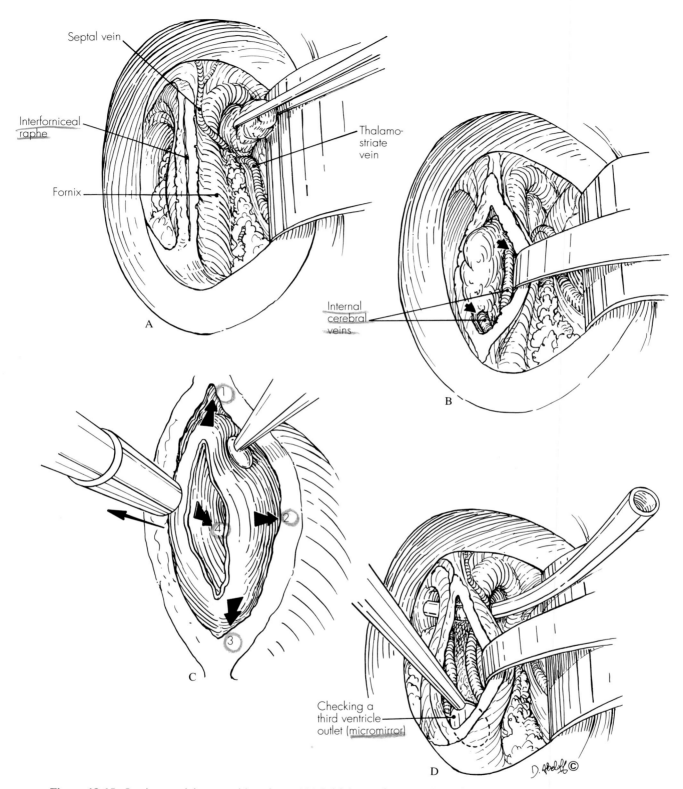

Figure 18-15. Lesion excision considerations. **(A)** Initial transforamenal manipulation to assess texture and excisability. **(B)** Development of raphe for dorsal exposure; internal decompression with identification of internal cerebral veins, general placement of microretractor system on right fornix; limit fornix incision to 2 cm extending from anterior foramen posteriorly to preserve hippocampal commisure. **(C)** Steps in capsular dissection. **(D)** Observation (micromirror) of patency of outlet orifices, para foramen of Monro, iter, hypothalamic floor (if pertinent).

cally, *standard microsurgical principles hold true in this region* as in others. In cystic lesions, aspiration is followed by wall dissection. In solid lesions, piecemeal central dissection followed by circumferential wall incision are aphorisms to be respected. In general, the more solid and adherent a lesion is, the greater the necessity for expansile exposures to aid in maneuvers for excision. Problems and potential complications relate to direct and indirect neurological injury (thalamic and hypothalamic surfaces) and vascular trauma (especially the internal cerebral vein in the diencephalic roof). Hemorrhage may be initiated by traction on the choroid plexus in the roof. *A constant danger in dissection is remote events.* All of the above may be largely avoided by meticulous and patient adherence to principles of microsurgical techniques and constant appreciation of the risks and breeches of discipline that make complications a reality. As decompression occurs, care must be taken not to overretract fornical and peripheral thalamic structures. Some retraction of the fornical bodies is necessary during intrafornical and subchoroidal exposures. We employed a thin, 5 mm blade tapered to 2 mm for gentle fornical retraction. It should be noted that during the stage of excision a secondary retractor is often employed on the contralateral cingulum and callosum. This is employed to maximize temporary view lines to the contralateral ventricle and foramen. Care must be taken to minimize pressure and time frames as mutism is considered to result from overretraction of cingulate structures bilaterally.

Stages of excision via the interfornical route include:

1. Internal decompression
2. Anterior dissection and excision
3. Lateral dissection and excision
4. Posterior dissection and excision
5. Inferior dissection and excision

Identification and protection of the internal cerebral veins is more difficult with small midventricular masses. We consider that there exists a true enhancement of dissection and exposure in larger lesions.

Inferior posterior dissection and excision should be gentle, as the basilar artery apex is adjacent to the region and, particularly in large (>2 cm) lesions, will be visualized at completion of the dissection.

Closure

Outlet occlusion of the lateral or third ventricular chambers is always a postoperative consideration. This may be guarded against at completion of dissection by inspection of all natural and divergent pathways, which are clearly appreciated by instrumentation being passed through the foramen of Monro. The posterior third ventricular outlet is visualized by direct inspection or mirror. Alternate flow paths include the callosotomy, septal window, and possibly the hypothalamic floor defect associated with the lesion's excision.

Hemorrhage is a constant risk, and a laborious and systematic hemostasis is imperative. We recommend layer by layer evaluation with the operating microscope to the superior cortical pial surface. We have found that the ependymal surface adjacent to the callosotomy (especially posteriorly) and abraded medial and paramedial cortical surfaces are areas of difficulty. The latter of the particular problems is technically initiated when extensive paramedian venous complexes are present on opening. Care must be taken with coagulation and hemastatic agents to ensure perfect hemastasis.

Avoidance of excessive *trapping of air* in the frontal fossa is important with dural closure. Care should be taken to displace air in situations of significant ventriculomegaly, in which there is a tendency for excessive trapping. A soft catheter may be placed in the subarachnoid space and led through the wound to

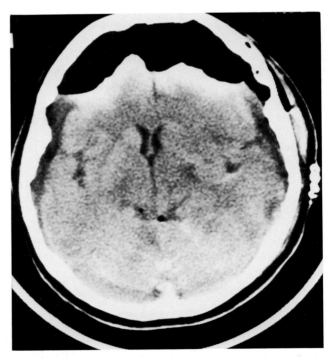

Figure 18-16. Postoperative CT scan with excessive frontal air; this risk may be avoided by proper intracranial fluid restoration and placement of a subarachnoid drain if required for gas decompression.

decompress the space and to avoid problems of tension pneumocephalis (Fig. 18-16).

Postoperative Problems

As has been noted (Table 18-14), the principal early concerns relate to the following:

1. Outlet construction
2. Hemorrhage
3. Pneumocephalus
4. Ventriculitis, meningitis
5. Memory loss

These issues may be guarded against intraoperatively but may occur during the early postoperative period. Simple decompression catheters will suffice to reduce excessive CSF and air, which occasionally are transient. Unfortunately, permanent shunting is sometimes necessary as diversion.

Intraventricular or other intracranial hemorrhagic events require exploration. They should be reduced by careful monitoring of early recovery systemic arterial blood pressures and the use of immediate sodium nitroprusside should the occasion require it. Hemorrhage in occipital horns is frequently visualized and is not problematic. Symptomatic and massive ventricular hemorrhage (as verified by imaging) requires complete ventricular lavage with body-temperature bacitracin-Ringer's lactate solution. Microscopic control of the hemorrhagic sources is followed by introduction of soft catheters to horn regions with gravity-assisted irrigation until clear. We rarely place a second ventricular catheter for lavage outflow as an alternative to direct exploration.

Ventriculitis is rarely encountered but may be heralded by mentation changes 3 days to several weeks postoperatively. CSF cells, sugar, and organism evaluation give the diagnosis. Intravenous agents, hardware removal, and vigilance are required for periods of 7 to 21 days. Infectious agents requiring intraventricular administration of antibiotics are rarely encountered. As previously noted, prophylactic antibiotics are employed routinely for at least 48 hours postoperatively. This practice has made ventriculitis-meningitis as an early clinical entity very rare in our experience of ventricular explorations.

Initial imaging during the postoperative period often shows bilateral or unilateral *subdural collections*. These rarely require surgical evacuation and usually resolve over 1 to 4 week time frames.

Memory loss for recent events may be noted in approximately one-third of patients and is dependent on numerous factors for its emergence but will generally improve in days, occasionally lasting several weeks or longer.

REFERENCES

1. Antunes J, Luis KM, Ganti SR: Colloid cysts of the third ventricle. Neurosurgery 7:450, 1980
2. Apuzzo MLJ: Surgery of masses affecting the third ventricular chamber: techniques and strategies. Clin Neurosurg 34:499, 1986
3. Apuzzo, MLJ, Chandrasoma PT, Zelman V et al: Computed tomographic guidance stereotaxis in the management of lesions of the third ventricular region. Neurosurgery 15:502, 1984
4. Apuzzo MLJ, Chikovani OK, Gott PS et al: Transcallosal interfornicial approaches for lesions affecting the third ventricle: surgical considerations and consequences. Neurosurgery 10:547, 1982
5. Apuzzo MLJ, Giannotta SL: Transcallosal interfornicial approach. p. 354. In Apuzzo MLJ (ed): Surgery of the Third Ventricle. Williams & Wilkins, Baltimore, 1987
6. Apuzzo MLJ, Zee CS, Breeze RE: Anterior and mid-third ventricular lesions: a surgical overview. p. 495. In Apuzzo, MLJ (ed): Surgery of the Third Ventricle. Williams & Wilkins, Baltimore, 1987
7. Backlund EO: Studies on craniopharyngiomas III. Stereotaxic treatment with intracystic Yttrium-90. Acta Chir Scand 139:237, 1973
8. Backlund EO, Johansson L, Surby B: Studies on craniopharyngiomas II. Treatment by stereotaxis and radiosurgery. Acta Chir Scand 138:749, 1972
9. Bosch DA, Rahn T, Backlund EO: Treatment of colloid cysts of the third ventricle by stereotactic aspiration. Surg Neurol 9:15, 1978
10. Cairns H, Mosberg WH: Colloid cyst of the third ventricle. Surg Gynecol Obstet 92:545, 1971
11. Carmel PW: Surgical syndromes of the hypothalamus. Clin Neurosurg 27:133, 1980
12. Ciric I: Colloid cysts of the third ventricle (Comment) Neurosurgery 7:455, 1980
13. Ciric I, Cozzens JR: Craniopharyngiomas: transsphenoidal method of approach—for the virtuoso only? Clin Neurosurg 27:169, 1980
14. Clar HE: Clinical and morphological studies of pituitary and diencephalic space-occupying lesions before and after operation, with specific reference to temperature regulation. Acta Neurochir 50:153, 1979
15. Damasio AR, Van Hoesen GW: Pathological correlates of amnesia and the anatomical basis of memory. p. 195. In Apuzzo MLJ (ed): Surgery of the Third Ventricle. Williams & Wilkins, Baltimore, 1987
16. Davis RL: Pathological lesions of the third ventricle and adjacent structures. p. 235. In Apuzzo MLJ (ed):

Surgery of the Third Ventricle. Williams & Wilkins, Baltimore, 1987

17. Dimond SJ, Scammel RE, Broadwers ETM et al: Functions of the centre section (trunk) of the corpus callosum in man. Brain 100:543, 1977

18. Ehni G: Transcallosal approaches to the anterior ventricular system (Comment). Neurosurgery 3:343, 1978

19. Ehni G: Interhemispheric and percallosal (transcallosal) approach to the cingulate gyri, intraventricular shunt tubes and certain deeply placed brain lesions. Neurosurgery 14:99, 1984

20. Ehni G, Ehni B: Considerations in transforaminal entry. p. 326. In Apuzzo MLJ (ed): Surgery of the Third Ventricle. Williams & Wilkins, Baltimore, 1987

21. Garretson HD: Commentary A. Memory in man: a neurosurgeon's perspective. p. 326. In Apuzzo MLJ (ed): Surgery of the Third Ventricle. Williams & Wilkins, Baltimore, 1987

22. Gazzaniga MS, Risse GL, Springer SP et al: Psychologic and neurologic consequences of partial and complete cerebral commis-rotomy. Neurology 25:10, 1975

23. Geffen G, Wash A, Simpson O et al: Comparison of the effects of trancortical and transcallosal removal of intraventricular tumors. Brain 103:773, 1980

24. Gordon HW, Bogen JE, Sperry RU: Absence of disconnexion syndrome in two patients with partial section of the neocommisures. Brain 94:327, 1971

25. Greenwood J: Paraphysical cysts of the third ventricle with report of eight cases. J Neurosurg 6:153, 1949

26. Greenwood J: Removal of foreign body (bullet) from the third ventricle. J Neurosurg 7:169, 1950

27. Gregorius FK, Hepler RS, Stern WE: Loss and recovery of vision with suprasellar meningiomas. J Neurosurg 42:68, 1975

28. Gutierrez-Lara F, Patino R, Italcim S: Treatment of tumors of the third ventricle: a new and simple technique. Surg Neurol 3:323, 1975

29. Hall WA, Lundsford LP: Changing concepts in the treatment of colloid cysts. An 11 year experience in the CT scan era. J Neurosurg 66:186, 1987

30. Hamer J: Removal of craniopharyngioma by subnasal transsphenoidal operation. Neuropediatrie 9:312, 1978

31. Harper RL, Ehni G: The anterior transcallosal approach to brain tumors. Adv Neurosurg 7:91, 1979

32. Heilman KM, Sypert GW: Korsakoff's syndrome resulting from bilateral fornix lesions. Neurology 27:490, 1977

33. Hirsch JF, Zovaou A, Renier D et al: A new surgical approach to the third ventricle with interruption of the striothalamic vein. Acta Neurochir 47:135, 1979

34. Hoffman, HJ, Hendrick EF, Humphreys RP: Management of craniopharyngioma. J Neurosurg 47:403, 1978

35. Horel JA: The neuroanatomy of amensia. A critique of the hippocampal memory hypothesis. Brain 101:403, 1978

36. Jeeves MA, Simpson DA, Geffer G: Functional consequences of the transcallosal removal of intraventricular tumors. J Neurol Neurosurg Psychiatry 42:134, 1979

37. Jefferson A, Assam N: The suprasellar meningiomas: a review of 19 years experience. Acta Neurochir (Suppl) 28:381, 1979

38. Julow J, Langi F, Hadja M et al: The radiotherapy of cystic craniopharyngioma with intracystic instillation of ^{90}Y sillicate colloid. Acta Neurochir 74:94, 1985

39. Kahn EA, Gosch HH, Seegar JF et al: Forty-five years experience with the craniopharyngiomas. Surg Neurol 1:5, 1973

40. Katz EL: Late results of radical excision of craniopharyngiomas in children. J Neurosurg 42:86, 1975

41. Kelly DL: Isodose colloid cysts of the third ventricle: a diagnostic and therapeutic problem resolved by ventriculoscopy. (Comment.) Neurosurgery 13:237, 1983

42. King TT: Removal of intraventricular craniopharyngioma through the lamina terminalis. Acta Neurochir 45:277, 1979

43. Kwan E, Wolpert SM, Smith SP et al: Radiology of third ventricular lesions. p. 262. In Apuzzo MLJ (ed): Surgery of the Third Ventricle. Williams & Wilkins, Baltimore, 1987

44. Lavyne MH, Patterson RH: Subchoroidal trans-velum interpositum approach. p. 381. In Apuzzo MLJ (ed): Surgery of the Third Ventricle. Williams & Wilkins, Baltimore, 1987

45. Laws ER: Transsphenoidal microsurgery in the management of craniopharyngioma. J Neurosurg 51:661, 1980

46. Laws ED, Kern EB: Complications of transsphenoidal surgery. Clin Neurosurg 23:401, 1976

47. Lipton JM, Rosenstein J, Sklar FH: Thermoregulatory disorders after removal of a craniopharyngioma from the third ventricle. Br Res Bull 7:369, 1981

48. Little JR, MacCarty CS: Colloid cysts of the third ventricle. J Neurosurg 39:230, 1974

49. Long DM, Chou SN: Transcallosal removal of craniopharyngiomas with the third ventricle. J Neurosurg 39:563, 1973

50. Long DM, Leibrock C: The transcallosal approach to the anterior ventricular system and its application in the therapy of craniopharyngioma. Clin Neurosurg 27:160, 1980

51. Matson DP, Crigler FJ: Management of craniopharyngioma in childhood. J Neurosurg 30:377, 1969

52. McClone DG, Raimondi AJ, Naidich JP: Craniopharyngiomas. Childs Brain 9:188, 1982

53. McKissock W: The surgical treatment of colloid cyst of the third ventricle. Brain 74:1, 1951

54. Mohadjer M, Teshman E, Mundinger F: CT—stereotaxic drainage of colloid cysts in the foramen of Monro and the third ventricle. J Neurosurg 67:220, 1987

55. Ono M, Rhoton AL, Peace D et al: Microsurgical anatomy of the deep venous system of the brain. Neurosurgery 15:621, 1984

56. Page RB: Commentary C. Diencephalic structures at risk in third ventricular surgery. p. 553. In Apuzzo MLJ (ed): Surgery of the Third Ventricle. Williams & Wilkins, Baltimore, 1987

57. Patterson JR, Leslie M: Colloid cyst of the third ventricle of the brain. Br Med J 1:920, 1935
58. Patterson RH: Subfrontal transsphenoidal and translamina terminalis approaches. p. 398. In Apuzzo MLJ (ed): Surgery of the Third Ventricle. Williams & Wilkins, Baltimore, 1987
59. Petrucci RJ, Buchheit WA, Woodruff GO et al: Transcallosal parafornical approach for third ventricle tumors: neuropsychologic consequences. Neurosurgery 20:457, 1987
60. Pollack IF, Lundsford LD, Lamovits TL et al: Stereotaxic intracavitary irradiation for cystic craniopharyngiomas. J Neurosurg 68:227, 1988
61. Poppen JL, Reyes V, Horrax G: Colloid cysts of the third ventricle. Report of seven cases. J Neurosurg 10:242, 1953
62. Powell MP, Torrens MJ, Thomsen JLG et al: Isodense colloid cysts of the third ventricle: a diagnostic and therapeutic problem resolved by ventriculoscopy. Neurosurgery 13:234, 1981
63. Reigal DH: Transcallosal approaches to the anterior ventricular system. (Comment) Neurosurgery 3:343, 1978
64. Rekate HL, Ruch J, Nulsen F et al: Needle biopsy of tumors in the region of the third ventricle. J Neurosurg 54:338, 1981
65. Rhoton AL, Yamamoto I, Pence DA: Microsurgery of the third ventricle. Part 2. Operative Approaches. Neurosurgery 8:357, 1981
66. Rivas JJ, Lobato RD: CT assisted stereotaxic aspiration of colloid cysts of the third ventricle. J Neurosurg 62:238, 1985
67. Rosenstein J, Symon L: Surgical management of suprasellar meningioma. Part 2: Prognosis for visual function following craniotomy. J Neurosurg 61:642, 1984
68. Rougerie J: What can be expected from the surgical treatment of craniopharyngiomas in children? Childs Brain 5:433, 1979
69. Shapiro K, Till K, Grant DN: Craniopharyngiomas in childhood. A rational approach to treatment. J Neurosurg 50:617, 1979
70. Shillito J: Craniopharyngiomas: the subfrontal approach or none at all? Clin Neurosurg 27:188, 1980
71. Shucart W: Anterior transcallosal and transcortical approaches. p. 303. In Apuzzo MLJ (ed): Surgery of the Third Ventricle. Williams & Wilkins, Baltimore, 1987
72. Shucart W, Stein B: Transcallosal approach of the interior ventricular system. Neurosurgery 3:339, 1978
73. Solero CC, Gromein S, Morello G: Suprasellar and olfactory meningiomas. Report on a series of 153 personal cases. Acta Neurochir 67:181, 1983
74. Sturm V, Rommel T, Strauss L: Preliminary results of intracavitory irradiation of cystic craniopharyngioma by means of stereotactically applied yttrium-90. Adv Neurosurgery 9:401, 1981
75. Suzuki J: Bifrontal anterior interhemispheric approach. p. 413. In Apuzzo MLJ (ed): Surgery of the Third Ventricle. Williams & Wilkins, Baltimore, 1987
76. Suzuki J, Katakura R, Mori T: Interhemispheric approach through the lamina terminalis to tumors of the anterior part of the third ventricle. Surg Neurol 22:157, 1984
77. Svien HS: Surgical experiences with craniopharyngiomas. J Neurosurg 23:148, 1965
78. Sweet W: Radical surgical treatment of craniopharyngioma. Clin Neurosurg 23:52, 1976
79. Sweet W: Recurrent craniopharyngiomas. Clin Neurosurg 27:206, 1980
80. Symon L, Jakubowski J: Transcranial management of pituitary tumors with suprasellar extension. J Neurol Neurosurg Psychiatry 42:123, 1979a
81. Symon K, Jakubouski J: Clinical features, technical problems and result of treatment of anterior parasellar meningiomas. Acta Neurochir (Suppl) 28:367, 1979b
82. Symon L, Rosenstein J: Surgical management of suprasellar meningioma. Part 1. The influence of tumor size, duration of symptoms and microsurgery on surgical outcome in 101 consecutive cases. J Neurosurg 61:633, 1984
83. Till K: Craniopharyngioma. Childs Brain 9:179, 1982
84. Tindall GT, Tindall SL: Pterional approach. p. 440. In Apuzzo MLJ (ed): Surgery of the Third Ventricle. Williams & Wilkins, Baltimore, 1987
85. Trescher JH, Ford FR: Colloid cyst of the third ventricle. Arch Neurol Psychiatry 37:759, 1932
86. Viale GL, Turtas S: The subchoroid approach to the third ventricle. Surg Neurol 14:71, 1980
87. Weiss MH: Transnasal transsphenoidal approach. p. 476. In Apuzzo MLJ (ed): Surgery of the Third Ventricle. Williams & Wilkins, Baltimore, 1987
88. Winston KR, Cavazzuti V, Antunes T: Absence of neurologic and behavioral abnormalities after anterior transcallosal operation for third ventricular lesions. Neurosurgery 4:386, 1974
89. Yamamoto I, Rhoton AL, Peace DA: Microsurgery of the third ventricle. Part 1: Microsurgical anatomy. Neurosurgery 5:334, 1981

19 Lateral Ventricular Masses

Joseph M. Piepmeier
Dennis D. Spencer
Kimberlee J. Sass
Timothy M. George

Mass lesions of the lateral ventricles present a unique surgical challenge. Tumors that arise in this location often are benign, grow at a slow rate, and reach a very large size before they are identified.[2,6,9,24,26,28,40,46,48,52] These lesions commonly receive their blood supply from branches of the choroidal vessels of both the anterior and posterior circulations.[1,3–5,10,31,39,41,52,54] They cause hydrocephalus by obstructing normal cerebrospinal fluid (CSF) pathways[40,47] or by overproduction of spinal fluid.[33,54] These characteristics and the relatively deep location of ventricular masses require careful consideration to determine the appropriate surgical management and to avoid complications. There is no surgical method that can eliminate all of the obstacles that occur in the treatment of these lesions. Operative techniques designed to address specific problems such as the lesion's size, location, or vascular supply may complicate the surgeon's ability to preserve neurological function or perform a complete resection.[48] Therefore, the surgeon must examine the relative advantages and disadvantages of a range of options for each patient to attain realistic surgical goals with a minimum risk of neurological impairment.

LITERATURE REVIEW

Mass lesions of the lateral ventricles are uncommon. Consequently, very few reports address the potential complications that may occur in their management.[40,45,48,51,52] The literature concerning these lesions focuses on a particular pathological diagnosis[2,7,10,15,18,19,22,24,26,28,30–33,39,41,47,53–56] or specific operative technique[8,11,21,23,35] and it provides little information regarding the potential problems associated with surgical treatment. In addition, because many of these reports contain small numbers of patients, it is difficult to establish relative risks for each complication. To assist in the evaluation of the complications that occur with this surgery we have examined 21 consecutive patients that were treated at Yale-New Haven Hospital between 1984 and 1990 and compared these results with earlier reports.[40] Our patient group consists of 15 males and 6 females ranging from 3 months to 73 years of age (average, 27 years). The majority of these lesions (86 percent) were tumors, and 78 percent of them were benign or low-grade neoplasms. The other lesions included a cavernous hemangioma, an arteriovenous malformation (AVM), and an epithelial cyst. The diagnoses are shown in Table 19-1.

Preoperative Findings

Surgical complications from any lesion can be, in part, predicted by the patient's preoperative status. Neurological deficits resulting from a lateral ventricular mass typically are vague and include headache, poor balance, and difficulty with memory.[26,40,52] Traditional localizing findings such as aphasia and agno-

Table 19-1. Lateral Ventricular Masses Treated at Yale 1984–1990

Diagnosis	No.
Choroid plexus papilloma	5
Malignant astrocytoma	2
Oligodendroglioma	2
Meningioma	2
Subependymoma	2
Ependymoma	1
Teratoma	2
Renal carcinoma	1
Mixed glioma	1
Cavernous hemangioma	1
Arteriovenous malformation	1
Epithelial cyst	1

Table 19-2. Incidence of Surgical Complications from Reported Series and the Yale Series for Patients with Mass Lesions of the Lateral Ventricles

Complication	Literature (%)	Yale Series (%)
Visual field deficit	20–64	9.5
Hemiparesis	8–30	4.8
Speech deficit	8–36	14.3
Subdural hematoma	11	9.5
Death	12–75	14.3
Seizures	29–70	19
Infection	Unknown	4.8
Incomplete resection	33–50	19
Persistent hydrocephalus	12–33	35

sia are rarely present. As the ventricular lesion enlarges, these symptoms progress and are associated with hyperreflexia, ataxia, visual problems, and, on occasion, seizures.[10,12,31] Preoperative neuropsychological testing can reveal a number of deficits in these patients including memory difficulties and impaired functioning on measures of intelligence for which speed of performance and facility with novel visual information are important task components. The performance IQ (PIQ) is more sensitive than the verbal IQ (VIQ) in detecting global changes in the brain. It is common to find a significant deficit in the PIQ compared with the VIQ in the preoperative evaluation regardless of the location of the mass within the ventricles.[40] This pattern of memory impairment and a relative deficiency in the PIQ is considered to be a result of hydrocephalus. Consequently, it is anticipated that surgical management may further impair the patient's cognitive function. Lateralization of motor or sensory findings generally is limited to patients with very large lesions or masses in the posterior ventricle associated with entrapment of the occipital and temporal horns.

Postoperative Deficits

While it is difficult to document the true frequency of postoperative complications, selected case reports include a description of the results of surgical management. A summary of these results is shown in Table 19-2.

A postoperative visual field loss appears to be one of the most common focal deficits, particularly with posterior ventricular or trigone lesions resected through a parietal or occipital approach. The relative incidence of this problem ranges between 20 and 64 percent for parietal incisions and near 100 percent for the occipital approach.[5,12,26] The most common deficit is an homonymous field loss. In our experience this occurred in two patients (9.5 percent) following a parietooccipital incision and an occipital lobectomy.

Hemiparesis frequently is observed during the immediate postoperative period following intraventricular surgery for trigone or midbody tumors. Permanent impairment in motor function occurs in 8 to 30 percent of reported patients.[6,8,12,40,45] In some small series all the patients sustained a permanent loss of motor function following surgery.[24] In our series one patient (4.8 percent) suffered a hemiparesis following the resection of a metastatic renal carcinoma in the trigone through the superior parietal lobule.

Potential deficits in speech function complicate the surgery for lesions in the ventricle of the dominant hemisphere.[17] There are few reports that document this problem, and speech function is difficult to measure in children. However, approximately 8 to 36 percent of patients sustain a permanent speech impairment.[12,13,40,45] In our experience three patients (14.3 percent) had a worsening of speech function following surgery. One of these patients had a superior parietal lobule incision and two patients had approaches through the middle frontal gyrus for lesions in the frontal horn of the dominant hemisphere. These latter two patients had postoperative speech apraxias associated with ideomotor and buccofacial apraxias.

Subdural hematoma and hygroma formation are significant problems, particularly in patients with preoperative ventricular enlargement[2,25,48] (Fig. 19-1). In a series of 38 patients, Tanaka[51] noted subdural fluid collections in 40 percent and persistent fluid collections in 24 percent. Symptomatic collections required surgical drainage in 11 percent. The risk of fluid collections was noted to be increased in patients with preoperative hydrocephalus whose tumors were removed through a transfrontal approach. In our se-

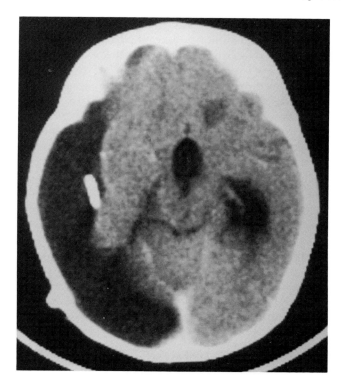

Figure 19-1. Postoperative CT scan of a 3-month-old boy following the resection of a large intraventricular teratoma. A large subdural fluid collection over the right hemisphere required shunting. Persistent ventricular enlargement also is present.

ries two patients (9.5 percent) required surgical treatment for a delayed chronic hematoma and a hygroma.

Mortality statistics vary widely, and the causes of death frequently are not provided. Within these limitations, the mortality for surgery on a lateral ventricular mass lesion ranges from 12 to 75 percent.[2,8,34,39,40,52] In the few cases in which the cause of death was determined, cerebral edema and massive brain swelling or intraventricular hemorrhage were the most common findings.[12,50] In one series of patients with meningiomas, all the deaths occurred when the tumor was removed *en bloc*.[10] Our mortality included three patients (14.3 percent) who had a postoperative intracerebral hemorrhage and two cases with fatal pulmonary emboli.

Postoperative seizures can occur in any patient who receives a craniotomy for removal of a mass lesion. There are no direct comparisons of operative techniques and the incidence of this problem. Postoperative seizures have been reported in 29 to 70 percent of patients managed with transcortical resections of their lesions.[10,26] The incidence of postoperative seizures following transcallosal surgery is un-

known, but it is likely to be significantly lower than this number. There was a 19 percent incidence of seizures in our patients who had transcortical surgery for their lesions. No seizures were noted in patients who had transcallosal surgery.

The incidence of postoperative infection for lateral ventricular lesions has not been reported. Our experience revealed one case of subdural empyema (4.8 percent).

Several other issues need to be addressed as postoperative problems that may not be clearly identified as complications. Incomplete surgical resection of the mass lesion occurs in 33 to 50 percent of cases.[2,8,20,32,34,40,45] In our experience subtotal resections occurred in four cases (19 percent), most frequently in cases of primary malignant brain tumors that lacked a clear demarcation from the surrounding brain.

Postoperative ventricular enlargement is noted frequently in spite of total tumor resection; the literature reports that 12 in 33 percent of patients require a ventricular shunt.[13,28,40,52] Our experience shows that 35 percent of the patients required shunts for persistent symptomatic hydrocephalus (Fig. 19-2). The im-

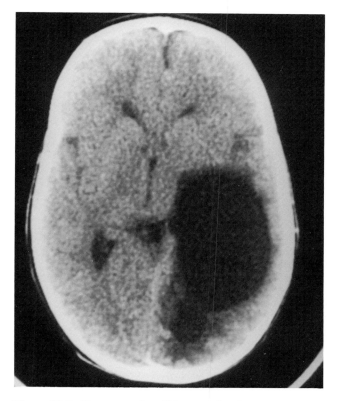

Figure 19-2. Postoperative CT scan of a 5-month-old boy following the resection of a large choroid plexus papilloma. Cystic dilatation of the trigone and temporal horn was treated with a ventriculoperitoneal shunt.

portance of persistent ventricular enlargement and its implications on neurological recovery are not well understood. Since many of the preoperative signs and symptoms of a ventricular mass lesion are similar to the problems associated with hydrocephalus, it is reasonable to assume that the treatment of hydrocephalus is an important part of overall surgical management.

OPERATIVE TECHNIQUE

Preoperative Evaluation

Preoperative evaluation of these patients is facilitated by detailed imaging studies with computed tomography (CT) and/or magnetic resonance imaging (MRI).[31,46] These studies can be imaged or reconstructed in axial, sagittal, and coronal planes to view the lesion from many angles (Figs. 19-3 to 19-6). Careful review of imaging studies can reveal important information concerning the size, location, and relative vascularity of the lesion.[1,10,41] However, large lesions may distort normal anatomy, and the

relationship of the mass to the third ventricle or the site of origin may not be determined clearly. Cerebral angiography also is important in the evaluation of these patients to examine the lesion's vascular supply and to determine changes in normal anatomical structures.[9] Angiography also is needed to demonstrate the venous drainage from the hemisphere into the superior sagittal sinus prior to interhemispheric dissection (Fig. 19-7).

The operative approaches to deep cerebral lesions within the ventricles require consideration of numerous factors. The basic principles that determine the success of the surgery include early access to the blood supply, minimal retraction for adequate exposure, piecemeal removal of large masses, and an understanding of the function of the surrounding anatomical structures. There are several alternatives for operative approaches to the lateral ventricle, and the optimal exposure of each lesion requires a balance of the benefits and liabilities of each (Fig. 19-8).

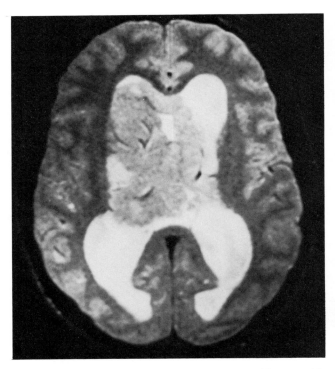

Figure 19-3. T₂-weighted MRI of a 30-year-old man with headaches and difficulty with motor control of the left arm. This mixed glioma originated from the ependyma of the frontal horn. The size and extension of this tumor indicate that a single operative approach may be insufficient for a total resection.

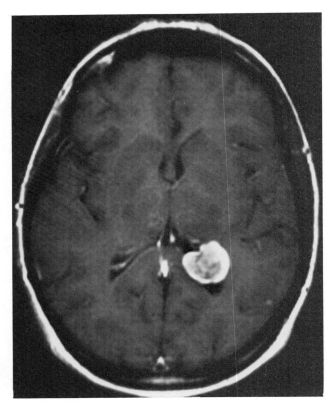

Figure 19-4. Gadolinium-enhanced MRI of a 37-year-old woman with a long history of headaches. This meningioma caused local distention of the left trigone but did not obstruct the ventricle. Although this lesion is somewhat posterior within the ventricle, approaching this lesion through the corpus callosum will reduce manipulation of the dominant hemisphere.

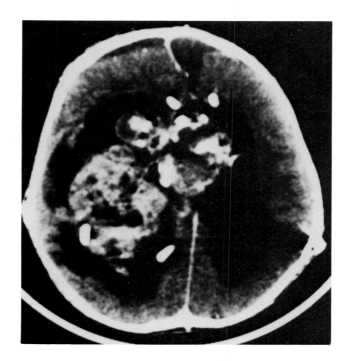

Figure 19-5. CT scan of a 3-month-old boy (same patient shown in Fig. 19-1). This large partially calcified teratoma caused massive ventricular distension and an increased head size. The white objects around the lesion are ventricular drainage catheters. Early access to the vascular supply is important in the preoperative planning for this infant.

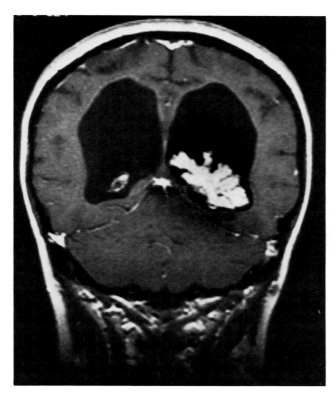

Figure 19-6. Sagittal, gadolinium-enhanced MRI of a 27-year-old woman who complained of headaches. This study reveals the typical appearance of a choroid plexus papilloma and massive ventricular enlargement. The enlarged ventricles can be used to the surgeon's advantage in planning the removal of this tumor.

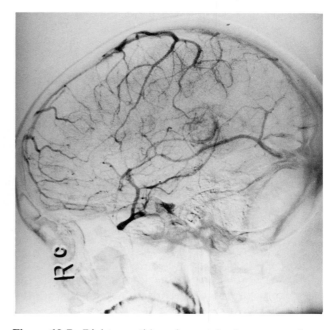

Figure 19-7. Right carotid angiogram in the venous phase from a 27-year-old woman with a right trigone meningioma. The study shows the vascular blush of the tumor. In addition, the relationship of the venous drainage from the hemisphere to the superior sagittal sinus with the tumor is clearly demonstrated. These findings can help to determine the optimal approach to the lesion (see text).

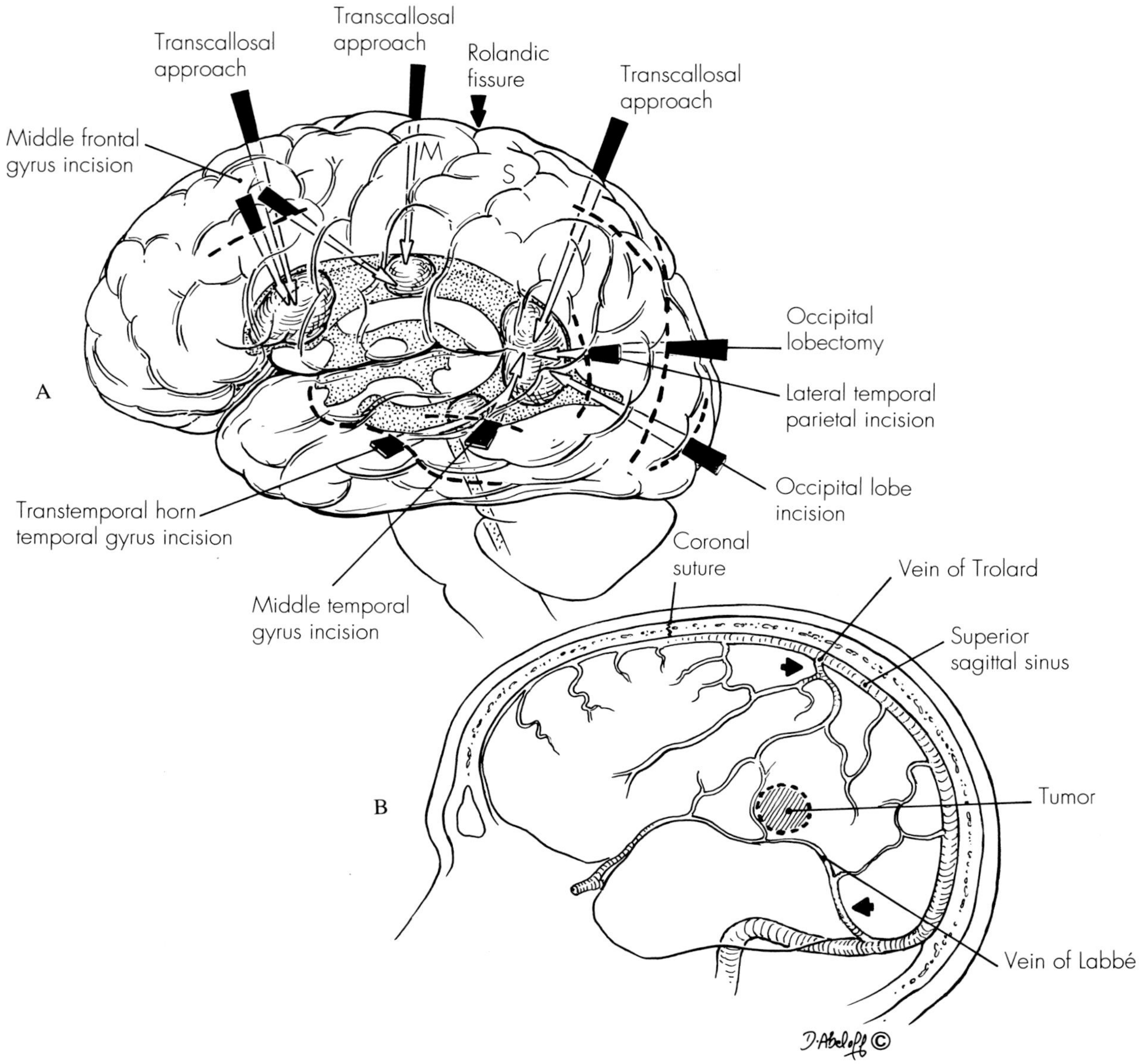

Figure 19-8. (A) Lateral illustration of the brain showing several options for surgical approaches to mass lesions throughout the lateral ventricles. *M*, motor; *S*, sensory. **(B)** Illustration of important venous drainage of the lateral hemisphere.

Temporal Lobe

The temporal horn of the lateral ventricle is the least likely site for a mass lesion compared with the other ventricular regions.[40,48] However, surgical approaches to this area can be utilized for access to the anterior choroidal artery. The three most commonly utilized avenues to access the temporal horn are at the temporoparietal junction, through the middle temporal gyrus, and by way of the transtemporal horn occipitotemporal gyrus. An approach through the temporoparietal junction will traverse the angular gyrus and result in dyslexia, agraphia, acalculia, and ideomotor apraxia in the dominant hemisphere.[12] In the nondominant hemisphere a similar approach causes very different problems including impaired memory for visual information, construction deficits, and neglect.[12,37] Incisions in this region must cross the optic radiations and will result in a visual field deficit.[12]

Approach to the temporal horn through the middle temporal gyrus can provide direct access to the lesion.[52] Variations in localization of the speech cortex in the dominant hemisphere make this a high-risk procedure without cortical stimulation to determine the limits of a safe resection.[13,38] In the nondominant hemisphere this may be an acceptable route.[12]

The transtemporal horn occipitotemporal gyrus approach has been developed for the resection of the hippocampus in the treatment of intractable seizures.[48] This provides exposure to the temporal horn and atrium and may be an acceptable alternative for lesions in this region. However, exposure of the temporal horn may result in a superior quadrant field deficit.

The temporal approach provides early access to the anterior choroidal artery but poor visualization of the posterior choroidal vessels until the lesion is almost completely resected.[48] Between 1984 and 1990 we had no experience with tumors confined to the temporal horn.

Scalp Incision

The temporal lobe is best exposed by an incision that starts 1 cm in front of the ear. In order to expose the inferior and anterior portions of the middle fossa, the incision should extend down to the base of the zygoma. The temporalis muscle can be mobilized from its attachment to the zygoma and greater wing of the sphenoid and reflected laterally to remove the muscle from the surgeon's line of approach.

Skull Opening

The temporal lobe is best exposed by a free bone flap. Removal of additional bone along the lateral temporal bone to the skull base will expand the surgeon's access to the inferior and middle temporal gyri. If mastoid air cells are entered, they should be closed with a generous use of bone wax.

Cortical Incision

Cortical incisions in the middle temporal gyrus should be preceded by measuring the distance from the tip of the lobe. Normally the temporal horn is approximately 3.5 cm from the temporal tip. An expanded temporal horn may be displaced and may change this distance. The exact distance can be determined by reviewing the preoperative imaging studies.

Parietal Lobe

Incisions through the parietal lobe provide direct access to lesions that reside at the trigone of the lateral ventricle.[48,52,56] A lateral parietal incision is contraindicated in the dominant hemisphere because of the very high risk of speech deficits.[12,40] The superior parietal lobule incision is the most commonly used in the parietal lobe.[10,40] However, exposure through this route poses a significant risk of acalculia and apraxia for the dominant hemisphere and visual-spatial processing problems as well as an homonymous hemianopia and hemiparesis with any significant retraction in either hemisphere.[12] This most often occurs when trying to expose a large lesion or when control of bleeding is a problem. Approaching a lesion through the parietal lobe places the vascular supply away from the surgeon's line of vision.[4] In our series, 10 patients had their lesions resected through superior parietal lobule approaches. The complications for this group include one hemiparesis, one hemianopia, and one death from an intracerebral hemorrhage.

Scalp Incision

The scalp should be opened to provide generous access to the parietal area; this is usually obtained by basing the scalp flap laterally with a generous base of vascularized tissue and extending the incision to the midline. Superficial landmarks including the parietal eminence, the parietal foramen, and the sagittal suture help to localize this region on the skull.

Skull Opening

Exposure of the parietal lobe should take into consideration the location of the vein of Trolard. Access to the ventricle should not be limited so that this vein receives retraction forces. The dura normally is opened toward the midline and reflected over the superior sagittal sinus without impeding its flow.

Cortical Incision

The superior parietal lobule is demarcated by the postcentral sulcus, the intraparietal sulcus, and the supramarginal gyrus. An incision in this region (Fig. 19-9) will place the line of dissection inferolaterally toward the ventricle. The incision should be sufficiently large to permit the use of a 2-cm retractor blade without tension. When the ventricle is opened, retraction forces should be minimized on the lateral white matter by gently elevating the brain rather than pushing it out of the way.

Occipital Lobe

Attempts to expose a lesion through the occipital lobe will ensure that the patient will sustain a permanent loss of an homonymous visual field.[10] This may

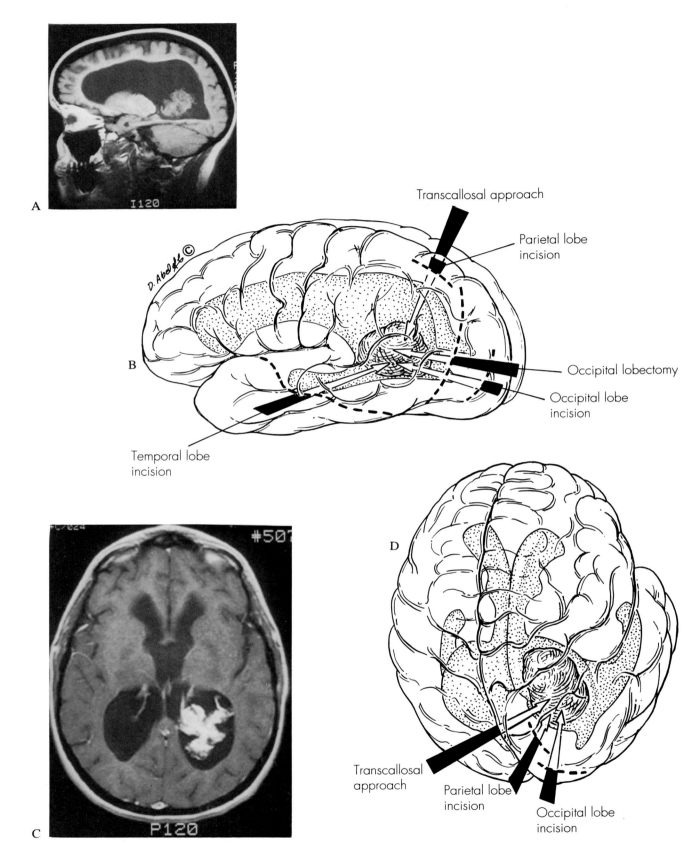

Figure 19-9. **(A)** Sagittal MRI illustrating a choroid plexus papilloma and hydrocephalus. **(B)** Illustration of possible approaches to this lesion. **(C)** Enhanced axial MRI of the same tumor. **(D)** Surgeon's view of the parietal approach to this lesion.

be acceptable, particularly when the same deficit is detected preoperatively and considered to be irreversible.[48] An occipital lobectomy can provide access to the entire ipsilateral ventricle but creates a long reach for lesions extending into the temporal horn or frontal horn. In addition, this exposure does not permit early access to the choroidal vessels and may require provisions for considerable blood loss for vascular lesions. The single patient in our series sustained an anticipated homonymous hemianopia following an occipital lobectomy for a large teratoma.

Scalp Incision

The incision for the occipital lobe typically is based on the occipital muscles to preserve the occipital artery.

Skull Opening

The craniotomy for the occipital lobe requires opening the skull near the superior sagittal sinus and the transverse sinus. We prefer to extend our opening up to these venous structures.

Cortical Incision

A lobectomy usually extends from the superior occipital gyrus to the tentorium. An incision in the occipital lobe (Fig. 19-9) typically is performed in the superior occipital gyrus, and dissection to the ventricle extends anterosuperiorly. This approach will cross the optic radiations and will usually result in loss of a visual field.

Frontal Lobe

Incisions through the middle frontal gyrus are one of the most often utilized routes to the anterior ventricle.[4,24,48] This is particularly helpful for tumors with a broad ependymal attachment in the frontal horn and permits access to the body of the ventricle. Significant speech problems may occur when this approach is used in patients with hydrocephalus and dominant hemisphere lesions even when Broca's area is undisturbed. Frontal incisions in either hemisphere also can result in attention deficits. Only three of our patients had their tumors removed through a middle frontal gyrus incision, and two of these had a speech apraxia associated with ideomotor and buccofacial apraxia following surgery in the dominant hemisphere.

Scalp Incision

Exposure of the frontal lobe typically requires extending the scalp incision into the temporal area or across to the opposite side to avoid a scar on the forehead.

Skull Opening

A free bone flap is easily obtained in the frontal area. The dura can become thin in older patients in the frontal area, and preservation of the dura may require additional burr holes to separate the dura from the inner table of the skull.

Cortical Incision

An incision in the middle frontal gyrus at the level of the coronal suture will place the surgeon's line of approach directly at the frontal horn and the foramen of Monro.

Corpus Callosum

Access to the lateral ventricles is easily provided through sectioning the corpus callosum. This route has been utilized increasingly for these lesions and provides a relatively safe access to all areas except the temporal horn and posterior lesions within the occipital horn.[21,40,45,48] Successful use of the transcallosal route requires careful patient selection since this surgery will result in some disconnection of the hemispheres.[14,27] Excluding neurological deficits attributable to surgical technique, the majority of postcallosotomy impairments are caused by the isolation of cortical centers or the disruption of critical callosal pathways in patients with anomalous cortical organization and those with specific neurological deficits.[20,29,36,42] These potential complications can be avoided by performing an intracarotid amytal procedure prior to transcallosal surgery.[44] This test can determine language dominance and memory function resident within each cerebral hemisphere. For example, sectioning of the splenium in patients with a dominant hemisphere homonymous hemianopia will cause alexia and visual agnosia.[29] Transcallosal surgery in left-handed, left-hemisphere speech-dominant and right-handed and right-hemisphere speech-dominant patients can cause agraphia and speech impairment.[43] Cerebral disconnection in left-hemisphere speech-dominant patients with right-hemisphere memory only or right-hemisphere speech-dominant patients with left-hemisphere memory only could result in a memory disorder.[43]

We have used the transcallosal approach for 10 lateral ventricular lesions; none of these patients suffered an increased focal neurological deficit. Complications in this group included 1 subdural hematoma and 1 infection. There were 2 deaths resulting from pulmonary emboli. In our experience transcallosal surgery is the preferred approach for a majority of lateral ventricular lesions.

Scalp Incision

An approach through corpus callosum requires access to the midline. This is obtained by extending the scalp incision across the midline so that the sagittal suture is easily visualized.

Skull Opening

The craniotomy should be extended to the midline so that the bone over the sagittal sinus does not obscure interhemispheric dissection. We prefer to place burr holes directly over the superior sagittal sinus. Alternatively, holes can be placed lateral to the sinus and the remaining bone removed with a ronguer.

Interhemispheric Dissection

Access to the corpus callosum (Figs. 19-10 and 19-11) requires preservation of medial draining veins.

The line of approach should avoid these veins as much as possible and still provide space for a 3-cm retractor blade. Arachnoid adhesions can become dense, particularly near the anterior cerebral arteries. When these adhesions obscure visualization, the operating microscope is necessary. The corpus callosum is identified by its relatively pale white color and the relative absence of subarachnoid vessels. A 1-cm or more incision can be obtained easily with gentle dissection through the fibers. A slight change in the angle of approach can result in opening the wrong lateral ventricle. This problem is easily corrected by identifying the septum pellucidum and redirecting the surgical angle.

Combined Approaches

Some lateral ventricular masses are too large to remove through a single operative approach and require the combination of transcortical and transcallosal exposure.[40] When the hemisphere is distended by tumor mass rather than by CSF, a transcortical incision and partial decompression may be needed to obtain sufficient relaxation to permit a safer interhemispheric dissection. In addition, portions of mass lesions with a broad ependymal attachment along the superior portion of the frontal horn may not be accessible from an interhemispheric approach.

Studies of patients that received corpus callosotomy for the treatment of epilepsy report a high fre-

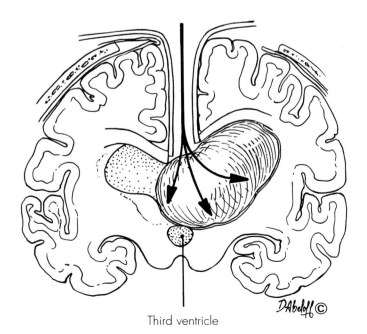

Third ventricle

Figure 19-10. Illustration of transcallosal approach to the lateral ventricular lesion. The superior portion of the mass should be delivered into the surgeon's line of view rather than retracting the hemisphere to expose it.

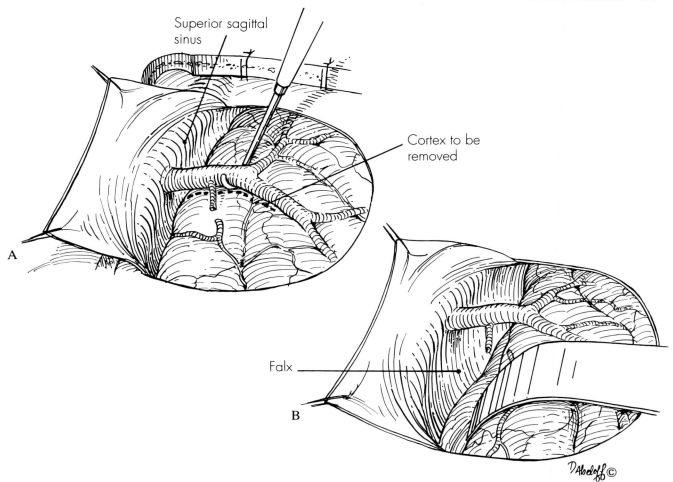

Figure 19-11. Illustration of techniques to preserve the medial veins draining into the superior sagittal sinus for interhemispheric dissection.

quency of neurological deficits in those who had evidence of a focal cortical lesion prior to surgery. Sass et al.[42,43] demonstrated that patients at risk for neurological deficits after callosotomy were those whose cortical lesions occurred during childhood, several years before cerebral disconnection. Certain early childhood injuries (e.g., illness, trauma) can cause the reorganization of cerebral function such that interhemispheric communication becomes more critical. In some cases of early childhood injury, both cerebral hemispheres contribute to speech or unilateral motor function. The disconnection of callosal pathways can disrupt speech and motor function. Combined lobectomy and callosotomy in adults did not appear to pose risks of neurological decline not implicitly inherent in either procedure alone.[43] Our evidence indicates that combined cortical incision and callosotomy can be performed safely in adults.[40] There are insufficient data to derive a conclusion regarding special risks for combined procedures in chil-

dren. Combined transcallosal and transcortical approaches were utilized in two patients in our series. Both patients tolerated this surgery well without sustaining any new permanent neurological deficits.

Scalp Incision

The use of combined approaches (Fig. 19-12) requires the exposure of a large area of the skull. This usually includes the exposure of the interhemispheric area as well as a transcortical avenue. As a rule, scalp incisions should cross the midline to access the corpus callosum and provide sufficient exposure for a transcortical approach in the same area. Combined approaches are most often used in the frontal area.

Skull Opening

The craniotomy encompasses the needs mentioned above for both the transcortical and transcallosal approaches.

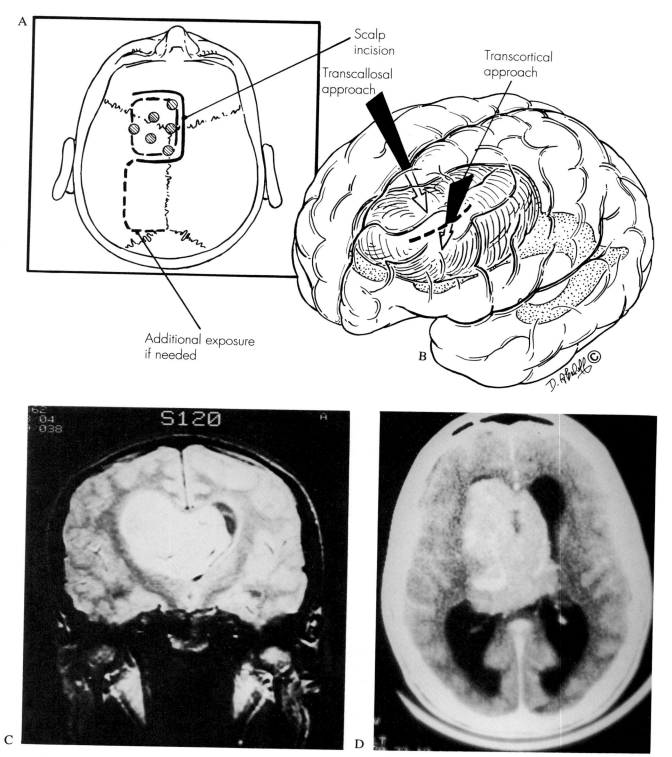

Figure 19-12. **(A)** Illustration of scalp incision and craniotomy for combined transcortical and transcallosal approach to a large ventricular mass. **(B)** Illustration of the surgeon's lines of view. **(C)** Coronal MRI and **(D)** axial CT images of a large tumor that required combined approaches for total removal.

Cortical Incision

The transcortical incision usually precedes the transcallosal approach to provide a decompression of a ventricle distended by tumor mass. This will permit a safer interhemispheric dissection with a relaxed hemisphere. The methods for performing these incisions are the same as those mentioned above.

PREVENTING COMPLICATIONS

The best method of avoiding postoperative complications is to anticipate the potential problems before they occur. This includes a careful assessment of the problems at each step and a surgical plan based on the potential for avoiding them. Rigid loyality to a particular operative technique will restrict the surgeon's ability to manage each patient in an optimal manner. The surgery should include sufficient flexibility in the operative exposure to permit alternative approaches and preparation for contingency plans when unforeseen problems arise.

Intraoperative Measures

Patient positioning on the operating table depends on the operative approach. The possibility of hemisphere collapse following the removal of large volumes of CSF virtually eliminates the use of the sitting position. However, gravity can be used to the surgeon's advantage, particularly during interhemispheric dissection by allowing the hemisphere to fall away from the falx.[48] Interhemispheric approaches to the corpus callosum can be facilitated by placing the patient in the lateral decubitus position with the involved hemisphere dependent. The falx can act as a retractor to hold the contralateral hemisphere out of the way while the involved hemisphere is gently retracted. Patient positioning should allow access for placement of a scalp incision and craniotomy that does not limit approach options. If an incision needs extension or if access to the opposite hemisphere is required, then provisions for these contingencies must be included.

The surgery for lateral ventricular lesions may require the patient to remain on the operating table for a prolonged period of time. Attention should be directed toward avoiding peripheral nerve compression such as the axilla (for the lateral decubitus position) or by tight restraining straps over the arms and legs. However, the patient must be securely fixed to the operating table preferably by a three-point pin head rest so that the table can be rotated to improve visu-

alization of the lesion. Elevation of the patient's head will improve venous drainage and help to control bleeding.

Placement of the bone flap is the next consideration. Careful review of the radiographs will help to place the bone flap and permit access to the preferred site for approach. In addition, access to the ventricle for insertion of a drainage catheter should be considered. If the catheter is left in position for gradual decompression of the ventricle, then its insertion should be away from the operative approach to decrease the risk of accidental removal. We prefer to extend the craniotomy to the midline for interhemispheric approaches. This procedure should be performed carefully to avoid injury to the superior sagittal sinus.

The next consideration is the site for cortical incision. The optimal corridor to the ventricles should not compromise neurological function through direct manipulation of eloquent cortical structures. Consequently, the shortest pathway to the lesion is not necessarily the best option. Some surgeons prefer to make incisions within the depths of a sulcus to limit cortical manipulation. While this technique is helpful for smaller subcortical lesions, the need to access large lesions deep in the brain may make this too confining. When an incision needs to be extended, the surgeon is obliged to follow the direction of the sulcus, which may limit exposure. The exposure should permit access to the lesion with the initial goal of interrupting the vascular supply to minimize blood loss. Since many of these lesions are over 7 cm in size and often extend into more than one region of the ventricle, the surgery requires patience to deliver the lesion into the field of view without excessive retraction. Constant attention to intraoperative bleeding will reduce the risk of loss of the plane of dissection between the mass and the ependymal surface. One of the most common causes of postoperative neurological deficits is excessive retraction to expose the mass or to stop bleeding. Ventricular distention from hydrocephalus and tumor mass will stretch the surrounding white matter tracts and reduce their resistance to injury from additional retraction. Immediate relaxation can be obtained by tapping the obstructed ventricle to remove spinal fluid. The fluid in an obstructed ventricle may contain a relatively high protein content, resulting in sluggish flow through a small-bore catheter.

Adequate brain relaxation is particularly important prior to interhemispheric dissection. Care should be taken to preserve adequate venous drainage into the superior sagittal sinus to avoid venous infarction.[40,45,48,50] Most often there are two or three large veins that serve the medial hemisphere, but there is no clear rule on which may be sacrificed. Our experience shows that the smallest anterior vein usually can be coagulated and transected if necessary. However, preoperative angiograms should be inspected to ensure that adequate venous outflow is preserved. These veins are most susceptible to avulsion at their insertion into the sinus. Injury at this site not only causes loss of the vein, but also opens the sinus. When necessary, stripping the vein from the cortical surface can reduce tension and allow greater access to the interhemispheric region.[49] Access to the corpus callosum and either lateral ventricle can be obtained on either the right or left side, and the decision

regarding placement of the craniotomy should, in part, be dictated by the anatomy of these medial veins[35,40,45] (see Fig. 19-7).

Deep lesions such as intraventricular masses require the use of the operating microscope. The advantages of improved illumination and magnification cannot be replaced by any other surgical technique. It is important to use the microscope at the appropriate time, since too early reliance can restrict the surgeon's field of view. Frequent orientation to the surrounding anatomy such as the thalamostriate vein, the septum pellucidum, and the foramen of Monro will prevent unwanted manipulation of inappropriately identified structures (Fig. 19-13). When bleed-

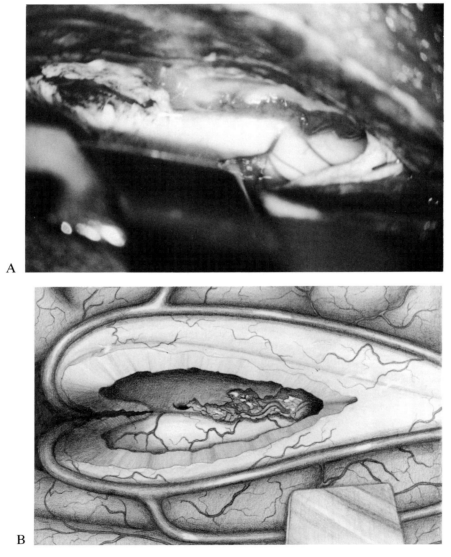

Figure 19-13. **(A)** Intraoperative photograph of a transcallosal exposure of the lateral ventricle. The choroid plexus can be seen entering the foramen of Monro. **(B)** Artist's drawing of an exposure similar to the one shown in Fig. A.

ing occurs during surgery is it helpful to protect the foramen of Monro with a cotton square to avoid obscuration of this structure and to prevent blood from pooling in the ventricles. After the lesion has been resected meticulous attention should be directed toward identifying and controlling any bleeding areas. Copious irrigation to remove residual blood that has collected in the ventricles will reduce the risk of postoperative ventricular obstruction and probably improved postoperative headache. When the foramen of Monro can not be cleared of obstruction a window can be opened in the septum pellucidum to untrap the ipsilateral ventricle.

Increased neurological deficits following surgical intervention commonly result from inadequate anticipation of the difficulty in removing a lesion from the lateral ventricles. Poor preparation can result in inadequate exposure, loss of control of intraoperative hemorrhage, and excessive retraction to access the mass. These problems can be minimized by resecting the exposed portion of the lesion and delivering the remainder of the mass into the field of vision. Early reports of lateral ventricular tumors that display the entire lesion as a gross pathological specimen clearly demonstrate why the surgery caused profound neurological deficits and high mortality.[5] When a mass lesion will not deliver into the operative field, alternative approaches can be used only if the surgeon is prepared.

Piecemeal resections will result in bleeding, and many times this can not be avoided.[41,48] The initial portions of tumor resection should be directed toward gaining access to the vascular supply in order to control blood loss as soon as possible. Significant blood loss should be anticipated for vascular lesions, and adequate blood replacement should be available to maintain stable vital signs. This is particularly important in infants, in whom a significant portion of the blood volume can be rapidly depleted. Exsanguination is a likely cause of the earlier reports of high mortality in infants with choroid plexus papillomas.[41,52]

The majority of ventricular mass lesions are benign or low-grade tumors, and complete removal can result in prolonged survival or cure. Consequently, total resection should be the goal of surgery. There are no specific indications for planning a subtotal resection. However, incomplete removal may be preferable when the site of attachment invades into deep structures such as the thalamus. When a subtotal resection is required, reduction in the size of the mass and removal of ventricular obstruction are important goals. Lesions with medial attachment may require the sacrifice of the ipsilateral fornix. Although the

literature concerning the dangers of fornix injury offers conflicting recommendations, a bilateral injury should be avoided.[16]

Once the lesion has been removed, additional attention to details will reduce the risk of postoperative problems. Removal of large ventricular masses and drainage of CSF can cause the hemispheres to collapse. Replacing air with warm irrigation fluid into the ventricle will reduce these problems. Incisions through the cortex or the corpus callosum should be covered with an absorbable hemostatic barrier such as Surgicel or Gelfoam to keep the fluid contained within the ventricles and to prevent subdural fluid collections. This material should not be allowed to fall into the ventricle and cause obstruction. These problems are presented in Table 19-3.

Postoperative Care

Many problems can complicate the care of a patient following the removal of a ventricular lesion. Elegant surgical procedures can be negated by inadequate monitoring and lack of anticipation of the potential issues that require continued observation. The initial postoperative management should be in an intensive care unit staffed by personnel trained to evaluate neurosurgical patients. When the patient awakens from anesthesia a careful neurological examination is required to establish a baseline for further evaluations. The level of consciousness is a critical part of this assessment. Any decline in neurological function or unexplained elevation in intracranial pressure should be aggressively investigated to determine a cause. These patients are at risk for hemorrhage, hydrocephalus, and subdural hematomas, particularly when a large lesion has been removed. It may be difficult to distinguish clinically between these problems, and imaging studies should be used liberally. The appropriate care of the patient depends on the findings from this testing.

The routine care of a postoperative patient includes the use of an intraventricular catheter, which will allow a method for monitoring intracranial pressure and serve as a warning that problems are developing. We obtain a CT scan after the first 24 hours to examine the surgical site and to evaluate for hemorrhage, ventricular size, and any residual tumor. This study is helpful for determining the anticipated postoperative course. Based on the findings from this study, the neurological examination, and the intracranial pressure, a decision can be made regarding mobilization out of bed and increasing the patient's activities. In the uncomplicated case the catheter is

Table 19-3.   Intraoperative Complications

Complication	Avoidance	Management
Cortical injury	Place bone flaps away from eloquent cortex. Precisely identify cortical anatomy. Preserve important draining veins. Limit cortical incisions to areas of safe access.	Replace retractors that compress the cortex. Reorient the approach to avoid cortical manipulation. Dissect veins from their pial attachment to reduce tension.
White matter injury	Minimize the forces from retractors. Avoid approaches that cross vital fiber tracts. Maintain control of bleeding. Deliver the lesion into the field of view.	Obtain additional relaxation of the hemisphere with osmotic diuretics, catheter drainage of CSF, and hyperventilation.
Excessive blood loss	Control bleeding. Approach lesions from the area of maximal blood supply.	Replace blood volume as needed to maintain an adequate blood volume and perfusion pressure.
Cerebral edema and brain swelling	Relax the hemisphere prior to deep dissection. Maintain adequate venous outflow through cortical veins and sinuses. Utilize preoperative steroids.	Administer intraoperative osmotic diuretics and reexamine arterial PCO_2. Elevate the patient's head. Examine for obstructions to venous outflow. Look for an intraoperative subdural hematoma.
Mortality	Select patients for surgery and operative approaches carefully. Anticipate the need for intraoperative blood replacement.	Control blood loss. Replace blood volume as needed. Avoid manipulating invasive lesions that extend into deep midline structures.

removed and the patient is mobilized on the third postoperative day. Patients who are restricted in their mobilization receive physical therapy in bed. They are treated with minidose subcutaneous heparin and antithromboembolic stockings. These measures are helpful but do not preclude the chances of pulmonary emboli.

Excessive drainage of CSF should be avoided since this may increase the risk of subdural formation before the brain has reexpanded. Management of a ventricular catheter requires that drainage be limited to small volumes to maintain an intracranial pressure between 10 and 15 mmHg. The patient's head should be maintained at 20 to 30 degrees elevation, and mobilization out of bed should proceed slowly until the intracranial pressure has stabilized. The goal is to maintain normal pressure without overdrainage or too low a pressure. Any operative procedure that enters the ventricular system creates the potential risk of CSF leakage.[12] This problem can be minimized by controlling elevated intracranial pressure caused by altered CSF absorption and circulation. The catheter requires careful attention to prevent infection and ventriculitis. The risk of contamination of the CSF increases with the length of time the catheter is in place and the number of times the catheter system is opened. Sterile technique for sampling of the spinal fluid including cell profile, glucose, protein, and culture can detect the signs of infection. Early intervention with antibiotic therapy and catheter removal or replacement are then needed.

Some postoperative problems can be anticipated based on prior experience with a surgical procedure. For example, patients will have a transient disconnection syndrome depending on the amount of the corpus callosum that is sectioned during transcallosal surgery.[40,43] The syndrome includes mutism, akinesia, apathy, unilateral weakness (leg more than arm), forced grasping, fixed gaze, disinhibition, incontinence, and right-left confusion. Varying amounts of this syndrome occur following major resections of the callosum, and the surgeon should be prepared to monitor them during the postoperative period.

Hydrocephalus is a common problem for patients with ventricular lesions, and ventricular enlargement frequently remains following resection of the mass.[40] It is unclear which patients would benefit from shunting and what part of the postoperative problems including speech, motor function, and cognitive abilities would improve faster by this intervention. Patients with persistent elevation in intracranial pressure and obstruction of CSF pathways are appropriate candidates for ventricular shunts. In addition, our experience suggests that enlarged ventricles and normal intracranial pressure may present a condition analogous to normal pressure hydrocephalus. We have seen significant improvement in cognitive and focal deficits in selected patients after shunting for this problem. While it is not possible to draw firm conclusions regarding the indications for shunting, it should be considered for patients with enlarged ven-

Table 19-4. Postoperative Complications

Complication	Avoidance	Management
Subdural hematoma	Mobilize the patient slowly. Avoid overdraining through the ventricular catheter.	Perform frequent imaging studies to detect extra-axial fluid collections. Keep head elevation to 20 degrees. Surgical drainage for symptomatic collections with mass effect.
Seizures	Use the transcallosal approach when possible. Minimize cortical manipulation.	Use anticonvulsant medication when necessary.
Hydrocephalus	Remove obstructing lesions at the foramen of Monro. Open the septum pellucidum. Irrigate blood from the ventricle.	Monitor intracranial pressure with a ventricular catheter. Follow ventricular size with imaging studies. Shunt patients for symptomatic persistent hydrocephalus.
Intracerebral hemorrhage	Pay meticulous attention to hemostasis. Gently irrigate away blood clots to make sure the bleeding has stopped.	Check the prothrombin time (PT), partial thromboplastin time (PTT) and platelet count, particularly if the patient has received many transfusions. Repeat imaging studies to determine the size and location of the hemorrhage. Surgically evacuate hemorrhage that has mass effect or is obstructing the ventricle.
Incomplete resection	Plan operative approaches to access the entire lesion. Maintain clear planes between the lesion and the ependyma. Frequently orient with surrounding anatomy to avoid missing some of the lesion.	Stage the operation when necessary or utilize an alternative approach.
Mortality	Carefully monitor the patient's neurological and hemodynamic status in an intensive care unit. Examine for deep venous thrombosis in patients restricted to bed rest.	Utilize the vascular catheter and imaging studies to determine a cause for neurological deterioration. Optimize cardiovascular function prior to removing monitoring devices.

tricles who do not achieve the anticipated recovery following intraventricular surgery.

The surgical management of lateral ventricular lesions has a relatively high risk for mortality and neurological morbidity. Complications can be minimized by anticipating potential problems at each step of surgery (Table 19-3). The importance of flexibility in surgery cannot be overstated. The surgeon should be prepared to redirect the approach to the lesion when needed. In selected cases this may require staging the resection in order to accomplish a total removal of the lesion. Careful attention to the small details such as patient positioning and craniotomy placement will reduce the risk of unintended injury. Following surgery close monitoring and rapid intervention to correct problems will improve the patient's chances of recovery (Table 19-4).

REFERENCES

1. Abbie AA: The clinical significance of the anterior choroidal artery. Brain 56:233, 1933
2. Afra D, Turoczy L, Deak G: Ependymomas extending into both lateral ventricles: CT-diagnosis and operability. Neurochirurgie 42:255, 1981
3. Bernasconi V, Cabrini GP: Radiological features of tumors of the lateral ventricles. Acta Neurochir 17:290, 1967
4. Bret P, Gharbi S, Cohadon F, Remond J: Les meningiomes du ventricule lateral. Neurochirurgie 35:5, 1989
5. Busch E: Meningiomas of the lateral ventricles of the brain. Acta Chir Scand 82:282, 1930
6. Collmann H, Kazner E, Sprung C: Supratentorial intraventricular tumors in childhood. Acta Neurochir (Suppl) 35:75, 1985
7. Eekhof JL, Thomeer RT, Bots GT: Epidermoid tumor in the lateral ventricle. Surg Neurol 23:189, 1985
8. Ehni G: Interhemispheric and pericallosal (transcallosal) approach to the cingulate gyri, intraventricular shunt tubes, and certain deeply placed brain lesions. Neurosurgery 14:99, 1984
9. Falk B: Radiologic diagnosis of intraventricular meningiomas. Acta Radiol 46:171, 1956
10. Fornari M, Savoiardo M, Morello G, Solero C: Meningiomas of the lateral ventricles. J Neurosurg 54:64, 1981
11. Fukushima T: Endoscopic biopsy of intraventricular tumors with the use of a ventriculofiberscope. Neurosurgery 2:110, 1978
12. Gassel MM, Davies H: Meningiomas in the lateral ventricles. Brain 84:605, 1961
13. Geffen G, Walsh A, Simpson D, Jeeves M: Comparison of the effects of transcortical and transcallosal re-

moval of intraventricular tumors. Brain 103:773, 1980

14. Goldstein MN, Joynt RJ, Hartley RB: The long-term effects of callosal sectioning. Arch Neurol 32:52, 1975

15. Hasuo K, Fukui M, Tamura S et al: Oligodendrogliomas of the lateral ventricle: computed tomography and angiography. J Comput Tomogr 11:376, 1987

16. Heilman KM, Sypert GW: Korsakoff's syndrome resulting from bilateral formix lesions. Neurology 27:490, 1977

17. Henderson VW, Friedman RB, Teng EL, Weiner JM: Left hemisphere pathways in reading. Neurology 35:962, 1985

18. Honda M, Kishikawa M, Nishimori I et al: Intraventricular neuroblastoma. A light and electron microscopic study and review of the literature. Pathol Res Pract 185:267, 1989

19. Ivan LP, Martin DJ, Mallya KB, Schneider E: Choroid plexus papilloma in a 4-month-old child: a case report. J Child Neurol 1:53, 1986

20. Jeeves MA, Simpson DA, Geffen G: Functional consequences in the transcallosal removal of intraventricular tumors. J Neurol Neurosurg Psychiatry 42:134, 1979

21. Jun CL, Nutic SL: Surgical approaches to intraventricular meningiomas of the trigone. Neurosurgery 16:416, 1985

22. Kamiya K, Inagawa T, Nagasako R: Malignant intraventricular meningioma with spinal metastasis through the cerebrospinal fluid. Surg Neurol 32:213, 1989

23. Kempe LG, Blaylock R: Lateral-trigonal intraventricular tumors. A new operative approach. Acta Neurochir 35:233, 1976

24. Kikuchi K, Kowada M, Mineura K, Uemura K: Primary oligodendroglioma of the lateral ventricle with computed tomographic and positron emission tomographic evaluations. Surg Neurol 23:483, 1985

25. Klein DM: Simultaneous subdural effusion and hydrocephalus in infancy. Surg Neurol 6:363, 1976

26. Kobayashi S, Okazaki H, MacCarty CS: Intraventricular meningiomas. Mayo Clin Proc 46:735, 1971

27. Ledoux JE, Risse GL, Springer SP et al: Cognition and commissurotomy. Brain 100:87, 1977

28. Lee KS, Kelly DL: Primary oligodendroglioma of the lateral ventricle. South Med J 83:254, 1990

29. Levin HS, Rose JE: Alexia without agraphia in a musician after transcallosal removal of a left intraventricular meningioma. Neurosurgery 4:168, 1979

30. Lobbato RD, Cabello A, Camena JJ et al: Subependymoma of the lateral ventricle. Surg Neurol 15:144, 1980

31. Mani RL, Hedgcock MW, Mass SI et al: Radiographic diagnosis of meningioma of the lateral ventricle. J Neurosurg 49:249, 1978

32. Marshall LF, Rorke LB, Schut L: Teratocarcinoma of the brain—a treatable disease? Childs Brain 5:96, 1979

33. Milhorat TH, Hammock MK, Davis DA, Fenster-

macher JD: Choroid plexus papilloma. Childs Brain 2:273, 1976

34. Nagib MG, Haines SJ, Erickson DL, Mastri AR: Tuberous sclerosis: a review for the neurosurgeon. Neurosurgery 14:93, 1984

35. Nehls DG, Marano SR, Spetzler RF: Transcallosal approach to the contralateral ventricle. J Neurosurg 62:304, 1985

36. Oepen S, Schultz-Wealing R, Zimmerman P et al: Long-term effects of callosal lesions. Acta Neurochirurg 77:22, 1985

37. Ogden JA: Dyslexia in a right-handed patient with a posterior lesion of the right cerebral hemisphere. Neuropsychologia 22:265, 1984

38. Ojemann GA: Individual variability in cortical localization of language. J Neurosurg 50:164, 1979

39. Pascual-Castroviejo I, Villarejo F, Perez-Higueras A et al: Childhood choroid plexus neoplasms. A study of 14 cases less than 2 years old. Eur J Pediatr 140:51, 1983

40. Piepmeier JM, Sass KJ: Surgical management of lateral ventricular tumors. p. 333. In Paoletti P, Takakura K, Walker M, Butti G, Pezzotta S (eds): Neuro-oncology. Kluver, Dordrecht, 1991

41. Raimondi AJ, Gutierrez FA: Diagnosis and surgical treatment of choroid plexus papillomas. Childs Brain 1:81, 1975

42. Sass KJ, Novelly RA, Spencer DD, Spencer SS: Postcallosotomy language impairments in patients with anomalous cerebral dominance. J Neurosurg 72:85, 1990

43. Sass KJ, Spencer SS, Westerveld M, Spencer DD: The neuropsychology of corpus callosum for epilepsy. p. 291. In Bennett TT (ed): The Neuropsychology of Epilepsy. Plenum, New York, 1992

44. Sass KJ, Westerveldt M, Novelly RA et al: Intracarotid amytal procedure findings predict postcallosotomy motor impairments in right hemisphere speech dominant epileptic patients, abstracted. Epilepsia 30:711, 1989

45. Shucart WA, Stein BA: Transcallosal approach to the anterior ventricular system. Neurosurgery 3:339, 1978

46. Silver AJ, Ganti SR, Hilal SK: Computed tomography of tumors involving the atria of the lateral ventricles. Radiology 145:71, 1982

47. Sima AA, Robertson DM: Subependymal giant-cell astrocytoma. J Neurosurg 50:240, 1979

48. Spencer DD, Collins WF, Sass KJ: Surgical management of lateral intraventricular tumors. p. 583. In Schmidek HH, Sweet W (eds): Operative Neurosurgical Techniques. Grune & Stratton, Orlando, FL, 1988

49. Sugita K, Kobayashi S, Yokoo A: Preservation of large bridging veins during brain retraction. J Neurosurg 57:856, 1982

50. Synek VM, Wilson JL, Macdonald GM, Synek BJ: Unusual scalp recorded somatosensory evoked potentials after removal of a large intraventricular meningioma. Clin Electroencephalogr 19:74, 1988

51. Tanaka Y, Sugita K, Kobayashi S et al: Subdural fluid collections following transcortical approach to intra- or paraventricular tumors. Acta Neurochir 99:20, 1989

52. de la Torre E, Alexander E, Davis C, Crandell DL: Tumors of the lateral ventricles of the brain. J Neurosurg 20:461, 1963

53. Townsend JJ, Seaman JP: Central neurocytoma—a rare benign intraventricular tumor. Acta Neuropathol 71:167, 1986

54. Turcotte JF, Copty M, Bedard F et al: Lateral ventricle choroid plexus papilloma and communicating hydrocephalus. Surg Neurol 13:143, 1980

55. Vaquero J, Cabezudo J, Leunda G et al: Primary carcinoma of the choroid plexus with metastatic dissemination within the central nervous system. Acta Neurochir 51:105, 1979

56. Wang AM, Power TC, Rumbaugh CL: Lateral ventricular meningioma. Comput Radiol 9:355, 1985

20 Cavernous Sinus Masses

Vinko V. Dolenc

The location of the cavernous sinus (CS), its internal anatomy, and its relation to the surrounding structures allow for numerous possible complications in surgical procedures for tumor and vascular pathology in this region. Complications related to surgery in and around the CS may be roughly divided into several categories: damage to the bony sinuses, cranial nerves, blood vessels, and brain. Other general complications may occur, such as postoperative hemorrhage, infections, embolism, etc.

In order to avoid opening the bony sinuses anteriorly and the middle and/or inner ear in the region of the pyramid, a thorough and detailed study of all available images is required, from skull x-ray films and computed tomography (CT) scans to magnetic resonance imaging (MRI). In the bony structures surrounding the CS, attention should be paid to the variations and changes, such as osteolysis, hyperostosis, calcifications, and ossifications, resulting from pathological processes in the CS. Prior to each operation in the CS, whether for vascular or tumor pathology, an angiographic study of the position and form of the internal carotid artery (ICA) throughout its entire course from the entry to the carotid canal in the petrous bone to the ophthalmic artery is required, as well as cross-flow studies. Last, but no less important, are the type, shape, size, and location of the lesion within or adjacent to the CS, and the relationship of this lesion to the bony structures, blood vessels, cranial nerves, and brain itself. An exact estimate of normal and pathological anatomy in a given case dictates the strategy of approach, the extent of exploration, and protective measures required in surgery of the CS.

POSITIONING OF THE PATIENT

The initial positioning of the patient on the operating table for surgery in and/or around the CS is in principle the same as that required for the pterional approach.[1] The patient lies supine with the head fixed in the Mayfield headrest and rotated 35 degrees in the opposite direction to the lesion. The head must lie along the axis of the body so that on rotation of the head to the side contralateral to the CS lesion the veins in the neck are not stretched on the side of the lesion and compressed on the contralateral side. The head must be deflected so that the orbitozygomatic junction on the side of the pathology is the highest point of the head (Fig. 20-1).

Since the entire operating table needs to be readjusted in the course of the operation to the Trendelenburg and anti-Trendelenburg positions, and also rotated to the left and to the right, it is necessary that the patient be fastened to the table preoperatively with one wide belt across the chest and another of similar width across the hips and pelvis. Only in this manner will the head and body move together during intraoperative repositioning of the table, thus avoiding additional stretching or compression of the veins in the neck.

CRANIOTOMY AND COMPLETE EPIDURAL EXPOSURE

The skin incision differs slightly from the pterional incision and extends in a semicircular line from the junction of the scalp and the forehead in the midline downward to in front of the tragus of the ear (Fig.

20-1). The concavity of the incision faces anteriorly. The skin flap, together with its subcutaneous tissue, is then peeled away from the fascia of the temporalis muscle and reflected anteriorly across the eye. The skin flap must be lifted as far as the orbital rim.[1-3] When this is not possible, it is necessary to continue the skin incision in the opposite direction beyond the midline, but on the scalp. This gives a more favorable working angle for exposure of the orbital rim. The temporal end of the skin flap should be made far enough dorsally at the tragus, so that the area dorsal to the superficial temporal and of course dorsal to the frontal branch of the facial nerve is reached.[18]

The muscle is incised immediately at its insertion, commencing behind the orbitozygomatic junction and extending in a dorsal direction to the posterior

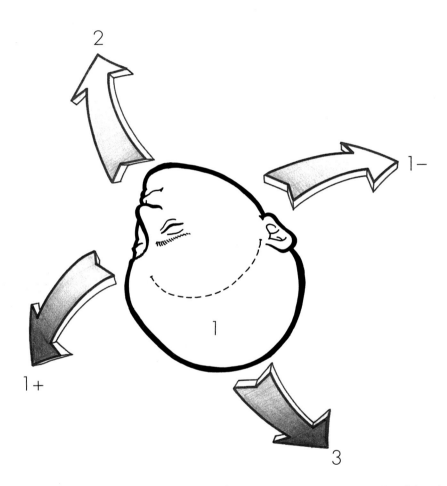

Figure 20-1. The initial position of the patient's head is indicated by the number 1. By tilting the table in the direction of the anti-Trendelenburg position ("head-up," indicated by the number 2), the lateral regions of the cavernous sinus in the middle cranial fossa can be more clearly seen. By tilting the table in the direction of the Trendelenburg position ("head-down," indicated by the number 3), the structures along the edge of the tentorium and along the medial edge of the CS can be visualized. With each degree of tilting of the table, the table must also be rotated to the left or to the right to allow better visualization of the region of the sella (position 1+), or of the pyramid (position 1−). By suitably positioning the head and the entire table, it is possible to reach each region of the CS with minimal or no retraction of the brain. The intraoperative repositioning of the table calls for small adjustments to the position of the microscope, thereby enabling the neurosurgeon to avoid awkward postures. Good mobility of the operating table thus not only protects the patient's brain but also relieves strain on the doctor's neck.

part of the temporalis muscle.[3] The other arm of the incision of the muscle runs in a downward direction parallel to the muscle fibers (i.e., caudally toward the ear). The temporalis muscle is then peeled off from the squama of the temporal bone, reflected laterally, and fixed with fish hooks. The periosteum is incised from the orbitozygomatic junction in a semicircle across the frontal bone and then in a dorsal direction and again in a lateral direction.[3] The frontal bone is thereby stripped of periosteum, but the insertion of the temporalis muscle is left intact. The first burr hole is made behind the orbitozygomatic junction, in an anteromedial direction, thus at the same time cutting into the orbit and the intracranial space.[3] Two additional burr holes are made, one temporobasally and the other frontodorsally. The bone flap is then excised. Using a craniotome, the bone is first cut frontally 2 to 3 mm behind the orbital rim. When it is not possible to cut from the burr hole behind the orbitozygomatic junction to the burr hole frontodorsally with the craniotome, the cut is stopped just above the orbit medially and commenced from the opposite side. Usually there is no difficulty in connecting the two dorsal burr holes. The next bone cut extends anteriorly from the burr hole, which is located temporobasally, toward the sphenoid wing. The sphenoid wing is resected, and the bone flap is elevated in its entirety and removed for the duration of the operative procedure.[3] During craniotomy it is possible to damage the periorbita, as well as the dura at any site around the bone cut, and, when the frontal sinus is larger than normal, there is a risk of opening the sinus in the bone frontally, behind the orbital rim (Fig. 20-2). In such cases watertight closure of the frontal sinus is essential at the conclusion of the operation. If the dura has been damaged, which often occurs in elderly patients in whom the dura is firmly adherent to the bone, watertight reconstruction is also necessary. Damage to the periorbita, with resultant bulging of fatty tissue, is treated by bipolar coagulation, resulting in retraction of the fatty tissue.

In the majority of cases the temporal bone cannot be adequately resected basally using the craniotome only, and therefore the temporal bone is additionally trimmed in the basal direction, using a rongeur. The dura is carefully peeled off the bone. Care should be taken not to damage the temporalis muscle, which must also be removed from the bone. Then follows additional trimming of the bone in a direction toward the base, with complete hemostasis being carried out on the dura and in the muscle using bipolar coagulation, and on the bone edges using bone wax.

The next step is the peeling of the dura from the orbit anterior and posterior to the sphenoid wing. Similarly, the periosteum is carefully peeled off from the inner surface of the orbit.

Subsequently, the orbital roof both anterior and posterior to the sphenoid wing is trimmed using a small rongeur. Dorsally the bone is removed as far as the foramen rotundum thus freeing the superior orbital fissure (SOF) in its entirety from the dorsal aspect. On the anterior aspect of the SOF, removal of the sphenoid wing is continued toward the anterior clinoid process (ACP) and still more medially to the optic canal. The procedure to this point can be carried out with the naked eye, although magnification is preferred. However, removal of the ACP and opening of the optic canal must be performed under magnification. Before commencing the opening of the optic canal and removal of the ACP it is necessary to examine the edges of the bone in the area from which the orbital roof was removed, due to the possibility of damaging the frontal sinus during removal of the bone medially and anteriorly. The bone edges should also be meticulously inspected for possible minor bleeding from the bone.

The ACP must never be removed in one piece; it must first be hollowed out with a high-speed diamond drill and only then can the thinned walls facing the SOF, optic nerve, and ICA be cut off and removed (Fig. 20-3). The separation of the dura from the ACP must be performed very carefully so as to avoid damage to the third cranial nerve on its lateral aspect, the ICA on its anterior and inferior aspects, or the optic nerve medially. Care must also be taken when drilling the ACP and even more so when drilling the lateral and dorsal walls of the optic canal, to avoid generating excessive heat, which would damage the optic nerve and the third cranial nerve. The drill is only rotated a few times, followed by a pause, and the drill tip must be constantly irrigated with saline. The optic canal is opened along its entire length on its lateral and dorsal aspects, while on its medial aspect great care must again be taken not to open the bony sinus. In the majority of cases this is the sphenoid sinus, but in some cases these are the dorsolateral ethmoid cells of a markedly enlarged ethmoid sinus. More often than on the medial aspect of the optic nerve, the sphenoid sinus is opened in the corner between the optic nerve and the anterior loop of the ICA, during removal of the optic strut between the ICA and the optic nerve. It is not necessary to emphasize that any accidental opening of the sinus must be closed in a watertight fashion.

If the ACP has been carefully removed in the manner described the wall of the CS should be preserved

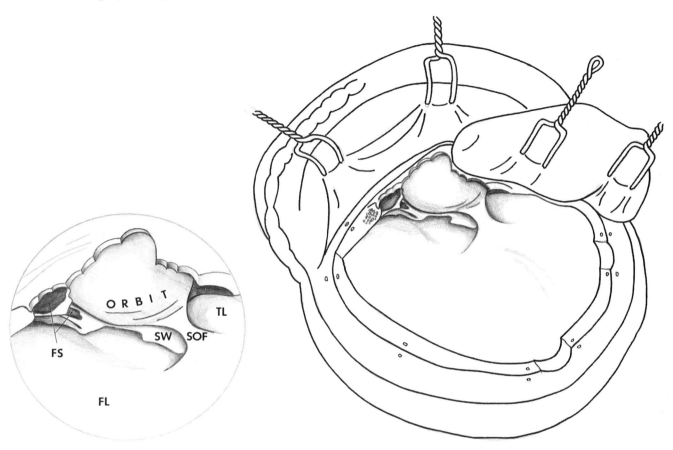

Figure 20-2. The roof of the orbit is removed on its anterior and dorsal aspects. The superior orbital fissure (*SOF*) is freed. Due to rotation of the head, the SOF is in the vertical direction. Posterior to the SOF lies the temporal lobe (*TL*), and medial to the SOF lies the sphenoid wing (*SW*). The dura over the frontal lobe (*FL*) is gently separated from the anterior and superior parts of the roof of the orbit. In the medial corner of the exposed orbital roof an enlarged frontal sinus (*FS*) can easily be entered, and for this reason, the extreme medial part of the cut of the orbital roof should be carefully checked, and, if the FS is opened, the holes should be sealed to prevent CSF leak.

undamaged in over 90 percent of cases, and hence no bleeding from the CS should occur (Fig. 20-4). Only when the tip of the ACP protrudes into the CS will a minor, insignificant venous bleeding occur upon removal of the tip of the ACP. The bleeding is controlled by inserting a small piece of Surgicel into the hole. Under no circumstances must one attempt to stop this bleeding by coagulation, nor any bleeding from the dura covering the third cranial nerve, or from the dura propria covering the optic nerve. Coagulation at these sites may damage the nerve(s). It is therefore preferable to achieve hemostasis using only Surgicel.

In the next phase, the operating table, together with the patient, is moved to the so-called anti-Trendelenburg position (i.e., the "head-up" position). In this manner a better view of the base of the middle cranial fossa is obtained (Fig. 20-1). The dura is then peeled from the temporal bone as far as the base, exposing the foramen rotundum, foramen spinosum, and foramen ovale (Fig. 20-5). The wall around the foramen rotundum is removed, thus exposing nerve V$_2$ in the canal (Fig. 20-5). The middle meningeal artery is cut after being coagulated immediately in front of the foramen spinosum, and the proximal stump is then pushed into the canal and sealed first

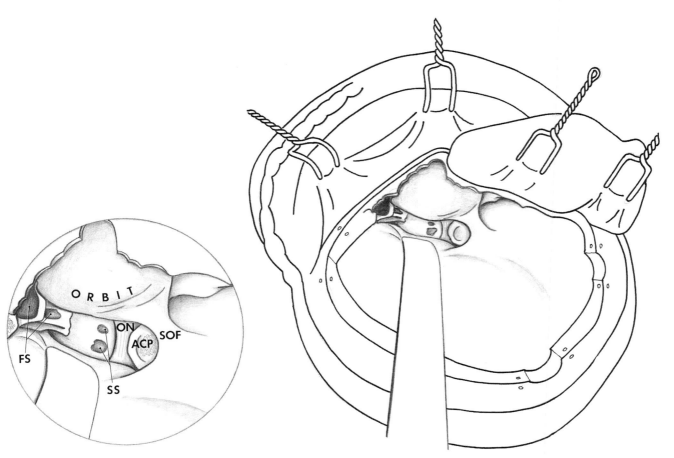

Figure 20-3. After the removal of the bone [the roof of the orbit posterolateral to the superior orbital fissure (*SOF*)], the last part of the sphenoid wing is removed. Once the peripheral end of the optic canal with the optic nerve (*ON*) is reached, it is of paramount importance not to continue trimming the bone using a rongeur. The last piece of the sphenoid wing should be hollowed out with a high-speed diamond drill, which should also be used to remove the lateral, dorsal, and medial walls of the optic canal. On the medial aspect of the ON, the sphenoid sinus (*SS*) may be entered. If so, it should be sealed watertightly. During drilling of the anterior clinoid process (*ACP*) and the walls of the optic canal, continuous irrigation with saline is mandatory.

with Surgicel and then with bone wax (Fig. 20-6). Thus it is possible for the dura to be further peeled away from the bone enabling clear exposure of the foramen ovale and the bony wall between the foramen ovale and foramen spinosum. The dura is then peeled from the anterior aspect of the pyramid, dorsal to nerve V_3 and the geniculate ganglion. Here special care must be given to the greater petrosal nerve, which must never be stretched, but must be sharply cut, in order to avoid damaging the geniculate ganglion with resultant loss of function of the facial nerve.[3] Once the dura has been removed from

the anterior aspect of the petrous bone posterior to nerve V_3 and the geniculate ganglion, these two structures are pushed even more anteriorly and the carotid canal in Glasscock's triangle is opened.[4] Here again great care must be taken not to damage the ICA or the eustachian tube when drilling the bone, since in 25 percent of patients the ICA is covered only by a thin bony layer or the bone is missing. To avoid such damage, drilling of the bone begins approximately 5 to 8 mm medial to the foramen spinosum, just behind nerve V_3. In no circumstances should drilling extend to the arcuate eminence posteriorly. If drilling is car-

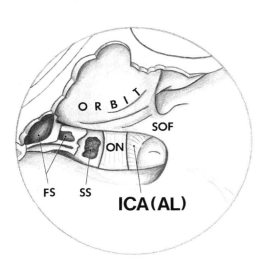

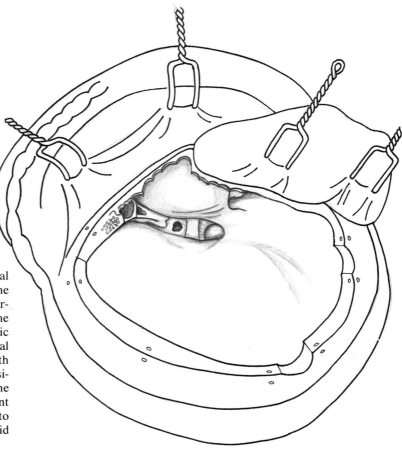

Figure 20-4. After complete removal of the orbital roof around the superior orbital fissure (*SOF*) and the anterior clinoid process (*ACP*), the internal carotid artery (*ICA*) is exposed at its anterior loop (*AL*). The optic nerve (*ON*) is exposed after removal of the optic strut on the lateral side and the wall of the optic canal posteriorly and medially. The ON is still covered with dura propria. On the medial aspect of the ON a possible hole in the sphenoid sinus (*SS*) and holes in the frontal sinus (*FS*) are indicated. It is of paramount importance to carry out careful drilling of the bone to avoid entering the bony sinuses and hence to avoid CSF leak.

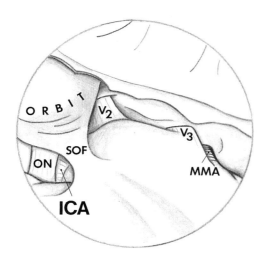

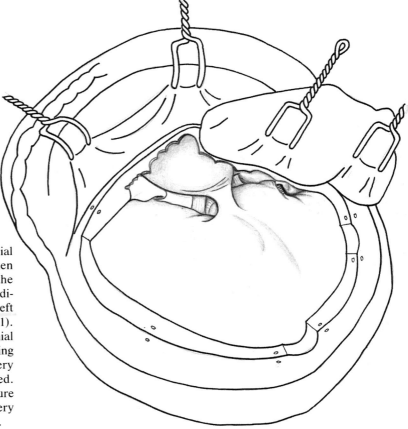

Figure 20-5. To reach the base of the middle cranial fossa and to visualize the foramen rotundum, foramen ovale, and foramen spinosum, it is necessary to tilt the table toward position 2 (in an anti-Trendelenburg direction—"head-up") and to rotate the table to the left (i.e., to reach position 2+, as indicated in Fig. 20-1). The epidural structures in the right middle cranial fossa, V₂ entering the foramen rotundum, V₃ entering the foramen ovale, and middle meningeal artery (*MMA*) entering the foramen spinosum are exposed. On the medial aspect, the superior orbital fissure (*SOF*), optic nerve (*ON*), and internal carotid artery (*ICA*) are seen. The dura has not yet been opened.

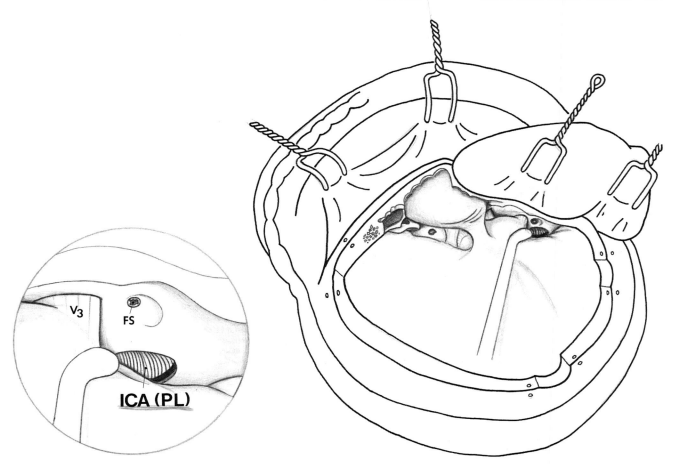

Figure 20-6. To achieve good visualization of the foramen spinosum and the anterior aspect of the petrous bone, it is necessary to tilt the table in the anti-Trendelenburg direction ("head-up") and then to rotate it to the left so that position 2+ is reached (Fig. 20-1). After cutting the middle meningeal artery (MMA), its proximal stump is coagulated and pushed into the foramen spinosum (*FS*), which is filled with Surgicel and bone wax. Behind V_3 entering into the foramen ovale, the dura is peeled off from the anterior aspect of the petrous bone and the carotid canal is opened using a high-speed diamond drill. In this manner, the posterior loop of the internal carotid artery (*ICA PL*) is visualized. Attention should be paid to the surrounding structures covered by bone lateral to the carotid canal (the eustachian tube) and posterior to the carotid canal (the inner ear).

ried out too dorsally, the inner ear will be reached, whereas if it is carried out too laterally, the tensor tympani muscle and the eustachian tube will be damaged. A mistake of the former kind will result in at least deafness and problems with balance while a mistake of the latter kind will lead to hearing problems and most probably also to cerebrospinal fluid (CSF) leak. After opening the carotid canal and exposing the ICA, the artery is dissected off from the inner side of the carotid canal in its entire circumference. As much of the bone as necessary is removed along and around the artery to enable placement of at least two temporary clips on the artery, or, when

necessary, anastomosis of the artery with the vein graft either end to side or end to end.

The epidural phase described, or the "general approach," is recommended in all cases in which it is anticipated that it will be necessary to open the entire CS, or when the ICA would hinder exploration of the CS. Complete exploration, as described above, is recommended if the surgeon has not sufficient experience in CS surgery, since if damage to the ICA occurs, and the ICA in the petrous bone has not been dissected free, and if it is not possible to place temporary clips proximally and distally, hemorrhage from the ICA is extremely difficult to control.

OPENING THE DURA

The dura is not opened until complete hemostasis has been achieved. The dura is incised in the shape of a letter Y, the incision beginning about 2 cm lateral to the lateral tip of the SOF and extending along the sylvian fissure to the lateral tip of the SOF.[3] The medial arm of the incision is continued medially along the SOF as far as the site of the base of the ACP, which has been removed. The incision then turns in an extreme medial direction and the dura is incised across the ICA and the optic nerve. The lateral arm runs from the lateral tip of the SOF around the CS in such a manner that about 2 to 3 mm of the dura is left around the sinus, and the incision is continued to the geniculate ganglion. The incision so shaped affords optimum protection of the brain when retraction is necessary, as the cortex is thus covered by dura during the operation, enabling better protection of the brain than any synthetic material. Such an incision of the dura also allows watertight closure after removal of the lesion from the CS. During incision of the dura, the incision on the medial side of the SOF can mistakenly be made right at the SOF, resulting in difficulties during closure due to the dura having been cut too closely to cranial nerves III, IV, and VI. It is not necessary to stress that incision of the dura over the ICA and optic nerve should be very carefully carried out so as to avoid damage to the ICA or optic nerve, particularly when the lesion (i.e., an aneurysm or a tumor) lies between or under the ICA and the optic nerve. When opening the dura laterally around the outer edge of the CS and around the temporal lobe, venous bleeding may sometimes present difficulties when there is rich drainage from the sylvian region in the direction of the CS. The possibility of such a complication must be anticipated so that any unnecessary blood loss can be avoided. When it is necessary to explore the entire CS, there is no other option apart from cutting these veins. However, when it is necessary to open only the medial part of the CS in the so-called anteromedial and paramedial triangles[3] (i.e., in the majority of pituitary tumors that only partly occupy the CS, in all carotid-ophthalmic aneurysms, and in smaller aneurysms in the region of the anterior loop of the ICA), the veins can be preserved by only cutting the dura medial to them and fixing it with stay sutures superiorly and laterally.

SPLITTING OF THE SYLVIAN FISSURE

In his book *Microneurosurgery,*[17] Yasargil states that the pterional approach is "useful for aneurysms of the anterior circulation and upper basilar artery, as well as for tumors of the orbital, retro-orbital, sellar, parasellar, chiasmatic, subfrontal, retroclival and prepontine areas." This statement holds true on condition that the sylvian fissure is split. Apart from petroclival tumors (meningiomas) and others (fifth nerve neurinomas), which may only partially invade the dorsal part of the CS (the inferolateral and dorsal parts of Parkinson's triangle),[3] all other vascular and tumorous lesions in the CS are so located that complete splitting of the sylvian fissure is required in order to provide good access. Splitting of the sylvian fissure is imperative in order to gain as much space as necessary without retraction of the frontal and temporal lobes, while at the same time allowing exposure of the entire intrathecal segment of the ICA, the entire segment of the middle cerebral artery (MCA) with all its branches, the anterior cerebral artery (ACA₁), the anterior communicating artery (ACoA), and the initial segments of the ACA₂, as well as the ACA₁ and ICA contralaterally (Fig. 20-7). Both optic nerves, chiasm, and the ipsilateral optic tract can also be seen. Also exposed are the pituitary stalk, diaphragm sellae, ipsilateral posterior clinoid process (PCP), dorsum sellae, and even contralateral PCP. Lateral to the ICA, complete splitting of the fissure provides good visualization of the third and even fourth cranial nerves, the tentorial edge and posterior communicating artery (PCA₁), the initial segment of the PCA₂, the superior cerebellar artery, the bifurcation of the basilar artery, and its upper segment, as well as the initial segments of the PCA₁ and superior cerebellar artery and the third cranial nerve contralaterally. In certain lesions, which do not necessarily occupy the whole CS but are located only in its anteromedial part, or even in the immediate vicinity of the CS, the above-mentioned structures are displaced, stretched, and/or encompassed by the lesion (large or giant carotid-ophthalmic aneurysms, pituitary tumors extending into the CS, with suprasellar and retrosellar extension, craniopharyngiomas, and meningiomas). By complete splitting of the sylvian fissure and simultaneous gentle retraction of the temporal lobe, it is possible to determine exactly the lateral expansion of the lesion, while its medial expansion can be determined by gentle retraction of the laterobasal region of the frontal lobe. Due to frequent overlapping of the frontal and temporal lobes it is risky and frequently impossible to split the sylvian fissure from the ICA along the MCA in a peripheral direction. It is much simpler and safer to split the sylvian fissure in the opposite direction (i.e., from the periphery toward the center). In this manner in the peripheral part of the sylvian fissure, where the veins are seen in the subarachnoid space, one of the cortical arteries is identified and followed into the depths. The frontal and temporal lobes are gently separated

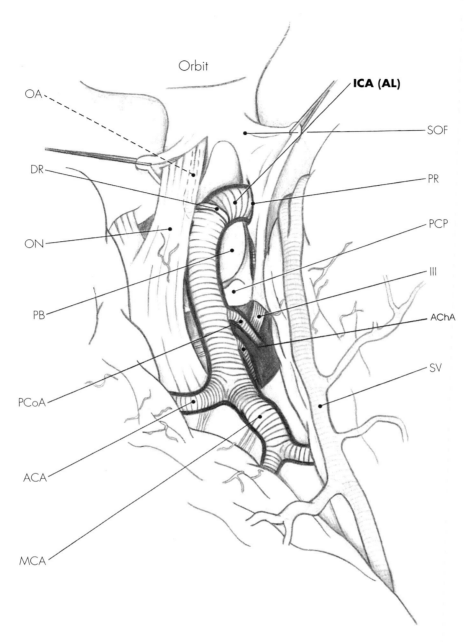

Figure 20-7. The sylvian fissure is split. The sylvian vein (*SV*) is preserved. The middle cerebral artery (*MCA*), anterior cerebral artery (*ACA*), and internal carotid artery (*ICA*), including its anterior loop (*AL*), ophthalmic artery (*OA*), posterior communicating artery (*PCoA*), and anterior choroidal artery (*AChA*) are visualized. The dural ring (*DR*) proximal to the ophthalmic artery is cut around the ICA, and the pituitary body (*PB*) and the proximal ring (*PR*) are visualized. Both optic nerves (*ON*s), chiasm, and right optic tract are visualized. On the lateral aspect of the posterior clinoid process (*PCP*), the third cranial nerve is visualized at its entry point into the wall of the CS. Wide and complete splitting of the sylvian fissure gives a good approach to the space between the ICA and chiasm, and to the lateral aspect of the ICA and PCoA and AChA toward the tentorial edge, exposing the third nerve, tentorial edge, and even the entry point of the fourth cranial nerve. To visualize all these structures it is necessary to retract very gently and lift the temporal lobe. Good access is also possible to the sella on both sides of the ICA, medially and laterally to it. Only complete splitting of the sylvian fissure, together with the removal of the anterior clinoid process and the cutting of the dural ring around the ICA, allow complete resection of the lesion in the sella, anteromedial part of the CS, retrosellar and suprasellar areas, and on the upper clivus, for which the removal of the dorsum sellae and PCP is also required. *N.B.:* It goes without saying that without removal of the ACP and complete cutting of the dural ring around and around the ICA, it is impossible to reach the floor of the sella.

using bipolar forceps and small pieces of cotton swabs are inserted into the cavity. The branches of the MCA are thus followed as far as the bifurcation of the MCA. Upon reaching the MCA trunk, the frontal and temporal lobes can easily be separated proceeding from the inside outward. The arachnoidea on the surface of the sylvian fissure and the fibrous tracts running across the MCA and its branches must be sharply cut. Splitting the sylvian fissure should be performed in such a manner so as to avoid any damage to the surface of the brain by laceration of the pia and to preserve all the cortical veins and arteries.

DISSECTION OF CRANIAL NERVES III TO VI AND THE ICA

Slight retraction of the temporal lobe in a lateral direction exposes the tentorial edge, the entry point of the third cranial nerve into the wall of the CS, and the entry point of the fourth cranial nerve under the tentorial edge into the lateral wall of the CS (Fig. 20-8). Both nerves can easily be traced in their course through the wall of the CS, dissected, and separated from the fibrous canal in such a manner that only the external layer of the canal is cut, the internal layer remaining intact. During dissection of the third and fourth nerves great care must be taken in the region of the SOF, where not only are these two nerves adjacent to one another but the fourth nerve even runs over the third nerve (Fig. 20-9). Dissection allows both nerves to be retracted in a medial or lateral direction (Fig. 20-10). Thus the CS can be entered in one of three ways, either through the anteromedial triangle, through the paramedial triangle, or through Parkinson's triangle.[3] These approaches allow exploration of the anterior loop of the ICA, the horizontal segment of the ICA, and even the medial loop of the ICA, as well as the whole area medial to these structures, after which the meningohypophyseal trunk is easily reached. It is not necessary to emphasize that during the removal of the tumorous or vascular lesion from the region around the anterior and medial loops, as well as from around the horizontal segment of the

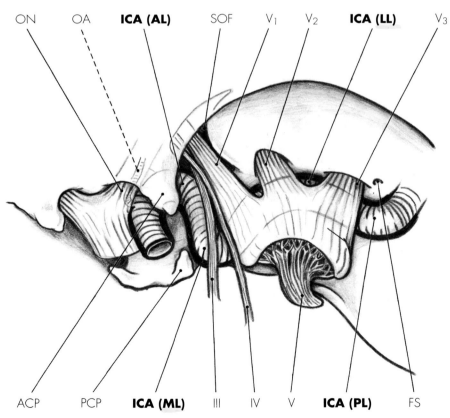

Figure 20-8. Schematic relation of the nerves [optic nerve (*ON*), oculomotor, trochlear, and trigeminal nerves] and the internal carotid artery (*ICA*) in its entire course from the carotid canal in the petrous bone to the intrathecal part, with all four loops—anterior (*AL*), medial (*ML*), lateral (*LL*), and posterior (*PL*)—together with adjacent bony structures.

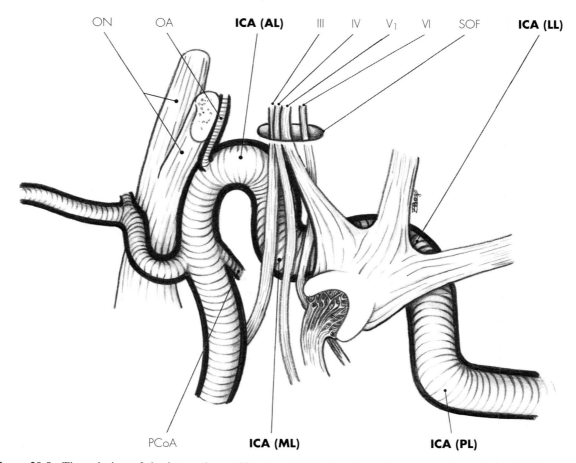

ON OA **ICA (AL)** III IV V₁ VI SOF **ICA (LL)**

PCoA **ICA (ML)** **ICA (PL)**

Figure 20-9. The relation of the internal carotid artery (*ICA*) along its entire course through the skull base from the petrous bone into the intradural space to cranial nerves III through VI running through the cavernous sinus (*CS*) or its lateral wall. All four loops of the ICA—anterior (*AL*), medial (*ML*), lateral (*LL*), and posterior (*PL*)—are visualized. The relationship of the optic nerve (*ON*) to the ophthalmic artery (*OA*) is presented. The entry points of cranial nerves II through VI as well as the exit points of these nerves are fixed and cannot be displaced or significantly changed by vascular or tumorous pathology of the CS. The cranial nerves therefore can be dissected from their entry to their exit points and then mobilized to either side (medially or laterally). In this manner, the triangle-shaped "windows" can be easily enlarged and/or shifted in a medial or lateral direction. Entering through these "windows" into the CS, the lesion can be removed and the nerves and the ICA dissected free.

ICA, and medial to these structures, it is of great advantage that the ICA in the carotid canal be dissected free so that temporary clips can be promptly placed, thus occluding flow through the ICA in the CS in the event of any unforeseen damage to the artery.

When the lesion is situated in the CS lateral to the horizontal segment of the ICA and dorsal to the segment of the ICA extending from the lateral to the medial loop, complete transsection of the tentorium must be performed posterior to the entry point of the fourth cranial nerve into the lateral wall of the CS. If the decision is made to cut the tentorium from its lateral aspect, the temporal lobe must be retracted in a medial and upward direction, which of course means that the brain must be retracted using considerable force. On the other hand, it is much easier to retract the temporal lobe gently in a lateral direction and lift it slightly from the lateral wall of the CS, thereby exposing the tentorial edge posterior to the entry point of the fourth cranial nerve. Transsection of the tentorium is then commenced perpendicular to the tentorial edge and proceeds toward the pyramid, across the fifth cranial nerve. On reaching the pyramid, behind the geniculate ganglion, the spatula is moved from the medial to the lateral side of the tem-

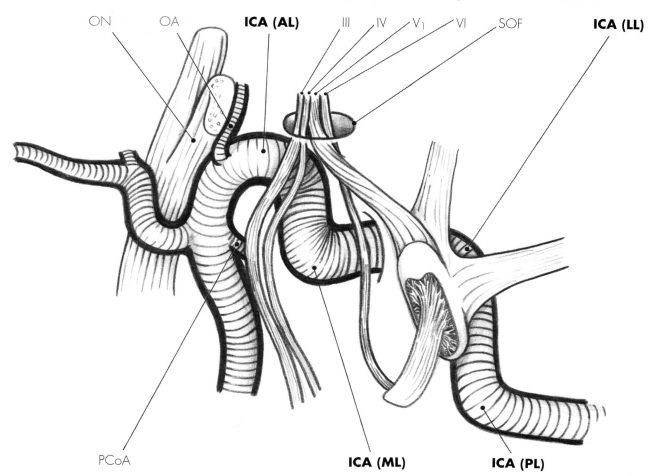

Figure 20-10. The central portion of the cavernous sinus (*CS*) with the medial loop of the internal carotid artery (*ICA*) can be reached via Parkinson's triangle by lifting and retracting the V_1 and geniculate ganglion (*GG*) laterally and dorsally, thus exposing the sixth nerve in its entire course from Dorello's canal to the superior orbital fissure (*SOF*). By retracting the third and fourth nerves medially, the medial aspect of the medial loop (*ML*) of the ICA as well as the segment of the ICA from is medial loop to its anterior loop (*AL*) can be well visualized. By rotating the operating table, all corners of the CS can be checked, and the lesion can be removed from the lateral ring of the ICA in the lateral corner of the CS, from Dorello's canal in the inferior corner of the CS, and then along the petroclinoid ligament to as far as the region of the sella and even from the sella itself.

poral lobe. With slight retraction on the lateral aspect, the margin of the tentorial cut can be ascertained. Hemostasis is then performed in the area of the upper petrous sinus, after which an additional dural incision is made near the geniculate ganglion and nerve V_3, and across the lateral triangle toward nerve V_2. This allows removal of the lateral wall (i.e., its external dural layer) by peeling it off from the geniculate ganglion, V_3, V_2, V_1, and the fourth cranial nerve, and from the tumor in the CS without forceful retraction of the temporal lobe. If the lesion has also invaded the posterior cranial fossa, the apex of the pyramid is drilled off.[5,6] In this manner the petroclinoid ligament is reached and, being in a more lateral location, retraction of the temporal lobe is not

necessary. Upon removal of the apex of the pyramid and exposure of the petroclinoid ligament, Dorello's canal is reached and the sixth cranial nerve is identified beneath the petroclinoid ligament, and then traced in a peripheral direction, proceeding from the dorsal aspect beneath the geniculate ganglion.[7,15,16] The geniculate ganglion and the fifth cranial nerve, together with the first branch of the trigeminal nerve, are then retracted dorsolaterally and the fifth nerve is followed across the ascending segment of the ICA from its lateral to its medial loop, and then further anteriorly along its horizontal segment from its medial to its anterior loop under V_1, and medial to the sixth cranial nerve.

The nature of the tumor and the size of the vascular lesion determine whether the lesion can be safely removed in toto, whether the ICA can be preserved patent, and whether the integrity of the nervous structures (nerves II through VI) can be preserved intact. In cases of extensive expansion of a tumor, usually a meningioma, into the posterior cranial fossa, when the apex of the pyramid must be drilled off as far as the internal auditory canal, damage to the seventh and eighth cranial nerves can occur, particularly if the tumor has grown into the canal.[5,6] In such instances it is preferable to operate in two stages. During the first stage, using a suboccipital approach, the tumor in the posterior cranial fossa is removed, the seventh and eighth cranial nerves dissected, and the sixth and fifth cranial nerves dissected to their entry points into the CS. In this manner the supratentorial stage involving complete removal of the remaining tumor is easier and safer.

When a tumor has infiltrated into the wall of the ICA, complete removal of the tumor from the artery is not possible without risking subsequent rupture of the ICA. There are therefore two options. A portion of the tumor can be left around the artery and later treated with γ-knife surgery, or a decision can be made to resect the diseased segment of the ICA and to implant a graft. Despite some recommended methods of grafting the ICA in the CS (and also when cross-circulation is not satisfactory), we are of the opinion that successful direct grafting is only possible (although carrying a certain risk) when the cross circulation is good and when the patient tolerates the balloon occlusion test preoperatively. This also holds true for large and giant aneurysms, traumatic aneurysms, and high-flow carotid cavernous fistulas (CCFs).

After complete removal of the lesion, vascular or tumorous, from the CS, minor venous hemorrhage is usually found to occur retrogradely from the inferior petrosal sinus via communication in the region of the clivus, as well as through the intercavernous sinuses in the sella and even from the veins along the ICA in the carotid canal, and from the orbital vein. These hemorrhages can easily be stopped with small pieces of Surgicel. In order to prevent postoperative venous hemorrhage as a result of dislocation of Surgical due to retrograde venous pressure occurring as a result of the patient's straining, it is important to introduce some sutures and form a mesh behind which Surgicel will be held in place and not be displaced due to increased venous pressure.

CLOSURE OF THE DURA

After the lesion has been removed from in and/or around the CS, the dura should be closed watertightly whenever possible. Only careful planning of the dural cut at the beginning of the operation will enable watertight resuturing of the dura. When the dura has been invaded by tumor it should also be resected to a greater or lesser extent; grafting with fascia lata or lio-dura is advisable. In addition, fibrin glue may be useful to close the dura watertightly from the epidural aspect. This is even more important when the bone is either damaged during surgery, or by trauma, or eroded by a tumorous or vascular lesion or by trauma. When the probability of CSF leak is very high, it is advisable to insert a lumbar drain for at least 7 days postoperatively.

DISCUSSION

In the last 20 years, the anatomy of the CS has been continuously studied and is well described.[7,10–14,16] Due to this new anatomical knowledge, successful surgery of the CS has been conducted since 1965.[1–3,5,6,8,9,11–13]

Despite a sound knowledge and understanding of the anatomy of the CS, postoperative sequelae are still numerous; some are very serious and in rare cases even life-threatening. The most frequent complications are pareses of cranial nerves III through VI. These occur in 80 percent of cases, but 90 percent improve within the first 3 months. An important complication is CSF leak, which usually results from accidental opening of the bony sinus during the operation. Only in a smaller number of cases is CSF leak due to changes in the bone caused by the lesion itself. A life-threatening complication is rupture of the ICA, which may occur either intra- or postoperatively due to damage to the artery during removal of the tumor from the wall of the artery. When the tumor is adherent to the wall of the artery, or has even infiltrated, it is preferable to leave part of the tumor around the artery, and treat the patient postoperatively with γ-knife surgery. On the other hand, if a radical approach is chosen, the artery must be resected together with the tumor and the artery is then reconstructed with a graft. This of course demands great experience. Rarer, although not insignificant, is the problem of hemorrhage from the venous channels after the tumor has been completely removed. If the venous channels are not well packed, fatal hemorrhage may occur postoperatively due to the extrusion of the hemostatic material during straining of the patient. It is therefore advisable that at the completion of surgery, after complete removal of the tumor, some sutures be placed from one side of the CS to the other, thus forming a mesh that will prevent the Surgicel from being extruded from the CS. Too tight a packing around the ICA in the CS may also be dangerous because it may cause stenosis and even occlusion of the ICA. It is thus necessary to remove all of the Surgicel from the CS at the end of the operation and then to replace it loosely, at the same time checking that the ICA is not compressed at any site and that the venous hemorrhage has been completely stopped. Possible damage to the optic nerve during surgery of the CS, due to opening of the optic canal, is of two types (i.e., purely mechanical and thermal). Both these complications can be avoided by careful removal of the wall of the optic canal.

Contusions, lacerations of the brain, and intracerebral hematomas can only be avoided by exerting gentle retraction during the operation. This is only possible if the sylvian fissure is completely split and separated enough to enable surgery in the CS to be carried out by gently retracting the temporal lobe in a lateral direction and removing the tumor from the medial side of the CS, after which the temporal lobe is gently retracted from the lateral side in a medial direction, allowing removal of the tumor from the lateral side of the CS. By gentle manipulation of the temporal lobe during CS surgery there is little probability that the patient will have epilepsy after surgery. However, patients require at least 3 to 6 months of antiepileptic prophylaxis after operations for tumors of the CS.

Incomplete removal of a benign tumor from the CS does not fall into the category of complications; however, it represents an incorrect assessment of the degree of difficulty of the operative procedure and a definitely higher percentage of possible complications during further surgery. In order to conduct operative procedures in the CS safely, not only is a theoretical knowledge of the anatomy of the parasellar region required, but also practice in the laboratory before live surgery.

REFERENCES

1. Dolenc VV: Direct microsurgical repair of intracavernous vascular lesions. J Neurosurg 58:824, 1983
2. Dolenc VV: A combined epi- and subdural direct approach to carotid-ophthalmic artery aneurysms. J Neurosurg 62:667, 1985
3. Dolenc VV: Anatomy and Surgery of the Cavernous Sinus. Springer-Verlag, New York, 1989
4. Glasscock ME: Exposure of the intra-petrous portion of the carotid artery. p. 135. In Hamberger CA et al

(eds): Disorders of the Skull Base Region. Proceedings of the Tenth Nobel Symposium. Almqvist & Wiksell, Stockholm, 1969
5. Kawase T, Toya S, Shiobara R et al: Skull base approaches for meningiomas invading the cavernous sinus. p. 346. In Dolenc VV (ed): The Cavernous Sinus. A Multidisciplinary Approach to Vascular and Tumorous Lesions. Springer-Verlag, New York, 1987
6. Kawase T, Toya S, Shiobara S et al: Transpetrosal approach for aneurysms of the lower basilar artery. J Neurosurg 63:857, 1985
7. Lang J: Middle cranial base anatomy. p. 313. In Sekhar LN et al (eds): Tumors of the Cranial Base. Diagnosis and Treatment. Futura, Mount Kisco, 1987
8. Lesoin F, Pellerin P, Autricque A et al: The direct microsurgical approach to intracavernous tumors. p. 323. In Dolenc VV (ed): The Cavernous Sinus. A Multidisciplinary Approach to Vascular and Tumorous Lesions. Springer-Verlag, New York, 1987
9. Mullan S: Treatment of carotid-cavernous fistulas by cavernous sinus occlusion. J Neurosurg 50:131, 1979
10. Parkinson D: Collateral circulation of cavernous carotid artery: anatomy. Can J Surg 7:251, 1964
11. Parkinson D: A surgical approach to the cavernous portion of the carotid artery. Anatomical studies and case report. J Neurosurg 23:474, 1965
12. Parkinson D: Carotid cavernous fistula: direct repair with preservation of the carotid artery. Technical note. J Neurosurg 38:99, 1973
13. Parkinson D: Surgical management of internal carotid artery aneurysms within the cavernous sinus. p. 837. In Schmidek HH et al (eds): Operative Neurosurgical Techniques. Indications, Methods and Results. Grune & Stratton, Orlando, FL, 1988
14. Taptas JN: The so-called cavernous sinus: a review of the controversy and its implications for neurosurgeons. Neurosurgery 11:712, 1982
15. Umansky F, Elidan J, Valarezo A: Dorello's canal: a microanatomical study. Neurosurgery 75:294, 1991
16. Umansky F, Nathan N: The cavernous sinus. An anatomic study of its lateral wall. p. 56. In Dolenc VV (ed): The Cavernous Sinus. A Multidisciplinary Approach to Vascular and Tumorous Lesions. Springer-Verlag, New York, 1987
17. Yasargil MG: Microneurosurgery. Vol. 1. Thieme Stratton, New York, 1984
18. Yasargil MG, Fox JL, Ray MW: The operative approach to aneurysms of the anterior communicating artery. p. 113. In Krayenbuhl H (ed): Advances and Technical Standards in Neurosurgery. Vol. 2. Springer-Verlag, New York, 1975

21 Brain Metastases

Douglas Kondziolka
L. Dade Lunsford

Despite advances in earlier recognition, more accurate localization, and more effective treatment, metastatic brain tumors continue to challenge the neurosurgeon's skill. As recently as 20 years ago, the surgical mortality after total removal of a brain metastasis was 8 percent; after partial removal, it was 18 percent, and after "biopsy only," 30 percent.[29] By the beginning of the 1990s, new developments in neuroimaging, anesthesia, microsurgical, and stereotactic techniques had enhanced our ability to diagnose brain metastases accurately and to treat them safely. The present challenge is to determine when, how, and by what method to treat the intracranial manifestation of a systemic disease, because experience has taught us that, "For intracranial metastatic tumors . . . any course of action—but particularly no treatment—results in a high mortality rate."[88]

Between 75,000 and 140,000 new intracranial metastases are diagnosed annually in the United States.[25,89] Because 45 to 65 percent of such patients have solitary tumors that might warrant surgery,[5,16,33,58,89] approximately 40,000 people/year will be examined for this purpose by neurosurgeons. This chapter will address current strategies both to manage and to avoid mismanagement of brain metastases. We will describe techniques for complication avoidance to make a proper diagnosis and to perform surgery, and we will present guidelines for recommending adjuvant therapies.

THE IMPORTANCE OF MAKING A DIAGNOSIS

Reliance on the Patient's History

In some patients with metastatic cancer, a newly recognized intracranial mass often is presumed to be part of the disease's "natural history." The new onset of one or more intracranial mass lesions in a patient with active extracranial cancer can appropriately be considered metastatic brain disease, providing that the imaging findings are typical for metastasis. In this setting, the clinical and imaging information alone can guide appropriate management.

There are four other clinical situations that represent examples of more complex diagnostic issues. First, the diagnosis of a new brain mass with only a *remote* history of cancer should alert the clinician to the possibility of a second primary benign or malignant tumor. For example, meningiomas are common tumors in older women, some of whom also have been treated remotely for breast cancer.[72] Consideration that the new tumor must be a metastatic breast deposit, rather than a new primary, could lead to erroneous and ineffective treatment. If the medical history elicits a past systemic malignancy, then staging of the disease becomes paramount, that is, location and number of other metastases and their suitability for treatment. The neurological history may reveal no symptoms for those lesions diagnosed during staging. In some patients, symptoms evolve rapidly, because many metastases cause focal neurological deficits associated with extensive regional brain edema and occasionally obstructive hydrocephalus. In contrast, prolonged, slowly progressive symptoms should suggest a diagnosis other than brain metastases (for example, a primary glial neoplasm).

Second, the diagnosis of a new solitary intracranial lesion in the absence of a known primary tumor, despite seemingly typical imaging findings, should not automatically be considered a metastasis. The differential diagnosis in this example will be discussed more thoroughly in sections below. In this instance, additional neuroimaging tests or histological confirmation should guide treatment. Third, atypical imaging findings may herald a wide variety of neoplastic, vascular, or infectious conditions, all of which warrant unique therapies. For example, septic emboli and their hemorrhagic, ischemic, or inflammatory sequelae can resemble multiple metastatic deposits. Fourth, the presence of an immunocompromised state places the patient at risk for a host of infectious or neoplastic processes ranging from fungal, parasitic, or granulomatous disease to lymphomas, some of which may resemble metastases on imaging studies.

The Value of a Thorough Examination

To avoid complications from mismanagement based on an improper presumptive diagnosis, every patient should have a comprehensive clinical investigation. The examination of a patient suspected of having metastatic brain disease should assess the neurological status of the patient, estimate the patient's suitability for surgery, and determine the overall degree of systemic cancer involvement. A conscientious general physical examination should involve abdominal palpation, rectal examination, lymph node survey, skin assessment, and retinal funduscopy in order to detect tumors not previously recognized. As part of this initial evaluation, we routinely obtain a chest roentgenogram and chest and abdominal computed tomography (CT) scans. These provide information mandatory to select the best site for obtaining a histological diagnosis, which proves invaluable to both the neurosurgeon and neuropathologist, should the brain mass be chosen as the logical site for biopsy.

Neuroimaging to Aid the Diagnosis

Neuroimaging recognition of small intracranial metastases is the next step and must include high-resolution cerebral CT, often supplemented by magnetic resonance imaging (MRI), to detect lesions that might go unnoticed by a poor quality or incomplete CT study.[47] CT should include a lateral electronic (scout) skull radiograph with marked axial image levels to aid bone flap placement if a craniotomy is performed subsequently. The role of cerebral angiography is limited to lesions whose differential diagnosis includes vascular abnormalities such as a vascular malformation or giant aneurysm. At present, contrast-enhanced MRI is the best study to detect small tumor deposits and to confirm whether a metastatic tumor is truly solitary,[11] although even MRI is not foolproof.[27] Metastatic tumors can develop adjacent to other intracranial tumors or fluid collections detected by CT or MRI.[91] Subdural hematomas can occur from subdural tumor deposits rather than from trauma,[1,7,44] and intraparenchymal hematomas can be caused by tumors.[42,54] Although intracranial metastases most commonly develop in the distal vascular territories of the anterior, middle, or posterior cerebral arteries,[40] they occasionally (and unexpectedly) also occur in the pineal region,[86] in the pituitary gland, and on cranial nerves.[82]

The Differential Diagnosis

Despite a thorough physical and imaging examination, most patients with a presumed metastatic brain tumor present a diagnostic challenge. Intra-axial tumors such as gliomas, primary central nervous system lymphomas, or primitive neuroectodermal tumors can all appear to be "metastatic"[9] (Fig. 21-1). Dural or intraventricular metastases often resemble meningiomas.[39,55,59,66] The clinical assessment and rapid onset of symptoms in patients with brain tumors (primary or secondary) can suggest the diagnosis of cerebrovascular disease (transient ischemic attack or stroke.[43] Brain imaging should follow the clinical assessment so that patients with tumors are not presumed to have had a stroke and receive anticoagulant therapy. On CT images, thrombosed aneurysms and resolving hematomas may enhance peripherally after administration of contrast (mimicking "ring-enhancing" metastases), and small angiographically visible or occult vascular malformations may appear as homogeneously enhancing lesions. MRI helps to characterize these lesions further by

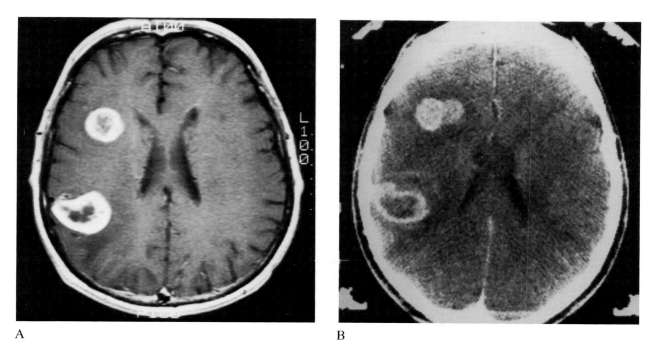

A   B

Figure 21-1. Contrast-enhanced **(A)** MRI and **(B)** CT scan showing multiple lesions that were considered to represent multiple brain metastases. However, stereotactic biopsy defined the diagnosis as multicentric glioblastoma multiforme.

demonstrating flow-void signal or mixed signal caused by hemosiderin, recent hemorrhage, or calcification.[69] MRI is also superior to CT for distinguishing lesions of vascular origin and should be performed whenever the diagnosis of brain tumor is not clearly established. Patchell and colleagues[63] described 54 patients who were considered to have a metastasis based on CT or MRI; in fact, 2 had glioblastomas, 2 had abscesses, 1 had an astrocytoma, and 1 had an inflammatory disorder.

Intracranial abscesses or granulomas are well circumscribed, often have peripheral enhancement and surrounding edema, and may be indistinguishable from metastatic tumors on the basis of imaging criteria. Although indium-111 leukocyte radionuclide brain scan has been reported to differentiate between metastases and abscesses (due to leukocyte uptake in pyogenic foci), Balachandran and coworkers[3] showed that even this test is nonspecific. Immunocompromised patients are prone to toxoplasmosis and viral and fungal infections, as well as intracranial malignancies. In the evaluation of patients with the acquired immunodeficiency syndrome (AIDS), antitoxoplasmosis therapy has been advocated before resorting to stereotactic biopsy. However, the high prevalence of neoplasia (particularly lymphoma) in patients with AIDS may warrant stereotactic biopsy

more frequently to guide appropriate management.[10] The differential diagnostic possibilities are summarized in Figure 21-2.

Potential Complications from an Erroneous Preoperative Diagnosis

Surgery performed to remove a presumed metastasis can be associated with unexpected problems if the lesion proves to be of vascular or infectious origin. For example, massive unanticipated hemorrhage might occur if the mass proved to be an aneurysm or arteriovenous malformation (AVM). Achieving hemostasis without the benefit of angiographic information can be especially vexing. Belief that an intracerebral hematoma is neoplastic in origin (e.g., melanoma) can lead to intraoperative catastrophe if the lesion is actually caused by an unrecognized preoperative coagulopathy. Adequate survey of blood coagulation (platelet count, prothrombin and partial thromboplastin times, and possibly bleeding time) can reduce this risk. Surgical resection of a metastatic tumor should be total, in contrast to abscess drainage with limited dissection of the abscess capsule. Because total extirpation of a brain abscess by craniotomy is rarely warranted, this potential compli-

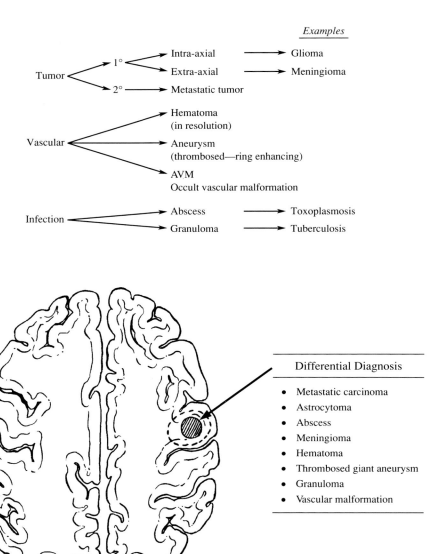

Figure 21-2. The differential diagnosis of a solitary brain lesion. The diagram illustrates one location at which multiple pathological entities must be considered in the differential diagnosis in order to guide management.

cation is best avoided by having a high index of suspicion or even by considering stereotactic biopsy as the first procedure.

Delayed complications from treatment based upon an incorrect preoperative diagnosis can be equally dangerous. For example, radiation therapy empirically administered to treat a mass lesion without a histological diagnosis can lead to incorrect primary treatment and can delay appropriate treatment of a brain abscess, encephalitis, paraneoplastic effects of a systemic cancer, or other tumor. For vascular lesions such as aneurysms and AVMs, the risk of hemorrhage remains unchanged after administration of fractionated radiation therapy.

RECENT HISTORY OF SURGERY FOR BRAIN METASTASES

Potential complications related to intracranial metastatic tumor surgery are related to tumor location, histological type, and surgical technique used. Operative mortality rates of 25 and 38 percent were reported for two large series performed prior to 1960.[74,77] A review of the series reported from 1971 to 1980 showed an operative mortality of 10 to 30 percent.[5,26,64,67,88] Horwitz and Rizzoli[36] cited a pre-CT era study that found a 16.8 percent postoperative mortality for supratentorial metastatic tumors and a 3.7 percent mortality after resection of cerebellar tumors. Postoperative complications were noted in 24 percent of patients reviewed by Haar and Patterson[29] in 1972. Increased neurological deficits, intracerebral hemorrhage, or wound infection were followed by a second procedure in one-third of these patients. In reviewing the literature to 1977, Posner[64] found that reoperation for hematoma or infection was necessary in 7 to 17 percent of patients. Sundaresan et al.[79] reported on the removal of 34 solitary metastatic tumors; intracerebral hematomas developed in two patients, and three others had increased deficits.

More recent reports (perhaps reflecting the benefits derived from CT imaging, microsurgical technique, and improved neuroanesthesia), indicate that the current overall 30-day mortality for metastatic brain tumor surgery varies from 2 to 6 percent.[62,63,79,87] In a 1980 report on a series of 33 patients, Galicich et al.[26] described four postoperative deaths that resulted from pulmonary embolism, hepatic failure, pneumonia, or growth of undetected brain metastases. Patients who had no evidence of systemic cancer had a 1-year survival rate of 81 percent and no operative morbidity or mortality. Although no clear correlation has been noted between

the histological tumor type and onset of surgical complications, Bremer and colleagues[8] reported intracerebral hemorrhage at the site of tumor resection in 7 of 17 (41 percent) patients with metastatic melanoma. In series performed before the use of high-resolution imaging, undetected tumor nodules occasionally led to massive postoperative edema and death.[8,36] Currently, such a risk should be very low.

The choice of surgical technique depends on the desired result. Tumor biopsy alone can establish a histological diagnosis (Fig. 21-3) but per se provides no therapeutic benefit. However, if the sole therapy intended after diagnosis is irradiation (either by fractionated or radiosurgical technique), biopsy may be satisfactory as the initial procedure. Indications for tumor resection potentially include an uncertain diagnosis, failure of nonsurgical therapy, a radiation "resistant" tumor,[5,56] and solitary tumor in a location acceptable for surgery. Tumor resection is performed to achieve the following goals: establish a diagnosis, remove the source of brain edema (Fig. 21-4), eliminate regional brain compression, and/or achieve cytoreduction. Surgical resection of solitary metastases appears to provide improved patient survival[5,18,21,26,39,52,53,57,62,67,79,80,85,87,90,92]; a randomized prospective trial indicated that resection followed by whole-brain radiotherapy improved survival and length of quality survival as compared to radiotherapy alone.[63]

STEREOTACTIC BIOPSY: CURRENT ROLE AND TECHNIQUES

Until the 1980s, high mortality rates for brain tumor biopsy were almost the rule. The excessive postoperative mortality rate associated with tumor biopsy in reports dating from the 1960s and 1970s is related to several factors: failure to use stereotactic technique, inadequate imaging to localize the target, the presence of multiple tumors, and poor preoperative medical or neurological condition, in essence making the patient a poor candidate for tumor resection. In 1963, Richards and McKissock[68] reported a 67 percent mortality rate after biopsy of metastatic tumors. Also, in their experience, the risk was higher after partial excision (45 percent) than after gross total excision (32 percent). By 1972, Haar and Patterson[29] reported mortality rates reduced to 30, 18, and 8 percent after biopsy, partial excision, and total excision, respectively. Currently, in properly selected patients, modern imaging-guided stereotactic biopsy is an accurate, highly diagnostic, and low-morbidity method to obtain histological confirmation of the tu-

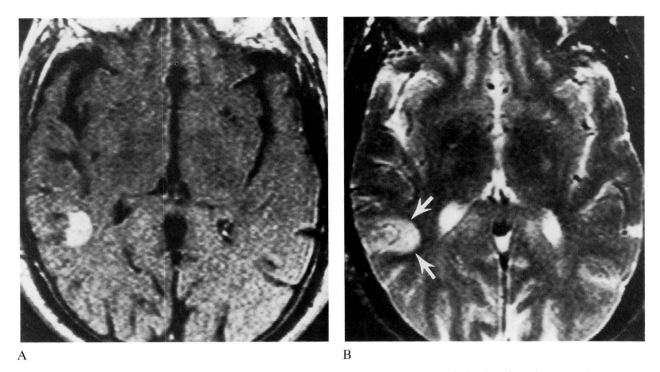

A   B

Figure 21-3. **(A)** T_1 spin-echo MRI with gadolinium-DTPA enhancement and **(B)** T_2 spin-echo MRI show a right parietal lobe lesion 6 years after the patient was treated for thyroid carcinoma. The tumor had only a small amount of surrounding edema (*arrows*). Stereotactic biopsy proved this tumor to be an anaplastic astrocytoma.

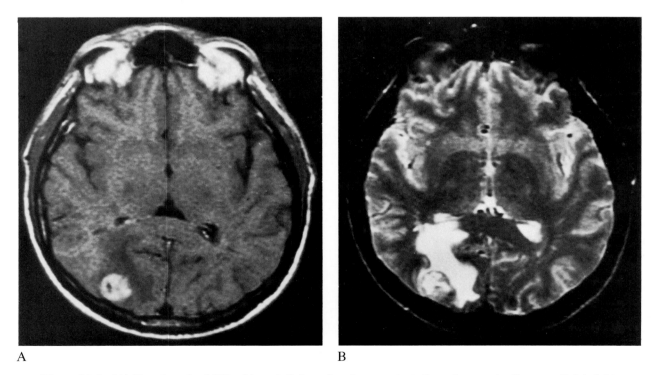

A   B

Figure 21-4. **(A)** T_1 spin-echo MRI with gadolinium showing a metastatic melanoma to the superficial right occipital lobe. **(B)** T_2 spin-echo MRI demonstrating marked surrounding edema.

mor type.[2,48] A review of our 10-year experience (Presbyterian University Hospital, Pittsburgh) with stereotactic biopsy in 35 patients with metastatic tumors showed no resultant morbidity or mortality. This series comprised 25 patients with lobar tumors, 5 with tumors of the basal ganglia or thalamus, and 5 with brainstem tumors.

The major potential complications related to stereotactic biopsy are three: the risk of an intracerebral hemorrhage, infection, and failure to obtain a diagnostic sample. Although tumor "seeding" along the tract of the stereotactic probe has been reported in a patient with pineoblastoma,[70] such a complication is almost unheard of after biopsy of metastases. The incidence of wound infection using the twist-drill approach is also negligible. We routinely administer a single intravenous dose of vancomycin (0.5 g) after stereotactic frame application and before biopsy, but we are not convinced that even this is necessary. In an effort to minimize potential complications related to general anesthesia, almost all patients undergo the procedure under local infiltration anesthesia supplemented with mild sedation. Children under the age of 14 and anxious or agitated adults receive general anesthesia. A preoperative coagulopathy is an absolute contraindication to biopsy; accordingly, blood clotting indices should be assessed in all patients before biopsy is performed.

The risk of biopsy-induced intracerebral hemorrhage is related to the tumor location and to the chosen probe trajectory (Fig. 21-5). In general, a trajectory should be selected that traverses the fewest pial surfaces, in order to avoid major cerebral arteries and veins. The precoronal approach (15 to 25 mm lateral to midline, 10 to 15 mm anterior to the coronal suture) provides the safest access to the majority of lesions within the frontal lobe, basal ganglia, thalamus, and suprasylvian region. Axial contrast-enhanced CT images should be obtained in all planes that the biopsy probe will traverse; these should be examined to identify any vessels that may cross this course. Coronal reconstructions enable one to visualize the longitudinal plane of the trajectory and to identify the ventricular system. The *exact* plane of the biopsy probe can be visualized on an oblique CT or MRI sequence by tilting the gantry (range of 40 degrees). We have used a specially designed CT program that superimposes our selected biopsy path on each consecutive axial CT slice (so that we can follow this path through the brain),[51] but careful attention to the axial or coronal CT images will provide similar information. To prevent dural laceration or dissection, a stop is placed on the drill bit to limit the depth of skull penetration to 10 mm. Additional

drilled increments of 1 to 2 mm are used to reach the epidural space while leaving the dura intact. A sharp biopsy probe is then inserted to penetrate the dura.

Instrument selection for stereotactic biopsy is determined first by safety and second by yield. For non-brainstem biopsies, we initially use the 1.8-mm Backlund spiral (Elekta Instruments, Tucker, GA), which removes a core of tissue but fails to extract vessels in most cases. Our second instrument is an aspiration needle (1.8 mm in outer diameter), which removes tissue with 2 to 3 cc of air suction. If no tissue is removed by these techniques (an infrequent occurrence), we advocate using a side-cutting suction/aspiration (Sedan type) probe. Although some authors advocate using biting instruments (such as 1-mm cupped flexible bronchoscopy forceps),[2] we do not use them because they can tear vessel walls.

Four locations present additional technical challenges to the surgeon. Avoidance of the greater number of bridging veins close to the superior sagittal sinus is mandatory at the parietooccipital cortex in order to prevent hemorrhage and/or venous infarction. As a result, we often employ a burr hole in this region to visualize the pial surface directly. The pia is cauterized and opened sharply, and the probe inserted into the brain under direct vision. For posterior occipital trajectories, we perform a twist-drill approach with the patient in a semisitting position. Lesions near or within the sylvian fissure region are associated with an increased risk of arterial hemorrhage. In similar fashion to the parietal approach, we perform a burr hole and visually inspect the brain surface prior to needle passage. This enables us to choose a stereotactic path to the target that avoids the middle cerebral artery branches of the temporal lobe and infrasylvian fissure. For tumors above the sylvian fissure, the precoronal approach is safer than the lateral convexity route.

Samples of tumors in the upper brainstem (midbrain and pons) are obtained by a precoronal trajectory to minimize the number of pial or ependymal surfaces crossed.[12] The approach passes the probe through the cerebral cortex, lateral ventricle, thalamus, and cerebral peduncle into the long axis of the brainstem (Fig. 21-6). In patients with hydrocephalus, it is important that little cerebrospinal fluid (CSF) be released prior to biopsy to reduce the possibility that the ventricular size (and possibly stereotactic coordinates) could change. In addition, a small aspiration needle (0.9 mm) is used initially to minimize the degree of tissue manipulation and potentially reduce the incidence of iatrogenic brainstem neurological deficits.

Stereotactic biopsy of lesions within the cerebel-

(A) Midbrain-Pons Location

Problems	Solutions
1. Hemorrhage	• Minimize pial surfaces crossed
	• Use transventricular route
	• Pass through long axis of brainstem
	• Small aspiration needle (0.9 mm)
2. Hydrocephalus	• Minimize CSF release prior to biopsy (coordinates may change)

(B & C) Parietooccipital Location

Problems	Solutions
1. Bridging veins	• Burr hole to inspect pial surface (no twist drill)
2. Posterior inferior occipital location	• Sit patient up for biopsy

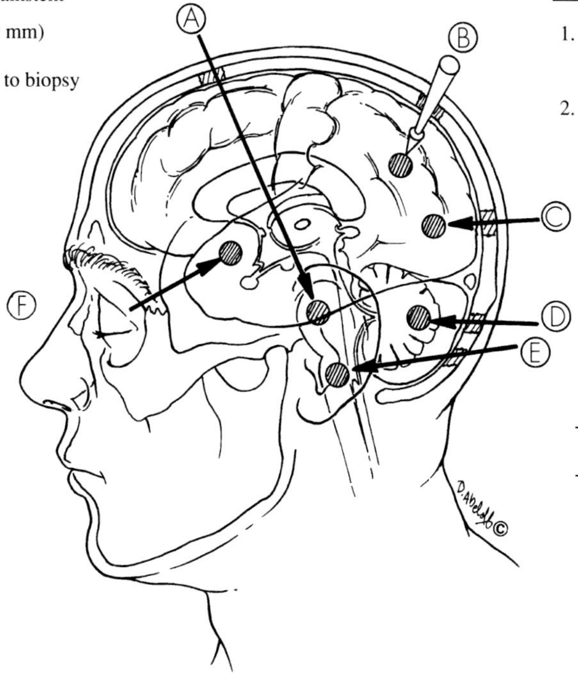

(D & E) Caudal Brainstem or Cerebellar Location

Problems	Solutions
1. Patient positioning	• Sitting upright
	• Prone position suitable under general anesthesia
2. Hemorrhage	• Laterally placed suboccipital burr hole
	• Choose a trajectory that is completely transparenchymal (not subarachnoid)
	• Avoid transtentorial puncture
	• Small aspiration needle for brainstem (0.9 mm)

(F) Temporal Lobe–Sylvian Location

Problems	Solutions
1. Hemorrhage (sylvian vessels)	• Burr hole to inspect brain surface prior to needle passage
	• Choose stereotactic path to avoid sylvian middle cerebral artery branches

Figure 21-5. Major complications and their solutions for different stereotactic biopsy approaches.

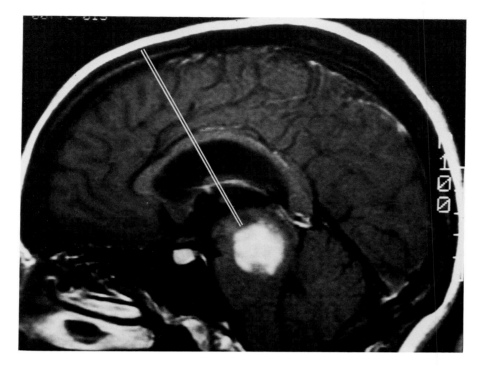

Figure 21-6. Sagittal contrast-enhanced MRI showing the stereotactic approach to a tumor of the midbrain and upper pons, using the precoronal entry point.

lum or caudal brainstem warrant special considerations. Access to the lateral pons or medulla is gained via the middle or inferior cerebellar peduncle, using a lateral probe insertion point. A transcerebellar trajectory is chosen via a lateral suboccipital twist drill approach, either with the patient in the semisitting position (under local anesthesia) or prone (under general anesthesia). In this way, transtentorial puncture is avoided. We again use a small aspiration needle (0.9 mm) or a 3-mm Sedan-type needle to minimize brainstem manipulation.

The use of these methods has avoided complications in the vast majority of stereotactic biopsies. Should intraoperative hemorrhage occur (with blood loss through the probe) only one maneuver should be performed: *The probe should be left in place and blood allowed to drain.* The probe should be periodically cleared by introducing the stylet and by rotating it. The bleeding will cease, often within 15 minutes. Hypertension, if present, should be controlled. No attempt should be made to cauterize with the tip of the needle or instill hydrogen peroxide through the cannula.[19] After bleeding stops, the probe should be removed slowly at 2-mm increments to ensure that bleeding has indeed ceased. After biopsy, a CT scan should be performed to determine whether any hematoma remains and whether observation alone or craniotomy is indicated, depending on the clinical result. In the event of intraventricular hemorrhage, an external ventricular drain can be placed stereotactically. Stereotactic coordinates of the frontal horn should be obtained before biopsy in patients with paraventricular tumors so that a drain can be placed quickly in the unusual event of hemorrhage. The placement of a ventricular drain also should be considered after brainstem biopsies if the aqueduct is judged to be compressed.

CRANIOTOMY AND RESECTION

The surgical resection of a metastatic brain tumor is usually straightforward and uneventful. A good technical result can be achieved with careful attention to standard neurosurgical principles and to the occasional difficulties that metastatic tumors present. Because certain intraoperative complications are intrinsic to particular locations, we have divided this discussion into tumors in three locations: the lateral cerebral convexity (Fig. 21-7), the medial cerebral hemisphere, and the cerebellum. In the section on tumors of the convexity we will address the general principles of metastatic tumor surgery, with reference to their application to tumors of the lateral cerebrocortical and subcortical region.

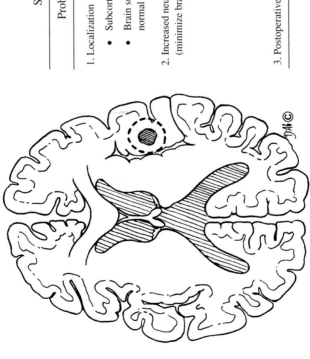

Supratentorial Lateral Convexity Tumors

Problems	Solutions
1. Localization	• Stereotactic guidance
• Subcortical location	• Intraoperative ultrasound
• Brain surface appears normal	
2. Increased neurological deficit (minimize brain manipulation)	• Stereotactic craniotomy
	• Electrophysiological studies intraoperatively
	• EEG
	• Motor-evoked potentials
	• Avoid prolonged retraction
3. Postoperative seizures	• Therapeutic anticonvulsant levels

Figure 21-7. Major complications and their solutions for supratentorial lateral convexity tumors.

Surgery for Lateral Convexity Tumors

In an attempt to reduce brain edema and prevent wound infection, systemic corticosteroids[41] are begun preoperatively and intravenous antibiotics[31] 1 hour before surgery. Although Cohen and coworkers[13] have recommended that prophylactic anticonvulsants be withheld until the first seizure in patients with brain metastases, we believe that therapeutic anticonvulsant levels should be attained in all patients before surgical resection. An indwelling urinary catheter is placed to monitor urinary output during surgery and in the immediately postoperative period. Under general endotracheal anesthesia, the patient is placed in rigid head fixation. An arterial $PaCO_2$ of 32 to 37 mmHg is desirable. This should be reduced further to the range of 25 to 32 mmHg if brain swelling becomes apparent during surgery. The head is elevated approximately 20 to 30 degrees above the heart to facilitate venous drainage, to lower intracranial pressure, and to provide a relaxed brain for surgery. Although some surgeons prefer to have the anesthesiologist administer mannitol at the beginning of the procedure (so that the brain will be maximally relaxed at the time of dural opening), we prefer to use an osmotic diuretic only if the brain continues to be tight at dural incision or brain dissection. It is easier to assess the degree of brain relaxation after tumor resection if osmotic diuretics have not been given.

Accurate tumor localization is one of the most important aspects of craniotomy for brain metastases. Dural metastases or tumors that extend to the pial surface are uncommon; as a result, most metastases are not visible after dural opening. A thorough review of the axial CT images aids tumor localization, in order to place the bone flap correctly. Transposition of information from the axial CT image (usually a transverse section in the orbitomeatal plane) to the lateral scalp or skull surface can be difficult. A number of simple maneuvers assist in planning. One technique is to identify the image that shows an obvious external landmark (such as the external auditory meatus) and then count CT images upward from this level. If the center of the tumor is five slices above the external auditory meatus (using 1-cm-thick slices), then the tumor is located 5 cm above the external ear canal in the orbitomeatal plane. Anterioposterior localization of the tumor in that plane can be determined by the relative distance of the tumor from the anterior and posterior skull surfaces. A second technique uses the lateral CT electronic radiograph. The CT software can localize all axial images on the lateral radiograph so that the tumor margin can be roughly outlined. This technique is not precise, because localizations performed on a flat, lateral skull film must be transposed to the curved convexity of the patient's scalp surface (this problem is greatest near the midline, where the head is most curved).

When the neurosurgeon is confronted by a normal brain surface and a hidden subcortical tumor, several techniques can be used for tumor localization. Close inspection of the pial surface may show a localized area of increased vascularity, arterialized veins,[20] or an expanded gyrus. All of these signs are indirect evidence of an underlying neoplasm. Gentle finger palpation may detect a subcortical firmness, indicative of underlying tumor. These techniques, although time-honored, are not always reliable. When a tumor's location is suspected based on surface examination, a brain needle can be passed for deep tissue "palpation" or biopsy. Alternatively, a small cortical opening can be made and a "limited dissection" performed until the lesion is reached. In order to reduce the likelihood of failure to discover the tumor (Fig. 21-8), the prudent surgeon should consider one of the following two techniques, even before cortical dissection.

Intraoperative ultrasonography can be used to localize some subcortical lesions. A radiologist or neurosurgeon experienced in ultrasound technology can manipulate the transducer to detect echogenic lesions that appear distinct from the surrounding brain. The ventricular system or falx provides an internal landmark to establish the tumor's location between two known references (the brain surface and the internal landmark). Using ultrasound, many lesions can be found, provided the craniotomy has been placed appropriately, but smaller tumors may escape even this method of detection. If this intraoperative method is unsuccessful, it is best to terminate the procedure. A metallic clip placed in the suspected area prior to dural closure will indicate the operative location in reference to the tumor location on a postoperative CT scan. The tumor then can be accurately located and removed during a second operation.

Stereotactic techniques offer an alternate and more precise guidance for craniotomy. Although stereotactic frame application and intraoperative CT scanning may slightly prolong surgery, they completely eliminate the problem of not finding a tumor at surgery. In most centers, the stereotactic frame is affixed under local anesthesia, followed by stereotactic CT scanning. The patient is then transferred to the operating room for craniotomy. Stereotactic guidance is most useful for small subcortical tumors that otherwise are occasionally impossible to find during craniotomy.[38]

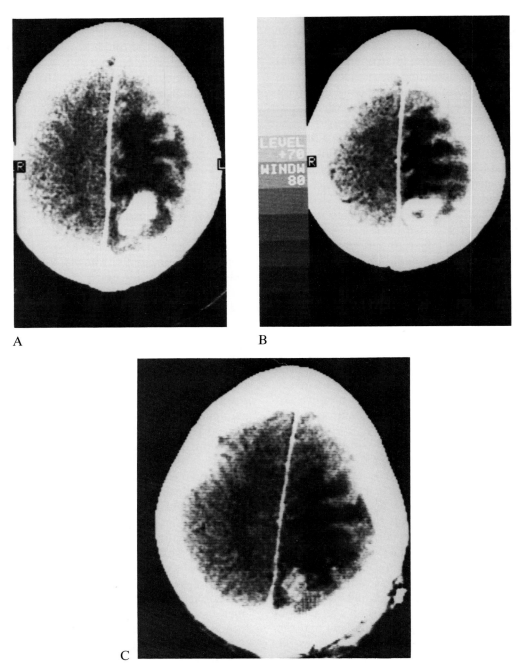

Figure 21-8. (A&B) Consecutive axial contrast-enhanced CT images of a left occipital tumor with hemispheric edema. At craniotomy, the tumor could not be identified despite multiple cortical incisions and dissections; neither intraoperative ultrasonography or stereotactic guidance were used. **(C)** A postoperative scan showed that the enhancing mass was smaller, but diagnostic tissue was not obtained. Three months later, the patient had another craniotomy for an enlarging tumor; metastatic adenocarcinoma of the lung was identified.

If stereotactic coordinates are obtained for the tumor margins, a precise limited bone flap can be planned to minimize exposure of the normal brain (Fig. 21-9). After exposure of the brain surface, a probe can be passed directly to the tumor (more recently, laser-beam probes have been used to facilitate stereotactic craniotomy), and dissection proceeds along the guided path. The use of stereotactic craniotomy was recently endorsed by Moore and coworkers[60] after obtaining successful results in nine patients with metastatic tumors; none of these patients had increased deficits despite location of their tumors in motor or speech areas. Kelly and associates[38] reported on the computer-assisted stereotactic resection of intracranial metastatic tumors in 44 patients, all of whom had a gross total removal. The series included 15 patients with superficial subcortical tumors, 23 with deep tumors, and 6 with lesions in the posterior fossa. They observed no operative mortality and only 7 percent operative morbidity in patients who underwent stereotactic resection. The potential for increased neurological deficits after tumor resection can be prevented, at least in part, by preoperative steroid administration, by a direct approach to the tumor (as previously discussed), by avoidance of prolonged brain retraction, and by minimizing brain

dissection. For lesions in critical brain locations, intraoperative electrophysiological (evoked potential) monitoring may help to avoid neurological deficits during surgical resection.

After localization of the tumor, removal is facilitated by identification of the plane between edematous brain tissue and the tumor margin. Metastatic brain tumors often appear grossly encapsulated and can be readily dissected from the surrounding brain.[67,77] However, the tumor-brain plane should not be considered absolute; biopsies of surrounding brain tissue (as much as 4 to 5 mm from the tumor "capsule") often have yielded microscopic deposits of tumor (D. Kondziolka, unpublished data). For small tumors, the brain is lined with consecutive cotton slabs, and the tumor is rolled slowly away from normal brain. Through the operating microscope, the plane can be readily identified and small neoplastic vessels cauterized. Grasping forceps can be used to hold the tumor firmly and roll it away from the brain as dissection proceeds. This technique lessens the need for small extracapsular incisions into normal brain tissue and minimizes the amount of normal brain exposed in the region surrounding the tumor. Thus, it is hoped, a neurological deficit from regional brain manipulation is avoided. For large tumors, the

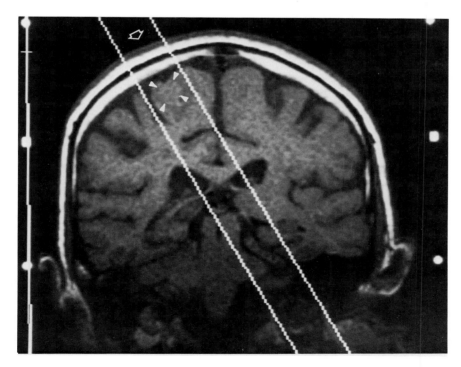

Figure 21-9. Coronal MRI of a metastatic tumor within the right precentral gyrus. The oblique lines identify the lateral margins of the tumor (*arrowheads*) during planning for stereotactic craniotomy via a limited bony and brain exposure (*arrow*).

ultrasonic aspirator assists internal debulking to reduce the amount of brain retraction and exposure. Bleeding is usually minimal once the entire tumor is removed. Careful attention to hemostasis in the tumor bed (with cautery, irrigation, peroxide, and multiple Valsalva maneuvers performed by the anesthetists) will reduce the likelihood of hematoma formation in the operative site. As the final step in brain hemostasis, we line the incised brain surface with surgical cellulose.

A standard craniotomy closure is performed with watertight dural closure, replacement of the bone flap, approximation of muscle if appropriate, and a two-layer scalp closure. A full head dressing is applied, and the patient is allowed to awaken at the end of an uneventful procedure. Intubation and hyperventilation (and possibly intracranial pressure monitoring) are continued into the immediate postoperative period if brain swelling was noted during surgery. Fluid replacement is maintained at 75 to 85 ml/h (less than maintenance) to reduce extracellular volume expansion and edema. Continuous electrocardiographic monitoring and frequent measurements of electrolytes, blood counts, arterial blood gases, and urinary output are performed in the recovery room and during the first 24 hours in a neurosurgical observation unit. Anticonvulsants and corticosteroids are continued. If neurological deterioration occurs in the postoperative period, serum levels of electrolytes, blood gases and anticonvulsants are drawn (specifically to check for hyponatremia, hypokalemia, hypoxia, or anticonvulsant toxicity), and CT scanning performed. Imaging evidence of increased brain edema warrants treatment with corticosteroids, osmotic diuretics, and possibly hyperventilation. Evidence of new intracranial hemorrhage at the operative site requires reexploration of the craniotomy.

Surgery in the Medial Hemisphere

The neurosurgical principles discussed above also apply to tumors located along the medial cerebral hemisphere. As with lateral convexity tumors, the head is elevated, but it is kept facing directly forward to prevent the opposite hemisphere from leaning into the interhemispheric exposure and to maintain orientation. The neck is slightly flexed or extended to keep the tumor in a superior position (the surgeon must always be able to place two or three fingers between the chin and neck).

Most tumors in this area are subcortical in location and do not directly abut the pial surface or project

into the interhemispheric fissure (Fig. 21-10). Again, the problem of tumor localization and bone flap planning are addressed by careful review of the CT scout film, use of stereotactic craniotomy, or intraoperative ultrasonography. Because the interhemispheric fissure is even more restricted than the convexity, localizing subcortical tumors can be even more troublesome.

Protection of the superior sagittal sinus and bridging veins is imperative (Fig. 21-11). Although these structures may be occluded if they drain the anterior frontal lobe, in more posterior locations their sacrifice can lead to venous infarction and resultant significant morbidity or mortality. To protect the sagittal sinus during craniotomy, burr holes should be placed on either side of the sinus, rather than directly over it. Careful dissection can then free the sinus from the overlying inner table of the skull prior to sawing and lifting of the craniotomy flap. Some surgeons prefer to fashion two burr holes directly over the sinus; this provides visualization and protection of the sinus, with adequate exposure of the medial convexity cortex but more restricted access into the interhemispheric fissure. Hemorrhage from inadvertent entry

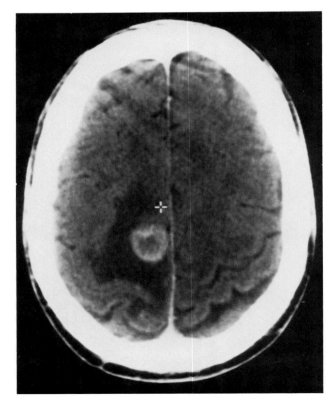

Figure 21-10. Contrast-enhanced CT scan showing a metastatic tumor within the subcortical medial parietal lobe.

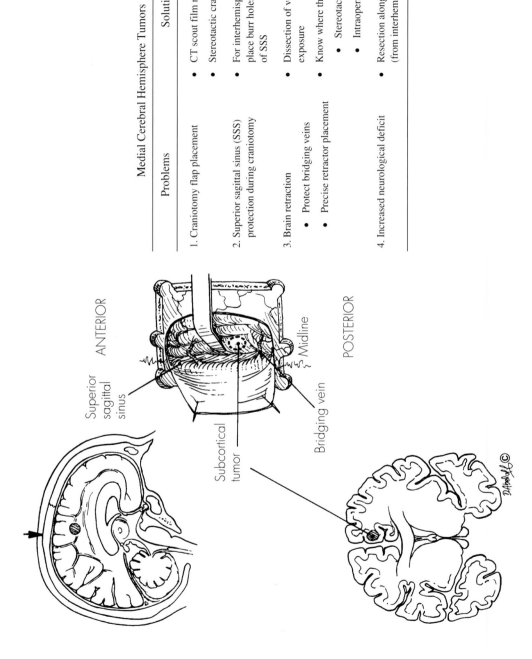

Medial Cerebral Hemisphere Tumors

Problems	Solutions
1. Craniotomy flap placement	• CT scout film review
	• Stereotactic craniotomy
2. Superior sagittal sinus (SSS) protection during craniotomy	• For interhemispheric approach, place burr holes on either side of SSS
3. Brain retraction	• Dissection of veins to increase exposure
• Protect bridging veins	• Know where the tumor is
• Precise retractor placement	• Stereotactic guidance
	• Intraoperative ultrasound
4. Increased neurological deficit	• Resection along shortest path (from interhemispheric fissure)

ANTERIOR

Superior sagittal sinus

Subcortical tumor

Midline

Bridging vein

POSTERIOR

Figure 21-11. Major complications and their solutions for surgical resection of tumors in the medial cerebral hemisphere.

of the sinus usually can be stopped by direct tamponade with Gelfoam (absorbable gelatin sponge) and cottonoid pads; suture repair is not often necessary. The sinus, falx, and opposite hemisphere dura should be protected with cotton slabs during the rest of the procedure. A horseshoe-shaped dural opening with the sinus as its base should be used to expose the brain; this technique keeps the two layers of dura together at the sinus and prevents bleeding from venous lacunae. The dural opening need not extend far laterally if the dissection will be limited to the interhemispheric fissure.

To facilitate brain retraction, bridging veins can be dissected laterally at their attachment to the brain. Hemorrhage from a torn bridging vein usually can be stopped by temporary compression, rather than cauterization and vein sacrifice. Brain retractors should be placed so as not to compromise venous drainage and yet provide optimal exposure. Knowledge of the tumor location permits precise retractor placement.

Medial hemisphere metastatic tumors are approached through the interhemispheric fissure or directly through the medial convexity cortex (in noncritical areas). In general, dissection should proceed along the shortest route to the tumor. A tumor 3 cm below the convexity cortical surface may be only 1 cm below the pial surface of the interhemispheric fissure. If preoperative imaging studies show that the best tumor trajectory lies through the medial cortical convexity, a parasagittal craniotomy that exposes the superior sagittal sinus may be unnecessary. If the tumor subsequently cannot be reached by the convexity approach, an additional parasagittal bone flap can provide further exposure. This situation can be avoided in advance by stereotactic craniotomy or by beginning the procedure with the interhemispheric-convexity exposure craniotomy in order to access both avenues of dissection. Closure and postoperative care are standard, as detailed earlier.

Surgery for Posterior Fossa Tumors

Operations for posterior fossa metastatic tumors have the potential for greater morbidity and mortality than that for tumors found in most lobar locations, both because of the tumors' proximity to the brainstem and their tendency to lead to hydrocephalus. Tumors of the brainstem proper are rarely candidates for surgical excision and may be more amenable to radiosurgery. Cerebellar tumors can be located primarily in the hemisphere or vermis and can grow to reach the fourth ventricle, cerebellar peduncles, or brainstem pia. Such tumors are usually intraparen-

chymal and do not often grow primarily in the subarachnoid cisterns or extend through the tentorium.

The regional surgical anatomy of the posterior fossa exposure and its attendant problems are shown in Figure 21-12. Because of the smaller confines of the posterior fossa and the lower risk of a new major deficit when traversing the cerebellum, tumor localization is less critical than for tumors in the supratentorial compartment. Small tumors (<1.5 cm) are occasionally difficult to find. Thus, preoperative imaging studies must be reviewed carefully. The tumor should be located in reference to visible external brain landmarks. For example, how far is the tumor from the midline? How far below the tentorium? How deep from the surface of the hemisphere? Certain tumors sometimes prove to be more superior and deeper than suspected, partly because of the angle of vision commonly used during posterior fossa craniectomy. With the neck flexed to expose the suboccipital region, the surgeon's line of vision proceeds from the midcerebellar level externally and travels inferiorly. Finding the superior tumor requires that the craniectomy reach the level of the transverse sinus and that the cerebellar dissection stay superior in a plane parallel to the tentorium.

A generous, rather than a limited, suboccipital craniectomy (including the foramen magnum) aids in midline tumor exposure and in providing tonsillar decompression in the event of tumor recurrence or increased intracranial pressure. Because of the poor long-term survival rate and the chance for local recurrence, craniotomy (as opposed to craniectomy) has little place in metastatic tumor surgery in the posterior fossa.

The presence of hydrocephalus should be recognized from the preoperative imaging studies. Before beginning the craniectomy exposure, consideration should be given to placement of an occipital or frontal burr hole, should rapid ventricular access for CSF diversion be necessary during or after surgery. We use this simple technique, even in patients without significant ventricular dilatation. An occipital burr hole has the advantage of being contained within the same shaved and prepared area as the craniectomy incision. Placed 7 cm above the inion and 3 cm lateral to the midline, the burr hole is drilled and the underlying dura cauterized but not opened. In most patients, a ventriculoperitoneal shunt is not necessary if the tumor causing the hydrocephalus is excised. However, if the tumor is not amenable to resection (e.g., brainstem, pineal region), a ventriculoperitoneal shunt may represent the only required surgical treatment.

In posterior fossa operations for midline or para-

Posterior Fossa Craniectomy and Cerebellar Tumors

Problems	Solutions
1. Tumor localization	• Generous craniectomy including foramen magnum
	• Imaging study review
2. Venous bleeding during craniectomy	• Exclude transverse sinuses from craniectomy if possible
	• Hemostatic clips for occipital and marginal sinuses as needed
3. ↑ICP	• Open cisterna magna
• Brain swelling	
• Tight dura	
4. Increased neurological deficit	• Midline approach via cerebellar vermis if possible
	• Protect fourth ventricle structures
5. Postoperative hemorrhage or edema	• Place occipital burr hole for rapid CSF access to lateral ventricle
	• Consider ventriculostomy

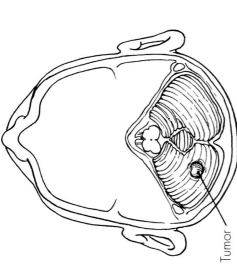

Tumor

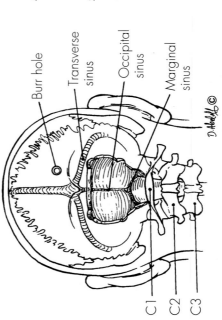

Burr hole

Transverse sinus

Occipital sinus

Marginal sinus

C1
C2
C3

D. Abeld ©

Figure 21-12. Major complications and their solutions for posterior fossa craniectomy and resection of cerebellar tumors.

median metastatic tumors, the risk of air embolism can be minimized by placing the patient in the prone, rather than the sitting position. Lateral tumors can be approached via a lateral suboccipital or retromastoid exposure. Pooling of blood in the surgical field is rarely a problem, because even vascular metastatic lesions are usually well encapsulated. To prevent venous bleeding during craniectomy, the transverse and sigmoid sinuses should not be exposed unless their visualization is necessary for tumor removal. During bony removal, an alert awareness of the location of the sinus can prevent major hemorrhage. Gentle use of a rongeur under the foramen magnum usually prevents the tearing of large veins that drain into the marginal sinus. Resecting the posterior arch of C1 often is not necessary, but if performed, close attention must be paid to protecting the extradural vertebral artery adjacent to the lateral aspect of the arch. Subperiosteal dissection with a finger (rather than with an elevator) effectively exposes the posterior arch and protects the artery. During opening of the dura, the occipital sinus in the midline, the marginal sinus under the foramen magnum, and venous lacunae within the lateral cerebellar convexity dura must be anticipated. A methodical piecemeal bone opening, followed by placement of hemostatic clips along the bleeding dural margins during dural opening, will prevent major blood loss. In some patients, a number of clips may be required, especially at the inferior midline. If the dura is especially tight during opening, a small incision into the dura over the cisterna magna to drain CSF will relax the brain effectively and facilitate further exposure. Routine drainage of CSF from the cisterna magna after dural opening provides regional brain relaxation prior to cerebellar dissection.

A straight, direct route should be taken to the tumor to minimize potential neurological deficits associated with tumor excision. Coagulation and incision into the cerebellar vermis provide a low-morbidity path to midline or paramedian lesions. Incisions of the vermis should spare the two normal veins that course down its surface; an incision often can be made between these two vessels. If exposed, the floor of the fourth ventricle should be protected by cottonoids, to prevent accumulation of blood, which can lead to postoperative hydrocephalus, or local irritation leading to postoperative nausea. A direct approach through the cerebellar hemisphere should be used for more lateral tumors. Circumferential tumor exposure, neoplastic vessel coagulation, and tumor resection or ultrasonic aspiration then should be performed.

The postoperative management of a patient after posterior fossa craniectomy entails the same standard neurosurgical principles as those applied to other patients. Postoperative vigilance can detect any deterioration in neurological status resulting from life-threatening hemorrhage. Reduction in heart rate, change in respiratory pattern, elevation in blood pressure, ipsilateral gaze paresis, or new focal weaknesses may herald deterioration into obtundity and coma and should alert the clinician to the possibility of posterior fossa hemorrhage, edema, infarction, or hydrocephalus. A spinal needle inserted through the previously placed burr hole provides life-saving CSF drainage and relief of intracranial pressure until more definitive measures are performed (e.g., reopening of the wound or placement of a formal ventriculostomy). When less rapid signs of deterioration are seen, an immediate CT scan should be performed, treatment then being dictated by the CT findings.

Shunt Placement

The placement of a shunt (usually ventriculoperitoneal) never should be considered innocuous. Although it is technically less challenging than many other procedures, the indications for CSF diversion should be weighed against predicted life expectancy and expected symptomatic benefit. Patients who have advanced systemic metastases or multiple brain metastases and a life expectancy of 1 month or less may not warrant any surgical procedure, including shunt placement. The indication for shunt placement in a patient with a metastatic brain tumor should be to treat symptomatic hydrocephalus resulting from tumor(s) not amenable to surgical resection.

Complications directly attributable to shunt placement include intracerebral hemorrhage, CSF or wound infection, thoracic or abdominal viscous laceration, shunt blockage, and subdural hematoma. Although relatively rare, upward herniation of the cerebellum has been reported to occur after lateral ventricular CSF diversion in patients with posterior fossa tumors.[73] This herniation can lead to new neurological deficits (often of ocular motility) from compression of brain tissue at the tentorial notch. Intratumoral hemorrhage also can occur after a major change in CSF pressure dynamics.[42,84,93] Aseptic technique, perioperative antibiotics, accurate insertion of the catheter into the frontal horn of the lateral ventricle, controlled passage of the connecting instrument, and adequate abdominal exposure will reduce or eliminate most of these complications. Most surgeons choose a medium-pressure system to prevent overdrainage. Patients are mobilized slowly over the first 3 days after insertion to reduce the incidence of low-pressure headache or CSF over-drainage.

Peritoneal seeding from malignant intracranial cells through the ventriculoperitoneal shunt system is a theoretical risk. We believe that this risk alone does not preclude shunt placement. The use of a millipore filter to prevent passage of malignant cells has been advocated,[35] but its role remains unclear. We do not use a CSF filter device routinely.

ADJUVANT THERAPY

Fractionated Radiotherapy

Fractionated external-beam radiotherapy is the most common treatment method used for patients with metastatic brain tumors. Conventional radiation doses of approximately 3,000 cGy delivered over 10 to 12 fractions are used regardless of specific number of tumors or their histological diagnosis.[17] Although treatment of all kinds generally is withheld when a patient is in a deteriorating terminal condition, radiotherapy can be offered to many patients as a noninvasive treatment method to prolong survival and hopefully improve quality of life. Hagen and colleagues demonstrated that radiation therapy provided better central nervous system tumor control than did conservative management[30]; nonetheless, the 1-year survival rates remain modest.[17,75,88,92]

Analysis of the 30-day morbidity and mortality after fractionated irradiation may provide more information about treatment failure than about treatment complications. Patchell et al.[63] reported that 17 percent of patients had complications, and 4 percent died during the first 30 days after conventional radiotherapy. Radiation-induced injuries of the brain have been detected in patients with extended survival.[52,79] For example, Lishner and colleagues[45] described late complications in 19 percent of 48 patients with lung cancer patients who received prophylactic CNS irradiation; dementia developed in two patients and focal deficits of motor or visual pathways developed in seven. Some of these patients also received chemotherapy. Despite such long-term complications, the authors concluded that prophylactic irradiation should still be used as part of the combined treatment approach in patients who responded well to treatment of their primary lung disease. Griffin and associates[28] also were able to define the benefit of prophylactic cranial irradiation in a series of patients with non-small cell lung cancer. DeAngelis and coworkers[15] observed radiation-induced dementia in 12 patients within 5 to 36 months of radiotherapy (whole-brain doses of 2,900 to 3,900 cGy were delivered in 10 fractions of 300 to 600 cGy). These patients had progressive cognitive dysfunction, ataxia, and urinary incontinence, yet had no evidence of tumor recurrence. The authors suggested that patients in good neurological condition with control of systemic disease should receive reduced doses per fraction of 120 to 200 cGy to a total dose of 4,000 to 4,500 cGy, to improve the safety of treatment in patients who might be expected to have a relatively long survival.

Management options are limited for complications related to whole-brain fractionated radiotherapy. If radiation-induced edema is present, a course of corticosteroid medication is appropriate. Shunting may correct symptoms arising from delayed onset of hydrocephalus. Unfortunately, most dementias and cranial neuropathies are not reversible. The delayed observation on imaging studies of contrast enhancement in the region of treatment or at the site of tumor does not always indicate radiation necrosis or tumor recurrence. Schnittker et al.[71] reported that the biopsy of a radiodense lesion at a site treated 26 months earlier by fractionated technique revealed nonspecific cells and reactive change without viable tumor.

To treat tumors that recur after radiotherapy, some institutions boost the original fractionated irradiation dose in an attempt to reduce tumor regrowth. Cooper and colleagues[14] studied the value of reirradiation in patients whose tumors recurred after receiving an initial 3,000 cGy whole-brain course. Following a second course of 2,500 cGy in 10 fractions, they noted "response" in 42 percent of patients; their mean survival was 5 months. Hazuka and Kinzie[32] reported on 44 patients who underwent reirradiation consisting of total whole-brain doses of 600 to 3,600 cGy delivered in fractions of 200 to 400 cGy. Mean survival after the second course was only 8 weeks. Because only 27 percent of patients showed improvement in neurological status or quality of life after the second treatment, they concluded that such retreatment was seldom worthwhile.

Brachytherapy

Brachytherapy has been used sparingly for the adjuvant treatment of brain metastases. The stereotactic implantation of a radioactive isotope is designed to deliver a localized boost to previously administered fractionated radiation therapy, while maintaining a fall-off in dose outside the imaging-defined tumor margin.[4] Brachytherapy generally is restricted to solitary supratentorial tumors that are less than 6 cm in diameter, do not cross the midline, and do not show subependymal tumor spread. Prados and colleagues[65] treated 14 patients with metastases treated using iodine-125 brachytherapy. They reported that patients survived a median of 80 weeks and suggested that brachytherapy may provide symptomatic improvement and longer survival. Most of their patients were treated at the time of tumor recurrence (4 to 16 months after initial treatment). Heros et al.[34] reported on three patients treated with iridium-195 (tumor dose of 6,000 cGy), noting long-term survival in two patients with breast cancer. One patient underwent resection of a mass at the site of brachytherapy; radionecrosis was found on histological examination. Because surgical resection is a valuable option for many patients with solitary brain metastases, the role of brachytherapy remains limited.

Complications from brachytherapy include intratumoral or intracerebral hemorrhage from catheter insertion and delayed radionecrosis (months after treatment).[4,65] Radiation necrosis is difficult to confirm with CT or MRI, but positron emission tomography may help in the future. In some patients, radionecrosis can be diagnosed only after biopsy. Resection may be necessary if corticosteroid therapy fails to control the surrounding edema.

Stereotactic Radiosurgery

In an attempt to deliver a tumoricidal focal boost of radiation, reduce hospital stays, avoid craniotomy, and prolong survival, we have used stereotactic radiosurgery in 42 patients with solitary brain metastases. Mean survival after radiosurgery in our initial review (first 3-year experience), was 9.3 months. Most patients had stabilization or improvement of their neurological symptoms.[11,49] Only three patients in this series demonstrated tumor growth and required later tumor resection. Reduction in the amount of surrounding edema (Fig. 21-13) was seen in most patients within 3 months; in a similar number of patients, the treated tumor disappeared completely (Fig. 21-14). In contrast to our experience with both vascular malformations and benign brain tumors, neither perilesional edema nor worsening of focal deficits has developed to date in any patient with a metastasis.[50] This difference in results may be due to the limited length of survival after treatment of metastases. We performed radiosurgery in combination with whole-brain radiation therapy in order to treat potential tumor deposits outside the imaging-defined tumor margin. Two of our patients, both with

renal cell carcinoma, refused to undergo fractionated radiotherapy.

Loeffler and associates[46] evaluated the radiosurgical treatment using a modified linear accelerator in 18 patients with a total of 21 intracranial metastases, most of which were recurrent. The median interval between radiotherapy and radiosurgery was 10 months. Although no new neurological deficits occurred in follow-up, four patients had increased deep white matter edema and exacerbation of deficits; corticosteroid therapy was successful for these complications. A small region of alopecia developed transiently in two patients after the treatment of peripheral lesions (dose to scalp was 400 cGy). We have reduced the occurrence of focal alopecia by injecting a 10- to 20-ml deposit of saline below the galea, to move the scalp further from even low radiation doses. Sturm and colleagues[78] reported that one patient died of increased edema and herniation 15 hours after linear accelerator radiosurgery for a cerebellar metastasis. This tumor was large (42-mm diameter) and had been treated with a dose of 25 Gy to the tumor margin, an excessive dose considering the tumor volume and location. It is hoped that dose-volume analyses,[22,23] currently being conducted at several centers, will reduce radiation-induced complications after radiosurgery.

Chemotherapy

A wide range of chemotherapy protocols have been used to provide additional treatment to patients with brain metastases. Acute complications related to chemotherapy are well known and include nausea and vomiting; subacute problems include pancytopenia, peripheral or cranial neuropathy, and specific organ dysfunction depending on the agent used. Treatment failure is related to poor central nervous system delivery,[24] a limited ability to penetrate the blood-brain barrier,[61] a high toxicity-effect ratio, or poor tumoricidal activity. In an attempt to overcome some of these limitations, blood-brain barrier modification and agent delivery with tumor-specific monoclonal antibodies have been used.[61] Intra-arterial chemotherapy has been given to treat malignant brain tumors.[37] Stewart and associates[76] assessed the effects after intra-arterial administration of BCNU, VM-26, and cisplatin combined with systemic chemotherapy. Manifestations of toxicity included myelosuppression (severe in 22 percent), moderate to severe pain (25 percent), nausea and vomiting (24 percent), transient neurological deficits (31 percent),

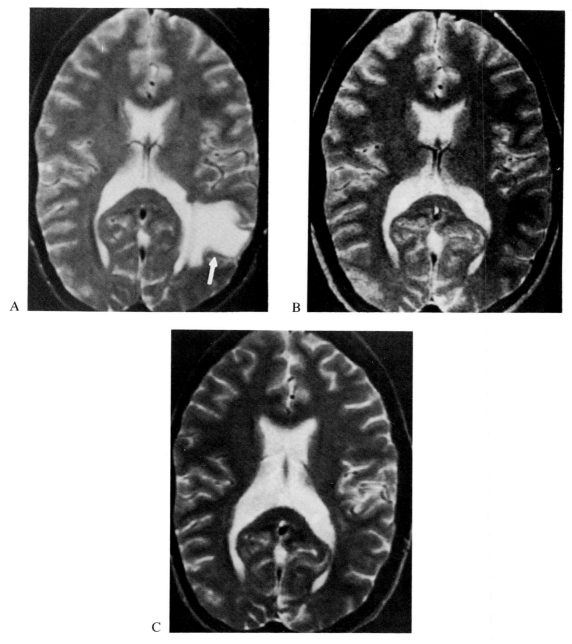

Figure 21-13. Serial MRI (T$_2$ spin-echo) **(A)** before, **(B)** 4 months after, and **(C)** 7 months after stereotactic radiosurgery for a left parietal metastatic melanoma. Resolution of the peritumoral edema (*arrow*) and normalization of the cortical sulcal pattern are demonstrated.

permanent neurological deficits (11 percent), and one instance of carotid occlusion. It is not known whether superselective catherization can reduce the incidence of complications seen with infraclinoid internal carotid arterial injections, especially to the optic nerve. The overall role of localized intra-arterial chemotherapy for metastatic tumors remains to be defined.

Intraventricular chemotherapy delivery using a ventricular reservoir system occasionally is used to treat patients with leptomeningeal metastases. Diffuse necrotizing leukoencephalopathy was noted in 9

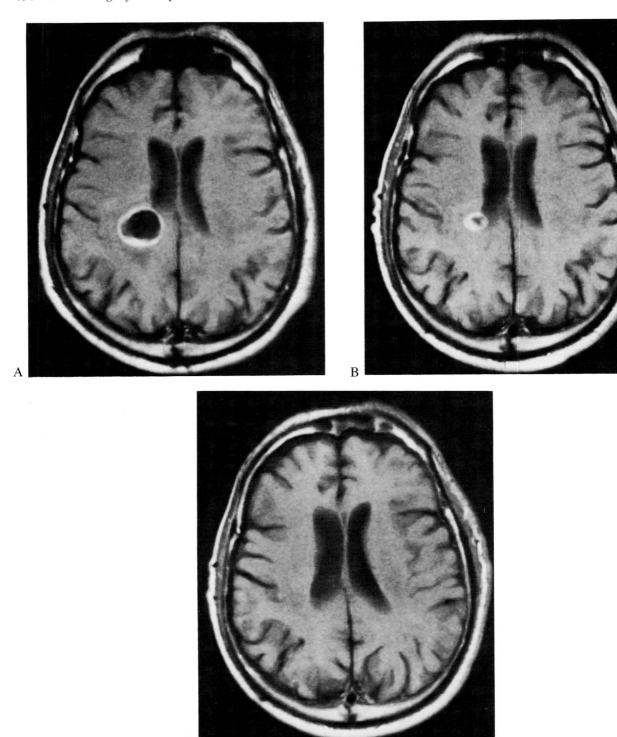

Figure 21-14. Serial MRI (T_1 spin-echo with gadolinium-DTPA) demonstrating a parietal tumor adjacent to the right lateral ventricle. **(A)** Stereotactic biopsy confirmed this to be a metastatic carcinoma of unknown origin. **(B)** The tumor was smaller 5 weeks after treatment, and **(C)** was completely gone 8 months after treatment, which consisted of radiosurgery (16 Gy to the tumor margin) combined with fractionated radiation therapy. The surrounding brain appears normal after treatment.

of 14 patients with meningeal carcinomatosis from breast cancer who survived for more than 4 months after receiving intraventricular methotrexate (including all of 4 patients who also received whole-brain radiation therapy).[6] A case of fatal methotrexate neurotoxicity was reported by ten Hoeve and Twijnstra.[83]

SUMMARY: MANAGEMENT STRATEGIES AND COMPLICATIONS

Limited options are available for patients who have multiple brain metastases. Commonly, the lesions are not anatomically contiguous such that a single craniotomy and local resection would suffice (Fig. 21-15). For patients in reasonably good clinical condition, whole-brain radiotherapy is an acceptable method for treating detected and as yet undetected tumor deposits. Although stereotactic radiosurgery has had limited use as a noninvasive treatment for multiple tumors,[46] perhaps it will have a greater role in carefully chosen patients. An algorithm for the management of patients with solitary brain metastases is presented in Figure 21-16. Patients in poor systemic and/or neurological condition who have a terminal prognosis should receive palliative care only. The administration of oral corticosteroid therapy in itself does not increase survival beyond 1 or 2 months.[5] However, it has proved effective in the short-term control of symptoms so that further treatment can be administered. On the other hand, prolonged steroid therapy can cause some major complications, notably Cushing syndrome, peptic ulcer disease and gastritis, hypertension, salt and water retention, impaired wound healing, and immunosuppression. The onset of proximal myopathy can be particularly devastating in a patient who is already compromised from tumor-related motor deficits. To avert these complications, steroid doses should be tapered or eliminated when symptoms stabilize.

Solitary brain metastases located in regions suitable for resection are often treated by craniotomy and excision followed by fractionated external-beam radiation therapy (3,000 cGy). This combination of treatments has been relatively effective in prolonging survival and maintaining quality of life.[63] The most significant complication after such treatment is delayed recurrent intracranial tumor, either at the site of previous resection or at a distant location. Recurrent solitary tumors can be treated again, either by surgical excision (if the patient remains in satisfactory neurological condition) or by repeated irradia-

tion. Stereotactic radiosurgery may be an excellent alternative to craniotomy as first-line treatment of solitary metastases and is probably a safer method of reirradiation because of its focused delivery with steep fall-off in dose outside the tumor margin. The repeated administration of localized fractionated radiation therapy can also be considered. Other adjuvant techniques such as systemic or intra-arterial chemotherapy or hyperthermia[81] should be performed as part of institutional protocols; their overall role requires further study.

Another potential complication after craniotomy and radiation therapy is the development of radiation necrosis in surrounding normal tissue. This complication has been detected most often in patients who survive more than 12 months after treatment. Although cerebral radionecrosis can be difficult to differentiate from recurrent tumor with conventional imaging, its presence can be suggested by positron emission tomography but can be confirmed only by tissue biopsy. Localized radionecrosis may require resection. Necrotic regions that are large or those in critical locations are treated by systemic corticosteroid therapy.

For tumors located in brain locations unsuitable for resection, or for those in patients who are medically unfit or who decline craniotomy, fractionated radiation therapy should be considered, up to a total dose of approximately 3,000 cGy. Various protocols add the use of localized boost radiation to the tumor, through the secondary use of either radiosurgery or brachytherapy. For solitary tumors less than 3 cm in diameter, we advocate boost radiosurgery, in a dose of 16 Gy (delivered to the tumor margin). In this setting, radiosurgery is used to achieve the additional local tumor control that craniotomy gives to fractionated irradiation (both prolonging survival and improving quality of life). For larger tumors, brachytherapy can be considered, although the proportion of patients who will benefit is unknown. Complications related to radiation treatment alone are similar to those that occur when administered after craniotomy. The problem of recurrent tumor can be addressed by surgical excision, additional radiosurgery, or a boost dose of radiation delivered by either fractionated technique or brachytherapy. Intracavitary irradiation for cystic tumors also has had a minor role in treating recurrent metastases.

Overall, the care of patients with brain metastases still remains a challenging field of therapy. Multimodality treatment including surgery, radiation therapy, radiosurgery, or chemotherapy may further improve survival. Astute clinicians will plan their treatment strategies carefully and anticipate common treatment

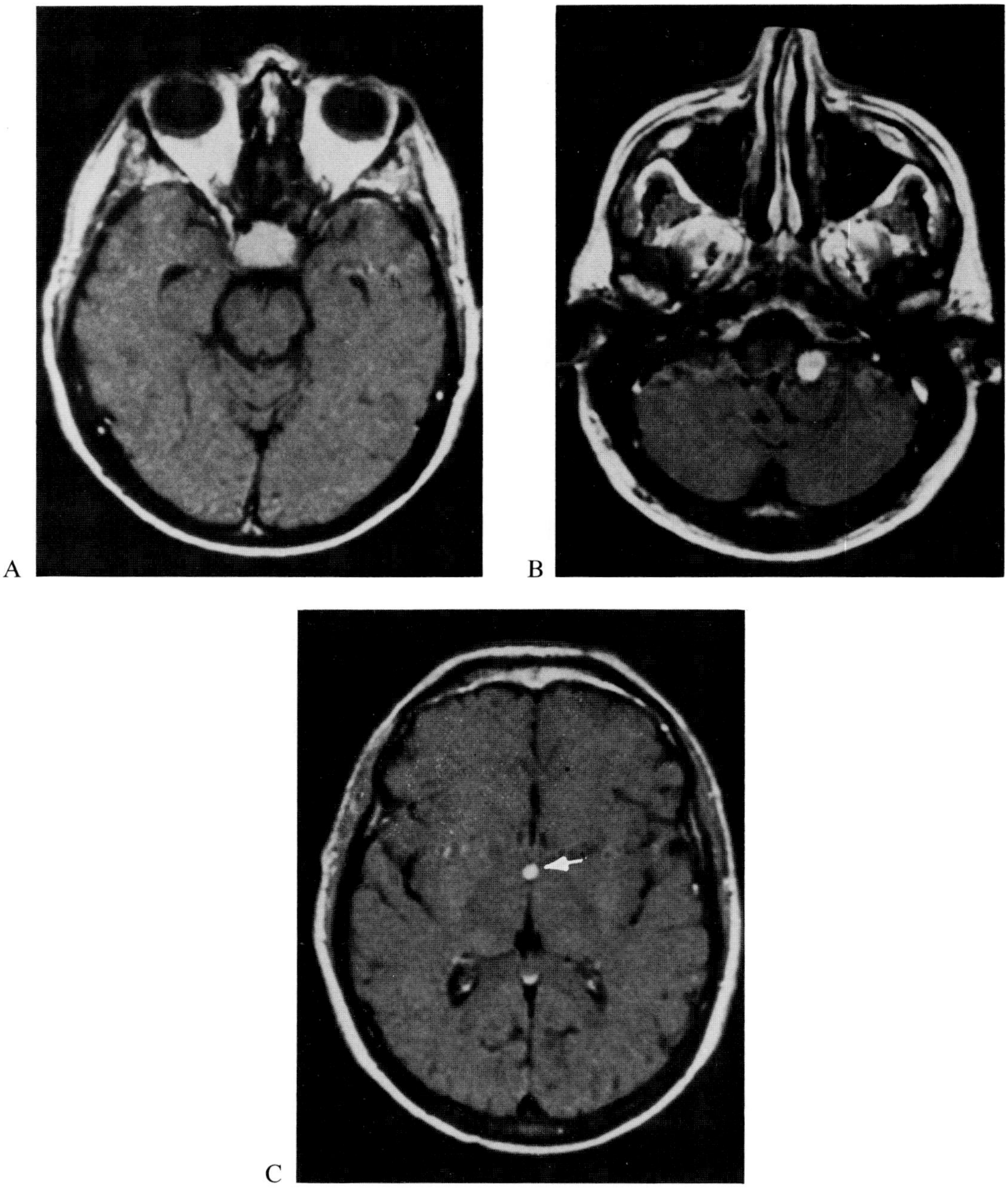

Figure 21-15. Multiple brain metastases: **(A)** Pituitary gland, **(B)** cerebellar peduncle, and **(C)** third ventricle. All were treated with stereotactic radiosurgery in a patient with renal cell carcinoma.

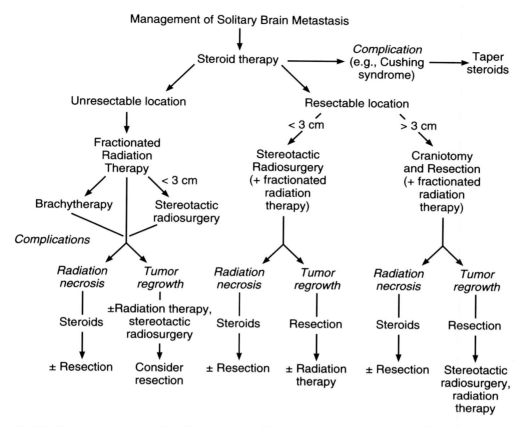

Figure 21-16. Management algorithm for patients with solitary brain metastases, including strategies for treating complications.

pitfalls, while remaining prepared to address management complications.

REFERENCES

1. Ambiavagar PC, Sher J: Subdural hematoma secondary to metastatic neoplasm. Cancer 42:2015, 1978
2. Apuzzo MLJ, Chandrasoma PT, Cohen DM et al: Computed imaging stereotaxy: experience and perspective related to 500 procedures applied to brain masses. Neurosurgery 20:930, 1987
3. Balachandran S, Husain MH, Adametz JR et al: Uptake of indium-111-labeled leukocytes by brain metastases. Neurosurgery 20:606, 1987
4. Bernstein M, Laperriere N, Leung P et al: Interstitial brachytherapy for malignant brain tumors: preliminary results. Neurosurgery 26:371, 1990
5. Black P: Brain metastases: current status and recommended guidelines for management. Neurosurgery 5:617, 1979
6. Boogerd W, Sande JJ, Moffie D: Acute fever and delayed leukoencephalopathy following low dose intraventricular methotrexate. J Neurol Neurosurg Psychiatry 51:1277, 1988
7. Braun EM, Burger LJ, Schlang HA: Subdural hematoma from metastatic malignant disease. Cancer 32:1370, 1973
8. Bremer AM, West CR, Didolkar MS: An evaluation of the surgical management of melanoma of the brain. J Surg Oncol 10:211, 1978
9. Chadduck WM, Roycroft D, Brown MW: Multicentric glioma as a cause of multiple cerebral lesions. Neurosurgery 13:170, 1983
10. Ciricillo SF, Rosenblum ML: Use of CT and MR imaging to distinguish intracranial lesions and define the need for biopsy in AIDS patients. J Neurosurg 73:720, 1990
11. Coffey RJ, Flickinger JC, Bissonette DJ et al: Radiosurgery for brain metastases using the cobalt-60 gamma unit: methods and results in 24 patients. Int J Radiat Oncol Biol Phys 20:1287, 1991
12. Coffey RJ, Lunsford LD: Stereotactic surgery for mass lesions of the midbrain and pons. Neurosurgery 17:12, 1985
13. Cohen N, Strauss G, Lew R et al: Should prophylactic anticonvulsants be administered to patients with newly diagnosed cerebral metastases? A retrospective study. J Clin Oncol 6:1621, 1988
14. Cooper JS, Steinfeld AD, Lerch IA: Cerebral metastases: value of re-irradiation in selected patients. Radiology 174:883, 1990
15. DeAngelis LM, Delattre Y, Posner JB: Radiation-induced dementia in patients cured of brain metastases. Neurology 39:789, 1989

16. Delattre Y, Krol G, Thaler HT et al: Distribution of brain metastases. Arch Neurol 45:741, 1988

17. Deutsch M, Parsons JA, Mercado R: Radiotherapy for intracranial metastases. Cancer 34:1607, 1974

18. Deviri E, Schachner A, Halevy A et al: Carcinoma of the lung with a solitary cerebral metastasis. Surgical management and review of the literature. Cancer 52:1507, 1983

19. Dolan EJ: Danger of use of hydrogen peroxide in stereotactic biopsies. Appl Neurophysiol 50:237, 1987

20. Feindel W, Perot P: Red cerebral veins. A report on arteriovenous shunts in tumors and cerebral scars. J Neurosurg 22:315, 1965

21. Fernandez E, Maira G, Puca A et al: Multiple intracranial metastases of malignant melanoma with long-term survival. J Neurosurg 60:621, 1984

22. Flickinger JC: An integrated logistic formula for prediction of complications from radiosurgery. Int J Radiat Oncol Biol Phys 17:879, 1989

23. Flickinger JC, Lunsford LD, Kondziolka D: Dose-volume considerations in radiosurgery. Stereotact Funct Neurosurg 57:99, 1991

24. Front D, Even-Sapir E, Iosilevsky G et al: Monitoring of Co-57-bleomycin delivery to brain metastases and their tumors of origin. J Neurosurg 67:506, 1987

25. Galicich JH, Sundaresan N: Metastatic brain tumors. p. 597. In Wilkins RH, Rengachary SS (eds): Neurosurgery. McGraw-Hill, New York, 1985

26. Galicich JH, Sundaresan N, Thaler HT: Surgical treatment of single brain metastases. Evaluation of results by computerized tomography scanning. J Neurosurg 53:63, 1980

27. Goldstein S, Neuwelt EA: Superior sensitivity of computed tomographic scanning to magnetic resonance imaging in metastatic neoplasia: two case reports. Neurosurgery 20:959, 1987

28. Griffin BR, Livingston RB, Stewart GR et al: Prophylactic cranial irradiation for limited non-small cell lung cancer. Cancer 62:36, 1988

29. Haar F, Patterson RH: Surgery for metastatic intracranial neoplasm. Cancer 30:1241, 1972

30. Hagen NH, Cirrincione C, Thaler HT et al: The role of radiation therapy following resection of single brain metastasis from melanoma. Neurology 40:158, 1990

31. Haines SJ: Efficacy of antibiotic prophylaxis in clean neurosurgical operations. Neurosurgery 24:401, 1989

32. Hazuka MB, Kinzie JJ: Brain metastases: results and effects of re-irradiation. Int J Radiat Oncol Biol Phys 15:433, 1988

33. Hendrickson FR, Lee MS, Larson M et al: The influence of surgery and radiation therapy on patients with brain metastases. Int J Radiat Oncol Biol Phys 9:623, 1983

34. Heros DO, Kasdon DL, Chun M: Brachytherapy in the treatment of recurrent solitary brain metastasis. Neurosurgery 23:733, 1988

35. Hoffman HJ, Hendrick EB, Humphreys RP: Metastasis via ventriculoperitoneal shunt in patients with medulloblastoma. J Neurosurg 44:562, 1976

36. Horwitz NH, Rizzoli HV: Postoperative Complications of Intracranial Neurological Surgery. Williams & Wilkins, Baltimore, 1982

37. Johnson DW, Parkinson D, Wolpert SM et al: Intracarotid chemotherapy with 1,3-bis(2-chloroethyl)-1-nitrosourea (BCNU) in 5% dextrose in water in the treatment of malignant glioma. Neurosurgery 20:577, 1987

38. Kelly PJ, Kall BA, Goerss SJ: Results of computed tomography-based computer-assisted stereotactic resection of metastatic intracranial tumors. Neurosurgery 22:7, 1988

39. Killebrew K, Krigman M, Mahaley MS et al: Metastatic renal cell carcinoma mimicking a meningioma. Neurosurgery 13:430, 1983

40. Kindt GW: The pattern of location of cerebral metastatic tumors. J Neurosurg 21:54, 1964

41. Kofman S, Garvin JS, Nagamani D et al: Treatment of cerebral metastases from breast carcinoma with prednisolone. JAMA 163:1473, 1957

42. Kondziolka D, Bernstein M, Resch L et al: Significance of hemorrhage into brain tumors: clinicopathological study. J Neurosurg 67:852, 1987

43. Kondziolka D, Bernstein M, Resch L et al: Brain tumors presenting as TIAs and strokes. Can Family Physician 34:283, 1988

44. Leech RW, Welch FT, Ojemann GA: Subdural hematoma secondary to metastatic dural carcinomatosis. J Neurosurg 41:610, 1974

45. Lishner M, Feld R, Payne DG et al: Late neurological complications after prophylactic cranial irradiation in patients with small-cell lung cancer: the Toronto experience. J Clin Oncol 8:215, 1990

46. Loeffler JS, Kooy HM, Wen PY et al: The treatment of recurrent brain metastases with stereotactic radiosurgery. J Clin Oncol 8:576, 1990

47. Lopez-Pousa S, Ojeda B, Lopez-Lopez JJ: The correlation between clinical symptomatology and computerized tomography in brain metastases secondary to breast and lung neoplasias. Comput Tomog 5:17, 1981

48. Lunsford LD, Coffey RJ, Cojocaru T et al: Image-guided stereotactic surgery: a 10-year evolutionary experience. Stereotact Funct Neurosurg 54+55:375, 1990

49. Lunsford LD, Flickinger JC, Coffey RJ: Stereotactic gamma knife radiosurgery: initial North American experience in 207 patients. Arch Neurol 47:169, 1990

50. Lunsford LD, Kondziolka D, Flickinger JC: Stereotactic radiosurgery: current spectrum and results. Clin Neurosurg 38:405, 1992

51. Lunsford LD, Listerud JA, Rowberg AH et al: Stereotactic software for the GE 8800 CT scanner. Neurol Res 9:118, 1987

52. Madajewicz S, Karakousis C, West CR et al: Malignant melanoma brain metastases. Review of Roswell Park Memorial Institute experience. Cancer 53:2550, 1984

53. Mandell L, Hilaris B, Sullivan M et al: The treatment of single brain metastasis from non-oat cell lung carcinoma. Cancer 58:641, 1986

54. Mandybur TI: Intracranial hemorrhage caused by metastatic tumors. Neurology 27:650, 1977

55. Mansfield JB: Dural invasion by Hodgkin's disease. Neurosurgery 11:808, 1982

56. Maor M, Frias AE, Oswald MJ: Palliative radiotherapy for brain metastasis in renal carcinoma. Cancer 62:1912, 1988

57. McCann WP, Weir BKA, Elvidge AR: Long-term survival after removal of metastatic malignant melanoma of the brain. J Neurosurg 28:483, 1968

58. Merchut MP: Brain metastases from undiagnosed systemic neoplasms. Arch Intern Med 149:1076, 1989

59. Meyer PC, Reah TG: Secondary neoplasms of the central nervous system and meninges. Br J Cancer 7:438, 1953

60. Moore MR, Black PM, Ellenbogen R et al: Stereotactic craniotomy: methods and results using the Brown-Roberts-Wells stereotactic frame. Neurosurgery 25:572, 1989

61. Neuwelt EA, Specht HD, Barnett PA et al: Increased delivery of tumor-specific monoclonal antibodies to brain after osmotic blood-brain barrier modification in patients with melanoma metastatic to the central nervous system. Neurosurgery 20:885, 1987

62. Patchell RA, Cirrincione C, Thaler HT et al: Single brain metastases: surgery plus radiation or radiation alone. Neurology 36:447, 1986

63. Patchell RA, Tibbs PA, Walsh JW et al: A randomized trial of surgery in the treatment of single metastases to the brain. N Engl J Med 322:494, 1990

64. Posner JB: Management of central nervous system metastases. Semin Oncol 4:81, 1977

65. Prados M, Leibel S, Barnett CM et al: Interstitial brachytherapy for metastatic brain tumors. Cancer 63:657, 1989

66. Pritchard PB, Martinez RA, Hungerford GD et al: Dural plasmacytoma. Neurosurgery 12:576, 1983

67. Ransohoff J: Surgical management of metastatic tumors. Semin Oncol 2:21, 1975

68. Richards P, McKissock W: Intracranial metastases. Br Med J 1:15, 1963

69. Rigamonti D, Dryer BP, Johnson PC et al: The MRI appearance of cavernous malformations (angiomas). J Neurosurg 67:518, 1987

70. Rosenfeld JV, Murphy MA, Chow CW: Implantation metastasis of pineoblastoma after stereotactic biopsy. J Neurosurg 73:287, 1990

71. Schnittker JB, Thomas HG, Johns RD et al: Late appearance of a radiodense lesion at the site of an irradiated metastasis: neuropathological findings. Neurosurgery 23:785, 1988

72. Schoenberg B, Christine BW, Whisnant JP: Nervous system neoplasms and primary malignancies of other sites. The unique association between meningiomas and breast cancer. Neurology 25:705, 1975

73. Schut L, Bruce DA, Sutton LN: Medulloblastomas. p. 758. In Wilkins RH, Rengachary SS (eds): Neurosurgery. McGraw-Hill, New York, 1985

74. Simionescu M: Metastatic tumors of the brain. A follow-up study of 195 patients with neurosurgical considerations. J Neurosurg 17:361, 1960

75. Sorensen JB, Hansen HH, Hansen M et al: Brain metastases in adenocarcinoma of the lung: frequency, risk groups, and prognosis. J Clin Oncol 6:1474, 1988

76. Stewart DJ, Grahovac Z, Hugenholtz H et al: Combined intraarterial and systemic chemotherapy for intracerebral tumors. Neurosurgery 21:207, 1987

77. Stortebecker TB: Metastatic tumors of the brain from a neurosurgical point of view. A follow-up study of 158 cases. J Neurosurg 11:84, 1954

78. Sturm V, Kober B, Hover KH et al: Stereotactic percutaneous single dose irradiation of brain metastases with a linear accelerator. Int J Radiat Oncol Biol Phys 13:279, 1987

79. Sundaresan N, Galicich JH, Beattie EJ: Surgical treatment of brain metastases from lung cancer. J Neurosurg 58:666, 1983

80. Sundaresan N, Sachdev VP, DiGiacinto GV et al: Reoperation from brain metastases. J Clin Oncol 6:1625, 1988

81. Tanaka R, Kim CH, Yamada N et al: Radiofrequency hyperthermia for malignant brain tumors: preliminary results of clinical trials. Neurosurgery 21:478, 1987

82. Taylor HG, Lefkowitz M, Skoog SJ: Intracranial metastases in prostate cancer. Cancer 53:2728, 1984

83. ten Hoeve RFA, Twijnstra A: A lethal neurotoxic reaction after intraventricular methotrexate administration. Cancer 62:2111, 1988

84. Vaquero J, Cabezudo JM, DeSola RG et al: Intratumoral hemorrhage in posterior fossa tumors after ventricular drainage. J Neurosurg 54:406, 1981

85. Vieth RG, Odom GL: Intracranial metastases and their neurosurgical treatment. J Neurosurg 23:375, 1965

86. Weber P, Shepard KV, Vijaykumar S: Metastases to pineal gland. Cancer 63:164, 1989

87. White KR, Fleming TR, Laws ER: Single metastasis to the brain. Surgical treatment in 122 consecutive patients. Mayo Clin Proc 56:424, 1981

88. Winston KR, Walsh JW, Fischer EG: Results of operative treatment of intracranial metastatic tumors. Cancer 45:2639, 1980

89. Wright DC: Metastatic brain tumors. Contemp Neurosurg 12:1, 1990

90. Yardeni D, Reichenthal E, Zucker G et al: Neurosurgical management of single brain metastasis. Surg Neurol 21:377, 1984

91. Zager EL, Hedley-White ET: Metastasis within a pituitary adenoma presenting with bilateral abducens palsies: case report and review of the literature. Neurosurgery 21:383, 1987

92. Zimm S, Wampler GL, Stablein D et al: Intracerebral metastases in solid-tumor patients: natural history and results of treatment. Cancer 48:384, 1981

93. Zuccarello M, Dollo C, Carollo C: Spontaneous intratumoral hemorrhage after ventriculoperitoneal shunting. Neurosurgery 16:245, 1985

$\mathcal{22}$ Visual System Tumors

Optic Gliomas

Robin P. Humphreys

LITERATURE REVIEW

The therapeutic choices for patients with gliomas of the visual system are to a large degree arbitrary and uncertain.[1,12] Treatment recommendations for such patients range from expectant observation to operative exploration and biopsy or nerve-tumor resection, to chemotherapy and irradiation adjunctive therapy, or to any combination of these. Much effort has thus been devoted to analyzing the specific treatment goals for these patients, so that the techniques of optic nerve tumor surgery and its complications have received less emphasis. Hence, some major reviews of this problem make no specific mention of operative complications.[1,4,8,11,12,13]

Those reports that document postoperative complications individually span years of experience. In retrospect, some authors acknowledge that mortality and severe complications occurred at times when operative and anesthetic techniques were far less sophisticated than at present. Deaths have occurred after optic nerve and chiasm tumor surgery, in one series reaching 25 percent.[6,9,10] The complications encountered after craniotomy for optic nerve tumor include all those that might be anticipated—postoperative visual deterioration, ptosis, strabismus, pulsating exophthalamos, meningitis, spinal fluid fistula, denervation of the ocular globe, ophthalmic artery injury and seizure disorder.[3,5,7,9,15] At the very least all patients will experience swelling of the eyelids, which resolves in 2 weeks,[3] and some will have postoperative ptosis or strabismus.[3,5,7] Denervation

of the globe is a rare complication but may necessitate later enucleation of the eye.[5]

This chapter reviews the complications associated with operative care for the patient with an optic nerve glioma. It is presumed that the tumor involves one optic nerve only and that operation is being undertaken because of completely failed vision or ipsilateral and/or progressive proptosis.

OPERATIVE TECHNIQUES

While preoperative neuroimaging will beautifully outline the tumor and its distortion of the optic nerve (Fig. 22-1), what may not be clear is the juxtaposition of the tumor with the ocular globe and its infiltrative relationship to the adjacent chiasm. Hence the surgeon in the preoperative counseling session may have to qualify the operative intent of "total tumor removal" by intraoperative decisions based on the visible and histopathological extent of the tumor. For example, when embarking on a course of action that will render the patient blind in one eye, the surgeon should be quite reluctant to sacrifice a portion of the chiasm or the contralateral crossing knee fibers, creating appropriate field defects relative to the other eye, simply to accomplish a complete removal of the tumor.

Computed tomography (CT) and magnetic resonance imaging (MRI) studies, in addition to detailing the features of the optic nerve and tumor, will show the optic canal and its size, the relationship of the

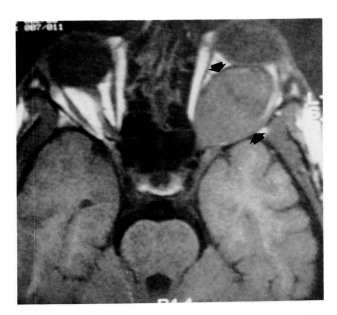

Figure 22-1. Axial MRI of optic nerve tumor (*arrows*) distorting globe and causing slight proptosis.

extraocular muscle cone to the tumor, the size and position of the ethmoid air cells, and the cavernous sinus. Tumor invasion of any of these structures should be recognized beforehand so that the hazards of cerebrospinal fluid (CSF) fistula and infection and untoward bleeding can be avoided.

Patients should be advised that immediately prior to anesthetic induction they will be asked to identify their "bad" eye to the operating team, especially if they do not have an obvious orbital or ocular deformity. The forehead can then be marked appropriately to confirm the side for craniotomy.

The neurosurgical approach to the optic nerve tumor is via a frontal craniotomy ipsilateral to the tumor and a subfrontal extradural and intradural exposure of the orbital roof, the optic canal, and the opticochiasmatic junction and adjacent carotid artery. The advantage of this exploration is that it permits resection of "tumor-bearing nerve from the globe to the chiasm" while preserving the globe for cosmesis.[5] Some right-handed surgeons may prefer to approach a left nerve tumor from the patient's right side, and such a maneuver may work; however, the initial exposure does threaten the right olfactory bulb in a situation such that the left bulb or tract may be jeopardized at a later stage in the dissection. In addition, an unnecessary amount of the chiasm and normal right optic nerve remain exposed during the dissection and tumor removal, leaving them vulnerable to damage by drying or by the passage of instruments.

The patient is best positioned supine with head held in the midaxial posture (Fig. 22-2A). Some surgeons when approaching the right parasellar structures prefer to rotate the head to the patient's left in the belief that such will bring the optic nerve and internal carotid artery "up into the field." Such a maneuver may distort the viewing of the usual anatomical planes and potentially camouflage the chiasm, which is now thrown backward out of view. It could also contribute to the skidding of bone removal instruments, which may take the orbitotomy and canal decompression more medial than was desired.

As the tumor exploration will require visualization of the chiasm and proximal portion of the opposite optic nerve, the surgeon must turn the craniotomy across the midline (Fig. 22-2B). Some surgeons may choose to include the supraorbital rim in the craniotomy too.[8] In any patient over 10 years of age, the craniotomy places the frontal air sinus in the flap, and so the usual maneuvers are carried out to isolate and cover the sinus with a pericranial flap at the conclusion, in order to minimize the risk of CSF leak and meningitis (Fig. 22-2C). However, what may not be apparent until after the fact is inadvertent violation of the ipsilateral posterior ethmoid air sinus during deroofing of the optic canal. These air cells are smaller and more partitioned than those of the frontal sinus and their entry lies close to the ultimate subfrontal and optic nerve dural sheath openings. Should the patient develop signs of CSF leakage postoperatively, with or without complicating meningitis, it must not necessarily be concluded that this has occurred because of problems with the frontal sinus only.

As the target of the procedure lies within the orbital cavity, it is tempting to expose the orbital roof by dissecting across it in the extradural plane. That maneuver is usually accomplished swiftly until the medial and posterior limits of the anterior fossa are reached. Sooner or later, the dura covering the pole or undersurface of the frontal lobe must be opened to expose the intradural portion of the optic nerve and the anterior clinoid process and superior margin of the optic foramen. The dural flap on the brain side can be placed between the brain and the retractor to act as additional protection against brain retractor pressure (Fig. 22-3A). Simultaneously, a decision must be made about the need to sacrifice the ipsilateral olfactory bulb or tract in order to achieve enough retraction of the frontal lobe.

With modern neuroimaging, optic nerve involvement by tumor will be apparent, although intracranial, intradural extension may not be clear. The surgeon is advised to inspect the optic nerve and chiasm

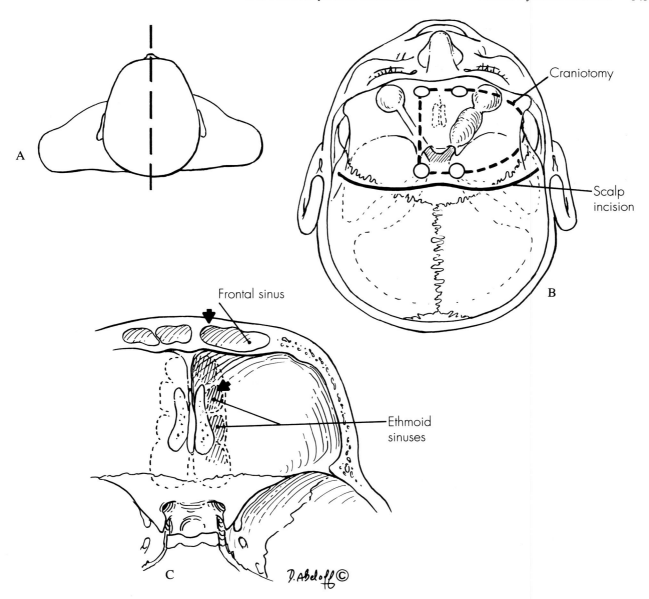

Figure 22-2. (A) Midaxial head positioning. **(B)** Transcoronal scalp flap and right frontal osteoplastic craniotomy taken across midline to the left. **(C)** The ethmoid air sinus is outlined. Its vulnerability during deroofing of the optic canal must be appreciated.

intradurally prior to the orbital exploration. The "lie" of the nerve and the course of the optic canal are determined, and if tumor is evident, the nerve may be sectioned adjacent to the chiasm. When the nerve is cut at the opticochiasmatic junction, the surgeon must remember that the plane of severance is at a right angle to the long axis of the nerve and *not* in the bicoronal dimension across the nerve (Fig. 22-3B). Furthermore, the cut should ideally be placed 6 mm or more beyond the opticochiasmatic junction in order to preserve the looping Willbrand knee fibers.[7]

A lesion affecting the optic nerve just in front of the chiasm may cause a temporal field defect with respect to the opposite eye in addition to the blindness present in the affected eye. The tumor that extends into the intracranial optic nerve may appear gray and "discolored,"[5] but in other cases it may only enlarge and distort the nerve and stretch its surface vasculature.

If the intradural, intracranial nerve appears normal, the orbital roof and optic canal are approached extradurally. While the dura is easily stripped from

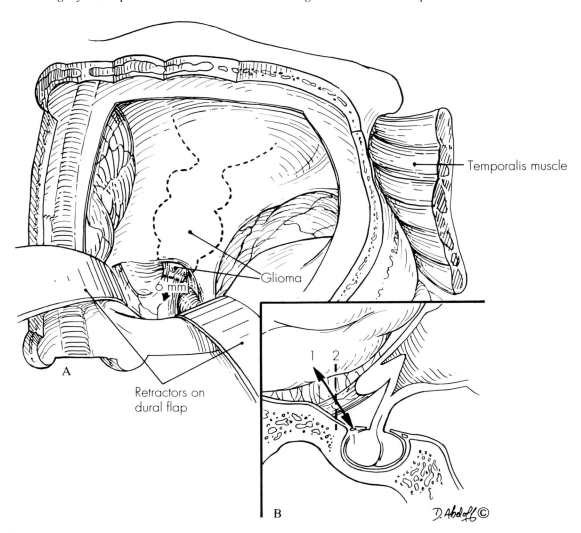

Figure 22-3. (A) Retractor on dural flap. The optic nerve is visualized and its lie determined. **(B)** The ultimate plane (1) of section of the optic nerve, at right angle to the long axis of the nerve, 6 mm anterior to the chiasm. Plane 2 represents an incorrect coronal section of the optic chiasm.

the floor of the anterior cranial fossa, it must be incised somewhere along the axis of the optic canal proceeding anteriorly from the optic foramen (Fig. 22-4A). The goal is not to remove the entire orbital roof but rather to remove just that part covering the optic canal even if it is expanded. The initial bony entry can be created with a miniature high-speed drill burr, but the surgeon is advised to beware of the heating and concussive/vibrating effect that it may create (Fig. 22-4B). The canal and orbital roof removal continues under the operating microscope with 1- and 2-mm antral punches (Fig. 22-4C). This is relatively easily and quickly accomplished.

From this point on, the somewhat complex normal anatomical configuration of the orbital contents,

blurred as it is through the periorbital and orbital fat, tends to be even more confusing because of distortion from the optic nerve mass. Muscle bundles are flattened, blanched, and pushed up or aside. Branches of cranial nerves are thinned and may be deviated; the surgeon's aim is to identify the frontalis nerve, which is a relatively broad band running about parallel to the optic nerve and on top of the levator palpebrae superioris and superior rectus muscles (Fig. 22-5A). In order to maintain continuity through the optic canal and foramen, the annulus of Zinn must be opened; this act may sacrifice the trochlear nerve (Fig. 22-5B), which sweeps close to the annulus from lateral to medial as it also crosses the levator and superior rectus muscles and reaches the par-

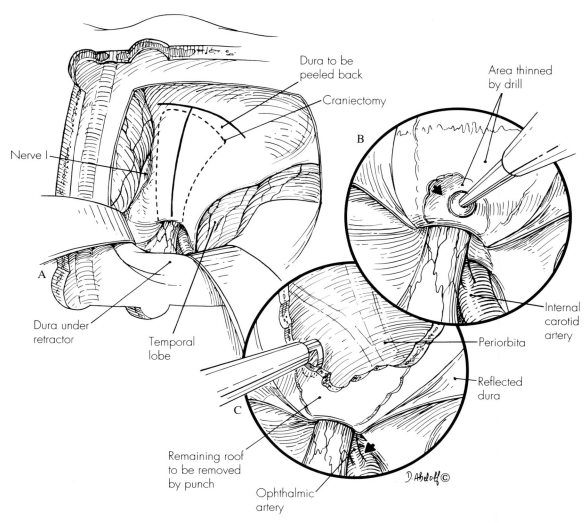

Figure 22-4. (A) The outline of the dural incision and orbital roof removal. **(B&C)** Methods for orbital roof bone removal.

asagittal plane and the superior oblique muscle. It is stated that there is no obvious functional or cosmetic impairment should the fourth nerve be sacrificed.[5]

The dissection through the periorbital fat can be frustrating, especially if the surgeon wishes to preserve the orbit and the structures contained within. As the nerves supplying the levator and superior rectus muscles proceed from lateral to medial, the medial side serves as the entrance to the optic nerve and tumor. However, the muscles may be sufficiently distorted that they are thinned and friable and not easily displaced. Retraction can be frustrating, and it may become necessary to divide the levator origin at the

annulus of Zinn (Fig. 22-6A). Microdissectors and retractors are used to withdraw the muscle bellies and develop a plane to the tumor sheath and optic nerve. The tumor can be further delineated with blunt dissection, and the surgeon should expect its outline to be irregular though smooth. As the exploration proceeds around the girth of the optic nerve tumor, a blunt microhook will assist in ventral dissection and confirm the site of union of the nerve and tumor with the globe. Once identified, the junction can be coagulated with bipolar forceps and the nerve sectioned (Fig. 22-6B). Branches of the ophthalmic artery that serve the nerve can be traced to it and divided after coagulation. The central retinal artery

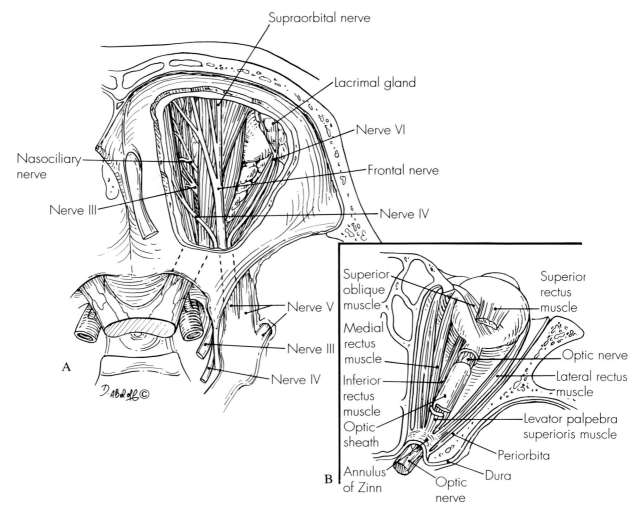

Figure 22-5. (A) Normal superior orbital anatomical structures visualized from above. **(B)** Relationship of annulus of Zinn to optic sheath.

enters the dura 8 to 15 mm behind the globe on the nerve's medial surface.[8]

If the tumor is sufficiently large and irregular that it cannot be easily removed, the mass can be reduced by laser vaporization or ultrasonic aspiration provided that the handpiece of the instrument can be easily introduced into the bony decompression. The tumor and nerve can then be removed as far back as the opticochiasmatic junction, either en bloc or as two separate portions, depending on whether or not the annulus has been opened. Immediately before its extraction, the chiasmatic end of the nerve should be tagged so that the pathologist can examine this portion for evidence of tumor that might have gained access to the chiasm. Once the tumor has been ex-

cised, the levator palpebrae is repaired with fine non-dissolvable suture material, and the periorbital structures closed as required. The dura over the canal is also repaired (Fig. 22-6C).

The surgeon must now make a decision about reconstruction of the bony defect in the orbital roof to prevent visible globe pulsation with proptosis. In some cases the surgeon may have decided in advance to have a craniofacial surgeon assist in the orbital roof exposure and reconstruction, although this is not usually required for the glioma of the optic nerve. As microscopic techniques increasingly permit a much more conservative, linear removal of the glioma from the roof of the optic canal, in many circumstances no roof reconstruction will be necessary.

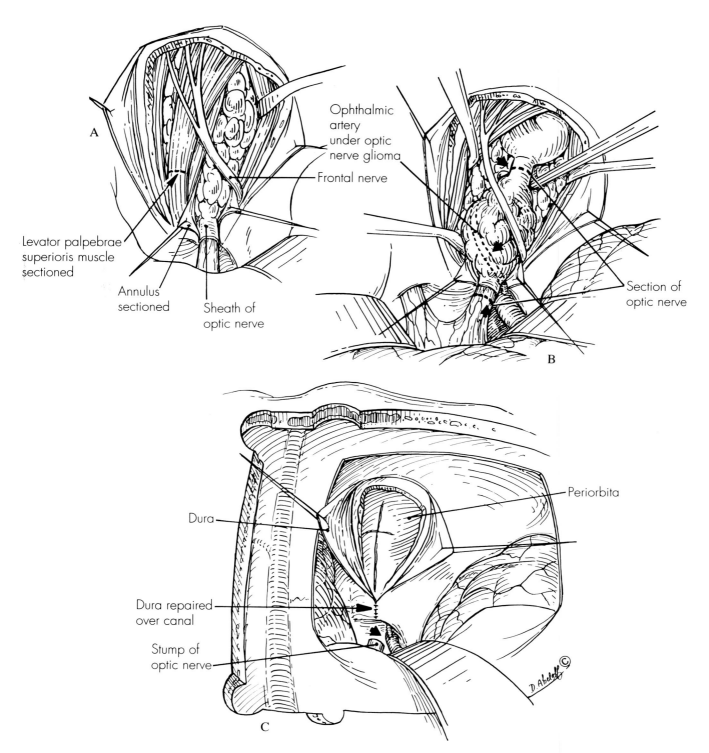

Ophthalmic
artery
under optic
nerve glioma

Frontal nerve

Levator palpebrae
superioris muscle
sectioned

Annulus
sectioned

Sheath of
optic nerve

Section of
optic nerve

Periorbita

Dura

Dura repaired
over canal

Stump of
optic nerve

D. Abeloff ©

Figure 22-6. (A) dissection proceeds medial to the optic nerve tumor. The annulus has been divided and the levator palpebrae sectioned. **(B)** The dissection proceeds about the tumor girth. The lines for nerve-tumor section are shown. **(C)** Dural wound repair after tumor removal.

If the defect is more extensive, a tantalum mesh screen can be molded and placed in the extradural space, although one must recognize the limitation introduced by such a maneuver with regard to postoperative MRI surveillance.

POSTOPERATIVE COMPLICATIONS

Complications of optic glioma surgery are listed in Table 22-1, along with strategies for their avoidance or management.

Early Complications

Eyelid Swelling

Most if not all patients will have periorbital ecchymosis and swelling for 3 to 5 days after surgery. This is the cost of the retracted transcoronal scalp flap and dissection around and beneath the supraorbital rims. It occurs independently of the tidiest of scalp hemostases and postoperative dressings and must resolve on its own. The only hazard that it potentially creates is the inability to test vision in the normal eye during the first few days; hence, the surgeon should en-

Table 22-1. Optic Glioma Surgery: Complication Avoidance and Management Techniques

Complication	Intraoperative Strategies	Early Postoperative Strategies	Late Postoperative Strategies
Wrong side surgery	Confirm side of surgery preinduction		
Ptosis	Levator palpebrae gentle retraction; if divided, neat repair at conclusion Use exposure to medial side of nerve	Wait for resolution	Consider ophthalmic sling repair
Strabismus	Gentle extraocular muscle retraction Identify course of trochlear nerve Use exposure to medial side of nerve	Wait for resolution	Corrective strabismus surgery
Visual deterioration	Be alert to plane of section of involved optic nerve relative to Willbrand knee fibers	As per intraoperative	Search for probable tumor recurrence in chiasmatic stump
Pulsating exophthalmos	Consider craniofacial techniques for nerve exposure and repair of orbital roof defect Placement of tantalum mesh over craniectomy	Wait	As per intraoperative strategy
CSF fistula	Be alert to violation of sinuses, especially posterior ethmoid Prepare pericranial flap Check dural integrity	Distinguish CSF leak from those of nasal secretion leaks and lacrimation Wait 6 weeks Search for and correct CSF fistula	Search for and correct CSF fistula
Meningitis	As per CSF fistula	Early diagnosis and treatment Search for CSF fistula	As per early postoperative strategy
Denervation of ocular globe	Be aware of position of nasociliary nerves	Globe protection	Ophthalmic assistance
Seizure disorder	Beware of brain retractor pressure and release retractor	Treat seizure Assess and treat hyponatremia CT of brain for hematoma/contusion and relieve where necessary	Treat seizure if more than two occurrences CT of brain for porencephaly
Anosmia	Protect olfactory nerve and tract, deciding which one if either should be sacrificed for exposure		
Recurrent tumor	Identify limits of tumor in nerve and know the resection margins Tag chiasmatic end of resected nerve	Decisions about tumor recurrence and need for repeat operation vis-à-vis adjunct treatments	As per early postoperative strategy

deavor to do this testing immediately after the patient awakens from anesthesia and before the swelling appears.

CSF Fistula and Meningitis

The appearance of an early postoperative CSF fistula with or without complicating meningitis indicates violation of one of the paranasal air sinuses. The surgeon will know if the frontal sinus was compromised and perhaps inadequately patched. It may be less clear, however, if the ethmoid air cells have been violated so that they now serve as the source of the leak. Once the meningitis (if present) is cured, coronal sections on CT imaging capably outline bony and sinus anatomy and can indicate the presence of CSF in the sinus. A reexploration of the operative wound with *intradural* fascial patch grafting is required to eradicate the fistula.

Seizures

An early postoperative convulsion may occur especially in children. This is usually a hazard of open craniotomy and brain retraction. Three early seizures are permitted before anticonvulsant treatment is instituted. Whether seizure happens early or late, CT scanning is required to search for frontal lobe contusion, hematoma, or porencephaly. At all times the surgeon should be aware of the pressure exerted on the frontal lobe by brain retractors.

Ptosis

Ipsilateral upper lid ptosis should be anticipated as an early postoperative complication. At the very least, it arises from dissection around or traction on the levator palpebrae muscle, and if that muscle should have to be sectioned and then repaired,[5] the occurrence of ptosis is a given. Regardless of the cause, substantial improvement generally occurs over the subsequent 6 to 12 months, but if it does not, corrective lid surgery can be performed by an ophthalmic surgeon.[2]

Impaired Vision in Contralateral Eye

The goal of the operative procedure described above is to remove a tumor-bearing optic nerve that has severely impaired or completely eradicated vision in the involved eye. Should the early postoperative evaluations show that vision in the opposite, previously unaffected eye is worse, the surgeon may be hard pressed for an explanation. The likeliest cause is a discrete field defect arising from section of Willbrand's crossing fibers in the diseased nerve. More substantial visual loss, for which there is no operative solution, has probably occurred on an ischemic basis. Obviously, follow-up CT or MRI examination is required.

Late Complications

Anosmia

For the reasons mentioned, the patient should be advised before surgery that unilateral anosmia may be an unavoidable complication of the operative exposure but that as long as it is unilateral there will be no overall interference with smell or taste.

Strabismus

Postoperative strabismus can have either a neurogenic or a muscular explanation. That is, the oculomotor or trochlear nerves or the muscles that they subserve may be stretched or otherwise damaged, especially if the tumor is large and dissection around its girth awkward. It has been suggested that long-lasting strabismus is an uncommon problem and that it usually improves.[3,5,7] The ophthalmologist should advise at a later stage whether corrective strabismus surgery will relieve the unimproved condition.

Incidentally there is no ocular prosthesis that is as satisfactory as the patient's own globe. Unless the tumor has spread into the eye, every effort is made during the tumor surgery to preserve the globe and its governing extraocular nerves and muscles to protect the patient's ocular cosmesis.

Pulsating Proptosis

Even though the optic nerve tumor bulk has been removed, intraorbital tissue swelling may account for continuing proptosis in the early days after operation. This resolves in a few weeks' time, perhaps to the extent that the globe becomes enophthalmic.

If in the longer term the globe remains proptotic and pulsates, this is related to transmitted cerebral pulsation through the defect in the orbital roof, which presumably was either left unrepaired or has eroded away. Given this continuing circumstance, the patient should declare just how troubling the problem is. Reparative craniofacial surgery with use of split calvarial bone grafts to reconstruct the bony defect can be offered as a solution, but only after follow-up imaging has confirmed that the proptosis is not due to tumor recurrence.

Denervation of the Ocular Globe

The nasociliary nerve crosses the optic nerve with the ophthalmic artery and runs obliquely beneath the superior rectus and superior oblique muscles. As it crosses the optic nerve, it gives rise to the long ciliary nerves, which are ultimately distributed to the ciliary body, iris, and cornea. These nervous structures are fine and almost covert, and their damage can result in insensitivity of the exposed epithelium of the cornea, which in turn may result in keratitis and perhaps the need for enucleation of the eyeball. Once again, the ophthalmologist must play an important role in the patient's follow-up.

Tumor Recurrence

Although the surgeon may have been convinced that the optic nerve resection margins were free of tumor at the time of operation, tumor may recur some time later. It can arise from the stump on the globe and grow substantially to once again occupy the orbit and optic canal. In this circumstance the decision for reoperation will be dictated by the histologic type of the original tumor, the cosmetic or symptomatic ocular disabilities, and the threat of tumor extension into the intracranial space. If instead, the tumor has arisen from the chiasm stump, it is likely that the chiasm is infiltrated and that further surgery has little to offer and adjuvant therapy should be considered.

Orbital Meningiomas and Other Tumors

Joseph C. Maroon
Michael Kazim
John S. Kennerdell

The complexities of diagnosis and management of orbital disease inherently increase the likelihood of complications. The wide variety of pathology with a limited spectrum of clinical presentations makes the diagnosis of orbital disease difficult at best. With the advent of noninvasive imaging ultrasound, high-resolution CT, and more recently, MRI, the indications for diagnostic orbitotomy have virtually vanished. With the knowledge of the anatomic location and the radiological characteristics of a mass, the surgeon has a far better chance of making the correct diagnosis and intervening appropriately. It is the objective of this chapter to clarify certain of the diagnostic uncertainties as well as to highlight those points of the surgical technique that are crucial in avoiding the most common complications.

TYPES OF TUMORS

The incidence of orbital tumors reported in any series varies with the source of the cases. Since the mid-1980s we have used a neurosurgery-ophthalmol-ogy team approach for the diagnosis and treatment of orbital lesions. We have evaluated and treated over 1,200 patients with orbital tumors. The incidence of the different tumors and pseudotumors as of 1990 is shown in Table 22-2.

DIAGNOSIS

To evaluate the patient with orbital disease we use a diagnostic "decision tree" based on the presenting signs and symptoms to simplify the diagnostic workup and to arrive at the appropriate therapeutic option (Fig. 22-7). We begin with a thorough history and a physical examination, which includes assessment of visual acuity, pupils, eye position, and ductions, Hertel measurements, and evaluation of the fundus. Visual fields are determined and ultrasonography is performed on all patients, and where appropriate a CT scan and/or MRI is obtained. The decision as to whether to obtain a CT scan or MRI can be complicated; however, it is based on a principal difference between the two imaging systems. In gen-

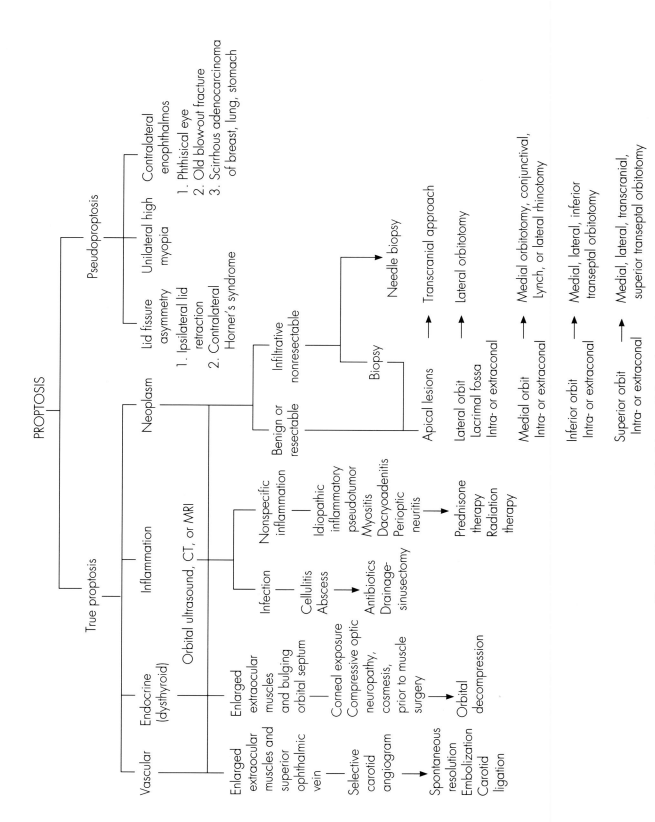

Figure 22-7. Diagnostic "decision tree" for patients with proptosis.

Table 22-2. Orbital Tumors and Pseudotumors,
1975–1990

Type of Neoplasm or Pseudotumor	No. Reported
Adenoid cystic carcinomas	10
Benign mixed lacrimal gland tumors	16
Dermoids/epidermoids	55
Hemangiomas	40
Hemangiopericytomas	12
Lymphangiomas	30
Meningiomas (orbital, 30; sphenoorbital, 141)	171
Metastatic tumors	40
Nonspecific orbital inflammation	105
Neurofibromas	29
Optic nerve gliomas	30
Rhabdomyosarcomas	11
Fibrous histiocytomas	3
Cholesteatomas	4
Venous varices	3
Liposarcomas	2
Lymphoid lesions	105
Mucoceles	56
Eosinophilic granuloma	6
Hematomas	12
Squamous cell carcinomas	6
Blue nevus	1
Basal cell carcinomas	25
Total	772

eral, CT scans are most useful in imaging bony abnormalities, while MRI is best for evaluating soft tissue densities. There are times when information from the two modalities is complementary, in which case both are used. In addition to the above mentioned studies, hematological determinations and fine-needle aspiration biopsy may be useful adjuncts. By using the decision tree of Fig. 22-7, orbital tumors can be diagnosed preoperatively with an 80 to 90 percent reliability.

Once it has been determined that a surgical lesion exists, it is essential to further explore the precise relationship of the tumor to the optic nerve in order to determine the least traumatic surgical approach for its removal.

The presenting sign for most of our patients is painless proptosis. Hemangiomas, neurofibromas, optic gliomas, meningiomas, dermoids, and dysthyroid orbitopathy account for the majority of these neoplasms. Painful proptosis suggests an orbital inflammatory process, which can be a nonspecific inflammation or can be due to infections, metastatic lesions, primary orbital malignancies, lymphoid lesions, rhabdomyosarcomas, and occasionally dysthyroid disease. Decreased visual acuity or visual field function without proptosis suggests a smaller but critically located orbital lesion. It may be a cir-

cumferential lesion compressing the optic nerve, such as meningioma, glioma, or neurofibroma, or it may be located deep in the orbital apex or in the intracanalicular space.

In spite of adherence to a systematic approach to these patients, several disease entities remain problematic. The classic lesion responsible for false negative orbital explorations is nonspecific orbital inflammation, which can present with painful proptosis, restriction of extraocular motility, and, when severe, impaired optic nerve function. However, no discrete mass is found on CT scan. Instead, most commonly there is increased fat intensity in the intraconal space or thickening of the extraocular muscles and tendons. There may be thickening or contrast enhancement of the sclera and optic nerve sheath, and the lacrimal gland may be discretely involved. The CT scan if carefully reviewed and on occasion a fine-needle aspiration biopsy can obviate the need for an exploratory orbitotomy. High-dose oral corticosteroid treatment can be both diagnostic and therapeutic, as this lesion is highly responsive.

Dysthyroid orbitopathy is another inflammatory process, which presents much the same picture as pseudotumor, from which it can often be distinguished by the presence of thyroid dysfunction. However, this is not always the case, as a small percentage of patients are euthyroid at the time of presentation. It is also common for the tendons to be spared enlargement in thyroid disease. In fact, one of the classical findings early in the development of CT was the "lollipop" sign, which is actually the tangential view of an enlarged inferior rectus muscle that had been mistaken for an inferior orbital mass. With the advent of coronal projections, this distinction has been less confusing. Figure 22-8 illustrates how large the muscle may become and how if unilateral, it could easily be mistaken for a neoplasm or pseudotumor.

An optic nerve meningioma produces annular enlargement of the nerve, which can cause it to be confused with an optic nerve glioma. With the advent of MRI techniques, these lesions can usually be distinguished, because meningiomas display hyperintensity of the subdural space whereas gliomas are more homogeneous. While this is generally the case, there have been notable exceptions that indicate the uncertainty of the radiologic diagnosis. Figure 22-9A illustrates a confirmed optic nerve meningioma in a 46-year-old woman, not to be confused with the typical optic glioma in a 6-year-old child shown in Figure 22-9B. In addition, meningiomas must be distinguished from fibrous dysplasia; age and location are useful parameters. Figure 22-10A shows a typical sphenoid

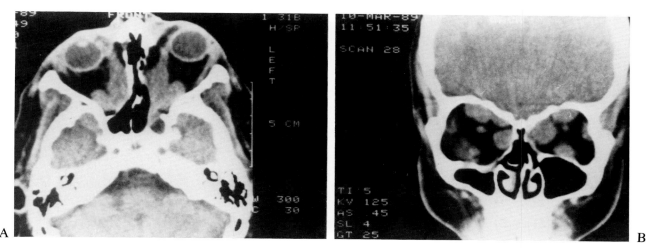

Figure 22-8. Dysthyroid ophthalmopathy, which can simulate a pseudotumor or neoplasm.

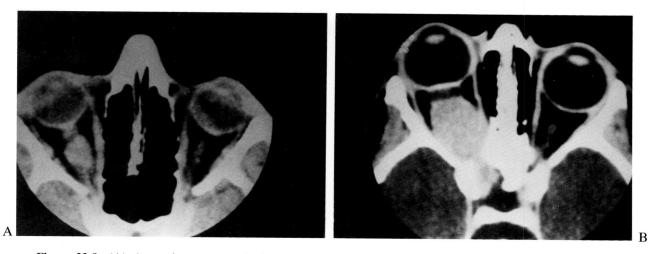

Figure 22-9. (A) An optic nerve meningioma in a 46-year-old woman. **(B)** An optic glioma with nerve enlargement in a 6-year-old child.

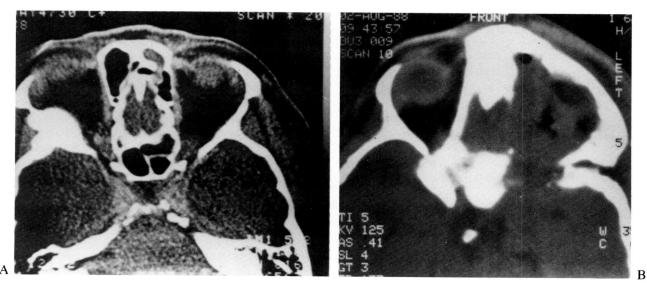

Figure 22-10. (A) Hyperostosis of a sphenoid wing meningioma in a middle-aged woman. **(B)** Dysplastic bone proliferation in a 10-year-old boy extending into the midline sinuses.

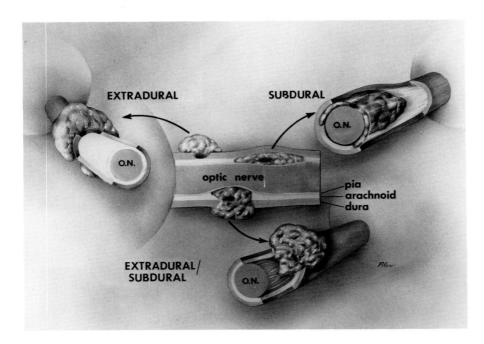

Figure 22-11. The origins of optic nerve meningiomas: extradural, subdural, and subdural with axial extension.

wing meningioma in a 46-year-old woman, and Figure 22-10B shows a hyperostatic fibrous dysplasia in a 10-year-old boy.

An optic nerve meningioma may originate in a subdural, extradural, or combined location. It may focally enlarge or may extend axially along the nerve to the intracranial compartment (Fig. 22-11). Our management of these lesions depends on the location, size, CT and/or MRI appearance of the tumor and the visual acuity and age of the patient. Table 22-3 summarizes our approach relative to location and visual acuity.

Finally, CT scans have also simplified the management of medial masses in the pediatric age group. Most of the discrete, solid, slowly growing orbital masses are dermoids, but the presence of an encephalocele in this region could result in disaster for the unprepared surgeon. A preoperative CT scan will also reveal the hemangiomas and the rhabdomyosarcomas that may confuse the clinical picture.

SURGICAL ANATOMY

A thorough understanding of orbital anatomy is essential to avoid complications regardless of the surgical approach taken. The difficulties of orbital anatomy stem from the highly compact three-dimensional space involved, which contains multiple crucial structures suspended in a sea of fat. Tumors that seem large and striking on a CT scan or MRI may be very obscure once the orbital span has been entered.

The surgical orbit is divided into four potential spaces: subperiosteal, extraconal, intraconal, and subtenon. The optic canal is formed by the union of two roots of the lesser wing of the sphenoid bone. The upper root of the lesser sphenoid wing forms the roof of the canal; the sphenoid sinus and the ethmoidal air cells border the optic canal medially, and the optic strut forms its inferior lateral border. The optic strut is a bony ridge joining the lesser wing to the body of the sphenoid bone. The optic canal is 5 to 20

Table 22-3. The Management of Optic Nerve Meningiomas According to Location and Visual Acuity

Location	Visual Acuity	Treatment
Mid to anterior	Stable	Observation
Mid to anterior	Progressive loss	Lateral microsurgical operation
Apical	Nearly normal or normal	Observation
Apical	Progressive Loss	Radiation and/or craniotomy
Apical	No light perception (or large tumor or intracranial extension)	Craniotomy

mm long, 4.5 mm wide, and 5 mm in average height (Fig. 22-12). The proximal opening is formed dorsally by the falciform process, a thick fold of dura overlying the optic nerve. The distal opening is elliptical, and its widest diameter is vertically oriented. Each optic nerve leaves the chiasm and travels about 15 mm through the intracranial subarachnoid space. The intracranial arachnoid continues as a discrete structure through the optic canal and fuses with the pia at the globe. At the orbital portion of the optic canal, the pia and arachnoid are fused dorsomedially and ventrally with the dura and the fibrous annulus of Zinn, thus tethering the optic nerve and partially occluding the subarachnoid space but not obliterating its continuity (Fig. 22-12).

The intracranial dura continues through the canal as a dural-periosteal layer and then separates into a dural layer, which forms the dura of the optic nerve, and a periosteal layer, which becomes the periorbita. At the orbital apex, the annulus of Zinn serves as the origin of five of the six extraocular muscles. The levator muscle arises from the upper medial margin of the annulus, while the superior rectus muscle lies immediately beneath the levator and arises from the superior portion of the annulus. More medially and inferiorly is the origin of the medial rectus muscle. The annulus of Zinn loops widely around the nerve, laterally and inferiorly, giving rise to the lateral rectus muscle, which has its origin from two narrow heads. The annulus of Zinn envelops the optic fora-

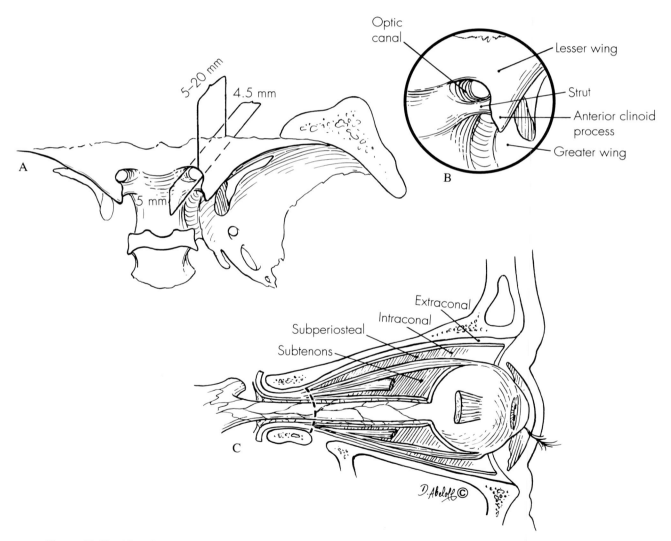

Figure 22-12. **(A)** The sphenoid wing and optic canal showing the variable dimensions of the optic canal. **(B)** Close-up of the optic canal and its anatomic boundaries. **(C)** Cross sectional view of the orbit illustrating the relationship of the muscles and optic nerve to various compartments.

men and the medial aspect of the superior orbital fissure.

The ophthalmic artery provides the major blood supply to the optic nerve. Its branches include the pial vessels and a major intraneural branch, the central retinal artery. The ophthalmic artery arises from the carotid artery just about the cavernous sinus and passes through the optic canal lateral and inferior to the optic nerve. As the ophthalmic artery enters the orbit, it assumes a more medial position, and 8 to 15 mm behind the globe it gives rise to the central retinal artery, which penetrates the medial midportion of the optic nerve to supply the retina. The intraorbital portion of the optic nerve derives its blood supply from the plexus in the pia mater, which is supplied by the ciliary arteries. The primary venous drainage of the orbit is through the superior and inferior ophthalmic veins. The superior orbital vein passes above the lateral rectus muscle and through the superior orbital fissure, draining into the cavernous sinus. The inferior orbital vein draws a network of channels on the medial wall and floor of the orbit.

Upon unroofing the orbit, the frontalis nerve is visible through the thin periorbita. Once the periorbita is opened, the frontalis nerve is seen overlying the levator and superior rectus muscles. In the same plane lies the trochlear nerve, which crosses from lateral to medial above the optic nerve. The optic nerve is approached medially between the dorsal superior rectus and the medial rectus muscle. This approach obviates potential trauma to the nerves passing through the oculomotor foramen. In the orbital apex, the optic nerve is approached laterally in order not to jeopardize its blood supply.

SURGICAL TECHNIQUE

Frontoorbitotemporal Craniotomy

The traditional approach to the orbit, used since the time of Walter Dandy, continues to be through a frontotemporal craniotomy. This exposure, however, requires at times undue brain retraction to obtain adequate exposure for intraconal and apical lesions of the orbit. We therefore designed a frontoorbitotemporal craniotomy approach, which provides excellent visualization of the orbital structures, including the apex, with minimal brain retraction. We also use this approach for midline basal tumors such as tuberculum sella meningiomas, craniopharyngiomas, and any lesion arising in the suprasellar area between the optic nerves. To obtain optimum results and minimize complications, there must

be strict adherence to certain surgical principles and an appreciation for the anatomical structure, as described below.

Skin Incision

We usually shave no more than 2 to 3 cm of the hair posterior to the hairline. Thus, to satisfy postoperative cosmetic concern, hair can be combed forward to hide the visible effects of surgery. If, however, one anticipates a defect in the ethmoid or superior wall of the sphenoid sinus, a more posterior skin flap should be elevated and a skin incision should be planned to provide for mobilization of the periosteum and galea, which can be placed over such a defect in the frontal fossa. Since we use a bicoronal skin incision, an appreciation of the normal anatomical position of the frontalis nerve is necessary to avoid frontalis nerve palsy. Finally, the supraorbital nerve is dissected in a subperiosteal fashion and wedged from the supraorbital notch to preserve sensation in the forehead.

Craniotomy Procedure

The craniotomy is performed by using two to three burr holes connected with the craniotome, as illustrated in Fig. 22-13. The frontal sinus is intentionally opened anteriorly through a burr hole that is low enough to permit use of an osteotome to detach the medial orbital rim from the nasion. This cut should not be too far posterior; otherwise, the trochlear apparatus will be interrupted. The orbital contents also must be protected with a brain ribbon when making the medial cut. The roof of the orbit is not transected, but the bone flap, when elevated, breaks in its thinnest portion, leaving the orbital roof attached to the bone flap (Fig. 22-14). There is no danger to the orbital contents since the elevation is anterior and superior. Appropriate precautions must be taken not to enter the sagittal sinus when making the medial trephine holes.

Upon elevating the bone flap, every precaution should be taken to maintain the dura intact, since a postoperative CSF leak can be a catastrophic complication. If the dura is torn upon exposure, it *must* be meticulously closed in a watertight fashion at the conclusion of the operation.

Once an opening has been made into the frontal sinuses, these sinuses must be managed to prevent infection and subsequent CSF leakage. At this point of the operation we exenterate the mucosa, fill the frontal sinus with bacitracin ointment, and occlude it from the operative field with cottonoid pledgets. Ex-

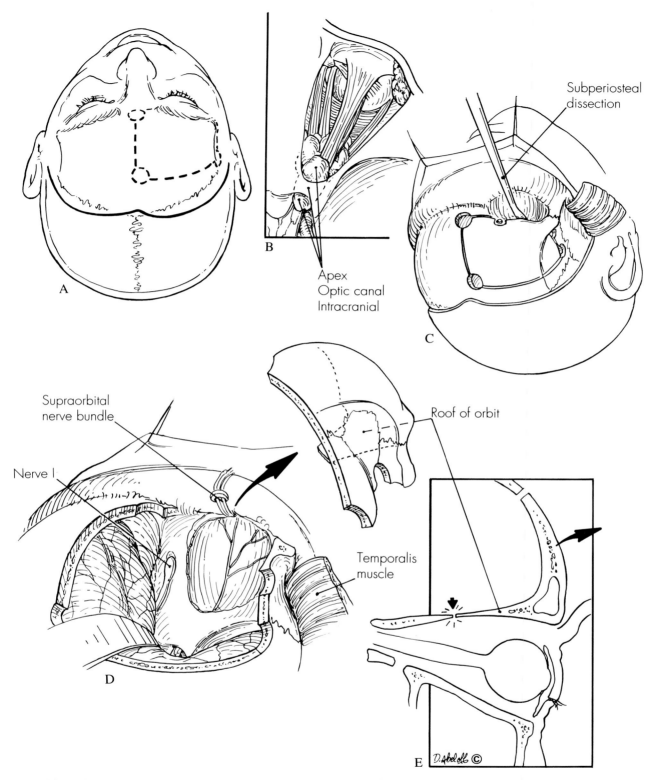

Figure 22-13. **(A)** Bicoronal skin incision and location of burr holes for frontoorbitotemporal craniotomy. **(B)** Orbit from above and the relationships of the optic nerve and muscles at the apex. **(C)** Technique for dissecting periorbital fascia from under the surface of the orbital roof preparatory to elevating the bone flap. **(D)** Exposure of the orbit after elevation of the bone flap and removal of the orbital roof. **(E)** CSF rhinorrhea through the frontal sinus anteriorly and the ethmoid sinus posteriorly will occur if these are not sealed properly at the completion of the operation.

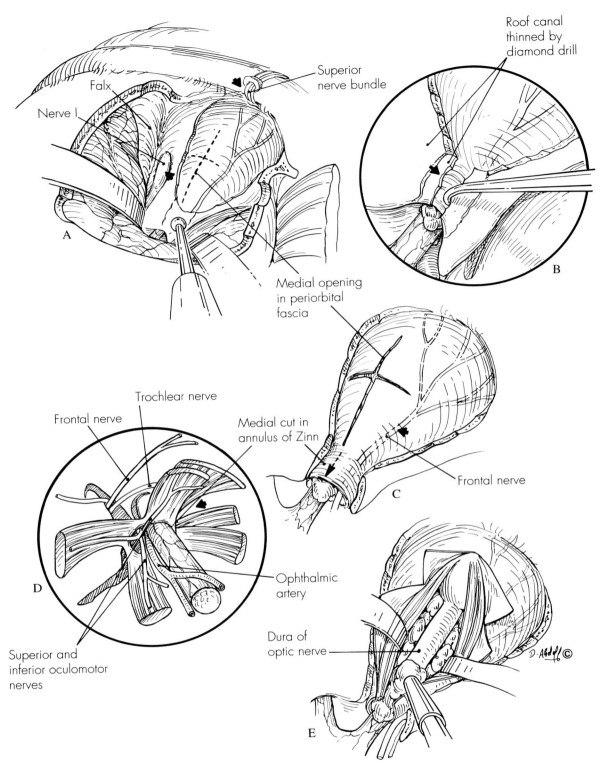

Figure 22-14. (A) Extradural approach and decompression of the orbit and optic canal with a diamond drill. The supraorbital and olfactory nerve are spared. **(B)** Extradural decompression of optic nerve (close-up). **(C)** Medial opening of the periorbital fascia to obviate injury to the superior rectus and levator muscles and structures in the superior orbital fissure. **(D)** The orbital apex showing the relationship of cranial nerves to the muscles, optic nerve, and superior orbital fissure. **(E)** Separation of muscles after opening the annulus of Zinn to expose the orbital apex tumor dorsal to the optic nerve.

tradural dissection is then performed to completely unroof the orbital space back to the optic canal. If the exposure is for a tumor in the middle or anterior portion of the orbit, more posterior bone removal is not required. If the tumor is in the apex, however, or in the optic canal itself, the entire orbital roof is excised and optic nerve decompression is carried out in an extradural manner. This requires considerable and at times tedious dissection posteriorly, particularly over the optic canal itself, with use of the operating microscope and a high-speed diamond drill.

In unroofing the optic canal extradurally, obvious care must be taken to avoid injury to the optic nerve. Rongeurs are never placed under the bone; rather, the canal roof is thinned with a diamond drill and then exposed with a small curette or nerve hook. There is a temptation to open the dura and incise that portion of it over the optic canal in order to unroof the canal in an intradural manner. This certainly can be done, but a defect is then created, which further necessitates an absolutely watertight closure of the dura, since this opening is sometimes difficult to repair.

Following exposure of the orbital contents and/or optic canal, the intraorbital tumor is localized by digital palpation or intraoperative ultrasound. When the tumor has been located, dissection is carried directly down to it with use of a two- or three-blade self-retaining system in order to avoid hand-held retractors in the orbit.

If the tumor is medial or dorsal or affects the optic nerve, the annulus of Zinn should be opened medial to the levator and superior rectus muscles to avoid injury to the occular motor nerve passing through the occular motor foramen lateral to these structures. An attempt is made to preserve the trochlear nerve, but this is not always possible. Dissection through the ubiquitous fat is best carried out bluntly with small dissecting instruments, but bipolar coagulation with irrigating forceps may be used to shrink the fat to obtain improved exposure.

The tumor is removed with microsurgical dissecting techniques, which may be facilitated by use of a carbon dioxide or sapphire tip laser. An optimal retracting instrument in the orbit is the ophthalmic cryoprobe, which is a 2- to 3-mm instrument that can be frozen to the surface of the tumor and used for retraction and dissection. After tumor removal, hemostasis must be obtained; otherwise, extremely disconcerting proptosis and chemosis will occur.

We have not found it necessary to replace the orbital roof with a prosthetic material in the closure in any of the over 200 cases in which we have used this technique. Globe pulsation may be noted for several days postoperatively, but this quickly subsides and is of no cosmetic significance. The sinuses are obliterated by first filling them with bacitracin ointment and then inserting muscle tissue taken from the temporalis muscle into the cavities. A galeal flap is mobilized and sutured over the muscle-filled sinus to the underlying dura. Fibrin glue is then placed around the borders to enhance the watertight seal. The dura is then closed meticulously in a watertight fashion and tested with Valsalva maneuvers to ensure that the seal is indeed watertight at the completion of the closure.

The bone flap is replaced and sutured, usually with four equidistant sutures. A cranioplasty to cover the holes and the saw cuts is then constructed with methyl methacrylate. The skin is then closed in layers in the usual fashion. A drain is not used if the sinus has been penetrated, since air can then be aspirated through the frontal sinuses and create a subgaleal pneumocephalus.

Postoperatively, patients routinely have mild to moderate periorbital ecchymosis and some swelling, which quickly subsides within 2 to 4 days. If there is a postoperative orbital hematoma, severe chemosis can occur, which must be treated with various ointments to prevent undue damage to the conjunctiva. If the technical details of this procedure are adhered to, patients usually can be discharged from the hospital 5 to 7 days postsurgery and show no evidence of brain retraction on subsequent MRIs or CT scans.

Incidence of Complications

The most significant complications from a frontoorbitotemporal approach include those listed in Table 22-4. The cerebral edema frequently associated with undue retraction necessitated by a standard Dandy type of frontotemporal craniotomy is avoided in the frontoorbitotemporal approach. The incidence of this complication in our series of over 200 cases was less than 2 percent. Injury to the frontoorbital nerve, best avoided by dissecting the nerve from the supraorbital notch, occurs in approximately 20 percent of cases. Even then, however, it does not cause significant disability. Optic neuropathy due to inadvertent retraction, vascular compromise, or heat transmission from laser or bipolar coagulation energy has occurred in less than 5 percent of our cases. This complication is avoided by meticulous surgical technique but at times may be unavoidable when tumors are intimately attached to the optic nerve or fill the optic foramen.

Pulsating proptosis or disfiguring enophthalmos occurs rarely. Indeed, in our series we have never

Table 22-4. Complications of Frontoorbitotemporal Craniotomy: Avoidance and Management

Complication	Avoidance	Management
Cerebral edema due to retraction	Frontoorbitotemporal instead of traditional frontotemporal approach	Osmotic diuretics, hyperventilation steroids, etc.
Frontal nerve avulsion	Dissect from supraorbital notch	None
CSF rhinorrhea	Watertight dural closure: muscle occlusion of sinuses, paracranial or galial graft	Reoperation with meticulous closure
Optic nerve injury	Use only microsurgical technique and diamond drill to unroof optic canal	Thorough decompression; possibly steroids
Injury to nerves in oculomotor foramen	Enter orbit medially between superior rectus and levator and the medial rectus	Nerve injury must be avoided
Postoperative ptosis	Avoid undue retraction of levator and superior rectus muscles	2 to 5 months for recovery
Central retinal artery occlusion with blindness	Extreme care in dissection medial to the nerve in the apex	None
Pulsating proptosis	Replacement of orbital roof attached to bone flap and watertight dural closure	Reoperation and repair if cosmesis unsightly
Postoperative chemosis and hematoma	Meticulous hemostasis at closure	Local conjunctival treatment with moist compresses and antibiotic ointment

had to repair such a condition; in the course of 1 or 2 months this has become self-limiting in all our cases. Conjunctival swelling and chemosis occur frequently and are best avoided with meticulous hemostasis. Even then, application of a firm compressive dressing with appropriate antibiotic and lubricating ointments to the conjunctiva is required and anticipated. The incidence of CSF rhinorrhea from opening the frontal sinus has been 3 percent in our series. Meningitis occurred in one patient, requiring reoperation and reclosure of the dura, which had not been completely sealed. This is a most serious complication and, again, is avoided by meticulous attention to closure of the frontal and ethmoid sinuses and watertight closure of the dura.

Lateral Microsurgical Approach

In 1889 Kronlein first proposed a lateral approach to the orbit. In 1953 the Kronlein incision was modified from a "horseshoe" osteoplastic type to a transverse incision, which extended 30 to 55 mm from the lateral canthus posteriorly. In 1976 we described our modification and advocated use of the operating microscope with a lateral approach to the orbit. The skin incision is a hockey stick incision, which is curved up to the lateral brow and then posteriorly along the line that would be covered by the earpiece of a pair of eyeglasses (Fig. 22-15). It does not proceed posteriorly more than 35 to 40 mm from the

lateral canthus; otherwise the frontalis nerve may be damaged. In addition, no further exposure is necessary for lateral approach to tumors in the superior, lateral, and inferior intraconal compartment. We no longer use a lateral canthal splitting incision because of the occasional complications occurring with reapproximation of the canthal ligament.

After the skin incision is made, the temporalis fascia but not the muscle is incised, beginning at the midportion of the frontozygomatic bone and extending posteriorly to the length of the skin incision. A curved incision is then made through the periosteum of the frontozygomatic bone. With a periosteal elevator, the periorbital fascia is removed from the inner surface of the lateral wall of the orbit, a malleable ribbon being used to protect the globe from injury. The muscle in the temporal fossa is then dissected subperiosteally but not cut and is then retracted posteriorly to expose the lateral orbital wall. The zygomatic artery and the meningeal branch of the lacrimal artery, which may be encountered during a subperiosteal dissection, are easily controlled with electrocautery or bone wax.

A reciprocating saw is used to excise the lateral rim of the lateral orbit just above the zygomaticofrontal suture line, and another cut is made approximately 1.5 cm below this. These two cuts are made while an assistant protects the intraorbital contents with a malleable brain retractor, which is inserted between the inner surface of the lateral wall of the

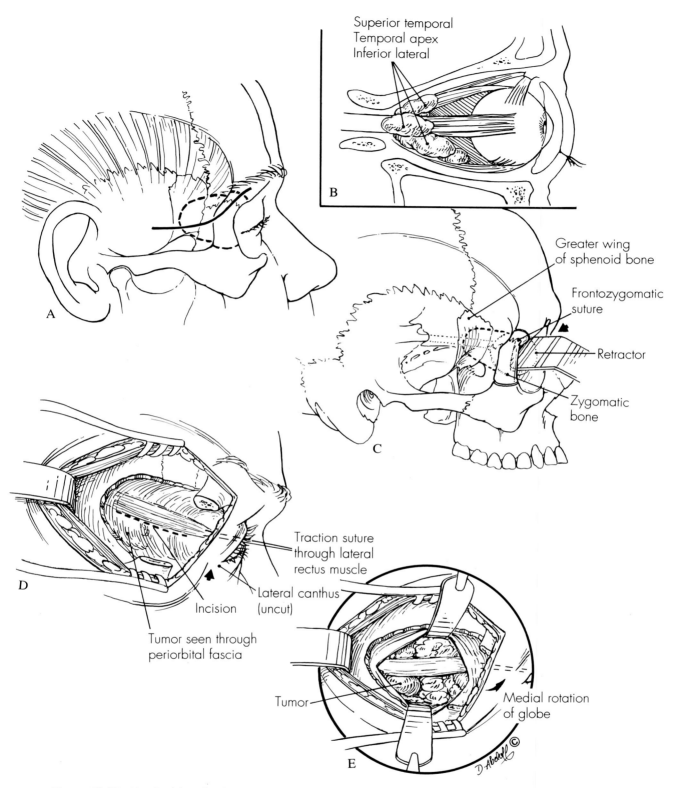

Figure 22-15. (A) Incision for lateral orbitotomy. **(B)** Exposure of orbital contents after bone removal, depicting lesions superolateral and inferior to the lateral rectus. **(C)** Self-retaining retractor inserted above the periorbital fascia to protect the globe while the orbital zygomatic arch is incised. **(D)** Completion of lateral orbitotomy, a traction suture is used to identify the lateral rectus muscle through orbital fat. **(E)** The lateral rectus muscle is retracted dorsally to expose the intraconal tumor.

orbit and the periorbital fascia. The saw cut must not be too high or it can enter the frontal fossa and lacerate the brain. A rongeur is next used to grasp the orbital rim and elevate and break the bone posteriorly at its attachment to the greater wing of the sphenoid. Additional bone is then rongeured away from the greater sphenoid wing.

If it is necessary to obtain more apical exposure in the orbit, additional bone is removed from the sphenoid bone with a high-speed air drill until dura is palpated. A small-angled rongeur is then used to remove additional bone. Obviously, considerable care is needed in this maneuver to avoid opening the dura and creating a CSF leak or damaging the brain. The vascularity of this bone is variable and frequently requires application of copious amounts of bone wax.

With the bone thus removed, the periorbital fascia and retrobulbar contents become visible. A traction suture to the lateral rectus muscle at its globe attachment allows one to identify the muscle through the periorbital fascia. Gentle palpation usually identifies tumors in the superior, lateral, or inferior intraconal compartment. An incision is then made in the periorbital fascia above or below the lateral rectus muscle depending on the location of the tumor. Dissection of the muscle itself is not carried out because of the adherent scar that may subsequently form and limit extraocular movement postoperatively. We use our specially designed self-retaining retractor to dissect through the fat in a fashion similar to that described for the frontoorbitotemporal approach. The fat is usually separated, not excised. The globe may be retracted gently anteriorly, and up to four self-retaining retractor blades may be used to expose a 1-cm tumor. The fine neural vascular structures in the lateral compartment of the orbit are carefully preserved. Tumors in the lateral intraconal compartment, such as hemangiomas, dermoids, or neurofibromas, may be grasped with a cryoprobe and delivered with little fear of injuring adjacent structures as microdissection techniques are used to separate surrounding tissue.

If the purpose of the operation is to remove a tumor attached to the optic nerve, proximal and distal exposure of the nerve is obtained. Exophytic or extradural tumors, such as meningiomas, are found by palpation and subsequent dissection. Usually these are easily dissected from the surrounding tissue and exposed. If the mass is large, ultrasonic aspiration or the carbon dioxide laser on low wattage is used to reduce its bulk and obtain proximal and distal exposure.

Once the mass is reduced, a plane may be seen between the normal dura and the tumor. This plane is exploited, and a tumor is removed from its dural attachment by microdissecting techniques. If no plane is seen, the dura of the optic nerve is incised, and an attempt is made to remove the tumor from the intradural compartment, provided that a CT scan does not show axial intracranial extension of the tumor. Obviously, there is a high risk of additional nerve damage, depending on manipulation, and of sacrifice of the vascular supply to the optic nerve. One cannot dissect safely on the posterior medial surface of the optic nerve without risking damage to the central retinal artery and consequent blindness. Perforating arteries that arise from the posterior ciliary arteries are normally seen on the lateral surface of the dura, and these may be sacrificed if it is necessary to open the dura to expose a subdural tumor. The blood supply to the retrolaminar portion of the optic nerve is primarily through the rich anastomotic vascular network located in the pia. With careful, tedious dissection, therefore, the lateral but not the medial dura surrounding the optic nerve may be excised with a moderate degree of safety.

Specifically with regard to optic nerve meningiomas, we have debulked or completely removed tumors that are primarily extradural and anteriorly attached to the optic nerve. Rarely, subdural tumors that are in the anterior portion of the nerve may be removed by incising the lateral dura and microdissecting the tumor from its arachnoidal plane. Those tumors that are subdural and that extend axially into the apical intracranial compartment are not approached for therapeutic purposes via a lateral microsurgical orbitotomy.

Once the intraorbital tumor has been removed, the periorbital fascia is reapproximated, and the lateral orbital rim is simply reinserted in its position. The bone is not wired or sutured in place. The fascia over the temporalis muscle is closed to maintain the lateral rim of the orbit in its position; in several hundred cases this has not been associated with any cosmetic problems. The skin is closed in a subcuticular fashion, and a firm compressive dressing is applied for 48 hours and then removed.

If complete hemostasis is not achieved, severe conjunctival and lid edema may occur and require either reoperation or extensive local treatment of the globe and cornea. A tarsorrhaphy is never performed because of the compressive effect on the cornea and globe that might occur if a hematoma were to develop.

Incidence of Complications

Complications associated with lateral microsurgical orbitotomy include retraction of the lateral angle of the eye when the lateral canthal ligament is transected, undue retraction on the lateral rectus muscle, and optic neuropathy (Table 22-5). The injury to the lateral canthal ligament is best avoided by making a hockey stick incision rather than a Berke straight lateral incision. When this is done, the incidence of lateral canthal dystopia is approximately 1 to 2 percent, depending on the degree of retraction and associated trauma to the lateral rectus muscle. Most patients will experience a period of double vision due to muscle edema. Fortunately, this generally resolves within several weeks. Injury to the optic nerve is dependent on the location of the tumor, the amount of retraction used, and the judiciousness with which bipolar and carbon dioxide laser energy is used. Our overall incidence of optic neuropathy following surgery through the lateral microsurgical approach has been approximately 4 percent. Blindness has occurred in only 2 of our over 400 cases; one was due to compromise of the central retinal artery and the other to undue retraction on the optic nerve itself. Chemosis has occurred postoperatively in approximately 15 to 20 percent of patients and is due to swelling of tissue and occasional postoperative hematoma, which is avoided by meticulous hemostasis.

Anteromedial Microorbitotomy

Tumors that lie in the intraconal space medial to the optic nerve are best approached through anteromedial microorbitotomy. A specially designed self-retaining retractor is used to facilitate this procedure (Fig. 22-16). As in all surgery, a lack of exposure increases the risk of complications. While this approach can successfully be used to approach the more anterior tumors, those lying posteriorly pose a greater technical challenge. When exposure is limited either by the position of the mass or by narrow lid fissure width, a lateral orbitotomy may be performed to further reflect the globe laterally.

The field is prepared and draped in the usual fashion. A small eyelid speculum is placed between the lids, and a 360-degree limbal peritomy is performed. Conjunctival relaxing incisions are made superior and inferior to the medial rectus muscle, which is isolated with a muscle hook. It is important to free the muscle from its attachments to the intermuscular septa and check ligaments. The muscle is imbricated near its insertion with a 6-0 double-armed Vicryl suture doubly locked at both ends and is then disinserted and retracted medially. A 4-0 braided suture is woven through the insertion and used to apply lateral traction to the globe.

The standard lid speculum is then replaced by the specially designed medial orbital self-retaining retractor. The enucleation spoon is used to cradle the globe laterally while the teeth of the retractor spread the conjunctiva and lids superiorly and inferiorly. The arms of the retractor can be mounted with malleable microretractors to maximize medial exposure by spreading orbital fat planes. The handle of the retractor is angled so that it rests on the temporalis muscle lateral to the orbit. With the retractor in place, the operating microscope with a 300-mm objective can be used. As dissection proceeds deeper in the intraconal compartment, the orbital fat is retracted superiorly and inferiorly with cottonoid pledgets and additional malleable retractors as needed.

Of paramount importance in orbital surgery is avoidance of trauma to the optic nerve, which can result from three major insults. Most common is pressure on the nerve, which may be caused by poorly positioned retractors or excessive retraction.

Table 22-5. Complications of Lateral Microsurgical Approach: Avoidance and Management

Complication	Avoidance	Management
Transection of frontalis branch of facial nerve	Limit incision to 40 mm from lateral canthal margin	None
CSF leak through wound	Microsurgical and diamond bit removal of greater wing of sphenoid and orbital roof when exposing dura of the frontotemporal area	Watertight closure of dura using sutures, Gelfoam, muscle, and/or fibrin glue
Postoperative fibrosis of lateral rectus	Avoid dissection and undue traction on muscle itself	Lysis of postoperative scar
Globe perforation	Avoid dissecting on globe itself or undue retraction	Repair hole and retinal tear
Visual impairment or blindness	Avoid dissection in posterior medial aspect of orbit, avoid retraction and manipulation of nerve itself	Possibly steroids
Postoperative chemosis and conjunctival swelling	Firm orbital dressing but no tarsorrhaphy	Compresses, antibiotic ointment steroids
Postoperative double vision	Gentle traction on lateral rectus muscle	None

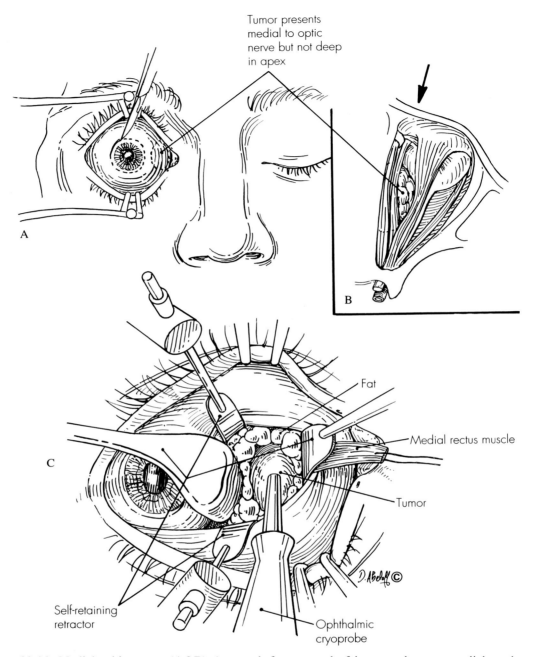

Tumor presents
medial to optic
nerve but not deep
in apex

A

B

Fat

Medial rectus muscle

Tumor

C

Self-retaining
retractor

Ophthalmic
cryoprobe

Figure 22-16. Medial orbitotomy. **(A&B)** Approach for removal of intraconal tumor medial to the optic nerve. **(C)** The cryoprobe attached to the medial orbital tumor for removal while the globe is retracted laterally after detaching the medial rectus muscle and reflecting it medially.

The use of the operating microscope aids visualization and thereby minimizes the danger of excessive retraction. The ophthalmic cryoprobe can greatly facilitate retraction and dissection (Fig. 22-17C). In addition, the specially designed retractor aids in achieving atraumatic exposure. In spite of this, the pupil should be inspected repeatedly, and if mydriasis is noted, all retractors should be removed and the eye returned to the primary position until the pupil constricts. Care must also be taken not to devascularize the nerve, either during the dissection or while removing or debulking the tumor. This complication can be minimized if the surgeon has a thorough knowledge of the vascular supply to both the nerve and globe. Finally, the nerve may suffer thermal injury through the use of cautery or a laser in an attempt to achieve hemostasis or to debulk a tumor. To avoid thermal injury, power settings should be kept as low as possible, and no energy source should be applied directly to the nerve. Bipolar cautery has been shown to be least damaging to the optic nerve and therefore should be used exclusively in the orbit.

At the conclusion of the intraconal dissection, it is essential to obtain hemostasis, as postoperative retrobulbar hemorrhage is catastrophic and can result in blindness.

The medial rectus muscle is reattached to the globe with the 6-0 Vicryl suture. Postoperative adduction palsy is most commonly the result of trauma to the medial rectus muscle. Postoperative edema can be minimized through careful operative technique limiting the pressure placed on the muscle with retractors. Muscle function generally returns within 1 month after surgery if this is the cause. Adduction palsy can also result from a muscle that has slipped from its insertion. This can be avoided by carefully placing the 6-0 Vicryl stitch through the muscle belly prior to disinsertion and into the sclera when reattaching the muscle. A too deeply placed scleral stitch should also be avoided as this may perforate the globe. Similar care must be taken when placing the scleral traction sutures. When a slipped muscle is suspected, surgery to reattach it should be undertaken immediately, as the difficulty of retrieving the muscle increases with the ensuing fibrosis.

The conjunctiva is closed with pursestring sutures, which are inserted through the conjunctiva near the limbus at the area of the superior and inferior conjunctival relaxing incision. After a lengthy procedure, conjunctival edema makes identification of the caruncle difficult. If care is not taken to properly place the caruncle during the closure, it is easy to either bury it in the closure or displace it laterally. In addition, the conjunctival closure must be accurate so as not to include Tenon's capsule. If a postoperative cyst is noted, it must be excised with careful closure of the conjunctiva. An antibiotic ointment is applied between the lids, and a firm dressing is applied.

Avoidance of Complications

The incidence of complication with anteromedial microorbitotomy have been few, although this is the least frequently used surgical approach for orbital tumors (Table 22-6). We have had one globe perforation in approximately 40 cases. This was a small perforation due to the use of a sapphire tip laser to remove a lymphangioma from the posterior aspect of the globe. One patient required reoperation because of double vision resulting from inadequate reattachment of the medial rectus muscle to the sclera. Chemosis and conjunctival edema occur in virtually 100 percent of these cases because of the perimeter incision in the conjunctiva itself, but these effects are usually adequately treated with an antibiotic steroid ointment and compresses.

Table 22-6. Complications of Anteromedial Microorbitotomy: Avoidance and Treatment

Complication	Avoidance	Management
Injury to the globe	Avoid undue retraction, perform lateral orbitotomy if traction required	Possibly steroids
Medial rectus palsy	Proper suturing for reattachment to globe, avoid trauma to muscle	Reoperation to correct problem
Optic neuropathy	Avoid pressure from improperly placed retractor, use microsurgical technique, avoid devascularizing nerve medially	IV steroids
Thermal injury to optic nerve	Use carbon dioxide laser and bipolar coagulation only when nerve is fully protected with wet cottonoids, never use unipolar cautery	IV steroids
Globe perforation	Meticulous placement of scleral stitch when reattaching medial rectus muscle, avoid traction on globe	Repair immediately with retinal surgeon
Chemosis and conjunctival edema	Meticulous conjunctival closure without injury to Tenon's capsule, antibiotic ointment, and firm pressure dressing	Topical steroids

REFERENCES

Optic Gliomas

1. Alvord EC Jr, Lofto S: Gliomas of the optic nerve or chiasm. Outcome by patients' age, tumor site, and treatment. J Neurosurg 68:85, 1988
2. Crawford JS (ed): The Eye in Childhood, by the Ophthalmic Staff of The Hospital for Sick Children, Toronto. Year Book Medical Publishers, Chicago, 1967, Ch. 15
3. Gabibov GA, Blinkov SM, Tcherekayev VA: The management of optic nerve meningiomas and gliomas. J Neurosurg 68:889, 1988
4. Heiskanen O: Raitta C, Torsti R: The management and prognosis of gliomas of the optic pathways in children. Acta Neurochir (Wien) 43:193, 1978
5. Housepian EM, Marquardt MD, Behrens M: Optic gliomas. p. 916. In Wilkins RH, Rengachary SS (eds): Neurosurgery. McGraw-Hill, New York, 1985
6. Iraci G, Gerosa M, Tomazzoli L et al: Gliomas of the optic nerve and chiasm. A clinical review. Childs Brain 8:326, 1981
7. Lloyd LA: Gliomas of the optic nerve and chiasm in childhood. Trans Am Ophthalmol Soc 71:488, 1973
8. Maroon JC, Kennerdell JS: Surgical approaches to the orbit. Indications and techniques. J Neurosurg 60:1226, 1984
9. Miller NR, Iliff WJ, Green WR: Evaluation and management of gliomas of the anterior visual pathways. Brain 97:743, 1974
10. Myles ST, Murphy SB: Gliomas of the optic nerve and chiasm. Can J Ophthalmol 8:508, 1973
11. Oxenhandler DC, Sayers MP: The dilemma of childhood optic gliomas. J Neurosurg 48:34, 1978
12. Tenny RT, Laws ER Jr, Younge BR et al: The neurosurgical management of optic glioma. Results in 104 patients. J Neurosurg 57:452, 1982
13. Udvarhelyi GB, Khodadoust AA, Walsh FB: Gliomas of the optic nerve and chiasm in children: An unusual series of cases. Clin Neurosurg 13:204, 1965
14. Wagener HP: Gliomas of the optic nerve. Am J Med Sci 237:238, 1959
15. Wong IG, Lubow M: Management of optic glioma of childhood: A review of 42 cases. p. 51. In Smith JL (ed): Neuro-ophthalmology. Vol. 6. CV Mosby, St Louis, 1972

Orbital Meningiomas and Other Tumors

16. Dandy WE: Orbital Tumors. Results Following the Transcranial Operative Attack. Oskar Priest, New York, 1941, p. 161
17. Housepian EM: Operative Neurosurgical Techniques. Vol. 1. Grune & Stratton, Orlando, 1981, p. 227
18. Housepian EM, Trokel SL, Jakobiec FO et al: Neurological Surgery. Vol. 2. WB Saunders, Philadelphia, 1982, p. 3024
19. Kennerdell JS, Dresner SC: The non-specific orbital inflammatory syndromes. Surv Ophthalmol 29:93, 1984
20. Kennerdell JS, Gardner TA: Tumors of the optic nerve. Curr Neuro Ophthalmol 2:17, 1990
21. Kennerdell JS, Maroon JC, Malton M, Warren FA: The management of optic nerve sheath meningiomas. Am J Ophthalmol 106:450, 1988
22. Kennerdell JS, Slamovits TL, Dekker A et al: Orbital fine-needle aspiration biopsy. Am J Ophthalmol 99:547, 1985
23. Maroon JC, Abla AA, Kennerdell JS, Garrity J: Tumors of the orbit. p. 1. In Wilkins RH, Rengachary SS (eds): Neurosurgery. McGraw-Hill, New York, 1988
24. Maroon JC, Kennerdell JS: Lateral microsurgical approach to intraorbital tumors. J Neurosurg 44:556, 1976
25. Maroon JC, Kennerdell JS: Surgical approaches to the orbit: Indications and techniques. J Neurosurg 60:1226, 1984
26. Rootman J (ed): Diseases of the Orbit. JB Lippincott, Philadelphia, 1988, p. 3

23 Intracranial Epidermoid Tumors

Don M. Long

Epidermoid tumors are congenital neoplasms that grow through desquamation of keratin, cholesterol, and cellular debris. The expansion usually conforms to available subarachnoid spaces.[5,74] Dermoid tumors are similar but have dermal elements. These tumors are histologically benign, but rare malignant degeneration does occur.[44]

Intracranial epidermoid tumors account for approximately 1 to 2 percent of all brain tumors. The most common intracranial locations are parachiasmal and in the cerebellopontine angle.[3,31] However, these tumors have been described within the third ventricle, in the lateral ventricles, especially the temporal horns, beneath the frontal lobe in the anterior fossa, and at the temporal tip in the middle fossa.[8,11,35,36,75] Small intradiploic tumors are often found near the pterion in infants.[18,32]

In the infratentorial space they have been described at the jugular bulb mimicking glomus tumor and on the clivus.[10,13,68] The fourth ventricle is a common location.[30,67] Tumors that are apparently within the parenchyma of the brainstem have been reported.[46,77] The cerebellopontine angle is the most common location, where they represent 7 percent of tumors.[4,30,40]

The natural history of the intracranial tumors is a slow relentless progression of symptoms.[5] They are not known to remain asymptomatic. Specific signs and symptoms depend upon the location of the tumor. Seizures are a common presenting symptom, but increased pressure is rare, even with intraventricular tumors.[35–37]

DIAGNOSIS

Magnetic resonance imaging (MRI) has revolutionized the diagnosis of these tumors,[14,23,42] and they are now diagnosed with virtual certainty before surgery, which was not the case in the past. Plain skull films do not usually show any abnormality with intracranial tumors. There may be nonspecific bony erosion locally, as first described by Cushing.[21] Intradiploic tumors present with an osteolytic, well-defined, usually sclerotic lesion.[19,22,53,78] Typically they are found in frontal, parietal, and occipital bones. Pneumoencephalography and angiography demonstrated only mass effect.[57] In that era most of these tumors were diagnosed only at exploration. The computed tomography (CT) scan can be quite misleading.[56] The typical picture is an irregular lucent area that looks like an irregularly enlarged subarachnoid space. It is difficult to tell the difference in many instances. The density of the contents of these tumors is similar to cerebrospinal fluid. The irregular outline of the apparent cavity is the best clue. A rare tumor has a capsule thick enough to be seen to aid in the diagnosis.[6,7,15,24,29,33,38,39,41,45,46] MRI has changed all of this uncertainty. There is no longer any confusion about the diagnosis. The MR signal characteristic of the cholesterol crystals is so distinctive that the diagnosis is usually made with virtual certainty. In T_1 images the epidermoid is well defined and separable from normal tissues; in T_2 images the tumors have high signal intensity (Figs. 23-1 and 23-2). They rarely enhance.[62,66,69,72,76] The tumor most likely to be

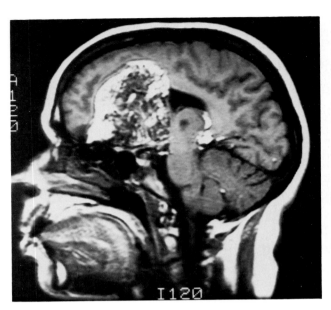

Figure 23-1. A huge suprachiasmatic and intraventricular epidermoid. Note the tumor in the aqueduct and fourth ventricle. The bright T₂ signal of fat and the matted appearance are typical.

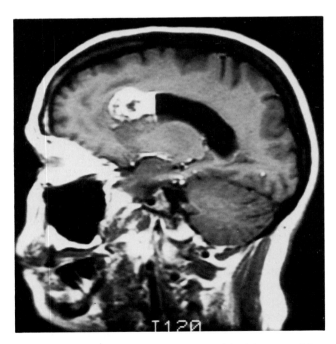

Figure 23-2. Intraventricular epidermoid with unusual fat-fluid level after leaking into the ventricle.

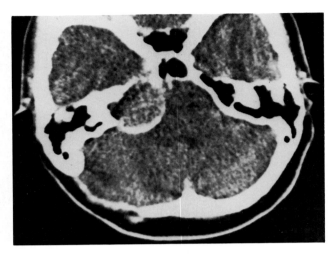

Figure 23-3. Cholesterol granuloma of the petrous apex often mistaken for intracranial epidermoid.

confused with epidermoid is the hamartomatous lipoma.[16,55] These tumors have a fat density that is virtually identical to the epidermoid. They do have a greater likelihood of having calcium within them, but not all are calcified. These lipomas are more likely to occur in the cerebellopontine angle and in the subchiasmatic space. Intramedullary lipomas are known and are almost as rare as the intramedullary epidermoid. Cholesterol granulomas of the petrous apex may mimic intracranial epidermoids (Figs. 23-3 and 23-4).

Clinical Diagnosis

The symptoms and signs of these tumors relate entirely to their location. There is nothing distinctive about the epidermoid except for the propensity for a meningitis-like syndrome to develop when the capsule ruptures and the cholesterol crystals reach the subarachnoid space.[20,25,52]

Supratentorial Tumors

The small intradiploic tumors are nearly always found in childhood by a mother who feels the lump in the pterional region. The small rubbery-feeling nodule is unlikely to be mistaken for anything else. Adults usually present with a painless, palpable mass. Treatment consists of total excision.

Patients with suprasellar tumors typically present with visual complaints.[8,54,64] The tumors may be indistinguishable from tuberculum meningiomas and pituitary tumors. Because they are less well defined, they are unlikely to cause a pure bitemporal field deficit. They are more like meningiomas in that the type of field deficit may be quite variable. The field defects tend to be irregular, not symmetrical, and depend upon where in the optic apparatus the pressure occurs. Optic atrophy from prolonged compres-

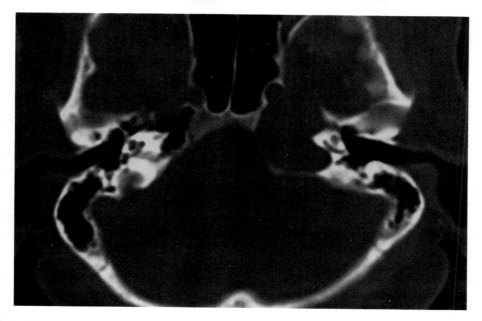

Figure 23-4. The diagnosis of petrous apex cholesterol granuloma is confirmed by bone windows, which show the erosion and ballooning of the right petrous bone.

sion is a common clinical finding. The optic canal may be enlarged from pressure. Unlike meningiomas these tumors do not effect the carotid system. They may invade or compress the cavernous sinus, producing various combination of extraocular muscle palsies. The third nerve is the most likely to be involved because of its exposed position.

Tumors of the trigeminal region manifest with facial pain and combinations of nerve palsies including cranial nerves III through VIII.[11,59]

Intraventricular tumors are usually asymptomatic. It is common for them to be discovered on a scan done for some unrelated symptom. When the tumor is large enough, hydrocephalus may result and the resultant symptoms of increased pressure are nonspecific[65,80] (Fig. 23-1).

Occasionally, one of these tumors will rupture into the ventricular or the subarachnoid space. A syndrome indistinguishable from meningitis will occur (Mollaret's meningitis)[17,20,25] (Fig. 23-2).

Infratentorial Tumors

Tumors of the cerebellopontine angle present in very much the same way as meningiomas in the same location.[48,60] Hearing loss, dizziness, trigeminal paresthesias, and facial synkinesis are all related.[9,63] If the tumors grow large enough, compression of the upper brainstem is possible, but significant brainstem compressive signs are very rare. Patients usually

have these tumors discovered during an investigation for hearing loss or vertigo.

Tumors that occur in the area of the jugular foramen manifest with lower cranial nerve dysfunction. Hoarseness and difficulty swallowing are the most common symptoms.[28] These tumors tend to have extensions into the foramen magnum and upper cervical cord. Pain in the distribution of the second cervical nerve root or upper cervical myelopathy can both occur.

Epidermoids of the fourth ventricle characteristically produce dramatic hydrocephalus. The symptoms are nonspecific and suggest only increased intracranial pressure, not the etiology.[30,67]

The tumors that occur within the brainstem have a protean presentation depending upon their location. The symptoms are suggestive of any other intramedullary lesion. The rarity of this presentation makes it difficult to state with any certainty what typical symptoms should be. There is nothing to suggest that these symptoms are different from any other intramedullary abnormality. Asymmetrical combinations of cranial nerve palsies and long tract signs occur.[46,77]

OPERATIVE TREATMENT

The goal of surgery is total removal.[81] These are curable tumors and the only real chance for this cure is the first operation. Recurrent tumors are notoriously difficult to treat and are virtually never curable in my experience. Technically speaking, these tumors are easy. They are soft and the contents are dislodged with suction or simple manual manipulation. While they surround vessels and nerves, they rarely invade. The real issue in surgery is the difficulty of removing every bit of capsule. If the entire capsule is not removed, recurrence is the rule. A review of published cases suggests that only 50 percent have been cured by conventional surgery. Microtechniques have improved the total removal rate. The second major problem with the initial surgery is the noxious nature of the cholesterol/keratin material that constitutes the bulk of the tumor. If this material escapes into the subarachnoid space, the result is striking meningitis that may be highly disabling and can produce permanent cranial nerve deficits. The technique of surgery has to minimize the possibility that the cholesterol crystals can be spread.[74]

Given these two general considerations, the surgery involved does not differ from that required for virtually any other mass lesion. I will describe surgery for the common tumors, those that are parasellar and those in the cerebellopontine angle, in detail. With minor modifications related to location, the same techniques can be employed for any of the other tumors. The rare tumor within the brainstem also requires separate discussion, as do intradiploic tumors.

Suprasellar and Parasellar Epidermoids

The operations are done under general anesthesia with the patient supine and the head turned (Fig. 23-5A). I prefer to have the zygoma parallel to the floor of the operating room because it is more comfortable for the surgeon. However, any angle of head turning beyond 45 degrees will be satisfactory. The microscope positioning is less comfortable for the surgeon, however. The routine pterional flap is planned.[49,51] I use an elongated question mark–shaped incision that follows the hairline from the midfrontal region down to the zygoma in front of the ear. The scalp flap is lifted separately, taking care to preserve the motor branch to the frontalis muscle anteriorly. There are two simple ways to handle the temporalis muscle. One is to turn the bone flap with muscle attached. This does not provide the low exposure that the parasellar tumors require in some instances, but it is perfectly acceptable for these tumors unless they are very large. The other method is to cut the temporalis at its insertion on the temporal bone, leaving a small

cuff for later repair. Then the temporalis scraped from the temporal and sphenoid bones, providing direct access to the base. This results in less temporal and frontal retraction and an excellent exposure along the sphenoid wing (Fig. 23-5B&C). The bone flap is cut with a single hole placed at root of the zygomatic process of the frontal bone just above the zygoma. A single hole here usually allows the bone flap to include frontal bone and temporal bone. The bone is broken across the base as low as possible to minimize the amount of bone that needs to be removed. The greater wing of the sphenoid is then drilled away until the surgeon has direct access to the base for positioning the microscope. I do not use spinal drainage, but mannitol 0.5 g/kg in a 20 percent solution is administered about the time the skin incision begins. This means that by the time the dura is ready to be opened, the brain will be relaxed. Because of the brain relaxation, I prefer to put dural retention sutures circumferentially at the bone edges to reduce epidural bleeding.

The dura can be opened in one of two ways. One possibility is to open the dura in a line parallel with the inferior bony margin, leaving about a 5-mm cuff for closure. This allows dura to remain over the frontal lobe and offers some protection during retraction. Another possibility is to open the dura over the frontal lobe with the base of the dural flap the base of the bony incision. This exposes more frontal and temporal lobe, but has the advantage of a smooth dural flap along the base, which effectively prevents the troublesome epidural oozing that often develops around the sphenoid bone resection. Epidural hemostasis is key at this point. There is nothing more annoying than a slow ooze that periodically obscures the field during the delicate dissection of the capsule. Since the intracranial operation is virtually without bleeding, it is very important to make certain there is no contamination of the operative field from outside. Packing with hemostatic agents, cottonoid, and retention sutures to control this bleeding are an essential part of the procedure.

There is one modification of the opening procedure sometimes required for especially large tumors. Occasionally a subfrontal exposure may be added to the pterional approach for tumors that are very large. In that case the skin incision is elongated to the midline or beyond just behind the hairline. A single burr hole is still used, but the bone flap is cut into the frontal bone further, staying clear of the frontal sinus. Otherwise the procedure remains the same as described (Fig. 23-6A).

Once the dura is opened, the frontal lobe should be elevated along the margin of the sphenoid wing until

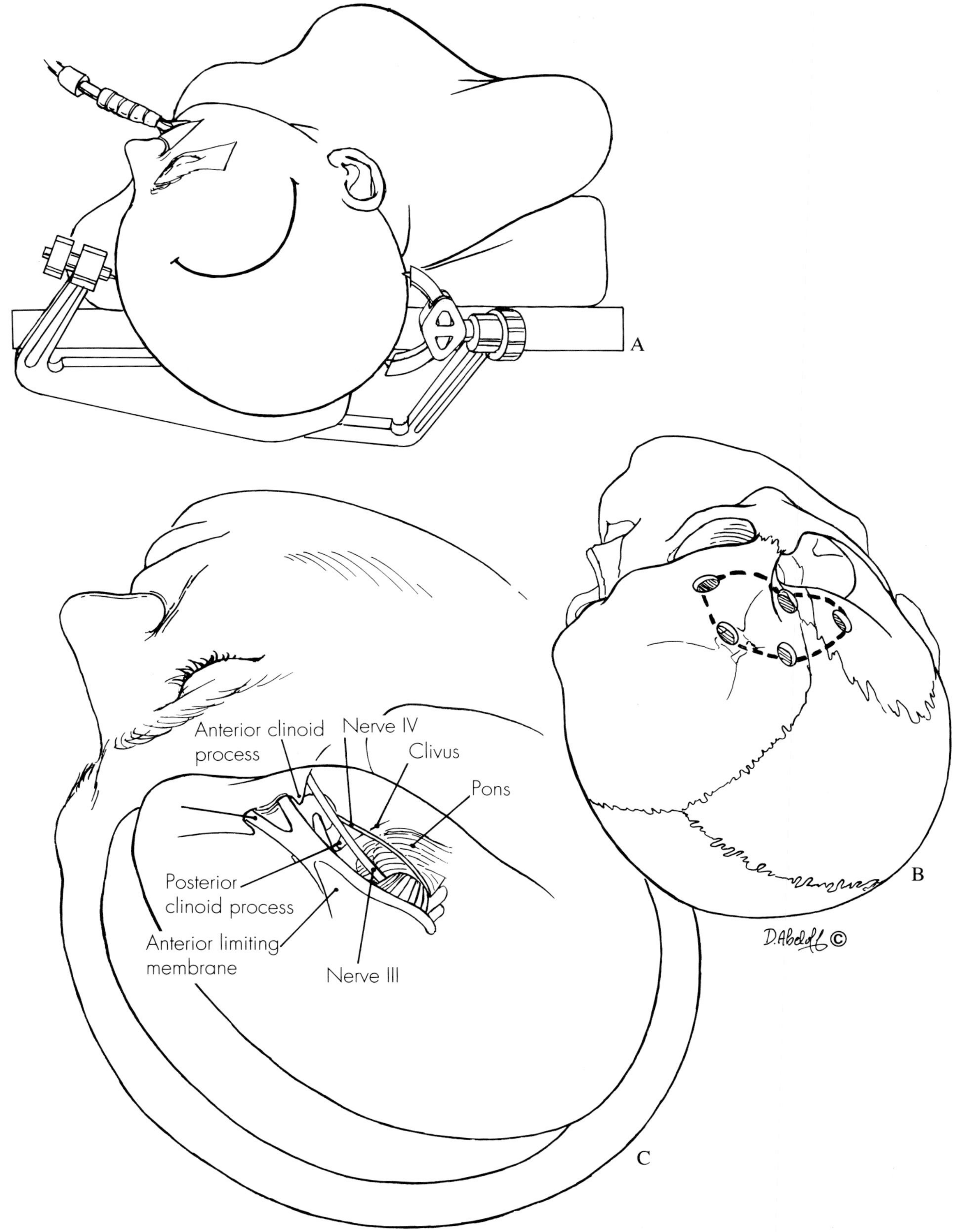
A
Anterior clinoid process
Nerve IV
Clivus
Pons
Posterior clinoid process
Anterior limiting membrane
Nerve III
B
D.Abdolf ©
C

Figure 23-5. **(A)** Position and limited pterional incision. **(B)** Bone flap outline with a posterior hole for temporal extension. **(C)** Schematic representation of the chiasm optic nerve, third nerve, and tentorial relationships, which will be key in the surgical dissection.

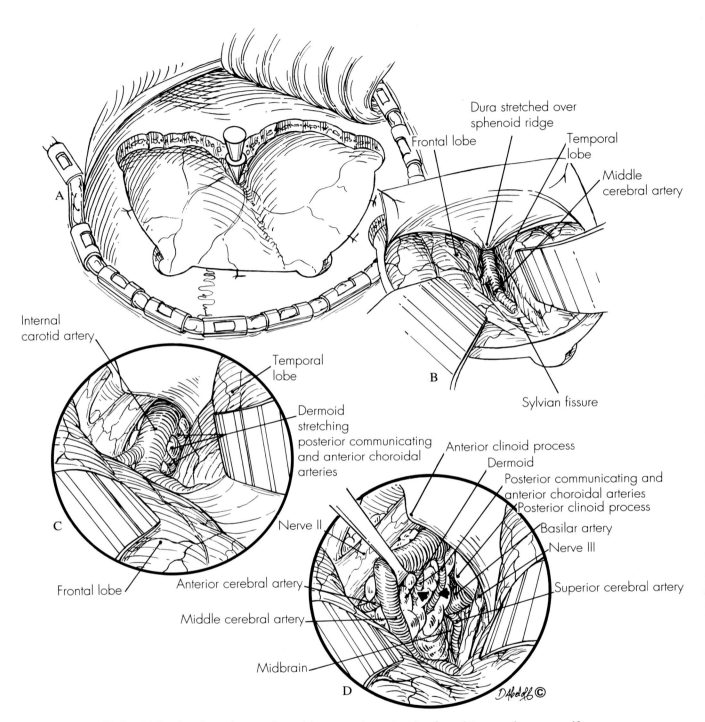

Figure 23-6. (A) Pterional craniotomy flap with a posterior extension for subtemporal exposure if necessary. **(B)** Division of the sylvian fissure and elevation of frontal and temporal lobes. **(C)** Exposure of the carotid artery with the tumor medial to it. **(D)** Elevation of the carotid artery to expose the posterior extent of the tumor surrounding the posterior communicating and anterior choroidal arteries. Note the extension of the tumor medial to the carotid beneath the optic nerve as well.

olfactory nerve, optic nerve, and carotid artery are visualized. Temporal lobe retraction may be required if the temporal lobe overhangs or if the tumor extends posteriorly. Remember the draining veins at the temporal tip that enter the petrosal sinus. They are easy to tear and should be coagulated if the retractors are going to stretch them. The key to a successful operation is to approach a pristine tumor unstained by blood in order to facilitate the capsular dissection (Fig. 23-6B).

Once the area of the chiasm is exposed, the retractors are put in place and the microscope brought into the field. The tumor is usually immediately apparent (Fig. 23-6C). The extent of the tumor is now well known from the imaging studies, and the approach can be planned in advance. The first step is dissection of arachnoid from the tumor surface and placement of retractors for optimum exposure of the tumor. I excise all this arachnoid since it is so difficult to tell what is tumor capsule and what is arachnoid. This will expose the tumor as far as possible. It is virtually impossible to remove anything but small tumors intact. However, if the tumor is only a few centimeters in size, it certainly is worthwhile trying to make an extracapsular dissection. The techniques involved are no different than those for any other tumor. These lesions tend to be densely adherent to surrounding structures, and it is better to remove all of the reactive arachnoid around them than to run the risk of leaving any capsule behind.

The more typical tumor is large and irregular in shape and infiltrates all of the subarachnoid space. The tumors fill and distort the subarachnoid space surrounding all vessels and nerves. The most important thing is to remember the anatomy and where the important structures are going to be located. It is probable they will not have been displaced significantly, but simply surrounded.

If the capsule is going to be entered, it is important to pack all of the surrounding subarachnoid space with cotton so that any lost crystals will not spread through those pathways. Another trick is to irrigate frequently, and if any cholesterol-filled cysts occur within the tumor, the whole area should be irrigated thoroughly as soon as the cyst contents begin to leak when the cyst is opened. This careful irrigation throughout is important to reduce the risk of the postoperative aseptic meningitis.

In the usual situation the tumor capsule will have to be opened at some convenient place (Fig. 23-6D). Where this is done depends entirely on the anatomy of the tumor. Gentle suction will usually suffice to remove the tumor content. Once the bulk of the material is gone, the next step is the tedious dissection

of the capsule. It is mandatory that every shred of capsule be removed if recurrence is to be prevented. Using high magnification, microtechniques are used to strip the capsule and thickened arachnoid from all of the structures. The capsule can be very adherent. Microscissors and round knives are often required to supplement blunt dissection. The tumor is usually down into the interpeduncular space. Great care must be taken here to prevent injury to the small perforators from the basilar apex and its branches. Remember that the pituitary stalk must be preserved (Fig. 23-7).

When all the tumor is out and all the capsule removed, the operative site should be irrigated again with saline until there is no hint of reactive material and then the wound can be closed.

Rarely, these tumors can actually invade the chiasm. How much manipulation within the chiasm is possible is a matter of judgment and cannot be prescribed. However, recurrence is virtually certain if total removal is not achieved.

Approach to Tumors within the Third and Lateral Ventricles

The operative approach used here depends upon the location of the tumor. Some of the larger suprasellar tumors extend through the lamina terminalis into the third ventricle. These tumors should be approached in the manner described and the mass removed by following its posterior extension into the ventricle. Fortunately, the intraventricular tumors usually strip off the walls of the ventricle without much adherence.

If the tumor is wholly within the ventricle, I prefer the transcallosal approach.[49,50] This operation has been described in detail elsewhere. It is done under general anesthesia with the patient in a supine position with the head elevated 15 to 30 degrees. A coronal incision at the level of the coronal suture is made and a bone flap turned from the midline to the right side one-third in front of the suture and two-thirds behind. It is not necessary for the flap to cross the midline unless there are bilateral extensions of the tumor. The dura is opened with the flap along the midline after appropriate dural retention sutures are placed. The flap should be based on the sagittal sinus and great care must be taken not to injure draining veins. An appropriate interhemispheric approach is chosen so that veins will not be disturbed. The right hemisphere is dissected free from the falx until the corpus callosum is seen. The anterior cerebral arteries need to be mobilized so that the approach can go

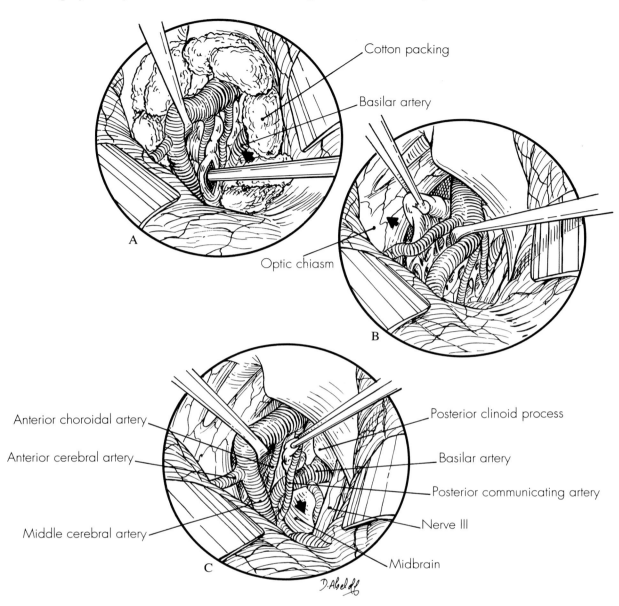

Figure 23-7. **(A)** The tumor is now entered, and the contents of the tumor capsule are being removed by aspiration. Note the cotton packed in the subarachnoid space, preventing spread of the tumor contents. (cotton packing not shown in Figs. B and C, for clarity). **(B)** The capsule is now resected free from the undersurface of the optic nerve chiasm. **(C)** The residual capsule is removed from the vessels.

through the corpus callosum between them. Splitting the corpus callosum will usually place the surgeon in the right ventricle. Visualize the septum pellucidum and the foramina of Monro, which can be localized by following the choroid plexus anteriorly. The exposure of the third ventricle can be obtained through the right foramen of Monro. Great care must be taken not to injure the fornix. It is acceptable to make an incision anterior to the foramen dividing the fornix on one side provided care is taken not to injure the op-

posite side. Access may also be gained by elevating the choroid at its insertion, the taenia choroidea. This allows the roof of the third ventricle to be lifted up and to the left side, exposing the tumor. Tumor removal is no different from that described above. It is particularly important not to allow any of this material to escape in the ventricular system, or catastrophic ventriculitis can occur. When all tumor is removed, a copious irrigation should follow. The wound is closed by restoration of anatomy.

Tumors of the lateral ventricle are approached in the same way. By dividing the septum, it is possible to explore the entire extent of either lateral ventricle by this approach, and it is generally not necessary to divide the corpus callosum posteriorly, which has the risk of injury to the transfer of visual information.

Approach to Tumors of the Middle Fossa and Cavernous Sinus

The surgical approach for these tumors is through a standard pterional operation.[49,51] Most tumors involving the middle fossa are at the temporal tip and underneath the temporal lobe in the region of the Gasserian ganglion. Their management consists of pterional subtemporal exposure with total removal following the principles that have been described. These tumors rarely present any problem. They can grow to enormous size because they are often mistaken for porencephalic cysts so they are not removed until growth is obvious. Nevertheless, their removal is straightforward. The tumors that involve the region of the cavernous sinus are more complex, but rarely present any real technical difficulties. They tend to spill over into the posterior fossa surrounding the third, fourth, and sixth nerves. This is the most difficult part of their removal. Their treatment is very much like a meningioma. Find the nerves on the posterior margin of the tumor and then gradually remove the tumor by gentle suction until the nerves are completely free. The tumors do invade the cavernous sinus, but the gentle suction extracts them without much problem. As with all of these tumors, the key to successful surgery is removal of the thickened arachnoid from around the nerves. This is the difficult part of the operation. Medially in the cavernous sinus the mass has usually just pushed dura medially and the removal of the capsule from this region is not difficult.

Infratentorial Epidermoids

The cerebellopontine angle is the typical place for the infratentorial epidermoid to occur. Because of the way these tumors grow, insinuating themselves around all the structures in the subarachnoid space, it is not uncommon for the tumor to have invaded other areas than that traditionally occupied by cerebellopontine angle tumors (Fig. 23-8). They grow into the region of the sixth nerve and the trigeminal canal as well as around into the interpeduncular space. They grow downward, involving the region of the jugular bulb, and can even spill into the cervical subarach-

noid space. MRI will virtually always show the extent of the tumor so the operation can be planned accordingly. The bony exposure is tailored to the particular part of the posterior fossa where the tumor is located. However, typically it is necessary to do an extensive removal from the tentorium to the foramen magnum. The exposure should not be limited unless the tumor is quite small.

The operations are done under general anesthesia with the patient supine and the head turned 45 to 60 degrees or in the park bench position with the head parallel to the floor.[49,71] The incision is a curvilinear elongated C at the mastoid occipital junction. The occipital bone is exposed and a craniectomy done to expose the transverse sinus superiorly and the sigmoid sinus laterally. Depending on the extent of the tumor the entire occipital bone may be removed unilaterally or the exposure may be more limited for smaller tumors. I begin the dural opening with a diagonal from the junction of the transverse with the sigmoid sinus extending to the medial inferior extent of the bony removal and then make another incision perpendicular to this line in its midpoint. The cerebellum is then gently retracted until the tumor is seen. Self-retaining retractors are important to protect the cerebellum from undue manipulation (Fig. 23-9).

The first step is to expose the tumor from top to bottom (Fig. 23-10A&B). It's very important to understand the anatomy before entering the tumor. It may be possible to see some or all of the cranial nerves, but they may also be totally obscured by the tumor. Identify the trigeminal canal, the porus acousticus, and the jugular bulb. Sometimes this can only be done by removing part of the tumor. First try to make the identification on the basis of bony landmarks and if this fails, use gentle suction to begin to remove the tumor contents. Remember that total removal is the key. As the contents of the tumor are delivered, watch carefully for cranial nerves and important vessels that are likely to be enfolded within the tumor (Fig. 23-10C&D). As the tumor contents are removed, the capsule can be dissected free from surrounding structures and gradually delivered. The capsule is usually thin enough that this has to be done piecemeal. The tumor is gradually removed, exposing cranial nerves laterally; then the more medial portions are removed, exposing the brainstem. I prefer to take the capsule off at the time I am removing tumor so that I do not forget some portion that is tucked away in a corner and easily left in place. The most difficult places for removal are typically at the junction of the fifth nerve with the pons and similarly at the junction of the seventh and eighth nerves.

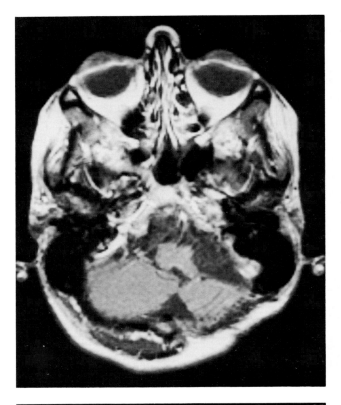

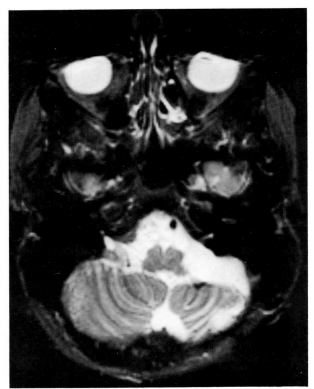

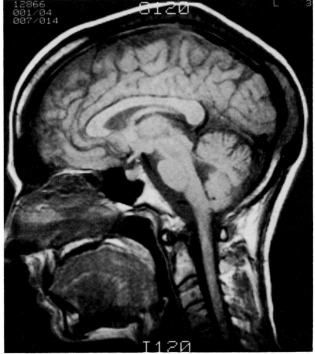

Figure 23-8. The typical lucent expansion of the subarachnoid space is seen on CT imaging. The tumor extended from the tentorium to C2.

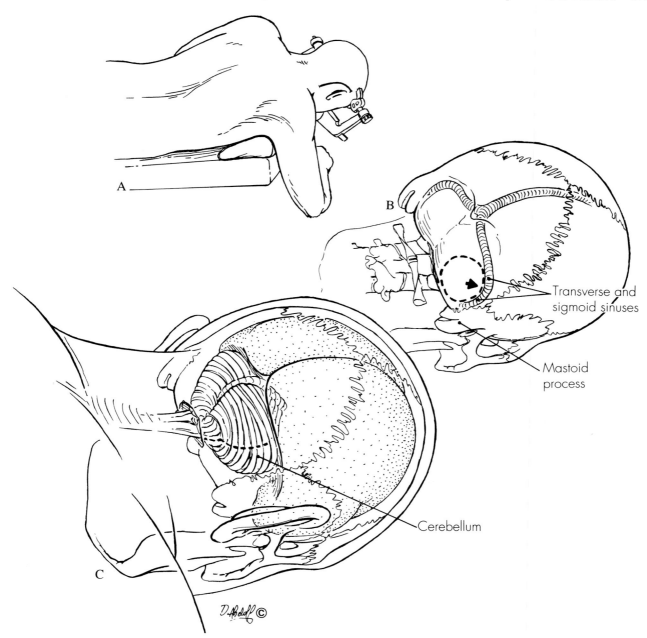

Figure 23-9. **(A)** The park bench position. The dependent arm is supported. **(B)** Schematic representation of the placement of the suboccipital craniectomy to allow access to the cerebellopontine angle. **(C)** The dural opening to permit retraction of the cerebellum for tumor exposure.

Since the tumors tend to surround the nerves, they can be on the underside, and it is easy to leave small scraps of capsule around the nerves. While every effort should be made to save hearing, it is still important to get these tumors out. Permanent cranial nerve deficits other than hearing loss are extremely uncommon. All of the major branches of the basilar are commonly surrounded by tumor, but fortunately the tumor is much softer than the arteries and their injury is unlikely (Fig. 23-11).

The ultrasonic dissector can be used, but generally gentle suction is all that is required, which minimizes the risk of vascular or nerve injury. With smaller tumors or as larger tumors are made smaller by intracapsular removal, it is important to dam the subarachnoid spaces wherever they appear, to keep the

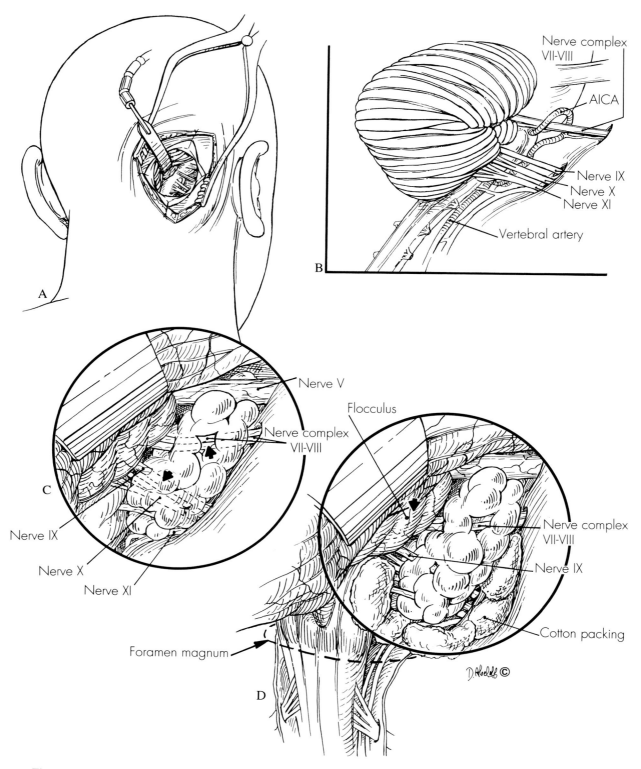

Figure 23-10. **(A)** Relationships of the cranial nerves in the cerebellopontine angle. Cranial nerves V, VII, VIII, IX, X, XI, and XII are typically surrounded by tumor. **(B)** The cerebellum is retracted to expose the angle and the tumor with the surrounding cranial nerves. *AICA,* anterior inferior cerebellar artery. **(C)** Schematic representation of the typical location of the tumor and of the cranial nerves passing through it, surrounded by tumor mass. **(D)** Before tumor is removed, cotton is packed to restrict access to the contents to the subarachnoid space. The tumor is then removed and the cranial nerves dissected free from residual tumor before the mass is excised.

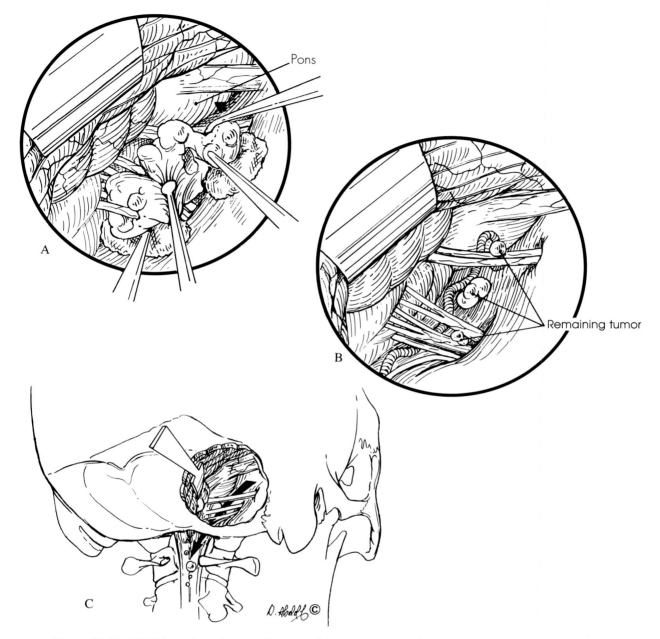

Figure 23-11. (A) Dissection of tumor from cranial nerves. **(B)** Residual tumor on nerves. **(C)** Seeding of cervical subarachnoid space with recurrent tumor. Remember to look!

cholesterol contents from reaching them. This is particularly true inferiorly, for you do not want this noxious material falling into the spinal canal. Regular irrigation with saline is important. Once the tumor is totally removed, thorough irrigation with a large amount of saline will reduce the risk of aseptic meningitis.

This basic surgical technique may be modified for smaller tumors according to their location. If the tu-

mors are only in the angle or only in the region of the fifth nerve, the craniectomy can be more limited and superiorly placed. For those that are wholly in the region of the jugular bulb, a lower exposure is necessary. However, these are minor variations, and the procedure described is satisfactory for virtually all of these tumors.

Remember that the cerebellopontine angle is the second place where primary epidermoid carcinoma can occur. These tumors are easily confused with meningioma or simple epidermoid. On imaging the keys are the extent of bony destruction that sometimes occurs and the enhancing character of the tumor. Typically these tumors have a mass in the cerebellopontine angle, but are en bloc along the whole base unilaterally, sometimes bilaterally. They cannot be cured surgically by any known technique. The usual goal is decompression of the brainstem with removal of as much tumor as possible. The tumors are soft, necrotic, and easily removed by suction. It is possible they might be amenable to radical excision with the sacrifice of multiple cranial nerves, but no one has reported a significant series using radical surgery. The most common approach is to remove the tumor mass compressing the brain and as much of the soft en bloc tumor as possible, and to follow this with radiation.

Fourth Ventricular Epidermoids

Occasionally one of these tumors occurs within the fourth ventricle.[30,67] It is approached like any other intraventricular tumor. I prefer general anesthesia in the prone position with a midline incision for bilateral craniectomy tailored to the size of the exposure necessary to remove the tumor. The dura of the posterior fossa is opened in a Y-shaped fashion and the tumor exposed by retracting the tonsils laterally. It may be necessary to split the vermis. This is true because it is important to see the entire tumor so that total removal is possible. Whenever possible, the tumor capsule should be dissected free from surrounding brain and the tumor removed as a single mass to avoid any contamination of the ventricle with its contents. Unfortunately, these tumors often grow large before they are detected and, as elsewhere, they insinuate themselves in all directions. In such a situation it is better to remove the tumor by suction and then dissect the remaining capsule and its contents free from surrounding wall. It actually is easier to get a total removal here than in the subarachnoid space because the definitions between brain and the tumor are not obscured by thickened arachnoid. It is important to surround the tumor completely with cotton, protecting the ventricle and the subarachnoid space from its contents. Copious irrigation should be employed. The most likely place for tumor to be left is the lateral foramina. Be especially careful where the tumor is adherent to the choroid plexus.

Once the tumor is out and you have irrigated much more than you think should be necessary, the wound is closed in anatomical layers, and no special care is required.

Intramedullary Infratentorial Tumors

Very rarely an epidermoid will be found within the substance of the brainstem.[46,77] It is more common for a fourth ventricular tumor to have eroded deep within the brainstem or for a cerebellopontine angle tumor to appear to have an intramedullary component. However, these true intramedullary tumors have been described. They are hard to distinguish preoperatively from the equally rare intramedullary lipoma. This would rarely make a difference in terms of the choice to operate or not, but it certainly is an important difference in terms of removal. The lipoma simply needs to be debulked. These epidermoid tumors are curable and invariably fatal if not removed.

The approach to the intramedullary tumor is dictated by the location of the tumor. The best rule to follow is to approach the tumor through the portion of the brainstem where it is closest to the surface. Operating through the floor of the fourth ventricle risks many important structures. Unless the tumor actually presents in the fourth ventricle, it is better to approach this kind of tumor laterally. However, if the scans demonstrate that the floor of the fourth ventricle is sufficiently thin, then an approach such as that described for the intraventricular tumor is reasonable.

In most other instances, it is better to approach laterally. These tumors, like cavernous angiomas, are clearly defined from the brainstem, and operating within the brainstem is not as hazardous as it is with the gliomas. If there is no place where the tumor has really approached the surface sufficiently close to make the exposure relatively safe, I prefer to enter the pons through the brachium pontis. The resultant cerebellar deficit is usually compensated for within a matter of months.

The basic techniques of managing these tumors are the same as described for all the others, but it is usually not possible to get the wide exposure that is desirable to visualize the entire capsule. As with any similar brainstem tumor, the mass can be debulked to limit manipulation of the brainstem and allow the capsule to be delivered through a very small opening. High magnification and blunt dissection of the capsule from the wall are key. The plane between brain and capsule is much easier to define than the plane between capsule and arachnoid, so these tumors can be teased free without remnants. Since there will always be recurrence if any of the tumor is left, it is very important to spend whatever time is required to remove the capsule completely. Again, as with all these tumors, copious irrigation and damming the subarachnoid space with cotton to prevent spread of the tumor contents is important.

Intradiploic Tumors

Intradiploic tumors are simple to cure. MRI defines them exactly. Most are within the skull, but extension to the subgaleal or extradural compartments occurs.[18,19,53,78] The flap should extend beyond cyst margins. The key is total removal of the cyst wall and the contents. Remove bone until it is certain no cyst remnants remain.[22,58] Drilling the margins back to normal bone is one good way to be sure exenteration is complete. Then replace bone with an acrylic cranioplasty. Cure is the rule.

Malignant Change in Epidermoid Tumors

Epidermoid carcinoma may mimic epidermoid tumor in two areas. One has been described in the cerebellopontine angle.[34,79] The other is at the region of the gasserian ganglion. Given MRI, it would be unusual to confuse the epidermoid carcinoma with epidermoid tumor now. The malignant tumors enhance and destroy bone most of the time, but may not, and the surgeon has to be prepared for the fact that malignancies can occur in these locations. Malignant epidermoid carcinomas in the other locations are rarely reported, suggesting that these two classes of tumors do not represent changed biological behavior, but rather two distinct neoplasms. Intradiploic tumors are known to undergo malignant degeneration, but this is unusual.[27,44,47,61]

PREVENTION OF COMPLICATIONS

There is only one complication unique to the epidermoid tumors. These tumors occasionally present with a meningitis-like syndrome following spontaneous rupture of the contents into the subarachnoid space or ventricle.[2,12,70,73] Spilling this inflammatory material during surgery or leaving residual tumor may result in a severe syndrome of septic meningitis that is indistinguishable from an overwhelming infection.

The syndrome usually begins a few days after surgery.[1] It is signaled by high temperature and intense local pain. Patients often become confused, and serious impairments of level of consciousness can occur. Localizing signs relate to the structures in the general vicinity. While this is primarily a meningeal reaction, blood vessels are not immune. I have been shown one case in which an inflammatory aneurysm was proved to have developed after the local reaction of this type. These patients are acutely ill and require immediate treatment to minimize long-term complications. First, it is necessary to be certain this is not bacterial meningitis. Lumbar puncture will demonstrate cloudy fluid filled with white cells both acute and chronic. The protein is high. The culture is obviously the key. When this type of tumor has been removed and such a meningitic reaction occurs, I prefer to treat promptly after lumbar puncture rather than waiting for the cultures to be reported. The risk of administering steroids to a patient with true meningitis is certainly less than the risk of leaving the aseptic reaction untreated.

Treatment of this complication is high-dose steroids.[17] In order to prevent it I give all patients with a suspected epidermoid a preoperative regimen of glucosteroids, and rather than discontinuing steroids promptly after satisfactory surgery, I continue the drug for 5 to 7 days and then taper it slowly over the next 3 or 4 days. The choice of steroids and the exact course is empiric. Should the aseptic meningitis syndrome occur in spite of the usual doses of steroids (dexamethasone 10 mg intravenously prior to surgery and 4 mg every 6 hours for 5 days before beginning a 3- to 4-day taper), the reaction is treated by increasing the steroid dose. Again, this dosage is empirical. I usually begin by doubling the standard doses. High-dose steroids will usually bring the reaction under control promptly. A lumbar puncture is performed to be certain that no infection is being missed, but the syndrome is so typical and the risk of this kind of overwhelming meningitis so small that it is unlikely the error will be made, except in unusual circumstances.[43]

The late complication of this reaction is adhesive arachnoiditis surrounding the cranial nerves in the area of surgery. Progressive deficits can occur with this form of arachnoiditis, but are rare. To prevent late reactions, continue steroids for 10 to 14 days and then gradually decrease them at a rate commensurate with maintaining the patient without symptoms.

The syndrome is distressing and always worrisome, but with steroids, it is unlikely that the reactions will be severe or the sequelae significant.

RECURRENT TUMORS

Diagnosis of recurrent epidermoid tumors has been made much easier by MRI.[14] CT scanning showed a lucent area hard to differentiate from cerebrospinal fluid. MRI shows the typical characteristics of cholesterol-laden fatty contents of the cyst, and the diagnosis is usually secure on the basis of imaging alone.

Surgical removal is the only therapy currently available. Since these tumors insinuate themselves into normal subarachnoid space and surround vessels and nerves without deforming them significantly, it is common for them to grow back to enormous size before they are discovered unless routine postoperative scans are done. Those in the suprasellar region that effect the anterior visual apparatus are usually discovered when smaller. Third and fourth ventricular tumors may be found early if they obstruct spinal fluid flow.

The key to prevention of recurrence is total removal at the first operation. Subsequent procedures are much less likely to result in cure of the tumor. The approaches used for these tumors are no different than for first operations.

There are two important general aspects that are the same as for the initial surgical procedure. The first is to be certain that the cholesterol crystals are not allowed to circulate in the subarachnoid space. They will incite a serious aseptic reaction, which may lead to progressive cranial nerve deficits. The real key to curative surgery is attention to the capsule. At the first operation, every effort must be made to remove every tiny piece of capsule. The problem is that the capsule is often very adherent to all surrounding structures and it can be a slow and tedious dissection to remove it. It is very hard to tell capsule from thickened arachnoid, so it is better to remove everything possible at the first operation rather than run a risk of recurrence.

Chiasmal Recurrence

The recurrence of epidermoid tumors in the region of the chiasm is rare. This is fortunate because reoperation is extremely difficult. Total removal of these tumors from the chiasmal area is much easier probably because they tend to cause visual symptoms earlier when they are small. When first seen the tumors may look very much like a craniopharyngioma, but the pearly appearance makes differentiation possible. Rarely, these tumors may recur in the suprachiasmatic space, where they can grow to a larger size before they are detected, and where total removal is more difficult. Even more rarely, they may occur in the region of the cavernous sinus where they are actually easier to remove than most other tumors involving the sinus and related structures.

Diagnosis of Recurrence

MRI makes diagnosis straightforward. The fatty characteristics of the tumor are typical, and early recurrence can be detected. It has been my rule to repeat MRI on a yearly basis following initial successful removal after proving total removal with a postoperative scan. When total removal has not been achieved, as evidenced by a negative postoperative scan, I recommend reoperation to remove the lesion totally. When recurrence of tumor is seen on routine follow-up, consideration of reoperation should be discussed with the patient immediately. It is always possible to wait to be certain that significant tumor will occur, but the natural history of these tumors is slow, steady progression and there is little value in procrastination. It may be difficult to decide to do such a formidable operation in a patient who is asymptomatic, but in whom the scan has become diagnostic for recurrent tumor. Serial scans with proof of growth settle the issue. In this situation repeat of the scans every 3 months is preferable so that growth is determined while the tumor is still small.

Yearly neuroophthalmological examinations including visual fields are routine in our follow-up to supplement the scan. In the days before MRI, the examination was the most accurate way to determine symptomatic recurrence. Now MRI is so successful that the examination may not be as useful for determination of recurrence of tumor. However, the second major complication of these tumors is dense adhesive arachnoiditis. The examination can be very useful in determining an early visual change secondary to arachnoiditis so that treatment can proceed before visual loss is severe.

Surgical Treatment

Once recurrence is established, reoperation is the only available treatment. I approach these tumors through a pterional route. Many surgeons use a subfrontal approach. The frontal flap can be extended to allow both a pterional and a subfrontal exposure. I prefer to approach these tumors from the nondominant side, but nearly always approach them from the side of previous surgery to protect the opposite frontal lobe. It is important to examine the MRI for frontal lobe injury. It is extremely important to avoid bilateral frontal lobe injury, and for that reason, I will tailor the approach to offer the least damage to normal frontal lobe. The exposure has no other special requirements. Once the adhesions are transected, it is possible to expose the chiasmal area by proceeding along the sphenoid wing to the carotid artery. The problem with these tumors is that dense adhesions may have formed secondary to chemical reaction in the original procedure and the resultant arachnoiditis can completely obliterate all of the anatomy, making it extremely difficult to identify the optic nerves. When this has not occurred, the removal of recurrent tumor is straightforward. Tumor is easily identified because it consists principally of the pearly cholesterol material. This can be removed easily by suction. The tedious part of the operation then is removal of all of the reactive arachnoid and identifiable tumor capsule. The thin capsule can be so closely applied to blood vessels, brain, and nerve that it is extremely difficult to remove the residual capsule with certainty. There is little concern about opening into subarachnoid space and spreading the noxious material at this point, but if normal subarachnoid channels are opened at any place, they should be occluded with cottonoid. Once the tumor is out, thorough irrigation until the fluid is completely clear will usually reduce the risk of aseptic meningitis.

It is common for the normal anatomy of the entire chiasmal area to be obliterated by arachnoiditis. In that case you must expose enough of the carotid artery to be certain about its location and then find the chiasm by the relationships. In this situation a broad exposure is important, so I usually add the subfrontal retractors to allow the orbital roofs and sphenoid planum to be exposed as well. This gives bony anatomy and orientation. Then the microdissection of the thickened arachnoid from the chiasmal structures can proceed under high magnification. It is difficult to overemphasize the care that must be taken. This is a tedious procedure that virtually always must be done with sharp instruments.

Sometimes it can be so difficult to identify the optic nerves and chiasm that it is better to begin from normal anatomy. In this situation the best plan is to identify the orbital roof, the location of the optic canal, and then drill away orbital roof and optic canal until normal nerve is discovered. This can be done bilaterally. Then the nerves can be followed back into the scar and the removal of the scar and recurrent tumor continues until the nerves are free of compression and all tumor is removed.

Chiasmal Arachnoiditis without Tumor Recurrence

An unusual complication of the removal of a subchiasmal epidermoid is the subsequent development of progressive adhesive arachnoiditis without obvious recurrent tumor.[73] In this situation MRI will not help because it is unlikely to demonstrate any significant abnormality. The hallmark of the problem is progressive, painless visual loss. Do not be reassured by a normal image when this occurs. It is because of this complication that we employ a combination of scans and visual examinations for long-term evaluation of patients after surgery. It can be difficult to decide to explore the chiasm when the MRI remains negative for recurrent tumor. Nevertheless, in most instances in which a visual deterioration occurs and is documented to be progressive, exploration is reasonable.

The approaches are exactly the same and the problem is no different than when there is recurrent tumor and dense adhesions. The goal is to remove the arachnoidal reaction completely from around the optic nerves. The surgical technique will depend upon the distortion of the anatomy. Sometimes the chiasm and optic nerves can be identified easily and the arachnoid removed with high magnification and sharp dissection. Sometimes there is simply a grayish-white mask covering the base completely, obliterating normal anatomy, and obscuring the nerves. In this situation it is better to identify the bony anatomy, find the optic canals, and remove orbital roof and optic canals until normal nerves are seen. Then, they can be traced back into the mass and the tissue removed.

It is key to do this in an atraumatic fashion. This means exceptionally high magnification, usually 10 to 16, and sharp dissection, which minimizes traction on the nerve. You must also avoid any injury to intrinsic blood vessels on the nerves or chiasm. When you finish, the optic nerves should have been circumferentially decompressed and chiasmal anatomy should be normal.

There is nothing known that will prevent the recurrence of the problem, but to date I have not seen a patient who deteriorated further or required additional surgery for arachnoiditis of any cause.

Recurrent Tumors of the Cerebellopontine Angle and Jugular Bulb

The diagnosis of recurrence is made by the appearance of new neurological deficits, usually changes in cranial nerve function, or by MRI. I obtain regular images on a yearly basis for all patients with epidermoid tumors so that recurrences will be found early.

These tumors can be approached by a unilateral retromastoid incision. I use a curvilinear incision like an elongated C. All the operations are done under general anesthesia in the park bench position. Occipital bone is removed as necessary for exposure of the recurrence and the dura is opened in a cruciate fashion with each flap raised off the cerebellum. The dura is usually adherent to the cerebellum and must be dissected free. Bipolar coagulation with fine forceps works well for this maneuver. When the cerebellum is retracted and the angle exposed, the tumor is usually seen immediately. The recurrent tumor has the same pearly glistening capsule so the tumor recurrence is simple to identify. However, the recurrences are not always a single mass. It is not uncommon for the recurrent tumor to be a series of discrete islands of tumor, each probably representing a small area where capsule was left. These are commonly on cranial nerves or adherent to the brainstem and are particularly found in those areas where capsular removal would have been most difficult. Taking them off the junction of the fifth, seventh, and eighth nerves with the brainstem is particularly difficult because of the lateral pontine veins. The large masses are easy to find, but it is important to explore the area thoroughly, retracting brainstem and lifting cranial nerves to look for small bits that could be missed only to recur again. Remember the cranial nerves commonly go through these tumors. It is wise to find the nerve where it is normal and follow it through the tumor. This is particularly important for the tumors that extend down into the area of the 9th, 10th, and 11th nerves, because these small nerves are very difficult to identify within the bulk of the tumor.

When the tumor recurrence is large enough that the cranial nerve anatomy is obscured, the best technique is gentle suction of the cholesterol crystals until the nerves are seen. This needs to be done under high magnification and slowly with great care until the nerves are identified.

Once the major mass of tissue is removed, the capsule should be manipulated away from nerves, vessels, and the brainstem. Because of the reaction incited by the tumor, the capsule is likely to be adherent, intermixed with thickened arachnoid, and very difficult to remove. Everything possible should be taken out. It is better not to create a major neurological deficit with one of these benign tumors, for even with incomplete removals, patients can go for years before recurrences occur.

The tumor will invest major blood vessels as well. The basilar can virtually always be seen on MRI so its location is clear. However, the major branches may be more difficult to define because of their circuitous courses. I do not use angiography. What is necessary is gentle removal of recurrent tumor with a clear picture of the anatomy at all times.

When all discernible tumor is removed, the area should be irrigated with saline thoroughly. The closure requires no special care. The patient must be watched postoperatively for the development of fever and signs of meningitis. When the process is aseptic, it is promptly relieved by steroids. However,

it is necessary to be certain the patient does not have a true postoperative infection before the steroids are employed. Fortunately, with care in occluding cerebrospinal fluid pathways during the surgery and thorough irrigation, it is very uncommon for the aseptic meningitis syndrome to occur.

These patients should be followed for recurrence on a yearly basis with MRI.

CONCLUSIONS

Epidermoid tumors are relatively rare and are now easily diagnosed.[82] They are more likely to be misdiagnosed as an expanded subarachnoid space or porencephalic cyst than anything else. Because they are insidious in growth, they often reach substantial size before symptoms occur.[26] The majority are either suprasellar or in the cerebellopontine angle. Once diagnosed, they should be removed if symptomatic. They gradually grow by desquamation and may reach enormous size. They are much easier to remove when they are small. The key to surgery is removal of the tumor with capsule intact when possible. When this is not possible, the contents should be evacuated and the capsule then dissected free no matter how tedious this exercise is. Leaving the capsule in place guarantees recurrence. Remember that blood vessels and cranial nerves are usually surrounded by these tumors rather than pushed to the side as they are with the more common meningiomas and schwannomas. Containing the desquamation so that it does not reach the ventricular surface or subarachnoid space is key to preventing the one serious complication of this tumor, the aseptic meningitis syndrome.

These tumors are curable. The best chance of cure is with the first operation; the surgeon should enter these operations with a commitment to the time and effort required for total tumor excision with preservation of all neurological structures.

REFERENCES

1. Abramson RC, Morawetz RB, Schlitt M: Multiple complications from an intracranial epidermoid cyst: case report and literature review. Neurosurgery 24:574, 1989
2. Achard JM, Lallement PY, Veyssier P: Recurrent aseptic meningitis secondary to intracranial epidermoid cyst and Mollaret's meningitis: two distinct entities or a single disease? A case report and a nosologic discussion. Am J Med 89:807, 1990
3. Alpers BJ: The cerebral epidermoids. Am J Surg 43:55, 1939
4. Altschuler EM, Jungreis CA, Sekhar LN et al: Operative treatment of intracranial epidermoid cysts and

cholesterol granulomas: report of 21 cases. Neurosurgery 26:606, 1990

5. Alvord ED, Jr: Growth rates of epidermoid tumors. Ann Surg 2:267, 1977
6. Amendola MA, Garfinkle WB, Ostrum BJ et al: Preoperative diagnosis of a ruptured intracranial dermoid cyst by computerized tomography—case report. J Neurosurg 48:1035, 1978
7. Arienta C, Zavanone M: Intracranial dermoid cysts. Diagnostic value of CT scan. Case reports. J Neurosurg Sci 27:111, 1983
8. Arseni C, Danaila L, Constantinescu A: Cranial and orbital epidermoid tumours. J Neurosurg Sci 19:139, 1975
9. Auger RG, Piepgras DG: Hemifacial spasm associated with epidermoid tumors of the cerebellopontine angle. Neurology 39:577, 1989
10. Bartal A, Razon N, Avram J et al: Infratentorial epidermoids. Acta Neurochir [Suppl] (Wien) 42:142, 1988
11. Baumann CHH, Bucy PC: Paratrigeminal epidermoid tumors. J Neurosurg 13:455, 1956
12. Becker WJ, Watters GV, de Chadarevian JP, Vanasse M: Recurrent aseptic meningitis secondary to intracranial epidermoids. Can J Neurol Sci 11:387, 1984
13. Berger MS, Wilson CB: Epidermoid cysts of the posterior fossa. J Neurosurg 61:214, 1985
14. Brant-Zawadzki M, Badami JP, Mills CM et al: Primary intracranial tumor imaging: a comparison of magnetic resonance and CT. Radiology 150:435, 1984
15. Braun IF, Naidich TP, Leeds NE et al: Dense intracranial epidermoid tumors. Computed tomographic observations. Radiology 122:717, 1977
16. Budka H: Intracranial lipomatous hamartomas (intracranial "lipomas"). A study of 13 cases including combinations with medulloblastoma, colloid and epidermoid cysts, angiomatosis and other malformations. Acta Neuropathol (Berl) 28:205, 1974
17. Cantu RC, Ojemann RG: Glucosteroid treatment of keratin meningitis following removal of a fourth ventricle epidermoid tumor. J Neurol Neurosurg Psychiatry 31:73, 1968
18. Ciappetta P, Artico M, Salvati M et al: Intradiploic epidermoid cysts of the skull: report of 10 cases and review of the literature. Acta Neurochir (Wien) 102:33, 1990
19. Constans JP, Meder JF, De Divitiis E et al: Giant intradiploic epidermoid cysts of the skull. Report of two cases. J Neurosurg 62:445, 1985
20. Crossley GH, Dismukes WE: Central nervous system epidermoid cyst: a probable etiology of Mollaret's meningitis. Am J Med 89:805, 1990
21. Cushing H: A large epidermal cholesterotoma of the parietotemporal region deforming the left hemisphere without cerebral symptoms. Surg Gynecol Obstet 34:557, 1922
22. Dan NG, Caspary EJ: Giant intracranial epidermoid tumour: a singular pearl? Aust NZ J Surg 46:243, 1976
23. Davidson HD, Ouchi T, Steiner RE: NMR imaging of congenital intracranial germinal layer neoplasms. Neuroradiology 27:301, 1985

24. Davis KR, Roberson GH, Taveras JM et al: Diagnosis of epidermoid tumor by computed tomography. Analysis and evaluation of findings. Radiology 119:347, 1976
25. de Chadarevian JP, Becker WJ: Mollaret's recurrent aseptic meningitis: relationship to epidermoid cysts. Light microscopic and ultrastructural cytological studies of the cerebrospinal fluid. J Neuropathol Exp Neurol 39:661, 1980
26. deSouza CE, deSouza R, daCosta S et al: Cerebellopontine angle epidermoid cysts: a report on 30 cases. J Neurol Neurosurg Psychiatry 52:986, 1989
27. Dubois PJ, Sage M, Luther JS et al: Case report. Malignant change in an intracranial epidermoid cyst. J Comput Assist Tomogr 5:433, 1981
28. Dykman TR, Montgomery EB, Jr, Gerstenberger PD et al: Glossopharyngeal neuralgia with syncope secondary to tumor. Treatment and pathophysiology. Am J Med 71:165, 1981
29. Fawcitt RA, Isherwood I: Radiodiagnosis of intracranial pearly tumours with particular reference to the value of computer tomography. Neuroradiology 11:235, 1976
30. Fiume D, Gazzari G, Spallone A, Santucci N: Epidermoid cysts of the fourth ventricle. Surg Neurol 29:178, 1988
31. Flemming JFR, Botterell EH: Cranial dermoid and epidermoid tumors. Surg Gynecol Obstet 109:403, 1959
32. Fornari M, Solero CL, Lasio G et al: Surgical treatment of intracranial dermoid and epidermoid cysts in children. Childs Nerve Syst 6:66, 1990
33. Gagliardi FM, Vagnozzi R, Caruso R, Delfini R: Epidermoids of the cerebellopontine angle: usefulness of CT scan. Acta Neurochir (Wien) 54:271, 1980
34. Garcia CA, McGarry PA, Rodriguez F: Primary intracranial squamous cell carcinoma of the right cerebellopontine angle: case report. J Neurosurg 54:824, 1981
35. Grant FC, Austin GM: Epidermoids: clinical evaluation and surgical results. J Neurosurg 7:190, 1950
36. Guidetti B, Gagliardi FM: Epidermoids and dermoid cysts. J Neurosurg 47:12, 1977
37. Hamel E, Frowein RA, Karimi-Nejad A: Intracranial intradural epidermoids and dermoids. Surgical results of 38 cases. Neurosurg Rev 3:215, 1980
38. Handa J, Okamoto K, Nakasu Y et al: Computed tomography of intracranial epidermoid tumours with special reference to atypical features. Acta Neurochir (Wien) 58:221, 1981
39. Hiratsuka H, Okada K, Matsunaga M et al: Diagnosis of epidermoid cysts by metrizamide CT cisternography. Neuroradiology 26:153, 1984
40. House JL, Brackmann DE: Cholesterolgranuloma of the cerebellopontine angle. Arch Otolaryngol Head Neck Surg 108:504, 1982
41. Hwang WZ, Hasegawa T, Ito H et al: Intracranial epidermoids—concerning the low absorption value on computerized tomography. Acta Neurochir (Wien) 78:33, 1985
42. Ishikawa M, Kikuchi H, Asato R: Magnetic resonance imaging of the intracranial epidermoid. Acta Neurochir (Wien) 101:108, 1989

43. Kohno K, Sakaki S, Nakano K et al: Brain abscess secondary to intracranial extradural epidermoid cyst. Surg Neurol 22:541, 1984
44. Komjatszegi S: Primary intracranial epidermoid carcinoma [letter]. J Neurosurg 52:440, 1980
45. Laster DW, Moody DM, Ball MR: Computerized cranial tomography of free intracranial fat in congenital tumors. Comput Tomogr 2:257, 1978
46. Leal O, Miles J: Epidermoid cyst in the brainstem: case report. J Neurosurg 48:811, 1978
47. Lewis AJ, Cooper PW, Kassel EE, Schwartz ML: Squamous cell carcinoma arising in a suprasellar epidermoid cyst. Case report. J Neurosurg 59:538, 1983
48. Lo WWM, Solti-Bohman LG, Brackmann DE, Gruskin P: Cholesterol granuloma of the petrous apex: CT diagnosis. 153:705, 1984
49. Long DM: Atlas of Operative Neurosurgical Technique. Vol. 1. Cranial Operations. Williams & Wilkins, Baltimore, 1989
50. Long DM, Chou SN: Transcallosal removal of craniopharyngiomas within the third ventricle. J Neurosurg 39:563, 1973
51. Long DM, Rhoton AL: The pterional approach in aneurysm surgery, Part II. p. 245. In Hopkins LN, Long DM (eds): Clinical Management of Intracranial Aneurysms. Raven Press, New York, 1982
52. Lunardi P, Missori P: Cranial and spinal tumors with meningitic onset. Ital J Neurol Sci 11:145, 1990
53. Lye RH, Pickard JD: Occipital 'sebaceous cysts'—a trap for the unwary. Br J Surg 67:333, 1980
54. MacCarty CS, Leavens ME, Love JG, Kernohan JW: Dermoid and epidermoid tumors in the central nervous system of adults. Surg Gynecol Obstet 108:191, 1959
55. Machen BC, Williams JP, Lum GB et al: Intracranial gyriform calcification associated with subarachnoid fat. J Comput Tomogr 10:385, 1986
56. Maulsby GO, Sheldon JJ, Leborgne JM, Altman DH: Intracranial dermoid cyst: diagnosis by computerized tomography. Am J Dis Child 134:420, 1980
57. Mikhael MA, Mattar AG: Intracranial pearly tumors: the roles of computed tomography, angiography, and pneumoencephalography. J Comput Assist Tomogr 2:421, 1978
58. Miller NR, Epstein MH: Giant intracranial dermoid cyst: case report and review of the literature on intracranial dermoids and epidermoids. Can J Neurol Sci 2:127, 1975
59. Miyazawa N, Yamazaki H, Wakao T, Nukui H: Epidermoid tumors of Meckel's cave: case report and review of the literature. Neurosurgery 25:951, 1989
60. Nagashima C, Takahama M, Sakaguchi A: Dense cerebellopontine epidermoid cyst. Surg Neurol 17:172, 1982
61. Nishiura I, Koyama T, Handa J, Amano S: Primary intracranial epidermoid carcinoma—case report. Neurol Med Chir (Tokyo) 29:600, 1989
62. Olson JJ, Beck DW, Crawford SC, Menezes AH: Comparative evaluation of intracranial epidermoid tumors with computed tomography and magnetic resonance imaging. Neurosurgery 21:357, 1987
63. Otsuka S, Nakatsu S, Matsumoto S et al: Epidermoid tumor presenting with trigeminal neuralgia and ipsilateral hemifacial spasm: a case report. Nippon Geka Hokan 58:245, 1989
64. Panagopoulos KP, el-Azouzi M, Chisholm HL et al: Intracranial epidermoid tumors. A continuing diagnostic challenge. Arch Neurol 47:813, 1990
65. Peyton WT, Baker AB: Epidermoid, dermoid and teratomatous tumors of the central nervous system. Arch Neurol Psychiatry 47:890, 1942
66. Rooney MS, Poon PY, Wortzman G: Magnetic resonance imaging of intracranial epidermoids: report of two cases. J Can Assoc Radiol 38:283, 1987
67. Rosario M, Becker DH, Conley FK: Epidermoid tumours involving the fourth ventricle. Neurosurgery 9:9, 1981
68. Sabin HI, Bordi LT, Symon L: Epidermoid cysts and cholesterol granulomas centered on the posterior fossa: twenty years of diagnosis and management. Neurosurgery 21:798, 1987
69. Savader SJ, Murtagh FR, Savader BL, Martinez CR: Magnetic resonance imaging of intracranial epidermoid tumours. Clin Radiol 40:282, 1989
70. Schwartz JF, Balentine JD: Recurrent meningitis due to an intracranial epidermoid. Neurology 28:124, 1978
71. Sekhar LN, Schramm VL, Jr, Jones NF: Subtemporal-preauricular infratemporal fossa approach to large lateral and posterior cranial base neoplasms. J Neurosurg 67:488, 1987
72. Stephenson TS, Spitzer RM: MR and CT appearance of ruptured intracranial dermoid tumors. Comp Radiol 11:5, 1987
73. Tomlinson BE, Walton JN: Granulomatous meningitis and diffuse parenchymatous degeneration of the nervous system due to an intracranial epidermoid cyst. J Neurol Neurosurg Psychiatry 30:341, 1967
74. Ulrich J: Intracranial epidermoids: a study on their distribution and spread. J Neurosurg 21:1051, 1964
75. Vaghi MA, Bruzzone MG, Visciani A, Passerini A: Intracranial tumors arising from the floor of the middle fossa. Ital J Neurol Sci 6:469, 1985
76. Vion-Dury J, Vincenteilli F, Jiddane M et al: MR imaging of epidermoid cysts. Neuroradiology 29:333, 1987
77. Weaver EN, Coulon RA: Excision of brain-stem epidermoid cyst. J Neurosurg 51:254, 1979
78. Wilson ES, Jr, Sheft DJ: Epidermoid tumor of the skull with intracranial pneumatocele. Case report. J Neurosurg 28:600, 1968
79. Wong SW, Ducker TB, Powers JM: Fulminating parapontine epidermoid carcinoma in a four-year-old boy. Cancer 37:1525, 1976
80. Yamakawa K, Shitara N, Genka S et al: Clinical course and surgical prognosis of 33 cases of intracranial epidermoid tumors. Neurosurgery 24:568, 1989
81. Yasargil MG, Abernathey CD, Sarioglu AC: Microneurosurgical treatment of intracranial dermoid and epidermoid tumors. Neurosurgery 24:561, 1989
82. Zhou LF: Intracranial epidermoid tumours: thirty-seven years of diagnosis and treatment. Br J Neurosurg 4:211, 1990

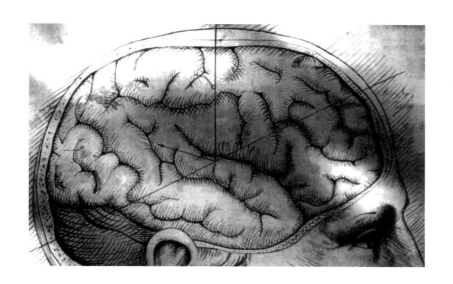

Supratentorial Procedures

Part 3: Vascular Disorders

24 The Ontogenetic and Phylogenetic Basis of Cerebrovascular Anomalies and Variants

Peter L. Mayer
E. Leon Kier

the more we know the more there is to know...
Harvey Cushing[88]

The topic of cerebrovascular variation has fascinated physicians and anatomists for centuries. It is a voluminous subject that encompasses not only the reports of anomalies but also the ontogenetic and phylogenetic studies and hypotheses through which these anomalies can be understood. The purpose of this chapter is to organize much of this literature into a synopsis, which can be used easily by the practicing clinician.

This chapter reviews the topic of cerebrovascular variation with emphasis on its phylogenetic and ontogenetic background. It is not intended as a review of the entire literature on cerebrovascular anomalies and variants; rather, it is hoped that this chapter will provide an understanding of the principles of variation for those interested in vascular neurosurgical disease, such as the neurosurgeon who is faced with a cerebrovascular anomaly and who wishes to understand it better or to find the available literature on it.

The chapter is divided into three parts. The first is a review of the phylogenetic background of human cerebral vasculature, including a brief discussion of the concepts of evolution and homology. A summary is presented of the cerebral vasculature of organisms thought to be similar to those of the direct human phylogenetic pathway, as demonstrated through comparative anatomy. In this first section it can be seen how the brain vasculature has changed as the brain has evolved. This concept is especially relevant to the understanding of human ontogeny, which "recapitulates" phylogeny to a remarkable degree. The next section is a summary of human cerebrovascular ontogeny, based mainly on the important human work of Congdon[78] and Padget[328] and supplemented by other cerebrovascular investigations using nonhuman embryos. Finally, the anatomy of the human brain vasculature is reviewed, with a discussion of the variations and anomalies associated with each arterial system. In this section the ontogenetic and phylogenetic backgrounds of reported anomalies are briefly discussed again for each system individually. Although this may seem redundant, in preparing the text it was felt that most readers would benefit from finding the pertinent background of each arterial system along with its description rather than having to look for the information in the longer first and second sections. Also in the third section, the anatomy of other species that is homologous with the given human arterial systems under discussion is often presented. The way different species use homologous anatomy (which has evolved from the same ancestral anatomy) to suit their particular needs adds a new dimension to the understanding of human arterial variation. Indeed, human cerebrovascular anomalies are often homologous with the normal anatomy of other species.

COMPARATIVE ANATOMY

The following definitions are important for the understanding of this section. They are taken mainly from Stahl,[413] Romer,[366] and Webster's Seventh New Collegiate Dictionary (Gove[151]).

A species is said to be *advanced* if, in reference to other existing species in its environment, its structure has been evolutionarily modified to give it an advantage. For example, the mackerel is advanced relative to another teleostean fish, the herring, because the mackerel's fins and jaws are modified to make it faster, more maneuverable, and better at grasping prey.

Primitive means "evolved long ago."[1]* Some living species, such as the sturgeon (a fish) or the *Sphenodon* (a reptile), probably evolved as species many hundreds of millions of years ago and have remained nearly or entirely unchanged since then. These species are primitive as compared with more advanced species within their orders. However, it should be noted that these species represent evolutionary success stories in longevity. Many more advanced species, indeed whole orders, have evolved and became extinct, while these species have remained unchanged. Terms such as primitive, progressive, and advanced should be used in the scientific sense only to avoid connotations about the intrinsic worth or value of a species.

A species is termed *progressive* or *specialized* if it possesses evolved features that improve upon an ancestral design in order to take advantage of conditions present in the environment. Species become progressive or specialized by evolving special anatomic structures. The fossil record shows that extremes of specialization may ultimately become detrimental, resulting in the decline of a species, especially if environmental conditions change to de-

stroy an ecological niche to which a species has become extremely specialized. In this case less specialized species may adapt to new environmental conditions better and survive longer.

The terms *lower* and *higher* are used to describe the relative position of a species in a phylogenetic hierarchy. For example, species whose orders evolved more recently are designated as higher (e.g., humans, order Primata), while species whose orders evolved longer ago are designated as lower (e.g., iguanas, order Reptilia). Again, one should use these terms in the scientific sense only, avoiding connotations about the intrinsic worth or value of a species.

Homology means "likeness in structure between parts of different organisms due to evolutionary differentiation from the same or a corresponding part of a remote ancestor."[151] Romer[366] defines homology as "the thesis that specific organs of living members of an animal group have descended, albeit with modification, slight or marked, from basically identical organs present in their common ancestor." Homology is determined by common ancestry, structural correspondence, or both. As discussed by Campbell and Hodos,[64] the first basis of homology is stronger, as structural resemblance may not necessarily be the result of inheritance from a common ancestor. Non-homologous resemblance, collectively called *homoplasy,* is seen in *parallelism* (the development of similar new characteristics by unrelated organisms in response to similarity of environment), *convergence* (independent development of similar characters by unrelated organisms owing to similarity of habits or environments), *analogy* (modification of structures with different developmental backgrounds to perform the same function), *mimicry* (the securing of some advantage by one organism that is due to a superficial resemblance to another among which it lives), and *chance similarity.*

Strict homology of structures in living organisms is very difficult to prove. Hypotheses concerning adult structural homologies may be strengthened by showing similarity in ontogenetic development. More often, however, homology is inferred if certain adult anatomic criteria can be met. In the case of blood vessels these criteria are not precisely defined. As with tests of homology that apply to other organs, Shellshear[401] attempted to roughly define the interspecies homology criteria for cerebral blood vessels as: (1) structures supplied, (2) relationship of arteries to cerebral topography, (3) anastomoses with other arteries, and (4) relationship of sympathetic nerves to the arteries. These criteria are used by most writers.

Comparative anatomy uses inductive reasoning to

---

* The term *primitive* is also used in embryology to mean "developed early in embryogenesis."

gain insight into biological evolution. In its broadest interpretation the study of comparative anatomy combines a broad base of information that includes anatomy, embryology, paleontology, physical anthropology, evolutionary theory, and taxonomy. Observing the way an organ is modified by different species to adapt it to their life-styles adds a new dimension to the understanding of that organ's morphology and evolution.

Ontogeny (the development of an individual organism) and phylogeny (the evolution of a genetically related group of organisms) are related, although it is now recognized that the nineteenth century biogenetic law "ontogeny recapitulates phylogeny" is figurative, not literal. It is unlikely that every ancestral morphology is "recapitulated" by the ontogeny of more advanced organisms. However, higher organisms did evolve from lower organisms, and the phylogenetic sequence of morphological changes that resulted in the morphology of a high organism is often strikingly reflected in the early developmental stages of that organism.

No living species belong to our direct phylogenetic pathway (phylesis). Rather, we share common ancestor species, now extinct, with all living species. Every living species, no matter how primitive, has adapted to its particular ecological niche to some degree thereby changing itself from its ancestor species.

Evolution is accomplished in one of two ways: when embryonic characteristics are added that change later embryonic stages or when embryonic characteristics already present undergo change in their rate of maturation.[150] Evolution can be relatively gradual or relatively rapid. Through survival of the fittest and/or by chance, preadapted† organs are used to modify a species' life-style. Once a new structure appears in a species' phylesis, it remains in all higher forms even if diminished functional need reduces the size of the structure.

Shellshear[400] observed that phylogenetically newer structures are generally supplied by blood vessels that branch from adjacent, phylogenetically older structures. Abbie[3] added that in extreme anatomic change, the source of blood supply to a new structure may shift to another source if it is hemodynamically expedient.

---

† *Preadaptation* is the term given to a structure that is later evolutionarily modified to create a new structure; however, it should be noted that this does not imply any sort of preordained order of progression.

OVERVIEW OF COMPARATIVE CEREBROVASCULAR ANATOMY

Studies of comparative cerebrovascular anatomy are important for several reasons. First, they have been important for the understanding of brain evolution.[3,399,408] Second, cerebrovascular variations have been used in the systematic classification of related species.[54–59,347] Finally, understanding how different species have used homologous structures to adapt to their particular life-styles adds another dimension to the understanding of human cerebrovascular variation.

The cerebral vasculature of many species has been studied. However, when deciding what vertebrates to study for an understanding of human anatomy, it is important to know what living species are most similar to those hypothetical species that were our ancestors. Table 24-1 indicates our hypothetical ancestors, as well as the fossil and living species thought to be most closely related to them. The table has been developed from several sources[209,219,366,413,471]; in the table, species discussed or mentioned in this chapter are indicated in boldface.

Protochordates

Protochordates, which are generally very small marine organisms that possess notochords, are thought to represent the ancestors of vertebrates. The best known example of this subphylum is the amphioxus (Fig. 24-1), although the nemertines are probably closer to our true phylogenetic pathway.[383]

The central nervous system (CNS) of amphioxus is essentially a spinal cord. It lacks specialized receptors and centers for olfaction, taste, lateral line system, labyrinthine system, and vision.[383] A pair of nerves exits the ventral surface of the cephalic end. Primitive hypophyseal structures are present. Dorsal and posterior to these, paired nerves enter, supplying sensory input from the head region. There is a grouping of neurons at the cranial end around the primitive third ventricle, probably representing a diencephalon. The ventricular system opens via an anterior neuropore to the water. Caudally, five paired, mixed nerves are present, associated with branchial arches. The midbrain and hindbrain are difficult to differentiate as they appear to be essentially a continuation of the spinal cord without typical landmarks. There is no cerebellar homologue.

The CNS of amphioxus has no intrinsic blood supply.[18] It is supplied with oxygen via diffusion from its

Table 24-1. Human Phylogenetic Pathway[a]

Hypothetical Species in Human Phylesis	Closest Representative	
	Fossil Species	Living Species
Protozoa	Many	Protozoa
Coelenterates	Many	Corals, hydra, jellyfish
Pterobranchs	Many	Rhabdopleurs
Filter feeders	Many	Tunicates, hemichordates
Protochordates	Many	Nemertines, **amphioxus**
Fish		
Jawless fish	Ostracoderms	**Lamprey, hagfish**
Arachaic jawed fish	Placoderms	
Higher fish		
Teleosts	Many	Perch, bass, carp
Cartilaginous fish	Many	**Sharks, rays,** skates, chimeras
Sarcopterygians	Rhipidistians, coelacanths, lungfish	Latimeria, **lungfish**
Amphibians	Labyrinthodonts, ichthyostegids, *Triadobatrachus*	None; modern **anurans, urodeles,** and Apodia very aberrant
Reptiles	Cotylosaurs, chelonia	**Turtles, alligators, lizards,** *Sphenodon*
Mammal-like reptiles	Therapsids, theriodonts	
Monotremes (egg-laying mammals)	Eozostrononts	Platypus, **spiny anteater**
Metatheria (marsupials)	*Alphadon, Aegialodon*	**Opossum, kangaroo**
Placental mammals		
Insectivores	*Erythrotherium, Kennalestes, Gypsonictops*	**Tree shews, hedgehogs, moles**
Primates		
Lower primates	*Purgatorius*, plesiadapoids, adapids, anaptomorphids, omomyids, lemurs, tarsoids	**Lemurs, lorises, goligos, tarsier**
New World monkeys	Omomyids	Marmosets, **cebids**
Old World monkeys	*Aeolopithecus, Parapithecus, Propliopthecus, Apidium, Cercopithecus*	**Macaques, baboons,** langur
Apes	*Dryopithecus, Proconsul,* pongids, *Ramapithecus, Oreopithecus*	Gorillas, **chimpanzees, orangutans, gibbons**
Hominids		
Australopithecus	Lucy	
Homo	*Homo habilis, Homo erectus*	
Homo sapiens	Cro Magnons, Neanderthals	**Modern human**

[a] Boldface indicates a species that is discussed or mentioned in the chapter.

somatic vasculature and presumably also its ventricles and ependymal processes.[382]

Cyclostomes

The lampreys (petromyzonts) and hagfish (myxinoids) are living primitive jawless fish, close to the phylogenetic pathway that led to higher vertebrates. Their brains are close to those of higher fish in complexity, and they have four distinctive, primitive meninges, containing a relatively rich plexus of blood vessels. In this class the first appearance of a primitive capillary net within the brain is noted.[18,84,85] The brains of cyclostomes like those of all submammalian vertebrates, are supplied almost entirely by paired internal carotid arteries,[104] of which each divides into larger caudal and smaller cranial branches. The caudal branches unite into a slender basilar artery in the

hagfish but remain as two separate basilar arteries in the lamprey. The remainder of the vasculature of the cyclostomes is essentially similar to that of higher fish.

Fish

The brain of *Squalus acanthias*, the dogfish shark, like that of all fish, is characterized by a large brainstem primarily concerned with controlling the coordinated, repetitive respiratory movements.[215] Also important in the brainstems of fish are connections for cutaneous and gustatory information.[138,335] Brain structures involved in special sensory and motor tasks are developed to a greater or lesser extent according to the life-style of the particular species. Most fish have prominent optic lobes representing the mesencephalic terminations of completely

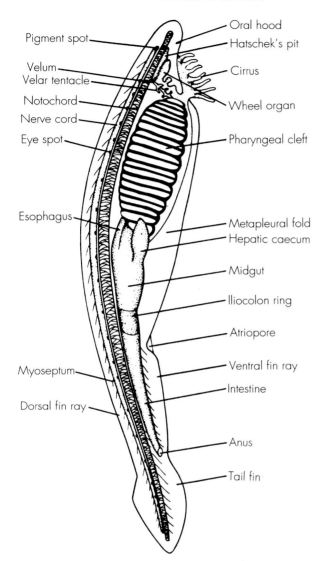

Pigment spot
Velum
Velar tentacle
Notochord
Nerve cord
Eye spot
Esophagus
Myoseptum
Dorsal fin ray

Oral hood
Hatschek's pit
Cirrus
Wheel organ
Pharyngeal cleft
Metapleural fold
Hepatic caecum
Midgut
Iliocolon ring
Atriopore
Ventral fin ray
Intestine
Anus
Tail fin

Figure 24-1. The protochordate amphioxus, the central nervous system of which is essentially a spinal cord (nerve cord). (From Kluge et al.,[219] modified from Crouch,[86a] with permission.)

crossed optic nerves.[3,138] The cerebellum of many fish is relatively large and complex, presumably reflecting their tridimensional movement.[366] The forebrain "hemispheres," including the basal nuclei, are very primitive, concerned essentially with the processing and relaying of olfactory information.[3,92,405–407] The ventral portion of the forebrain, including the olfactory centers and more primitive striatum (paleostriatum) is more primitive than the dorsal, which includes the pyriform and hippocampal

areas and more advanced striatum. A band of fibers, the interlobar commissure, connects the dorsal portions of the forebrain hemispheres. It is probably homologous with the hippocampal commissure of higher vertebrates.

Fish respire via gills (Fig. 24-2A–D). The afferent blood supply to the gills comes from the heart via ventral aortae, while oxygenated blood leaves the gills via dorsal aortae to distribute to the head and body.[209,219,366,471] A branch of the anterior dorsal aorta (homologue of the internal carotid artery of higher vertebrates) known as the *orbital artery* (homologue of the stapedial artery of higher vertebrates) branches from the anterior dorsal aorta at the level of the hyomandibular bone (homologue of the stapes) to supply the face and jaw via supraorbital, infraorbital, and mandibular divisions (Fig. 24-3A). More distally, an ophthalmic artery branches from the anterior dorsal aorta to supply the eye.

The brain of *Squalus* is supplied exclusively by paired anterior dorsal aortae, or internal carotid arteries[3,104,138] (Fig. 24-4). Each branches into a thin anterior or cranial and a large posterior or caudal division. The anterior division branches further into medial and lateral olfactory arteries, which supply the forebrain structures. The medial olfactory branch of the anterior division of the internal carotid artery (ICA) is homologous with portions of the human anterior cerebral artery (ACA), while the lateral olfactory artery is homologous with portions of the human middle cerebral artery (MCA). The lateral aspect of the telencephalon, the primordium pyriformis, is supplied by the lateral olfactory artery. The primitive basal nuclear complex, the paleostriatum, is supplied from both the medial and lateral olfactory arteries by a series of arterioles, which penetrate the ventrolateral surface of the brain along a fissure known as the *endorhinal* fissure. These are the early homologues of the lenticulostriate arteries of humans.

The posterior division of the ICA in most fish is larger than the anterior and appears to be the direct continuation of the ICA. Proximal branches of the caudal division include diencephalic and hypophyseal arteries, at least one cerebellar branch on each side, and large, paired, tectal arteries, which supply the optic lobes. More caudally, the posterior divisions of both sides unite to form a single basilar artery in the ventral midline of the brainstem. This artery of the dogfish shark tapers as it runs caudally along the medulla oblongata, providing numerous branches to brainstem centers. It may have loops or fenestrations, which presumably reflect its formation from paired embryonic primordia as in many other vertebrates. In this regard it is worth noting that the

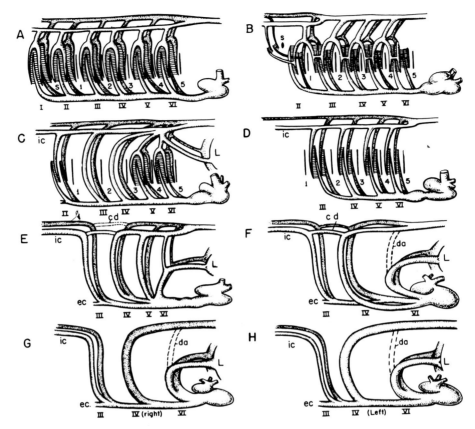

Figure 24-2. Diagrams of the aortic arch system of various vertebrates, left lateral view. Sequential embryonic changes of the human aortic arch and neck arteries recapitulate to some extent the sequence of phylogenetic changes of these vessels. **(A)** Hypothetical ancestor of vertebrates; **(B)** primitive fish (shark); **(C)** lungfish; **(D)** higher fish (teleost such as perch); **(E)** amphibian (salamander); **(F)** reptile (lizard); **(G)** bird; **(H)** mammal. Roman numerals, aortic arches; Arabic numerals, gill slits; *cd*, carotid duct (ductus caroticus); *da*, ductus arteriosus (embryonic); *ec*, external carotid artery; *ic*, internal carotid artery; *L*, lung; *s*, spiracular slit. (From Romer,[366] with permission.)

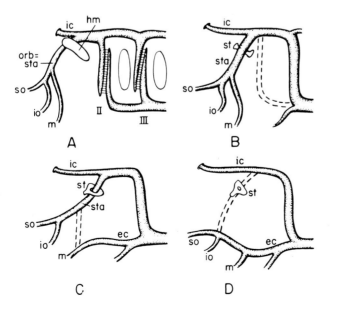

Figure 24-3. Diagram demonstrating the phylogenetic changes of the stapedial artery, left lateral view. The hyomandibular bone of fish is homologous with the stapes and the orbital artery is homologous with the stapedial artery. **(A)** Dorsal aorta and orbital arteries in a fish. **(B)** Internal carotid and stapedial arteries in a reptile. **(C)** Internal carotid and stapedial arteries in a rat. **(D)** Internal carotid and stapedial arteries in a human. Roman numerals, aortic arches; *ec*, external carotid artery; *ic*, internal carotid artery; *io*, infraorbital artery; *hm*, hyomandibular bone; *m*, maxillary artery; *orb*, orbital artery; *so*, supraorbital artery; *st*, stapes bone; *sta*, stapedial artery. (From Romer,[366] with permission.)

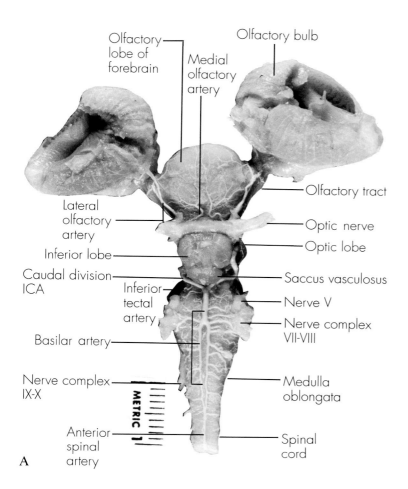

Olfactory lobe of forebrain

Olfactory bulb

Medial olfactory artery

Olfactory tract

Lateral olfactory artery

Optic nerve

Inferior lobe

Optic lobe

Caudal division ICA

Saccus vasculosus

Inferior tectal artery

Nerve V

Nerve complex VII-VIII

Basilar artery

Nerve complex IX-X

METRIC

Medulla oblongata

Anterior spinal artery

Spinal cord

A

Figure 24-4. Brain of a dogfish shark (*Squalus acanthias*), arterial system injected with barium gelatin. The medial and lateral olfactory arteries are homologous with the anterior and middle cerebral arteries of higher vertebrates. Olfaction is the dominant sensory input to the forebrain, as evidenced by the large size of the olfactory apparatus. **(A)** Ventral view; **(B)** left lateral view.

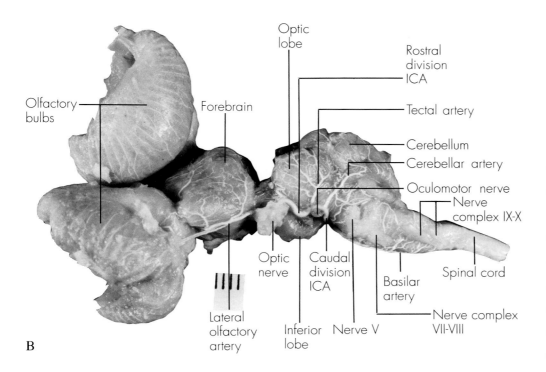

Optic lobe

Rostral division ICA

Olfactory bulbs

Forebrain

Tectal artery

Cerebellum

Cerebellar artery

Oculomotor nerve

Nerve complex IX-X

Optic nerve

Caudal division ICA

Spinal cord

Basilar artery

Lateral olfactory artery

Inferior lobe

Nerve V

Nerve complex VII-VIII

B

697

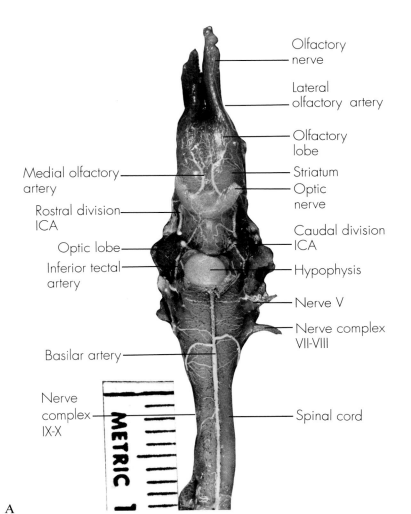

A

Figure 24-5. Brain of a frog (amphibian), arterial system injected with barium gelatin. The medial and lateral olfactory arteries are homologous with the anterior and middle cerebral arteries of higher vertebrates. Note that the forebrain is no larger in diameter than the hindbrain. **(A)** Ventral view; **(B)** left lateral view.

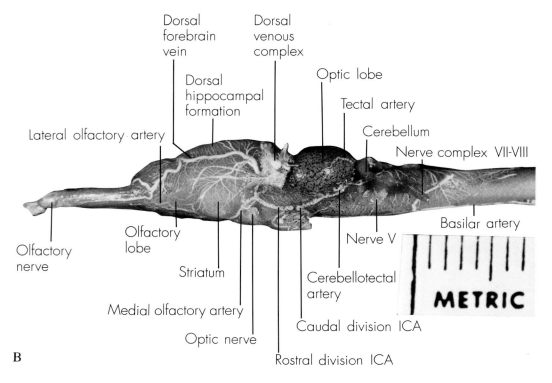

B

caudal ICA divisions of rays do not form a basilar artery at all but rather unite in an anastomotic plexus at the spinomedullary junction.[104]

Amphibians

Phylogenetically the living amphibians are a relative mystery.[3,209,219,366,413,471] The fossil record of these small, fragile tetrapods is very limited and fragmentary. Furthermore, their structures are so specialized as compared with their more generalized ancestral condition that even the study of their ontogeny has revealed almost no information about their phylesis. The living amphibians represent the end of a long side branch rather far from the direct phylogenetic pathway of higher vertebrates. Nonetheless, these species are the only living representatives of the important phylogenetic link between fish and reptiles. Amphibians represent a huge evolutionary step away from fish; they suspend their body from legs and breathe air to live on land.

The amphibian has evolved a relatively larger forebrain than that of fish, although it appears still to be predominantly olfactory in nature.[178,215] The primordia of the hippocampal system is located on the dorsomesial aspect of the hemisphere, with the primordium pyriformis located dorsolaterally and the primordial striatum located ventrally. The optic lobes are relatively smaller, as is the cerebellum, which is considered by some to resemble the human cerebellum in an early embryonic stage.[18]

The amphibian brain (Figs. 24-2E, 24-5, and 24-6A) is supplied exclusively by paired ICAs. However, the rostral and caudal divisions of the intracranial ICA are now of approximately equal caliber, reflecting the increasing importance of the forebrain, even at this still primitive stage.[3,104,138] The rostral division of the ICA again divides into medial and lateral olfactory branches, which supply the structures of the forebrain. In both *Necturus* and frog, the medial olfactory artery mainly supplies the more primitive anteromedial olfactory region, with branches entering the primitive interhemispheric fissure to supply the structures of the mesial and anterior telencephalon. These regions include the septal nuclei, anterior portions of the primordium hippocampi, medial and ventral parts of the paleostriatum, and ventral portions of the amygdaloid nuclei. The medial olfactory artery is the forerunner of the ACA of higher vertebrates.

The larger lateral olfactory artery supplies most of the dorsolateral and posterior dorsomedial portion of the telencephalon, including the majority of the primordium hippocampi, the primordia pyriformis, and the dorsal and lateral parts of the striatal and amyg-

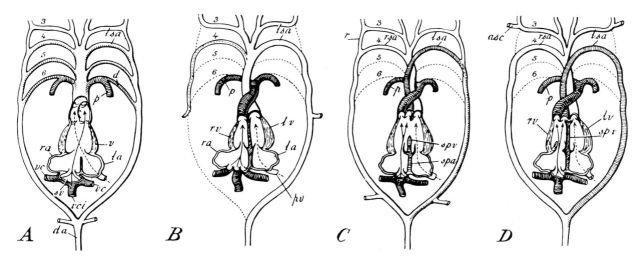

Figure 24-6. Diagrams of ventral view of heart and aortic arch systems of various vertebrates. Sequential embryonic changes of the human aortic arch and neck arteries recapitulate to some extent the sequence of phylogenetic changes of these vessels. **(A)** Amphibian. **(B)** Mammal. **(C)** Typical reptiles. **(D)** Crocodile (a reptile). Solid arrows, venous blood flow; broken arrows, oxygenated blood flow (from lungs); shaded vessels contain venous blood in whole or in part; *asc*, anterior subclavian artery; *d*, ductus arteriosus; *da*, dorsal aorta; *la*, left atrium; *lsa*, left systemic arch; *lv*, left ventricle; *p*, pulmonary artery; *pv*, pulmonary vein; *r*, ductus caroticus; *ra*, right atrium; *rsa*, right systemic arch; *rv*, right ventricle; *spa*, interatrial septum; *spv*, interventricular septum; *sv*, sinus venosus; *v*, ventricle; *vc*, anterior vena cava; *vci*, posterior vena cava. (From Romer,[366] modified from Goodrich,[148a] with permission.)

daloid nuclei. However, these latter areas are supplied by perforating branches, which may originate from both the medial and lateral olfactory arteries. The lateral olfactory artery is the early homologue of the MCA of higher vertebrates.

The arteries considered homologous with the posterior cerebral arteries (PCAs) of higher vertebrates are represented by diencephalic and tectal arteries in amphibians. As in fish, there is no supply to the forebrain from the caudal division of the ICA. It should be noted that the vascular supply to the small cerebellum, as seen in Fig. 24-5, is via what may be called the *cerebellotectal artery*.

Reptiles

The forebrain of reptiles, now the largest subdivision of the brain, shows a great relative increase in size as compared with that of fish and amphibians. This is primarily due to the enlargement of the basal nuclei.[3,86,92,178,215,405–408] These nuclei consist of a large paleostriatum covered by an invagination of the pyriform cortex known as the *hypopallium*.[408] The paleostriatum is homologous with a portion of the globus pallidus of mammals, while the hypopallium is the homologue of parts of the caudate nucleus, putamen, and claustrum (the neostriatum). The striatal complex takes the form of a large mass of tissue, which compresses the lateral ventricles.[215] A new "general" cortex of neopallium is also noted for the first time in phylogeny. This small but important area of the reptilian brain is thought to be the forerunner of the mammalian neocortex. It is found on the anterodorsal surface of the cerebral hemisphere and is separated medially from the hippocampal structures by the rhinal fissure and laterally from the pyriform lobe structures by the endorhinal fissure.[408] The olfactory system is prominent, being still apparently the main sensory input to the telencephalon. The optic lobes are relatively large, as in amphibians and fish. There are still no significant corticospinal or cerebellar systems.

The entire intracranial circulation of reptiles (Figs. 24-2F, 24-3B, 24-6C&D and 24-7) is supplied, as in fish and amphibians, by paired ICAs, which branch into rostral and caudal divisions. The arteries of the forebrain of reptiles are more clearly homologous with those of humans.[104,138] The ACA, homologue of the medial olfactory artery of fish and amphibians, is the direct continuation of the rostral division of the ICA. It runs along the ventromedial aspect of the telencephalon and into the interhemispheric fissure. Significant branches take a recurrent course over the

olfactory tubercle to anastomose ventrolaterally with similar branches of the MCA. The main segment of the ACA runs dorsomesially, where it anastomoses with the PCA to supply the anterior portions of the hippocampal formation and the neopallium. In addition, recurrent branches of the ACA supply perforating arteries to the paleostriatum (Fig. 24-8A). These are the homologues of the medial lenticulostriate arteries and recurrent artery of Heubner of humans and other mammals.[3,138,399] The MCA of the reptile, homologous with the lateral olfactory artery of fish and amphibians, is a branch of the cranial division of the ICA. In the reptile a segment of the main trunk of the MCA runs in the endorhinal fissure, supplying perforating branches to the hypopallium, which are homologous with the lateral lenticulostriate arteries of mammals within the anterior perforated substance.[3,138,399] Inferomedial branches of the MCA anastomose with the recurrent branches of the ACA over the olfactory tubercle, as just described, and lateral branches join the PCA to supply the general cortex.

The PCAs may arise from the rostral division, the caudal division, or the bifurcation of the ICA.[3,60–62,138,216] Posteriorly, these vessels are hidden under the posterior bulges of the telencephalon, which now touch the optic lobes. The PCA sends its first branches mainly to the optic lobe, mesencephalon, diencephalon, and pineal gland. It then continues over the posterior aspect of the hemisphere into the interhemispheric fissure, turning rostrally to course anteriorly to the olfactory bulbs. The PCAs of reptiles supply the hippocampal and parahippocampal areas, the choroid plexus of the third and lateral ventricles, and the general cortex. Over this latter area the PCA enters into an anastomotic plexus with branches of the ACA and MCA. It should be noted that it is branches of the diencephalic and tectal arteries that are annexed for supply of the cerebrum as the cerebrum becomes larger in the reptilian order. These branches have "become" the PCA as a secondary hemodynamic expedient, while the arteries to the diencephalon and mesencephalon are now branches of the PCA.[3]

A phylogenetically important artery (or sometimes an anastomotic group of arteries), known as the inferior cerebral artery, is present in reptiles. This has been considered by several authors to be the early homologue of the stem of the anterior choroidal artery.[1,3,138] However, Burda has shown that in many reptiles another branch, the small lateral choroidal branch of the cranial division of the ICA supplies the choroid plexus as well.[60–62]

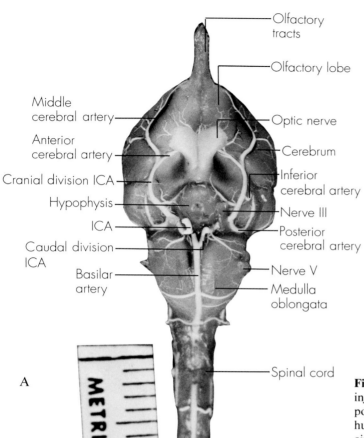

A

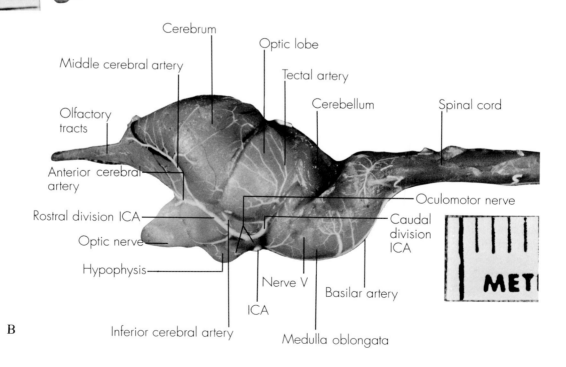

B

Figure 24-7. Brain of an iguana (reptile), arterial system injected with barium gelatin. The cerebrum is the largest portion of the brain and the arterial homologues of the human brain arteries are more clearly recognized. Note the circulus arteriosus (of Willis). **(A)** Ventral view; **(B)** lateral view.

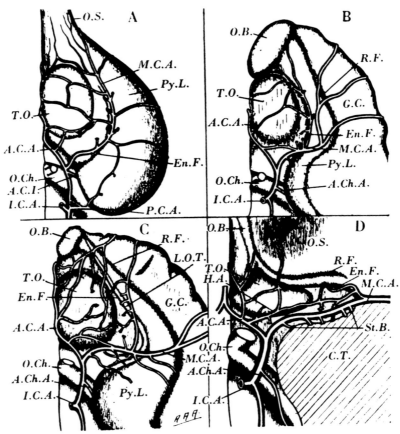

Figure 24-8. Diagrams of the comparative anatomy of the anterolateral basal perforation zone (anterior perforated substance) and the arteries that cross it. The variable anterior cerebral artery (ACA) and middle cerebral artery (MCA) supply of the basal ganglia is present throughout phylogeny. This is clarified when one notes that the entorhinal fissure is "pulled" laterally and "folded" on itself as the forebrain enlarges in phylogeny to become the anterior perforated substance. The reciprocal relationship between the ACA and MCA and the recurrent artery of Heubner in the supply of this region is also seen in the ontogeny of these vessels (see Figs. 24-15 to 24-18 and 24-50). **(A)** Left ventral aspect of forebrain of *Sphenodon*, a primitive reptile. **(B)** Left ventral aspect of forebrain of a marsupial, a primitive mammal. **(C)** Left ventral aspect of forebrain of a kuru, an ungulate similar to a sheep. **(D)** Left side of anterior perforated substance of a monkey. *A.C.A.*, anterior cerebral artery; *A.C.I.*, inferior cerebral artery; *A.Ch.A.*, anterior choroidal artery; *C.T.*, cut surface of temporal lobe; *G.C.*, general cortex; *En.F.*, endorhinal fissure; *H.A.*, recurrent artery of Heubner; *I.C.A.*, internal carotid artery; *L.O.T.*, lateral olfactory tract; *M.C.A.*, middle cerebral artery; *O.B.*, olfactory bulb; *O.Ch.*, optic chiasm; *O.S.*, olfactory stalk; *P.C.A.*, posterior cerebral artery, *Py.L.*, pyriform lobe; *R.F.*, rhinal fissure; *St.B.*, striate branches; *T.O.*, tuberculum olfactorium. (From Abbie,[3] with permission.)

The caudal division of the ICA in reptiles may be smaller or larger than the rostral. In most reptiles a single basilar artery is formed by the two caudal divisions after the latter have given rise to large posterior cerebral and mesencephalic or tectal arteries to the midbrain and optic lobes and cerebellar arteries to the cerebellum. The cerebellar arteries are homologous with the superior cerebellar arteries of mammals. The basilar artery tapers and becomes continuous with one or more anterior spinal arteries.

A cerebrovascular variation is noted in some snakes, in which one or the other ICA is much smaller than the other. In this case the cranial and caudal ICA divisions are also asymmetric in size, although the rest of the vessels on the brain are of equal size.[138] Also in snakes, a pair of large vessels branch from the extracranial ICAs of both sides and enter the cranium with the first cervical nerves to anastomose with the basilar artery.[104,138]

In turtles and probably in all reptiles, the stapedial

artery (Fig. 24-3B) is a major branch of the ICA.[8,60–62] Indeed, the brain of reptiles is so small as compared with the size of the head that the ICA is better described as a branch of the stapedial artery.

Monotremes

Monotremes comprise an order of primitive mammals that represents in some respects the transition from reptiles to placental mammals, although these mammals are not thought to be close to the direct phylesis of higher mammals. The only living monotreme species include the duck-billed platypus (*Ornithorhynchus anatinus*) and the spiny anteaters or echidnas (*Tachyglossus* and *Zaglossus*) of Australia and New Guinea. They are hairy and exothermic, features that place them in the mammalian class. However, these species have limited capacity for thermoregulation[413] and are oviparous (i.e., they lay eggs).

The brains of monotremes are intermediate between those of reptiles and placental mammals. The telencephalon includes a relatively large area of neopallium, including a corticospinal system with internal capsule, cerebral peduncles and pyramidal tracts, and hippocampal and anterior commissures, but no corpus callosum.[405–407] The cerebellum has also evolved and with it the pons. However, the olfactory structures are still very large, possibly still constituting the greatest sensory input to the brain. The vascular structures of the brain of the spiny anteater have been reviewed by Shellshear.[401]

The monotreme brain possesses the hallmark of the mammalian cerebrovascular system: it is supplied by true vertebral arteries caudally in addition to ICAs rostrally.[104,141] Presumably the vertebral arteries evolved from segmental cervical arteries as a means to supplement the brain circulation via the basilar artery as the cerebrum and cerebellum enlarged. However the evolution of the vertebral artery has been little studied.

Relatively small, paired ICAs in these species are still best described as dividing intracranially into rostral and caudal divisions. Each rostral division then branches into ACAs and MCAs. The ACAs, which are often of unequal caliber, unite to the anteroventral portion of the interhemispheric fissure to form an unpaired ACA. This vessel branches to supply the olfactory structures, septal area, and anterior neopallium. Branches of the ACA enter the homologue of the anterior perforated substance (the endorhinal fissure, called by Shellshear[401] the arcuate fissure). One or more conspicuous recurrent branches to the endorhinal fissure originate from the azygous segment of the ACA to supply the perforating branches before anastomosing with an anterior branch of the MCA. This recurrent artery appears to be homologous with the recurrent artery of Heubner in humans.

The MCA supplies the lateral portions of the olfactory structures, the pyriform lobe, and the greater part of the neopallium. An anterior branch runs in the endorhinal fissure, providing perforating branches to the basal ganglia, as just noted.

Shellshear[401] names the caudal branch of the ICA the posterior communicating artery, as is the customary nomenclature in higher mammals. It anastomoses with the basilar artery. Interestingly, the brain of the echidna is probably perfused primarily via the very large vertebral and basilar arteries, which are considerably larger than the ICAs. The cranial end of the basilar artery branches into two large trunks at the level of the interpeduncular cistern. Shellshear, with this in mind, described these trunks as the origins of the PCAs. This is the usual anatomical but phylogenetically inaccurate description in higher vertebrates, since the PCAs evolved earlier than the vertebral arteries and were originally perfused via the ICAs. Each PCA supplies the tectum, lateral midbrain, majority of the thalamus, majority of the hippocampus (which is mainly dorsal to the thalamus in the interhemispheric fissure), dorsal (hippocampal) commissure, and posterior aspect of the cerebral cortex.

From the basilar artery arise cerebellar arteries, which are probably homologous to the superior cerebellar artery of higher mammals. An internal auditory artery is also noted. Anterior spinal arteries arise from each vertebral artery just rostral to the posterior inferior cerebellar arteries.

Marsupials

Marsupials are primitive mammals that do not lay eggs but have only a rudimentary placenta. Young are born very immature and are nurtured for a long time in the specialized marsupium or pouch. One species, the opossum *Didelphis virginiana*, thrives in North America. Most marsupials are found in the southern Pacific (e.g., in Australia).

Like the brain of the spiny anteater, that of the marsupial is primitive as compared with that of higher mammals, with large olfactory structures and pyriform lobes.[3,153,405–407] A relatively large neopallium is present, but the corpus callosum is lacking, although there are dorsal (hippocampal) and anterior commissures. The cerebellum is similar in advancement to that of the spiny anteater.

As with all mammalian brains at some stage in their development, the marsupial brain is supplied by paired ICAs and vertebral arteries (Fig. 24-9). From the distal ICA, branches supply the median eminence, hypophysis, hypothalamus, mammillary bodies, and tuber cinereum. The ICAs divide in this mammal into larger anterior than posterior divisions. This is similar to the usual human anatomy, in which the posterior communicating artery (homologue of the caudal division of the ICA) is usually smaller than the ICA or basilar artery. Also as in the human, the MCAs appear to be the direct continuations of the ICA, being larger than the ACAs. The latter supply the olfactory structures and remain separated (without an anterior communicating artery) within the interhemispheric fissure. Included in a group of vessels that enter the anterior perforated substance of marsupials is a relatively large recurrent branch[3] (Fig. 24-8B). These perforating vessels supply the anterior portions of the basal ganglia. The ACAs anastomose dorsomedially with the PCAs to supply the hippocampal formation.

The MCAs of marsupials appear to be the predominant suppliers of the neopallium. They also supply the large pyriform cortex and send a large lenticulostriate branch with several perforating rami through the endorhinal fissure to supply the posterolateral portions of the basal ganglia and amygdala. The anterior choroidal artery arises in these mammals from either the MCA or the large lenticulostriate branch. It attains a typically mammalian configuration in that it courses along the optic tract to the lateral geniculate body, supplying blood to these structures a well as to the choroid plexus of the lateral ventricle, crus cerebri, posterior limb of the internal capsule, ventrolateral nucleus of the thalamus, pyriform cortex, and the medial globus pallidus. The anterior choroidal artery anastomoses with branches of the MCA and PCA over the pyriform cortex; with branches of the PCA at the level of the lateral geniculate body, crus cerebri, and choroid plexus of the lateral ventricle; and with branches of the ACA, MCA, and PCA on the surface of the optic chiasm.[3]

Paired vertebral arteries reach the brain via the foramen magnum. They unite into a single basilar artery, which may have loops or fenestrations. The small posterior communicating arteries probably indicate that the majority of blood supply to the PCAs and hindbrain is delivered via the vertebrobasilar system. The posterior communicating arteries supple-

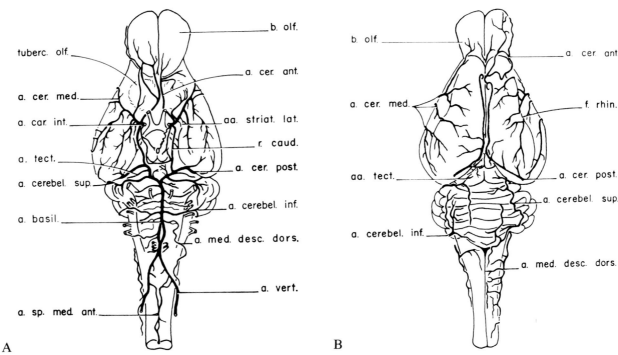

Figure 24-9. Diagrams of the brain of an opossum, a primitive mammal (marsupial). Note the absence of an anterior communicating artery and the presence of a basilar artery fenestration. The PCA supplies the (dorsal) hippocampal formation and anastomoses with the ACA anteriorly. Note the dorsal position of the rhinal fissure, which in the human is on the inferior surface of the temporal lobe. The cerebral cortex is supplied by branches of the ACA, PCA, and MCA. **(A)** Ventral view; **(B)** Dorsal view. (From Gillilan,[141] with permission.)

ment the ICAs in supplying branches to the mammillary bodies and tuber cinereum.

The PCAs course around the midbrain, enter the posterior interhemispheric fissure, and then course rostrally along the (dorsal) hippocampus. As already noted, they unite anteriorly with branches of the ACA. The PCAs supply branches to the hypothalamus, cerebral peduncles, midbrain, tectum, thalamus, choroid plexus of the third and lateral ventricles, pineal region, hippocampus, and neopallium. The latter structure also is supplied by cortical branches of both the MCA and ACA, forming an anastomosing plexus, as in all higher vertebrates.

The cerebellum is supplied by the basilar artery via superior and inferior[142] or anterior inferior[467] cerebellar arteries.

Primates

In primate phylesis the brain undergoes a massive expansion, characterized by a dominance of the cerebral cortex. The cortex becomes a massive neural integration (association) structure, where input from the environment can be added to memory to produce complex behaviors, thoughts, and emotions and greatly enhance the ability to learn. The cortex expands frontally, posteriorly, and lateroventrally, becoming folded and convoluted in higher primates. As the cortex enlarges, the pyriform lobe takes an extreme anteroventral position, becoming nearly hidden by the temporal lobes. Within the anlage of the hippocampal formation a massive neocortical commissure, the corpus callosum, develops. The hippocampal formation, which includes the temporal lobe structures, the fornix system, and the supracallosal gray matter and tracts (paraterminal body, indusium griseum, gyrus fasciolaris, and medial and lateral longitudinal striae), is greatly reduced in relative size. The cerebral cortex extends posteriorly to the extent that it completely covers the midbrain and cerebellum.

Primate (e.g., human) cerebral cortex mass increases relatively more than the size of the head. This is due partly to a limit in the size of the head at birth for passage through the human birth canal. The cerebrum therefore has to fold or invaginate somewhat, which results in the formation of the basal perforation zone, insula, choroidal fissures, tela choroidea of the third ventricle, and cortical sulci and gyri. This folding is reflected in the characteristic S-shaped course delineated by the lenticulostriate arteries and perforating branches of the recurrent artery of Heubner, as seen in the anteroposterior (AP) view of the cerebral angiogram.[214]

The earliest representatives of the primate order were probably small animals represented most closely by living species of tree shrews (Tupaiids). These mammals share a similar ecological niche and body habitus with many members of the rodent and insectivore‡ orders. They are differentiated from the insectivores and rodents partly on the basis of their tooth and jaw structures.[413] However, in the smallest and most primitive primates, as in insectivores and rodents, cerebrovascular anatomy, especially the anatomy of the ICA, external carotid artery (ECA) and stapedial artery, takes on particular importance as a means for the systematic classification of these animals.[58,79] This is further discussed below in the sections on carotid and stapedial artery anomalies.

The vascular anatomy of the human brain is probably familiar to most readers. The cerebrovascular anatomy of other primates is essentially identical to that of the human except as individual vessels reflect the relative proportions of cerebral structures. Details of the cerebrovascular anatomy of humans and other primates can be found in numerous publications[30,31,112,139–141,200,202,243,316,377,384,385,400,417] and therefore will not be further described here.

Other Placental Mammals

Although nonprimate mammals are not very close to the phylogenetic pathway of humans, their cranial vascular anatomy is often relevant to the understanding of human cerebrovascular anomalies and variants. As will be seen, many human variations bear close resemblance to the normal anatomy of various animals.

Details of the cerebrovascular anatomy of many species are available, including members of the following orders: rodents,[54–58,104] lagomorphs (rabbits),[104,125] carnivores (e.g., cats[93,104,144,199] and dogs[96,97,104,123,125,144]), perissodactyls (odd-toed ungulates, including equids, tapirs, and rhinoceroses),[104,110,143] and artiodactyls (even-toed ungulates such as pigs, goats, sheep, and bovids).[104,123,125,143] The particulars of the various anatomical arrangements will not be described in detail except as they relate to particular human cerebrovascular variations described below.

It should be noted that the brains of many mam-

---

‡ Insectivores are an order of placental mammals including shrews, moles, and hedgehogs, the members of which are believed to be similar to the ancestral species of most or all of the modern orders of placental mammals.

mals, including many carnivores, artiodactyls, and cetaceans (sea mammals) are supplied via extracranial and/or intracranial vascular retia. The *rete mirabile* is a complex structure, a description of which is beyond the scope of this chapter. A thorough review of the rete mirabile is presented by McFarland et al.[286] in their study of the extremely specialized cerebrovascular supply of the dolphin.§ The purpose of the rete mirabile is uncertain, but it is employed in some mammals for the supply of the brain, orbit, limbs, and/or testicles. Theories about the function of retia include temperature regulation,[23] pulse pressure damping,[286] cerebral blood flow regulation,[109,110,143,286] and intracranial pressure and/or volume regulation.[110]

ONTOGENY OF HUMAN CEREBRAL VASCULATURE

The embryonic period of development is characterized by those processes that result in the differentiation of the fundamental tissues and organ systems of the organism. The fetal period is defined as the time from the end of the embryonic period until birth.[253] Thus, the duration of the embryonic period is somewhat arbitrary; in humans it corresponds roughly to the first trimester of pregnancy.

Embryos of apparently the same gestational age may be different in size owing to individual variation and inaccuracy of measurements and menstrual history. Nonetheless, all embryos conform to a relatively predictable progression of morphological changes.[253,325,328,421] Steps in this progression correspond roughly to the size of the embryo, the number of somites, and the estimated gestational age (EGA). Embryo size is usually given in millimeters as crown-rump length (CRL) or crown-heel length, although the latter is more often used for fetuses than for embryos. The commonly used classification developed by Streeter et al.[421] and O'Rahilly[325] divides the progression of embryonic development into 23 stages or horizons.

Streeter[420] subdivided the embryonic development

of the cerebral vasculature into five morphological periods. Padget[328] divided cerebrovascular ontogeny into seven periods and added an eighth to include the fetal and adult configuration. The end of the seventh embryonic stage corresponds to the time at which the stems of origin of all adult arteries can be identified.

Many publications have been devoted to descriptions of various aspects of human cerebrovascular development.[11,78,111,116,142,159,200,214,218,265,328,420,460,462] Other authors have studied the cerebrovascular development of nonhuman organisms in an effort to gain insight through studies that cannot be performed on human material.[104,115,116,141,179,255,266,273,274,296–298,373–375,422,449]

It is not known to what extent cerebrovascular development is programmed genetically or adapts passively as the rest of the brain develops. Streeter[420] believed that cerebrovascular development was totally without genetic programming. The brain vasculature is continuously shaped according to the needs of the embryonic brain at every moment,[420] capillary formation and resorption being prominent components of the process.[273,274,449] As blood flows in the developing nervous system and as the organism grows, certain channels become progressively more important (i.e., larger). Apparently once vessels reach a critical size, they can no longer be reabsorbed but persist into adulthood. Any changes in the brain that affect its permanent vasculature may result in the modification of vascular channels, but their presence remains.[420]

The most striking morphological features of the early embryonic head and neck are the pharyngeal arches. The first two pairs appear in the 2.5- to 3.5-mm CRL, 13 to 20 somite, stage IX, 23- to 24-day EGA embryo. As the first arches partially involute, the next appear. A total of six pharyngeal arches ultimately appear as the embryonic substrate for much of the head and neck, although the fifth is small and transient or absent. Each pharyngeal arch consists of a bar of mesodermal supporting tissue (future cartilage and bone), associated muscle, a main artery, and a cranial nerve. The arches are separated externally by deep ectodermal invaginations or clefts and internally by reciprocal, endoderm-lined pouches, which nearly meet the clefts. The pharyngeal arches are homologous with the branchial arches of fish and amphibians, which become gills in these lower vertebrates. The vasculature of gills evolved into major segments of the carotid, subclavian, aortic, and pulmonary arterial systems of higher vertebrates (compare Figs. 24-2 and 24-6 with Figs. 24-10 to 24-18). The arteries of the branchial arches are synonymously called *aortic, branchial,* or *pharyngeal arch* arteries.

---

§ In the Cetacea internal carotid and vertebral arteries are present during early embryonic development but later regress completely. The spinovascular and cerebrovascular supply in the dolphin is via a massive and highly innervated thoracospinal-cranial-ophthalmic rete mirabile, supplied by intercostal and posterior thoracic arteries. No circle of Willis is present, but homologues of the anterior, middle and posterior cerebral arteries emerge from the rete intracranially.

The following summary of human vasculature embryology is taken mainly from Padget's monumental study.[328] Padget studied, described, and drew the cerebral vasculature from reconstructions of sectioned human embryos. Her work supplemented and elaborated work by Congdon[78] on the aortic arches. Other information on cerebrovascular embryology has come from animal studies. The descriptions below are an amalgamation and summary of these data.

The first differentiated vascular tissue probably develops in situ, as primordial angioblastic cell islands within the embryonic yolk sac and body, around the beginning of the third week of gestation, as noted by Sabin[373–375] in the chick and pig. The angioblastic cell islands coalesce by extensions of cytoplasm and expand through cell division, cell growth, and the formation of new angioblasts, forming angioblastic cords. The centers of the continuously growing cords may then undergo liquefaction while the outer cells remain fused, producing large, interconnecting endothelial cell channels in an irregular plexus.[373–375,449] (Alternatively, Manasek[266] has provided evidence for lumen formation by secretory products being forced between angioblasts, which are fixed to each other by intercellular junctions.) It is thought that primordial blood cells are also formed in situ within this angioblastic tissue.[375,420]

In this very early precirculatory period embryonic vessels cover the central nervous system in the form of an extensive capillary plexus.[115,116,273,274,373,420,449] The simple vessels are composed of endothelial cells joined by tight junctions and surrounded by a thin, incomplete basal lamina. They grow actively by sprouting and advancing basal lamina-deprived filopodia into the surrounding tissue.[273,274] Primitive paired aortae and a large, ventral hindbrain channel develop in situ from the capillary plexus.[78,116,141,179,328,374,420] It is not known what factors initiate the differentiation of the arterial, venous, and capillary tissue compartments at the time that blood circulation is established.

Around the time that the anterior neuropore closes in the 3-mm CRL, 20-somite, stage XI, 23- to 25-day EGA embryo, the already prominent head plexus is supplied by the primitive ICA rostrally and the primitive trigeminal artery caudally. The internal carotid and trigeminal arteries are branches or continuations of the first arch of the paired dorsal aortae.¶

¶ The term *dorsal aorta* refers to the homologous dorsal aortae of fish, which receive blood from the ventral aortae via the gills; the ventral aorta homologue in humans is the aortic sac, from which the CCA and initial portions of the ECA and ICA originate.

Vascularization of the embryonic brain follows a caudal to rostral progression, starting at the myelencephalon and ascending along the metencephalon, mesencephalon, diencephalon, striatum, and telencephalon.[274,420,422]

The primitive hindbrain channel breaks up into a plexus of primordial vessels. Some of these apparently become veins to receive blood from the head plexus and drain into the anterior cardinal vein (future internal jugular/superior vena cava system).[373,420] Others apparently become arteries, forming the bilateral longitudinal neural arteries, the primordia of the basilar artery.[328] Sabin[373] has noted that the chick heart begins to beat at the stage of 9 or 10 somites, but that this does not result in circulation of blood, presumably because there is not yet a completed circuit. Actual circulation in the chick probably begins at the 15- to 16-somite stage, which may correlate with the early part of the stage described here for the human.

Just before the neural tube closes, in the stage XII, 21- to 29-somite, 3- to 5-mm CRL, 24- to 26-day EGA embryo, two bilateral longitudinal neural arteries (plexuses) have formed along nearly the entire ventrolateral extent of the brain (Fig. 24-10). These paired plexuses are the primordia of the basilar artery and run, ventromedial to all the cranial nerve root primordia, from the prominent trigeminal roots rostrally to the first cervical nerve root primordia caudally. At the cervical end, the bilateral longitudinal neural arteries become smaller and merge with similar bilateral plexuses along the ventrolateral aspect of the spinal cord.[78,142] At several points prominent arterial anastomoses join the dorsal aortae (future ICAs) to the bilateral longitudinal neural arteries (future basilar artery).[142,296,328,373] They are named for adjacent neural structures and include the primitive trigeminal, otic, and hypoglossal arteries, which are adjacent to the trigeminal ganglion, otic vesicle and hypoglossal nerve roots, respectively. The trigeminal artery is the largest of these and persists for the longest time in the embryonic period.[328]

Anastomoses also connect the dorsal aortae to the bilateral ventrolateral neural/spinal plexuses between each and every somite, as described by Padget[329] (Fig. 24-11). Later, throughout the spine the somites divide such that each vertebral body (centrum) is formed by the fusion of the caudal half of the somite above and the rostral half of the somite below. However, the rostral portion of the first somite remains unpaired; known as the *proatlas*, it forms the rostral end of the odontoid process. The anastomosis between the dorsal aorta and the bilateral ventrolateral neural/spinal plexus that lies between the last two occipital somites is the *primitive*

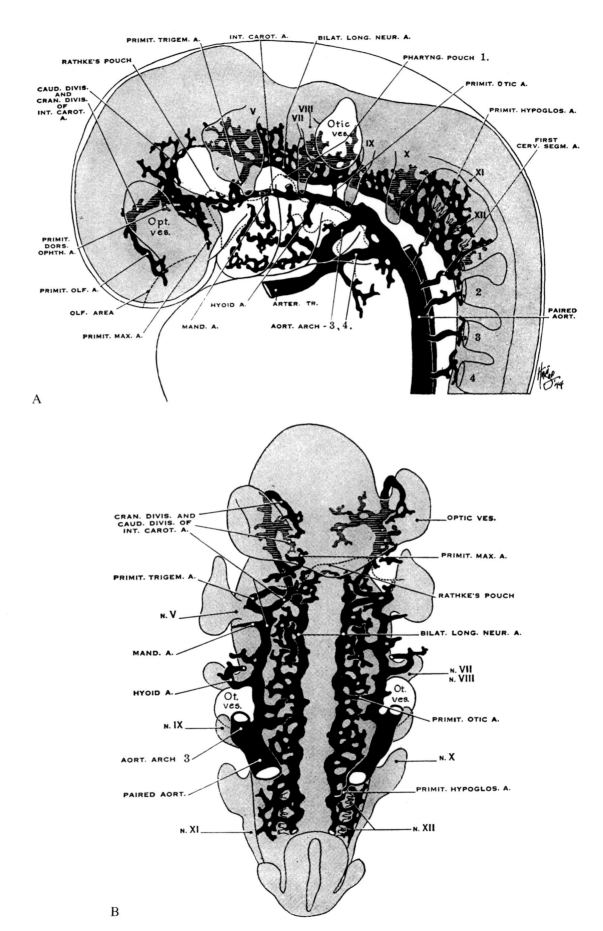

Figure 24-10 (A&B) (*Figure continues.*)

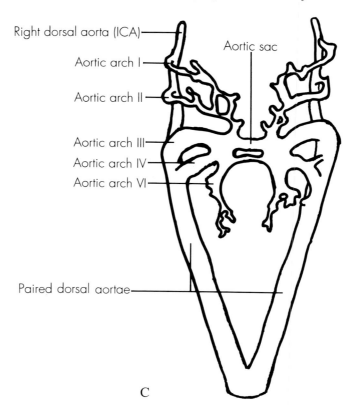

Figure 24-10 (*Continued*). Diagrams of the cerebral arterial system and aortic arches of a human embryo. The bilateral longitudinal neural arteries are supplied by the primitive trigeminal, otic, hypoglossal, and proatlantal intersegmental arteries, as the posterior communicating and vertebral arteries have not yet formed. Note the multiple aortic arches in various stages of formation and regression. (**A**) Lateral view of a 4-mm CRL embryo. (**B**) Ventral view of a 4-mm CRL embryo. (**C**) Ventral view of the aortic arches of a 4-mm CRL embryo. (Figs. A and B from Padget,[328] with permission; Fig. C modified from Congdon,[78] with permission.)

hypoglossal artery; that between the last occipital and the first cervical somite is known as the *proatlantal intersegmental artery;* and the six in the cervical region are called *cervical intersegmental arteries.*

Also at this stage the cranial extension of the dorsal aorta (the future internal carotid artery) becomes most prominently supplied by the third aortic arch as the first and second pharyngeal arches partially involute along with their vessels. Maintaining their dorsal connection with the internal carotid artery, the arteries of the first and second arches become the primitive mandibular and hyoid arteries, respectively. At the base of the forebrain a branch of the internal carotid artery forms the primitive maxillary artery. Other tiny branches form an anastomotic plexus around Rathke's pouch, connecting the two ICAs.

The most cranial segment of the ICA bifurcates into a cranial (or rostral or anterior) and a caudal (or posterior) division, "recapitulating" phylogeny. These are the future ACA/MCA and posterior communicating artery/PCA systems, respectively. The cranial division of the internal carotid artery is smaller than the caudal at this stage, which is suggestive of primitive vertebrates. The cranial division terminates in a plexus medial to the optic vesicle, supplying the prosencephalon and olfactory structures.

The caudal division supplies the diencephalon and mesencephalon, the latter of which is being forced by the constraints of the skull into a flexure. The caudal division of the ICA does not yet appear to anastomose significantly with the future basilar artery primordia (the bilateral longitudinal neural arteries)—thus, there is no posterior communicating artery.

In the early part of the next stage, the stage XIV, 5- to 7-mm CRL, 29- to 34-day EGA embryo now possesses a definitive posterior communicating artery connecting the caudal division of the ICA with the still paired bilateral longitudinal neural arteries (Fig. 24-12). However, by the end of this stage the basilar artery has formed, although the exact process of its formation from the bilateral longitudinal neural arteries is not clear—it appears to be a type of fusion process.[78,115,116,296,328,373]

Padget[328] draws attention to a plexus of vessels dorsal and parallel to the bilateral longitudinal neural arteries, which she calls the *primitive basilovertebral anastomosis.* These vessels form an important anastomotic plexus between the developing basilar, vertebral, and proatlantal intersegmental arteries, sending branches to supply the lateral and dorsal hindbrain. The primitive basilovertebral anastomosis will become the hemispheric branches of the anterior

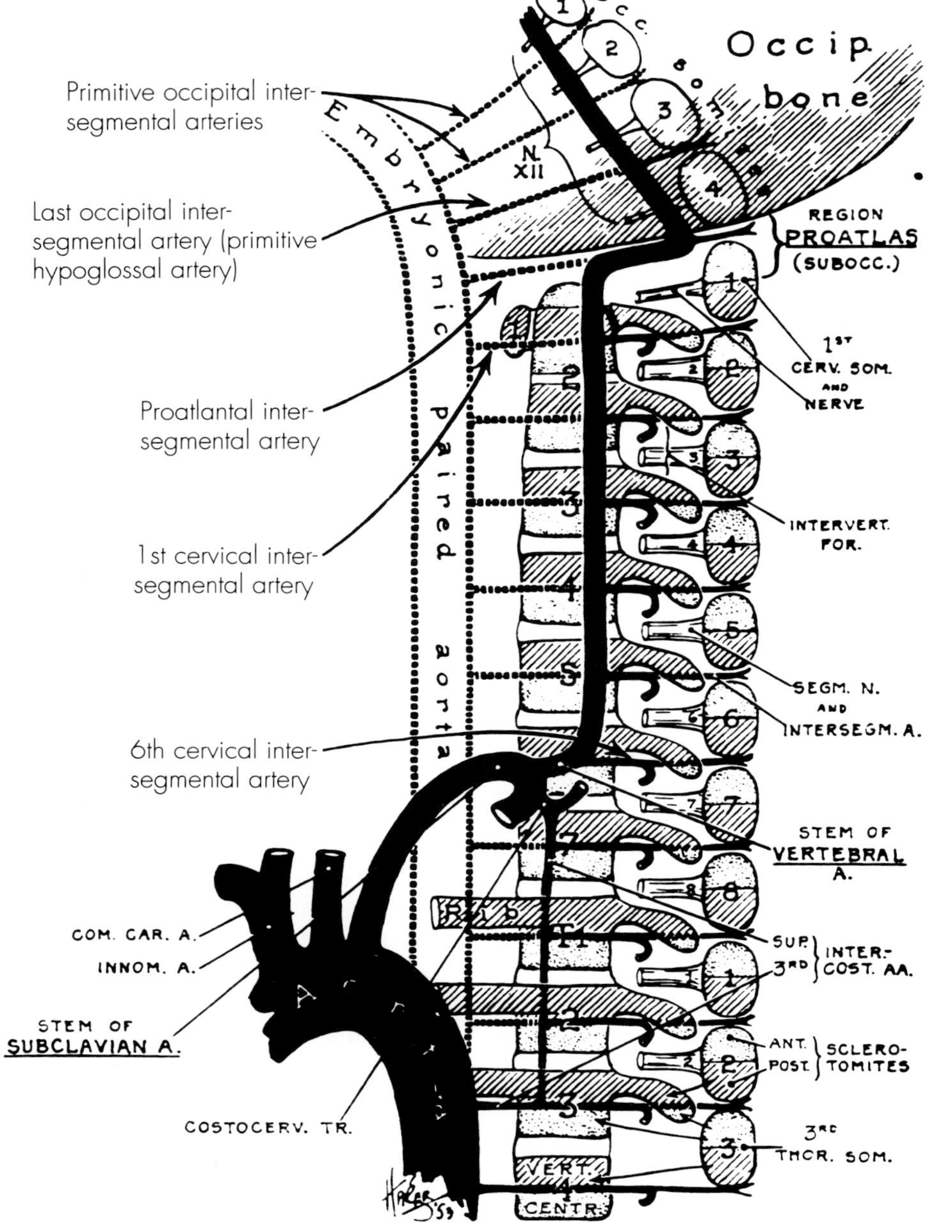

Figure 24-11. Semischematic diagram demonstrating the precise relationships and nomenclature of the embryonic cervical intersegmental arteries, subclavian artery, vertebral artery, primitive hypoglossal artery, proatlantal intersegmental artery, cervical nerves, cervical vertebrae, and embryonic cervical somites. Note that the persistent proatlantal intersegmental artery is between the occiput and C1, the first cervical intersegmental artery is at the level of the second cervical nerve, etc. (Modified from Padget,[329] with permission.)

and posterior inferior cerebellar arteries (AICA and PICA, respectively). This plexus also forms part of the primitive hypoglossal artery anastomosis.[306]

With further enlargement of the posterior communicating artery, the primitive trigeminal, otic, hypoglossal, and proatlantal intersegmental arteries regress. A segment of the proatlantal intersegmental artery normally persists as the horizontal, suboccipital segment of the vertebral artery. Padget[328] notes that in some embryos the primitive trigeminal artery may persist on one side for some time as the dominant anastomosis with the basilar artery, in which case the posterior communicating artery on the side ipsilateral to that trigeminal artery will be relatively smaller. It is possible that the common adult asymmetry of the posterior communicating arteries has its beginning here, as suggested by Gillilan.[142]

At this stage it becomes clear that the origin of the ICA is the third aortic arch. The dorsal end of the primitive mandibular artery (first arch) and the ventral end of the primitive hyoid artery (second arch) dwindle, along with the segment of the dorsal aorta connecting the third and fourth aortic arches. This latter segment of the dorsal aorta is known as the *ductus caroticus*. With regression of the ductus caroticus, the cerebral circulation becomes completely separated from the systemic circulation.

The primitive hyoid artery retains its dorsal connection with the ICA, forming a conspicuous ICA branch there. This is the anlage of the embryonic stapedial artery, which is important for the formation of much of the future ophthalmic artery and ECA systems.

Also at this stage, an arterial supply to the eye can be identified in the form of a primitive dorsal ophthalmic artery arising from the ICA. Furthermore, a pair of relatively large vessels in the ventral segment of the first two aortic arches is developing; these are the ventral pharyngeal arteries,[78] which extend from the origin of the third aortic arch cranioventrally to supply portions of the first two pharyngeal arches. These vessels will contribute to the formation of the ECA system.

The next phase in the vascular development of the very small embryo reveals major development of the vertebral arteries. This occurs in the stage XVI, 7- to 12-mm CRL, 32- to 37-day EGA embryo by enlargement of rostrocaudal anastomoses between consecutive cervical intersegmental arteries, with simultaneous dwindling of their aortic origins (Fig. 24-13). The proatlantal intersegmental artery separates from the ICA but maintains continuity with the plexus on the lateral aspect of the hindbrain, thus allowing for the future vertebrobasilar continuity.[179,297] The process progresses in a rostral to caudal direction.

Also at this stage a prominent branch of the cranial division of the ICA, the anterior choroidal artery, courses upon the primordial diencephalon and into the developing choroidal fissure. This fissure is noted for the first time as the telencephalic vesicles begin to "evaginate" from the prosencephalon. Further anteriorly the supply to the ocular structures has become more complex with the development of a primitive ventral ophthalmic artery, which anastomoses with the primitive dorsal ophthalmic artery via shared branches. The ventral ophthalmic artery itself appears to be a branch of the ACA.

The earliest branches of what may be called an MCA are noted more rostrally along the cranial division of the ICA. The future ACA is the termination of the cranial division of the ICA. A few, small, mesially directed branches are noted, but the main segment of the ACA forms the large primitive olfactory artery, recalling the condition in lower vertebrates. Padget[328] states that the primitive olfactory artery represents the future medial striate arteries and recurrent artery of Heubner.

The caudal division of the ICA, now a large posterior communicating artery, has two large branches, the diencephalic and mesencephalic arteries. The PCA is not present at this time; it will develop from branches of the diencephalic, mesencephalic, and anterior choroidal arteries and of the MCA. The superior cerebellar artery is the main artery supplying the structures of the developing cerebellum superior to the fourth ventricle. Other cerebellar branches are not present, but there are numerous branches supplying the pons and medulla from the basilar artery.

In stage XVII 12- to 14-mm CRL, 34- to 40-day EGA embryo, the right dorsal aorta begins to regress[78,328] (Fig. 24-14). The hyoid artery gives rise to its important stapedial branch, coursing characteristically through the primordial stapes. The stapedial artery anastomoses with the distal segment of the ventral pharyngeal artery to supply the first and second pharyngeal bars, thus taking over much of the territory of the primitive mandibular artery (artery of the first aortic arch). Barry[28] clearly illustrates that the common carotid arteries are formed from the ventral aortic root between the third and fourth aortic arches (Fig. 24-15). The proximal segment of the ICA develops from the third aortic arch, and the stem of the external carotid artery is formed from the ventral pharyngeal artery.

The primitive olfactory artery possesses a significant mesially directed branch, which enters the primordial interhemispheric fissure. There is also a plexiform anterior communicating artery complex at

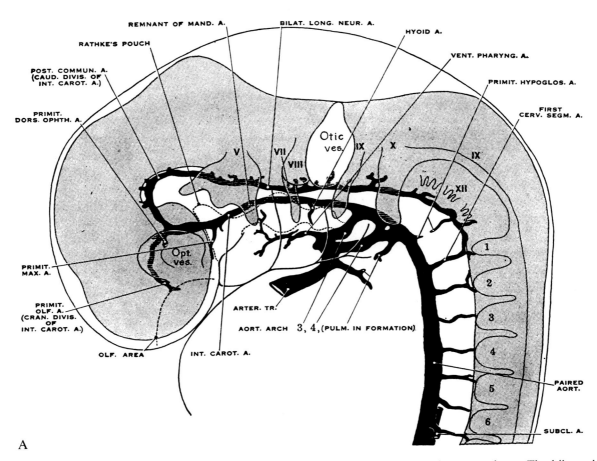

A

Figure 24-12. Diagrams of the cerebral arterial system and aortic arches of a human embryo. The bilateral longitudinal neural arteries are supplied by the posterior communicating and proatlantal intersegmental arteries. Note that the (paired) bilateral longitudinal neural arteries are in the early process of fusion to become the basilar artery. **(A)** Lateral view of a 5.3-mm CRL embryo. (*Figure continues.*)

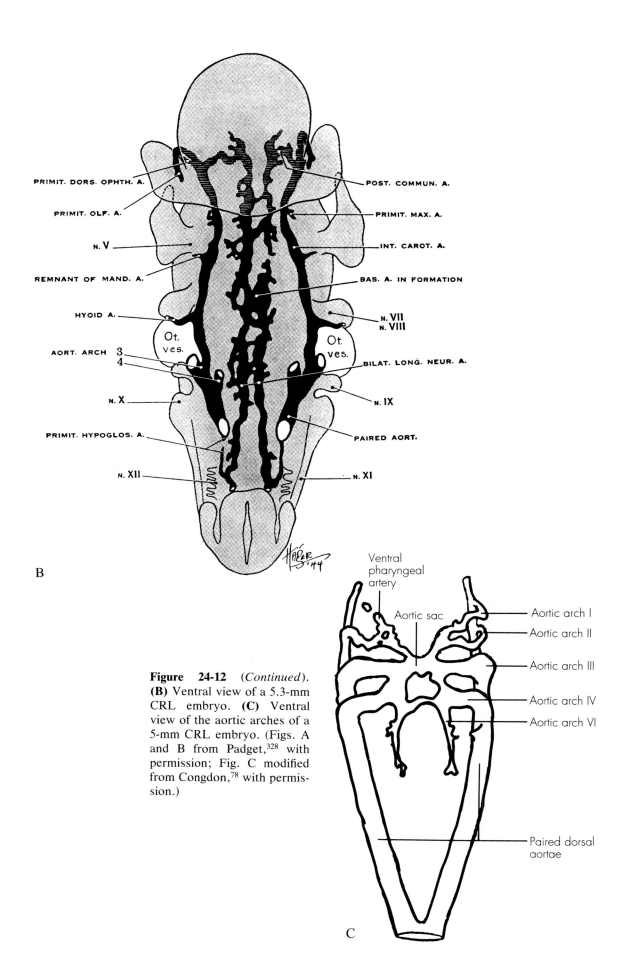

B

PRIMIT. DORS. OPHTH. A.

PRIMIT. OLF. A.

N. V

REMNANT OF MAND. A.

HYOID A.

AORT. ARCH 3
4

N. X

PRIMIT. HYPOGLOS. A.

N. XII

POST. COMMUN. A.

PRIMIT. MAX. A.

INT. CAROT. A.

BAS. A. IN FORMATION

N. VII
N. VIII

BILAT. LONG. NEUR. A.

N. IX

PAIRED AORT.

N. XI

Ot. ves.

Ot. ves.

Figure 24-12 (*Continued*). **(B)** Ventral view of a 5.3-mm CRL embryo. **(C)** Ventral view of the aortic arches of a 5-mm CRL embryo. (Figs. A and B from Padget,[328] with permission; Fig. C modified from Congdon,[78] with permission.)

Ventral pharyngeal artery

Aortic sac

Aortic arch I

Aortic arch II

Aortic arch III

Aortic arch IV

Aortic arch VI

Paired dorsal aortae

C

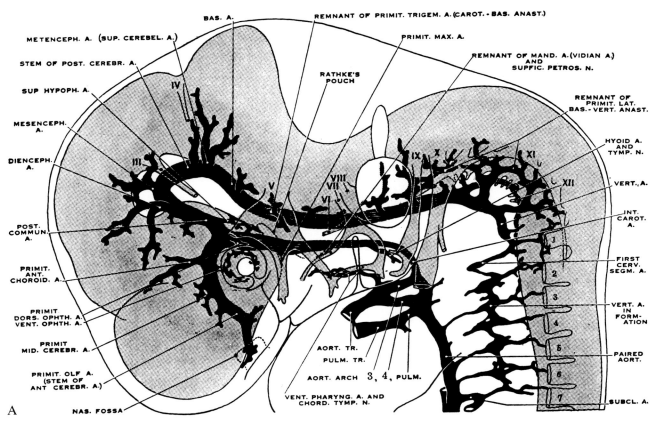

Figure 24-13. Diagrams of the cerebral arterial system and aortic arches of a human embryo. The telence-phalic supply is mainly from the medial olfactory and anterior choroidal arteries. The vertebral artery is forming by enlargement of anastomoses between adjacent cervical intersegmental arteries. The ICA fills via the third and fourth aortic arches, suggestive of a reptilian phylogenetic stage. **(A)** Lateral view of a 9-mm CRL embryo. (*Figure continues.*)

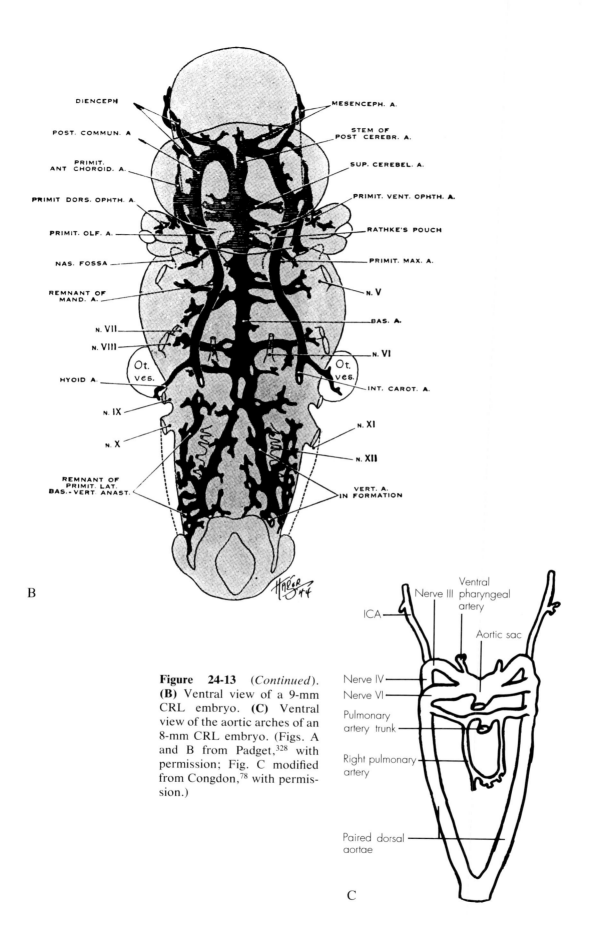

B

Figure 24-13 (*Continued*). **(B)** Ventral view of a 9-mm CRL embryo. **(C)** Ventral view of the aortic arches of an 8-mm CRL embryo. (Figs. A and B from Padget,[328] with permission; Fig. C modified from Congdon,[78] with permission.)

DIENCEPH

MESENCEPH. A.

POST. COMMUN. A

STEM OF POST CEREBR. A.

PRIMIT. ANT CHOROID. A.

SUP. CEREBEL. A.

PRIMIT DORS. OPHTH. A.

PRIMIT. VENT. OPHTH. A.

PRIMIT. OLF. A.

RATHKE'S POUCH

NAS. FOSSA

PRIMIT. MAX. A.

REMNANT OF MAND. A.

N. V

N. VII

BAS. A.

N. VIII

N. VI

HYOID A.

Ot. ves.

Ot. ves.

INT. CAROT. A.

N. IX

N. X

N. XI

N. XII

REMNANT OF PRIMIT. LAT. BAS.-VERT. ANAST.

VERT. A. IN FORMATION

ICA

Nerve III

Ventral pharyngeal artery

Aortic sac

Nerve IV

Nerve VI

Pulmonary artery trunk

Right pulmonary artery

Paired dorsal aortae

C

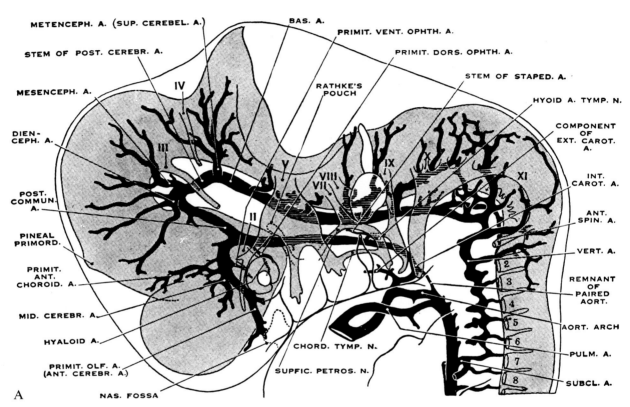

Figure 24-14. Diagrams of the cerebral arterial system and aortic arches of a human embryo. The MCA is a branch of the rostral division of the ICA. The PCA is represented by branches of the diencephalic and mesencephalic arteries only, with no telencephalic supply. The vertebral artery is forming from anastomoses between adjacent cervical intersegmental arteries. **(A)** Lateral view of a 12.5-mm CRL embryo. (*Figure continues.*)

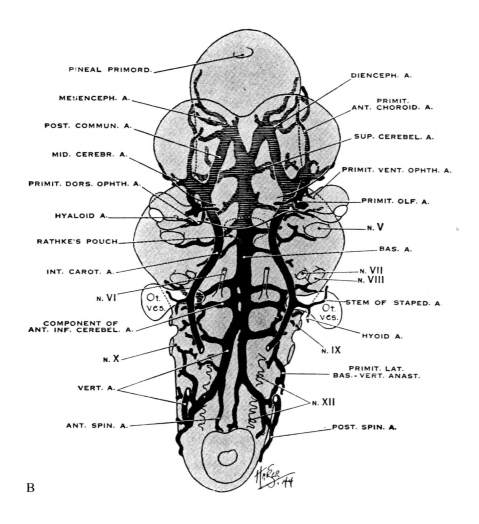

B

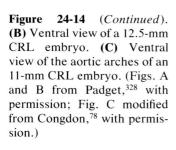

Figure 24-14 (*Continued*).
(B) Ventral view of a 12.5-mm
CRL embryo. **(C)** Ventral
view of the aortic arches of an
11-mm CRL embryo. (Figs. A
and B from Padget,[328] with
permission; Fig. C modified
from Congdon,[78] with permission.)

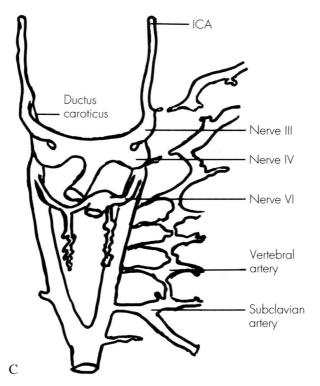

C

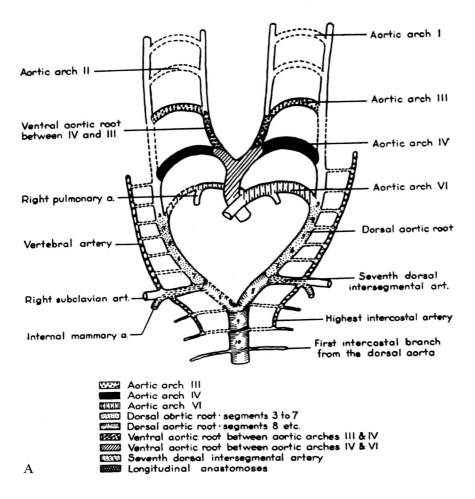

Aortic arch I

Aortic arch II

Aortic arch III

Ventral aortic root between IV and III

Aortic arch IV

Aortic arch VI

Right pulmonary a.

Dorsal aortic root

Vertebral artery

Seventh dorsal intersegmental art.

Right subclavian art.

Highest intercostal artery

Internal mammary a.

First intercostal branch from the dorsal aorta

Aortic arch III	
Aortic arch IV	
Aortic arch VI	
Dorsal aortic root · segments 3 to 7	
Dorsal aortic root · segments 8 etc.	
Ventral aortic root between aortic arches III & IV	
Ventral aortic root between aortic arches IV & VI	
Seventh dorsal intersegmental artery	
Longitudinal anastomoses	

A

Figure 24-15. Diagrams of the developmental changes of the embryonic aortic arches, ventral view. The common carotid artery and the most proximal portions of the ECA and ICA are formed from the third aortic arch. **(A)** Aortic arch system corresponding to human embryos of approximately 10-mm CRL. **(B)** Aortic arch system corresponding to human embryos of approximately 16-mm CRL (cf. Fig. 24-16C) (*Figure continues.*)

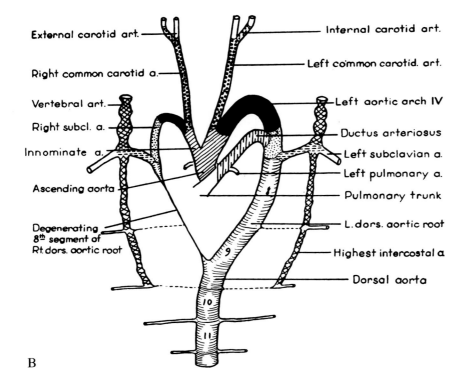

External carotid art.

Internal carotid art.

Right common carotid a.

Left common carotid. art.

Vertebral art.

Left aortic arch IV

Right subcl. a.

Ductus arteriosus

Innominate a.

Left subclavian a.

Left pulmonary a.

Ascending aorta

Pulmonary trunk

Degenerating 8th segment of Rt. dors. aortic root

L. dors. aortic root

Highest intercostal a.

Dorsal aorta

B

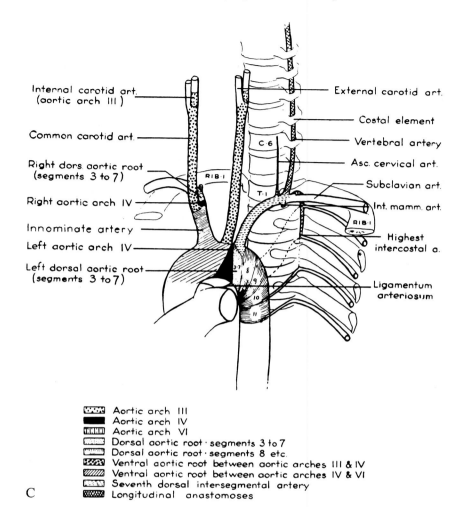

Figure 24-15 (*Continued*). **(C)** Adult proximal aorta and great vessels. (From Barry,[28] with permission.)

Internal carotid art. (aortic arch III)

Common carotid art.

Right dors. aortic root (segments 3 to 7)

Right aortic arch IV

Innominate artery

Left aortic arch IV

Left dorsal aortic root (segments 3 to 7)

External carotid art.

Costal element

Vertebral artery

Asc. cervical art.

Subclavian art.

Int. mamm. art.

Highest intercostal a.

Ligamentum arteriosum

C6

RIB-1

T-1

RIB-1

C

▨ Aortic arch III
■ Aortic arch IV
▥ Aortic arch VI
▢ Dorsal aortic root · segments 3 to 7
▨ Dorsal aortic root · segments 8 etc.
▨ Ventral aortic root between aortic arches III & IV
▨ Ventral aortic root between aortic arches IV & VI
▢ Seventh dorsal intersegmental artery
▨ Longitudinal anastomoses

the close of this stage. However, the telencephalic vesicles are still mainly covered by only a capillary plexus, as the vascularization of the brain, especially the telencephalon, follows a caudal to rostral progression that parallels its development.[273,274,422]

The anterior choroidal artery is a large branch of the cranial division of the ICA, perhaps reflecting a large energy requirement of the choroid plexus, even at this stage.[214,230] This may be related to a function of the embryonic choroid plexus in providing nutrients to the developing telencephalon via diffusion through the cerebrospinal fluid (CSF).[111,218]

In the stage XVIII to XIX, 16- to 18-mm CRL, 40- to 43-day EGA embryo, the stapedial artery is at its state of maximal development (Fig. 24-16). It has two divisions, the ventral or maxillomandibular division and the dorsal or supraorbital division. The former anastomoses with and later forms a large portion of the ECA system, and the latter enters the orbit to supply its extraocular structures. Orbital branches of the supraorbital division of the stapedial artery in-

clude the supraorbital, frontal, and anterior ethmoidal arteries, which accompany the supraorbital, frontal, and nasociliary nerves, respectively. Although not specifically indicated by Padget, the other orbital branches such as the supratrochlear, dorsal nasal, palpebral, posterior ethmoidal, and zygomatic branches of the adult ophthalmic artery are certainly also derived from the supraorbital division of the stapedial artery. These stapedial artery branches will be annexed by the ophthalmic artery in subsequent stages. One other ocular branch, the lacrimal artery, forms in the final embryonic stage (see below), derived partly from the stapedial and partly from the ophthalmic artery. The adult origin of the ophthalmic artery is noted at this stage caudal to the optic nerve and lateral to Rathke's pouch. This possibly represents a relocation of the primitive dorsal ophthalmic origin by caudal migration.

The primitive mandibular branch of the ICA, the artery of the first aortic arch, becomes the Vidian artery (artery of the pterygoid canal). The primitive

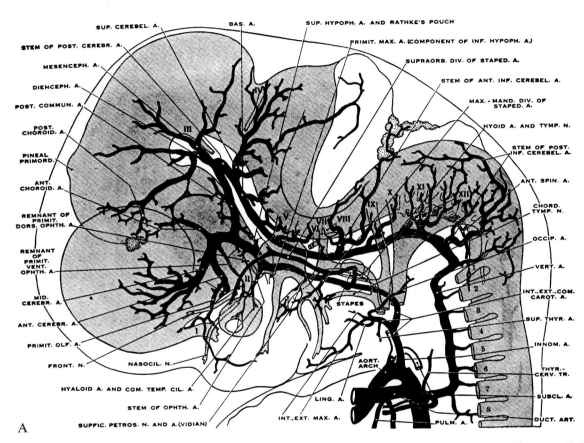

Figure 24-16. Diagrams of the cerebral arterial system and aortic arches of a human embryo. The stapedial artery courses through the stapes to supply the face and orbit. A branch of the diencephalic artery is involved in the supply of the choroid plexus. The primitive olfactory artery is involved in the formation of the lenticulostriate vessels and the recurrent artery of Heubner. The superior cerebellar artery is at a stage of greater relative maturity than the AICA or PICA and is physically separated from these arteries by the pontine flexure. The right dorsal aorta is regressing. **(A)** Lateral view of an 18-mm CRL embryo. (*Figure continues.*)

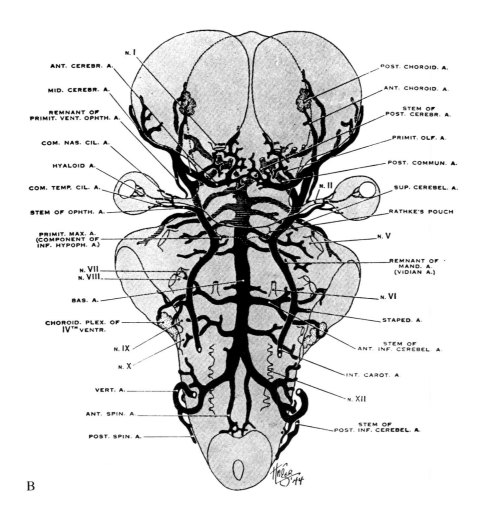

B

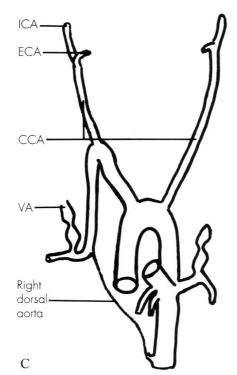

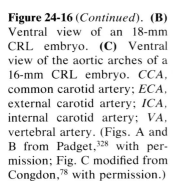

Figure 24-16 (*Continued*). **(B)** Ventral view of an 18-mm CRL embryo. **(C)** Ventral view of the aortic arches of a 16-mm CRL embryo. *CCA,* common carotid artery; *ECA,* external carotid artery; *ICA,* internal carotid artery; *VA,* vertebral artery. (Figs. A and B from Padget,[328] with permission; Fig. C modified from Congdon,[78] with permission.)

C

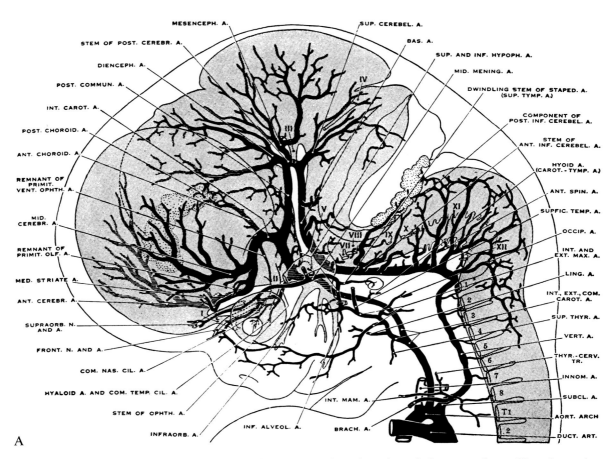

Figure 24-17. Diagrams of the cerebral arterial system and aortic arches of a human embryo. The telencephalon is the largest portion of the brain. The choroid plexus is supplied by branches of the ACA and the anterior choroidal, posterior communicating, and diencephalic (posterior cerebral) arteries. The plexiform anterior communicating artery completes the circle of Willis anteriorly. The stapedial artery is annexed by the external carotid and ophthalmic arteries as its internal carotid stem regresses. **(A)** Lateral view of a 24-mm CRL embryo. (*Figure continues.*)

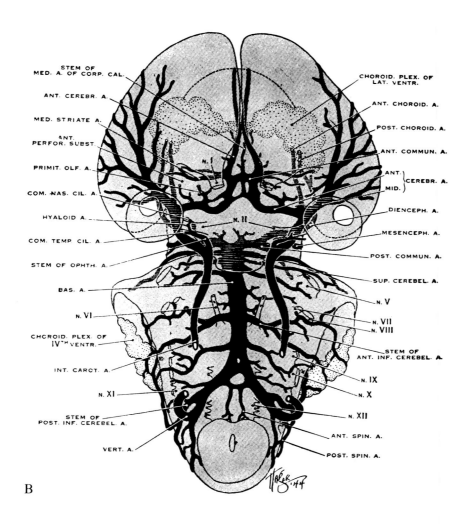

B

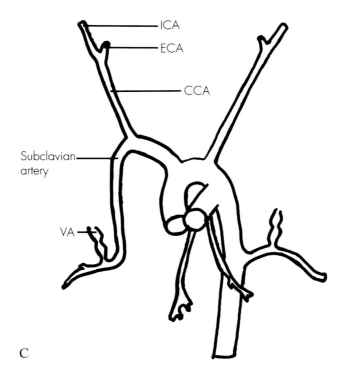

Figure 24-17 (*Continued*). **(B)** Ventral view of a 24-mm CRL embryo. **(C)** Ventral view of the aortic arches of an 18-mm CRL embryo. (Figs. A and B from Padget,[328] with permission; Fig. C modified from Congdon,[78] with permission.)

C

maxillary branch of the ICA becomes the inferior hypophyseal artery, supplying the posterior pituitary. The ECA system also completes its development; its (internal) maxillary branch will soon anastomose with and take over supply of the maxillo-mandibular division of the stapedial artery, forming the definitive maxillary artery.

Cranially, the mesial branch of the primitive olfactory artery (the ACA) is larger than the lateral, true terminal segment that supplies the region of the inferior forebrain (the recurrent artery of Heubner). The telencephalon has grown and with it the MCA. The choroid plexus is supplied by prominent anterior and posterior choroidal arteries, which anastomose within the developing choroidal fissure.

Caudally, two large arteries, the arteries of the diencephalon and mesencephalon, nearly dominate the cerebral vasculature. The future telencephalic distribution of the PCA will result from the confluence and enormous late growth of branches of these and the posterior and anterior choroidal arteries and the MCA. Furthermore, the PCA will soon be supplied in large part from the vertebrobasilar system, as a secondary expedience, as the cerebrum grows massively over the hindbrain. The development of the PCA and its shift in source of supply from the anterior to the posterior circulation "recapitulates" its phylogeny.

The superior cerebellar artery is the main supplier of the cerebellum superior to the fourth ventricle. Several branches arise from the basilar artery to supply the brainstem and the large choroid plexus of the fourth ventricle. The vertebral arteries are well defined, originating from the subclavian arteries, as the heart has begun to descend into the chest. Anterior spinal branches of the vertebral arteries can also be identified.

In the next to last embryonic phase of cerebrovascular development (stages XX and XXI, 18- to 24-mm CRL, 43- to 48-day EGA) the structures of the face become more clearly human in their appearance, and the head lifts up from the chest (Fig. 24-17). With the extreme folding of the brain at the mesencephalic and pontine flexures, the brain also has a more adult configuration.

The stapedial artery divides into several segments, which become important portions of various other arterial systems. At the stapes, the stapedial artery regresses. The proximal segment, arising from the ICA (i.e., the hyoid artery with the stapedial branch), persists as the small and variably present caroticotympanic branch of the petrous ICA. The segment that remains immediately distal to the stapes becomes the superior (anterior) tympanic branch of the

(internal) maxillary artery. This segment presumably also forms the inferior tympanic branch of the ascending pharyngeal artery. The ventral or maxillomandibular division of the stapedial artery, as noted, forms a large portion of the ECA system, including the infraorbital and inferior alveolar arteries. The dorsal or supraorbital division of the stapedial artery becomes the middle meningeal artery system. That segment lying between the stapes and the foramen spinosum becomes the tiny superficial petrosal artery.[123,183,300,353]

The supraorbital division of the stapedial artery also contributes, along with the dorsal and ventral ophthalmic arteries, to the formation of an arterial ring encircling the optic nerve. The dorsal and ventral ophthalmic arteries anastomose with the definitive ophthalmic artery, which appears to be a new and independent branch of the ICA. The stem of the definitive ophthalmic artery later migrates to its adult supraclinoid internal carotid artery location.

The anterior cerebral arteries supply the mesial surfaces of the cerebral hemispheres in the now definitive interhemispheric fissure and send one or more branches to the choroid plexus of the lateral ventricle in the region of the foramen of Monro. From the anterior communicating artery the median artery of the corpus callosum supplies the commissural plate of the primitive corpus callosum. The developing recurrent artery of Heubner and medial striate arteries, as previously noted, represent the terminus of the primitive olfactory artery.

In the hindbrain the AICA and PICA are still very plexiform, paralleling the still very rudimentary developmental state of the inferior cerebellum. However, the superior cerebellar artery is well developed.

Padget[328] defines the last phase of embryonic vascular development as that time at which the definitive stems of all major adult arterial trunks can be identified (Fig. 24-18). This corresponds roughly to the end of the first gestational trimester (stage XXII and XXIII, CRL 27 to 40+ mm, EGA 50+ days) and signifies the onset of the fetal phase of development. It should be noted that neural organization of the CNS, especially the telencephalon, is still very rudimentary at the end of the embryonic period.[253]

The definitive ophthalmic artery attains its adult form with the regression of the medial or cranioventral portion of the arterial ring encircling the optic nerve. The supraorbital division of the stapedial artery dwindles at the orbital margin, leaving the lacrimal, supraorbital, supratrochlear, dorsal nasal, palpebral, ethmoidal, and zygomatic arteries as branches of the ophthalmic artery. These remnants

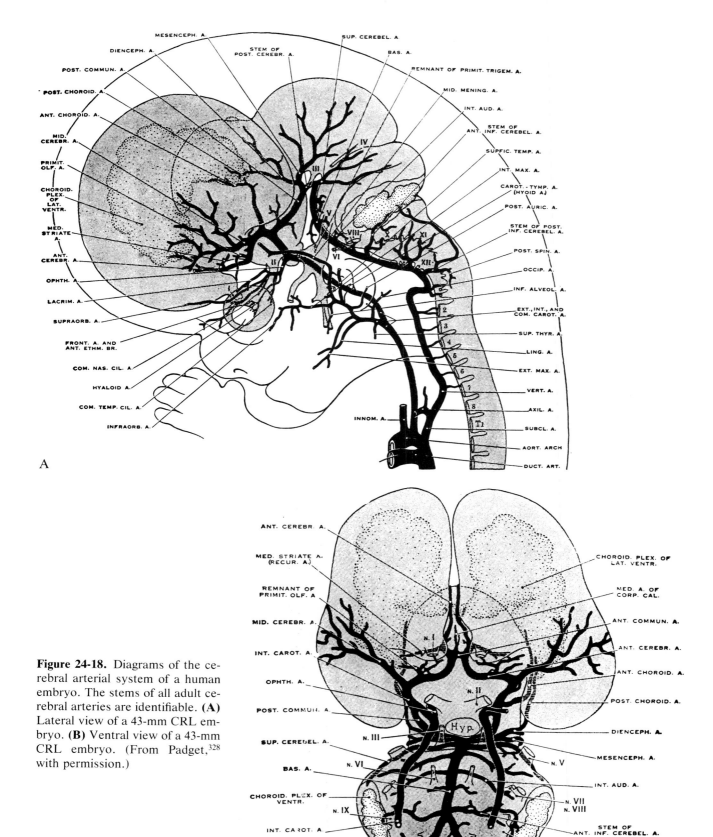

Figure 24-18. Diagrams of the cerebral arterial system of a human embryo. The stems of all adult cerebral arteries are identifiable. **(A)** Lateral view of a 43-mm CRL embryo. **(B)** Ventral view of a 43-mm CRL embryo. (From Padget,[328] with permission.)

of the stapedial artery provide important anastomoses via the orbit for the ECA and ICA systems. In addition, the middle meningeal artery, along with its anterior or recurrent meningeal branch, is derived from the supraorbital division of the stapedial artery. The anterior meningeal branch enters the orbit via the superior orbital fissure to anastomose with the lacrimal artery, providing another potential anastomosis between the ECA and ICA systems. The hyaloid artery (central artery of the retina) and the common temporal ciliary arteries are derived from the primitive dorsal ophthalmic artery, while the common nasal ciliary artery is the remnant of the primitive ventral ophthalmic artery.

The median artery of the corpus callosum persists at this stage and often into adulthood and may become rather prominent as an accessory or median ACA. Chief supply of the choroid plexus of the lateral and third ventricles comes from the posterior choroidal arteries, with only the temporal horns supplied by the anterior choroidal artery. Extensive anastomoses exist between the posterior and anterior choroidal arteries within the choroid plexus. Moreover, an ACA branch to the choroid plexus may also persist into adulthood.[214] Also noted at this stage are the superior hypophyseal arteries to the anterior pituitary, originating from the supraclinoid ICA and the posterior communicating arteries.

The cerebral arteries of the neonate are essentially comparable with those of the adult except for differences in relative proportion (Fig. 24-19). Tables 24-2 and 24-3 summarize the homologous arteries found in the embryo and adult.

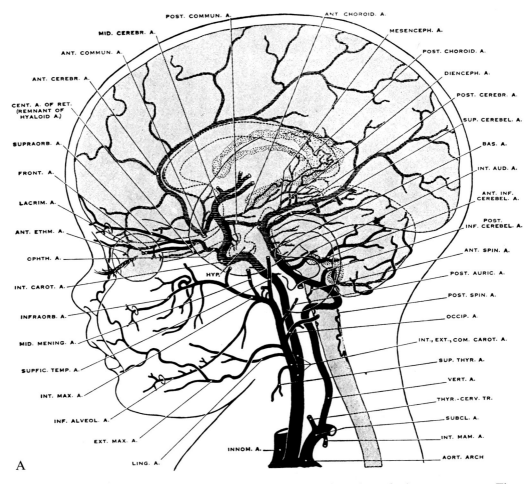

A

Figure 24-19. Diagrams of the cerebral arterial system and aortic arches of a human neonate. The cerebral arteries of the neonate are comparable with those of the adult except for differences in relative proportions. The definitive aortic arch results partly from the descent of the heart into the chest and changes in the pharynx. **(A)** Lateral view. (*Figure continues.*)

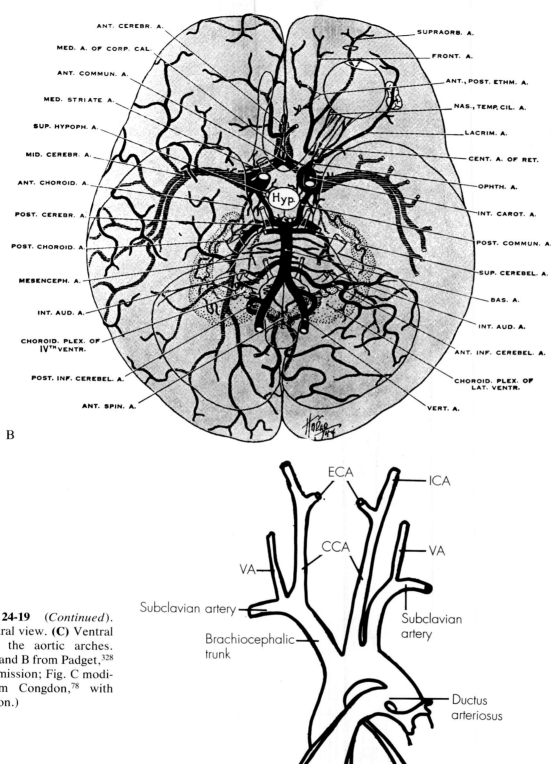

ANT. CEREBR. A.

MED. A. OF CORP. CAL.

ANT. COMMUN. A.

MED. STRIATE A.

SUP. HYPOPH. A.

MID. CEREBR. A.

ANT. CHOROID. A.

POST. CEREBR. A.

POST. CHOROID. A.

MESENCEPH. A.

INT. AUD. A.

CHOROID. PLEX. OF IVᵀᴴ VENTR.

POST. INF. CEREBEL. A.

ANT. SPIN. A.

SUPRAORB. A.

FRONT. A.

ANT., POST. ETHM. A.

NAS., TEMP. CIL. A.

LACRIM. A.

CENT. A. OF RET.

OPHTH. A.

INT. CAROT. A.

POST. COMMUN. A.

SUP. CEREBEL. A.

BAS. A.

INT. AUD. A.

ANT. INF. CEREBEL. A.

CHOROID. PLEX. OF LAT. VENTR.

VERT. A.

Hyp.

B

ECA

ICA

VA

CCA

VA

Subclavian artery

Subclavian artery

Brachiocephalic trunk

Ductus arteriosus

C

Figure 24-19 (*Continued*). **(B)** Ventral view. **(C)** Ventral view of the aortic arches. (Figs. A and B from Padget,[328] with permission; Fig. C modified from Congdon,[78] with permission.)

Table 24-2. Embryonic Arteries of the Brain and Their Known or Presumed Adult Homologues

Embryonic Artery	Adult Artery
Aortic sac	Segments of aortic arch, pulmonary trunk, brachiocephalic trunk, pulmonary arteries, common carotid artery, ECA
Dorsal aortae	Aorta, ICA, ductus arteriosus
Ventral aortae (ventral pharyngeal arteries)	Much of external carotid artery system
Aortic arch 1 (primitive mandibular artery)	Vidian artery (artery of the pterygoid canal) (may be ICA and/or ECA origin in adult), segments of maxillary artery (annexed mainly by primitive stapedial artery and thus ECA)
Aortic arch 2 (primitive hyoid artery)	Caroticotympanic branch of ICA
Stapedial branch	Maxillary artery and branches; middle meningeal, inferior alveolar, and infraorbital arteries; lacrimal, supraorbital, supratrochlear, dorsal nasal, palpebral, ethmoidal and zygomatic branches of ophthalmic artery; anterior (recurrent) meningeal branches middle meningeal arteries
Aortic arch 3	Common carotid artery, proximal segments of ICA and ECA
Aortic arch 4	Aortic arch and left subclavian artery (left arch 4), right subclavian artery (right arch 4)
Aortic arch 6	Pulmonary arteries
Primitive maxillary artery	Inferior hypophyseal arteries
Primitive ventral ophthalmic artery	Common nasal ciliary arteries
Primitive dorsal ophthalmic artery	Hyaloid artery (central retinal artery), common temporal ciliary artery
Rostral division of ICA	Anterior cerebral, middle cerebral, and anterior choroidal arteries; lenticulostriate arteries; recurrent artery of Heubner,
Caudal division of ICA	Posterior communicating artery, P_1 segment of posterior cerebral artery
Diencephalic artery, mesencephalic artery	Posterior cerebral artery, superior cerebellar artery
Bilateral longitudinal neural arteries	Basilar artery, superior cerebellar arteries
Primitive lateral–basilovertebral anastomosis	AICAs, PICAs
Cervical intersegmental arteries	Vertebral arteries, subclavian arteries
Proatlantal intersegmental artery	Horizontal, suboccipital segment of vertebral arteries

Abbreviations: AICA, anterior inferior cerebellar artery; ECA, external carotid artery; ICA, internal carotid artery; PICA, posterior inferior cerebellar artery

HUMAN CEREBROVASCULAR ANOMALIES AND VARIANTS

Cerebral Angioarchitecture

The vascular anatomy of the CNS has been the subject of intensive study for centuries.[77] Accepted modern anatomic descriptions, concepts, and nomenclature generally date from only as far back as the mid- or late nineteenth and early twentieth centuries.[30,31,73,112] Prior to this, although some anatomic descriptions were accurate by modern standards, other areas were understood incompletely or described incorrectly[484] (Fig. 24-20).

Unlike any other organ, the CNS is supplied only by arteries that penetrate from its surface.[84,85,460,462] Penetrating vessels enter at right angles to the CNS surface, branching to supply a continuous capillary network throughout their roughly orthogonal course toward the nearest ventricle.[75,111,113,224,255,273,274,282,299, 314,384–386,422] There may or may not be significant numbers of arteriole to arteriole anastomoses within the CNS parenchyma; their presence is supported by some authors[13,75,111,113,170,208,224,255,273,274,314] and refuted by others.[113,119,299] However, functionally at least, penetrating arterioles are considered end arteries insofar as an acute arteriolar occlusion will result in a more or less well demarcated CNS infarction. Shellshear[400] cited John Hunter as the person who introduced the concept of end arteries. Perforating arterioles are relatively constant in both their sites of penetration of the CNS surface[492] and their territory of supply.[1–3,30,31,401] The perforating arteries, generally unnamed, have been called *arteries of sup-*

Table 24-3. Adult Cerebral Arteries and Their Known or Presumed Embryonic Homologues

Adult Artery	Embryonic Artery
Common carotid artery	Aortic arch 3
ECA	Ventral pharyngeal artery, aortic sac
ICA	Aortic arch 3, dorsal aorta
Caroticotympanic artery	Stapedial branch of hyoid artery (aortic arch 3)
Vidian artery	Primitive mandibular artery (aortic arch 2)
Inferior hypophyseal artery	Primitive maxillary artery
Ophthalmic artery	Primitive dorsal and primitive ventral ophthalmic arteries, supraorbital division of stapedial artery
Maxillary artery	Maxillomandibular division of stapedial artery
Middle meningeal and recurrent meningeal arteries	Supraorbital division of stapedial artery
Accessory meningeal artery	?Maxillomandibular and supraorbital divisions of stapedial artery
Artery of foramen rotundum	?Maxillomandibular and supraorbital divisions of stapedial artery
Recurrent artery of Heubner, medial and lateral lenticulostriate arteries	Rostral division ICA, primitive olfactory artery
ACA	Rostral division ICA
MCA	Rostral division ICA
Anterior choroidal anterior	Anterior choroidal artery
PCA	Diencephalic and mesencephalic arteries
Posterior communicating artery; P_1 segment of PCA	Caudal division ICA
Superior cerebellar artery	Superior cerebellar artery, mesencephalic artery
AICA	Lateral basilovertebral anastomosis
PICA	Lateral basilovertebral anastomosis
Basilar artery	Bilateral longitudinal neural arteries
Vertebral artery	Cervical intersegmental arteries 1–6, proatlantal intersegmental artery
Origin of subclavian artery	Cervical intersegmental artery 6
Aortic arch	Aortic arch 4
Pulmonary artery, ductus arteriosus	Aortic arch 6

Abbreviations: AICA, anterior inferior cerebellar artery; ACA, anterior cerebral artery; ECA, external carotid artery; ICA, internal carotid artery; MCA, middle cerebral artery; PCA, posterior cerebral artery; PICA, posterior inferior cerebellar artery.

ply[399–402] or *nutrient arteries*[137,139] as opposed to the large, muscular *arteries of distribution*[399–402] or *conducting arteries*[137,139] that supply the arterioles. These latter vessels are the anatomically named arteries, and they are relatively variable in their course. It is with the variations and anomalies of the origins and distributions of these larger arteries that the present chapter is concerned.

Anomalies and Variants in General

When referring to vascular anatomical patterns that are different from standard or classical descriptions, the terms *anomaly* and *variation* or *variant* often are used interchangeably. Strictly speaking, *anomaly* means "abnormality" and perhaps should be used to refer to a given anatomical configuration that is pathological. *Variation,* on the other hand, connotes a more harmless anatomical configuration, which is merely different from what is usual or expected. However, the semantic difference between these terms is often not appreciated or adhered to, so that the words have become essentially synonymous, and throughout this chapter they will be so used. It will be indicated specifically when an anatomical arrangement appears to be pathological.

Cerebrovascular anomalies are usually found incidentally at angiography or autopsy, often with no clinical significance. However, multiple cerebrovascular anomalies are occasionally found in the same patient.[105, 114, 123, 168, 229, 230, 284, 291, 318, 333, 339, 348, 446, 470,488] Moreover, cerebrovascular anomalies have been reported with other congenital anomalies, such as aortic arch anomalies,[122,301,311,357] multiple cerebral aneurysms,[225] cerebral arteriovenous malformations,[7,135,196,451] moyamoya disease,[226] anomalies of the nervous system and/or supporting structures,[107,162,163,280,281,429,443] and anomalies of other organs.[146,186,281,311,450] This suggests that in some cases a vascular anomaly is the result of a more global developmental problem, perhaps genetic or humoral.

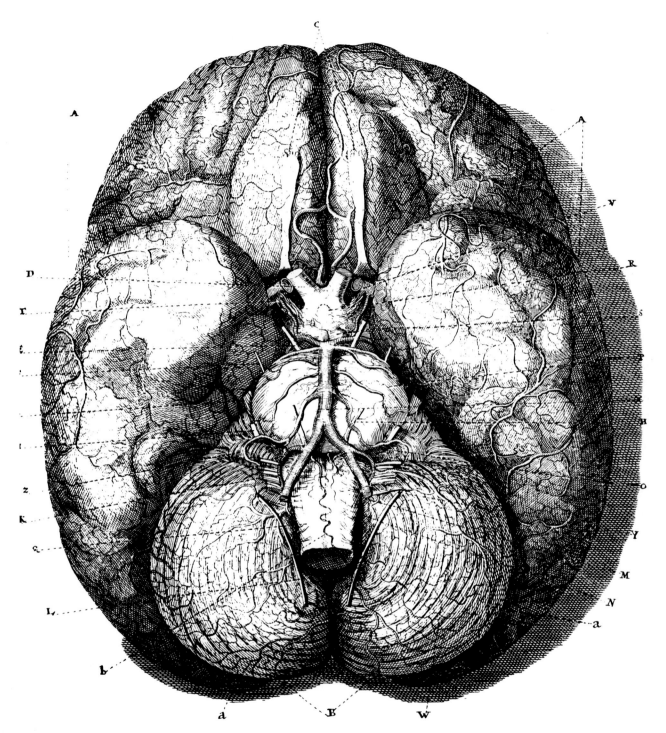

Figure 24-20. Cerebral arterial circulation injected with colored wax or mercury. This drawing from the seventeenth century is the earliest known detailed study of the angioarchitecture of the brain. (From Ruysch,[372] with permission.)

All cerebral arteries at one time exist as a capillary plexus.[78,115,116,179,273,274,328,373-375,420,449] From the primordial plexus, certain channels become dominant or preferred, many of these being the vessels that eventually become known as the normal, named arteries. The normal anatomy is relatively consistent among individuals, providing the basis for the classical descriptions of the vessels found in textbooks and classical reports.[30,31,73,74,112,202,300,316,377,384,385,417,419] However, in any individual the dominant channels that emerge from the primordial plexus may occasionally be different from the "normal." This concept can be used to understand all cerebrovascular variations.

Adjacent and/or anastomotic arteries and arterial systems share a reciprocal relationship in both their stems of origin and territories of supply rather than being sharply demarcated. The territory classically described as normal for a given artery usually represents its average, or sometimes its maximal, territory. However, in a given individual the area of supply of a particular artery or arterial system may be very large or very small. When large, it will be seen to have taken over the territory of adjacent arteries, and that of the adjacent arteries will be correspondingly reduced. Conversely, if a particular artery is small or absent, the "lost" territory will be seen to be supplied by the adjacent and/or anastomotic arterial systems.

Development from a primordial plexus is the basis for the anomalies known as *multiplications* (duplications, triplications, etc.), *fenestrations,* and *fusions.* Multiplications and fenestrations have been described for all arteries and represent essentially the same type of anomaly. When the multiplied arterial segment is short and the duplicate vessels reanastomose, it is generally called a fenestration, while long multiplied segments that do not reanastomose or that reanastomose at a great distance from their point of departure are more often referred to as duplications, triplications, etc. Any artery may occasionally develop as multiple or fenestrated channels even if its most common condition is single, because of the potential for various numbers of dominant channels to develop in the primordial plexus from which the artery arises. Conversely, arterial trunks that are normally adjacent may occasionally develop as a common stem, which then ramifies to supply the various distributions. A duplicated artery will be seen to supply some portion of the territory of the normal artery, while the normal vessel will be seen to be lacking that portion of its territory. Fenestrations are particularly common in arteries that are known to develop as the result of fusion of paired embryonic channels. Multi-

plications, fusions, and fenestrations are usually not clinically significant except that the proximal portions of fenestrations have been associated with aneurysm formation.[16,40,43,65,220,293,457,490,492,494]

It should be noted that several authors have discussed the vascular anatomy of the brain in terms of *segmentalization* or *metamerization.*[228-230,399-402] The concept is that the earliest CNS is simply a nerve cord, supplied by segmental or metameric vessels, which are not different from those in any other part of the body and are serially homologous with the segmental supply of the spinal cord (the primitive caroticobasilar and caroticovertebral arteries of the early embryo are considered by some to be these segmental arteries at the level of the brainstem and diencephalon). Later, as the brain develops and enlarges, arterial anastomoses form between segments to supply the expanding tissue. As the cerebral and cerebellar hemispheres develop further, branches of these *intersegmental* anastomoses grow to supply this tissue; these branches are termed *suprasegmental.* However, owing to the somewhat speculative nature of this concept, this chapter limits this terminology mainly to the vertebral artery, which clearly develops from spinal segmental vasculature.

Carotid Arteries

Anatomy

Cervical Segment

The right common carotid artery arises from the brachiocephalic trunk and bifurcates at C3-C4 or C4-C5 into the ECA and ICA at the level of the upper margin of the thyroid cartilage.[74,261,300,404] The left common carotid artery arises from the aortic arch between the origins of the brachiocephalic trunk and the left subclavian artery, bifurcating also at approximately C4-C5. The cervical segment of the ICA courses upward, anterior to the transverse processes of the first three cervical vertebrae and lateral to the ECA to enter the carotid canal via its opening in the inferior surface of the petrous bone.

Petrous Segment

Within the carotid canal, the petrous segment of the ICA may supply several small branches to surrounding structures.[312,336,340,352,353] One of these is the phylogenetically and ontogenetically significant caroticotympanic branch to the tympanic cavity via a tiny foramen in the carotid plate. Although this tiny branch has been described thoroughly by Nager and Nager,[312] this vessel is not generally found in injection studies.[340,352] Other petrous branches include the artery of the pterygoid canal (Vidian artery) and the periosteal branches.

Cavernous Segment

The ICA exits the carotid canal at the foramen lacerum and enters the cranial cavity. After a short extracavernous, epidural segment, it enters the cavernous sinus, where it assumes a characteristic S-shaped course. Parkinson and Shields[338] state that the cavernous sinus has no distinct inferior boundary, which is contrary to the description of Wallace et al.,[472] who state that the entrance to the cavernous sinus is marked by a band-like dural impression. The branches of the cavernous ICA constitute a relatively complex topic. They have been studied extensively owing to their hemodynamic, surgical, ontogenetic, and phylogenetic significance.

Several authors have examined the branches of the cavernous ICA in reference to other intracranial structures or pathology.[283,390,415] Parkinson[336] established the standard neurosurgical nomenclature. As angiographic and microsurgical techniques developed, the role of the cavernous branches in intracranial pathology were analyzed in greater and greater detail.[166,173,189,267,268,321,381,472] The anatomy of these branches was found to be much more variable than indicated by Parkinson's description. For this reason Lasjaunias and coworkers[229,235,237,483] and Tran-Dinh[452] have not used Parkinson's nomenclature, proposing or using alternatives. However, this chapter will continue to use the nomenclature of Parkinson, as it will be most familiar to the majority of readers.

The first (i.e., most proximal) and largest branch of the cavernous ICA is the meningohypophyseal trunk, from which the tentorial, dorsal meningeal, and inferior hypophyseal arteries arise. The tentorial branch gives rise to small branches to cranial nerves III and IV, a branch to the roof of the cavernous sinus, and branches to the falx and tentorium. The artery to the tentorium often goes by the eponym *artery of Bernasconi and Cassinari*, after the authors who described the vessel in relation to tentorial meningiomas.[39,70] The dorsal meningeal branch supplies branches to the clivus and to cranial nerve VI, and the inferior hypophyseal branch supplies branches to the dura of the sella floor, posterior clinoid process, dura of the cavernous sinus, and posterior lobe of the hypophysis, and it anastomoses with its opposite counterpart.

Lasjaunias and his co-workers[229,235,237,483] believe that the branches usually attributed to the meningo-

hypophyseal trunk are derived from separate embryonic arteries, namely the primitive trigeminal and primitive maxillary arteries, although the evidence for this is not certain. In support of this belief, Lasjaunias and co-workers have shown that in their studies branches usually attributed to the meningohypophyseal trunk arise from a common origin in only 10 percent of cases. More often, these branches originate along the medial and lateral aspects of the ascending segment of the cavernous ICA, or they may form variable branching patterns.

The next branch of the cavernous ICA is the artery of the inferior cavernous sinus (Fig. 24-21). Lasjaunias and his associates[66,228–230,235–238,483] have called this the *inferolateral trunk* and believe that it is derived from the primitive dorsal ophthalmic and stapedial arteries. This important vessel was noted by Parkinson[336] to supply the gasserian ganglion and

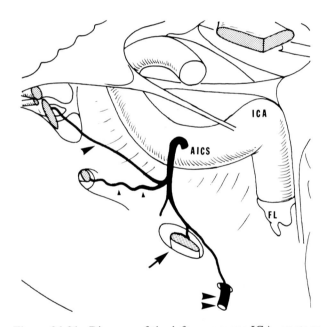

Figure 24-21. Diagram of the left cavernous ICA, posterosuperolateral view, showing the artery of the inferior cavernous sinus. This cavernous ICA branch may anastomose with several branches of the maxillary artery. Note that these anastomoses represent potential routes for cerebral embolization from the ECA system. *AICS,* artery of the inferior cavernous sinus (also called inferolateral trunk by Lasjaunias and co-workers); *FL,* foramen lacerum; *ICA,* cavernous segment of internal carotid artery; single large arrowhead, recurrent (anterior) meningeal branch of middle meningeal artery (coursing through left superior orbital fissure); small arrowheads, artery of the foramen rotundum; arrow, foramen ovale with accessory meningeal artery; double large arrowheads, middle meningeal artery (via foramen spinosum). (Modified from Lasjaunias et al.,[237] with permission.)

anastomose with the main trunk of the middle meningeal artery. Branches of the artery of the inferior cavernous sinus may also anastomose with the recurrent branch of the middle meningeal artery, accessory meningeal artery, and artery of the foramen rotundum. In addition, a branch to the pterygoid canal (vidian artery) may, rarely, branch from the artery of the inferior cavernous sinus to anastomose with a vidian branch of the internal maxillary artery (although the vidian branch of the ICA more commonly arises from the petrous segment). Finally, some authors have also described an anastomosis of the ascending pharyngeal artery with the artery of the inferior cavernous sinus via the foramen lacerum.[233,239,353,483]

The last group of branches from the cavernous ICA are known as capsular arteries. They supply the dura of the sella turcica, anastomosing with their counterparts of the opposite side. The anatomy of the capsular branches has been described in detail by McConnell[283] in reference to the blood supply to the pituitary.

De la Torre and Netsky[96] and later Lasjaunias and co-workers[66,229,230,235–238,483] have studied and discussed the normal and anomalous anatomy of the branches of the cavernous ICA in numerous publications. They have made important contributions to the understanding of the anatomic variations of this arterial system based on the ontogeny and comparative anatomy of the vasculature. Branches of the cavernous ICA (i.e., the meningohypophyseal trunk, artery of the inferior cavernous sinus, capsular branches and persistent primitive trigeminal artery) form potential anastomoses with branches of numerous other arterial systems, including the maxillary artery (middle meningeal artery and its anterior or recurrent meningeal branch, accessory meningeal artery, artery of the foramen rotundum), the ascending pharyngeal artery (branch to the foramen lacerum, hypoglossal branch, clival branches), and the trigeminal (gasserian) branch of the AICA (probably the remnant of the embryonic trigeminal artery). Variations of the vessels in this region can be understood as persistence or enlargement of certain anastomoses, with regression of hypoplasia of others, as discussed below. Furthermore, these variations are often homologous with the normal anatomy of various mammals.

Supraclinoid Segment

Medially to the anterior clinoid process and inferiorly to the optic nerve, the ICA exits the cavernous sinus. The supraclinoid or paraclinoid segment of the ICA is that part extending from its exit from the cavernous sinus to its terminal bifurcation into the ACA and MCA. The terminal end lies inferior to the anterior perforated substance, just inferomedial to the limen insulae. This segment is subarachnoid. Together, the cavernous and supraclinoid segments of the ICA are referred to as the *carotid siphon*. Major branches of the supraclinoid ICA include the ophthalmic, posterior communicating and anterior choroidal arteries, in caudal to rostral sequence. Smaller branches of the supraclinoid segment of the ICA to the region of the optic chiasm and infundibulum have been studied by Gibo et al.[136]

Ontogeny

The common carotid arteries and carotid bifurcations are remnants of the embryonic aortic sac and the third aortic arch. The most proximal segment of the ICA represents the third aortic arch, and the remainder of this artery represents the dorsal aorta superior to this arch. The second aortic arch, the hyoid artery, becomes the hyoid-stapedial system. Its ICA remnant is represented by the caroticotympanic artery and probably portions of the other intratympanic vessels. The artery of the first arch, the primitive mandibular artery, becomes the artery of the pterygoid canal (vidian artery). It is presumed that the branches of the cavernous ICA are ontogenetically related to the embryonic stapedial artery in a manner similar to that of the petrous ICA branches. This is because of known anastomoses between these systems (e.g., maxillary artery branches with cavernous ICA branches). However, the ontogeny of the cavernous internal carotid artery branches is not known.[338]

The ECA is formed by annexation of the arteries of the pharyngeal arches and much of the embryonic stapedial artery is formed from the ventral pharyngeal artery which is derived from the aortic sac of the human embryo and represents the ventral aorta of lower vertebrates.

Phylogeny

Fish and larval amphibians oxygenate their blood via gills, which are supplied by ventral aortae and drain via dorsal aortae. The dorsal aortae then conduct oxygenated blood to the brain and body. The evolutionary changes that led to lungs and a four-chambered heart and that changed the aortic arch system of lower vertebrates into the craniofacial, cervical, and thoracic vessels of higher vertebrates are complex topics, relevant to the understanding of human craniofacial vasculature (Figs. 24-2 and 24-6). However, they are beyond the scope of this chapter.

The brains of all submammalian vertebrates are supplied exclusively by paired ICAs. The basilar artery is present in these organisms, representing the (usually anastomosed) caudal divisions of the ICAs. The brains of submammals are so small that the ICAs are sometimes minute as compared with the vessels that supply the jaws, face, and head.

The brains of all mammals are supplied by paired ICAs and vertebral arteries at some time in development. Along the phylogenetic pathway that leads to humans there is a tendency to increasing relative size of the ICAs and decreasing relative size of the ECAs and stapedial arteries.

Anomalies and Variants

Lie[257] in 1968 published a thorough review of the congenital anomalies of the extracranial carotid arteries.

Multiplications

Developmentally, the ICA arises from a plexus of channels, as already stated. Duplications and fenestrations of the extracranial[168,217,443] as well as the intracranial[149,152,494] ICA presumably reflect this plexiform ontogeny. No vertebrate is known to normally possess multiple ICAs on one side.

Internal Carotid Artery Branches and Absence of External Carotid Artery

Normally there are no branches of the cervical ICA.[74,300] However, Havelius and Hindfelt[175] found minute branches of the cervical ICA near the skull base in 18 percent of cadaver arteries studied. These vessels were thought to supply the periadventitial sympathetic nerve plexus of the ICA and/or the proximal extracranial course of the lower cranial nerves. These authors suggested a possible role for these branches in the etiology of some cases of Horner's syndrome and jugular foramen syndrome.

ECA branches may, rarely, arise anomalously from the cervical segment of the internal carotid artery.[257,317,378,443,447] In addition, Kwak et al.[227] have reported an anomalous origin of the posterior meningeal artery from the cervical ICA. Teal et al.[447] have described a case of cervical ICA origin of the PICA. In both cases the anomalous artery was normally a branch of the vertebral artery. These anomalies represent a persistent proatlantal intersegmental artery (see below).

Ontogeny. The mechanism by which ECA branches arise from the ICA would appear to represent failure of the ventral pharyngeal arteries to form. As a result those branches of the embryonic aortic arches that would normally regress at their dorsal ends as their more ventral connection with the ventral pharyngeal artery strengthens would, in the absence of this artery, persist as branches of the dorsal aorta and hence of the ICA.

Lateral Position of the External Carotid Artery

Anomalous lateral position of the ECA has been reported by several authors[46,161,168,257,404,446] and probably occurs more frequently than reported. The ICA normally branches from the dorsolateral aspect of the common carotid artery,[404] while the ECA arises from its anteromedial side. Dorsomedial origin of the ICA from the common carotid artery may be more common on the right than on the left.[404]

Ontogeny. Normally, the origin of the ECA develops from the ventral pharyngeal artery near the midline. It then migrates slightly laterally to assume its usual position, arising from the carotid bifurcation anteromedial to the ICA. Lie[257] has proposed that excessive migration causes the ECA to assume an anomalous dorsolateral position relative to the ICA. However, Smith and Larson[404] suggest the possibility of rotation of the arteries during development, while Teal et al.[447] believe that most reported cases are acquired lesions, secondary to arteriosclerosis.

Separate Origins of External and Internal Carotid Arteries

Separate origins of the ECA and ICA from the aorta constitute a rare anomaly,[52,122,257,363] which is sometimes associated with other major and minor vascular anomalies. This association suggests a more global developmental abnormality in some cases, perhaps humoral or genetic.

Ontogeny. Separate origins of the ECA and ICA probably represent regression of the third aortic arch with persistence of the segment of dorsal aorta between the third and fourth arches (the ductus caroticus).[257] In this way the ICA would arise from the fourth arch (i.e., the aorta), and the ECA would arise from the common carotid artery in its usual location (i.e., the third arch).

Level of Bifurcation of Carotid Arteries

As already noted, the carotid arteries most often bifurcate at C3-C4 or C4-C5. Rarely, the bifurcation is in the thorax, and may be as low as T3.[378,466,492] The carotid bifurcations are usually not at the same level in a given individual.[404]

Ontogeny. A short common carotid artery (i.e., low bifurcation) may be the result of persistence of the ductus caroticus (that segment of the dorsal aorta between the third and fourth aortic arches), with involution of the distal segment of the third aortic arch and secondary migration of the ECA onto the common carotid artery.[257,297] This mechanism would be similar to that which results in a separate ICA and ECA arising from the aorta, but with secondary migration of the ECA to form a short common carotid artery. Alternatively, the common carotid artery may simply fail to elongate as the heart descends into the chest.[297]

Tortuosity

Tortuosities of the carotid arteries, also known as or related to dolichoectasia, kinking, coiling, looping, etc., are poorly defined phenomena (Fig. 24-22),[4,121,251,257,345,477] which most likely represent a group of separate but related entities. Leipzig and Dohrmann[251] reported that 92 percent of known cases have occurred in women. However, Abraham[4] reported no sex difference. Tortuosity may be unilateral but is more often bilateral.

Physicians first gained interest in tortuosity anomalies when they were implicated as the cause of fatal hemorrhage during surgery for tonsils and adenoids.[35,63,69,206,287,326] Later, ICA tortuosity was examined as potentially contributing to the etiology of some cases of cerebrovascular insufficiency.[477] In addition, several authors have reported cases of entrapment of the hypoglossal nerve in the neck secondary to an ICA loop.[324,393,457] Also, although most reports of ICA tortuosity relate to the cervical segment, the siphon may also be tortuous. In this case the supraclinoid ICA may erode the sphenoid sinus, thereby becoming subject to injury during sphenoid sinus surgery.[198] Surgery to correct a tortuous ICA has been performed in adults as well as in children.

The etiology of arterial tortuosity, especially the looping or coiling types, is thought to be mainly developmental, whereas kinking and aneurysmal dilatation are considered more likely to be acquired. Support for the congenital nature of these anomalies comes from their high incidence in children and

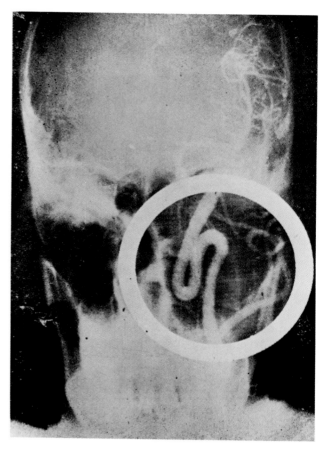

Figure 24-22. Right common carotid arteriogram, AP view, demonstrating extreme ICA tortuosity. Note absence of atherosclerosis or aneurysmal dilatation. The etiology of this anomaly is unknown. (From Abraham,[4] with permission.)

fetuses[63,257] and their association with other vascular anomalies, including contralateral absence of the ICA and separate origins of the ECA and ICA.[52,114,311,446] Clearly, however, degenerative processes may change the anatomy of the carotid arteries. For example, in aortic arch disease the arch may elevate, forcing the carotid arteries to bend.[251]

Ontogeny. The ontogenetic basis of carotid artery tortuosity is not well understood. Kelly,[206] citing diagrams by Quain, indicates that at the junction of the third aortic arch (the origin of the internal carotid artery) with the dorsal aorta, a pronounced bend is formed. This bend can also be seen in the diagrams of Congdon[78] and Padget[328] (see Figs. 24-10 and 24-12 to 24-18). As development proceeds, the heart descends into the chest, the carotid arteries lengthen, and the bend straightens. If the straightening is incomplete,

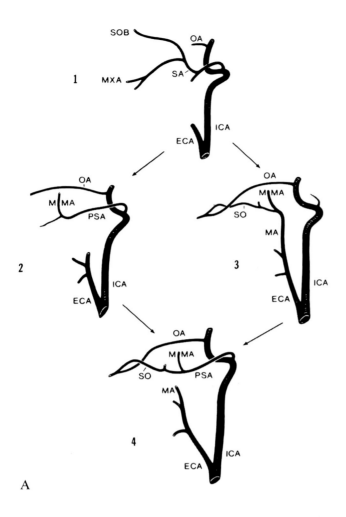

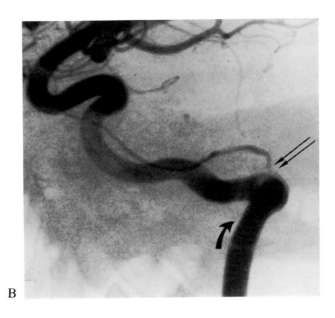

A

B

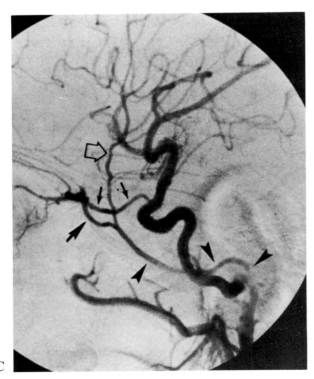

C

Figure 24-23. Anomalies of the embryonic stapedial artery, I. The supraorbital division of the embryonic stapedial artery forms the middle meningeal and recurrent meningeal arteries and the lacrimal branch of the ophthalmic artery. This provides the ontogenetic basis for numerous adult craniofacial vascular variations involving the middle meningeal, recurrent meningeal, and ophthalmic arteries. **(A)** Diagrams indicating some vascular variations due to persistence of various portions of the embryonic stapedial artery. (*1*) Normal stapedial artery of a human embryo of approximately 12-mm CRL (cf. Fig. 24-16). (*2*) Middle meningeal artery arising from the petrous ICA via the so-called persistent stapedial artery. (*3*) Persistence of the supraorbital division of the embryonic stapedial artery reflected in the shared supply of the orbital structures with the ophthalmic artery. (*4*) Persistent stapedial artery supplying the middle meningeal artery and sharing the supply of the orbit with the ophthalmic artery. *ECA*, external carotid artery; *ICA*, internal carotid artery; *MA*, maxillary artery; *MMA*, middle meningeal artery; *MXA*, maxillomandibular division of stapedial artery; *OA*; ophthalmic artery; *PSA*, persistent stapedial artery; *SA*, stapedial artery; *SO*, recurrent meningeal branch of middle meningeal artery coursing through superior orbital fissure; *SOB*, supraorbital branch of stapedial artery. **(B)** Persistent stapedial artery. Internal carotid arteriogram. Stenvers view demonstrating the middle meningeal artery (double arrows) arising from the petrous ICA (curved arrow). It is not known whether the vessel actually passes through the stapes. See item 2 in Fig. A. **(C)** Common carotid arteriogram, lateral view, demonstrating persistent stapedial artery. The anomalous vessel arises from the petrous portion of the ICA (arrowheads) and bifurcates into the middle meningeal artery (open arrow) and recurrent meningeal artery (*arrow*). The latter vessel courses through the superior orbital fissure to anastomose with the ophthalmic artery. See item 4 in Fig. A. (Figs. A and C modified from Marano et al.,[269] with permission; Fig. B from Lasjaunias et al.,[236] with permission.)

tortuosity may result. In support of this hypothesis Fields et al.[121] have observed that the initial curve of a tortuous ICA is almost always anteromedial, corresponding approximately to the direction of the embryonic bend, and that the glossopharyngeal nerves relates similarly to the embryonic and adult bends.

Persistent Stapedial Artery and Middle Meningeal Artery

Cerebrovascular anomalies that involve the middle meningeal artery, anterior or recurrent meningeal artery, caroticotympanic artery, maxillary artery (including its accessory meningeal and foramen rotundum branches) and the lacrimal branch of the ophthalmic artery all involve the *embryonic stapedial artery,* from which all these vessels are derived. These anomalies include

1. Petrous ICA origin of the middle meningeal artery (Fig. 24-23A&C) and/or the ophthalmic artery[12,107,157,183,228,229,236,257,269,288,378,416,443] (Fig. 24-23A&B). In the case of the latter anomaly, the vessel supplying the ophthalmic artery courses through the superior orbital fissure. Because of their petrous ICA origin, these anomalies are most often referred to as *persistent stapedial artery.*
2. Petrous ICA filling from the ascending pharyngeal artery.[50,89,184,228,229,234,236,263,285,303,356,426] This presumably occurs via an enlarged anastomosis between the caroticotympanic branch of the ICA and the inferior tympanic branch of the ascending pharyngeal artery in the middle ear. It is one form of so-called aberrant ICA in the middle ear (Fig. 24-24).**
3. Middle meningeal artery filling from the ascending pharyngeal artery via the middle ear.[228,236]
4. Ophthalmic artery origin of the middle meningeal artery and middle meningeal artery origin of the ophthalmic artery.[12,32,133,154,177,228,229,236,257,288,304,371,443,478] These anomalies occur via the anastomosis between the recurrent meningeal branch of the middle meningeal artery and the lacrimal branch of the ophthalmic artery.

5. Cavernous ICA origin of the middle meningeal and/or ophthalmic arteries.[66,166,177,189,223,228–230,235–238,241,452,483] In the former case the anastomosis is between the inferior branch of the cavernous sinus and the middle meningeal artery; in the latter there is an additional anastomosis between the recurrent branch of the middle meningeal artery and the lacrimal branch of the ophthalmic artery (Fig. 24-25). It should be noted that the ophthalmic and/or middle meningeal artery may also contribute to the supply of the cerebral circulation via the same anastomoses, especially in cases of acquired absence of the ICA (i.e., stenosis or occlusion) or high-flow states. These are discussed below in the section on ICA absence.
6. Cavernous ICA filling via maxillary artery branches (accessory meningeal artery and the artery of the foramen rotundum). This is analogous to filling of the cavernous ICA by the ophthalmic and middle meningeal arteries in cases of proximal ICA absence, as mentioned. These are discussed below in the section on ICA absence.
7. Basilar artery origin of the middle meningeal or ophthalmic artery[12,228–230,394,469] (Fig. 24-26). The anomalous vessel arises between the superior and anterior inferior cerebellar arteries and, in the case of basilar artery origin of the ophthalmic artery, courses through the superior orbital fissure.

Ontogeny. The ontogeny of the embryonic stapedial artery is complex, as described extensively by Padget.[328] The embryonic stapedial artery is a branch of the hyoid artery, the artery of the second arch of the dorsal aorta. At one time in embryogenesis the stapedial artery supplies a very large territory, including much of the developing orbit and face via its large supraorbital and maxillomandibular divisions. Later, the second arch dwindles at the level of the stapes, leaving only the tiny caroticotympanic artery as its remnant. The orbital branches of the supraorbital division of the stapedial artery are annexed by the ophthalmic artery, with the remainder of that division annexed by the ECA system as the middle meningeal artery system (including the recurrent meningeal artery). The normally present adult anastomosis between the recurrent branch of the middle meningeal artery and the lacrimal branch of the ophthalmic artery represents persistence of the anastomosis between the supraorbital division of the stapedial artery and the ophthalmic artery.

The maxillomandibular division of the embryonic stapedial artery is annexed by the ECA in the supply of the face and jaw structures, becoming the (internal) maxillary and facial (external maxillary) arteries. Finally, the accessory meningeal artery and the artery of the foramen rotundum are probably remnants

---

** In this case the cervical portion of the ICA is absent, and the "anomalous" ICA is actually the enlarged inferior tympanic branch of the ascending pharyngeal artery, persistently anastomosed with the equally enlarged caroticotympanic branch of the petrous ICA. The rest of the intracranial ICA is present and normal. In this anomaly the carotid canal is not present in the petrous bone. These cases can be discriminated from cases of ICA erosion of the carotid plate, which can also result in the ICA lying within the tympanic cavity. In the latter cases the ICA artery assumes a normal course in the neck, and a carotid canal can be demonstrated in the petrous bone by computed tomography (CT) or plain tomography.

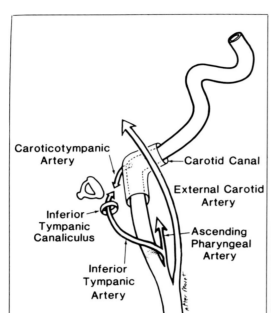
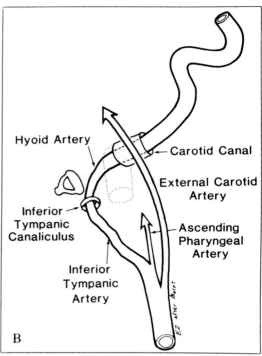

Figure 24-24. Anomalies of the embryonic stapedial artery, II. **(A)** Normal anatomy. **(B)** Anomalous condition. The ascending pharyngeal artery appears to be a branch of the ICA. Diagrams demonstrate absence of the right cervical ICA with persistence of the intracranial ICA, lateral view. Although the cervical ICA is absent, its petrous portion is reconstituted via an enlarged intratympanic anastomosis between the inferior tympanic branch of the ascending pharyngeal artery and the caroticotympanic branch of the ICA (remnant of the embryonic hyoid or stapedial artery). This anomaly appears to be homologous with the cerebral blood supply of many mammals in which the extracranial ICA is normally small or absent. (From Lo et al.[263] after Moret et al.,[302] with permission.)

of anastomoses between the supraorbital and maxillomandibular divisions of the stapedial artery.

In addition to what is known about the ontogeny of the stapedial artery and its derivatives from studies of vertebrate embryos, it is presumed that anastomoses also exist between this vessel and the inferior branch of the cavernous ICA, the ascending pharyngeal artery, and the primitive trigeminal artery. This presumption is based on the observed cerebrovascular anomalies described above. This concept has been developed best by Lasjaunias and coworkers.[66,229,230,235–238,241,302–304,483] Thus, persistence of various combinations of these known and presumed embryonic anastomoses, with regression of others, provides the ontogenetic basis for all the variations listed above:

1. Middle meningeal and/or ophthalmic artery origin from the petrous ICA artery (persistent stapedial artery) represents persistence of the main trunk and parts of the supraorbital division of the embryonic stapedial artery.
2. Petrous ICA filling from the ascending pharyngeal artery (aberrant ICA in the middle ear) represents enlargement of a normally minute, persistent, embryonic anastomosis between the ascending pharyngeal artery and the stem of the stapedial artery.
3. Middle meningeal artery filling from the ascending pharyngeal artery via the middle ear represents a persistent embryonic anastomosis between the ascending pharyngeal artery and the stem of the stapedial artery, with normal regression of the most proximal segment of the stem.
4. Ophthalmic artery origin from the middle meningeal artery and middle meningeal artery origin from the ophthalmic artery represent a normally small, persistent, embryonic anastomosis between a segment of the superior division of the stapedial artery (that part that becomes the recurrent meningeal artery) and the lacrimal branch of the ophthalmic artery.
5. Cavernous ICA origin of the middle meningeal and/or ophthalmic arteries and cavernous ICA filling from meningeal and/or ophthalmic arteries involve a presumed embryonic anastomosis between the supraorbital division of the stapedial artery (i.e., the future middle meningeal and recurrent meningeal arteries) and the artery of the inferior cavernous sinus.

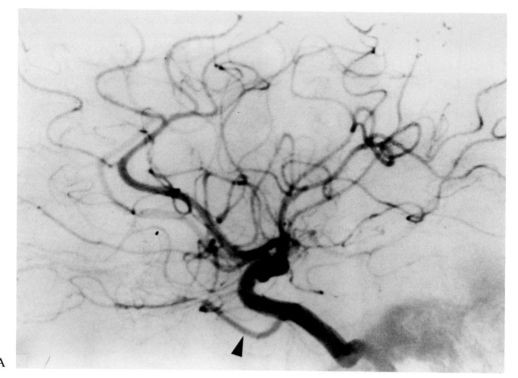

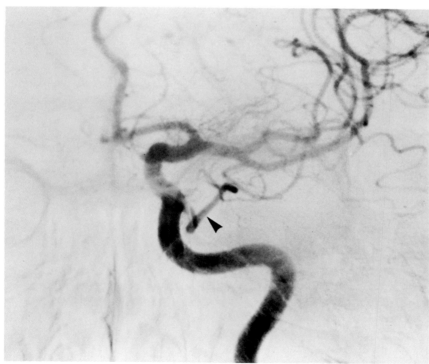

Figure 24-25. Anomalies of the embryonic stapedial artery, III. Internal carotid arteriograms demonstrating cavernous internal carotid origin of the ophthalmic artery. The anomalous ophthalmic artery (*arrowhead*) arises from the inferior branch of the cavernous ICA, courses through the superior orbital fissure, and anastomoses with the lacrimal branch of the ophthalmic artery. Cf. Fig. 24-21. **(A)** Lateral view. **(B)** Anteroposterior view.

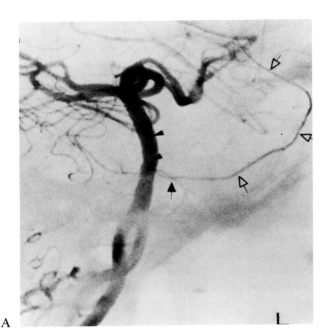

A   L

Figure 24-26. Anomalies of the embryonic stapedial artery, IV. These anomalies involve persistence of presumed embryonic anastomoses between the supraorbital division of the stapedial artery, the primitive trigeminal artery, the middle meningeal artery, the recurrent meningeal artery, and the inferior cavernous branch of the ICA. **(A)** Vertebral arteriogram, lateral view, demonstrating basilar artery origin (*arrowheads*) of the middle meningeal artery (*open arrows*). This represents a persistent anastomosis between the supraorbital division of the embryonic stapedial artery and the primitive trigeminal artery. **(B)** Vertebral angiogram, lateral view, demonstrating basilar artery origin (*single arrowhead*) of the ophthalmic artery. The vessel courses through the superior orbital fissure (*double arrowheads*). This represents a persistent embryonic anastomosis between the stapedial artery and the trigeminal artery. Supply of the ophthalmic artery is via the anastomosis between its lacrimal branch and the recurrent (anterior) branch of the middle meningeal artery. (Fig. A from Seeger and Hemmer,[394] with permission; Fig. B from Lasjaunias and Berenstein,[230] with permission.)

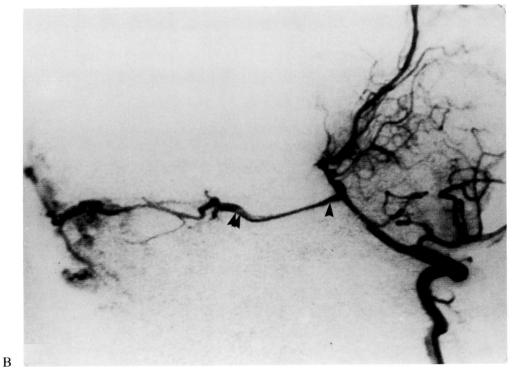

B

6. Cavernous ICA filling via maxillary artery branches (accessory meningeal artery and the artery of the foramen rotundum) are analogous to that from the meningeal and/or ophthalmic artery, noted above. These anomalies represent presumed embryonic anastomoses between the maxillomandibular division of the stapedial artery (future maxillary artery and branches), the supraorbital division of the stapedial artery (future middle meningeal and recurrent meningeal arteries), and the artery of the inferior cavernous sinus.

7. Basilar artery origin of the middle meningeal or ophthalmic arteries represents a presumed embryonic anastomosis between the supraorbital division of the stapedial artery (future recurrent meningeal artery) and the primitive trigeminal artery.

Phylogeny. The phylogenetic significance of the anastomoses between the main trunk of the middle meningeal artery, the recurrent branch of the middle meningeal artery, the accessory meningeal artery, the artery of the foramen rotundum, and the lacrimal branch of the ophthalmic artery is that these anastomoses, anomalous in the human, are homologous with the normal circulation of many mammals. These mammalian variations are listed in Table 24-6 and discussed below in the section on ICA absence.

In fish the orbital artery homologous with the stapedial artery of higher vertebrates branches from the ICA at the level of the hyomandibular bone, the homologue of the stapes (see Fig. 24-3). In fish this artery is a large vessel that supplies the jaws and face.

The stapedial artery as a major adult vessel is present in reptiles, variably present in small mammals, and absent in all larger mammals. Conroy[79] hypothesized that in evolution a critical size of the masticatory apparatus may have been reached beyond which the stapedial artery could not supply enough blood, the size of the artery being constrained by the size of the obturator foramen of the stapes through which it passes. The phylogeny of the stapedial artery is further discussed below in the section on ophthalmic artery anomalies.

It is worth noting that the stapedial artery has been employed as an aid in the systematic classification of certain mammals.[54–58] For example, primitive representatives of the primate order (tree shrews) share a similar ecological niche and body habitus with many species in the insectivore and rodent orders. These species are partly differentiated on the basis of the amount of annexation or lack thereof of the stapedial artery system by the ICA and/or ECA system. In other words, analysis of the anatomy of the stapedial artery, ICA, and ECA provides a means for the systematic classification of these externally similar mammals. This has been important in the identification of the presumed earliest representatives of the primate order. The same vascular relationships have been employed in the subclassification of members of the carnivore[59] and other orders.

Absence of the Carotid Artery

One of the more commonly reported congenital anomalies of the ICA in humans is its complete or partial absence.[33,105,114,117,122,123,146,160,163,186,195,225,229,238, 250,257,308,311,318,339,348,351,396,409,414,441,443,456,470,483,489,492] Lie[257] has provided a good review of these anomalies, differentiating between agenesis and aplasia of the ICA. *Agenesis* implies the failure of the ICA to develop, whereas *aplasia* implies secondary loss or in-

complete development of the vessel. In aplasia, a fine remnant of the ICA persists or a segment of the distal artery remains while proximal segments do not develop.[238] It might be more accurate to call the first type of aplasia *atresia* (lacking a lumen) or to refer to both types as *hypoplasia* (incomplete formation). Absence of a carotid canal in the petrous portion of the temporal bone by CT or plain tomography or by postmortem examination is felt to support a diagnosis of agenesis. Conversely, the presence of infraorbital and alveolar arteries favors aplasia, since these are branches of the embryonic stapedial artery, itself a transient branch of the developing ICA.[122,257] Perhaps this spectrum of developmental deficiencies in the formation of the ICA would be best referred to generically as *dysgenesis*.

As just noted, dysgenesis may involve only a segment of the ICA.[229,238] With this type of anomaly, a distal segment of ICA remains, but all segments proximal to it are missing. For example, if the petrous segment of the ICA is absent but the cavernous segment is present (filled, for example, via branches of the maxillary artery), the supraclinoid segment will also be present but the cervical segment will be absent. The routes by which the remaining segments of the ICA are reconstituted in cases of segmental dysgenesis are listed in Table 24-4.

In most cases of ICA dysgenesis, even bilateral dysgenesis, blood reaches the hemisphere ipsilateral to the dysgenetic ICA through the circle of Willis (Fig. 24-27). However, with an absent ICA and an incompetent circle of Willis, the next most common alternate route to reconstitute the anterior circulation is via the ophthalmic artery from the ECA system. This occurs anteriorly via craniofacial ECA branches to the ethmoidal, dorsal nasal, palpebral, supraorbital, and supratrochlear branches of the ophthalmic artery and posteriorly via the lacrimal branch of the ophthalmic artery.[90,121,154,176,229,241,257,279,362,370,440] A list of these branches is found in Table 24-5.

In addition to the anastomoses that involve the orbit, other routes that may be involved in the reconstitution of the intracranial ICA with an absent cervical segment involve branches of the maxillary artery. These are represented by anastomoses from the middle meningeal artery, the accessory meningeal artery, and the artery of the foramen rotundum to the inferior branch of the cavernous ICA, and from the artery of the pterygoid canal (vidian artery) to the petrous ICA.[9,10,33,51,105,106,121,123,163,176,229,237,257,271, 354,483,491] However, it is much more common to find these vessels recruited in cases of acquired ICA absence (e.g., atherosclerotic occlusion) or hig-flow states than in ICA dysgenesis (see below).

Table 24-4.   Persistent Embryonic Routes of Vascular Reconstitution in
Segmental Dysgenesis of Internal Carotid Artery

Segment of Adult ICA that Is Dysgenetic	Corresponding Dysgenetic Embryonic Artery	Segment of Adult ICA that Is Reconstituted	Persistent Embryonic Artery or Enlarged Branch Reconstituting Remaining Distal ICA Segment	Name of Corresponding "Persistent" Adult Vessel
Low cervical	?Proximal segment of aortic sac, ventral aorta, or aortic arch 3	Cervical	Cervical intersegmental artery	Persistent cervical intersegmental artery (from vertebral artery)
Cervical	Aortic sac, ventral aorta, aortic arch 3, dorsal aorta to level of primitive maxillary artery	Petrous	Stapedial or hyoid artery	Superior (anterior) or inferior tympanic to caroticotympanic artery (persistent stapedial artery) (from ECA)
			Mandibular artery	Vidian artery (from maxillary branch of ECA)
			Otic artery	Persistent primitive otic artery (from basilar artery)
Cervical + petrous	As above, plus dorsal aorta/ICA to level of foramen lacerum	Cavernous	Plexus around Rathke's pouch	Transsellar intracavernous intercarotid anastomosis, (? inferior hypophyseal, capsular or medial clival arteries) (from contralateral ICA)
			Trigeminal artery	Persistent primitive trigeminal artery (from basilar artery)
			Ascending pharyngeal artery	Foramen lacerum branch of ascending pharyngeal artery (from ECA)
Cervical + petrous + cavernous	As above plus dorsal aorta/ICA to level of anterior clinoid	Supraclinoid	Ophthalmic artery system, supraorbital division of stapedial artery	Ophthalmic artery via recurrent meningeal artery (from ECA)
		Caudal division of ICA		Posterior communicating artery (from basilar artery)

Abbreviations: ECA, external carotid artery; ICA, internal carotid artery.

Another ECA branch, the ascending pharyngeal artery, may also supply the intracranial ICA by several potential routes. Branches of the ascending pharyngeal artery may pass through the foramen lacerum or the foramen magnum to anastomose directly with the cavernous or paraclinoid ICA.[229,233,234,237,257,354,443,483] In addition, the inferior tympanic branch of the ascending pharyngeal artery may anastomose with the caroticotympanic branch of the petrous ICA in the middle ear (discussed above in the section on stapedial artery anomalies and shown in Fig. 24-24).

Other anastomoses that may become important in the supply of the brain lacking an ICA are persistent caroticobasilar and caroticovertebral anastomoses (e.g., persistent primitive trigeminal or hypoglossal arteries). These anomalies are more often found in

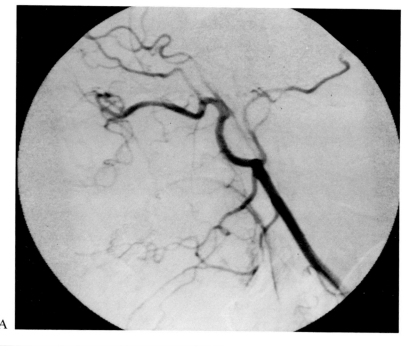

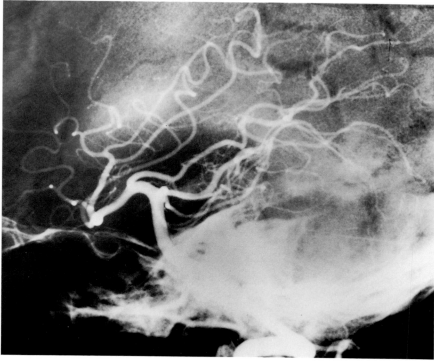

Figure 24-27. Angiograms demonstrating a case of dysgenesis of the ICA with reconstitution of the anterior circulation via the circle of Willis. This is homologous to the route of cerebral blood supply of some mammals that normally lack ICAs. **(A)** Left "common" carotid artery injection, lateral view. The ICA is absent. **(B)** Vertebral artery injection, lateral view. The left MCA fills from the posterior circulation via a large P_1 segment and posterior communicating artery. (The right MCA and both ACAs filled from the right ICA, and there was an aneurysm of the right ophthalmic artery.)

Table 24-5. Branching Patterns and Anastomoses of Ophthalmic and External Carotid Arteries

Artery/Branch	Foramen	Anastomoses	Usual Supply	Associated Nerves
Ophthalmic Artery System				
Lacrimal artery Zygomatic branch	Zygomaticotemporal foramen, zygomaticofacial foramen	Deep temporal branch of maxillary artery, Transverse facial and zygomaticoorbital branches of superior temporal artery	Lacrimal glands, lids, conjunctivae, cheek, zygoma	Lacrimal nerve
Recurrent meningeal branch (anterior meningeal artery)	Superior orbital fissure	Middle meningeal artery, artery of inferior cavernous sinus	Anterior fossa dura	
Supraorbital artery	Supraorbital foramen	Frontal branch of superior temporal artery, angular branch of facial artery	Ocular meninges, forehead, frontal sinus	Supraorbital nerve, frontal nerve
Posterior ethmoidal artery	Posterior ethmoidal canal	Sphenopalatine branch of maxillary artery, middle meningeal artery	Posterior ethmoidal air cells, anterior fossa dura	
Anterior ethmoidal artery	Anterior ethmoidal canal	Sphenopalatine branch of maxillary artery, middle meningeal artery	Anterior and middle ethmoidal air cells, frontal sinus, anterior fossa dura, lateral wall and dorsum of nose	Nasociliary nerve
Superior/inferior medial palpebral branches	Medial orbital rim	Zygomaticoorbital branch of superior temporal artery, angular branch of facial artery	Lids, nasolacrimal duct	
Supratrochlear artery	Medial orbital rim	Same as supraorbital artery	Forehead	Supratrochlear nerve
Dorsal nasal artery	Medial orbital rim	Angular and lateral branches of facial artery	Dorsum of nose	
External Carotid Artery System				
Ascending pharyngeal artery Inferior tympanic branch of ICA	Tympanic canaliculus	Caroticotympanic branch of petrous ICA	Medial wall of tympanic cavity, tympanic membrane	Tympanic branch of IX
Meningeal branches	Jugular foramen, foramen lacerum, anterior condyloid foramen, stylomastoid foramen	Meningohypophyseal and inferior branches of cavernous ICA, posterior meningeal branch of vertebral artery	Dura mater	Cranial nerves IX, X, XI, XII
Foramen lacerum branch	Foramen lacerum	Middle meningeal artery, inferior branch of cavernous ICA		
Prevertebral branches		Muscular branches of vertebral artery	Cervical muscles; sympathetic, vagus, and hypoglossal nerves	

(Continued)

Artery/Branch	Foramen	Anastomoses	Usual Supply	Associated Nerves
External Carotid Artery System				
Facial artery				
Lateral nasal branch	Medial orbital rim	Dorsal nasal branch of ophthalmic artery	Ala and dorsum of nose	
Angular branch	Medial orbital rim	Dorsal nasal branch of ophthalmic artery	Ala and dorsum of nose	
Occipital artery				
Mastoid branch	Stylomastoid foramen	Middle meningeal artery	Mastoid air cells, diploë, middle fossa dura	Cranial nerve VII
Meningeal branches	Jugular foramen, hypoglossal (condyloid) foramen	Middle meningeal artery	Posterior fossa dura	Cranial nerves IX, X, XI, XII
Occipital and muscular branches	Parietal foramen, foramen magnum	Middle meningeal artery, vertebral artery	Posterior fossa dura	
Superficial temporal artery				
Zygomaticoorbital branch	Zygomaticofacial foramen, medial orbital rim	Lacrimal and palpebral branches of ophthalmic artery	Orbicularis oris muscle	
Frontal branch	Superior orbital rim, supraorbital foramen	Supraorbital and supratrochlear branches of ophthalmic artery	Forehead	
Maxillary artery				
Anterior (superior) tympanic branch	Petrotympanic fissure	Caroticotympanic branch of ICA	Tympanic membrane	Cranial nerve IX
Middle meningeal artery	Foramen spinosum, (superior orbital fissure, foramina of greater sphenoidal wing)	Recurrent meningeal branch of lacrimal branch of ophthalmic artery, posterior meningeal branch of vertebral artery, inferior branch of cavernous ICA	Cranial nerve V ganglion, cranial nerve V and VII roots, middle fossa dura, tensor tympani muscle and canal	Sympathetic nerves, gasserion ganglion, cranial nerve VII roots
Accessory meningeal artery	Foramen ovale	Inferior branch of cavernous ICA	Facial muscles, V_3, cranial nerve V ganglion, middle fossa dura	V_3, gasserion ganglion
Artery of foramen rotundum	Foramen rotundum	Meningohypophyseal branch of cavernous ICA	V_3, middle fossa dura	V_3
Anterior deep temporal branch	Foramina of zygoma and greater sphenoid wing	Lacrimal branch of ophthalmic artery	Temporalis muscle	
Infraorbital artery, facial branch	Medial orbital rim	Dorsal nasal branch of ophthalmic artery	Anterior and medial face	V_2
Vidian artery (artery of pterygoid canal)	Pterygoid canal	Caroticotympanic branch of petrous ICA, Vidian branch of cavernous ICA	Auditory tube, sphenoid sinus, tympanic cavity	Greater petrosal nerve
Sphenopalatine branch	Anterior and posterior ethmoidal canals	Anterior and posterior ethmoidal branches of ophthalmic artery	Nasal cavity, ethmoidal, frontal, maxillary, sphenoid sinuses	V_2, sphenopalatine ganglion

Abbreviations: ICA, internal carotid artery; V_2, maxillary nerve; V_3, mandibular nerve.

the presence of congenital vertebral or basilar artery hypoplasia, with blood flow from the anterior to the posterior circulation, but the reverse flow may also occur. These anomalies are discussed below. Finally, a perisellar or transsellar intracavernous intercarotid anastomosis may reconstitute the cavernous segment of the ICA when the petrous and cervical segments are congenitally absent.[114,117,186,195,257,351,409,414,456] (Fig. 24-28).

It should be noted that the vessels supplying the brain in the absence of the ICA, whether arising from the ECA, contralateral ICA, or vertebrobasilar ar-

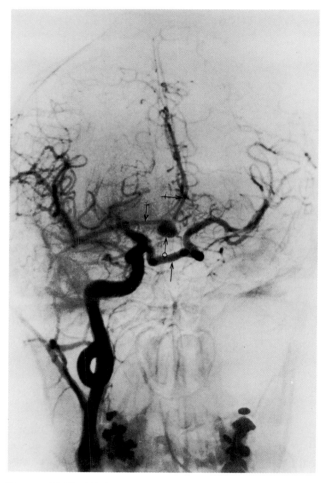

Figure 24-28. Right common carotid arteriogram, AP view, demonstrating filling of the left ICA via a large intercarotid, intracavernous, transsellar anastomosis (*arrow*). This anomaly may represent enlargement of an embryonic channel around Rathke's pouch or enlargement of inferior hypophyseal or capsular arteries. A similar large vessel is present in horses, and smaller examples may be found in carnivores. *Crossed arrows,* filling of both A$_2$ segments from right A$_1$ segment; *arrows with circle,* anterior communicating artery aneurysm. (From Huber,[186] with permission.)

tery systems, may themselves produce emboli to the nervous system.[26,51,121,154,229,307,309] These phenomena have obvious implications for complication avoidance during surgical and angiographic procedures.

Ontogeny. The cause of ICA dysgenesis is unknown. However, there may normally be asymmetry of the diameter of the ICAs of the two sides, especially when a segment of the circle of Willis is hypoplastic and one ICA supplies a greater proportion of the brain than the other.[250]

The ontogenetic basis for the reconstitution of the anterior circulation in cases of ICA dysgenesis represents a fundamental principle of cerebrovascular variation: If a given arterial system is small or absent, its usual territory will be supplied by an adjacent and/or anastomotic system. Thus, if a segment of the ICA is dysgenetic, embryonic anastomoses that may normally regress must remain patent to furnish blood to the remaining segments. These anastomoses, as described above, include branches of the ECA, ophthalmic artery, and contralateral ICA systems (cf. Table 24-5). In addition, the vertebrobasilar system may furnish blood via the circle of Willis.

Some of the persistent embryonic anastomoses involved in the reconstitution of the anterior circulation in cases of ICA dysgenesis are known from embryonic investigations. These include (1) anastomoses between the anterior or recurrent branch of the middle meningeal artery and the lacrimal branch of the ophthalmic artery; (2) anastomoses of craniofacial branches of the external carotid artery with the ophthalmic artery via the orbit; (3) anastomoses of the vidian branch of the maxillary artery via the pterygoid canal; and (4) primitive caroticobasilar and caroticovertebral anastomoses. In addition, the transsellar intracavernous intercarotid anastomoses may represent persistence of embryonic channels around Rathke's pouch, as described by Padget.[328] However, other anastomoses, not specifically described in ontogenetic studies, are presumed from adult human anatomy or from comparative anatomy. These include anastomoses between (1) the inferior branch of the cavernous ICA and the maxillary artery (middle meningeal, recurrent meningeal, accessory meningeal, and foramen rotundum branches) and (2) the inferior branch of the cavernous ICA and the ascending pharyngeal artery (inferior tympanic, foramen lacerum, and clival branches). In addition, it is thought that the transsellar intracavernous intercarotid anastomoses may represent hypertrophied inferior hypophyseal or capsular arteries, which are known to anastomose the ICAs of the two sides in the adult. However the ontogeny of the cavernous branches of the ICA is unknown.[338]

Phylogeny. The phylogenetic significance of the anomalous routes of supply to the brain in the absence of the ICA is that they are homologous with the normal anatomy of many mammals. These include carnivores (e.g., cats[59,93,104,144,199] and dogs[59,96,97,104,123,125,144]), perissodactyls (odd-toed ungulates, e.g., horses and rhinoceroses[104,110,143]), artiodactyls (even-toed ungulates, e.g., pigs, sheep, and bovids[104,123,125,141,143]), and primitive primates.[6,58,80,104] Interestingly, in bovids, sheep, and elephants (and probably all the species discussed here), the extracranial ICA is present in the fetus but absent in the adult.[110,143]

In the above species the extracranial ICA is small or absent, but the intracranial ICA is present. The intracranial ICA becomes "reconstituted" by branches of the ECA (e.g., the maxillary and ascending pharyngeal arteries) and then passes through the cavernous sinus to supply the circle of Willis, or the anterior circulation may be supplied entirely from the posterior circulation via the circle of Willis. The human homologies of these arteries may be surmised from the foramina through which they pass in the particular animal. Table 24-6 lists these arteries and their presumed human homologies.

Acquired Internal Carotid Absence and High-Flow States. As already noted, acquired forms of common carotid or ICA absence (e.g., from atherosclerotic, angiographic, or surgical occlusion) are similar to the congenital forms insofar as the same potential collateral routes of supply to the ICA are involved.[24,26,121,127,154,176,229,257,271,294,307,330,354,362,387,410,440] Generally, however, in cases of dysgenesis one main vessel carries the bulk of the flow, while in acquired absence and high-flow states numerous small vessels usually share the task via several different routes. If a great number of small vessels are involved, the angiographic appearance is sometimes referred to as a rete mirabile, owing to its superficial resemblance to that structure in some animals[90,121,257,472]

As in ICA dysgenesis, vessels supplying the brain in acquired ICA absence and high-flow states may produce nervous system emboli. Moreover, vascular steal syndromes may occur in this setting.[26,51,66,121,154,229,307,309]

Persistent Caroticobasilar and Caroticovertebral Anastomoses

Persistent caroticobasilar and caroticovertebral anastomoses are some of the most commonly reported cerebrovascular anomalies. They include persistent cervical intersegmental, proatlantal intersegmental, primitive hypoglossal, primitive otic, and primitive trigeminal arteries. Lie[257] reviewed much of the literature of these anomalies (Fig. 24-29).

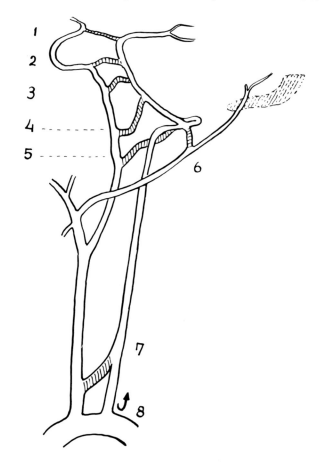

Figure 24-29. Persistent fetal caroticobasilar and caroticovertebral anastomoses. Semischematic diagram of normal and anomalous anastomoses between the carotid and vertebrobasilar arterial systems. (*1*) Posterior communicating artery; (*2*) persistent primitive trigeminal artery; (*3*) persistent primitive otic artery; (*4*) persistent primitive hypoglossal artery; (*5*) persistent proatlantal intersegmental artery; (*6*) occipital artery to vertebral artery anastomosis via muscular branch at C1; (*7*) persistent cervical intersegmental artery; (*8*) aortic arch. (From Lie,[257] with permission.)

Caroticobasilar and caroticovertebral anastomoses persist when their patency is required for the maintenance of blood supply to a portion of the cerebral circulation. For example, most of those that persist are found in the setting of unilateral or bilateral vertebral artery hypoplasia or basilar artery hypoplasia, with hypoplasia of the posterior communicating arteries or P_1 segments as well.[44,357,439,454] There may, rarely, be bilateral persistent embryonic arteries[41,203,439] or two different persistent embryonic arteries on the same side.[451] Most often the direction of blood flow in these persistent embryonic anastomoses is from the carotid to the vertebrobasilar circulation. Occasionally however, this direction is re-

Table 24-6. Routes of Blood Supply to Intracranial Internal Carotid Artery in Mammals With Absent or Small Extracranial Internal Carotid Arteries and their Human Homologies

Order/Genus	Arterial Anatomy	Foramen	Human Arterial Homology
Carnivora			
Dog	MA → ICA	Rotundum-ovale	AMA, AFR → AICS
	MA → ICA*	SOF	RMA → AICS
	MMA → ICA*	Spinosum	MMA → AICS
	APA → ICA	Lacerum	APA → AICS
Cat	MA → rete → ICA	Rotundum	AFR → AICS
	MA → rete → ICA	Ovale	AMA → AICS
	MA → rete → ICA*	SOF	RMA → AICS
	OccA → APA → rete → ICA*	Lacerum	APA → AICS
Artiodactyla			
Pig	MA → rete → ICA	Rotundum	AFR → AICS
	MA → rete → ICA	Ovale	AMA → AICS
	MA → rete → ICA	SOF	RMA → AICS
	APA → ICA*	Lacerum	APA → AICS
Sheep	MA → rete → ICA	Rotundum	AFR → AICS
	MA → rete → ICA	Ovale	AMA → AICS
	MA → rete → ICA*	SOF	RMA → AICS
	APA → ICA	Lacerum	APA → AICS
	MMA → ICA*	Spinosum	MMA → AICS
Cow	MA → rete → ICA	Rotundum	AFR → AICS
	MA → rete → ICA	Ovale	AMA → AICS
	MA → rete → ICA*	SOF	RMA → AICS
	MMA → ICA	Spinosum	MMA → AICS
	OccA → rete → ICA*	ACF	?APA → ?PPHA/PPTA
Perissodactyla			
Equids	APA → ICA*	Lacerum	APA → AICS, MHT, or CTA
Tapirs Rhinoceroses	OccA → VA		
Primata			
Loris	APA → ICA*	Lacerum	APA → AICS, MHT, or CTA
Galigo			

Abbreviations: ACF, anterior condyloid foramen; AFR, artery of the foramen rotundum; AICS, artery of the inferior cavernous sinus; AMA, accessory meningeal artery; APA, ascending pharyngeal artery; CTA, caroticotympanic artery; ICA, internal carotid artery; MA, maxillary artery; MHT, meningohypophyseal trunk; MMA, middle meningeal artery; OccA, occipital artery; PPHA, persistent primitive hypoglossal artery; PPTA, persistent primitive trigeminal artery; rete, rete mirabile; RMA recurrent (anterior) meningeal artery; SOF, superior orbital fissure; VA, vertebral artery; *, dominant supply route to intracranial ICA.

versed in ICA dysgenesis.[212,256,319,427] Furthermore, carotid to vertebrobasilar flow may reverse direction in the setting of acquired absence of the ICA.[238,256]

Persistent embryonic caroticobasilar anastomoses are usually asymptomatic, and are found incidentally at angiography or autopsy, although they are frequently associated with aneurysms. Rarely they may cause symptoms, which include facial and pharyngeal pain syndromes,[207,289,305] hemifacial spasm,[207] diplopia,[289] and posterior circulation ischemia second-

ary to carotid atherosclerosis.[149,333,346,350,418,423,473] This latter phenomenon has obvious implications for complication avoidance during carotid endarterectomy, angiography, and other procedures that involve the ICAs. However, it may be possible to occlude a persistent embryonic caroticobasilar or caroticovertebral anastomosis with no ill effects.[95]

Phylogeny. The phylogeny of persistent embryonic caroticobasilar and caroticovertebral anastomoses is obscure, since no adult vertebrate is known to possess them normally. Their presence in the embryos of some mammalian species has been observed, however, including the rabbit,[104] the pig,[373] and the rat.[298] In addition, de La Torre et al.[97] have noted the presence of a persistent primitive trigeminal artery in one adult dog that they studied. The comparative embryology of submammalian vertebrates might be useful in the further delineation of the origins of the embryonic caroticobasilar and caroticovertebral anastomoses.

Persistent Cervical Intersegmental Artery

Anatomy. The persistent cervical intersegmental artery is a caroticovertebral anastomosis in the neck (Fig. 24-30). It is most commonly represented

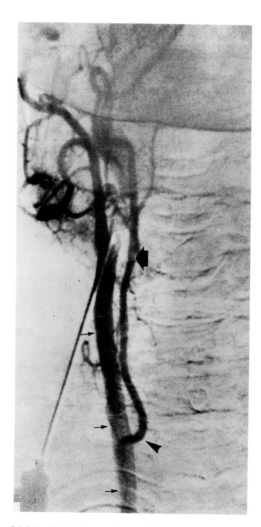

Figure 24-30. Right internal carotid arteriogram, AP view, demonstrating a persistent cervical intersegmental artery (*arrowhead*). This is most often represented by the common carotid artery (*small arrows*) origin of the vertebral artery (*large arrow*). (From Bernardi and Dettori,[37] with permission.)

by the vertebral artery arising from the internal or common carotid artery or from the aortic arch.[14,37,205,257,331,337] The identification of a persistent cervical intersegmental artery is strengthened by the demonstration of the anomalous vessel passing through the foramen transversarium of a cervical vertebra.[257]

Ontogeny. A cervical intersegmental artery in the adult represents persistence of one of the embryonic cervical intersegmental arteries. Normally the ventral (carotid) ends of these vessels regress while their dorsal (vertebral) ends anastomose, thus forming the vertebral artery.[78,328] The segment of the vertebral artery proximal to a persistent cervical intersegmental artery is generally absent, which results in the ICA origin of the vertebral artery. Indeed, the hypoplasia of the lower vertebral segment is presumably the reason for the persistence of the embryonic anastomosis.

Persistent Proatlantal Intersegmental Artery

Anatomy. The persistent proatlantal intersegmental artery is a rare but well described anomaly[14,44,187,228,229,249,257,264,328,329,332,355,425,439,454] (Fig. 24-31). Its angiographic differentiation from the persistent primitive hypoglossal artery has been clearly described.[14,187,257] The artery usually originates from the cervical ICA at a level between the bodies of the second and fifth (usually second or third) cervical vertebrae. It then ascends in the neck anterior to the cervical transverse processes, curving posteriorly just superior to the atlas. The persistent proatlantal intersegmental artery usually runs lateral to the ICA. The vessel then takes a horizontal course over the transverse process of the atlas, which is identical to the normal course of the horizontal segment of the vertebral artery. It then enters the skull through the foramen magnum to become the basilar artery. A persistent proatlantal intersegmental artery may be more common on the right side.[332]

It would perhaps be most accurate to describe the proatlantal intersegmental artery as only that segment of the artery that arises from the ICA and runs to the point beyond which its course is indistinguishable from that of the normal vertebral artery. The demonstration of the PICA or anterior spinal artery branching from the intracranial segment of the vessel, as in the case reported by Tanaka et al.,[439] supports this view.

Occasionally a so-called persistent proatlantal intersegmental artery arises from the ECA. However this probably simply represents enlargement of an anastomosis between muscular branches of the occipital and vertebral arteries at C1 or C2, with agene-

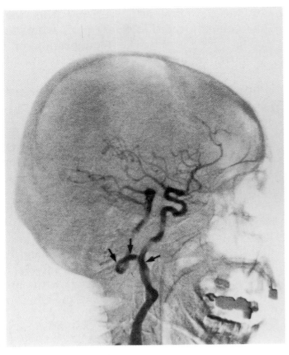
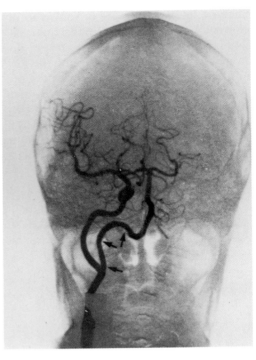

A   B

Figure 24-31. Right common carotid arteriogram demonstrating persistent proatlantal intersegmental artery (*arrows*). The artery takes a horizontal course over the transverse process of the atlas, identical to the normal course of the horizontal portion of the vertebral artery, and enters the skull through the foramen magnum to become the basilar artery. **(A)** Lateral view. **(B)** AP view. (From Tsukamoto et al.,[454] with permission.)

sis of the cervical vertebral artery inferior to the anastomosis (see Fig. 24-33).

The cases described by Teal et al.[447] and Kwak et al.[227] of a PICA and a posterior meningeal artery arising from the high cervical ICA probably represent proatlantal intersegmental arteries ending directly as branches of the vertebral artery. These are similar to the vertebral artery itself ending as a PICA.

Ontogeny. The proatlantal intersegmental artery is the most cranial of seven cervical intersegmental arteries found in very early embryos. The carotid end of this artery, like those of the lower six, normally dwindles as the vertebral artery is formed. However, the proatlantal intersegmental artery normally persists somewhat longer in development than either the other cervical intersegmental arteries or the other embryonic caroticobasilar and caroticovertebral anastomoses, and for a time it apparently supplies significant blood flow to the embryonic basilar artery primordia.[78,297,298,328] Eventually, the carotid end of the proatlantal intersegmental artery does regress, but the greater part of this artery persists as the horizontal segment of the vertebral artery. If the carotid end of the proatlantal intersegmental artery does not regress, the adult anomaly results. The proatlantal intersegmental artery shares a close functional rela-

tionship with the vertebral, occipital arteries, and primitive hypoglossal arteries, as discussed below.

Persistent Primitive Hypoglossal Artery

Anatomy. Cases of the persistent primitive hypoglossal artery have been reported by numerous authors[7,14,19,48,68,94,121,135,149,203,213,257,280,306,310,345,346,357, 397,411,418,423,468,474,493] (Fig. 24-32). Literature reviews have been published by Lie[257] and Resche et al.,[357] and angiographic diagnostic criteria have been outlined by Lie,[257] Anderson and Sondheimer,[14] and Brismar.[48]

The persistent primitive hypoglossal artery arises from the ICA at a level between the first and fourth cervical vertebrae, usually between the first and second. Thus, it usually arises somewhat higher than the persistent proatlantal intersegmental artery. The vessel then ascends with some tortuosity to enter the skull via the hypoglossal canal (anterior condyloid foramen). Intracranially the anomalous artery can be said to become the basilar artery. The persistent primitive hypoglossal artery may unite intracranially with the (usually hypoplastic) vertebral artery from the opposite side and may occasionally be joined by a hypoplastic vertebral artery ipsilaterally as well. The artery widens the hypoglossal canal, as noted by CT and plain tomography.[149,397]

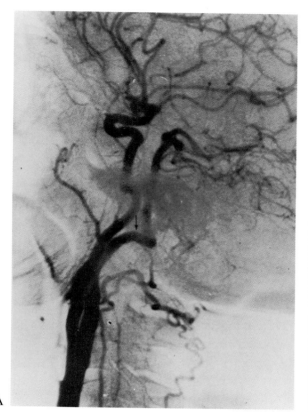
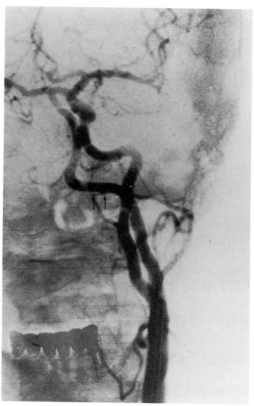

A

B

Figure 24-32. Left common carotid arteriogram demonstrating persistent primitive hypoglossal artery (*arrows*). The artery enters the skull via the anterior condyloid (hypoglossal) foramen to become the basilar artery. **(A)** Lateral view. **(B)** AP view. (From Stern et al.,[418] with permission.)

Lie presented four criteria necessary for the angiographic diagnosis of the persistent primitive hypoglossal artery: the artery is a large branch of the cervical ICA arising opposite the first to third cervical vertebrae; it enters the posterior fossa via the hypoglossal canal; the basilar artery fills only distal to it; and the posterior communicating arteries are absent. However, as has been shown by Brismar,[48] these criteria are not always fulfilled. To diagnose a persistent primitive hypoglossal artery, it is probably sufficient to demonstrate a prominent, anomalous vessel that arises from the ICA and enters the posterior fossa via the hypoglossal canal to supply the vertebrobasilar system.

Ontogeny. The persistent primitive hypoglossal artery represents the most inferior of several embryonic, caroticobasilar, intersegmental arteries of the occipital somites that normally involute very early in ontogeny. Morris and Moffat[306] pointed out that in some cases the persistent primitive hypoglossal artery may actually anastomose with the primitive lateral basilovertebral anastomosis (the primordia of the PICA and AICA) rather than with the vertebral or basilar artery directly.

Anatomical Relationship of the Proatlantal Intersegmental, Hypoglossal, Occipital, and Vertebral Arteries. A relationship exists between the proatlantal intersegmental, occipital, and vertebral arteries, as evidenced by their combined involvements in various vascular anomalies (Fig. 24-33). Many of these anomalies involve a normally present but small anastomosis between the cervical segment of the occipital artery and a muscular branch of the vertebral artery at C1 or C2. These anastomoses are best known from their demonstration in the setting of vertebral artery stenosis or occlusion when they become dilated in the development of collateral flow to the brain[121,320,387,410,440] (see Fig. 24-35).

Often a given anomaly is discussed in the literature with use of various nomenclatures. However, all these vascular anomalies are variations of the same arterial systems. They include

1. Vertebral artery origin of the occipital artery[228,229,240,294,315] (Fig. 24-33B)

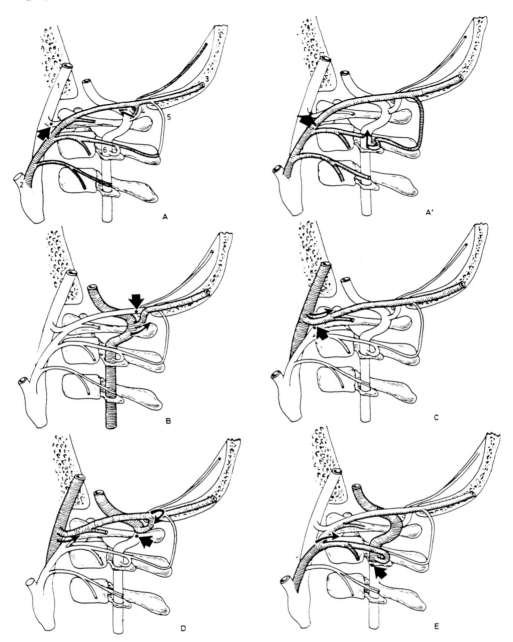

Figure 24-33. Diagrams demonstrating variations involving the ICA, ECA, vertebral artery, occipital artery, and persistent proatlantal intersegmental artery. View of left lateral aspect of craniocervical junction. Often the same anomaly is described in the literature with various nomenclatures. However, it can be seen that all these vascular anomalies are variations of the same arterial systems. Note that some of these human anomalies are homologous with the normal anatomy of other mammals. **(A&A′)** Normal anatomy. The occipital artery, a branch of the ECA, anastomoses with muscular branches of the vertebral artery superior to the transverse process foramina of C1 and C2. **(B)** The occipital artery is a branch of the vertebral artery at C1. **(C)** The occipital artery is a branch of the ICA. **(D)** The occipital artery arises from the persistent proatlantal intersegmental artery. **(E)** So-called ECA origin of the vertebral artery or ECA origin of the persistent proatlantal intersegmental artery (see Fig. 24-29). Large arrows with dots, point of embryonic arterial regression; small arrows, persistent or enlarged embryonic anastomoses. (*1*) ICA; (*2*) ECA; (*3*) occipital artery; (*4*) anastomosis between occipital artery and muscular branches of vertebral artery at C1; (*5*) portion of posterior cervical muscular supply shared by occipital artery and vertebral artery at C1; (*6*) anastomosis between occipital artery and muscular branch of vertebral artery at C2. (From Lasjaunias et al.,[240] with permission.)

2. ICA origin of the occipital artery[228,229,240,317,447] (Fig. 24-33C)
3. Occipital artery origin of the persistent proatlantal intersegmental artery[228,229,240,264,453] and persistent proatlantal intersegmental artery origin of the occipital artery[14,228,229,240,249,425] (Fig. 24-33D)
4. ECA origin of the vertebral artery[124,158,228,229,240] and persistent proatlantal intersegmental artery arising from the external carotid artery[14,228,229,240,249,315,355,380] §§ or from the carotid bifurcation[332] (Fig. 24-33E)

The hypoglossal artery also communicates with the carotid, vertebral, and occipital arterial systems, as evidenced by the following anomalies. Suzuki et al.[425] reported an anomaly in which a persistent proatlantal intersegmental artery and a persistent primitive hypoglossal artery arose from a common trunk, apparently a branch of the cervical ICA. Moreover, the occipital artery arose from the persistent proatlantal intersegmental artery. Furthermore, Morris and Moffat[306] described an anomaly in which a persistent primitive hypoglossal artery gave rise to the occipital artery. Finally, the ascending pharyngeal artery, which often shares a common trunk with the occipital artery, normally supplies a meningeal branch to the posterior fossa via the hypoglossal canal.[229,240]

Ontogeny and Phylogeny in Relation to the Persistent Proatlantal Intersegmental, Occipital, Hypoglossal, and Vertebral Arteries. Neither the ontogeny nor the phylogeny of the occipital artery nor its relationship with the persistent proatlantal intersegmental, persistent primitive hypoglossal, or vertebral artery has been extensively studied. Adams[6] studied the occipital artery and its relationship to the carotid arteries in birds and reptiles (these species do not possess vertebral arteries, which are found only in mammals). He hypothesized hat the mammalian occipital artery is homologous with the ventral subclavian artery of birds and reptiles (a branch of the ICA). Lasjaunias et al.[240] offered an analysis of the ontogeny of the occipital artery based mainly on their adult human arteriographic experience. They hypothesized that the occipital artery represents segments of the proatlantal and first cervical intersegmental arteries, initially originating from the ICA and secondarily annexed by the ECA. However, a better understanding of the variations of these arteries will require a phylogenetic and ontogenetic study of their relationships, particularly during the stages of formation and vascularization of the occipital and cervical somites.

The comparative anatomy of the carotid, vertebral, and occipital arteries has been described for several mammalian species, further indicating a relationship between these arterial systems. For example, in the domestic cat the occipital artery is prominent but does not supply any intracranial structures.[144] However in the dog, another carnivore, the inferior branch of the occipital artery anastomoses with the ipsilateral vertebral artery to form the cerebrospinal artery. The cerebrospinal arteries of each side in turn unite to supply the basilar and anterior spinal arteries.[15,144] In the horse the vertebral arteries are major suppliers of the brain and are almost exclusively supplied by the occipital arteries, while the cervical segments of the vertebral arteries are very small.[109,143] In the pig the vertebral arteries do not enter the head at all but end as the occipital arteries to supply the scalp.[143] In the sheep small branches of the vertebral arteries supply some of the blood to the brain, but most of vertebral artery flow is to the occipital arteries. In cattle small vertebral arteries supplement the occipital arteries, which are the dominant supplier of the brain via a rete mirabile.[123,143] Moreover, the occipital arteries in bovids enter the skull via the hypoglossal canals.

Persistent Primitive Otic Artery. The persistent primitive otic artery is the rarest of the persistent embryonic caroticobasilar and caroticovertebral anastomoses. Only one possible case had ever been reported when Lie[257] reviewed these anomalies in 1968. Since then there have been other reports.[107,203,451,487] The persistent primitive otic artery arises from the petrous ICA in the carotid canal, enters the intracranial cavity via the internal auditory meatus, and anastomoses with the basilar artery.

Because of the rarity of these reports and the lack of certainty regarding the identification of persistent primitive otic arteries reported, Lasjaunias and Berenstein[230] have expressed doubt as to the existence of this vessel at all, stating that the reported cases probably represent variations of persistent primitive trigeminal arteries.

Persistent Primitive Trigeminal Artery
Anatomy. The most common of the persistent embryonic caroticobasilar and caroticovertebral anastomoses that have been reported is the persistent primitive trigeminal artery (Fig. 24-34). Many hundreds of reports can be found in the literature.[7,32,34,41,53,72,76,95,107,120,128,134,156,174,180,181,192,196,203,207,211,223,226,229,230,256,257,281,289,301,305,319,328,333,338,345,350,379,380,389,392,418,427,439,440,442,451,457,473,486–488,492] Lie[257] estimates that this anomaly is found once in every 500 to 1,000 angiograms.

The anatomy of the persistent primitive trigeminal

---

§§ The case reported by Samra et al.[380] is probably that of a persistent proatlantal intersegmental, not a persistent primitive hypoglossal artery as they stated.

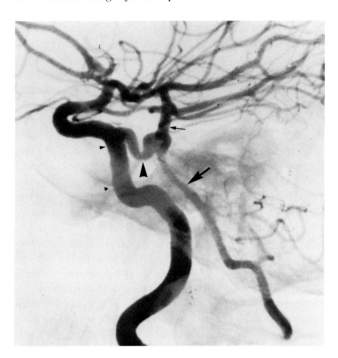

Figure 24-34. Internal carotid arteriogram (*small arrowheads*), lateral view, demonstrating persistent primitive trigeminal artery (*arrowhead*). Note that the vertebral artery (*large arrow*) is relatively hypoplastic as compared to the basilar artery (*small arrow*). The persistent primitive trigeminal artery is the largest of the embryonic caroticobasilar anastomoses and persists for the longest time in ontogeny.

artery has been described by several authors,[257,338,389] This artery arises from the proximal segment of the cavernous ICA[338] and either penetrates the dorsolateral aspect of the sella trucica to emerge on the superior clivus or runs along the lateral aspect of the sella medial to the gasserian ganglion. The persistent primitive trigeminal artery anastomoses with the basilar artery between the superior cerebellar artery and the AICA to supply some or all of the posterior fossa, usually in the setting of basilar or bilateral vertebral artery hypoplasia. Rarely, a persistent primitive trigeminal artery anastomoses directly with a hemispheric branch of the superior cerebellar artery[223,442] or the AICA or PICA without anastomosing with the basilar artery.[34,72,76,107,174,192,392]

As discussed in the section on anomalies involving the embryonic stapedial artery, the ophthalmic or middle meningeal artery may, rarely, arise from the basilar artery. The origin of the anomalous vessel is between the superior cerebellar artery and the AICA. This is presumed to represent a persistent embryonic anastomosis between the embryonic trigeminal ar-

tery and the recurrent meningeal or middle meningeal artery.

Ontogeny. Of the embryonic caroticobasilar anastomoses, the trigeminal artery is the largest and persists for the longest time. It provides most of the blood to the basilar artery primordia prior to the development of the posterior communicating and vertebral arteries. Presumably, these facts account for the more frequent persistence of this artery as compared with other persistent embryonic caroticobasilar and caroticovertebral anastomoses.

Cases of a persistent primitive trigeminal artery supplying the cerebellar arteries directly presumably indicate an embryonic connection with the primitive basilovertebral anastomosis of Padget,[328] from which the hemispheric rami of the cerebellar arteries develop. This is analogous to the anastomosis between the primitive hypoglossal artery and the primitive basilovertebral anastomosis discussed by Morris and Moffat.[306]

Ophthalmic Artery

Anatomy

The ophthalmic artery is normally the first major branch of the supraclinoid ICA. Its origin is usually subdural.[177] The artery enters the optic canal, coursing into the orbit inferior to the optic nerve. Within the orbit the artery then makes a dorsolateral bend around the nerve to lie on the superior aspect of the nerve. A description of the detailed branching pattern of the ophthalmic artery is beyond the scope of this chapter, but such a description can be found in several standard anatomic texts[74,177,300] The branches of the ophthalmic artery are summarized in Table 24-5.

Many anomalies of the ophthalmic artery are discussed elsewhere in this chapter. These include cavernous ICA origin of the ophthalmic artery and supply of the cavernous ICA via the ophthalmic artery (sections on anomalies of the embryonic stapedial artery and absence of the ICA); middle meningeal artery origin of the ophthalmic artery and origin of middle meningeal artery from ophthalmic artery (section on anomalies involving the embryonic stapedial artery); and basilar artery origin of the ophthalmic artery (section on persistent stapedial artery).

Other reported anomalies of the ophthalmic artery origin include ACA origin[172,230] and posterior communicating artery origin.[123] Fisher's[123] case of posterior communicating artery origin of the ophthalmic artery was in the setting of ICA agenesis. Presumably the supraclinoid segment of the ICA was present, and the ophthalmic artery arose from it normally; this would appear as if it had arisen from the posterior communicating artery.

Ontogeny

The ontogeny of the ophthalmic artery is highly complex. The early embryonic blood supply to the optic cup comes from two transient branches of the ICA known as the ventral and dorsal ophthalmic arteries. Later, the embryonic stapedial artery, another ICA branch, contributes to the supply of the optic structures by its large superior division, which along with the dorsal and ventral ophthalmic arteries forms an arterial ring around the optic nerve. Soon, the ventromedial segment of the arterial ring, the stems of the ventral and dorsal ophthalmic arteries, and portions of the supraorbital division of the stapedial artery regress. As these regressions occur, the definitive stem of the ophthalmic artery develops by annexation of the branches of the other arteries. The definitive ophthalmic artery later migrates to the adult supraclinoid location.

Branches of the supraorbital division of the embryonic stapedial artery include the supraorbital, frontal, and anterior ethmoidal arteries, as well as (probably) the supratrochlear, dorsal nasal, palpebral, posterior ethmoidal, and zygomatic arteries. The central artery of the retina and the common temporal ciliary arteries are derived from the primitive dorsal ophthalmic artery, while the common nasal ciliary artery is derived from the primitive ventral ophthalmic artery. The lacrimal artery forms partly from the stapedial and partly from the definitive ophthalmic artery. When the supraorbital division of the stapedial artery regresses at the orbital margin, its branches persist, forming important potential anastomoses between the ECA and ICA systems via the ophthalmic artery.

The ACA origin of the ophthalmic artery is described by Lasjaunias and co-workers[230,483] as persistence of the embryonic ventral pharyngeal artery. Although from the diagrams of Padget,[328] it does appear that the ventral ophthalmic artery arises from the ACA, the complexity of the development of the ophthalmic system, with migration of the various ophthalmic stems, makes this ontogenetic homology far from certain. A demonstration of the primitive ventral ophthalmic artery coursing through the optic canal primordium would strengthen this hypothesis. However, the orbital and cranial foramina and fissures were not indicated in Padget's work.[328]

Phylogeny

The arterial supply to the orbital structures for several species of embryonic and adult submammals has been partially studied.[8,60–62,366] The details of the branching patterns, foramina of entry into the cranial cavity, and anastomoses with other arteries are lacking in these studies, which were primarily concerned with the arteries of the brain, so that the human homologies of these arteries are not entirely certain. Furthermore, the nomenclature used by different authors is not consistent. Nonetheless, the information available is sufficient to permit some deductions.

In fish a branch known as the orbital artery (homologue of the stapedial artery) arises from the dorsal aorta (ICA) at the level of the hyomandibular bone (evolutionary precursor of the stapes). This vessel supplies the extracranial structures of the head via supraorbital, infraorbital, and the mandibular branches. The supply to the eyeball is via a more distal branch of the ICA.

In reptilian embryos[60–62] the orbital artery, a prominent branch of the ICA at the level of the stapes that is probably homologous to the stapedial artery of higher vertebrates, supplies the posterolateral aspect of the primordial orbit. It shares in the supply of the developing eye structures with a branch of the anterior division of the ICA known as the anterior orbital artery. Later in development, the anterior orbital artery disappears, and the eye is supplied from a different vessel, the ophthalmic artery. The ophthalmic artery branches from the anterior division of the ICA more proximally than the earlier anterior orbital artery. The origin of the ophthalmic artery is just proximal to the lateral choroidal artery (homologue of the anterior choroidal artery).

Adult reptiles may or may not possess an ophthalmic artery (i.e., a branch of the ICA that supplies the eye via the optic canal).[8,60–62] In those species without one, the eye is apparently supplied by the orbital (stapedial) artery. Moreover, it appears that in several reptilian species the supply of the eye and orbit is shared by the ophthalmic and stapedial arteries.

In the dog the (internal) ophthalmic artery branches from the ACA.[96,97,144,197] It enters the orbit on the dorsomedial aspect of the optic nerve via the optic foramen and anastomoses within the orbit with the external ophthalmic artery, a branch of the maxillary artery. The maxillary artery in the dog is presumably derived from the stapedial artery, as in humans and other mammals. Gillilan[144] states that the external ophthalmic artery in the dog is homologous with the anterior or recurrent meningeal branch of the middle meningeal artery in humans. A demonstration of the artery coursing through the superior orbital fissure would strengthen this homology, although it is probably correct. Lasjaunias and co-workers[230,237,483] state that the internal ophthalmic artery in the dog is homologous with the primitive ventral ophthalmic artery of the human. However, as noted above, this is not certain.

Vertebrobasilar System

The anatomy and embryology of the human vertebrobasilar system has been described by many authors.[17,74,78,126,142,223,230,257,270,300,315,328,391,419,430,492] In addition, development of the vertebrobasilar system has been examined in the fetal rat by Moffat[296] and in the fetal rabbit by Gillilan.[142]

Vertebral Artery

Anatomy

The vertebral artery arises from the subclavian artery deep in the neck, and in approximately 90 percent of cases it enters the foramen transversarium of C6. In most other cases this artery enters the foramen transversarium of C5; less often it enters at C7 and least often at C4 or higher.[17,223,229,450] The vertebral artery then passes vertically upward through the transverse process foramina of the other cervical vertebrae. The vessel is accompanied by the vertebral venous plexus and sympathetic nerves. At the atlas the artery makes a characteristic horizontal bend to course posteromedially in a groove on the superior surface of the posterior arch. It then makes another characteristic superior bend as it passes through the posterior atlanto-occipital membrane. Krayenbuhl et al.[223] have stated that these bends are necessary for movements of the head, although this hypothesis has been disputed by Penning.[343] The vertebral artery enters the cranial cavity via the foramen magnum, where it becomes subarachnoid. The arteries of either side are asymmetric in more than 90 percent of cases, the left generally being larger than the right.[223,391,419] They join at the pontomesencephalic junction to become the basilar artery, although the level of their junction may be about 1 cm above or several centimeters below this point.[419]

Branches of the vertebral artery in the cervical region include muscular, meningeal and radicular. Muscular branches form anastomoses with several branches of the ECA (e.g., the ascending pharyngeal and occipital arteries), with the ascending and deep cervical arteries, and with muscular and radicular branches of the opposite vertebral artery. Along with other arteries of the neck, these anastomoses form important potential routes for collateral flow to the brain in cases of subclavian and vertebral artery occlusion and dysgenesis[17,121] (Fig. 24-35). Other branches of the vertebral artery include the PICAs (see below) and the anterior spinal arteries.

Ontogeny

The vertebral arteries form by enlargement of anastomoses between adjacent cervical intersegmental arteries, with regression of the carotid ends of these vessels. A more dorsal portion of the cervical intersegmental artery below anastomoses with a more ventral portion of the cervical intersegmental artery above, forming for a time a zigzag pattern of anastomoses. The sixth cervical intersegmental artery forms the stem of the subclavian and vertebral arteries. The highest cervical intersegmental artery, which courses between the atlas and the occiput and is called the proatlantal intersegmental artery, becomes the horizontal segment of the vertebral artery.

Phylogeny

The vertebral arteries are absent in all submammals but are present in even the most primitive mammals. The mammalian telencephalon and cerebellum, as compared with those of more primitive vertebrates, are enormous relative to the size of the rest of the brain. Furthermore, the evolutionary expansion of the telencephalon in early mammals is largely posterior over the brainstem and cerebellum. Blood supply to the posterior telencephalon was derived from expansion of the territories of the diencephalic and mesencephalic arteries, which were branches of the posterior division of the ICA and the basilar artery. The vertebral arteries presumably evolved to supplement the supply of the telencephalon and cerebellum.

Anomalies and Variants

The anomalies of the persistent cervical intersegmental artery, persistent proatlantal intersegmental artery, and persistent primitive hypoglossal artery are discussed above in the section on carotid artery anomalies.

Multiplication

Anatomy. Vertebral artery multiplication anomalies (i.e., fenestration and duplication) have been reported by numerous authors[67,162,167,169,171,221,222,229,231, 295,315,359,359,419,433,445,446,450,470,487,492] (Fig. 24-36). Lasjaunias and co-workers[229,231] have differentiated between vertebral artery *fenestrations*, in which the multiplied vessels remain inside the vertebral canal,

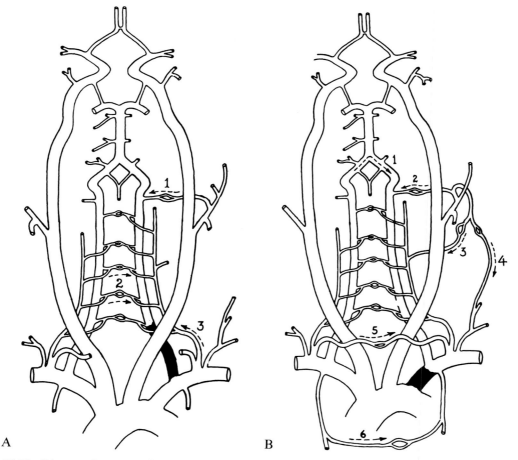

Figure 24-35. Diagram demonstrating some potential pathways for collateral flow to the brain in the setting of proximal vertebral artery or subclavian artery occlusion. The intraspinal anastomoses between the vertebral arteries probably are derived from cervical intersegmental arteries. **(A)** Vertebral artery occlusion. *(1)* Anastomosis between occipital and vertebral arteries; *(2)* intraspinal (radicular) vessels anastomosing with vertebral and ascending cervical arteries of both sides; *(3)* anastomosis between ascending cervical and vertebral arteries. **(B)** Subclavian artery occlusion. *(1)* Vertebral to vertebral artery anastomosis; *(2)* anastomosis between occipital and vertebral arteries; *(3)* anastomosis between thyrocervical trunk (ECA) and ascending cervical artery; *(4)* anastomoses between ECA and deep cervical (costocervical) arteries; *(5)* anastomosis between inferior thyroid arteries; *(6)* anastomosis between internal mammary arteries. (From Fields et al.,[121] with permission.)

and *duplication,* in which one of the vessels leaves the vertebral canal to enter the spinal canal at C1 or C2. Tokuda et al.[450] noted anomalies of the vertebral artery at C1 and C2 in 0.7 percent of vertebral angiograms, often associated with Klippel-Feil syndrome. They have advised caution in performing cervical punctures in view of the relatively high incidence of these vascular anomalies.

Ontogeny. The cervical intersegmental arteries that anastomose to produce the vertebral artery probably also form the vertebral radicular spinal arteries. These vessels enter the neural foramina at every cervical level to supply the intraspinal plexuses. The

duplicated, intraspinal vertebral segment may represent a radicular spinal artery entering the C1 or C2 neural foramen.[450]

Dysgenesis

Anatomy. The vertebral arteries are usually asymmetric. Unilateral hypoplasia (i.e., extreme narrowing of one vertebral artery) is less common,[32,126, 223,231,310,419,487] and complete agenesis is very rare.[492] Occasionally a small vertebral artery ends directly as the PICA.[32,306,492]

Hypoplasia of one vertebral artery and its branches may be compensated by anastomotic arterial systems at each level of the artery's course, in-

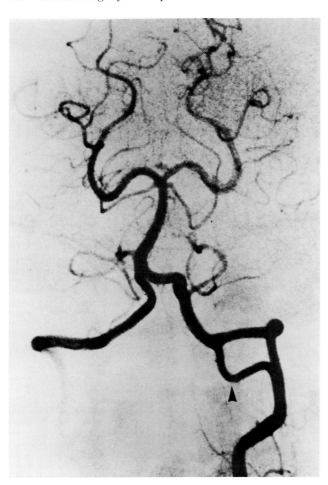

Figure 24-36. Left vertebral arteriogram, AP view, demonstrating fenestration or segmental duplication of the vertebral artery. The duplicated segment (*arrowhead*) may represent a segment of a persistent cervical intersegmental artery at C2. (From Kowada et al.,[222] with permission.)

cluding occipital, ascending pharyngeal, deep cervical, ascending cervical, and contralateral vertebral arteries in the neck and contralateral vertebral artery and ipsilateral AICA intracranially. In bilateral vertebral artery hypoplasia, the basilar artery most commonly fills via the circle of Willis from the anterior circulation. Filling of the posterior circulation by persistent embryonic caroticobasilar and caroticovertebral anastomoses is very rare, although conversely, the presence of persistent caroticobasilar and caroticovertebral anastomoses is almost always associated with unilateral or bilateral vertebral artery hypoplasia or basilar artery hypoplasia.

Phylogeny. As has already been reviewed, the cerebral circulation is supplied without vertebral arteries in all submammals. This is also the case with several

mammals. In other mammals vertebral arteries are minute. Most likely those mammals lacking vertebral arteries as adults possess them in fetal life but lose them secondarily by a process analogous to that of ICA regression in the bovids. Perhaps further study of these species would shed some light on the mechanisms of vertebral arterial dysgenesis and arterial dysgenesis in general.

Tortuosity. The vertebral artery may be tortuous in both children and adults[223] and may erode portions of the bony vertebrae.[22,27,81,108,132,188,260,323,388] The etiology of vertebral artery tortuosity is unknown. It is probably a result of the zigzag pattern that the vertebral artery assumes during its development.[328]

Basilar Artery

Anatomy

The basilar artery courses upward along the ventral pons, which it grooves. It begins inferiorly at the level of the pontomedullary junction and ends superiorly at the level of the interpeduncular fossa. It may terminate as much as 1 cm below or above the upper border of the pons.[419] At its superior end it divides to become the P_1 segments of the PCAs. Basilar artery tortuosity is normal with increasing age. Proximally the basilar artery is generally convex, curving away from the larger vertebral artery, and is often S-shaped. Major branches of the basilar artery include the anterior inferior and superior cerebellar arteries. In addition, the basilar artery supplies numerous smaller lateral pontine branches. One of these may be the labyrinthine or internal auditory artery to the inner ear, although this vessel may be a branch of the AICA, superior cerebellar artery, or PICA.[479] Finally, the basilar artery provides midline perforating arteries to the pons along its entire course, and the basilar tip (i.e., the most superior aspect) furnishes vessels to the posterior basal perforation zone (posterior perforated substance).

Ontogeny

The basilar artery develops from paired primordial plexuses, known as the bilateral longitudinal neural arteries, which course anteromedial to all the cranial nerve roots of the brainstem. At first these vessels are supplied almost exclusively by the embryonic trigeminal arteries. Later, posterior communicating arteries and other caroticovertebral and caroticobasilar anastomoses supply the basilar artery primordia. Finally, the vertebral arteries develop, the caroticovertebral and caroticobasilar anastomoses regress, and the bilateral longitudinal neural arteries unite to form a single basilar artery.

Phylogeny

A basilar artery is present in all vertebrates, although in all submammals and in several mammalian species it is supplied only from the anterior circulation, as previously discussed. In many species the basilar artery is fenestrated or duplicated for some or all of its length (see below) and may be tortuous, as in the dog.

Anomalies and Variants

Multiplication

Anatomy. The basilar artery appears to be the most common site of intracranial artery fenestration, called by some *segmental duplication*.[16,40,43,65,162,231,419,434,445,487] It is thought to occur in approximately 1 percent of the population and is found in 5 percent of all autopsies. The entire length of the basilar artery may be duplicated, but this is extremely rare.[492]

Basilar artery fenestration is most common in the proximal part of the artery, at the junction of the vertebral arteries.[65,231,434,445] In these cases the AICA or PICA may arise from the fenestration. These anomalies are usually clinically silent. However, there appears to be a high incidence of aneurysm formation at the proximal end of the fenestrated segment, probably due to a defect of the arterial wall[16,40,43,65] (Fig. 24-37). Furthermore, hemodynamic disturbance with turbulent flow in the fenestrated segment may result in basilar artery thrombosis.[40]

Ontogeny. As already discussed, the basilar artery develops from paired primordial vessels, the bilateral longitudinal neural arteries. Incomplete unification of these vessels provides the ontogenetic basis for fenestrations and duplications. It is presumably because of this unique ontogeny that the basilar artery is the most common site of arterial multiplication.

Phylogeny. The basilar arteries of the lamprey (a primitive jawless fish) and the ray (a type of shark) are paired for their entire length, and that of the dog-fish shark is paired for most of its length. The brains of embryonic reptiles reveal completely paired basilar arteries, which in some species persist into adulthood but in others fuse to form an unpaired vessel. In addition, the basilar artery has been observed to be fenestrated in numerous vertebrates, including monotremes, marsupials, horses, and cattle. Finally, the basilar artery of the black-faced spider monkey has been shown by Watts[476] to be paired throughout

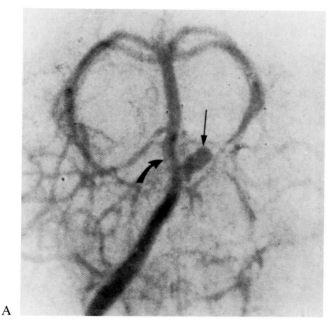
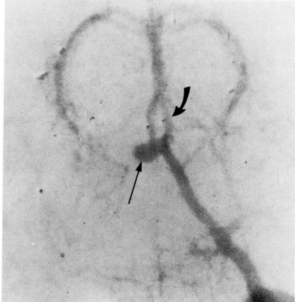

A B

Figure 24-37. The basilar artery is the most frequent site of intracranial arterial fenestration because the basilar artery forms by fusion of initially paired primordia. Usually these anomalies are asymptomatic, but aneurysm formation may occur at the proximal portion of the fenestration. **(A)** Right vertebral arteriogram, AP view, demonstrating an aneurysm (*straight arrow*) at the proximal end of a basilar artery fenestration (*curved arrow*). **(B)** Left vertebral arteriogram in same patient, AP view, demonstrating a second aneurysm (*straight arrow*) at the proximal end of the basilar artery fenestration (*curved arrow*). (From Campos et al.,[65] with permission.)

its entire length, the two vessels being joined at several points by transverse anastomoses. The basilar arteries of the rabbit,[104,141] pig,[373] and rat,[296,298] have been shown, like that of the human, to develop from paired primordia.

Dysgenesis. Hypoplasia of a short or long segment of the basilar artery has been reported rarely, and complete agenesis is extremely rare.[232,492] Perhaps this is because the potential circulatory alternatives are limited, which causes the embryo or fetus possessing such anatomy to be nonviable. In support of this idea, Szdzuy and Lehmann[428] have reported two cases of hypoplasia of the distal basilar artery combined with small vertebral arteries, both in young patients with symptoms of brainstem ischemia. These cases are extremely unusual in that the congenital vascular anomalies were causing ischemic symptoms primarily (i.e., without atherosclerosis, compression, thrombosis, etc.)

If a segment of the basilar artery is hypoplastic, the segment superior to the narrowing is most often supplied from the anterior circulation via the posterior communicating arteries, while the segment inferior to the narrowing is supplied by the vertebral arteries. These anomalies are not usually associated with persistent primitive caroticobasilar or caroticovertebral anastomoses, although the presence of such a persistent anastomosis is almost always associated with unilateral or bilateral vertebral artery or basilar artery hypoplasia.

The causes of basilar artery dysgenesis are not known. No known vertebrate lacks a basilar artery.

Cerebellar Arteries

The detailed gross and microsurgical anatomy of the cerebellar arteries has been described by many authors.[74,129,140,142,165,182,262,270,278,300,313,403,419,431,492]

Ontogeny

The superior cerebellar artery develops considerably earlier than and widely separated from the inferior cerebellar arteries. The latter develop from the lateral basilovertebral anastomosis. According to Padget[328] "wide variations in the origin and course of branches of the basilar and vertebral arteries . . . are explained chiefly by the late retention of different remnants of the lateral basilovertebral anastomosis." This observation provides the ontogenetic basis for the reciprocal variability of the AICA and PICA (Fig.

24-38). The earlier maturation of the superior cerebellar artery and its wide separation from the inferior cerebellar arteries is reflected in its more constant origin and distribution.

Phylogeny

The cerebella of fish, amphibians, reptiles, and even primitive mammals are supplied by a single pair of cerebellar arteries, which is probably most closely homologous with the human superior cerebellar artery. Marsupials and most nonprimate placental mammals possess two cerebellar artery pairs, which appear to be homologous with the superior cerebellar arteries and the AICAs or PICAs of higher primates. Higher primates possess three pairs of cerebellar arteries.

Posterior and Anterior Inferior Cerebellar Arteries

Anatomy. The PICA is the largest and usually the most distal branch of the vertebral artery. This vessel supplies the medulla oblongata, posteroinferior cerebellum, the majority of the choroid plexus of the fourth ventricle, and the posterior spinal cord via the posterior spinal arteries.

The AICA arises from the inferior or middle third of the basilar artery. Its main trunk runs in the cerebellopontine angle cistern. It furnishes blood to the rostrolateral medulla oblongata, caudolateral pons, anteroinferior cerebellum, and lateral portion of the choroid plexus of the fourth ventricle. In addition, it often supplies the inner ear via its internal auditory or labyrinthine branch. However, the internal auditory artery may arise independently from the basilar artery or from the superior cerebellar artery or the PICA.[479]

Anomalies and Variants. The exact site on the vertebral artery at which the PICA arises is variable. The origin may normally be anywhere from the proximal intracranial segment of the vertebral artery to its termination at the basilar artery. Occasionally the PICA may share a common trunk with the AICA at the point where the vertebral arteries join.[419] Rarely, the PICA arises from the vertebral artery extracranially; its extracranial origin at the level of the second or first cervical vertebra has been reported by several authors.[118,230,231,450,492] In these cases the anomalous PICA is said to enter the spinal canal at the level of

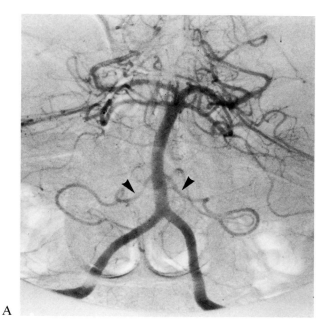

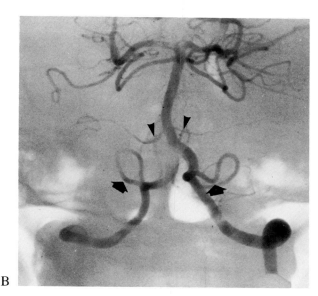

Figure 24-38. Angiograms demonstrating the reciprocal relationship between the ipsilateral AICA and PICA. This is a reflection of their development from the same embryonic plexus, the lateral basilovertebral anastomosis. **(A)** Vertebral arteriogram, AP view, demonstrating large AICAs (*arrowheads*) with absent PICAs. **(B)** Vertebral arteriogram, AP view, demonstrating large PICAs (*arrows*) and smaller AICAs (*arrowheads*) (cf. Fig. 24-17).

its origin, and there may be a duplicate PICA on the same side arising from the normal location. This anomaly appears to be similar to one type of vertebral artery duplication, discussed above, in which the duplicated vertebral artery segment at C1 or C2 courses into the spinal canal to reanastomose with the "normal" artery at the foramen magnum. The PICAs of the two sides may arise at similar or different points from their respective vertebral arteries.

The anomaly of a persistent primitive trigeminal or hypoglossal artery supplying the PICA directly without anastomosing with the basilar artery is discussed above in the section on persistent embryonic caroticobasilar and caroticovertebral anastomoses. The PICAs may occasionally be fenestrated or duplicated and may be absent entirely. The vertebral artery may occasionally end as the PICA without joining the basilar artery.

Like the PICA, the AICA may arise from its parent artery at variable locations, although in 95 percent of cases it arises from the lower or middle third of the basilar artery.[419] Occasionally the AICAs of either side arise from markedly different points along the basilar artery. The AICAs may, rarely, be duplicated or fenestrated, and may be absent entirely.

As noted above, the sizes and distributions of the hemispheric portions of the ipsilateral AICA and PICA are reciprocally related[71,129,140,142,214,262,270,278,313,419,431] (Fig. 24-38). This is so common that hypoplasia or absence of one AICA or PICA with reciprocal enlargement of the ipsilateral PICA or AICA, respectively, should probably be considered normal variance. Much less commonly, one AICA or PICA supplies the distribution of its contralateral counterpart, although there are anastomoses between the two PICAs and the two superior cerebellar arteries upon the vermis.[140,142] A markedly reciprocal relationship between the inferior (anterior or posterior) and superior cerebellar arteries does not exist.[165,182,230,419]

Superior Cerebellar Artery

Anatomy. The superior cerebellar artery origin is the most constant of the cerebellar artery origins; this artery arises from the superior end of the basilar artery, just proximal to the origins of the PCAs. The proximal segment of the artery courses within the perimesencephalic cistern and then branches to supply the superolateral pons, midbrain, and superior cerebellum. The superior cerebellar artery may fre-

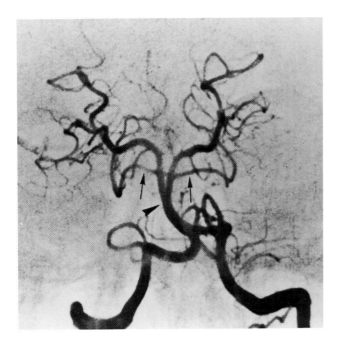

Figure 24-39. Vertebral arteriogram, AP view, demonstrating low bifurcation of the basilar artery (*arrowhead*) with superior cerebellar arteries arising from the P₁ segments (*arrows*) This most likely represents incomplete embryonic fusion of the paired basilar artery primordia. (From Krayenbuhl et al.,[223] with permission.)

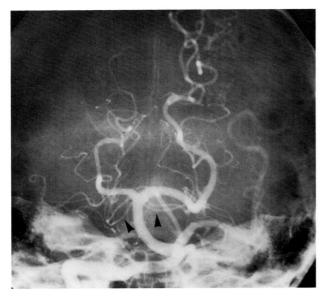

Figure 24-40. Vertebral arteriogram, AP view, demonstrating duplicated superior cerebellar arteries bilaterally (*arrowheads*). Multiplication anomalies are the result of artery formation from an embryonic plexus.

quently provide the origin for the internal auditory artery. The superior cerebellar artery anastomoses with branches of the PCA upon the midbrain and with the PICA upon the vermis.

Anomalies and Variants. As already noted, the superior cerebellar arteries are much less variable than the inferior cerebellar arteries both in their sites of origin from their parent artery and in their areas of distribution. Occasionally, the superior cerebellar artery may arise from the P₁ segment of the PCA; this is especially likely when the PCAs bifurcate from the basilar artery at a relatively low level, presumably owing to incomplete fusion of the paired embryonic basilar artery primordia (Fig. 24-39). Frequently, the superior cerebellar artery may be duplicated (Fig. 24-40), and rarely, it may be triplicated.[214] The origin of the superior cerebellar arteries from the P₁ segment of the PCA may be seen in several other mammals such as lagomorphs (rabbits), dogs, and marsupials.

Circle of Willis, Basal Perforating Arteries, and Cerebral Artery Stems

The circle of Willis has been studied by many authors.[104,137,155,204,244,245,292,327,349,360,419,487] The literature on the gross and microsurgical anatomy of these arteries and especially their perforating branches is enormous owing to their implication in the pathophysiology of adult and neonatal intracerebral hemorrhage and subcortical infarction[5,20,21,25,73,98–103,224, 282,299,314,334,365,437,438,461,481,497] and also to their involvement in aneurysms of the circle of Willis.[204,327] An understanding of their anatomy is essential for the avoidance of complications during aneurysm surgery.

Circle of Willis

Anatomy

Padget[327] proposed a classification scheme for description of the normal circle of Willis: the ACA is one-half the size of the internal carotid artery; the anterior communicating artery is one-half to two-thirds the size of the ACA; the posterior communicating artery is one-half the size of the PCA; and the PCA is one-half the size of the basilar artery. The frequency of "normal" circles of Willis in cadaver studies ranges from 20 to 50 percent[327,360] with variations from the normal approximately twice as common in cases with aneurysms[327] (Fig. 24-41). Up to 85 percent of cerebral aneurysms are found on those arteries that are the most variable.[137,204,327] Overall, 75 percent of circles of Willis show one, two, or three communicating arteries to be hypoplastic or show asymmetry of the ACA or PCA segments.[292] Wollschlaeger and Wollschlaeger[487] have suggested that knowledge of the variations of the circle of Willis may help to distinguish between hypoplasia and spasm on angiograms. However, the circle of Willis shows such frequent variability and is so often asymmetric that this distinction may still be difficult.

Ontogeny

A completed basal arterial circle forms very early in ontogeny. In the embryo and early fetus the calibers of the vessels of the circle of Willis are generally equal. However, in the later fetus and adult they are highly variable.[155,214,244,245,292,487] The circle of Willis in the 20- to 40-week fetus already shows asymmetry more commonly than symmetry.[292]

Phylogeny

De Vriese[104] thoroughly reviewed the comparative anatomy of the basal arterial circles of other vertebrates (Fig. 24-42). All vertebrates possess arterial anastomoses that link the ICAs of both sides. However the ''circle'' is incomplete or open anteriorly in many submammals inasmuch as there is no anterior communicating artery in some fish, amphibians, birds, and reptiles. Nonetheless, some reptiles do possess a complete basal arterial circle.[60–62,138] In submammals the brain is supplied exclusively by ICAs, whereas all mammalian species possess vertebral arteries at some time in their development. It is worth noting that the basal arterial circle of snakes and birds may be markedly asymmetric.[138] It appears that the basal arterial circle of all mammals is complete or closed, although the anterior portion (i.e., the region of the human anterior communicating artery) may be very small or plexiform as in cats[93,144,199] and cattle.[143] The most common form of the circle of Willis in mammals is one in which the ACA is fused or azygous[104,141,143,144,254,476] (Fig. 24-43; cf. Fig. 24-47).

Inferences

The causes of circle of Willis variability are unknown. As stated by Lazorthes et al.,[245] the variations seem to have no meaningful pattern. Most authors reporting on the circle of Willis do not address this issue. De Vriese[104] noted the variability but thought that it must have been an artifact of her injec-tion procedure. Guérin et al.[155] and Lazorthes and co-workers[244,245] hypothesized that variations arise from adptation to head movement in the fetus and adult, with differential compressions of various elements of the circle. However, the evidence supporting this hypothesis is not clear.

Phylogenetically, a group of arterial anastomoses at the base of the brain, often forming a complete loop (''circle''), is very old. It would therefore seem that this structure is somehow significant, perhaps endowing an evolutionary advantage to the species possessing it. Presumably a species possessing an anastomotic arterial circle supplying the brain could survive longer (i.e., to reproductive age) despite an occlusion of some portion of the circle or of one of the arteries supplying it. The factors governing the preservation of a basal arterial circle throughout phylogeny would be inherited (i.e., genetically based).

However, development of the vasculature of the individual organism is characterized by constant adjustments in the routes of blood flow. Some vascular channels are produced that eventually become superfluous, while others become more important as the brain develops and changes its morphology. Any vessels not required for the relatively direct transport of blood to a given structure tend to regress or disappear. Presumably the factors that modify developing arteries in this way are humoral, produced by endothelium or other vascular cells in response to pressure, flow, or pulsation.

The balance between these apparently opposing phylogenetic and ontogenetic factors would be expected to result in variability of the size of any artery that is important for an evolutionarily significant anastomosis (for the species) but yet is not directly required for the flow of blood to the brain (in the individual). The arteries of the circle of Willis clearly fit these criteria.

Basal Perforating Arteries

Anatomy

Territories of Supply. The basal perforation zone includes the anterior perforated substance, limen insulae, inferior portion of the choroidal fissure, and posterior perforated substance. The basal perforating arteries supply the basal ganglia, internal capsule, external capsule, claustrum, extreme capsule, hypothalamus, chiasm, infundibulum, hypophysis, amygdala, hippocampus, septal region, thalamus, and periventricular white matter and choroid plexuses of

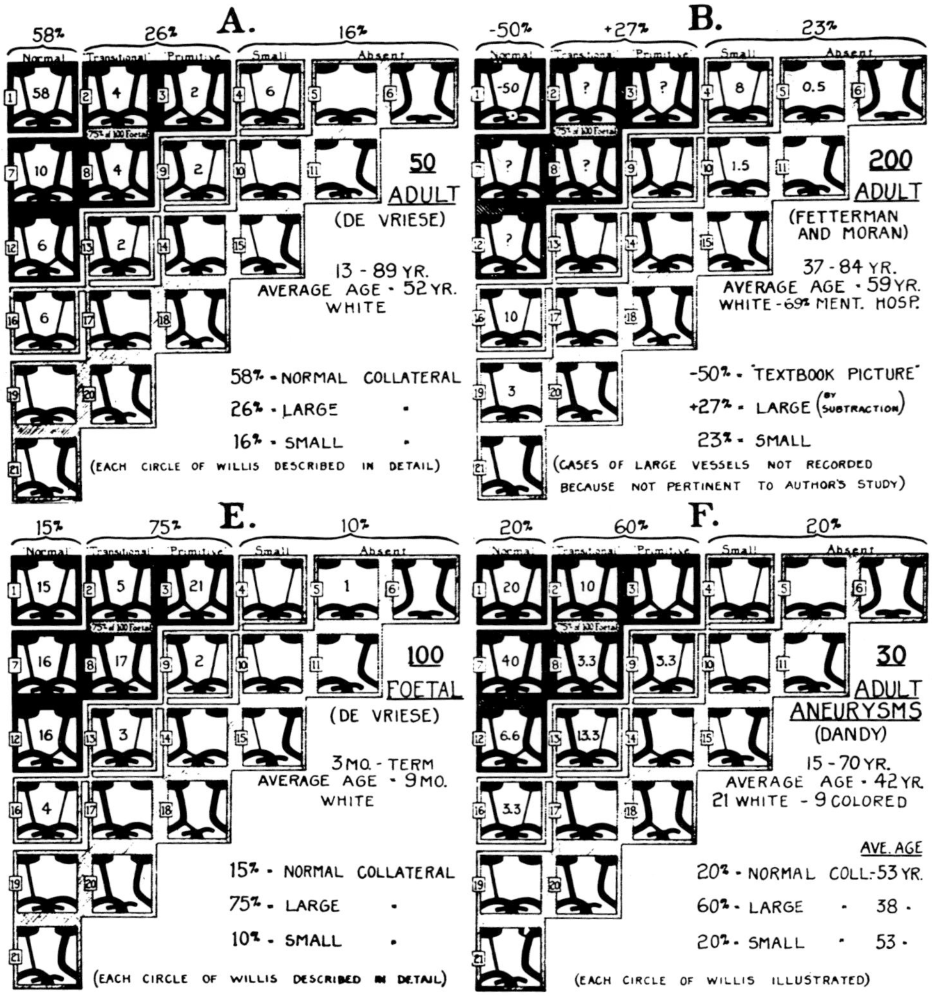

Figure 24-41. Diagrams of variations in the circle of Willis, exclusive of the ACA–anterior communicating artery complex, in several published series, as compiled, diagrammed, and summarized by Padget. (From Padget,[327] with permission.) (*Figure continues.*)

the third and lateral ventricles. The more external portions of this area (e.g., external capsule, claustrum, extreme capsule) may receive some "overlapping" blood supply from short and long medullary arteries penetrating from the insula, which makes these areas somewhat less susceptible to infarction.[299] However, the more central areas of the basal ganglia and thalamus have no such multiple supply. Indeed, the lenticulostriate and thalamoperforating arteries are classical end arteries, a phenomenon that has provided a reproducible ischemic stroke model in animals.[47,495]

Vasculature. The basal perforating arteries can be divided into two types: (1) the relatively large arteries of the basal ganglia (lenticulostriate) and thalamus (thalamoperforating), whose termination is deep; and (2) the relatively small vessels to the hypothalamus, infundibular region, and chiasmatic region, whose termination is superficial. This discussion will mainly concern the former.

The arteries of the basal perforation zone are telencephalic (basal ganglia, septal nuclei) and diencephalic (hypothalamus, thalamus). It is worth noting that the sites of origin of the basal perforating vessels anatomically merge with each other despite the embryologically disparate structures they supply.

Basal perforating arteries arise from the internal carotid, anterior cerebral, anterior communicating, anterior choroidal, middle cerebral, posterior communicating, posterior cerebral, and basilar arteries. They conform to a homotopic anatomical arrange-

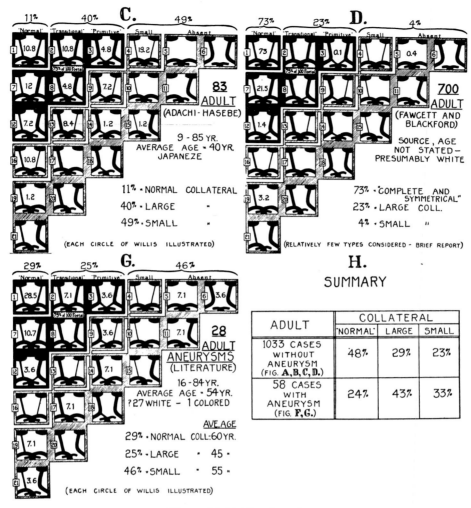

Figure 24-41 (*Continued*).

ment in both their sites of origin and areas of supply.[87,201,202,246-248,276,277,369,377,417,480,492] Those entering the anterior portion of the basal perforation zone arise from the anteromedial portions of the circle of Willis (i.e. from the ACA and the anterior communicating artery), including the recurrent artery of Heubner. These vessels supply the deep anteromedial cerebral structures, including the head of the caudate nucleus, anterior putamen, anterior globus pallidus, and anterior limb and genu of the internal capsule. Those entering the lateral portion of the basal perforation zone arise mainly from the proximal third and occasionally from the middle third of the horizontal segment of the MCA and from the anterior choroidal artery. The basal perforating branches of the MCA[277] are usually known as the *lenticulostriate arteries*. Together the arteries of the lateral basal perforation

zone supply the lateral deep structures, including most of the putamen, globus pallidus, and body of the caudate nucleus. Occasionally these arteries may arise from a single trunk with many branches (Fig. 24-44). The anterior choroidal artery, which courses through the lateral aspect of the basal perforation zone, including the choroidal fissure, also supplies the posterior portion of the lentiform nucleus, the posterior limb of the internal capsule, and even a posteroinferolateral part of the thalamus, including a variable supply to the lateral geniculate body.[1,2] The greater part of the thalamus is supplied by thalamoperforating arteries, which enter the posterior and posterolateral portions of the basal perforation zone. These vessels stem from the posterior communicating artery, the P_1 segment of the PCA, and the "tip" of the basilar artery. They supply the inferior por-

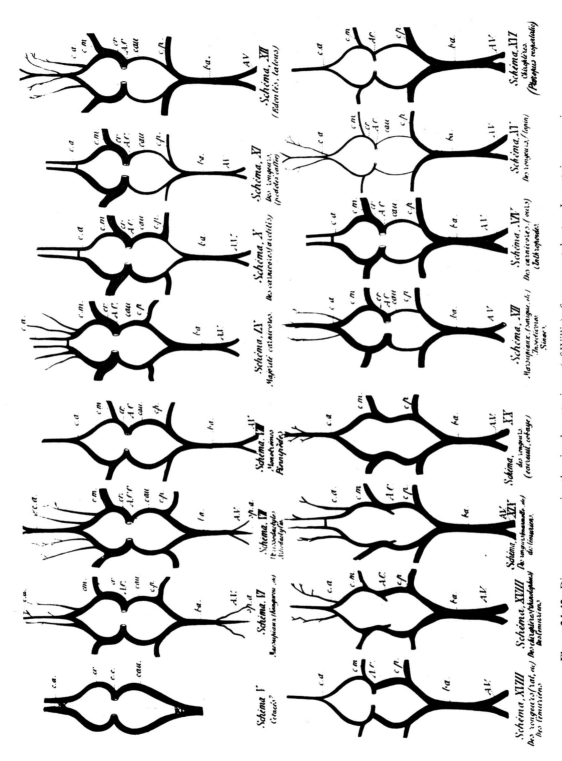

Figure 24-42. Diagrams comparing the circulus arteriosus (of Willis) of some vertebrates. In certain marsupials and ungulates (schemas VI and VII), vertebral arteries are vestigial and the basilar artery tapers to become the anterior spinal artery. The absence of vertebral arteries in cetaceans (whales, dolphins, and porpoises, schema V), marsupials (schema VI), and ungulates (schema VII) is a secondary phenomenon insofar as the embryos of these species do possess vertebral arteries. Note the variability of the ACA/anterior communicating artery complexes and the posterior communicating arteries in the numerous mammalian orders shown, suggestive of the normal variability found in humans (cf. Fig. 24-46). (From De Vriese[104] with permission.)

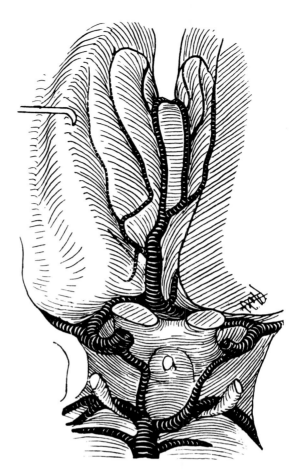

Figure 24-43. Diagram of the circulus arteriosus (of Willis) in a chimpanzee. Note the azygous ACA A_2 segment, which bifurcates into two pericallosal arteries on the dorsal surface of the corpus callosum. This is similar to the anatomy occasionally seen in the human azygous ACA (cf. Fig. 24-47). (From Watts,[476] with permission.)

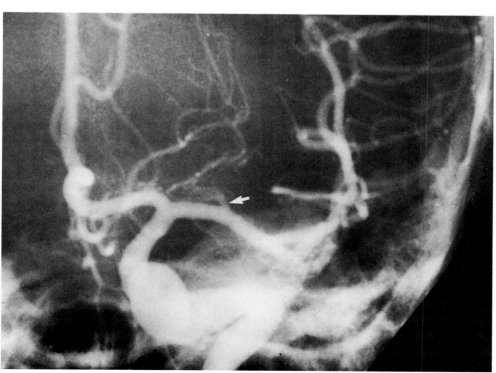

Figure 24-44. Left internal carotid arteriogram, AP view, showing anterolateral basal perforating arteries (lenticulostriate arteries) arising from a common trunk (*arrow*) from the proximal MCA.

tions of the thalamus. The superior thalamus is supplied by the medial and lateral posterior choroidal arteries, which are branches of the PCA.

Adjacent arteries of the basal perforating zone share in a reciprocal relationship for their territories of supply. The area of supply of any given artery may be very great or very small. If great, the artery branches to supply the territory of the adjacent artery or arteries, which will be reciprocally reduced, and vice versa.

Ontogeny

The ontogeny of the basal perforating arteries is not as well known as that of the main cerebral arterial trunks. This is because generally only larger trunks can be observed in tiny embryos. However, it is possible to deduce some of the development of these vessels.

Two important concepts will help to understand the developmental anatomy of the basal perforating arteries. First, the developing brain is supplied by blood vessels penetrating the brain substance over its entire surface. The basal perforating arteries are therefore not different from any other cerebral nutrient arteries, except in that they originate more proximally along the arteries of the brain base. Second, the early embryonic brain can be thought of as a hollow tube covered by a capillary plexus. In early development the striatal and diencephalic areas initially occupy large portions of the surface. Later the cerebral cortex expands massively, almost completely enveloping the striatum and diencephalon. As this occurs, the arteries of the striatum and diencephalon slowly become "bundled" together at the base of the brain. Only a basally situated hiatus in the cortical surface, the basal perforation zone, allows the nutrient arteries supplying these areas access to their territories. This process is reflected in the characteristic S-shaped course of the lenticulostriate arteries, which can be appreciated on the AP view of a cerebral angiogram[214] (Fig. 24-45). Further details about the ontogeny of the basal perforating arteries are discussed in the sections that follow.

Phylogeny

The reciprocity that exists between the arteries that provide the basal perforating vessels is a reflection of their phylogenetic background. In fish and some amphibians a series of arterioles arise from the medial and lateral olfactory arteries, which are ho-

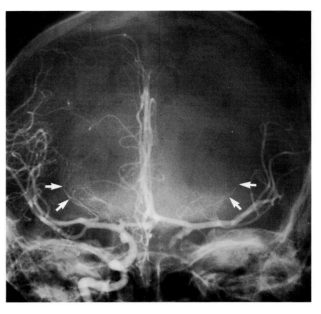

Figure 24-45. Right common carotid arteriogram, AP view, demonstrating the characteristic S shape of the lenticulostriate arteries (*arrows*). This is produced by a ventrolateral "folding" of the cerebral cortex over the basal ganglia during ontogeny.

mologous with the ACA and MCA of higher vertebrates, to penetrate the striatal region along the endorhinal fissure, which is roughly homologous with the anterior perforated substance. In some frog species (amphibians), a striatal common trunk branches from the medial olfactory artery, the homologue of the ACA of higher vertebrates, to supply the primordium amygdalae and striatal region. In reptiles several branches of the MCA course into the endorhinal fissure to supply the striatal and amygdaloid complexes.

The lenticulostriate arteries in the monotremes and marsupials branch from the ACA and MCA to enter the anterior perforated substance. One of those from the ACA is a recurrent branch, the homologue of the recurrent artery of Heubner.

In higher mammals the anatomy of the basal perforation zone resembles that of humans, and a comparison of these vertebrates reflects the balance between the ACA, MCA, and anterior choroidal arteries. In the cat the lenticulostriate arteries originate from both the ACA and the MCA. In horses, cattle, pigs, and sheep, the lenticulostriates arise from the MCA, from the rostral division of the ICA, or from the rete mirabile, and often from a single common trunk with numerous branches.

Cerebral Artery Stems

Anterior Cerebral and Anterior Communicating Arteries

Asymmetry of A_1 segments is very common; one A_1 segment may be absent or extremely hypoplastic.[104,194,230,259,344,487,492] When this occurs, the anterior communicating artery allows passage of blood to the A_2 segment from the contralateral ICA. Yasargil[492] points out that an A_1 segment that is aplastic by angiography is rarely completely absent at surgery. The size of the anterior communicating artery increases proportionally with the difference in size of the A_1 segments.[292,344] Rarely, the A_1 segment may be duplicated[230,344] or fenestrated.[193,220,230,291,293,445,487,490,492]

The anterior communicating artery complex, the most common site of aneurysm formation, is arguably the most common site of arterial variation[104,147,148,194,254,292,327,344,419,455,487,492] (Fig. 24-46). It is often doubled, tripled, or plexiform; rarely, it is absent entirely.[455] Milenkovic et al.[292] found that the anterior communicating artery was fenestrated, duplicated, or triplicated in 44 percent of fetal brains. Indeed, the "normal," anterior communicating artery is found in only a minority of cases.

The A_2 segments (i.e., proximal pericallosal arteries) are also highly variable. One pericallosal artery is often dominant. Variations include azygous (unpaired)[91,104,147,148,230,252,258,292,344,419,428,429,455,487,492] (Fig. 24-47) as well as triple[104,147,148,194,230,344,419,455,492] A_2 segments. An azygous ACA segment may be relatively short, as when the ACAs are fused just at the point of the anterior communicating artery, or it may be quite long. Because of this complicated anatomy, it has been recommended that the region the maximum possible exposure be provided via an interhemispheric approach when performing aneurysm surgery.[424]

A very unusual ACA anomaly is a large ACA arising from the ICA and coursing between the optic nerves[29,45,49,130,190,210,230,284,291,292,323,364,368,395,398,447] (Fig. 24-48). The vessel often supplies an azygous A_2 segment and is often associated with a duplicate A_1 segment that courses lateral to the optic nerve. Frequently associated are other congenital vascular and/or nervous anomalies. Odake[323] has suggested that this anomaly be referred to as *carotid-anterior cerebral artery anastomosis*. Another rare anomaly of the ACA is ACA origin of the ophthalmic artery.[172,230]

Ontogeny. The anterior communicating artery develops from plexiform channels that connect the primitive ACAs within the interhemispheric fissure. Also, a central artery to the genu of the corpus callosum can be identified throughout ontogeny, representing the basis for one or three A_2 segments.

With regard to the development of the anomalous carotid-ACA anastomosis, Moffat[298] showed that, in the rat, the carotid-ACA anastomosis represents persistence of the primitive maxillary artery. (This hypothesis was also suggested but not developed by Brismar et al.[49]) Moffat showed that the primitive maxillary artery participates in the formation of a complete arterial ring around the optic nerve, anastomosing with a recurrent branch of the primitive medial olfactory artery (primordial ACA). This anatomic configuration is very similar to that of the human embryo as drawn by Padget[328] (see Figs. 24-10, 24-12, and 24-13), except that in the human the ring is not entirely complete. In the rat the ventral aspect of the arterial ring normally regresses, resulting in the familiar anatomy in which the ACA and MCA originate from the ICA bifurcation, posterolateral to the optic chiasm. However, in 2 percent of rat embryos, Moffat noted that the dorsal rather than the ventral aspect of the perioptic arterial ring had regressed, resulting in an anomaly in which the primitive maxillary artery (a branch of the ICA) passed ventral to and between the optic nerves to supply the primitive olfactory artery. This is clearly homologous with the rare carotid-ACA anastomosis described above. Thus, if occasionally in the human embryo a complete arterial ring were formed around the optic nerve by the primitive maxillary artery and the recurrent branch of the primitive medial olfactory artery, with persistence of the ventral segment of the ring, this would result in the anomalous carotid-ACA anastomosis.

ACA origin of the ophthalmic artery is discussed above in the section on ophthalmic artery anomalies.

Phylogeny. The comparative anatomy of the ACA is discussed above in the section on comparative anatomy of the circle of Willis, and that relating to the ACA origin of the ophthalmic artery is discussed above in the section on ophthalmic artery anomalies.

Posterior Communicating Artery and P_1 Segment of Posterior Cerebral Artery

The relative sizes of the posterior communicating artery and the P_1 segment of the PCA are roughly inversely related, and their variation is very common. When the PCA originates from the ICA (so-called fetal-type posterior communicating artery,

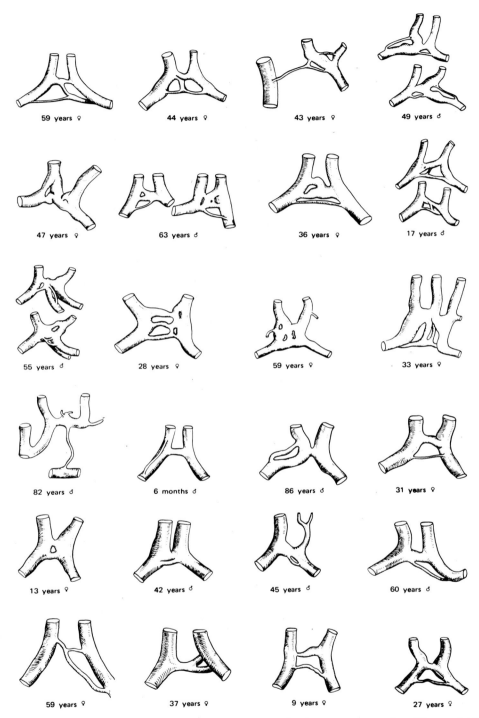

Figure 24-46. Diagrams of variations in the anterior communicating artery complex. The variability of the anterior communicating artery complex has its ontogenetic basis in its formation from plexiform channels (see Figs. 24-15 to 24-17). Plexiform anterior communicating artery complexes are seen in other mammals as well. (From Yasargil,[492] with permission.)

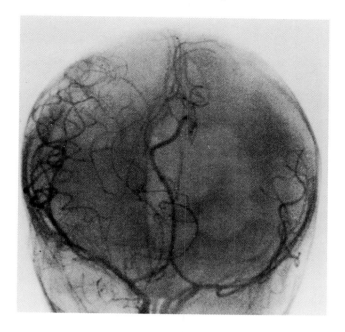

Figure 24-47. Right internal carotid arteriogram with cross-compression in an infant, AP view, demonstrating a long azygous ACoA. The artery is displaced to the right by a large porencephalic cyst; hydrocephalus is also present. Ontogenetically an azygous ACoA probably represents enlargement of the anterior artery of the corpus callosum or the ACA branch to the choroid plexus. An azygous ACA is found in many vertebrates (cf. Fig. 24-43). (From Szdzuy et al.,[429] with permission.)

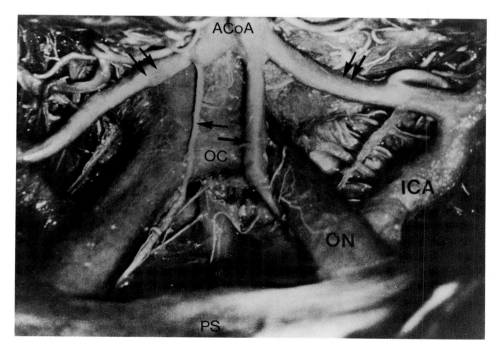

Figure 24-48. Cadaver dissection. Superoanterior view of anomalous vessels forming anastomoses between the ICAs and the anterior communicating artery (*ACoA*) bilaterally. The anomalous vessels (single arrows) course between the optic nerves (*ON*). The anomalous vessel on the cadaver's left is larger than that on its right. Note that the A_1 segments are duplicated, with "normal" A_1 segments lateral to the optic nerves (double arrows). This anomaly has been shown to represent a persistent embryonic anastomosis between the primitive maxillary artery and the ACA. The same anomaly can be seen in the rat. *OC*, optic chiasm; *PS*, planum sphenoidale. (Modified from Lasjaunias and Berenstein,[230] with permission.)

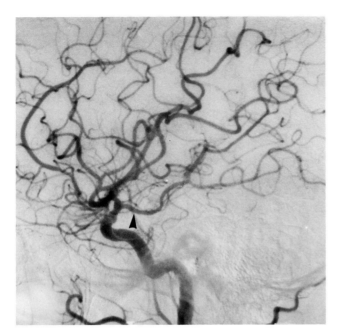

Figure 24-49. So-called fetal posterior communicating artery. Right common carotid artery angiogram, lateral view. The PCA fills via a widely patent posterior communicating artery (*arrowhead*). This variation does not actually represent persistence of a fetal (or more correctly, embryonic) stage, but rather a secondary alteration, due to hemodynamic factors.

Fig. 24-49 and see below), the P_1 segment is generally hypoplastic. Conversely, when the PCA arises from the basilar artery, the posterior communicating artery, the posterior communicating artery is hypoplastic[104,185,244,245,272,327,360,376,419,465,487,492,496] However, this ACoA/P_1 relationship is best considered as a continuous spectrum of normal variability.

The size of the posterior communicating artery is highly variable, although it is rarely entirely absent.[42,419,492] A relatively large and constant branch of the posterior communicating artery, known as the premamillary artery, supplies the cerebral peduncles, optic tracts, and posteriolateral portion of the basal perforation zone.[341,342] Reported posterior communicating artery variants (other than hypoplasia and so-called fetal type) include origin of the posterior communicating artery from the ophthalmic artery in the optic canal,[42] posterior communicating artery duplication[42,492] and fenestration,[487,492] and three posterior communicating arteries on one side.[42] The anomalous posterior communicating artery origin from the anterior choroidal artery is discussed below in the section on the anterior choroidal artery.

Anomalies of the P_1 segment of the PCA include its absence or extreme hypoplasia[104,194,292,419,492,496] and duplication.[291] Furthermore, one branch of a double PCA may arise from the posterior communicating artery, with the other arising from the basilar artery.[36,419,487]

An unusual anomaly was reported by Wismer[485] in which both PCAs arose from the right supraclinoid ICA, with only a posterior temporal branch arising from the left supraclinoid ICA. In this case the basilar artery was dysgenetic above the superior cerebellar arteries.

It should be noted that the term *fetal posterior communicating artery* is a misnomer. This term is used to refer to a widely patent posterior communicating artery, by which the PCA fills largely or exclusively from the ICA, the P_1 segment being hypoplastic. This terminology presumably is based on the idea that the posterior communicating arteries of embryos are usually as large as any other segment of the circle of Willis supplying blood to the PCAs from the ICA. However, in early embryos the P_1 segments are equally as large as the posterior communicating arteries, with which they most likely share equally in the supply of the PCAs. The variation of a large posterior communicating artery and a hypoplastic P_1 segment does not actually represent persistence of any embryonic stage. Rather, this variation is a vascular secondary alteration, probably due to hemodynamic factors, as discussed above in the section on the circle of Willis.

Ontogeny. Because of the usually smaller diameter of the posterior communicating artery as compared with the PCA, the latter is most often thought of as arising from the basilar artery. However, the PCA develops from the posterior division of the ICA, reflecting its phylogenetic background. Williams[482] has shown that the sympathetic nerve fibers innervating the PCA arise from the carotid rather than the vertebrobasilar plexus, a finding that supports this concept.

The human PCA develops through annexation of much of the territories of the primitive anterior choroidal, posterior choroidal, diencephalic, and mesencephalic arteries. Its large, early embryonic mesencephalic distribution is dwarfed later in ontogeny as the cerebral hemispheres grow.

The case reported by Wismer[485] appears to represent simultaneous hypoplasia of both the basilar artery above the superior cerebellar artery and the left posterior communicating artery. Most of the left PCA territory then became supplied by the right ICA (via the right posterior communicating artery and bilaterally patent P_1 segments). The small posterior temporal branch of the left supraclinoid ICA most likely represents a branch of the left anterior choroidal artery (see below).

Phylogeny. The PCA cannot be found in the brains of fish. It is represented in this stage as a branch of the caudal division of the ICA, which mainly supplies the optic lobes (i.e., mesencephalon). In reptiles the PCA is present and large. It may branch from either the rostral or caudal division of the ICA and courses in the space between the forebrain and the optic lobes. The PCA supplies the choroid plexus of the lateral ventricles in primitive reptiles, although a lateral choroidal branch from the rostral division of the ICA can be found in more advanced reptiles. Also in reptiles, the PCAs of either side meet in the posterior aspect of the interhemispheric fissure, where they anastomose with the ACAs to supply the hippocampal structures.

In mammals the cortical distribution of the PCA clearly dominates its territories of supply, in many mammals becoming a branch of the basilar artery that is supplied by the phylogenetically "new" vertebral arteries. The PCA's tectal, hippocampal, and choroidal supply is maintained, however, as are the anastomoses with the other arterial systems.

It can be seen how the variability of the PCA's origin and its reciprocal participation in the supply of the hippocampus (with the ACA, MCA, and anterior choroidal arteries), choroid plexus (with the anterior choroidal artery), and mesencephalon (with the superior cerebellar artery) are reflections of its phylogenetic background.

Internal Carotid Artery and Accessory Middle Cerebral Artery

Fenestrations of the ICA bifurcation have been rarely reported.[149,152] These incidentally noted anomalies are thought to reflect development from a primordial plexus. The anomaly of an accessory MCA arising from the ICA is discussed in the next section.

Recurrent Artery of Heubner and Accessory Middle Cerebral Artery

The recurrent artery of Heubner arises from the lateral aspect of the ACA, usually at the level of the anterior communicating artery. Its origin is from the A_2 segment slightly more often than from the A_1 segment.[147,148,275] It follows a characteristic "recurrent" course adjacent to the proximal ACA, terminating at

the limen insulae. Occasionally there are multiple recurrent arteries of Heubner.[147,194,275,369,455,480]

The recurrent artery of Heubner supplies perforating branches to the anterior and lateral portions of the basal perforation area. In this respect it has a reciprocal relationship with perforating (lenticulostriate) branches of the proximal ACA and MCA[3,147,230,369,459,480,492] (Fig. 24-50). Thus when the recurrent artery of Heubner is absent, branches to the anterolateral basal perforation zone will arise from the ACA and MCA and vice versa. The extreme example of the latter phenomenon is the so-called accessory MCA (Fig. 24-51). In this variant a "duplicate" or "accessory" MCA arises from either the distal ICA or the ACA, passes to the limen insulae, and irrigates a portion of the MCA territory[194,230,361,412,419,435,444,458,459,475,492] When an accessory MCA is present, the recurrent artery of Heubner is often absent, and perforating branches arise from the accessory artery, although occasionally a more typical recurrent artery of Heubner may also be found on the same side as[435,458] or arising from[194] an accessory MCA. This merely testifies to the number of potential variations that these overlapping systems may reveal.

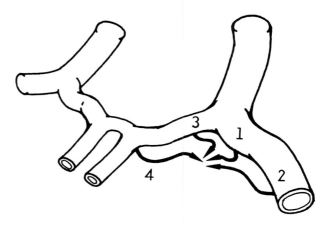

Figure 24-50. Diagram including the potential origins of the arteries of the anterolateral basal perforation zone, left superoanterior view. A reciprocal relationship exists between the branches of the ACA and MCA in the region of the anterolateral basal perforation zone (anterior perforated substance). The perforating branches may arise from the proximal MCA, the proximal ACA, and/or the recurrent artery of Heubner. This relationship has its basis in the ontogeny and phylogeny of these vessels (see figs. 24-8 and 24-15 to 24-18). (*1*) proximal MCA trunk; (*2*) distal MCA trunk; (*3*) proximal A_1 segment; (*4*) ACA opposite anterior communicating artery. (From Yasargil,[492] with permission.)

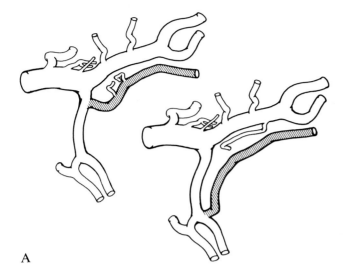

A

Figure 24-51. The recurrent artery of Heubner and the "accessory" MCA are the same artery, which may vary greatly in size. **(A)** Diagrams demonstrating two types of accessory MCA, left superoanterior view. *(left)* Origin at ICA-ACA junction; *(right)* origin from ACA opposite anterior communicating artery (usual origin of recurrent artery of Heubner). **(B)** Left ICA angiogram, AP view, showing left "accessory" MCA arising from ACA opposite anterior communicating artery *(large arrows)*. Note the recurrent artery of Heubner *(small arrows)* on the right side (Fig. A from Yasargil,[492] with permission.)

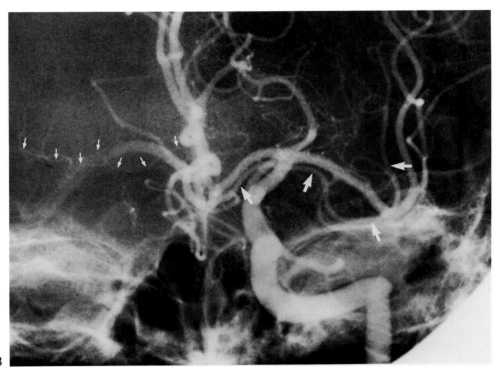

B

Ontogeny. The recurrent artery of Heubner (and the lenticulostriate arteries) represents the early termination of the primitive rostral division of the ICA (the primitive medial olfactory artery). Later, the ACA and MCA systems develop from plexiform branches of the rostral division of the ICA. Variability in the branching pattern that emerges from the early vascular plexus provides the ontogenetic basis for the reciprocal relationship between the ACA, MCA, and recurrent artery of Heubner. The development of these arteries of the anterolateral basal perforation zone results in the occasional development of an accessory MCA or a duplicated recurrent artery of Heubner.

Phylogeny. In submammalian vertebrates, branches from the ACA and MCA enter the endorhinal fissure (roughly homologous with the anterior perforated substance) to supply perforating branches to the primordial striatal and amygdaloid regions. As noted in reptiles and all higher vertebrates, one or several ACA branches course upon the anteroinferior surface of the brain to anastomose with reciprocal branches of the MCA (see Fig. 24-8). Perforating arteries to the endorhinal fissure arise from both the ACA and MCA and from the basal anastomotic branches between them.

Anterior Choroidal Artery

The anterior choroidal artery may possess a small, intermediate, or large distribution and may be represented by one, two, or three separate trunks. Although its territory is usually relatively small, it may contribute to the supply of the optic tract, posterior limb of the internal capsule, lateral geniculate body, portions of the optic radiations, portions of the corpora striata, uncus, temporal lobe cortex, amygdaloid nucleus, anterior hippocampus, cerebral peduncle, and substantia nigra. It anastomoses with the posterior communicating artery and proximal PCA in the ambient cistern, with the medial and lateral posterior choroidal arteries in the choroidal fissure, and with branches of the PCA or posterior communicating artery over the lateral geniculate body[1,2,30,31,82,83,131,145,230,358,432,448,492] (Fig. 24-52). If its cortical

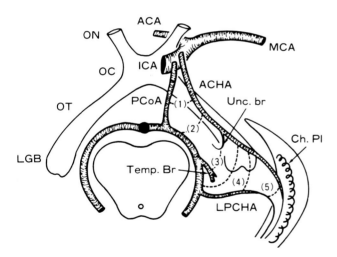

Figure 24-52. Diagram illustrating sites of potential anastomoses of the anterior choroidal artery with the posterior communicating artery and PCA. A reciprocal relationship exists between both the sites of origin and the territories of distribution of the anterior choroidal artery and the PCA in the region of the choroidal fissure and posteroinferomedial temporal lobe. This is a reflection of the ontogeny and phylogeny of this region. (*1*) Anastomosis with posterior communicating artery over optic tract; (*2*) anastomosis with PCA over cerebral peduncle; (*3*) anastomosis over pyriform cortex with temporal and hippocampal branches of PCA; (*4*) anastomosis with branches of PCA over lateral geniculate body; (*5*) anastomosis with posterior choroidal branches of PCA within choroid plexus of third and lateral ventricles. (From Takahashi et al.,[436] with permission.)

territory provides blood to portions of the temporal and occipital cortex, the usual branches of the PCA and/or MCA will be reciprocally reduced. This explains the following phenomena: (1) posterior communicating artery arising from the anterior choroidal artery; (2) anterior choroidal artery arising from the MCA or posterior communicating artery; and (3) origin of the anterior choroidal artery from the ICA proximal to the origin of the posterior communicating artery[34,145,164,230,265,291,358,376,432,448,492,496] (Fig. 24-53).

Ontogeny. The primitive anterior choroidal artery is at one stage the largest branch of the cranial division of the embryonic ICA. It courses upon the primordial diencephalon on its way into the developing choroidal fissure. The relatively large size of the anterior choroidal artery in the early embryo may reflect a large energy requirement of the choroid plexus, perhaps related to a function of the embryonic choroid plexus in providing nutrients to the developing telencephalon via diffusion through the CSF.

On the surface of the embryonic telencephalon and diencephalon and in the region of the developing choroidal fissure, the anterior choroidal artery anastomoses with adjacent arteries (i.e., the primordia of the MCA, posterior communicating artery, and PCA). These adjacent anastomotic arterial systems will share in a reciprocal relationship for the supply of the structures of the region, providing the ontogenetic basis for the reported anomalies.

Phylogeny. In reptiles the inferior cerebral artery, a branch of the cranial division of the ICA, courses along the optic tract to supply the optic tract, amygdala, and paleostriatum (forerunner of the corpus striatum). This represents the phylogenetic precursor of the stem of the anterior choroidal artery of higher vertebrates. The inferior cerebral artery of reptiles terminates by anastomosing with branches of the PCA over the primitive homologue of the lateral geniculate body. However, the inferior cerebral artery does not itself supply branches to the choroid plexus, as the temporal horns of the lateral ventricles have not yet developed. In the more advanced reptiles an anterior or lateral choroidal artery is found, which resembles even more closely that of mammals. The artery in the crocodile supplies the optic tract, lateral geniculate body, amygdaloid nucleus, and ventromedial paleostriatum before anastomosing with branches of the PCA.

In primitive mammals (marsupials) the anterior choroidal artery arises from the ICA and passes along the optic tract to the lateral geniculate body, supplying branches to the amygdaloid region and diencephalon. Over the surface of the lateral genicu-

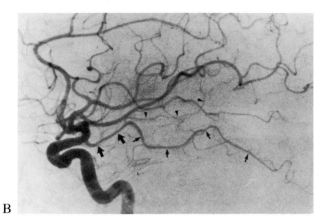

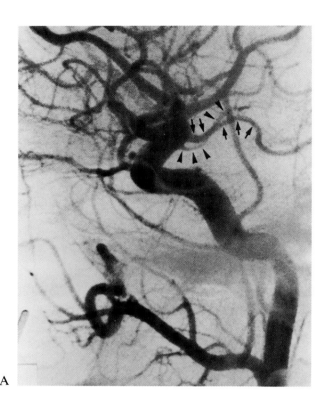

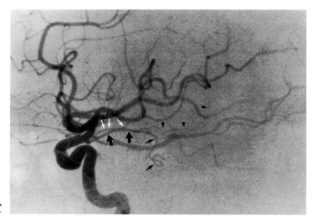

A   C

Figure 24-53. A reciprocal relationship exists between the territories of distribution of branches of the anterior choroidal and posterior communicating artery/PCA in the region of the choroidal fissure and posteroinferomedial temporal lobe. In the extreme case this may result in complete supply of the PCA territory by the anterior choroidal artery, with complete supply of the anterior choroidal artery territory by the PCA. **(A)** Common carotid arteriogram, lateral view, anterior choroidal artery (*arrowheads*) arising proximal to posterior communicating artery (*arrows*). **(B)** Left internal carotid arteriogram, lateral view, demonstrating a single branch of the supraclinoid ICA (*large arrows*), which bifurcates into the anterior choroidal artery (*arrowheads*) and PCA (*small arrows*). **(C)** Right internal carotid arteriogram, lateral view, demonstrating anterior choroidal artery (*large arrows*) bifurcating into a posterior temporal branch (*small black arrows*), usually a branch of the PCA, and a choroidal branch (*black arrowheads*). Note that another choroidal branch may be present from the proximal anterior choroidal artery (*white arrows*). (Fig. A from Hara et al.,[164] with permission; Figs. B and C modified from Takahashi et al.,[432] with permission.)

body, numerous anterior choroidal artery branches anastomose with branches of the PCA. Small branches from both the anterior choroidal artery and the PCA, predominantly the latter, supply the choroid plexus.

In higher mammals the anterior choroidal artery attains its "final" configuration. Its choroidal supply is limited to only the anterior part of the inferior horn of the lateral ventricle, while branches of the PCA (i.e., the lateral and medial posterior choroidal arteries in humans) supply the majority of the choroid plexus of the lateral and third ventricles. However,

the anterior choroidal artery remains an important artery for the supply of structures that have been "folded" into the region of the choroidal fissure by the expanding cerebral cortex. These include portions of the medial temporal lobe, corpora striata, internal capsule, and thalamus. The territory of supply of the anterior choroidal artery is adjacent to and reciprocal with parts of those of the MCA (lateral lenticulostriate arteries, medial temporal branches) and the posterior communicating artery and PCA (thalamoperforating arteries, choroid plexus of lateral ventricle).

World hystricomorphs, and in bathyergoids, with special reference to the systematic classification of rodents. Acta Anat (Basel) 80:516, 1971

58. Bugge J: The cephalic arterial system in the insectivores and the primates with special reference to the macroscelidoidea and tupaioidea and the insectivore-primate boundary. Z Anat Entwickl Gesch 135:279, 1972

59. Bugge J: The cephalic arterial system in carnivores, with special reference to the systematic classification. Acta Anat (Basel) 101:45, 1978

60. Burda DJ: Development of intracranial arterial patterns in turtles. J Morphol 116:171, 1965

61. Burda DJ: Embryonic modification of lacertilian intracranial arteries. Am J Anat 118:743, 1966

62. Burda DJ: Developmental aspects of intracranial arterial supply in the alligator brain. J Comp Neurol 135:369, 1969

63. Cairney J: Tortuosity of the cervical segment of the internal carotid artery. J Anat 59:87, 1924

64. Campbell CBG, Hodos W: The concept of homology and the evolution of the nervous system. Brain Behav Evol 3:353, 1970

65. Campos J, Fox AJ, Vinuela F et al: Saccular aneurysms in basilar artery fenestration. AJNR 8:233, 1987

66. Capo H, Kupersmith MJ, Berenstein A et al: The clinical importance of the inferolateral trunk of the internal carotid artery. Neurosurgery 28:733, 1991

67. Carella A, Lambert P, Federico F et al: Double fenestration of the extracranial vertebral artery. Neuroradiology 15:193, 1978

68. Carginin C, Benedetti A, Curri D et al: A case of persistent hypoglossal artery. Neurochirurgia (Stuttg) 19:231, 1976

69. Carmack JW: Aberrant internal carotids and their relation to surgery of the pharynx. Laryngoscope 39:707, 1929

70. Cassinari V, Bernasconi V: Aspects angiographiques des meningiomes de la faux du cerveau. Neurochirurgie 12:451, 1966

71. Castroviejo P: Vascular changes in cerebellar developmental defects. Neuroradiology 16:58, 1978

72. Chambers AA, Lukin R: Trigeminal artery connection to the posterior inferior cerebellar arteries. Neuroradiology 9:121, 1975

73. Charcot JM, Bouchard C: Nouvelles recherches sur la pathologie de l'hémorrhage cérébrale. Arch Physiol Norm Pathol 1:110, 643, 1868

74. Clemente CD (ed): Gray's Anatomy of the Human Body. 30th Ed. Lea & Febiger, Philadelphia, 1985

75. Cobb S: The cerebral circulation. XIII. The question of "end-arteries" of the brain and the mechanism of infarction. Arch Neurol Psychiatr 25:273, 1931

76. Cobb SR, Hieshima GB, Mehringer CM et al: Persistent trigeminal artery variant. Carotid-anterior inferior cerebellar artery anastomosis. Surg Neurol 19:263, 1983

77. Cole FJ: A History of Comparative Anatomy. Macmillan, London, 1944, p. 305

78. Congdon ED: Transformation of the aortic-arch system during the development of the human embryo. Contrib Embryol 14:47, 1922

79. Conroy GC: A study of cerebral vascular evolution in primates. In Armstrong E, Falk D (eds): Primate Brain Evolution: Methods and Concepts. Plenum, New York, 1982, p. 247

80. Conroy GC, Packer DJ: The anatomy and phylogenetic significance of the carotid arteries and nerves in strepsirhine primates. Folia Primatol 35:237, 1981

81. Cooper DF: Bone erosion of the cervical vertebrae secondary to tortuosity of the vertebral artery. Case report. J Neurosurg 53:106, 1980

82. Cooper IS: Surgical alleviation of parkinsonism: Effects of occlusion of the anterior choroidal artery. J Am Geriatr Soc 2:691, 1954

83. Cooper IS: Surgical occlusion of the anterior choroidal artery in parkinsonism. Surg Gynecol Obstet 99:207, 1954

84. Craigie EH: The comparative anatomy and embryology of the capillary bed of the central nervous system. Res Publ Assoc Res Nerv Ment Dis 18:3, 1938

85. Craigie EH: Vascular patterns of the developing nervous system. p. 28. in Waelsch (ed): Biochemistry of the developing nervous system: Proceedings of the First International Neurochemical Symposium. Academic Press, New York, 1955

86. Crosby EC: The forebrain of *Alligator mississippiensis*. J Comp Neurol 27:325, 1917

86a. Crouch JE: Anatomy of the Lower Chordates. Mayfield Publishing, Mountain View, CA, 1960

87. Crowell RM, Morawetz RB: The anterior communicating artery has significant branches. Stroke 8:272, 1977

88. Cushing H: The Medical Career. Dartmouth College Press, Hanover, NH 1929, p. 24

89. Damsma H, Mali WPTM, Zonneveld FW: CT diagnosis of an aberrant internal carotid artery in the middle ear. J Comput Assist Tomogr 8:317, 1984

90. Danziger J, Bloch S: The value of the external carotid circulation in the assessment of intracranial disease. Clin Radiol 26:261, 1975

91. Danziger J, Bloch S, Van Rensburg MJ: Agenesis of the corpus callosum associated with an azygos anterior cerebral artery, a lipoma and porencephalic cyst. S Afr Med J 46:739, 1972

92. Dart RA: A contribution to the morphology of the corpus striatum J Anat 55:1, 1920

93. Davis DD, Story HE: The carotid circulation in the domestic cat. Field Mus Nat Hist (Zool Ser) 28:5, 1943

94. Debaene A, Farnarier P, Dufour M et al: Hypoglossal artery, a rare abnormal carotid-basilar anastomosis. Neuroradiology 4:233, 1972

95. Debrun GM, Davis KR, Nauta HJ et al: Treatment of carotid cavernous fistulae of cavernous aneurysms

associated with a persistent trigeminal artery: report of three cases. AJNR 9:749, 1988

96. De la Torre E, Netsky MG: Study of persistent primitive maxillary artery in human fetus: Some homologies of cranial arteries in man and dog. Am J Anat 106:185, 1960

97. de la Torre E, Netsky MG, Meschan I: Intracranial and extracranial circulations in the dog: Anatomic and angiographic studies. Am J Anat 105:343, 1959

98. De Reuck J: The human periventricular arterial blood supply and the anatomy of cerebral infarctions. Eur Neurol 5:321, 1971

99. De Reuck J, Chatta AS, Richardson EP: Pathogenesis and evolution of periventricular leukomalacia in infancy. Arch Neurol 27:229, 1972

100. De Reuck J, Crevits L, de Coster W et al: Pathogenesis of Binswanger chronic progressive subcortical encephalopathy. Neurology 30:920, 1980

101. De Reuck J, Schaumburg HH: Periventricular atherosclerotic leukoencephalopathy. Neurology 22:1094, 1972

102. De Reuck J, van der Eecken HM: The arterial angioarchitecture in lacunar state. Acta Neurol Belg 76:142, 1976

103. De Reuck J, van der Eecken HM: Periventricular leukomalacia in adults: Clinicopathological study of four cases. Arch Neurol 35:517, 1978

104. De Vriese B: Sur la signification morphologique des artères cérébrales. Arch Biol 21:357, 1905

105. Dilenge D: Bilateral agenesis of internal carotid artery. Can Assoc Radiol J 26:91, 1975

106. Dilenge D, Geraud G: Accessory meningeal artery. Acta Radio Suppl (Stockh) 347:63, 1975

107. Dilenge D, Heon M: The internal carotid artery. p. 1202. In Newton TH, Potts DG (eds): Radiology of the Skull and Brain. CV Mosby, St. Louis, 1974

108. Dory MA: CT demonstration of cervical vertebral erosion by tortuous vertebral artery. AJNR 6:641, 1985

109. Du Boulay G, Darling M: Autoregulation in external carotid artery branches in the baboon. Neuroradiology 9:129, 1975

110. Du Boulay G, Kendall BE, Crockard A et al: The autoregulatory capability of Galen's rete cerebri and its connections. Neuroradiology 9:171, 1975

111. Duckett S: The establishment of internal vascularization in the human telencephalon. Acta Anat (Basel) 80:107, 1971

112. Duret H: Recherches anatomiques sur la circulation de l'encephale. Arch Physiol Norm Pathol 1:60, 1874

113. Duvernoy HM, Delon S, Vannson JL: Cortical blood vessels of the human brain. Brain Res Bull 7:519, 1981

114. Elefante R, Fucci G, Granata F et al: Agenesis of the right internal carotid artery with an unusual transsellar intracavernous intercarotid connection. AJNR 4:88, 1983

115. Evans HM: On the development of the aortae, cardinal and umbilical veins, and the other blood vessels of vertebrate embryos from capillaries. Anat Rec 3:498, 1909

116. Evans HM: The development of the vascular system. In Kiebel F, Mall FP (eds): Manual of Human Embryology. JB Lippincott, Philadelphia, 1912

117. Faivre J, Vallee B, Carsin M et al: Agenesis of the cervical and petrosal portions of the left internal carotid artery. With reconstitution of the cavernous portion through a transsphenoidal intercarotid anastomosis. J Neuroradiol 5:133, 1978

118. Fankhauser H, Kamano S, Hanamura T et al: Abnormal origin of the posterior inferior cerebellar artery. Case report. J Neurosurg 51:569, 1979

119. Fay T: The cerebral vasculature. Preliminary report of study by means of roentgen ray. JAMA 84:1727, 1925

120. Fields WS: The significance of persistent trigeminal artery. Carotid-basilar anastomosis. Radiology 91:1096, 1968

121. Fields WS, Bruetman M, Weibel J: Collateral circulation of the brain. Monogr Surg Sci 2:183, 1965

122. Fife CD: Absence of the common carotid. Anat Rec 22:115, 1921

123. Fisher AGT: A case of complete absence of both internal carotid arteries with a preliminary note on the developmental history of the stapedial artery. J Anat 48:37, 1914

124. Flynn RE: External carotid origin of the dominant vertebral artery. Case report. J Neurousrg 29:300, 1968

125. Francke JP, Clarisse J, Dhellemmes P et al: The arterial circle of the base of the brain and its feeding vessels in certain mammals. J Neuroradiol 4:271, 1977

126. Francke JP, Di Marino V, Pannier M et al: The vertebral arteries (arteria vertebralis). The V3 atlanto-axoidial and V4 intracranial segments-collaterals. Anat Clin 2:229, 1981

127. Fredy D, Hugonet P, Missir O et al: Obstruction of the cerebral blood vessels in the neck. Haemodynamic problems. Bosniak's plexus. J Neuroradiol 5:203, 1978

128. Freitas PE, Aquini MG, Chemale I: Persistent primitive trigeminal artery aneurysm. Surg Neurol 26:373, 1986

129. Fujii K, Lenkey C, Rhoton AL: Microsurgical anatomy of the choroidal arteries: Fourth ventricle and cerebellopontine angles. J Neurosurg 52:504, 1980

130. Fujimoto S, Murakami M: Anomalous branch of the internal carotid artery supplying circulation of the anterior cerebral artery. Case report. J Neurosurg 58:941, 1983

131. Furiani J: The anterior choroidal artery and its blood supply to the internal capsule. Acta Anat (Basel) 85:108, 1973

132. Gabrielsen TO: Size of vertebral artery and of foramen transversarium of axis: An anatomic study. Acta Radiol 9:285, 1969

133. Galligioni F, Pellone M, Bernardi R et al: Further

observations of the meningeal branch of the lacrimal artery. Four additional cases. AJR 101:22, 1967

134. Garza-Mercado R, Cavazos E: Persistent trigeminal artery associated with intracranial arterial aneurysm. Neurosurgery 14:604, 1984

135. Garza-Mercado R, Cavazos E, Urrutia G: Persistent hypoglossal artery in combination with multifocal arteriovenous malformations of the brain: Case report. Neurosurgery 26:871, 1990

136. Gibo H, Lenkey C, Rhoton AL: Microsurgical anatomy of the supraclinoid portion of the internal carotid artery. J Neurosurg 55:560, 1981

137. Gillilan LA: Significant superficial anastomoses in the arterial blood supply to the human brain. J Comp Neurol 112:55, 1959

138. Gillilan LA: A comparative study of the extrinsic and intrinsic arterial blood supply to brains of submammalian vertebrates. J Comp Neurol 130:175, 1967

139. Gillilan LA: The arterial and venous blood supplies to the forebrain (including the internal capsule) of primates. Neurology 18:653, 1968

140. Gillilan LA: The arterial and venous blood supplies to the cerebellum of primates. J Neuropathol Exp Neurol 28:295, 1969

141. Gillilan LA: Blood supply to primitive mammalian brains. J Comp Neurol 145:209, 1972

142. Gillilan LA: Anatomy and embryology of the arterial system of the brain stem and cerebellum. p. 24. In Vinken PJ, Bruyn GW (ed): Handbook of Clinical Neurology. Vol. 2. North-Holland, Amsterdam, 1972

143. Gillilan LA: Blood supply to brains of ungulates with and without a rete mirabile caroticum. J Comp Neurol 153:275, 1974

144. Gillilan LA: Extra- and intra-cranial blood supply to brains of dog and cat. Am J Anat 146:237, 1976

145. Goldberg HI: The anterior choroidal artery. p. 1628. In Newton TH, Potts DG (eds): Radiology of the Skull and Brain. CV Mosby, St. Louis, 1974

146. Goldstein SJ, Lee C, Young AB et al: Aplasia of the cervical internal carotid artery and malformation of the circle of Willis associated with Klippel-Trenaunay syndrome. Case report. J Neurosurg 61:786, 1984

147. Gomes F, Dujovny M, Umansky F et al: Microsurgical anatomy of the recurrent artery of Heubner. J Neurosurg 60:130, 1984

148. Gomes F, Dujovny M, Umansky F et al: Microanatomy of the anterior cerebral artery. Surg Neurol 26:129, 1986

148a. Goodrich ES: On the classification of the reptilia. Proc Roy Soc Lond [Biol] 615:261, 1916

149. Goulao A, Mauricio JC: A case of persistent hypoglossal intersegmental artery: Angiographic and CT study. Neuroradiology 29:102, 1987

150. Gould SJ: Ontogeny and Phylogeny. Belknap-Harvard, Cambridge, MA, 1977

151. Gove PB (ed): Webster's Seventh New Collegiate Dictionary. G&C Merriam, Springfield, MA, 1970

152. Grand W: Microsurgical anatomy of the proximal middle cerebral artery and the internal carotid artery bifurcation. Neurosurgery 7:215, 1980

153. Gray PA: The cortical lamination pattern of the opposum, *Didelphys virginiana.* J Comp Neurol 37:221, 1924

154. Grossman RI, Davis KR, Taveras JM: Circulatory variations of the ophthalmic artery. AJNR 3:327, 1982

155. Guérin J, Gouaze A, Lazorthes G: Le polygone de Willis de l'enfant et les facteurs de son modelage. Neurochirurgie 22:217, 1976

156. Guillaume J, Jauzac P, Roulleau J: Artère trigeminée primitive. A propos de six observations. Ann Radiol (Paris) 22:522, 1979

157. Guinto FC, Garrabrant EC, Radcliffe WB: Radiology of the persistent stapedial artery. Radiology 105:365, 1972

158. Hackett ER, Wilson CB: Congenital external carotid-vertebral anastomosis. A case report. AJR 104:86, 1968

159. Hamilton WJ, Boyd JD, Massman HW: Human Embryology. Williams & Wilkins, Baltimore, 1952, p. 159, 315

160. Handa J, Matsuda I, Nakasu S et al: Agenesis of an internal carotid artery: Angiographic, tomographic and computed tomographic correlation. Neuroradiology 19:207, 1980

161. Handa J, Matsuda M, Handa H: Lateral position of the external carotid artery. Report of case. Radiology 102:361, 1972

162. Handa J, Teraura T, Imai T et al: Agenesis of the corpus callosum associated with multiple developmental anomalies of the cerebral arteries. Radiology 92:1301, 1969

163. Hanson MR, Price RL, Rothner AD et al: Developmental anomalies of the optic disc and carotid circulation. A new association. J Clin Neuro Ophthalmol 5:3, 1985

164. Hara N, Koike T, Akiyama K et al: Anomalous origin of anterior choroidal artery. Neuroradiology 31:88, 1989

165. Hardy DG, Peace DA, Rhoton AL: Microsurgical anatomy of the superior cerebellar artery. J Neurosurgery 6:10, 1980

166. Harris FS, Rhoton AL: Anatomy of the cavernous sinus. A microsurgical study. J Neurosurg 45:169, 1976

167. Hasegawa T, Ito H, Hwang WZ et al: Single extracranial-intracranial duplication of the vertebral artery. Surg Neurol 25:369, 1986

168. Hasegawa T, Kashihara K, Haruhide I et al: Fenestration of the internal carotid artery. Surg Neurol 23:391, 1985

169. Hasegawa T, Kubota T, Ito H et al: Symptomatic duplication of the vertebral artery. Surg Neurol 20:244, 1983

170. Hasegawa T, Ravens JR, Toole JF: Precapillary arteriovenous anastomoses: "Thoroughfare channels" in the brain. Arch Neurol 16:217, 1967

171. Hashimoto H, Ohnishi H, Yuasa T et al: Duplicate origin of the vertebral artery: Report of two cases. Neuroradiology 29:301, 1987

172. Hassler W, Zenter J, Voigt K: Abnormal origin of the ophthalmic artery from the anterior cerebral artery: Neuroradiological and intraoperative findings. Neuroradiology 31:85, 1989

173. Hasso AN, Bentson JR, Wilson GH et al: Neuroradiology of the sphenoidal region. Radiology 114:619, 1975

174. Haughton VM, Rosenbaum AE, Pearce J: Internal carotid artery origins of the inferior cerebellar arteries. AJR 130:1191, 1978

175. Havelius U, Hindfelt B: Minor vessels leaving the extracranial internal carotid artery. Possible clinical implications. J Clin Neuro Ophthalmol 5:51, 1985

176. Hawkins TD: The collateral anastomoses in cerebrovascular occlusion. Clin Radiol 17:203, 1966

177. Hayreh SS: The ophthalmic artery. Normal gross anatomy. p. 1333. In Newton EH, Potts DG (ed): Radiology of the Skull and Brain. CV Mosby, St Louis, 1974

178. Herrick CJ: The morphology of the forebrain in amphibia and reptilia. J Comp Neurol 20:413, 1910

179. Heuser CH: The branchial vessels and their derivatives in the pig. Contrib Embryol 15:121, 1923

180. Higashida RT, Halbach VV, Mehringer CM et al: Giant cavernous aneurysm associated with trigeminal artery: Treatment by detachable balloon. AJNR 8:757, 1987

181. Hinck VC, Gordy PD: Persistent primitive trigeminal artery. One type of persistent carotid-basilar anastomosis. Radiology 83:41, 1964

182. Hoffman HB, Margolis MT, Newton TH: The superior cerebellar artery. Normal gross and radiographic anatomy. p. 1809. In Newton TH, Potts DG (eds): Radiology of the Skull and Brain. CV Mosby, St. Louis, 1974

183. Hogg ID, Stephens CB, Arnold GE: Theoretical anomalies of the stapedial artery. Ann Otol Rhinol Laryngol 81:860, 1972

184. Howard D: The internal carotid artery in relation to middle ear surgery. Clin Otolaryngol 7:381, 1982

185. Hoyt WF, Newton TH, Margolis MT: The posterior cerebral artery. Embryology and developmental anomalies. p. 1540. In Newton TH, Potts DG (eds): Radiology of the Skull and Brain. CV Mosby, St. Louis, 1974

186. Huber G: Intracranial carotid anastomosis and partial aplasia of an internal carotid artery. Neuroradiology 20:207, 1980

187. Hutchinson NA, Miller JDR: Persistent proatlantal artery. J Neurol Neurosurg Psychiatry 33:524, 1970

188. Hyyppa SE, Laasonen EM, Halonen V: Erosion of cervical vertebrae caused by elongated and tortuous vertebral arteries. Neuroradiology 7:49, 1974

189. Inoue T, Rhoton AL, Theele D et al: Surgical approaches to the cavernous sinus: A microsurgical study. Neurosurgery 26:903, 1990

190. Isherwood I, Dutton J: Unusual anomaly of anterior cerebral artery. Acta Radiol 9:345, 1969

191. Ito J, Maeda H, Inoue K et al: Fenestration of the middle cerebral artery. Neuroradiology 13:37, 1977

192. Ito J, Takeda N, Suzuki Y et al: Anomalous origin of the anterior inferior cerebellar arteries from the internal carotid artery. Neuroradiology 19:105, 1980

193. Ito J, Washiyama K, Kim CH et al: Fenestration of the anterior cerebral artery. Neuroradiology 21:277, 1981

194. Jain K: Some observations on the anatomy of the middle cerebral artery. Can J Surg 7:134, 1964

195. Janicki PC, Limbacher JP, Guinto FC: Agenesis of the internal carotid artery with a primitive transsellar communicating artery. AJR 132:130, 1979

196. Jayaraman A, Garofalo M, Brinker RA et al: Cerebral arteriovenous malformation and the primitive trigeminal artery. Arch Neurol 34:96, 1977

197. Jewell PA: The anastomoses between internal and external carotid circulations in the dog. J Anat 86:83, 1952

198. Johnson DM, Hopkins RJ, Hanafee WN et al: The unprotected parasphenoidal carotid artery studied by high-resolution computed tomography. Radiology 155:137, 1985

199. Kamijyo Y, Garcia JH: Carotid arterial supply of the feline brain. Applications to the study of regional cerebral ischemia. Stroke 6:361, 1975

200. Kaplan HA: Embryology and anatomy of the blood vessels of the brain. p. 5. In Fields WS (ed): Pathogenesis and Treatment of Cerebrovascular Disease. Charles C Thomas, Springfield, IL, 1961

201. Kaplan HA: The lateral perforating branches of the anterior and middle cerebral arteries. J Neurosurg 23:305, 1965

202. Kaplan HA, Ford DH: The Brain Vascular System. American Elsevier Publishing, New York, 1966

203. Karasawa J, Kikuchi H, Furuse S et al: Bilateral persistent carotid-basilar anastomoses. AJR 127:1053, 1976

204. Kayembe KNT, Sasahara M, Hazama F: Cerebral aneurysms and variations in the circle of Willis. Stroke 15:846, 1984

205. Keller HM, Imhof HG, Valavanis A: Persistent cervical intersegmental artery as a cause of recurrence of a traumatic carotid-cavernous fistula: Case report, with emphasis on Doppler ultrasound diagnosis. Neurosurgery 10:492, 1982

206. Kelly AB: Tortuosity of the internal carotid artery in relation to the pharynx. J Laryngol Otol 40:15, 1925

207. Kempe LG, Smith DR: Trigeminal neuralgia, facial spasm, intermedius and glossopharyngeal neuralgia with persistent carotid basilar anastomosis. J Neurosurg 31:445, 1969

208. Kennedy JC, Taplin GV: Shunting in cerebral microcirculation. Am Surg 33:763, 1967

209. Kent GC: Comparative Anatomy of the Vertebrates. CV Mosby, St. Louis, 1983, p. 451

210. Kessler L: Unusual anomaly of the anterior cerebral artery. Arch Neurol 36:509, 1979

211. Khodadad G: Persistent trigeminal artery in the fetus. Radiology 121:653, 1976

212. Khodadad G: Trigeminal artery and occlusive cerebrovascular disease. Stroke 8:177, 1977

213. Khodadad G: Persistent hypoglossal artery in the fetus. Acta Anat (Basel) 99:477, 1977b

214. Kier EL: The fetal cerebral arteries: A phylogenetic and ontogenetic study. p. 1089. In Newton TH, Potts DG (eds): Radiology of the Skull and Brain. CV Mosby, St. Louis, 1974

215. Kier EL: The cerebral ventricles: A phylogenetic and ontogenetic study. p. 2787. In Newton TH, Potts DG (eds): Radiology of the Skull and Brain. CV Mosby, St. Louis, 1977

216. Kier EL: Comparative anatomy of the third ventricular region. p. 37. In Apuzzo MLJ (ed): Surgery of the Third Ventricle. Williams & Wilkins, Baltimore, 1987

217. Killien FC, Wyler AR, Cromwell LD: Duplication of the internal carotid artery. Neuroradiology 19:101, 1980

218. Klosovskii BN: The Development of the Brain and its Disturbance by Harmful Factors. MacMillan, New York, 1963

219. Kluge AG, Frye BE, Johansen K et al: Chordate Structure and Function. Macmillan, New York, 1977

220. Korosue K, Kuwamura K, Okuda Y et al: Saccular aneurysm arising from a fenestrated anterior cerebral artery. Surg Neurol 19:273, 1983

221. Kowada M, Takahashi M, Gito Y et al: Fenestration of the vertebral artery: Report of 2 cases demonstrated by angiography. Neuroradiology 6:110, 1973

222. Kowada M, Yamaguchi K, Takahashi H: Fenestration of the vertebral artery with a review of 23 cases in Japan. Radiology 103:343, 1972

223. Krayenbuhl H, Yasargil MG, Huber P: Cerebral Angiography. Thieme, Stuttgart, 1982, p. 36

224. Kuban KCK, Gilles FH: Human telencephalic angiogenesis. Ann Neurol 17:539, 1985

225. Kunishio K, Yamamoto Y, Sunami N et al: Agenesis of the left internal carotid artery, common carotid artery, and main trunk of the external carotid artery associated with multiple cerebral aneurysms. Surg Neurol 27:177, 1987

226. Kwak R, Kadoya S: Moyamoya disease associated with persistent primitive trigeminal artery. Report of two cases. J Neurosurg 59:166, 1983

227. Kwak S, Nagashima T, Kobayashi S: Anomalous origin of the posterior meningeal artery from the internal carotid artery. Neuroradiology 19:103, 1980

228. Lasjaunias P: Craniofacial and Upper Cervical Arteries. Williams & Wilkins, Baltimore, 1981

229. Lasjaunias P, Berenstein A: Surgical Neuroangiography. Vol. 1. Functional Anatomy of Craniofacial Arteries. Springer-Verlag, Berlin, 1987, pp. 1, 245

230. Lasjaunias P, Berenstein A: Surgical Neuroangiography. Vol. 3. Functional Vascular Anatomy of Brain, Spinal Cord and Spine. Springer-Verlag, Berlin, 1990, p. 89

231. Lasjaunias P, Braun JP, Hasso AN et al: True and false fenestration of the vertebral artery. J Neuroradiol 7:157, 1980

232. Lasjaunias P, Manelfe C, Roche A et al: Segmental aplasia of the basilar artery in man. J Neuroradiol 6:127, 1979

233. Lasjaunias P, Moret J: The ascending pharyngeal artery: Normal and pathological radioanatomy. Neuroradiology 11:77, 1976

234. Lasjaunias P, Moret J: Normal and non-pathological variations in the angiographic aspects of the arteries of the middle ear. Neuroradiology 15:213, 1978

235. Lasjaunias P, Moret J, Doyon D et al: Collaterales C5 du siphon carotidien: Embryologie, correlations radio-anatomiques, radio-anatomie pathologique. Neuroradiology 16:304, 1978

236. Lasjaunias P, Moret J, Manelfe C et al: Arterial anomalies at the base of the skull. Neuroradiology 13:267, 1977

237. Lasjaunias P, Moret J, Mink J: The anatomy of the inferolateral trunk (ILT) of the internal carotid artery. Neuroradiology 13:215, 1977

238. Lasjaunias P, Santoyo-Vasquez A: Segmental agenesis of the internal carotid artery: Angiographic aspects with embryological discussion. Anat Clin 6:133, 1984

239. Lasjaunias P, Theron J: Radiographic anatomy of the accessory meningeal artery. Radiology 121:99, 1976

240. Lasjaunias P, Theron J, Moret J: The occipital artery. Anatomy, normal arteriographic aspects, embryologic structure. Neuroradiology 15:31, 1978

241. Lasjaunias P, Vignaud J, Hasso AN: Maxillary artery blood supply to the orbit: Normal and pathological aspects. Neuroradiology 9:87, 1975

242. Lazar ML, Bland JE, North RR et al: Middle cerebral artery fenestration. Neurosurgery 6:297, 1980

243. Lazorthes G: Vascularisation et Circulation Cerebrales. Masson, Paris, 1961

244. Lazorthes G, Gouaze A, Santini JJ et al: Le modelage du polygone de Willis. Role des compressions des voiess artérielles d'apport dans les mouvements de la colonne cervicale et de l'extremité céphalique. Neurochirurgie 17:361, 1971

245. Lazorthes G, Gouaze A, Santini JJ et al: The arterial circle of the brain (circulus arteriosus cerebri). Anat Clin 1:241, 1979

246. Lazorthes G, Salamon G: The arteries of the thalamus: An anatomical and radiological study. J Neurosurg 34:23, 1971

247. Lazorthes G, Salamon G: Etudes anatomique et radio-anatomique de la vascularisation artérielle du thalamus. Ann Radiol (Paris) 14:11, 1971

248. Leeds NE: The striate (lenticulostriate) arteries and the artery of Heubner. p. 1527. In Newton TH, Potts DG (ed): Radiology of the Skull and Brain. CV Mosby, St. Louis, 1974

249. Legre J, Tapias PL, Nardin JY et al: Embryonic inter-

segmental anastomosis between the external carotid and vertebral arteries. J Neuroradiol 7:97, 1980

250. Lehrer HZ: Relative calibre of the cervical internal carotid artery. Normal variation with the circle of Willis. Brain 91:339, 1968

251. Leipzig TJ, Dohrmann GJ: The tortuous or kinked carotid artery: Pathogenesis and clinical considerations. A historical review. Surg Neurol 25:478, 1986

252. LeMay M, Gooding CA: The clinical significance of the azygos anterior cerebral artery (A.C.A.). AJNR 98:602, 1966

253. Lemire RJ, Loeser JD, Leech RW et al: Normal and Abnormal Development of the Human Nervous System. Harper & Row, Hagerstown, MD, 1975

254. Lesem WW: The comparative anatomy of the anterior cerebral artery. Post-Graduate 20:455, 1905

255. Lewis OJ: The form and development of the blood vessels of the mammalian cerebral cortex. J Anat 91:40, 1957

256. Lewis VL, Cail WS: Persistent trigeminal artery with internal carotid artery occlusion. Neurosurgery 13:314, 1983

257. Lie TA: Congenital Anomalies of the Carotid Arteries. Excerpta Medica Foundation, Amsterdam, 1968

258. Lightfoote JB, Grusd RS, Nalls G: Azygos anterior cerebral artery mimicking an anterior communicating artery aneurysm. AJNR 10:S72, 1989

259. Lin JP, Kricheff II: Normal anterior cerebral artery complex. p. 1391. In Newton TH, Potts DG (eds): Radiology of the Skull and Brain. CV Mosby, St. Louis, 1974

260. Lindsey RW, Piepmeier J, Burkus JK: Tortuosity of the vertebral artery: An adventitious finding after cervical trauma. A case report. J Bone Joint Surg [Am] 67:806, 1985

261. Lippert H, Pabst R: Arterial Variations in Man. Classification and Frequency. JF Bergmann, Munich, 1985

262. Lister JR, Rhoton AL, Matsushima T et al: Microsurgical anatomy of the posterior inferior cerebellar artery. Neurosurgery 10:170, 1982

263. Lo WWM, Solti-Bohman LG, McElveen JT: Aberrant carotid artery: Radiologic diagnosis with emphasis on high-resolution computed tomography. Radiographics 5:985, 1985

264. Lui CC, Liu YH, Wai YY et al: Persistence of both proatlantal arteries with absence of vertebral arteries. Neuroradiology 29:304, 1987

265. Mall FP: On the development of the blood-vessels of the brain in the human embryo. Am J Anat 4:1, 1905

266. Manasek FJ: The ultrastructure of embryonic myocardial blood vessels. Dev Biol 26:42, 1971

267. Manelfe C, Tremoulet M, Roulleau J: Etude arteriographique des branches intracaverneuses de la carotide interne. Neurochirurgie 18:581, 1972

268. Manelfe C, Tremoulet M, Roulleau J: Les collaterales intracaverneuses de la carotide interne. 2. etude angiographique. Ann Radiol (Paris) 17:267, 1974

269. Marano GD, Horton JA, Gabriele OF: Persistent embryologic vascular loop of the internal carotid, middle meningeal, and ophthalmic arteries. Radiology 141:409, 1981

270. Margolis MT, Newton TH: The posterior inferior cerebellar artery. p. 1710. In Newton TH, Potts DG (eds): Radiology of the Skull and Brain. CV Mosby, St. Louis, 1974

271. Margolis MT, Newton TH: Collateral pathways between the cavernous portion of the internal carotid and external carotid arteries. Radiology 93:834, 1969

272. Margolis MT, Newton TH, Hoyt WF: The posterior cerebral artery. Gross and roentgenographic anatomy. p. 1551. In Newton TH, Potts DG (eds): Radiology of the Skull and Brain. CV Mosby, St. Louis, 1974

273. Marin-Padilla M: Early vascularization of the embryonic cerebral cortex: Golgi and electron microscopic studies. J Comp Neurol 241:237, 1985

274. Marin-Padilla M: Embryology. p. 23. In Yasargil MG (ed): Microneurosurgery. Vol. IIIA. Stuttgart, Thieme, 1987

275. Marinkovic S, Milisavljevic M, Kovacevic M: Anatomical bases for surgical approach to the initial segment of the anterior cerebral artery. Microanatomy of Heubner's artery and perforating branches of the anterior cerebral artery. Surg Radiol Anat 8:7, 18, 1986

276. Marinkovic S, Milisavljevic M, Kovacevic M: Interpeduncular perforating branches of the posterior cerebral artery. Surg Neurol 26:349, 1986

277. Marinkovic SV, Kovacevic MS, Marinkovic JM: Perforating branches of the middle cerebral artery. Microsurgical anatomy of their extracerebral segments. J Neurosurg 63:266, 1985

278. Martin RG, Grant JL, Peace D et al: Microsurgical relationships of the anterior inferior cerebellar artery and the facial-vestibulocochlear nerve complex. Neurosurgery 6:483, 1980

279. Marx F: An arteriographic demonstration of collaterals between internal and external carotid arteries. Acta Radiol 31:155–160, 1949

280. Matsumura M, Nojiri K, Yumoto Y: Persistent primitive hypoglossal artery associated with Arnold-Chiari type I malformation. Surg Neurol 24:241, 1985

281. Matsumura M, Wada H, Nojiri K: Persistent primitive trigeminal artery, cavum septi pellucidi, and associated cerebral aneurysm in a patient with polycystic kidney disease: Case report. Neurosurgery 16:395, 1985

282. Mayer PL, Kier EL: The controversy of the periventricular white matter circulation: A review of the anatomic literature. AJNR 12:223, 1991

283. McConnell EM: The arterial blood supply of the human hypophysis cerebri. Anat Rec 115:175, 1953

284. McCormick W: A unique anomaly of the intracranial arteries of man. Neurology 19:77, 1969

285. McElveen JT, Lo WWM, El Gabri TH et al: Aberrant internal carotid artery: Classic findings on computed

tomography. Otolaryngol Head Neck Surg 94:616, 1986

286. McFarland WL, Jacobs MS, Morgane PJ: Blood supply to the brain of the dolphin, *Tursiops truncatus*, with comparative observations of special aspects of the cerebrovascular supply of other vertebrates. Neurosci Biobehav Rev 3:suppl 1, 1979

287. McKenzie W, Woolf CI: Carotid abnormalities and adenoid surgery. J Laryngol Otol 73:596, 1929

288. McLennan JE, Rosenbaum AE, Haughton VM: Internal carotid origins of the middle meningeal artery. The ophthalmic-middle meningeal and stapedial-middle meningeal arteries. Neuroradiology 7:265, 1974

289. Merry GS, Jamieson KG: Operative approach to persistent trigeminal artery producing facial pain and diplopia. J Neurosurg 47:613, 1977

290. Michoty P, Moscow NP, Salamon G: Anatomy of the cortical branches of the middle cerebral artery. p. 1471. In Newton TH, Potts DG (eds): Radiology of the Skull and Brain. CV Mosby, St. Louis, 1974

291. Milenkovic Z: Anastomosis between internal carotid artery and anterior cerebral artery with other anomalies of the circle of Willis in a fetal brain. J Neurosurg 55:701, 1981

292. Milenkovic Z, Vucetic R, Puzic M: Asymmetry and anomalies of the circle of Willis in fetal brain. Microsurgical study and functional remarks. Surg Neurol 24:563, 1985

293. Minakawa T, Kawamata M, Hayano M et al: Aneurysms associated with fenestrated anterior cerebral arteries. Report of four cases and review of the literature. Surg Neurol 24:284, 1985

294. Miyachi S, Negoro M, Sugita K: The occipital-vertebral anastomosis as a collateral pathway: hemodynamic patterns. Case report. Surg Neurol 32:350, 1989

295. Mizukami M, Tomita T, Mine T et al: Bypass anomaly of the vertebral artery associated with cerebral aneurysm and arteriovenous malformation. J Neurosurg 37:204, 1972

296. Moffat DB: The development of the hind-brain arteries in the rat. J Anat 91:25, 1957

297. Moffat DB: Developmental changes in the aortic arch system of the rat. Am J Anat 105:1, 1959

298. Moffat DB: The embryology of the arteries of the brain. Ann R Coll Surg Engl 30:368, 1962

299. Moody DM, Bell MA, Challa VR: Features of the cerebral vascular pattern that predict vulnerability to perfusion or oxygenation deficiency: An anatomic study. AJNR 11:431, 1990

300. Moore KL: Clinically Oriented Anatomy. Williams & Wilkins, Baltimore, 1980

301. Moore TS, Morris JL: Aortic arch vessel anomalies associated with persistent trigeminal artery. AJR 133:309, 1979

302. Moret J, Delvert JD, Lasjaunias P: Blood supply of the ear and cerebellopontine angle. Vascular territories of the tympanic cavity. J Neuroradiol 9:215, 1982

303. Moret J, Delvert JC, Lasjaunias P: "Abnormal" vessels in the middle ear. J Neuroradiol 9:227, 1982

304. Moret J, Lasjaunias P, Theron J et al: The middle meningeal artery. Its contribution to the vascularisation of the orbit. J Neuroradiol 4:225, 1977

305. Morita A, Fukushima T, Miyazaki S et al: Tic douloureux caused by primitive trigeminal artery or its variant. J Neurosurg 70:415, 1989

306. Morris ED, Moffat DB: Abnormal origin of the basilar artery from the cervical part of the internal carotid and its embryological significance. Anat Rec 125:701, 1956

307. Mosmans PCM, Jonkmam EJ: The significance of the collateral vascular system of the brain in shunt and steal syndromes. Clin Neurol Neurosurg 82:145, 1980

308. Moyes PD: Basilar aneurysm associated with agenesis of the left internal carotid artery. J Neurosurg 30:608, 1969

309. Mueller RL, Hinck VC: Thyrocervical steal. AJR 101:128, 1967

310. Murayama Y, Fujimoto N, Matsumoto K: Bilateral persistent primitive hypoglossal arteries associated with a large ruptured aneurysm on one side. Surg Neurol 24:498, 1985

311. Murotani K, Hiramoto M: Agenesis of the internal carotid artery with a large hemangioma of the tongue. Neuroradiology 27:357, 1985

312. Nager GT, Nager M: The arteries of the human middle ear, with particular regard to the blood supply of the auditory ossicles. Ann Otol Rhinol Laryngol 62:923, 1953

313. Naidich TP, Kricheff II, George AE et al: The normal anterior inferior cerebellar artery. Anatomic-radiographic correlation with emphasis of the lateral projection. Radiology 119:355, 1976

314. Nelson MD, Gonzalez-Gomez I, Gilles FH: The search for human telencephalic ventriculofugal arteries. AJNR 12:215, 1991

315. Newton TH, Mani RL: The vertebral artery. p. 1659. In Newton TH, Potts DG (eds): Radiology of the Skull and Brain. CV Mosby, St. Louis, 1974

316. Newton TH, Potts DG (eds): Radiology of the Skull and Brain. CV Mosby, St. Louis, 1974

317. Newton TH, Young DA: Anomalous origin of the occipital artery from the internal carotid artery. Radiology 90:550, 1968

318. Nezu N, Ninchoji T, Kitanaka H et al: A case of congenital absence of the left internal carotid artery. Comput Med Imaging Graph 8:355, 1984

319. Nielsen PB, Jonson M: Persistent primitive trigeminal artery demonstrated by vertebral arteriography. AJR 101:47, 1967

320. Nierling DA, Wollschlaeger PB, Wollschlaeger G: Ascending pharyngeal-vertebral anastomosis. AJR 98:599, 1966

321. Nuza AB, Taner D: Anatomical variations of the intracavernous branches of the internal carotid artery with reference to the relationship of the internal ca-

rotid artery and sixth cranial nerve. A microsurgical study. Acta Anat (Basel) 138:238, 1990

322. Obayashi T, Furuse M, Tanaka O et al: Tortuous vertebral artery simulating extradural spinal tumor. Neurochirurgia (Stuttg) 29:96, 1986

323. Odake G: Carotid-anterior cerebral artery anastomosis with aneurysm: Case report and review of the literature. Neurosurgery 23:654, 1988

324. Olivier A, Scotti G, Melancon D: Vascular entrapment of the hypoglossal nerve in the neck. Case report. J Neurosurg 47:472, 1977

325. O'Rahilly R: Developmental Stages in Human Embryos. Part A. Embryos of the First Three Weeks (Stages 1 to 9). Carnegie Institution, Washington, 1973

326. Osguthorpe JD, Adkins WY, Putney FJ et al: Internal carotid artery as source of tonsillectomy and adenoidectomy hemorrhage. Otolaryngol Head Neck Surg 89:758, 1981

327. Padget DH: The circle of Willis. Its embryology and anatomy. p. 67. In Dandy WE (ed): Intracranial Arterial Aneurysms. Comstock, Ithaca, NY, 1944

328. Padget DH: The development of the cranial arteries in the human embryo. Contrib Embryol 32:205, 1948

329. Padget DH: Designation of the embryonic intersegmental arteries in reference to the vertebral artery and subclavian stem. Anat Rec 119:349, 1954

330. Pakula H, Szapiro J: Anatomical studies of the collateral blood supply to the brain and upper extremity. J Neurosurg 32:171, 1970

331. Palmer FJ: Origin of the right vertebral artery from the right common carotid: Angiographic demonstration of three cases. Br J Radiol 50:185, 1977

332. Palmer FJ, Philips RL: Persistent proatlantal artery arising from the common carotid bifurcation. Aust Radiol 22:226, 1978

333. Palmer S, Gucer G: Vertebrobasilar insufficiency from carotid disease associated with a trigeminal artery. Neurosurgery 8:458, 1981

334. Pape KE, Wigglesworth JS: Hemorrhage, Ischemia and the Perinatal Brain. Spastics International Medical Publications, JB Lippincott, Philadelphia, 1979, p. 11

335. Papez JW: Comparative Neurology. Thomas Y. Crowell, New York, 1929, pp. 80, 457

336. Parkinson D: Collateral circulation of cavernous carotid artery: Anatomy. Can J Surg 7:251, 1964

337. Parkinson D, Reddy V, Ross RT: Congenital anastomosis between the vertebral artery and internal carotid artery in the neck. Case report. J Neurosurg 51:697, 1979

338. Parkinson D, Shields CB: Persistent trigeminal artery: Its relationship to the normal branches of the cavernous carotid. J Neurosurg 39:244, 1974

339. Pascaud JL, Vigneu P, Hummel P et al: Absence partielle de carotide interne avec anastomose intercarotidenne trans-sellaire. Nouvelle observation et revue de la littérature. J Radiol 63:37, 1982

340. Paullus WS, Pait TG, Rhoton AL: Microsurgical exposure of the petrous portion of the carotid artery. J Neurosurg 47:713, 1977

341. Pedroza A, Dujovny M, Artero J et al: Microanatomy of the posterior communicating artery. Neurosurgery 20:228, 1987

342. Pedroza A, Dujovny M, Cabezudo-Artero J et al: Microanatomy of the premamillary artery. Acta Neurochir (Wien) 86:50, 1987

343. Penning L: Functional Pathology of the Cervical Spine. Williams & Wilkins, Baltimore, 1968, p. 50

344. Perlmutter D, Rhoton A: Microsurgical anatomy of the anterior cerebral-anterior communicating-recurrent artery complex. J Neurosurg 45:259, 1976

345. Perryman CR, Gray GH, Brust RW et al: Interesting aspects of cerebral angiography with emphasis on some unusual congenital variations. AJR 89:372, 1963

346. Pinkerton JA, Davidson KC, Hibbard BZ: Primitive hypoglossal artery and carotid endarterectomy. Stroke 11:658, 1980

347. Presley R: The primitive course of the internal carotid artery in mammals. Acta Anat (Basel) 103:238, 1979

348. Priman J, Christie DH: A case of abnormal internal carotid artery and associated vascular anomalies. Anat Rec 134:87, 1959

349. Puchades-Orts A, Nombela-Gomez M, Ortuno-Pacheco G: Variation in form of circle of Willis: Some anatomical and embryological considerations. Anat Rec 185:119, 1976

350. Quencer RM, Simon J: Transient bilateral occipital lobe ischemia: Microembolization through a trigeminal artery. Neuroradiology 18:273, 1979

351. Quint DJ: Boulos RS, Spera TD: Congenital absence of the cervical and petrous internal carotid artery with intercavernous anastomosis. AJNR 10:435, 1989

352. Quisling RG: Intrapetrous carotid artery branches: Pathological application. Radiology 134:109, 1980

353. Quisling RG, Rhoton AL: Intrapetrous carotid artery branches: Radioanatomic analysis. Radiology 131:133, 1979

354. Quisling RG, Seeger JF: Ascending pharyngeal artery collateral circulation simulating internal carotid artery hypoplasia. Neuroradiology 18:277, 1979

355. Rao TS, Sethi PK: Persistent proatlantal artery with carotid-vertebral anastomosis. J Neurosurg 43:499, 1975

356. Reilly JJ, Caparosa RJ, Latchaw RE et al: Aberrant carotid artery injured at myringotomy. Control of hemorrhage by a balloon catheter. JAMA 249:1473, 1983

357. Resche F, Resche-Perrin I, Robert R et al: The hypoglossal artery. A new case report. Review of the literature. J Neuroradiol 7:27, 1980

358. Rhoton AL, Fujii K, Fradd B: Microsurgical anatomy of the anterior choroidal artery. Surg Neurol 12:171, 1979

359. Rieger P, Huber G: Fenestration and duplicate origin of the left vertebral artery in angiography. Report of three cases. Neuroradiology 25:45, 1983

360. Riggs HE, Rupp C: Variation in form of circle of Willis. Arch Neurol 8:8, 1963

361. Ring BA: Normal middle cerebral artery. p. 1442. In Newton TH, Potts DG (eds): Radiology of the Skull and Brain. CV Mosby, St. Louis, 1974

362. Robbins JP, Fitz-Hugh GS, Craddock WD: Arterial collateralization after common carotid ligation. Ann Otol Rhinol Laryngol 82:257, 1973

363. Roberts LK, Gerald B: Absence of both common carotid arteries. AJR 130:981, 1978

364. Robinson LR: An unusual human anterior cerebral artery. J Anat 93:131, 1959

365. Roman GC: Senile dementia of the Binswanger type: A vascular form of dementia in the elderly. JAMA 258:1782, 1987

366. Romer AS: The Vertebrate Body. WB Saunders, Philadelphia, 1970

367. Roofe PG: The endocranial blood vessels of *Amblystoma tigrinum.* J Comp Neurol 61:257, 1935

368. Rosenorn J, Ahlgren P, Ronde F: Pre-optic origin of the anterior cerebral artery. Neuroradiology 27:275, 1985

369. Rosner SS, Rhoton AL, Ono M et al: Microsurgical anatomy of the anterior perforating arteries. J Neurosurg 61:468, 1984

370. Rovira M, Jacas R, Ley A: The collateral circulation in thrombosis of the internal carotid artery and its branches. Acta Radiol 50:101, 1958

371. Royle G, Motson R: An anomalous origin of the middle meningeal artery. J Neurol Neurosurg Psychiatry 36:874, 1973

372. Ruysch F: Epistola Problematica. Amsterdam, 1696, plate 13

373. Sabin FR: Origin and development of the primitive vessels of the chick and of the pig. Contrib Embryol 6:61, 1917

374. Sabin FR: Preliminary note on the differentiation of angioblasts and the method by which they produce blood-vessels, blood-plasma and red blood-cells as seen in the living chick. Anat Rec 13:199, 1917

375. Sabin FR: Studies on the origin of blood-vessels and of red blood-corpuscles as seen in the living blastoderm of chicks during the second day of incubation. Contrib Embryol 36:213, 1920

376. Saeki N, Rhoton L: Microsurgical anatomy of the upper basilar artery and the posterior circle of Willis. J Neurosurg 46:563, 1977

377. Salamon G: Atlas of the Arteries of the Human Brain. Sandoz Editions, Paris, 1971

378. Salamon G, Faure J, Raybaud C et al: External carotid artery. I: Normal external carotid artery. p. 1246. In Newton TH, Potts DG (eds): Radiology of the Skull and Brain. CV Mosby, St. Louis, 1974

379. Saltzman GF: Patent primitive trigeminal artery studied by cerebral angiography. Acta Radiol 51:329, 1959

380. Samra K, Scoville WB, Yaghmai M: Anastomosis of carotid and basilar arteries. Persistent primitive trigeminal artery and hypoglossal artery: Report of two cases. J Neurosurg 30:622, 1969

381. Santini JJ, Laffont J, Gouaze A: Les collaterales intracaverneuses de la carotide interne. 1. Etude anatomique. Ann Radiol (Paris) 17:265, 1974

382. Sarnat HB, Campa JF, Lloyd JM: Inverse prominence of ependyma and capillaries in the spinal cord of vertebrates: A comparative histochemical study. J Anat 143:439, 1975

383. Sarnat HB, Netsky MG: Evolution of the Nervous System. Oxford University Press, New York, 1981

384. Saunders RLCH, Feindel WH, Carvalho VR: X-ray microscopy of the blood vessels of the human brain. Part 1. Med Biol Illus 15:108, 1965

385. Saunders RLCH, Feindel WH, Carvalho VR: X-ray microscopy of the blood vessels of the human brain. Part 2. Med Biol Illus 15:234, 1965

386. Scharrer E: Arteries and veins in the mammalian brain. Anat Rec 78:173, 1940

387. Schechter MM: The occipital-vertebral anastomosis. J Neurosurg 21:758, 1964

388. Schimmel DH, Newton TH, Mani J: Widening of the intervertebral foramen. Neuroradiology 12:3, 1976

389. Schmid AH: Persistent trigeminal artery. An autopsy report. Neuroradiology 7:173, 1974

390. Schnurer LB, Stattin S: Vascular supply of intracranial dura from internal carotid artery with special reference to its angiographic significance. Acta Radiol 1:441, 1963

391. Scialfa G, Ruggiero G, Salamon G et al: Post mortem investigation of the vertebrobasilar system. Acta Radiol Suppl (Stockh) 347:259, 1975

392. Scotti G: Anterior inferior cerebellar artery originating from the cavernous portion of the internal carotid artery. Radiology 116:93, 1975

393. Scotti G, Melancon D, Olivier A: Hypoglossal paralysis due to compression by a tortuous internal carotid artery in the neck. Neuroradiology 14:263, 1978

394. Seeger JF, Hemmer JF: Persistent basilar/middle meningeal artery anastomosis. Radiology 118:367, 1976

395. Senter HJ, Miller DJ: Interoptic course of the anterior cerebral artery associated with anterior cerebral artery aneurysm. J Neurosurg 56:302, 1982

396. Servo A: Agenesis of the left internal carotid artery associated with an aneurysm on the right carotid syphon. Case report. J Neurosurg 46:677, 1977

397. Shapiro R: Enlargement of the hypoglossal canal in the presence of a persistent hypoglossal artery. Radiology 133:395, 1979

398. Sheehy JP, Kendall BE, Thomas GT: Infraoptic course of the anterior cerebral artery associated with a pituitary tumor. Surg Neurol 20:97, 1983

399. Shellshear JL: The basal arteries of the forebrain and their functional significance. J Anat 55:27, 1920

400. Shellshear JL: The arteries of the brain of the orangutan. J Anat 61:167, 1927

401. Shellshear JL: A study of the arteries of the brain of the spiny anteater (*Echidna aculeata*) to illustrate the principles of arterial distribution. Philos Trans R Soc Lond [Biol] 218:1, 1929

402. Shellshear JL: The arterial supply of the cerebral cortex in the chimpanzee (*Anthropopithecus troglodytes*). J Anat 65:45, 1930

403. Shrontz C, Dujovny M, Ausman JI et al: Surgical anatomy of the arteries of the posterior fossa. J Neurosurg 65:540, 1986

404. Smith D, Larsen JL: On the symmetry and asymmetry of the bifurcation of the common carotid artery. A study of bilateral carotid angiograms in 100 adults. Neuroradiology 17:245, 1979

405. Smith GE: Some problems relating to the evolution of the brain. Lecture I. Lancet 1:1, 1910

406. Smith GE: Some problems relating to the evolution of the brain. Lecture II. Lancet 1:147, 1910

407. Smith GE: Some problems relating to the evolution of the brain. Lecture III. Lancet 1:221, 1910

408. Smith GE: A preliminary role on the morphology of the corpus striatum and the origin of the neopallium. J Anat 53:271, 1919

409. Smith RR, Kees CJ, Hogg ID: Agenesis of the internal carotid artery with an unusual primitive collateral. Case report. J Neurosurg 37:460, 1972

410. Sole-Llenas J, Planas M: Occipital-vertebral anastomosis in a case of middle cerebral artery occlusion. Neuroradiology 1:88, 1970

411. Springer TD, Fishbone G, Shapiro R: Persistent hypoglossal artery associated with superior cerebellar artery aneurysm. Case report. J Neurosurg 40:397, 1974

412. Stabler J: Two cases of accessory middle cerebral artery, including one with an aneurysm at its origin. Br J Radiol 43:314, 1970

413. Stahl BJ: Vertebrate History: Problems in Evolution. Dover, New York, 1985

414. Staples GS: Transsellar intracavernous intercarotid collateral artery associated with agenesis of the internal carotid artery. Case report. J Neurosurg 50:393, 1979

415. Stattin S: Meningeal vessels of the internal carotid artery and their angiographic significance. Acta Radiol 55:329, 1961

416. Steffen TD: Vascular anomalies of the middle ear. Laryngoscope 78:171, 1968

417. Stephens RB, Stilwell DL: Arteries and Veins of the Human Brain. Charles C Thomas, Springfield, IL, 1969

418. Stern J, Correll JW, Bryan N: Persistent hypoglossal artery and persistent trigeminal artery presenting with posterior fossa transient ischemic attacks. Report of two cases. J Neurosurg 49:614, 1978

419. Stopford JSB: The arteries of the pons and medulla oblongata. J Anat 50:131, 1916

420. Streeter GL: The developmental alterations in the vascular system of the brain of the human embryo. Contrib Embryol 8:5, 1918

421. Streeter GL, Heuser CH, Corner GW: Developmental horizons in human embryos: Age groups XI–XXIII. In Embryology Reprint. Carnegie Institute of Washington, DC, 1951

422. Strong LH: The early embryonic pattern of internal vascularization of the mammalian cerebral cortex. J Comp Neurol 123:121, 1964

423. Sutherland GR, Donaldson AA: Persistent hypoglossal artery complicated by internal carotid artery stenosis. Clin Radiol 23:222, 1972

424. Suzuki J, Mizoi K, Yoshimoto T: Bifrontal interhemispheric approach to aneurysms of the anterior communicating artery. J Neurosurg 64:183, 1986

425. Suzuki S, Nobechi T, Itoh I et al: Persistent proatlantal intersegmental artery and occipital artery originating from internal carotid artery. Neuroradiology 17:105, 1979

426. Swartz JD, Bazarnic ML, Naidich TP et al: Aberrant internal carotid artery lying within the middle ear. High resolution CT diagnosis and differential diagnosis. Neuroradiology 27:322, 1985

427. Szdzuy D, Lehmann R: Persistent trigeminal artery in vertebral angiography. Neuroradiology 2:100, 1971

428. Szdzuy D, Lehmann R: Hypoplastic distal part of the basilar artery. Neuroradiology 4:118, 1972

429. Szdzuy D, Lehmann R, Nickel B: Common trunk of the anterior cerebral arteries. Neuroradiology 4:51, 1972

430. Takahashi M: The basilar artery. p. 1775. In Newton TH, Potts DG (eds): Radiology of the Skull and Brain. CV Mosby, St. Louis, 1974

431. Takahashi M: The anterior inferior cerebellar artery. p. 1796. In Newton TH, Potts DG (eds): Radiology of the Skull and Brain. CV Mosby, St. Louis, 1974

432. Takahashi M, Arii H, Tamakawa Y: Anomalous arterial supply of temporal and occipital lobes by anterior choroidal artery: Angiographic study. AJNR 1:537, 1980

433. Takahashi M, Kawanami H, Watanabe N et al: Fenestration of the extracranial vertebral artery. Radiology 96:359, 1970

434. Takahashi M, Tamakawa Y, Kishikawa T et al: Fenestration of the basilar artery. Report of three cases and review of the literature. Radiology 109:79, 1973

435. Takahashi S, Hoshino F, Uemura K et al: Accessory middle cerebral artery: Is it a variant form of the recurrent artery of Heubner? AJNR 10:563, 1989

436. Takahashi S, Suga T, Kawata Y et al: Anterior choroidal artery: Angiographic analysis of variations and anomalies. AJNR 11:719, 1990

437. Takashima S, Armstrong DL, Becker LE: Subcortical leukomalacia. Arch Neurol 35:470, 1978

438. Takashima S, Tanaka K: Development of cerebrovascular architecture and its relationship to periventricular leukomalacia. Arch Neurol 35:11, 1978

439. Tanaka Y, Hara H, Momose G et al: Proatlantal intersegmental artery and trigeminal artery associated with an aneurysm. Case report. J Neurosurg 59:520, 1983

440. Tatelman M: Pathways of cerebral collateral circulation. Radiology 75:349, 1960

441. Teal JS, Naheedy MH, Hasso AN: Total agenesis of the internal carotid artery. AJNR 1:435, 1980

442. Teal JS, Rumbaugh CL, Bergeron RT et al: Persistent carotid-superior cerebellar artery anastomosis: A variant of persistent trigeminal artery. Radiology 103:335, 1972

443. Teal JS, Rumbaugh CL, Bergeron RT et al: Congenital absence of the internal carotid artery associated with cerebral hemiatrophy, absence of the external carotid artery, and persistence of the stapedial artery. AJR 118:534, 1973

444. Teal JS, Rumbaugh CL, Bergeron RT et al: Anomalies of the middle cerebral artery: Accessory artery, duplication, and early bifurcation. AJR 118:567, 1973

445. Teal JS, Rumbaugh CL, Bergeron RT et al: Angiographic demonstration of fenestrations of the intradural intracranial arteries. Radiology 106:123, 1973

446. Teal JS, Rumbaugh CL, Bergeron RT et al: Lateral position of the external carotid artery: A rare anomaly. Radiology 108:77, 1973

447. Teal JS, Rumbaugh CL, Segall HD et al: Anomalous branches of the internal carotid artery. Radiology 106:567, 1973

448. Theron J, Newton TH: Anterior choroidal artery: I. Anatomic and radiographic study. J Neuroradiol 3:5, 1976

449. Tilney F, Casamajor L: The development of the hemal channels in the central nervous system of the albino rat. Anat Rec 11:425, 1917

450. Tokuda K, Miyasaka K, Abe H et al: Anomalous atlantoaxial portions of vertebral and posterior inferior cerebellar arteries. Neuroradiology 27:410, 1985

451. Tomsick TA, Lukin RR, Chambers AA: Persistent trigeminal artery: Unusual associated abnormalities. Neuroradiology 17:253, 1979

452. Tran-Dinh H: Cavernous branches of the internal carotid artery: Anatomy and nomenclature. Neurosurgery 20:205, 1987

453. Tsai FY, Mahon J, Woodruff JV et al: Congenital absence of bilateral vertebral arteries with occipital-basilar anastomosis. AJR 124:281, 1975

454. Tsukamoto S, Hori Y, Utsumi S et al: Proatlantal intersegmental artery with absence of bilateral vertebral arteries. J Neurosurg 54:122, 1981

455. Tulleken CAF: A study of the anatomy of the anterior communicating artery with the aid of the operating microscope. Clin Neurol Neurosurg 80:169, 1978

456. Udzura M, Kobayashi H, Taguchi Y et al: Intrasellar intercarotid communicating artery associated with agenesis of the right internal carotid artery: Case report. Neurosurgery 23:770, 1988

457. Ueda T, Wakisaka G, Kinoshita K: Fenestrations of the middle cerebral artery associated with aneurysms. AJNR 5:639, 1984

458. Umansky F, Dujovny M, Ausman J et al: Anomalies and variations of the middle cerebral artery: A microanatomical study. Neurosurgery 22:1023, 1988

459. Umansky F, Gomes FB, Dujovny M et al: The perforating branches of the middle cerebral artery. J Neurosurg 62:261, 1985

460. Van den Bergh R: La vascularization artérielle intracérébrale. Acta Neurol Psychiatr Belg 61:1013, 1961

461. Van den Bergh R: Centrifugal elements in the vascular pattern of the deep intracerebral blood supply. Angiology 20:88, 1969

462. Van den Bergh R, vander Eecken H: Anatomy and embryology of cerebral circulation. Prog Brain Res 30:1, 1968

463. Van der Eecken HM: The Anastomoses between the Leptomeningeal Arteries of the Brain: Their Morphological, Pathological and Clinical Significance. Charles C Thomas, Springfield, IL, 1959

464. Van der Eecken HM, Adams R: The anatomy and functional significance of the meningeal arterial anastomoses of the human brain. J Neuropathol Exp Neurol 12:132, 1953

465. Vincentelli F, Caruso G, Grisoli F et al: Microsurgical anatomy of the cisternal course of the perforating branches of the posterior communicating artery. Neurosurgery 26:824, 1990

466. Vitek JJ, Reaves P: Thoracic bifurcation of the common carotid artery. Neuroradiology 5:133, 1973

467. Voris HC: The arterial supply of the brain and spinal cord of the Virginian opossum (*Didelphis virginiana*). J Comp Neurol 44:403, 1928

468. Wackenheim A: Asymetrie de la face et des artères vertébrales. A propos d'un cas de persistence unilaterale de l'artère hypoglosse. Acta Radiol 13:268, 1972

469. Waga S, Okada M, Yamamoto Y: Basilar-middle meningeal arterial anastomosis. Case report. J Neurosurg 49:450, 1978

470. Wakai S, Watanabe N, Inoh S et al: Agenesis of internal carotid artery presenting with oculomotor nerve palsy after minor head injury. Neurosurgery 20:794, 1987

471. Wake MH (ed): Hyman's Comparative Vertebrate Anatomy. University of Chicago Press, Chicago, 1979

472. Wallace S, Goldberg HI, Leeds NE et al: The cavernous branches of the internal carotid artery. AJR 101:34, 1967

473. Waller FT, Simons RL, Kerber C et al: Trigeminal artery and microemboli to the brain stem. Report of two cases. J Neurosurg 46:104, 1977

474. Wardwell GA, Goree JA, Jimenez JP: The hypoglossal artery and hypoglossal canal. AJR 118:528, 1973

475. Watanabe T, Togo M: Accessory middle cerebral artery. Report of four cases. J Neurosurg 41:248, 1974

476. Watts JW: A comparative study of the anterior cerebral artery and the circle of Willis in primates. J Anat 68:534, 1933

477. Weibel J, Fields WS: Tortuosity, coiling, and kinking of the internal carotid artery. I. Etiology and radiographic anatomy. Neurology 15:7, 1965

478. Weinberg PE, Patronas NJ, Kim KS et al: Anomalous

origin in the ophthalmic artery in a patient with amaurosis fugax. Arch Neurol 38:315, 1981

479. Wende S, Nakayama N, Schwerdtfeger P: The internal auditory artery (embryology, anatomy, angiography, pathology). J Neurol 210:21, 1975

480. Westberg G: The recurrent artery of Heubner and the arteries of the central ganglia. Acta Radiol 1:949, 1963

481. Wigglesworth JS, Pape KE: An integrated model for haemorrhagic and ischaemic lesions in the newborn brain. Early Hum Dev 2:179, 1978

482. Williams DJ: The origin of the posterior cerebral artery. Brain 59:175, 1936

483. Willinsky R, Lasjaunias P, Berenstein A: Intracavernous branches of the internal carotid artery (ICA). Comprehensive review of their variations. Surg Radiol Anat 9:201, 1987

484. Willis T: Cerebri anatomia nervorumque descriptio et usus. J Fletcher, London, 1684

485. Wismer GL: Circle of Willis variant analogous to fetal type primitive trigeminal artery. Neuroradiology 31:366, 1989

486. Wollschlaeger G, Wollschlaeger PB: The primitive trigeminal artery as seen angiographically and at postmortem examination. AJR 92:761, 1964

487. Wollschlaeger G, Wollschlaeger PB: The circle of Willis. p. 1171. In Newton TH, Potts DG (eds): Radiology of the Skull and Brain. CV Mosby, St. Louis, 1974

488. Wolpert SM: The trigeminal artery and associated aneurysms. Neurology 16:610, 1966

489. Worthington C, Olivier A, Melanson D: Internal carotid artery agenesis: Correlation by conventional and digital subtraction angiography, and by computed tomography. Surg Neurol 22:295, 1984

490. Yamada T, Inagawa T, Takeda T: Ruptured aneurysm at the anterior cerebral artery fenestration. Case report. J Neurosurg 57:826, 1982

491. Yamanaka C, Hirohata T, Yoshimoto H et al: Basilar bifurcation aneurysm associated with bilateral internal carotid occlusion. Neuroradiology 29:84, 1987

492. Yasargil MG: Microneurosurgery. Vol. 1. Thieme, Stuttgart, 1984

493. Yeh H, Heiss JD, Tew JM: Persistent hypoglossal artery associated with basilar artery aneurysm. Neurochirurgia (Stuttg) 30:158, 1987

494. Yock DH: Fenestration of the supraclinoid internal carotid artery with rupture of associated aneurysm. AJNR 5:634, 1984

495. Yonas H, Wolfson SK, Cook EE et al: Selective lenticulostriate arterial occlusion. A reproducible model of primate focal cerebral ischemia. Surg Neurol 25:545, 1986

496. Zeal AA, Rhoton AL: Microsurgical anatomy of the posterior cerebral artery. J Neurosurg 48:534, 1978

497. Zimmerman RD, Flemming CA, Lee BCP: Periventricular hyperintensity as seen by magnetic resonance: Prevalence and significance. AJNR 7:13, 1986

25 General Overview and Principles of Neurovascular Surgery

Thoralf M. Sundt, Jr.

Perhaps as is true with virtually all aspects of neurological surgery, 95 percent of how a patient recovers from an operative procedure is related to what takes place in the operating room. Neurovascular surgery is particularly unforgiving—there is no margin for error. In dealing with blood vessels running to and within the brain, surgeons should bear in mind that their major responsibilities are related to preservation of flow through major arteries; prevention of emboli; protection of vital perforating vessels; avoidance of severe brain retraction; adequate exposure of the pathology, whether intra- or extracranial; and protection of the brain from periods of ischemia during the operation itself. Neurovascular surgery can be conveniently divided into three categories: extracranial occlusive vascular disease, intracranial aneurysms, and bypass procedures for occlusive or hemorrhagic vascular disease. This chapter discusses the general principles outlined above in each of these three categories of operative procedures.

EXTRACRANIAL OCCLUSIVE VASCULAR DISEASE—CAROTID ENDARTERECTOMY

Indications

It is beyond the scope of this chapter to discuss in detail the indications for a carotid endarterectomy. However, to place in perspective the techniques that are discussed, it is necessary to refer to this aspect of the operation to provide a frame of reference for the prevention of complications and for their management.

The primary indication for a carotid endarterectomy is a transient ischemic attack in a patient with a high-grade carotid stenosis. In patients with lesser degrees of stenosis an ulcer crater often heals spontaneously, and sometimes it is difficult to be certain that the mild stenosis identified on the angiogram is causally related to the ischemic event. Thus, in general terms, carotid endarterectomies at the Mayo Clinic are reserved for people with high-grade carotid stenosis (80 to 90 percent with a deep ulcer crater, corresponding to a 1- to 2-mm residual lumen by the criteria employed at Massachusetts General Hospital). Elderly patients with asymptomatic stenoses are observed, whereas patients with a very high-grade stenosis who are physiologically young and free of severe vascular disease in other parts of the body are given the option of undergoing angiography for possible surgery or having the lesion followed with noninvasive studies while they are taking aspirin. Patients who have recovered from a small stroke and still have a patent carotid artery are in some instances good candidates for surgery.

Monitoring

There is now little doubt that monitoring with a continuous electroencephalogram (EEG) throughout the operative procedure decreases the frequency of complications—the difference is totally analogous to the difference in flying with and without instruments. In approximately 10 to 15 percent of patients, blood flow will fall below the critical level required for adequate hemispheric perfusion with carotid occlusion.[7] An endarterectomy performed in haste is doomed to failure and major complications.

Operative Exposure

Adequate exposure of the carotid bifurcation is mandatory in patients undergoing a carotid endarterectomy. All too frequently complications related to this operation are directly attributable to a failure on the part of the surgeon to adequately expose the distal internal carotid artery. There has in the past been some argument about a transverse incision versus a longitudinal curvilinear incision; we prefer the latter (Fig. 25-1). In the hands of very experienced surgeons a transverse incision may perhaps be acceptable. The transverse approach does result in less scarring from the skin incision, but all too frequently it fails to provide the room necessary for distal exposure of the internal carotid artery or for proximal exposure of a thickened common carotid artery with

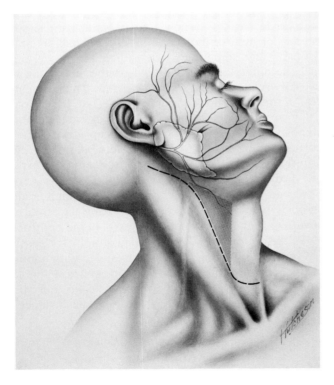

Figure 25-1. Carotid triangle is outlined by a shaded area. The conventional skin incision overlies the posterior margin of the triangle. (By permission of Mayo Foundation.)

diffuse atherosclerosis extending well below the carotid bifurcation.

The surgeon should be prepared to extend the incision either superiorly or inferiorly. Thus it is necessary to prepare the skin well above the level of the tragus of the ear. When necessary, the skin incision can be extended superiorly by skirting the earlobe and ascending in the pretragal crease to the superior border of the zygoma[7] (Fig. 25-2).

With far distal exposures, the superficial cervical fascia is incised and the posterior border of the parotid gland is exposed and elevated. The anterior-inferior surface of the auricular cartilage is followed deep to its "pointer," the triangular projection of cartilage at its medial limit. The temporoparotid fascia is incised between the mastoid process and the posterior margin of the parotid gland and the facial nerve found subjacent to the fascia. With a finger placed on the mastoid tip and directed anteriorly forward, the cartilaginous "pointer," and the palpable junction between the external auditory meatus (the tympanomastoid suture) all point to the main trunk of the seventh cranial nerve. Once the main trunk is identified, the lower division and marginal mandibular nerve that form the upper limit of the deep dissection can be traced forward by sharp dissection and elevated safely by using the mobilized parotid tissues as a "bundle"[5] (Fig. 25-3).

Preservation of Cranial Nerves

There are five cranial nerves that must be protected during this operative procedure. Not all these cranial nerves are identified during the procedure itself, but all can be injured indirectly from traction. These nerves include the facial, glossopharyngeal, vagus, spinal accessory, and hypoglossal. Knowledge of the functional anatomy of each of these nerves helps to prevent their injury.

Facial Nerve

The facial nerve exits from the stylomastoid foramen and ascends superiorly in the parotid gland itself. It lies deep to the digastric muscle. Damage to this nerve can be avoided by maintaining the dissection in the fascia around the parotid gland and then identifying the nerve by the methods indicated above prior to tracing it out into the parotid gland.

Glossopharyngeal Nerve

The glossopharyngeal nerve is primarily a sensory nerve carrying motor fibers to only one insignificant muscle, the stylopharyngeus muscle. It carries sen-

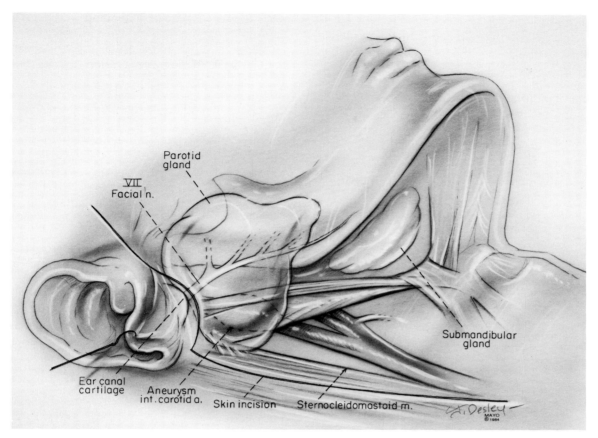

Figure 25-2. The skin incision follows the leading border of the sternocleidomastoid muscle and ascends to a point just behind the lobe of the ear. In the lower quarter of the postauricular sulcus, it drops to the bottom of the ear, skirts the earlobe, and then ascends in the pretragal skin crease to the superior border of the zygoma. (By permission of Mayo Foundation.)

sory fibers to the palate and soft pharynx so that damage to branches of this nerve superiorly result in sensory alterations to the pharynx and thus interfere with swallowing. Small filaments from the ninth and tenth cranial nerves to the pharynx are often identified as extending medially and deep to the internal carotid artery itself.

Vagus Nerve

The vagus nerve descends as a single trunk in the carotid sheath between the internal carotid artery and the jugular vein. This nerve carries motor fibers to the pharynx and larynx, and damage to the parent trunk or to its branches results in considerable dysphagia. It is usually not difficult to preserve the trunk of the vagus nerve and those filaments ultimately destined for the recurrent laryngeal nerve with it. The superior laryngeal nerve leaves the parent trunk of the nerve just above the carotid bifurcation, where it runs medial to the external carotid artery to enter the

larynx deep to the superior thyroidal artery. Preservation of this nerve is not difficult and it is readily identified.

More difficult to preserve are the motor branches to the pharynx, which leave the nerve and follow a course deep and medial to the internal carotid artery well above the origin of that vessel from the common carotid artery. These are very small filaments, and it is often very difficult to preserve them. Although they have been described in anatomical texts as running in the tissue plane posterior to the internal carotid artery, several small branches originating from the vagus nerve have been found in some of our patients anterior to the internal carotid artery. When possible, it is advisable to preserve any filaments arising from the vagus nerve, whether they run anterior or posterior to the internal carotid artery. In those cases in which an aneurysm is present in the internal carotid artery, we have left these filaments intact and then mobilized the internal carotid artery anteriorly to them after the vessel has been resected

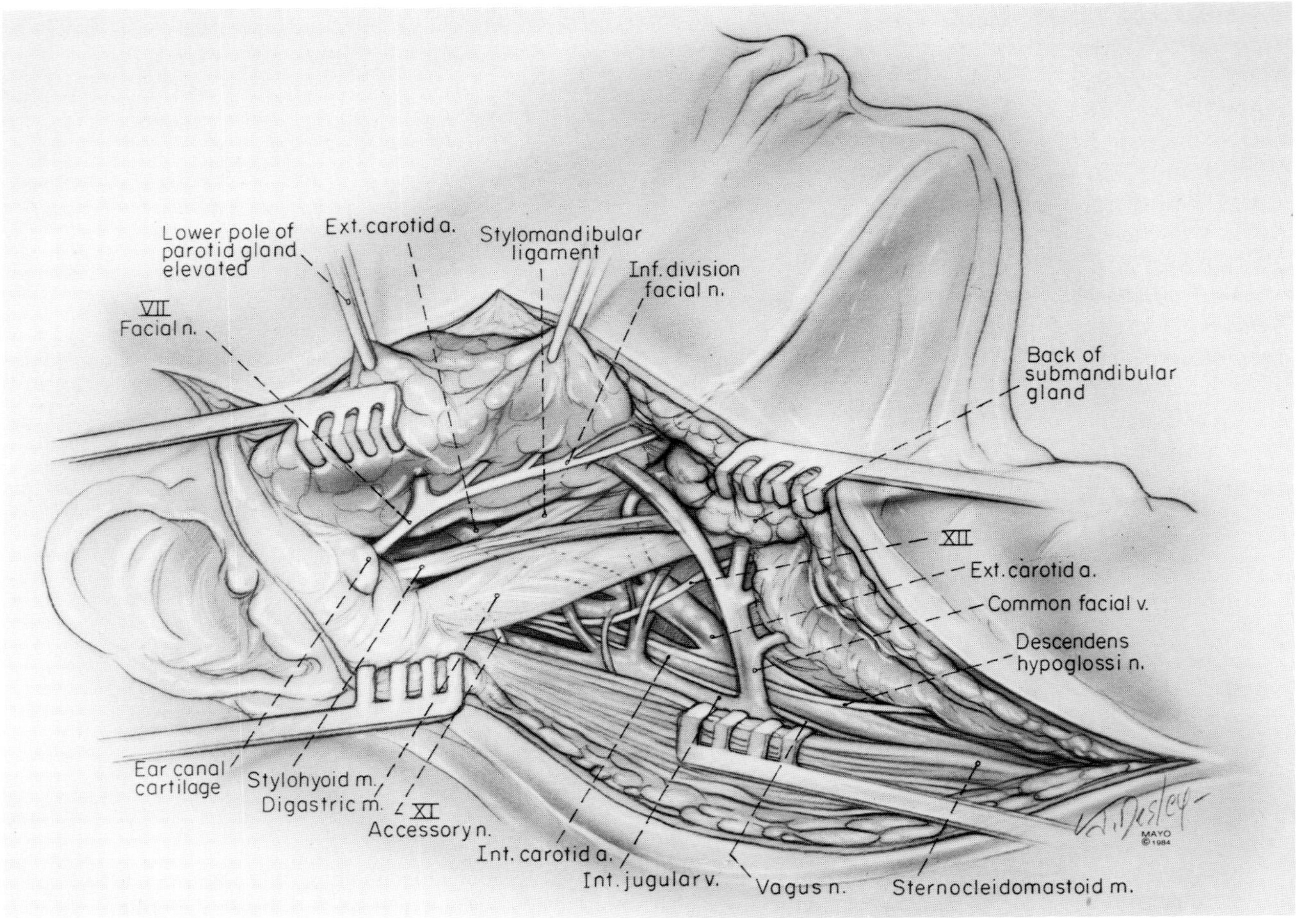

Figure 25-3. The lower pole of the parotid gland has been mobilized and retracted anteriorly and superiorly after the superficial, deep, and temporoparotid fasciae have been incised. The dissection is then carried along the anterior border of the cartilage of the external ear canal and the anterior surface of the mastoid process. The posterior belly of the digastric muscle is exposed. The deep cervical veins are divided by bipolar coagulation, and the distal internal carotid artery is exposed to the level of the styloid process. The carotid body and the carotid sinus should be injected with Xylocaine to avoid troublesome fluctuations in blood pressure. (By permission of Mayo Foundation.)

in preparation for the interposition vein graft. When a carotid body tumor is present, it is usually possible to work the nerve superiorly. In patients with a high bifurcation or a distal extension of an atherosclerotic plaque, these nerves are not usually involved, as the pathology seldom extends to the level of their origin.

Spinal Accessory Nerve

The spinal accessory nerve is identified adjacent to the vagus nerve, where it descends anterior to the jugular vein and then disappears from view under the border of the sternocleidomastoid muscle. It is not difficult to preserve this nerve, and it is only necessary to remember its anatomical course in order to identify it and keep it out of harm's way.

Hypoglossal Nerve

The hypoglossal nerve can be mobilized superiorly after the descendens hypoglossus has been resected. It is usually tacked temporarily to the parotid fascia in order to elevate it well out of the surgical field. The plexus of veins surrounding this nerve is best divided with a bipolar coagulator. The muscular branch of the occipital artery going to the sternocleidomastoid muscle should be doubly ligated with suture and divided. Coagulation techniques should not be relied upon to arrest bleeding from this artery, and if it does bleed after it has been divided following coagulation, damage can be inflicted on the nerve as a result of the dissection required to reexpose the bleeding point.

Endarterectomy

After the carotid artery has been exposed, the patient is given 5,000 units of heparin and the vessels are occluded in the following order: common carotid, external carotid, and finally internal carotid. The external and internal carotid arteries are occluded with temporary Sugita clips and the common carotid artery with a Fogarty clamp.

A bold incision is made in the common carotid artery with the tip of a No. 11 blade knife (Fig. 25-4). This incision is extended with Potts scissors well beyond the distal level of the plaque.[7] It is necessary to carry the incision 1 cm or so beyond what appears to be the upper demarcation point of the plaque. It is absolutely imperative that a clean endarterectomy be

achieved and that there be no lip of intima distally to serve as a source of emboli or dissection[3,4,6,10,11] (Fig. 25-4). On occasion the intima is quite thick distally and difficult to separate from the wall of the artery with a good demarcation point. In such instances a small nip in the tip of the intima will allow the surgeon to tear the plaque from the wall of the artery. The intima tends to tear transversely, and once the tear is initiated with the microscissors, it is possible to achieve a clean transverse tear (Fig. 25-5).

On occasion a tail or tongue of plaque extends superiorly on the posterior wall in a true subendothelial layer. This can usually be removed without extending the arteriotomy. The surgeon should merely lift the plaque away from the wall of the intima and follow it with a small dissector superiorly. It is seldom

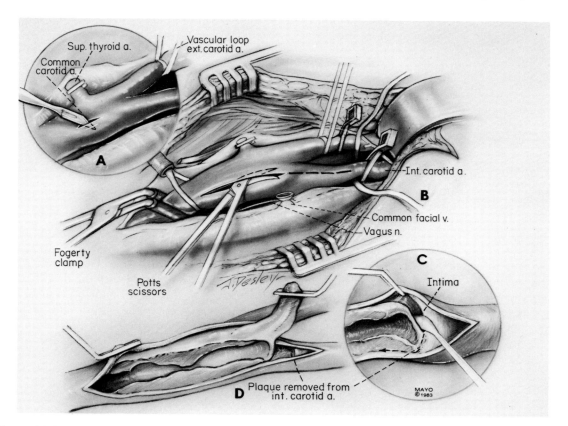

Figure 25-4. (**A**) With the common, external, and internal carotid arteries occluded, the common carotid artery is opened with a bold incision made with the tip of a No. 11 blade knife. Trial occlusions are to be avoided. (**B**) The arteriotomy is extended with Potts scissors until the distal limit of the plaque on the posterior wall of the internal carotid artery is visualized. If the EEG remains normal and collateral flow is adequate (as judged by backbleeding, stump pressures, or if available, cerebral blood flow measurements) a shunt will not be required. (**C & D**) Nevertheless, the plaque is routinely removed from the internal carotid artery initially so that a shunt can be placed easily if necessary. Usually there is a clear break point between the plaque and the normal distal intima. However, on occasion there is a smooth transition between the plaque and distally thickened intima. In these cases separation of the plaque from the distal vessel can be facilitated by creating a small incision in the intima of the artery and tearing the plaque away in a circumferential fashion. (By permission of Mayo Foundation.)

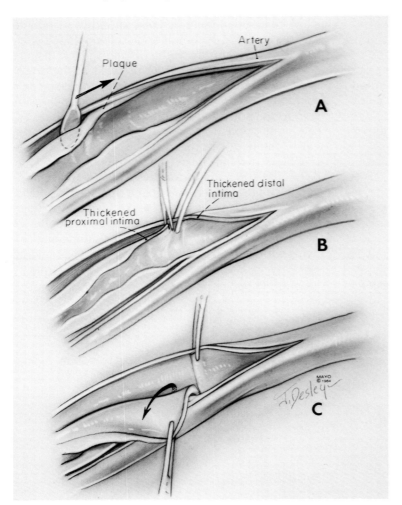

Figure 25-5. In cases in which the distal plaque blends imperceptibly with thickened intima, the limit of the dissection is determined by surgical judgment. (**A**) A breakpoint between the plaque with its intimal tail and the distal intima can be achieved by taking advantage of the intima's tendency to tear transversely. (**B**) The microscissors are laid flush with the surface of the vessel as the proximal plaque and intima are retracted away from the vessel wall. (**C**) The edge of the intima at its point of attachment is incised by creating a tear point, which is developed by grasping the vessel wall just distal to the tear point with forceps in one hand and the proximal plaque and intima with forceps in the other hand. Traction against countertraction produces a transverse tear in the intima with no free flap. (By permission of Mayo Foundation.)

necessary to tack the wall of the artery with sutures. On occasion, however, the intima will be thick distally, and although it is adherent to the wall where the dissection was terminated, one obtains the impression that the ledge is too thick for good healing and that it would be well to smooth this junction point with tack sutures. In these instances double-arm 6-0 Prolene sutures are used with the needle placed from the interior to the exterior for both limbs of the suture. In this manner the suture can be placed precisely and there is not risk of dissecting the intima from the wall of the artery (Fig. 25-6).

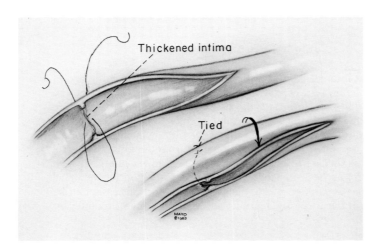

Figure 25-6. On occasion there will be a thickened spot on the intima distally, which should be secured by a tack suture or two. These should be passed from the inside of the vessel to the outside with use of double-armed sutures in order to minimize the risk of separating the intima from the vessel. If the proximal plaque and intima have been torn away from the vessel wall as described in Figure 25-5, it is rare that more than one or two tack sutures are required. A repair with a patch graft helps to control the distal intima. (By permission of Mayo Foundation.)

Shunt Placement

A shunt is used when monitoring procedures indicate that it is necessary.[7] Cases can be divided into four groups on the basis of occlusion flows and severity of EEG changes:

1. 0 to 5 ml/100 g/min and nearly isoelectric EEG: ± 3 percent of cases (always shunted)
2. 5 to 9 ml/100 g/min and severe EEG changes: 8 to 9 percent of cases (shunted, but not immediately)
3. 10 to 15 ml/100 g/min and moderate EEG changes: 15 percent of cases (usually shunted)
4. 15 to 20 ml/100 g/min with questionable EEG changes or preexisting deficit: 20 percent of cases (often shunted)

The tolerance of the brain to ischemia depends on the severity of the ischemia and the presence or absence of preexisting neuronal damage. On occasion a shunt must be inserted immediately, but in most instances it is possible to remove the plaque from the internal carotid artery as described previously and then place the shunt (Figs. 25-7 and 25-8). Shunts are available in three sizes and both the internal and ex-ternal (loop) configuration (these shunts are available through V. Mueller, Inc., McGaw Park, IL).

Closure of the Arteriotomy

We prefer to close the arteriotomy with a saphenous vein patch graft obtained from the saphenous vein at the ankle.[7] A primary closure often results in a very fine looking endarterectomy, but unfortunately the risk of postoperative occlusion is much higher with a primary closure than with a vein patch graft. If a vein patch graft is not available, our second choice is a Gortex graft.

A saphenous vein patch graft is sewn into place with a 5-0 running double-arm Prolene arterial suture (Figs. 25-9 and 25-10). Initially the distal suture is placed at the apex of the graft to anchor the graft to the most distal point of the arteriotomy (Fig. 25-9). The suture is the most important one in the suture line, and it must be placed accurately. The suture should purchase 1 mm of graft and 1 mm of artery. It is easier for a right-handed surgeon to first close that

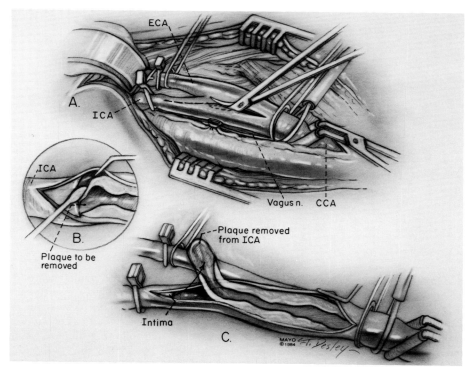

Figure 25-7. Ebersold's method of shunt placement. (**A**) The arteriotomy is extended from the common carotid artery (CCA) into the internal carotid artery (ICA) well beyond the level of the distal end of the plaque by using Pott's arterial scissors. The common carotid artery is occluded with a soft-shoed Fogarty clamp and the internal and external carotid arteries (ECA) with small intracranial vascular aneurysm clips. (**B**) Plaque is removed from the distal internal carotid artery and separated from normal intima by a circular tear under direct visualization with a small spatula. (**C**) The distal limit of plaque is reflected so that ample room will be present to insert the distal end of shunt. (*Figure continues.*)

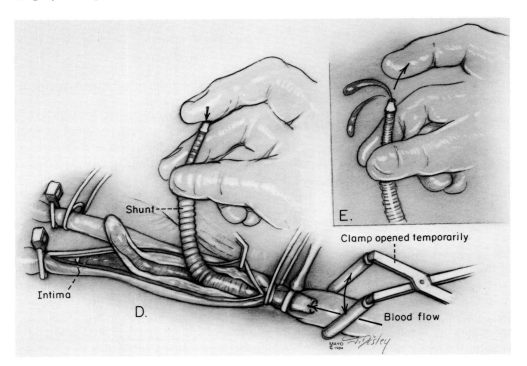

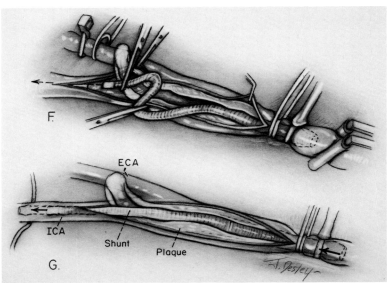

Figure 25-7 (*continued*). (**D**) The proximal end of the shunt is inserted into the common carotid artery, and the tourniquets are brought up snugly around the proximal end of the shunt. Before inserting the shunt into the common carotid artery and while the artery is still occluded, it is advisable to clear the stump of the common carotid artery of all blood by use of a small sucker. The residual blood frequently contains small particles of atherosclerotic material, which have floated into the area following the arteriotomy. (**E**) The Fogarty clamp is temporarily opened and the shunt cleared of blood. Pre-wetting the shunt with saline helps to prevent entrapment of air bubbles. (**F**) The distal end of the shunt is now inserted into the endarterectomized internal carotid artery. Most patients require medium-sized shunts, and it is seldom necessary to place a distal tourniquet when using the internal shunt. However, in some patients there is some bleeding around the shunt, which requires slight pressure from the vessel loop; this can be achieved by single strands placed on either side of the loop, which are brought together and approximated with a vascular clip. (**G**) The remaining portion of the endarterectomy is now completed, and the vessel is repaired with a saphenous vein patch graft. (By permission of Mayo Foundation.)

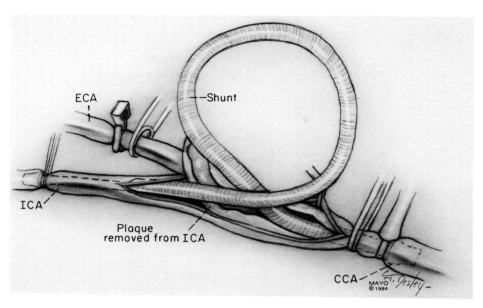

Figure 25-8. The use of the Sundt external or loop shunt differs somewhat from the internal shunt in that the distal end of the shunt must be secured with a tourniquet to prevent its dislodgement from the internal carotid artery. In all other respects the placement of this shunt is similar. (By permission of Mayo Foundation.)

Figure 25-9. (**A**) The vessel is repaired with a saphenous vein patch graft. (**B**) The initial closure is begun distally with a double-armed 5-0 Prolene suture. For right-handed surgeons, the lateral wall of the vessel is closed initially when performing a right carotid endarterectomy and the medial wall when performing a left carotid endarterectomy. Thus, the suture goes from the vein to the artery, which is particularly important for that portion of the vessel still containing normal intima. (**C**) After the first 2 to 3 cm of the vessel has been closed on one side, the opposite side is closed to a similar length. (**D**) Here it is necessary to backhand the sutures until the portion of the vessel containing normal intima has been closed, whereupon the direction may be reversed to facilitate and expedite the closure. (By permission of Mayo Foundation.)

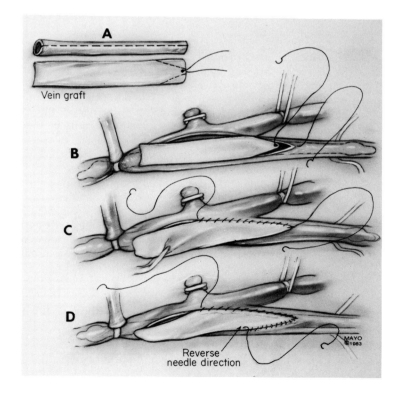

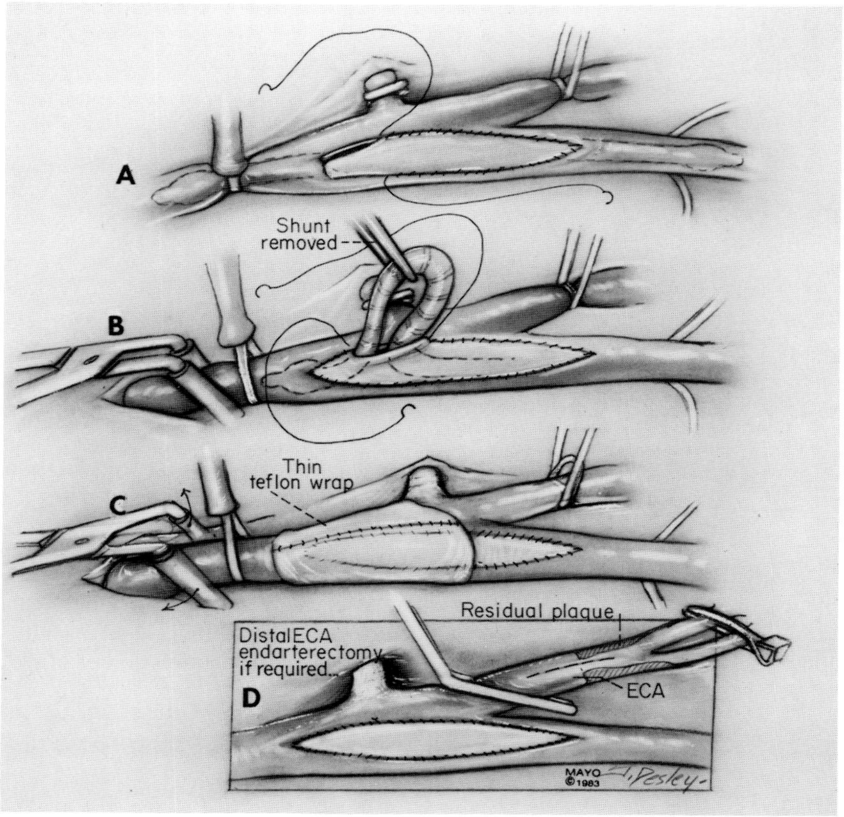

Figure 25-10. (**A**) Proximally the vein is shaped to smoothly taper into the common carotid artery, and then it is affixed to the base point of the arteriotomy with a double-armed 5-0 Prolene suture. The first several sutures on either side of this vein should incorporate the full thickness of the common carotid artery, and they should be passed from vein to artery in order to help affix the thickened intima. (**B**) The shunt is withdrawn prior to final closure of the arteriotomy. Although not shown in the figure, removal of the shunt is facilitated by passing a large suture loosely around the shunt at some point in the procedure while it is still widely exposed. The arteriotomy is then closed from both ends. Before tying the final knot, back bleeding is permitted from the internal carotid artery. The internal carotid artery is then closed, and flow is restored by removing the clamp from the common carotid artery and allowing flow from that vessel to pass into the external carotid artery. After 20 to 30 seconds of flow to be sure that all air is removed from the bifurcation site, the clip is removed from the internal carotid artery. (**C**) The vein graft is reinforced with a thin sheath of Teflon fabric. (**D**) In patients in whom an easily palpable temporal artery pulse is not present, the external carotid artery is temporarily occluded with a small vascular clamp and a separate arteriotomy made in that vessel. Invariably, an elevated ledge of intima will be identified at the distal limit or breakpoint of the plaque; this is sharply resected. The external carotid artery is usually closed primarily, as the arteriotomy is quite short. (By permission of Mayo Foundation.)

side of the graft in which a forehanded stitch will be used. Thus, for a right-handed surgeon the lateral distal one-third of the arteriotomy is closed vein-to-artery with a simple running suture when surgery is performed on the right carotid artery, and the medial wall is similarly closed in surgery on the left carotid artery. The first three to four sutures must be precisely placed so that there is a good taper of the vein and so that the vein is not bulging and aneurysmal (Fig. 25-9). This arrangement is best secured by plac-

ing gentle traction on the vein with the needle on each pass. The opposite wall is then closed using a backhand stitch for the first few stitches until the vein has been secured to that portion of the artery where intima remains (characteristically the arteriotomy is extended 1 cm beyond the limit of the endarterectomy). Once the vein has been secured to the portion of the vessel with normal intima, the direction of the suture is changed, and the remaining portion of the arteriotomy is closed with an overhand running suture; the surgeon should be very careful to have all sutures parallel to one another with an equal purchase of artery and vein.

After the distal half of the graft has been sewn into place, the proximal end of the graft is shaped and tapered. This end is then sewn in place to the wall of the common carotid artery according to the general principles outlined previously. One must be certain that the suture goes from the inside to the outside in that portion of the vessel with preserved intima, as it is possible to create intimal instability in a thick-walled artery by passing the needle from the outside to the inside in areas where the intima is particularly thick (Figs. 25-9 and 25-10). Each suture should purchase a full thickness of intima.

Aneurysm formation in the vein is a possible complication associated with the use of a vein graft. This is more likely to occur in that portion of the repair with the largest vessel circumference, as the total tangential shearing stress is greatest here. Accordingly, we have routinely reinforced the common carotid artery with a thin sheet of Teflon[7] (Fig. 25-10).

External Carotid

Unfortunately, the carotid plaque often extends diffusely into the external carotid artery from the bifurcation rather than terminating sharply as it often does in the internal carotid artery. Unless one is able to visually identify the demarcation point of the plaque after it has been severed from the external carotid artery and is certain that there is no lip of intima, it is necessary to make a separate incision in the external carotid artery and to sever the plaque from the wall of the vessel as described above for the internal carotid artery. In most instances the external carotid artery is reconstructed with a saphenous vein patch graft in the manner described for the common and internal carotid arteries.[7] Currently we open approximately 50 percent of external carotid arteries for resection of the plaque with patch grafting. A stump of an external carotid artery can be a dangerous source of future embolization, and we have seen this in three patients.

Tortuous or Elongated Internal Carotid Artery with Angulation or Kinking

In approximately 5 percent of our cases we have found it necessary to shorten by plication or resection a segment of the internal carotid artery in order to achieve a better reconstruction and to avoid kinking in the vessel after flow has been restored. Although it is often possible to predict from the preoperative angiogram whether a vessel will require a resection, not infrequently after removal of the plaque the surgeon will find a thin-walled, elongated bed, which if reconstructed without resection will lead to kinking.

There are several methods or techniques for shortening the vessel if the surgeon feels this is indicated.[7] If only a relatively short segment of the wall is to be excluded, an end-to-end plication without resection is a useful technique (Fig. 25-11). If a greater length (3 cm or more) must be excluded, a segmental resection will be necessary (Fig. 25-12). If a very long segment must be excised, it is best to ligate and divide the external carotid artery and to place the anastomosis at the proximal limit of the endarterectomy (Fig. 25-13) because vessels in which a long length must be resected invariably have very thin, degenerated walls. In these cases it is very difficult to avoid a transverse ridge at the site of the anastomosis owing to the thinness of the vessel wall and the failure to resect enough vessel because of interference from the origin of the external carotid artery. Placing the anastomosis at the proximal end of the endarterectomy prevents a ridge, as the segment proximal to the anastomosis has a thick wall.

Embolic Complications

Perhaps the worst complication that can occur during a carotid endarterectomy is an intracranial embolism. Acute occlusions can in large measure be prevented with saphenous vein patch grafting, and intraoperative ischemia can be prevented with proper monitoring techniques and shunting. Prevention of intracranial embolic complications is dependent on meticulous technique in handling the vessel prior to its opening and thereafter if a shunt is required, on careful attention to the proximal common carotid artery, where debris often floats into the stump of the opened vessel, "lying in wait" to be discharged intracranially with the placement of a shunt. Therefore before a shunt is placed, it is absolutely imperative that the surgeon examine the proximal stump of the common carotid artery regardless of the severity of the EEG change and to deliberately and very carefully remove all cholesterol or atheromatous material that may be floating freely in the bed of the opened vessel.[7] In our experience, we have noted that an embolus has usually occurred from this source rather than with manipulation of the vessel prior to occlu-

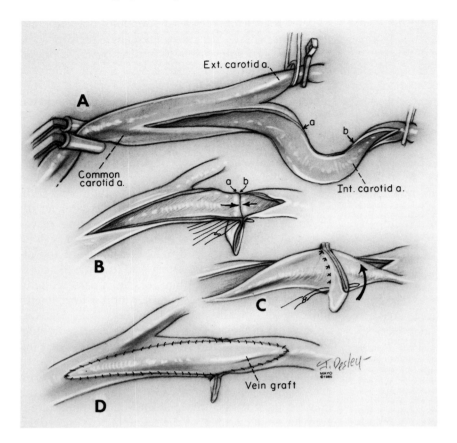

Figure 25-11. End-to-end plication technique for reconstructing a relatively short segment of tortuous vessel. Interrupted sutures provide a more precise anastomosis. A running suture tends to purse-string the anastomosis and causes ridges in the vessel wall. As indicated in Figure 25-12, if a shortening procedure is undertaken, one must draw both segments tightly to prevent aneurysmal outpouching of the proximal segment. If there is a thick distal intima, the plication can be placed at the distal end point of the endarterectomy in order to minimize the shelf. The arteriotomy should be extended well beyond the point of the plication. (By permission of Mayo Foundation.)

sion. Nevertheless, the latter also occurs and is a risk factor that should be considered very carefully.

In our experience the risk of intracranial embolization during a carotid endarterectomy approximates 1 percent. If an embolic complication occurs, it is invariably reflected by the EEG. An emergency embolectomy is indicated if angiography reveals a major occlusion (Fig. 25-14).

ANEURYSMS

It is self-evident that a detailed and thorough knowledge of normal neurovascular anatomy is an indispensable qualification for the aneurysm surgeon. The combination of a subarachnoid hemorrhage and a large aneurysm frequently distorts and obliterates normal structures, so that the origin, projection, and base of an aneurysm are obscured. A complete understanding of the relationships of major structures to one another and to perforating vessels gives the surgeon the confidence to create planes of dissection and to isolate the base of the aneurysm for clipping.

A readily identifiable reference point in the surgical field permits the surgeon to relate major anatomical structures to one another and to formulate a plan for reconstruction of the aneurysm with preservation of the vital perforating arteries. In the anterior circulation the optic nerve is the most readily identifiable reference point. For aneurysms in and around the caput of the basilar artery, the third cranial nerve serves this purpose. For lesions of the basilar trunk or the vertebral artery, the lower cranial nerves are useful benchmarks. Knowledge of the interrelationships of these cranial nerves to the major vessels permits the surgeon to develop planes of dissection and to work proximally and distally along major vessels to the pathology.

Positioning of Patient

With few exceptions, the patient is placed supine, with the head positioned as dictated by the location of the aneurysm. With most anterior circulation aneurysms, this approximates a 30-degree turn of the head. Exaggerated hyperextension or severe lateral rotation positions are to be avoided. These are usually unnecessary, as appropriate microscopic techniques make it possible to achieve ample room through arachnoidal planes with only minimal brain

Figure 25-12. A vessel may be elongated or tortuous as a result of medial thinning and stretching, which is caused by degeneration of the media due to a thick-walled plaque. Endarterectomy in such a vessel tends to produce an acute kink in the artery, usually beyond the distal limit of the repair, when flow is restored. This kink can serve as a source of occlusion. One must be cautious not to resect too much of the vessel, as the end-to-end anastomosis will also shorten the vessel somewhat. However, failure to resect enough of the vessel is associated with the risk of an aneurysmal outpouching of the segment proximal to the suture line, since the end-to-end anastomosis produces a transverse ridge if the vessel is inadequately shortened. A thrombus will form in this aneurysm and serve as a source of emboli. (By permission of Mayo Foundation.)

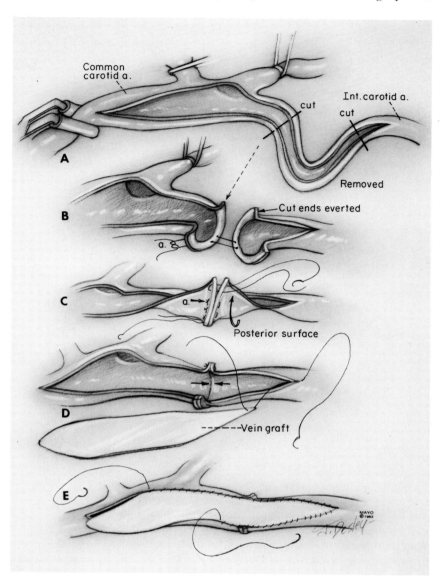

Surgical Approaches

Virtually all anterior circulation aneurysms can be approached pterionally, an approach popularized by Yasargil.[12] Exceptions include aneurysms arising at the division of the anterior cerebral artery into the pericallosal and callosal marginal branches and small mycotic aneurysms on distal branches of the middle cerebral artery. The bifrontal craniotomy is seldom employed today. Not only does this carry the risk of damage to the olfactory nerves, but also, of course, it creates the problem of a direct opening into the fron-

retraction. Rigid skull fixation in a three-point head rest is, of course, mandatory.

tal sinus, which must be sealed with a pericranial flap.

Accessibility and the difficulty in approaching aneurysms of the posterior circulation have necessitated a number of craniotomies.[8] The modified pterional approach is used for aneurysms arising at the caput of the basilar artery, where the caput is above the dorsum of the sella. This approach carries with it the disadvantage of not visualizing a low caput of the basilar artery. The subtemporal approach is used for aneurysms arising at the caput of the basilar artery in which the bifurcation of the basilar artery is low (i.e., below the dorsum sellae).[1]

For most aneurysms arising from the trunk of the basilar artery, we employ a posterior subtemporal approach. In this approach the tentorium is incised

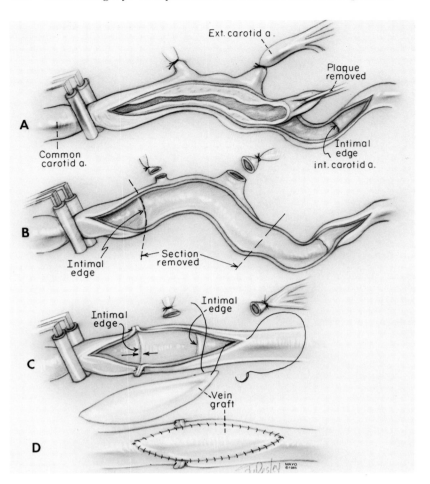

Figure 25-13. In cases in which a long length of vessel must be resected, it is advisable to ligate and divide the external carotid artery. The segmental resection is then performed more proximally than indicated in Figure 25-12. The anastomosis is placed at the proximal end of the endarterectomy. This prevents any ridging and aneurysmal outpouching as the vessel proximal to the anastomosis has a thick wall. (By permission of Mayo Foundation.)

parallel to the petrous bone, and the surgeon is then able to visualize the entire course of the basilar artery from its origin to its bifurcation. A far lateral inferior suboccipital approach is used for some lower basilar trunk and midline vertebral artery aneurysms.

A suboccipital approach is used for aneurysms arising from the vertebral artery at the origin of the posterior-inferior cerebellar artery.[2] These patients are usually placed in the sitting position. For aneurysms arising from the vertebral artery where it pierces the dura, the aneurysm is most readily exposed through a small midline suboccipital approach with the patient in the sitting position. In these patients the posterior-inferior cerebellar artery invariably takes its origin quite low on the vertebral artery. Last, there is a group of aneurysms arising from the distal posterior-inferior cerebellar artery that are approached through a midline suboccipital approach. During the operation these patients are placed in the sitting position, with appropriate monitoring for air emboli.

Brain Retraction

With few exceptions, only one blade of a self-retaining retractor is necessary for adequate exposure of saccular aneurysms and most giant aneurysms. Use of only one blade is safer, not only in terms of not tearing small vessels but also in terms of inflicting less tissue damage from retraction than results with use of two blades, as the natural retractability of the brain is not restrained. Use of two blades can result in stretching and tearing of tissue and often prevents the compensatory displacement and expansion of the brain in nonretracted areas, which is possible when only one retractor blade is used. Skillful brain retraction is as important for the aneurysm surgeon as is abdominal retraction for the general surgeon and in fact is one of the keys to successful aneurysm surgery. Some very experienced surgeons, such as Yasargil, have advanced the state of the art to a point at which brain retraction is so minimal that it might better be referred to as *brain retention*. Nev-

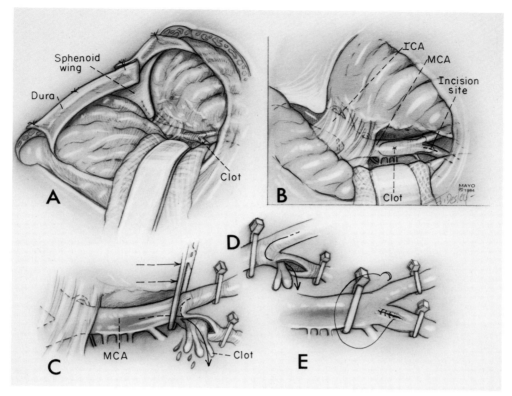

Figure 25-14. Operative sequence. (**A**) The middle cerebral artery is exposed through a pterional craniotomy. (**B**) In this example the embolus involves the main trunk, extending proximally to the lenticulostriates. (**C**) Temporary clips are placed on divisions distal to the embolus. The arteriotomy is preferably made in one of the middle cerebral artery (MCA) branches as opposed to the main trunk. (**D**) With the sequential removal of clips, antegrade and retrograde flow is used to remove both the proximal and distal portions of the embolus. (**E**) The arteriotomy is closed with running or interrupted 9-0 or 10-0 monofilament sutures. (By permission of Mayo Foundation.)

ertheless, for most surgeons a certain degree of brain retraction is necessary for adequate exposure of lesions of the circle of Willis.

We have preferred the brain retractor originally described by Yasargil and have used this almost exclusively for the past 15 years. Thus we have little experience with the more elaborate Greenburg and Sugita retractors, which are equally good or perhaps even better.

Use of the Yasargil retractor is illustrated in Figure 25-15. Note that the flexible arm is positioned in such a manner that it is supported by the head at point A (Fig. 25-15). The fixation device, which attaches the flexible arm to the operating table, is placed relatively close to the table to avoid excessive looping of the arm. The Yasargil retractor is attached to the operating table on the side opposite the craniotomy, and thus for the surgeon there is minimal interference from the retractor arm.

The mechanics of the Yasargil retractor are such that a standard routine should be adopted in placing the retractor in its proper position for the operation. The malleable retractor, seated in the fixation jaws at the distal tip of the flexible arm, is held in the approximate location in which it will be used during the operation. The universal joint affixing the bar to the operating table is loosened, and the bar is moved proximally and distally to a position such that the flexible arm traverses the distance between the malleable retractor and the fixation head without distortion. The bar is then secured in place. Next, the head of the bar is loosened so that it can be rotated clockwise or counterclockwise to adjust the flexible arm further and to determine the position at which the loosened configuration of this arm follows a smooth course and the contour of the skull. This is an important step in the establishment of a firm, reliable support for the fulcrum of the retractor. Thereafter, the

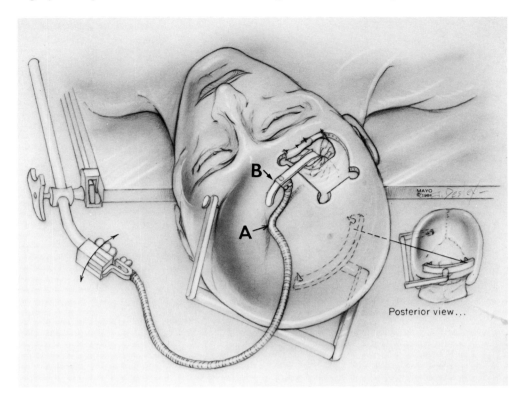

Figure 25-15. Schematic illustration of recommended positioning for the Yasargil retractor. The retractor is attached to the table on the side opposite to that of the craniotomy. The head of the bar of the fixation device to which is attached the flexible arm of the retractor is placed relatively close to the operating table in order to avoid excessive tortuousity in the flexible arm. The head can then be rotated to the direction for the flexible arm that will give it the desired configuration. It is important that the flexible arm follow a natural course when loosened that will closely approximate its position when tightened in order to avoid excessive torque. The support rendered to the flexible arm at point A gives considerable additional strength to the retractor, which not only increases the life of the retractor but, more importantly, the precision of the instrument. The malleable retractor can then be rotated around point B for fine adjustments after the flexible arm has been positioned. When used properly, the retractor not only retains the brain but elevates it slightly, thus opening up the arachnoidal cisterns and facilitating the dissection of the arachnoidal membranes. (By permission of Mayo Foundation.)

optimum tension is created in the flexible arm to hold it in place. It is not necessary to have a great deal of tension in the flexible arm (if properly positioned); in fact, this would interfere with precision control of the instrument. The tension in the flexible arm should only be sufficient to secure the arm where it is placed and prevent a drift. Excessive tension results in distortion of the flexible arm and lack of control.

It is important that the flexible arm of the retractor be positioned so that it has firm support on the scalp (point A in Fig. 25-15). This allows rotation of the malleable retractor at point B, the point at which the retractor is attached to the flexible arm. With experience, it is seldom necessary to readjust the alignment of the flexible arm throughout the operation, al-

though it is loosened and tightened many times as the dissection progresses and the brain is elevated progressively to open the subarachnoid cisterns.

Various types of fabrics to cover the brain and protect it during retraction have been tried at the Mayo Clinic. We have decided that the safest and most effective brain retraction can be achieved by placing a large piece of Surgicel over the area of the brain that will be retracted and overlaying this with a large piece of cottonoid. This provides the necessary friction to permit the retractor to elevate the brain and open the cisterns. With irrigation at the conclusion of the procedure, the Surgicel usually floats free from the brain, but adherent points are left in place. It is important that brain retraction be directed out from the wound and that the cisterns be opened rather than compressed. The free body diagram in Figure 25-15 illustrates this principle: to achieve this direction of retraction, the retractor must be supported at point A, and there must be sufficient friction between the brain and its protective cottonoid and the self-retaining brain retractor.

In general terms, the brain in older patients is stiffer and tolerates retraction poorly, whereas the brain in younger patients is more pliable and elastic. Fortunately (at least for the aneurysm surgeon), most older patients have a certain degree of atrophy, which makes it a great deal easier to open the subarachnoid spaces and identify the aneurysm. In fact, in many cases brain retraction in the older patient is very minimal and not necessary except to restrain certain structures from the surgical field. Younger patients have little atrophy, and the brain fills the calvarium so that exposure is achieved with appropriate but gentle retraction. There seems to be a certain degree of deformation memory, in that the brains in younger patients tend to remain displaced after a period of gentle retraction and, unless damaged, do not tend to refill the space created by retraction, at least for the hour or so required for the surgery itself. It is our experience that obesity is associated with a full or tight brain. In obese patients normal fissures are often obliterated and the dissections are more difficult.

Division of Arachnoid

For the knowledgeable surgeon sharp dissection is safer than blunt dissection. For right-handed surgeons the suction unit is held in the left hand with a small cotton pad over the tip of the sucker, which allows the instrument to serve as a small retractor and to provide countertension to the instrument that will be held in the right hand, which will be either a knurled, round handle for a No. 11 blade knife or a small dissector. Knowledge of the cisterns and the arachnoidal planes will facilitate the dissection, and these are considered subsequently in the appropriate chapters. The dissection should be carried initially as close to the base of the aneurysm as possible while the dome of the aneurysm is avoided in order to minimize the risk of premature rupture (Fig. 25-16). With few exceptions, aneurysms have usually ruptured from the dome or from near the dome unless a daughter sac is identifiable near the base. Once the arachnoid has been opened, the cotton pad is removed from the end of the suction tip so that blood can be aspirated from the appropriate or involved arachnoidal cisterns. Thereafter, the cottonoid is replaced over the tip of the suction unit so that the aneurysm can gradually be worked away from the perforating vessels and a plane of dissection can be created for the aneurysm clip.

Figure 25-16. The brain retractor should not only retract the brain slightly but should elevate it from the wound, thus opening the cisterns and permitting greater safety for sharp dissection of the arachnoid with the tip of a No. 11 blade knife or arachnoid dissector. The retractor should not be positioned to compress the area of the aneurysm, as this will congest the surgical field and increase the risk of injury to vital perforating vessels. (By permission of Mayo Foundation.)

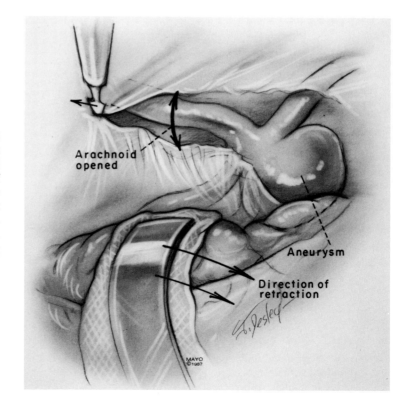

Suction Units

A variable suction unit (Fig. 25-17) is necessary for the atraumatic dissection and exposure of an aneurysm. Variable suction which is necessary to prevent injury to the aneurysm, resulting in its premature rupture, is provided by a tear-shaped side port in the suction handle rather than by a small single opening; this allows the surgeon to control precisely the amount of suction by varying the opening in this orifice.

The tip of the suction unit should be made blunt and smooth by fitting it with either a small metal or a Teflon cap. Suction tips must be changed frequently to be certain that damaged and irregular tips are not used, as these are dangerous and can result in injury to small vessels and to the aneurysm itself. Obviously, a variety of sizes and lengths should be available to the surgeon. A No. 5 suction tip is used for the bulk of the procedure, but of course should the aneurysm rupture, the tip must be changed rapidly.

Temporary Clipping

It has been found that temporary clipping is preferable to prolonged periods of hypotension; thus it is seldom necessary to reduce the systemic blood pressure below a mean of 60 mmHg.[8] With appropriate barbiturate protection, major vessels can be occluded rather safely for 10 to 15 minutes at normal tension. With longer periods of occlusion, the surgeon runs the risk of ischemic damage, which varies from patient to patient and vessel to vessel.

Preparation of Aneurysm for Clipping

Major and perforating vessels in and around the base of the aneurysm have to be identified prior to clipping, so that when the clip is applied to the aneurysm, these vessels can be kept free from harm and readily available for temporary clipping in case the aneurysm ruptures. An aneurysm clip should never

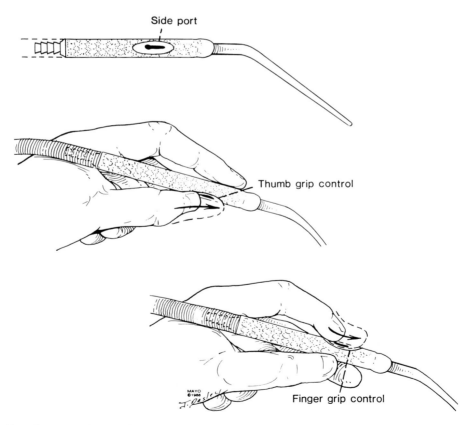

Figure 25-17. Microvascular suction unit for aneurysm surgery should be provided with a tear-shaped side port or opening, which permits precise regulation of the amount of suction. The unit illustrated has a knurled handle to which the suction tip is attached in a rotatable joint, so that the suction tip can be directed at the surgeon's angle of preference. (By permission of Mayo Foundation.)

be placed across an aneurysmal base before the planes for passage of the clip have been created with an aneurysm dissector.

Saccular Aneurysms

The general approach to saccular aneurysms is illustrated in Figure 25-18. The arachnoid overlying the area of the aneurysm is incised with the tip of a No. 11 blade knife with the brain placed on slight tension with a self-retaining retractor, which opens the cistern and places the arachnoid on a stretch.[8]

The surgeon needs to have precise knowledge of the anatomy and a basic understanding of the cisterns in order to facilitate this step in the procedure. In general, it is wise to identify and perhaps even to isolate for temporary clipping the major vessel proximal to the aneurysm. The dissection is carried distally to identify the base of the aneurysm. Under modest hypotension, the base of the aneurysm is then dissected away from perforating vessels. A small cottonoid placed on the end of a suction tip can be used for gently mobilizing the sac of the aneurysm away from vital perforating vessels, which should be visualized

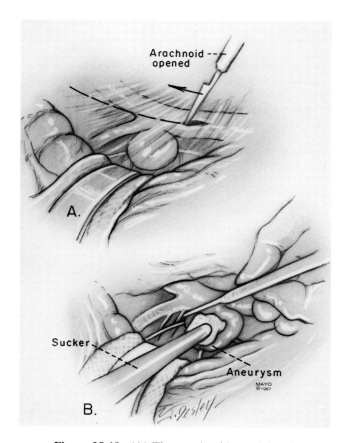

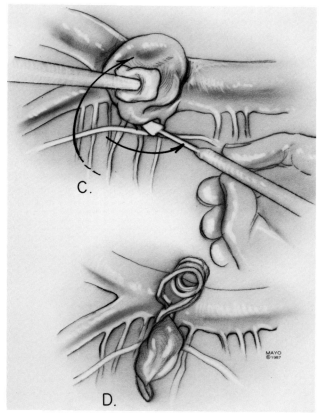

Figure 25-18. (**A**) The arachnoid overlying the saccular aneurysm is incised with the tip of a No. 11 blade knife and the dissection carried proximally to identify the parent artery for possible temporary clipping should the aneurysm rupture. (**B**) The walls of the aneurysm are then dissected from surrounding perforating vessels with a small aneurysm dissector or spatula. Under hypotension the aneurysmal sac can be deformed slightly and its volume reduced by compression with a blunt instrument such as a suction unit placed over a cotton paddy. (**C**) The aneurysm should be mobilized in all directions if possible in order to identify perforating vessels that are near its origin and that might be incorporated by a misplaced clip. (**D**) The aneurysm is occluded with an aneurysm clip that is appropriate for the size of the aneurysm. As small a clip as possible should be used for saccular aneurysms to facilitate the identification of perforating vessels after the aneurysm has been repaired. As the clip is placed across the base of the aneurysm, the surgeon should bear in mind that enough tissue is necessary to bridge the gap in the wall of the artery created by the aneurysm and thus that the clip should not be placed so close to the parent artery that the sac will tear with the compression by the clip. Such a tear invariably occurs at a base of the aneurysm, requiring the use of a clip graft. (By permission of Mayo Foundation.)

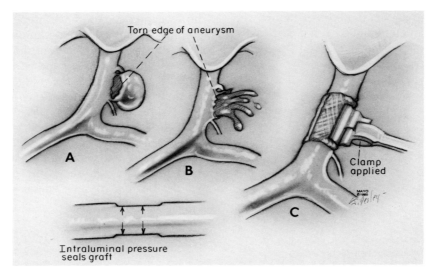

Figure 25-19. Repair of a hole in the wall of a vessel by using a clip graft. This clip should not be used except as a last resort as it carries the risk of damaging perforating vessels. However, this is, of course, far preferable to sacrificing a major vessel when there is a tear in its wall, which usually cannot be sutured as the hole is in such a position that it is difficult for the surgeon to rotate a needle and approximate the edges of the artery. Attempts at suturing holes in the walls of major vessels in and around the areas of aneurysms are often fraught with hazard and not infrequently result in more damage to the parent artery than was present before suturing was attempted. The appropriate size clip graft should be used for the specific artery that is damaged. In general terms, a 3.0- or 3.5-mm diameter clip graft is appropriate for most carotid arteries, but a 4.0-mm graft can be used for large vessels. The length of the clip graft (2.5, 5, or 7 mm) is determined by the length of the tear in the parent artery. (By permission of Mayo Foundation.)

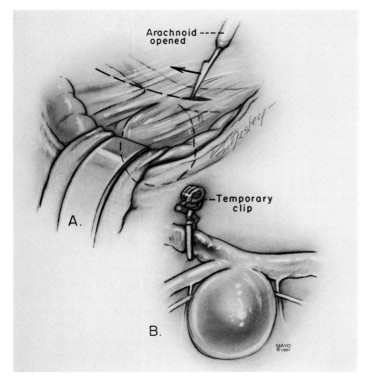

Figure 25-20. (**A**) The repair of a globular aneurysm. The arachnoid is incised with the tip of a No. 11 blade knife to expose the parent artery proximal to the site of the aneurysm. (**B**) A temporary clip is placed on the proximal artery to soften the aneurysm and increase the safety of its dissection from surrounding structures. (*Figure continues.*)

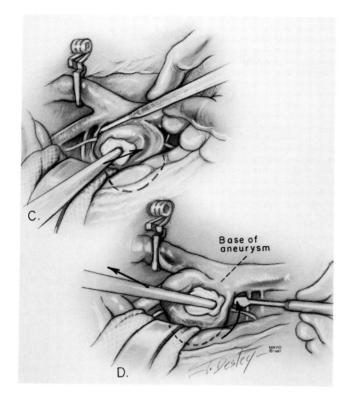

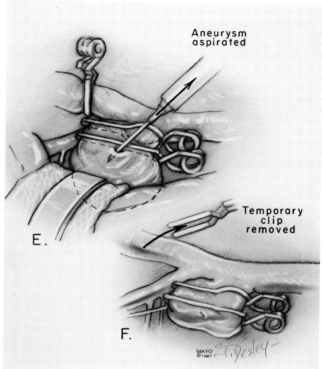

Figure 25-20 (*continued*). (**C**) The aneurysm is gently compressed with a cottonoid held in place with a suction unit as an aneurysm dissector is worked around the periphery of the lesion to separate perforating arteries from the walls of the aneurysm. (**D**) It is necessary that the dissection be carried circumferentially around the aneurysmal base to identify all perforating vessels in the region of the aneurysm. (**E**) Globular aneurysms usually have a thick base and thus are not often occludable with a single aneurysm clip. Drake's tandem clipping technique is particularly applicable for globular aneurysms. The first clip placed across the base of the aneurysm is an aperture clip, which allows the tips of the aneurysm clip to closely approximate and occlude the far wall of the aneurysm. This leaves a gap in the proximal portion of the neck, which is occluded by a second clip placed parallel to the first clip. (**F**) In globular aneurysms it is usually necessary to leave a small cuff of the base of the aneurysm present. This is somewhat exaggerated in the operative sketch above, but nevertheless it illustrates the point. It is necessary to leave a small cuff of aneurysmal base in order to avoid encroachment upon the lumen of the parent artery. After clipping has been achieved, the temporary clip is removed. Attempts to repair the aneurysm should not be undertaken until the aneurysm has been softened by either hypotension or proximal clipping. Thick-walled globular aneurysms tend to displace aneurysm clips proximally onto the parent artery. Thus it is necessary to have a strong clip available for the repair of these types of aneurysms. (By permission of Mayo Foundation).

before the clip is placed. It is important that the clip be placed on the aneurysmal sac at a distance that will allow approximation of the base of the aneurysm without tearing the aneurysm—that is, a clip should not be placed directly against the wall of the parent vessel where the aneurysm arises, as some tissue needs to be available for approximation. If the clip closes on the aneurysmal sac too close to the parent artery, it will tend to tear at the base, creating an uncomfortable situation, with a hole in a major artery. This can be repaired with a clip graft as illustrated in Figure 25-19, but this procedure carries with it the risk of damaged perforating vessels and should not be used except as a last resort.

Globular Aneurysms

The general methods and techniques used for the repair of globular aneurysms are illustrated in Figure 25-20. The technique differs slightly from that used for saccular aneurysms in that the wall of the aneurysm is invariably larger and generally has a relatively thick wall. In these cases the primary problem relates to total obliteration of the base of the aneurysm with preservation of the lumen in the parent artery.[8]

The general method of exposure for saccular aneurysms is also used for globular aneurysms, but in this case it is necessary not only to identify but also to isolate for temporary clipping the major vessel proximal to the site of the aneurysm. The aneurysm is then worked away from perforating vessels and prepared for clipping. A small dissector and spatula are used to create planes around the base of the aneurysm for the aneurysm clip, during which time the aneurysm is maneuvered and mobilized, with the tip of the suction unit separated from the aneurysm by a small cotton pledget. In some cases the aneurysm is so adherent to adjacent structures that it is difficult to mobilize and maneuver it and therefore perforating vessels on the far wall will not be visualized until after clipping of the aneurysm. Nevertheless, it is necessary that these vessels ultimately be visualized.

With few exceptions, globular aneurysms have a thick-walled base and also a wide neck, so that the surgeon has to be careful not to allow the aneurysm clip to encroach upon the lumen of the parent artery. This complication is most likely to occur if the surgeon attempts to clip the aneurysm under its full perfusion pressure without hypotension or temporary clipping. In such cases the aneurysm clip will often be "pumped" proximally onto the parent artery as the aneurysm redistends. To prevent this complication, temporary clipping should be used, and although only clipping of the proximal vessel is illustrated in Figure 25-20, at times it is necessary to occlude temporarily the major vessels exiting near the base of the aneurysm to gain total control of the lesion. The aneurysm clip should be placed at a point that will allow occlusion of the dome and most of the base but will permit flow through the parent artery. Thus, in many instances it is necessary to leave a small cuff of aneurysmal base to prevent encroachment upon the lumen of the parent artery by the aneurysm clips. Drake's tandem clipping technique (Fig. 25-20) is ideal for these situations in that the use of an aperture clip proximally allows good occlusion of the major base of the aneurysm but also some distension of the parent artery at the point where the aneurysm arose, while preventing stenosis from the clips. The use of aperture clip as the proximal clip in tandem clipping permits the tips of the blades to close on the aneurysmal sac and not be held apart by a thick-walled proximal base. Aneurysm clips are designed so that their tips will close first, and this is sufficient for thin-walled small aneurysms but is insufficient for thick-walled large aneurysms. The second clip in tandem with the proximal aperture clip occludes that portion of the base of the aneurysm filling through the area of the aperture.

Giant Aneurysms

Giant aneurysms differ from globular and saccular aneurysms not only in wall thickness but also commonly by the presence of thrombotic material. The surgeon should not attempt to repair a giant aneurysm without identifying the major vessels entering and exiting this lesion, as temporary occlusion of these arteries will be necessary to achieve good microvascular reconstruction.[8,9] In many instances it is necessary to have a bypass present before the aneurysm is occluded, as is illustrated in Figure 25-21. The period of temporary occlusion of a giant aneurysm that is necessary for thrombectomy and reconstruction varies from 15 minutes to 1 or 1½ hours. Thus, during the period of occlusion appropriate

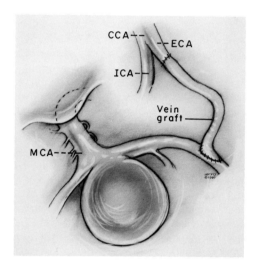

Figure 25-21. Protection by a saphenous vein bypass graft or temporal artery pedicle to the middle cerebral artery is advisable for giant aneurysms when they are located at a vulnerable point in the circulation (e.g., at the bifurcation of the carotid artery). In order to sustain adequate flow distal to the point of the aneurysm, a vein graft must be placed into a relatively large vessel such as one of the M_2 segments of the middle cerebral artery or an anterior temporal artery. The latter vessel works quite well for a temporary bypass graft and avoids the risk of injury to a major limb of the middle cereral artery. However, if the surgeon believes it is unlikely that flow through the giant aneurysm can be maintained after its repair, the vein graft should be placed into one of the major limbs of the middle cerebral artery, as the larger the recipient vessel, the greater the long-term patency of the vein. The temporal artery is anastomosed to a cortical vessel. (By permission of Mayo Foundation.)

measures should be taken to protect the brain. This includes not only protection by barbiturates and hypertension during occlusion but also placement of a vein bypass graft distally when necessary. In the middle cerebral complex, if it is believed that reconstruction is probably going to be achievable, the vein bypass graft can simply be placed in the anterior temporal branch of the middle cerebral artery, which eliminates the risk of injury to one of the major limbs of this artery in cases in which the giant aneurysm arises from the carotid artery or the proximal middle cerebral artery.

After the major vessels in and around the base of the giant aneurysm have been identified and temporarily occluded, the aneurysm is opened with the tip of a No. 11 blade knife at a good distance from its base (Fig. 25-22). The surgeon should avoid opening the giant aneurysm close to the base, as this will interfere with the clipping and reconstruction of the aneurysmal base and minimize the amount of tissue available for clipping. After the aneurysm has been opened, the plane of dissection is rapidly created between the wall of the aneurysm and the thrombus. The clot is removed by gentle dissection. With few exceptions the clot is laminated, so that planes of dissection are easily created. In particularly large giant aneurysms, some of the distal clotted material can be allowed to remain for removal after reconstruction of the base. No attempts should be made to remove the sac of the giant aneurysm except in selected cases of giant middle cerebral artery aneurysms in which excision is necessary to reconstruct the major vessels at the aneurysm base. Removing the sac of a giant aneurysm arising from the carotid, anterior communicating, basilar, or vertebral arteries is fraught with hazard, as these sacs are intimately adherent to vital perforating vessels.

In most instances, the sac can be reconstructed after the clot has been removed, as illustrated in Figure 25-22. However, in these cases it is frequently necessary to reinforce the primary clip with one or more booster clips to be certain that the base of the aneurysm has been firmly occluded. As is the case with globular aneurysms, a small cuff of aneurysmal base is frequently allowed to remain to prevent encroachment upon or narrowing of the lumen of the parent artery.

SAPHENOUS VEIN BYPASS GRAFTS

Saphenous vein bypass grafts for otherwise inoperable aneurysms of the intracavernous portion of the internal carotid artery remain a viable alternative, which surgeons should keep in mind and retain in their armamentaria. In our experience aneurysms arising from the distal or anterior loop of the internal carotid artery in the cavernous sinus can usually be repaired by direct clipping. However, as the aneurysm approaches the carotid canal in the cavernous sinus or actually involves the carotid canal in the bony portion of the petrous bone, it becomes fusiform and seldom can be repaired by direct clipping.

Our experience with saphenous vein bypass grafts to either the M_2 segment or the intracranial resected stump of the internal carotid artery has in general been good, although we recognize that this is less satisfactory than direct clipping of the aneurysm or balloon occlusion of a saccular component of an aneurysm arising in the cavernous sinus.[9]

Preparation of the Vein

Meticulous preparation of the vein is essential and is one of the most important aspects of the operative procedure. Techniques for the preparation of the saphenous vein graft and the principles involved have been previously reviewed in detail.[7]

The technical aspects of vein harvesting and preparation are crucial to the long-term success of saphenous vein bypass grafts in any location. On the neurosurgical service at the Mayo Clinic, a segment of the long saphenous vein is usually harvested from the distal leg rather than from the thigh in order to achieve a better diameter match between the vein and the recipient vessel. The skin incision is made one fingerbreadth anterior to the medial malleolus, where the vein is readily identifiable (Fig. 25-23 A & B). The incision is then carried proximally as needed, with care taken to remain directly over the vein in order to avoid creating any skin flap. Such flaps can slough and become major wound problems.

In our experience the vein, when distended, must measure at least 5 to 8 mm in diameter, as smaller veins have had a high rate of occlusion. Veins larger than 1 cm in diameter are disproportionately large at the distal anastomosis and are theoretically more prone to thrombosis secondary to slower flow, as described by Poiseuille's law. If the distal vein is too small or is unusable because of varicosities or other structural flaws, the proximal saphenous vein can be located in the groin and taken distally. The vein can be found near the fossa ovalis two fingerbreadths laterally from and two fingerbreadths below the lateral margin of the pubic tubercle. The incision is made from this part distally and aimed for the medial aspect of the tibial plateau. The vein should always be followed back to the fossa to confirm its identity.

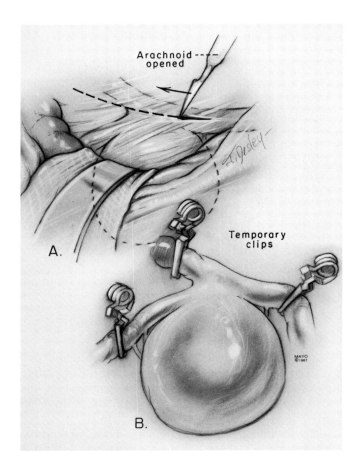

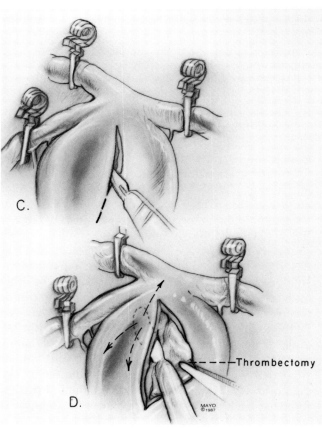

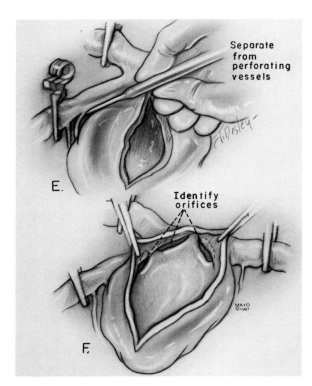

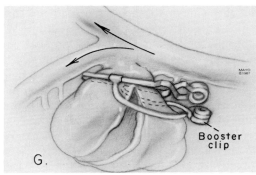

Figure 25-22. (**A**) The arachnoid is opened along the base of the giant aneurysm to expose the major arteries entering and leaving the lesion. (**B**) Temporary clips are then placed on the major vessels to decompress the aneurysm. (**C**) The aneurysm is opened with the tip of a No. 11 blade knife. (**D**) A clot along the wall of the aneurysm is removed by gentle dissection. These clots are usually laminated and are easily dissected away from the wall of the aneurysm. (**E**) After the aneurysm has been decompressed, its walls and margins are infolded to identify perforating vessels near its base. (**F**) The interior of the aneurysm is then inspected to identify the points of entrance and exit of the major arteries. In some cases this can be readily determined by external inspection of the aneurysm, and thus this step is not necessary. Also, in some cases the surgeon's angle of vision is such that the interior of the aneurysm cannot be inspected. (**G**) The base of the aneursym is occluded with a large, heavy-duty straight clip, which is reinforced with one or more booster clips. A small cuff of aneurysmal base is permitted to remain unclipped in order to prevent encroachment upon the lumen of the parent arteries by the aneurysm clips. (By permission of Mayo Foundation.)

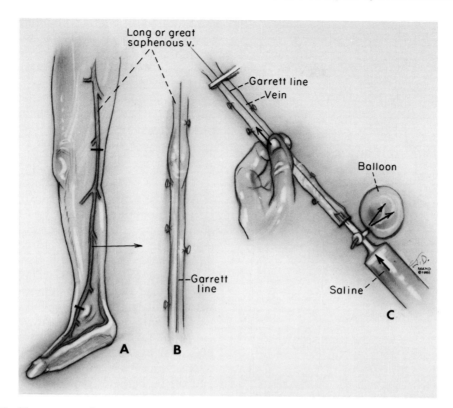

Figure 25-23. The great saphenous vein is harvested from the leg or thigh. There is considerable variability from patient to patient in the size of this vessel and in the number of branches. Small branches are ligated with 5-0 Prolene stick-ties and large branches with 3-0 silk stick-ties. Sometimes it is preferable to close large tributary vessels with a running 5-0 suture rather than to ligate the vessel with a larger suture, as the simple ligation with a tie sometimes distorts the lumen of the vein. The Garrett orientation line should be placed in the adventitia of the vein before it is harvested, as there is frequently a 360- to 720-degree rotation of the vein with distension after it is harvested. The proper orientation at that time cannot be determined. The vein is distended with the Shiley distension kit to 200 mmHg. The vein is worked between the index finger and thumb under cold saline solution until the vasospasm is overcome. It is preferable to leave the vein in situ after the tributaries have been ligated and to harvest it only after exposure of the intracranial recipient vessel and the cervical carotid arteries. (By permission of Mayo Foundation.)

After the skin has been incised, a delicate layer of areolar tissue can be identified overlying the vein. This tissue can be torn away from the vein by using the scissors with a spreading motion. While this is, no doubt, the quickest way to isolate the vein, one runs the risk of avulsing the tiny branches that lie within this layer. It is preferable to incise this tissue sharply 0.5 cm from the vein wall (Fig. 25-24). This will leave stumps of these small branches that are of sufficient length to be ligated after the vein has been removed from the leg. Large branches are ligated doubly with 3-0 or 4-0 silk free ties. Smaller branches may be similarly tied or may be closed with 5-0 Prolene stick ties. Holes made by avulsed branches may be repaired with a 7-0 Prolene mattress stitch. If simple ligation of a particularly large tributary will inordinately distort the lumen, the junction can be oversewn with a running 5-0 or 7-0 Prolene suture.

Prior to removing the vein, a 5-0 Prolene suture is placed in the adventitia of the vessel as an orientation line. We refer to this as a *Garrett line*, after the vascular surgeon from whom this technique was learned.[7] This is an extraordinarily important step in the procedure, as a vein tends to rotate with distension after it is harvested from the leg, and unless its proper orientation is identified in situ, there will be a rotation to the vein that cannot be corrected thereafter and that will predispose the vein to twisting and kinking. It is preferable to place the Garrett line before mobilizing and ligating the branches of the vein.

We prefer to mobilize the entire length of vein from one end to the other and then leave the vein in situ

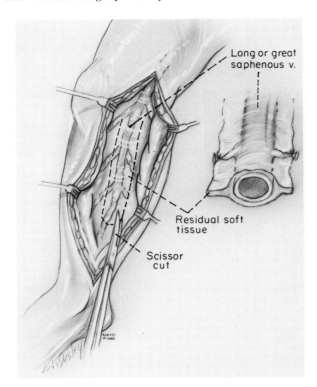

Figure 25-24. The vein should be harvested by incising the connective tissue surrounding the vessel several millimeters from the wall. This minimizes the handling of the vein itself and thereby minimizes both trauma and vasospasm. This technique also provides adequate room for subsequent ligation of any small branches that are missed while explanting the vessel. (By permission of Mayo Foundation.)

until it is ready to be transposed. In this manner flow is preserved through the vein for as long as possible. The vein is kept moist with saline packs.

At the time of harvesting, the vein is hydrodistended with a Shiley catheter distension system (Fig. 25-23C). This system has a bulb that distends at 200 mmHg and thus prevents overdistension and fracture of the vein wall from too much pressure. An early cause for graft occlusion in our series was overdistension of the vein. The vein is worked between the index finger and thumb until the spasm in it has been overcome, at which time the vein can be carefully inspected for any unligated branches.[7]

Cervical Exposure of Carotid Arteries

The carotid arteries are exposed as they are for an endarterectomy. However, the dissection is in general carried a bit higher, the incision being extended superiorly and anterior to the tragus of the ear. The parotid gland is mobilized anteriorly and superiorly to give good exposure to the distal external or/and internal carotid arteries. On occasion it is necessary in patients with a high bifurcation to identify the seventh nerve near its point of exit from the stylomastoid foramen and to trace it somewhat distally. Details of this technique have been described previously.[7]

Tunnel for Graft

A No. 20 French argyle trocar catheter is inserted into the temporalis muscle and passed over the zygoma through the deep layer of subcutaneous tissue anterior to the tragus of the ear, where it is then directed deep to the parotid gland to exit in the neck at the upper end of the cervical incision. One must be careful not to injure the superficial temporal artery with the sharp trocar of the catheter; for this reason, we frequently use a blunt heavy guide similar to that employed for shunt procedures. The distal end of the plastic sleeve is now opened by rotating the trocar over a No. 20 blade knife. The excision of this distal end of the catheter exposes the trocar, to which is now attached a No. 2-0 silk suture. The trocar is then withdrawn through the sleeve, bringing with it the suture.

Vein distension is maintained throughout by using the Shiley system and heparinized saline with an aneurysm clip at the most distal end of the vein. It is important to keep the vein moist during this portion of the procedure. The vein is then straightened according to the Garrett line, and the distal end of the vein graft is attached to the 2-0 silk suture and brought through the argyle catheter while maintaining vein distension. The argyle sleeve is then withdrawn over the vein. In this manner one is able to accurately place the vein graft without kinking, rotation, or injury. The path of a completed graft is illustrated in Figure 25-25.

Distal Anastomoses

For the distal anastomosis the surgeon has the option of placing the vein into the stump of the internal carotid artery or into one of the two M_2 segments of the middle cerebral artery. The selection of the recipient vessel is largely related to the anatomy of the aneurysm and to the quality and length of the internal carotid artery distal to the aneurysm. Crossflow also bears on this selection. In general terms, if the patient has adequate crossflow and the internal carotid artery is of good quality distal to the aneurysm, it is

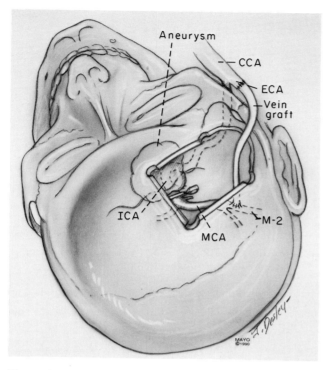

Figure 25-25. Completed vein graft coursing from the external carotid artery just distal to the bifurcation of the common carotid artery to a major limb of the middle cerebral artery. The vein follows a path that runs deep to the parotid gland and the deep cervical fascia of the high cervical area. It lies deep to the superficial temporal artery. It takes a course over the zygoma, where it pierces the temporalis muscle and then enters the cranial cavity through a small opening in the squamous portion of the temporal bone. (By permission of Mayo Foundation.)

better to place the vein graft into the stump of the internal carotid artery.[9] However, if there is inadequate crossflow, one of the M_2 segments should be used as the recipient vessel. As indicated below, patients tolerate temporary occlusion of one of the M_2 segments of the middle cerebral artery quite well for limited periods, and thus when a patient has virtually no crossflow from one hemisphere to the other or from the posterior to the anterior circulations, it is unwise to interrupt flow through the internal carotid artery until an alternate source of flow has been established.

End-to-End to Internal Carotid Artery

The anastomosis between the stump of the internal carotid artery and the distal end of the saphenous vein is best performed with interrupted 8-0 monofilament nylon sutures. The recipient internal carotid artery is unilaterally spatulated after it has been resected as far proximal in the cavernous sinus as possible. This artery is traced proximally past the anterior loop to the point where it takes its origin from the fusiform aneurysm; here it is sharply resected from the wall of the aneurysm, mobilized laterally, and spatulated (Fig. 25-26). The vein graft is in turn spatulated, and the two vessels are sewn end-to-end with interrupted sutures. The initial suture is from the apex of the venotomy to the distal end of the large spatulated portion of the internal carotid artery (Fig. 25-27). The anastomosis is then completed with 18 to 20 interrupted monofilament nylon sutures.

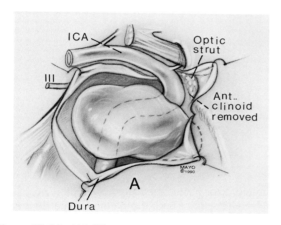
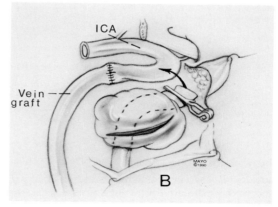

Figure 25-26. (**A**) Giant aneurysm involving the internal carotid artery proximal to the anterior loop of that vessel in the cavernous sinus. These aneurysms are often fusiform, which makes it difficult to reconstruct by clipping alone. (**B**) The aneurysm has been opened and found not to have a wall that could be converted to a channel for blood. Accordingly, the internal carotid artery has been divided from the distal sac of the aneurysm and rotated so that it could be sewn end-to-end to a vein graft coming from the stump of the cervical internal carotid artery. (By permission of Mayo Foundation.)

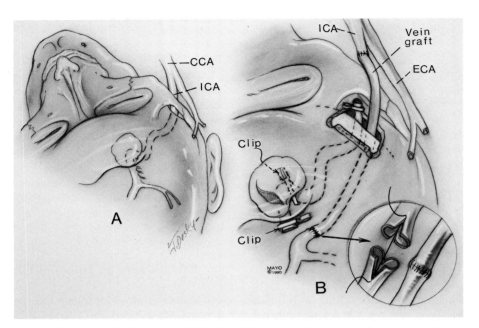

Figure 25-27. A saphenous vein bypass graft is placed between the stump of the cervical internal carotid artery and the intracranial internal carotid artery proximal to the origin of the ophthalmic artery. The distal vessels are fish-mouthed and anastomosed end-to-end using interrupted 8-0 monofilament nylon sutures. The proximal anastomosis is accomplished by using a running 6-0 Prolene suture after both the internal carotid artery and the vein graft have been spatulated. The vein follows a path deep to the parotid gland and superficial temporal artery to course over the zygoma and then through the temporalis muscle to enter the cranial cavity through a small opening in the squamous portion of the temporal bone. (By permission of Mayo Foundation.)

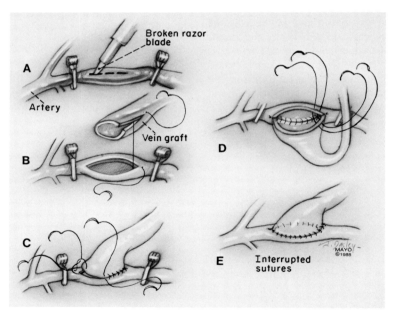

Figure 25-28. (**A**) The recipient vessel is opened with a broken razor blade. An adequate length is necessary to accept the spatulated vein. (**B**) The first suture is placed at the apex of both the spatulated incision in the vein and the proximal end of the arteriotomy in the artery. (**C**) The anastomosis is accomplished with multiple interrupted 8-0 sutures. These sutures must be placed close together in order to prevent bleeding because of the mismatch in the thickness in the wall of the vein in the artery. (**D**) The far side of the anastomosis is completed initially and then the near side. (**E**) Ordinarily 20 to 25 interrupted sutures are required for most anastomoses between the saphenous vein and the M_2 segment of the middle cerebral artery or the P_2 segment of the posterior cerebral artery, the vessel to which the vein is most commonly anastomosed. (By permission of Mayo Foundation.)

M₂ Segment of the Middle Cerebral Artery

An end-to-side anastomosis between the vein graft and the M₂ segment of the middle cerebral artery is used in those instances in which temporary occlusion of the internal carotid artery results in a sudden change of the EEG, indicating that it is necessary to preserve flow through the internal carotid artery until an alternate source of flow to the middle cerebral group has been provided. The anastomosis to the M₂ segment of the middle cerebral artery is performed as indicated in Figure 25-28. Usually the larger of the two M₂ segments of the middle cerebral artery is selected for this anastomosis. In general terms, patients tolerate temporary occlusion of one of the M₂ segments of the middle cerebral artery quite well for the 30 to 45 minutes required for this anastomosis.[7] Again, interrupted sutures are preferred over a running suture.

Proximal Anastomosis

There is a tendency to underestimate the proximal anastomosis, but this is based on an incorrect perception.[7] It is extraordinarily important that a strong pulse be present in the vein graft after flow is restored, and if a strong pulse, similar to that palpable in the carotid artery, is not present, the graft must be taken down and the anastomosis redone. Blood flow through the graft (determined by an electromagnetic flowmeter) is largely related to the distal runoff, whereas the quality of the pulse is related to the vein and to the construction of the proximal anastomosis. Several variations in the proximal anastomosis have been used.

End-to-End to Stump of External Carotid Artery

End-to-end anastomosis to the stump of the external carotid artery is our preferred proximal anastomosis and is used routinely whenever this artery has an adequate caliber and length.[7] Fortunately, in most instances this proves to be the case. The anastomosis is constructed with 12 to 14 interrupted 6-0 Prolene sutures, both the vein and the artery being fish-mouthed (Fig. 25-29). In cases in which the external carotid artery or the saphenous vein graft is smaller than average, it is sometimes necessary to enlarge the anastomosis with a roof-patch graft (Fig. 25-30).

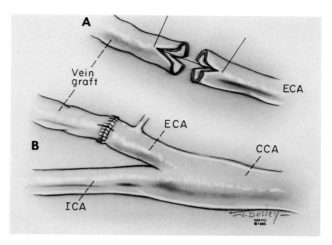

Figure 25-29. End-to-end anastomosis between the vein graft and the stump of the external carotid artery. The vein graft and external carotid artery are both fish-mouthed, and then the anastomosis is completed with 12 to 14 interrupted 5-0 or 6-0 Prolene sutures. This is currently our most common type of construction for the proximal anastomosis. (By permission of Mayo Foundation.)

End-to-End to Stump of Internal Carotid Artery

End-to-end anastomosis to the stump of the internal carotid artery is used for bypassing giant aneurysms of this artery. The internal carotid artery is divided just distal to its bulb at a point where it matches in caliber the distended vein graft. The anastomosis is thereafter carried out as described for the external carotid artery (Fig. 25-31).

End-to-Side to Common Carotid Artery

Not infrequently, the external carotid artery is of such poor quality or so heavily involved with atherosclerosis that it is necessary to place the anastomosis end-to-side to the common carotid artery. This anastomosis can be placed at the origin of the artery or more inferiorly. In several cases it has been necessary to complete a standard endarterectomy of the common and internal carotid arteries in order to free the external carotid artery from atherosclerosis. In these cases, we have found with experience that it is wise to patch-graft the site of the anastomosis in order to create a bulb at the origin of the vein graft[7] (Fig. 25-32).

Complications

One of the complications of a saphenous vein bypass graft is the development of a subdural hygroma, usually on the third to fourth day following the sur-

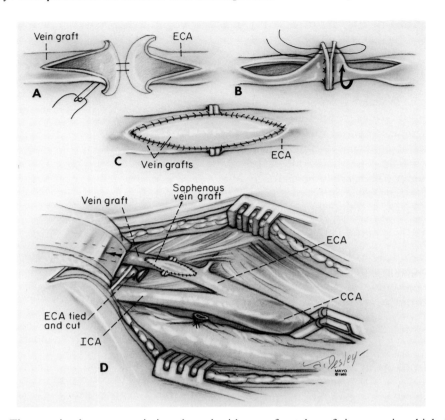

Figure 25-30. The proximal anastomosis is enlarged with a roof-patch graft in cases in which the external carotid artery or the saphenous vein is smaller than average. We have redone an anastomosis acutely on the table in cases in which the graft pulse appears to be inadequate. Placement of a roof-patch graft in these instances has usually resulted in a very significant improvement in the quality of the pulse and, we believe, in the long-term patency of the graft. (By permission of Mayo Foundation.)

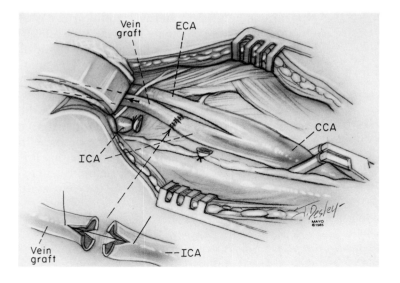

Figure 25-31. Proximal anastomosis between saphenous vein and stump of internal carotid artery in a patient with a giant aneurysm undergoing internal carotid artery ligation with a simultaneous interposition saphenous vein graft. The bulb of the internal carotid artery is preserved for the anastomosis. The vein graft and the internal carotid artery are both fish-mouthed and then sewn end-to-end with 12 to 14 interrupted 5-0 or 6-0 sutures. (By permission of Mayo Foundation.)

Figure 25-32. On occasion it is necessary to perform an endarterectomy in the common internal and external carotid arteries in cases in which there is significant stenosis of the external carotid artery. The external carotid artery cannot be reconstructed without also performing an endarterectomy in both the common and internal carotid arteries, and therefore a shunt is routinely employed in these cases as it is not possible to monitor the patients with cerebral blood flow measurements and EEGs in these situations. Following endarterectomy the external carotid artery is usually divided just distal to its origin and the saphenous vein graft sewn to the stump of the external carotid artery with interrupted sutures. Both the saphenous vein and the margin of the external carotid artery are spatulated; the site of the anastomosis is then enlarged with a saphenous vein roof patch, as illustrated in Figure 25-30. (By permission of Mayo Foundation.)

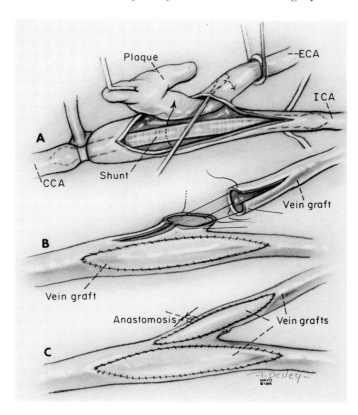

gery. These hygromas are not as frequent with grafts into the anterior circulation as with grafts into the posterior circulation, but nevertheless they do occur. The surgeon should be alerted to this possible complication and be prepared to place a subdural-peritoneal or a subdural-atrial shunt. These subdural hygromas can develop under considerable pressure, and they are not a complication that should be ignored or managed by temporizing measures.

REFERENCES

1. Drake CG: The treatment of aneurysms of the posterior circulation. Clin Neurosurg 26:96, 1979
2. Heros RC: Lateral suboccipital approach for vertebral and vertebrobasilar artery lesions. J Neurosurg 64:559, 1986
3. Ojemann RG, Crowell RM: Surgical Management of Cerebrovascular Disease. Williams & Wilkins, Baltimore, 1983
4. Patterson RH: Technique of carotid endarterectomy. p. 177. In Smith RR (ed): Stroke and the Extracranial Vessels. Raven Press, New York, 1984
5. Pearson BW, Sundt TM Jr: Exposure of the distal internal carotid artery. p. 298. In Sundt TM Jr (ed): Occlusive Cerebrovascular Disease: Diagnosis and Surgical Management. WB Saunders, Philadelphia, 1987
6. Robertson, JT, Auer NJ: Extracranial occlusive disease of the carotid artery. p. 1559. In Youmans JR (ed): Neurological Surgery. Vol. 3. WB Saunders, Philadelphia, 1982
7. Sundt TM Jr: Occlusive Cerebrovascular Disease: Diagnosis and Surgical Management. WB Saunders, Philadelphia, 1987
8. Sundt TM Jr: Surgical Techniques for Saccular and Giant Intracranial Aneurysms. Williams & Wilkins, Baltimore, 1990
9. Sundt TM Jr, Piepgras DG, Fode NC, Meyer FB: Giant intracranial aneurysms. Clin Neurosurg 37:116, 1990
10. Thompson JE: Surgery for Cerebrovascular Insufficiency (Stroke): with Special Emphasis on Carotid Endarterectomy. Charles C Thomas, Springfield, IL, 1968
11. Wylie EJ, Ehrenfeld WK: Extracranial Occlusive Cerebrovascular Disease: Diagnosis and Management. WB Saunders, Philadelphia, 1970
12. Yasargil MG: Microneurosurgery. Vol. 2. Clinical Considerations, Surgery of the Intracranial Aneurysms and Results. George Thieme Verlag, Stuttgart, 1987

26 Aneurysm Clip Design, Selection, and Application

Shigeaki Kobayashi

Yuichiro Tanaka

Various kinds of complications may occur in the clipping surgery of cerebral aneurysms. Table 26-1 lists complications related to clipping procedures used in our series of approximately 1,000 aneurysms. Complications may occur in the aneurysm itself, in the parent artery and branches, or in the neural tissues. Complications at the aneurysm include (1) residual neck caused by incomplete clipping; (2) slip-out of a clip, which may occur with small or wide-based aneurysms; and (3) laceration at the neck. Complications in the parent artery and branches consist of (1) stenosis of the parent artery due to inappropriate clipping or slip-in of a clip; and (2) branch occlusion due to inadvertent clipping. Complications relating to neural tissues include (1) accidental clipping of cranial nerves; and (2) compression of neural structures by the clip head.

These complications may occur in various situations; some, however, tend to occur in special situations and could be avoided by appropriate strategies. Such complications are related to the site and size of an aneurysm, to the approach route, to whether or not the aneurysm has ruptured; and to whether surgery is acute or delayed. Of these factors the site and size of an aneurysm are the main concerns in this chapter, in which we introduce measures based on our experience for avoiding complications related to the clipping procedure.

Table 26-2 lists some of our techniques to avoid the above-mentioned complications, namely techniques useful before application of a clip to gain better visu-

alization of the aneurysm neck and surrounding structures, methods of clip selection, methods of clip application, and techniques to be used after clipping.

In our practice we use Sugita's multipurpose head frame and tapered spatulas connected to a self-retaining retractor for retraction.[7] This system fine, delicate, steady, and exact retraction of brain, vessels, neural structures, and the aneurysm itself. Sugita's clips are used in the majority of cases.

TECHNIQUES USED BEFORE CLIPPING FOR BETTER VISUALIZATION OF THE ANEURYSM NECK AND SURROUNDING STRUCTURES

It is essential to expose the aneurysm neck and surrounding structures as widely as possible for safe and successful clipping while maintaining minimum brain retraction. Inadequate visualization of the neck may lead to several complications, such as residual neck, stenosis of the parent artery, or accidental clipping of perforating arteries and cranial nerves. First of all, selection of a proper approach route and minimal yet sufficient retraction of the brain before undertaking clipping are the most important to avoid these complications. In this section we describe several technical points to facilitate better visualization of the aneurysm neck when part of the aneurysm or the neck is exposed in the operating field.

Table 26-1. Complications Related to Aneurysm Clipping

Complications at the aneurysm
    Residual neck
    Slip-out of clip blades
    Laceration at neck
Complications in the parent artery and branches
    Stenosis of parent artery
    Occlusion of branch and perforating artery
Complications involving neural tissues
    Accidental clipping of cranial nerve
    Compression of neural tissue by clip head

Table 26-2. Techniques and Clip Selection to Avoid Complications

Technique	Illustration
Techniques used before applying clip for better visualization of aneurysm neck and surrounding structures	
Retraction of cranial nerve	Fig. 26-1
Retraction of artery or aneurysm	Fig. 26-2
Rotation of parent artery	Figs. 26-3, 26-4
Use of microsurgical mirror	Fig. 26-5
Tentative clipping	Fig. 26-6
Step clipping	
Alternate clipping	
Temporary clipping	Fig. 26-7
Suctioning of blood from aneurysm	Fig. 26-7
Selection of clip	Figs. 26-7, 26-8
Application of clip	
Multiple clipping	Figs. 26-9 to 26-11
Tandem clipping	
Counterclipping	
Other variations	
Formation clipping	Figs. 26-12, 26-13
Branch artery formation	
Parent artery formation	
Aneurysm formation	
Booster clipping	Fig. 26-14
Booster clip	
Duplication clipping	
Shank clipping	Fig. 26-10
Compression clipping	Fig. 26-15
Rotation advance	Fig. 26-16
Applicator changing	Fig. 26-17
Dissection with clip blade	Fig. 26-18
Techniques used after clipping	
Reinforcement of clipping with wrapping material	Fig. 26-19
Removal of brain to provide room for clip head	Fig. 26-20
Placement of cushion between clip head and neural tissue	

Retraction of Cranial Nerves

Retraction of cranial nerves is occasionally required to expose the neck of an aneurysm, especially in the case of a large or giant aneurysm of the internal carotid artery (see Case Study 1, Fig. 26-1). At that time removal of the roof of the optic canal and the anterior clinoid process facilitates mobilization of the optic nerve and internal carotid artery and lessens the risk of injuring the optic nerve when retracted.[4] When retracting the optic nerve, the intermittent retraction principle should be followed by, for instance, alternately retracting the nerve for 10 minutes and releasing it for 5 minutes.[1,16] When retracting the nerve, blanching of the vessels adjacent to the optic nerve is a warning sign that the pressure is excessive. Removing part of the bony structure in the base of the skull, such as the anterior or posterior clinoid process and the petrous pyramid, also has the advantage of providing room for inserting the clip blades. Placing a Silastic sheet between the optic nerve and the tip of a spatula is recommended to avert direct damage to the optic nerve. In our practice the optic and trigeminal nerves most often can be directly retracted with impunity. Retraction of cranial nerves III, VI, and VIII should best be avoided.

Case Study 1

This 66-year-old woman suffered a subarachnoid hemorrhage (SAH) 70 days before surgery (Fig. 26-1). The angiogram showed a giant aneurysm of the left internal carotid artery, probably located between the origins of the ophthalmic and posterior communicating arteries.

Operation

The sylvian fissure was opened widely through a left frontotemporal craniotomy. The optic nerve, which had become thin over the aneurysm, was unroofed and the anterior clinoid process carefully removed. The carotid dural ring was incised and the dural covering dissected; the cavernous sinus was, partly opened thereby, and bleeding from the sinus was controlled with Oxycel packing. We found it difficult to dissect the aneurysm from the optic nerve because of the high intraluminal pressure. The cervical carotid artery was temporarily occluded with a vessel tape, and the ophthalmic, posterior communicating, and distal carotid arteries were temporarily clipped for about 10 minutes under mannitol protection. The optic nerve was retracted medially with a tapered brain retractor after carefully dissecting it from the aneurysm to widely expose the neck and body. Three ring clips were successfully applied in tandem fashion (see Fig. 26-9).

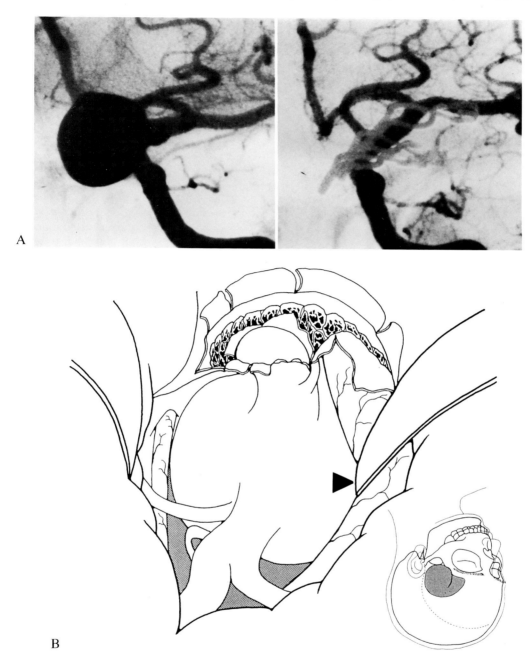

Figure 26-1. (**A**) Pre- and postoperative lateral angiograms of Case Study 1 patient, showing a giant aneurysm of the left internal carotid artery. Three ring clips are placed in tandem fashion. (**B**) Schema of the operation in Case Study 1, showing direct retraction of the optic nerve (*arrowhead*). The optic nerve is retracted medially with a tapered brain retractor after being carefully dissected from the aneurysm to widely expose the neck and body.

Direct Retraction of Aneurysm

Direct retraction of the aneurysm is often instrumental in securing the space for dissection and application of a clip, especially in the case of a large or giant aneurysm (see Case Study 2, Fig. 26-2).[12] Direct retraction of the aneurysm itself can be performed without temporarily clipping the parent artery; the procedure is more effective, of course, when it is carried out with temporary clipping. A 2-mm tapered spatula is most frequently used for retraction. The spatula should be applied to a part of the aneurysm with an apparently thick wall, and the retraction should proceed in a direction that does not produce

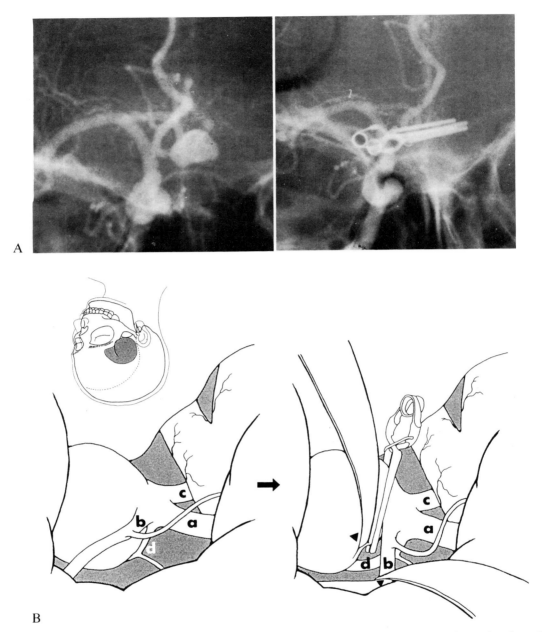

Figure 26-2. (A) Pre- and postoperative anteroposterior angiograms of Case Study 2 patient, showing a large aneurysm at the anterior communicating artery. Two straight clips are applied in this duplication clipping procedure. **(B)** Schema of the operation in Case Study 2, showing direct retraction of the aneurysm and artery (*arrowhead*). Dissection of the right A_2 segment of the anterior cerebral artery is performed with two spatulas placed on the aneurysm and the distal A_2. *a*, right A_1; *b*, right A_2; *c*, left A_1; *d*, left A_2.

an untoward shearing force on the aneurysm. The holding pressure of our retraction system (spatula and self-retaining retractor connected to the multi-purpose head frame) is sufficient to allow pulsatile motion of the spatula when it is holding an aneurysm; the spatula can be positioned exactly and kept from shifting while in place.

Case Study 2

This 38-year-old man suffered an SAH a day prior to the operation (Fig. 26-2). A large 15-mm aneurysm was found at the anterior communicating artery, pointing left laterally and anteriorly on the angiogram.

Operation

A right frontotemporal craniotomy was performed. The right A_1 segment of the anterior cerebral artery was traced distally after opening the sylvian fissure; the left A_1 segment was found in the fossa between the right A_1 segment and the chiasm. As the right gyrus rectus was partially removed by suction, the right A_2 segment was found; it has been stretched by the underlying tense aneurysm body. With direct retraction of the body of the aneurysm, the left A_2 segment was found in the fossa. The most difficult part of the whole procedure was separating the right proximal A_2 segment from the aneurysm neck. A temporary clip was applied to both A_1 segments, and further dissection of the right A_2 segment was begun with two spatulas placed on the aneurysm and the distal A_2 segment. A straight clip was applied to the neck. Puncture of the aneurysm body showed that occlusion of the neck was incomplete, possibly owing to unevenness of the inner surface of the neck. Therefore another straight clip was applied distal to the first clip to reinforce that clip (see Fig. 26-14B & C for duplication clipping).

Rotation of the Parent Artery

Rotation of the parent artery by direct retraction makes it possible to expose in the operating field an aneurysm located behind the parent artery on the side opposite to that used in the approach (see Case Studies 3 and 4, Figs. 26-3 to 26-5). A tapered spatula with a 2-mm wide tip is necessary to perform this

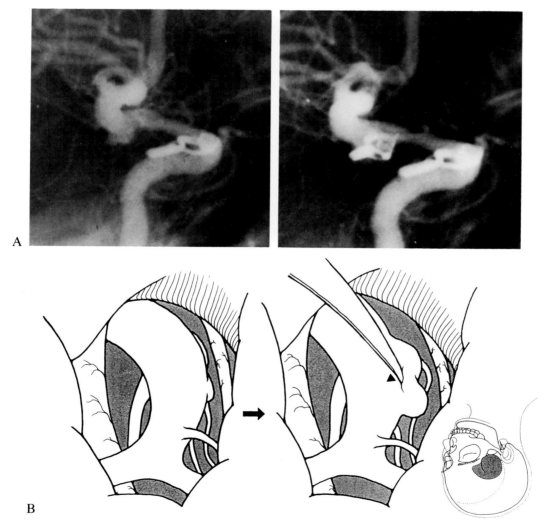

Figure 26-3. (**A**) Pre- and postoperative lateral angiograms of Case Study 3 patient, showing an aneurysm of the right internal carotid artery. (**B**) Schema of the operation in Case Study 3. Direct retraction to rotate the parent artery facilitates better visualization of the aneurysm (*arrowhead*).

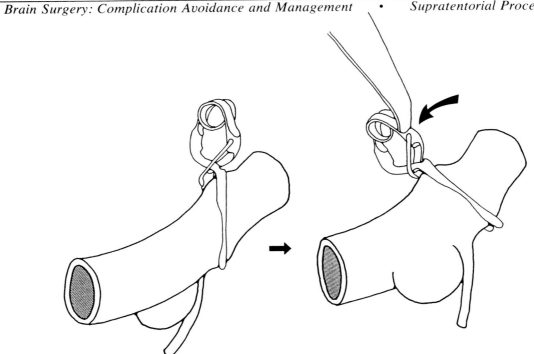

Figure 26-4. Indirect rotation method used to rotate the artery with the tip of spatula on a temporary clip (*curved arrow*).

procedure. Care should be taken not to cause premature rupture of the aneurysm when its dome is adherent to the surrounding structures. The parent artery can also be retracted indirectly by placing the tip of a spatula on the head of the temporary clip placed on the parent artery near the aneurysm (Fig. 26-4). In both cases the spatula is held by a self-retaining retractor connected to the multipurpose head frame.

Case Study 3

This 64-year-old man had suffered an SAH, and clipping of the left internal carotid artery aneurysm had been performed within 24 hours (Fig. 26-3). The nonruptured aneurysm of the right internal carotid artery was operated on 54 days after the first operation.

Operation

The sylvian fissure was opened as wide as possible through a right frontotemporal craniotomy. The proximal portion of the internal carotid artery was secured for possible temporary clipping. A cherry spot–like daughter aneurysm was found, which was continuous with the whitish bulge at the origin of the posterior communicating artery. This bulge could be called an aneurysmal dilatation rather than an infundibular dilatation, but two small perforating arteries were found to originate from it. All these findings

were obtained by using the direct retraction method to rotate the parent artery. A straight miniclip was placed, and the retractor was carefully removed.

Microsurgical Mirror

A microsurgical mirror is useful to confirm the position of the clip blade and small arteries behind the aneurysm to avoid accidentally clipping small branches and leaving residual neck (see Case Study 4, Fig. 26-5).[8] The mirror is available in different diameters ranging from 3 to 5 mm. When necessary, the mirror is held by a self-retaining retractor so that the surgeon can continue using both hands for the procedures.

Case Study 4

This 26-year-old woman had an SAH 13 days before the operation (Fig. 26-5). The angiogram showed a small aneurysm located dorsolaterally at the origin of the posterior communicating artery.

Operation

The aneurysm was semicircular and located dorsolaterally in the segment between the origins of the posterior communicating and anterior choroidal arteries. The aneurysm complex was dissected during a short period of temporary clipping of the parent ar-

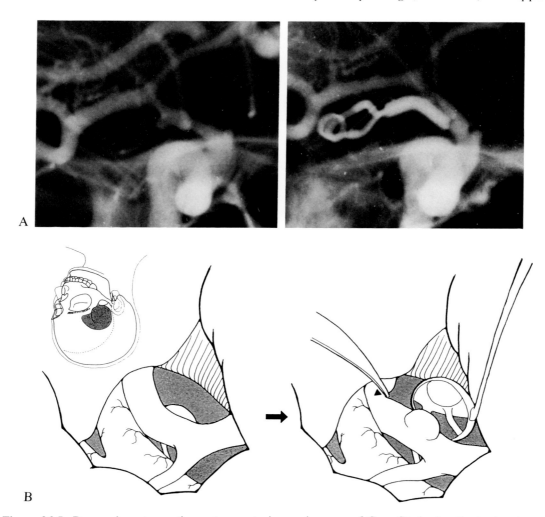

Figure 26-5. Pre- and postoperative anteroposterior angiograms of Case Study 4 patient, showing a small aneurysm located dorsolaterally at the origin of the posterior communicating artery. (**B**) Schema of the operation in Case Study 4. The proximal portion of internal carotid artery is pressed and retracted medially with the tip of a 2-mm spatula (*arrowhead*). A microsurgical mirror is helpful to confirm the origin of the posterior communicating and anterior choroidal arteries before application of a clip.

tery. Finally, the proximal portion of the internal carotid artery was pressed and retracted medially with the tip of a 2-mm spatula, causing counterclockwise rotation of the aneurysm, which was clipped with an L-shaped clip. Because the aneurysm was wide-based, the parent artery showed some stenosis when the clip was so placed as to include the whole aneurysm. The microsurgical mirror was helpful to confirm the origin of the posterior communicating and anterior choroidal arteries.

Tentative Aneurysm Clipping

Tentative aneurysm clipping is defined as a method in which a clip is placed on the body of an aneurysm before a permanent clip is applied; this differs from *temporary* clipping, in which the parent artery is temporarily occluded to facilitate aneurysm dissection and/or permanent clipping. Tentative clipping is a useful technique to prevent premature rupture of the aneurysm during dissection between the aneurysm and either the parent or the branch artery before placement of a permanent clip on the aneurysm neck (Fig. 26-6). This technique is also useful for reducing the volume of a large or giant aneurysm to provide space for further dissection and for insertion of clip blades. Tentative clipping include two variations, step clipping and alternate clipping. In step clipping the first clip is applied to the body or dome of an aneurysm, a permanent clip is then placed exactly on the neck after adequate dissection around the neck has been performed, and finally the first clip is re-

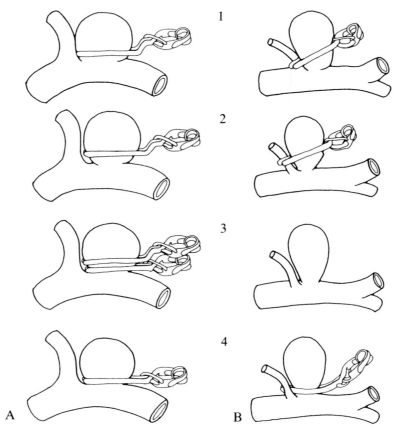

Figure 26-6. Diagrammatic representation of tentative clipping, defined as a method in which a clip is applied on the body of the aneurysm before applying a permanent clip. Tentative clipping includes two variations, (**A**) step clipping and (**B**) alternative clipping. *1,* application of first clip (**A & B**); *2,* dissection around the neck (**A & B**); *3,* application of the second clip (**A**) and removal of the first clip (**B**); *4,* removal of the first clip (**A**) and application of the second clip (**B**).

moved. This is essentially a variant of tentative clipping followed by permanent clipping; the series of clippings may be repeated until the final satisfactory clip is placed. In the step clipping procedure, the direction of the first clip blades is usually the same as that of the second permanent clip so that the first clip can be left until the second clip is placed; a bayonet clip is recommended for use as the first clip to avoid difficulty in inserting the second clip. When it is, difficult to place the first clip in the same direction as a second one, the second clip is placed after removing the first clip (alternate clipping); this procedure entails some risk of premature rupture of the aneurysm but allows more freedom for placing the final clip. There is a risk of embolus release from the aneurysm during tentative clipping, but this rarely occurs unless the aneurysm is extremely large or has ruptured during the procedure or the time for tentative clipping is prolonged.

Temporary Clipping and Blood Suctioning

Temporary clipping and/or suctioning of blood from the aneurysm is a method to reduce aneurysmal tension before application of a permanent clip (see Case Study 5, Fig. 26-7). Relaxation of aneurysmal tension before clip application has the advantages of preventing slip-off of clip blades in case of a large aneurysm, facilitating the checking perforators behind the aneurysm, and allowing easy dissection of the neck from the surrounding structure. When adequate relaxation of the aneurysm is not obtained by temporary clipping, puncture of the aneurysm is an effective means of reducing its size. Single puncture and suction of the aneurysmal contents is not always effective if arterial branches such as the posterior communicating or anterior choroidal artery are present in the segment of the parent artery occluded by the temporary clips. In such a situation continuous suctioning under negative pressure is helpful to maintain the slack aneurysm. Our puncture needle is so constructed that blood does not spill into the field when the stylet is removed. The puncture needle can be held in place by the flexible arm of the self-retaining retractor while the surgeon continues to work in the field.

SELECTION OF CLIP

Selection of an appropriate clip for each aneurysm is one of the most important decisions for successful clipping. The surgeon should keep in mind the need to select the best clip before the final clip application. Appropriate clipping is ordinarily possible with a regular clip from the standard clip set or a combination of clips if necessary. However, specially designed clips are occasionally needed for very unusual shaped aneurysms to avoid leaving residual neck or because of an unusual anatomical relationship between the aneurysm and parent artery in a narrow operating field. Figures 26-7 and 26-8 show some newly designed clips.[4,10]

Case Study 5

This 48-year-old woman had complained of failing vision in the left eye. A giant aneurysm measuring 2.5 cm was found on the carotid angiogram (Fig. 26-7).

Operation

With the sylvian fissure opened, an aneurysm was visualized in the ventral side of the internal carotid artery. The anterior clinoid process was then removed extradurally, with the intradural findings as the landmarks. The dura was opened from the intradural side, the carotid dural ring was opened, and the proximal carotid artery was secured. Under temporary clipping of the internal carotid artery, the aneurysm was punctured in the retrocarotid side with the puncture needle and dissected from the surrounding brain. Several attempts were made with different combinations of different types of clips under temporary occlusion or proximal clipping of the parent artery. Finally, a ring clip with leftward bent blades and a right-angled ring clip with straight 5-mm blades were applied in crosswise fashion (see Fig. 26-9). The greatest difficult was in avoiding stenosis and kinking for the distal neck, which had become narrowed by the pressure of the underlying giant aneurysm. The second clip was not placed flush with the parent artery for fear of causing stenosis or occlusion of that

artery. The postoperative angiogram showed a dog ear in the distal neck; the parent artery was patent.

Case Study 6

This 39-year-old man had suffered an SAH, and clipping of an aneurysm at the A_2-A_3 junction of the left anterior cerebral artery had been performed previously. This time surgery was performed on an unruptured aneurysm at the ophthalmic segment of the left internal carotid artery (Fig. 26-8).[5]

Operation

A left frontotemporal craniotomy was made. The sylvian fissure was separated, care being taken not to overly retract the frontal lobe, as we had suspected that the dome of the aneurysm would be adherent to the base of this lobe. The aneurysm was found to originate from the dorsal wall of the internal carotid artery in its ophthalmic segment and to be pressing upon the optic nerve, which had been slightly shifted frontally. The dura over the optic nerve and internal carotid artery was cut and reflected back, and the anterior clinoid process was then removed. The body of the aneurysm was double-domed, located dorsally just distal to the dural penetration. By carefully retracting the frontal lobe base and also the optic nerve, the aneurysm was dissected free of them despite the adhesion. The domes of the aneurysm were united at the top of the dorsum of the internal carotid artery. With the cervical carotid artery temporarily occluded for about 5 minutes at a time, attempts were made to occlude the aneurysm with different clips. Finally a newly designed reverse-curve L-shaped clip was used to occlude the two aneurysms from the opposite side of the optic nerve in order to prevent the clip from compressing the optic nerve. This clip was originally designed specifically for aneurysms at the A_2-A_3 junction of the anterior cerebral artery.

CLIP APPLICATION

Multiple Clipping

Multiple clipping is necessary for wide-neck and unusual-shaped aneurysms.[9,11] (see Figs. 26-1, 26-7, 26-10, and 26-13). Tandem or counterclipping is commonly used for these aneurysms (Fig. 26-9). In *tandem* clipping the clips are placed with their blades in the same direction, whereas in counterclipping the blades of two clips are oppositely placed in either a facing or a crosswise fashion. How to arrange the clips depends on the relationship between the neck

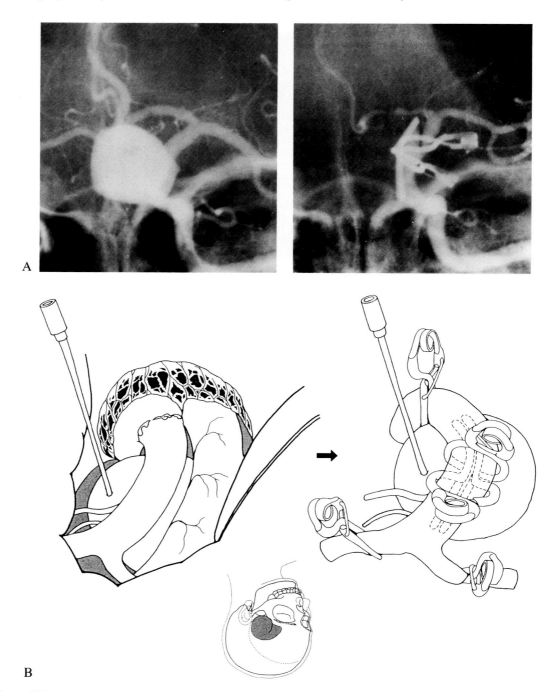

Figure 26-7. (**A**) Pre- and postoperative anteroposterior angiograms of Case Study 5 patient, showing a giant aneurysm of the left internal carotid artery. A ring clip with blades bent to the left and a right-angled ring clip are applied with care to keep the original curve of the parent artery. (**B**) Schema of the operation in Case Study 5. Temporary clipping and continuous suctioning of blood from the aneurysm reduce the aneurysm tension before application of permanent clips.

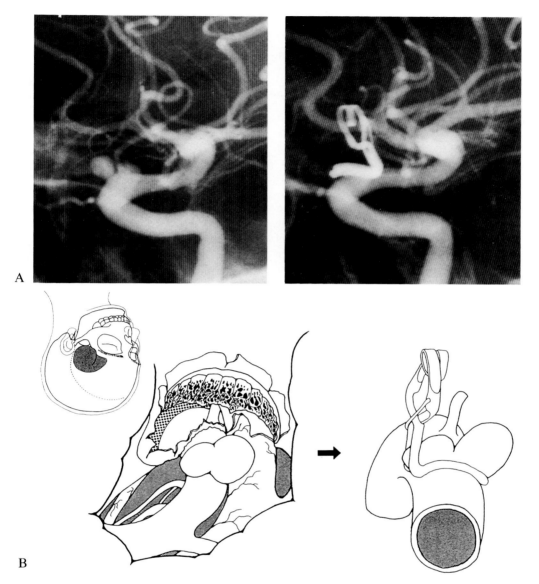

Figure 26-8. (**A**) Pre- and postoperative lateral angiograms of Case Study 6 patient, showing an aneurysm at the ophthalmic segment of the left internal carotid artery. (**B**) Schema of the operation in Case Study 6. The body of the aneurysm is double-domed. A newly designed reverse-curve L-shaped clip is used to occlude the two aneurysms from the opposite side of the optic nerve to prevent the clip from compressing the nerve.

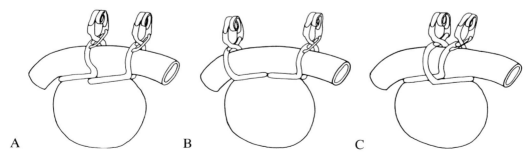

Figure 26-9. Multiple clipping, a method in which the aneurysm neck is occluded with more than two clips, includes many variations. (**A**) Tandem clipping and (**B & C**) counterclipping are commonly used for a large or giant internal carotid artery aneurysm. Counterclipping can be carried out in (**B**) facing or (**C**) crosswise fashion.

and surrounding tissues. It is important to keep in mind that the aneurysm and parent artery are related three-dimensionally and not as seen in a single angiographic view. Hemodynamic alteration may occur after clipping when the neck is wide. Clipping of a wide-neck aneurysm may straighten the parent artery, causing kinking of its distal branches and hence hypoperfusion (see Case Study 7, Fig. 26-10). A combination of clips with short blades is one of the methods of avoiding such a complication. However, multiple clipping with straight blades still may cause deformity of the parent artery; in order to prevent this, use of a ring clip with sideways bent blades is recommended (see Case Study 5, Fig. 26-7). Another complication related to multiple clipping is *clip junctional leakage*, which is bleeding from the aneurysm wall at the junctional portion of two or more clips (see Case Study 8, Fig. 26-11). This complication occasionally occurs in the area of the junction between a proximal blade end in the fenestrated clip and a blade of another clip because the jaw portion of the blade is not sharply rectangular, as well as because the aneurysm complex is three-dimensional.

Case Study 7

This 61-year-old women (Fig. 26-10), who had noticed a visual disturbance 2 months earlier, was diagnosed with upper bitemporal quadrantoanopsia. The angiogram showed a giant aneurysm at the left carotid siphon.

Operation

Two-thirds of the proximal carotid artery was located behind the optic nerve. The roof of the optic canal and a medial portion of the anterior clinoid were drilled off. The neck of the aneurysm was in the segment between the ophthalmic and the posterior communicating arteries. With elevation of the optic nerve and temporary occlusion of the internal carotid artery between the cervical carotid and distal intracranial carotid arteries, the entire aneurysm body was easily dissected. A ring clip with the longest blades was tentatively positioned on the distal portion of the aneurysm. Two angled ring clips and a bayonet clip were then placed on the neck, and the tentative clip was removed. The postoperative angiogram showed straightening of the distal portion of the internal carotid artery, causing kinking of the proximal portion of the left middle cerebral artery. A computed tomography (CT) scan showed a low-density area in the left caudate head, which may well have been caused by hypoperfusion in the region of the middle cerebral artery.

Case Study 8

This 62-year-old woman (Fig. 26-11) suffered an SAH 1 day before surgery. A large aneurysm was found in the right middle cerebral artery by angiography.

Operation

The neck and part of the body of the aneurysm were easily exposed, and then the M_1 segment was found. The ascending frontoparietal artery was traced back to the neck portion; a branch was found to originate from the ascending frontoparietal artery at the neck, which was coursing beneath the aneurysm body with strong adhesion. The angular artery, which was found deep in the temporal side, was carefully dissected with direct retraction of the aneurysm. Under temporary clipping of the parent artery, a bayonet clip was applied, with its shank portion including the bulging neck; this was not satisfactory. Multiple clipping was then tried several times without success, the procedure being complicated by bleeding from the junctional points of three clips. Finally, a bayonet clip was successfully applied after the aneurysm had been completely dissected from the arteries and brain.

Formation Clipping

Formation clipping is a multiple clipping technique whereby a branch or parent artery is reconstructed with the wall of the aneurysm. Furthermore, formation clipping can be applied to the body or dome of an aneurysm to make the shape of the aneurysm more suitable for final clipping (Fig. 26-12). Formation clipping is different from tentative clipping, in which the first clip is finally removed before or after application of a permanent clip (Fig. 26-6). Branch formation clipping is applied for an aneurysm whose branch arises directly from the aneurysm body (see Case Study 9, Fig. 26-13). When the aneurysm is so large that the parent artery is distended as part of the aneurysmal wall (see Case Studies 1 and 7, Figs. 26-1 and 26-10), formation clipping with a fenestrated clip to reconstruct a parent artery segment is usually necessary.

Case Study 9

This 54-year-old woman had suffered an SAH 5 weeks previously. Angiograms showed an aneurysm protruding laterally from the right vertebral artery at the level of the right posterior inferior cerebellar artery (PICA) (Fig. 26-13).

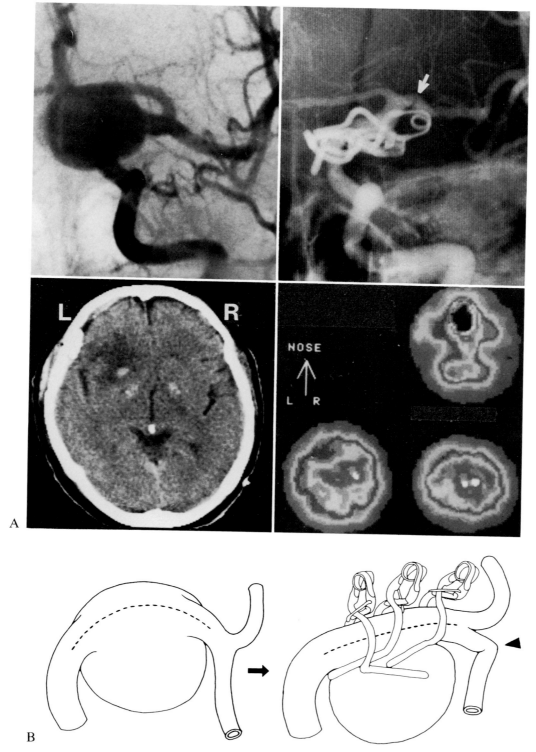

Figure 26-10. (**A**) A preoperative anteroposterior angiogram (*left*) of Case Study 7 patient, showing a giant left internal carotid artery aneurysm. A postoperative angiogram (*right*) reveals straightening of the distal portion of the internal carotid artery, causing kinking of the proximal portion of the left middle cerebral artery (*arrow*). A CT scan shows a low-density area in the left caudate head. A singe-photon emission computed tomogram (SPECT) demonstrates decreased blood flow in the region of the left middle cerebral artery. (**B**) Schema of the operation in Case Study 7. Multiple clipping is performed to occlude the internal carotid artery aneurysm. Three ring clips with straight blades caused straightening of the parent artery, resulting in kinking of the middle cerebral artery (*arrowhead*).

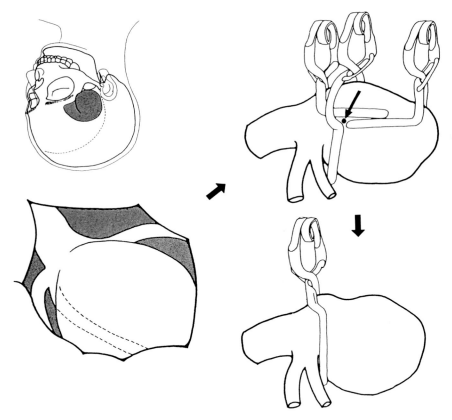

Figure 26-11. Schema of the operation in Case Study 8. A large aneurysm at the right middle cerebral artery is clipped by the multiple clipping method. Bleeding occurs at the point where three clips meet (*thin arrow*). Finally a bayonet clip is placed. Shank clipping, a method that uses an angled portion of the bayonet clip, is often effective for occluding a large aneurysm at the middle cerebral artery.

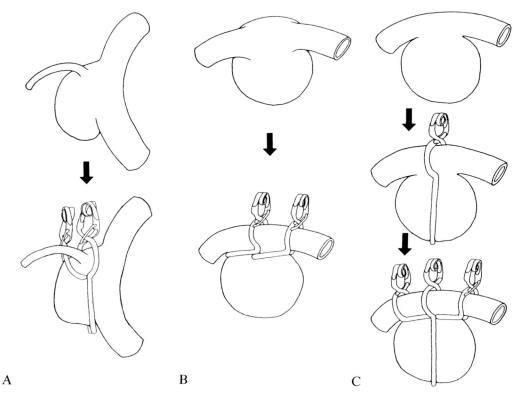

A   B   C

Figure 26-12. Diagrammatic representation of formation clipping. (**A**) Branch artery formation; (**B**) parent artery formation; (**C**) aneurysm formation.

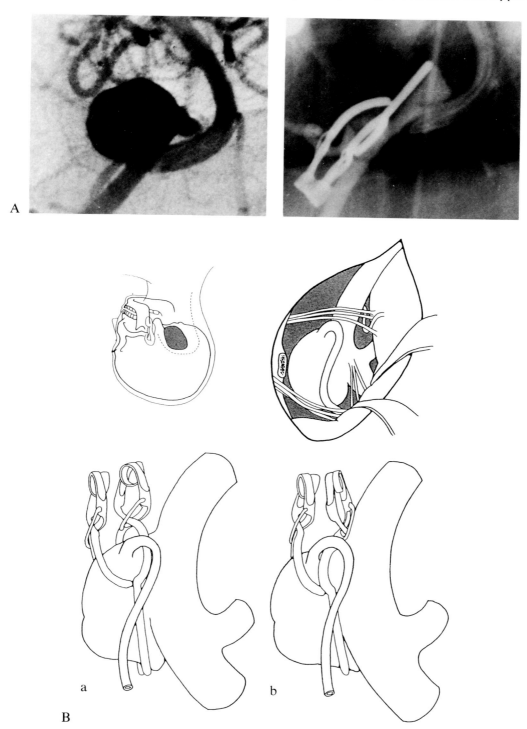

Figure 26-13. (**A**) A preoperative anteroposterior angiogram (*left*) of Case Study 9 patient, showing a large aneurysm protruding laterally from the right vertebral artery at the level of the PICA. An angiogram after the first operation (*right*) reveals that the proximal PICA segment was successfully reconstructed by the formation clipping method, while a small portion of the body remained distally. (**B**) Schema of the operation in Case Study 9. The PICA is found originating from the wall of the aneurysm. (*a*) A proximal portion of this artery is reconstructed with formation clipping with use of a straight ring clip and a curved clip in the first step. (*b*) In the second step the straight clip is replaced by a bayonet ring clip to occlude the residual portion of the aneurysm.

Operation

A right lateral suboccipital craniectomy was made with the patient in the lateral position. All the parent arteries of the bilateral vertebral and basilar trunk were cleanly exposed with moderate retraction of the medulla. The location of the PICA posed a serious problem, as it was branching from the aneurysm body. Initially the aneurysm neck and the PICA were tentatively clipped with a large straight clip while the bilateral vertebral arteries were temporarily clipped. A bayonet ring clip was positioned for this purpose to preserve the PICA. However, the large portion of the aneurysm in the distal side remained unclipped. The eminence of the jugular foramen was drilled off to create a space for the clip applicator. A straight ring clip with 9-mm blades was applied on the neck and the residual neck was occluded with a curved clip. The postoperative angiogram showed that the PICA was patent. Because the distal neck was not completely clipped, a second surgery was performed to replace the straight ring clip with a bayonet ring clip.

Booster Clipping

Booster clipping is a technique to reinforce the initial clipping by use of an additional, specially designed "booster" clip, which is placed on the blades of the primary clip (Fig. 26-14). Another method is duplication clipping, which reinforces the primary clipping with an additional clip placed either parallel or vertical to the primary clip. In parallel clipping it is best to place the second clip rather quickly before the first clip can be dislocated by high intraluminal pressure. One of the parallel clips may be a ring clip with

straight blades when an atheromatous uneven neck wall prevents complete closure of the aneurysm neck. Another point to remember before reinforcing is that the aneurysm may not have been sufficiently dissected.

Shank Clipping

The bayonet clip was originally designed to provide improved visualization of the neck during the clipping procedure. The angled portion of the bayonet is useful for clipping an unusual-shaped aneurysm, especially one that extends proximally to involve the bifurcation of the parent artery (see Case Study 8, Fig. 26-11). Shank clipping is used most often for middle cerebral artery aneurysms and occasionally for aneurysms in other locations.

Compression Clipping

For a broad-based and relatively small aneurysm, compression with clip blades against the wall of the parent artery where the neck arises is necessary to avoid leaving residual neck (see Case Study 10, Fig. 26-15). At the same time countercompression from the opposite wall of the parent artery with a silver dissector may be helpful.

Case Study 10

A 66-year-old woman had undergone the first clipping operation for left middle cerebral and ophthalmic artery aneurysms 2 months earlier (Fig. 26-15). The postoperative angiogram showed slippage of the clip for the ophthalmic artery aneurysm.

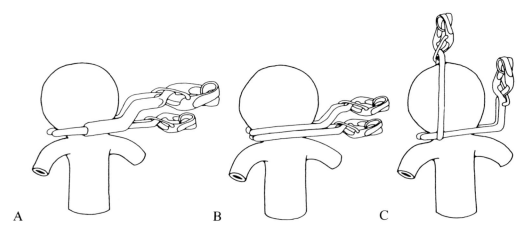

Figure 26-14. Schema of booster clipping. (**A**) A booster clip is placed on the blades of a regular straight clip. (**B & C**) Duplication clipping.

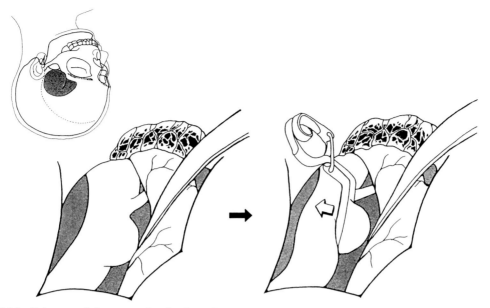

Figure 26-15. Schema of the operation in Case Study 10, showing the compression clipping method (*open arrow*). This method is effective for a broad-based and relatively small aneurysm.

Operation

With the intention of reclipping the ophthalmic artery aneurysm, the previous left frontotemporal craniotomy was reopened. Without opening the sylvian fissure, the internal carotid artery was approached. Dissection was performed around the previously placed clip between the internal carotid artery and the optic nerve. Adhesion around the aneurysm was moderate. The clip, which had slipped over to the proximal side of the neck and was holding only a small section of connective tissue, was easily removed. A bent clip was successfully placed with the clip blades pressing against the wall of the internal carotid artery to prevent slippage.

Rotation Advance

Rotation advance is a method for applying an L-shaped ring clip (Fig. 26-16). Rotation of the clip applicator is required to advance the tip of the clip blade deep enough for a large aneurysm located on the ventral side of the C_2-C_3 portion of the internal carotid artery.

Applicator Changing

A clip applicator may be changed during the clipping procedure (Fig. 26-17). The Sugita clip applicator is available with three different head angles (0, 15, and 30 degrees). In the narrow operating field for clipping, it is occasionally difficult to perform the clipping procedure with only a single applicator. Therefore, a clip may be tentatively applied to the aneurysm with one applicator and then adjusted with another applicator having a different head angle. A multijoint applicator is sometimes useful for this purpose. If the view of the operating field is blocked by the applicator, changing the axis of the microscope would be helpful in obtaining a suitable view of the local site.

Dissection with Clip Blades

In an extremely narrow and deep operating field, complete dissection around the neck is sometimes difficult. In that situation clipping is performed by advancing the clip blades in a closing and releasing maneuver, thus creating a space for clip blades wide enough to allow appropriate placement (Fig. 26-18). If the aneurysm ruptures during the procedure, the clip is immediately closed, and further measures can be taken as needed. This may be better than risking a major bleeding in a deep narrow field.

TECHNIQUES USED AFTER CLIPPING

Some additional procedures are required to prevent slippage of a clip and laceration of the aneurysm neck after clipping. Multiple clipping and booster

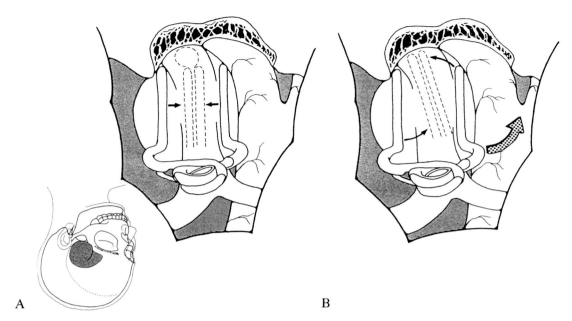

Figure 26-16. Schema of rotation advance (**B**), which is a method of applying an L-shaped ring clip for the aneurysm on the ventral side of the C$_2$-C$_3$ portion of the internal carotid artery. (**A**) This method is effective in that it avoids leaving residual neck.

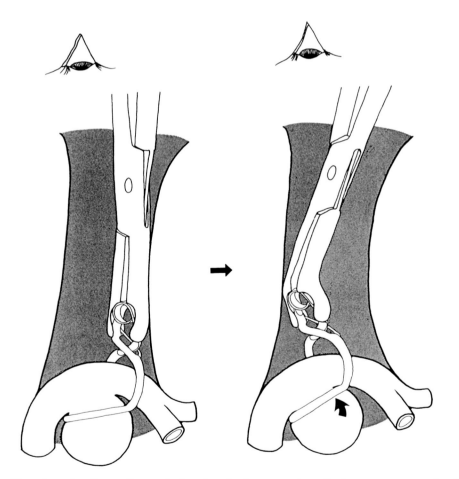

Figure 26-17. Changing of a clip applicator during the clipping procedure. In the narrow operating field a clip is tentatively applied to the aneurysm by one applicator and then adjusted (*curved arrow*) by another applicator with a different head angle.

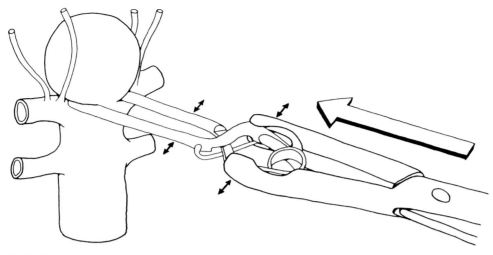

Figure 26-18. In dissection with clip blades the blades are advanced in a closing and releasing maneuver (*small arrows*), which creates a space wide enough to allow appropriate placement. This method is useful for an aneurysm presenting in an extremely narrow and deep operating field.

clipping are methods to prevent slip-out or slip-in of clip blades in a large or giant aneurysm when adequate closing pressure is not achieved by a single clip. Slippage of the clip may also occur when the aneurysm is very small. The technique described below for Case Study 11 augments the clipping force to avoid slip-out of a clip in the case of a small aneurysm (Fig. 26-19).

Another occasional cause of clip slip-out is pressure exerted by the brain surface on the clip head after clipping is completed and retractors on the brain are removed. This may also result in laceration of the aneurysm neck. Such a complication can be avoided by the method described for Case Study 12 (Fig. 26-20).

Inadvertent compression of cranial nerves by the clip is one of the complications to be avoided. One should be reminded of the possibility of such a complication when the nerve is directly retracted to facilitate clipping. Placement of a cushion between the clip head and the neural structure is one technique to reduce the risk of nerve injury when the compression is unavoidable.

Reinforcement of Clipping with Wrapping Material

Case Study 11

An incidental aneurysm in the left anterior cerebral artery was found on angiographic examination of a 60-year-old man (Fig. 26-19). The aneurysm appeared wide-based on the angiogram.

Operation

The sylvian fissure was widely separated and an aneurysmal dilatation was found in the A_1 segment just distal to the distal bifurcation of the internal carotid artery. All these parent arteries appeared sclerotic, with a bright yellowish color. On exploration it was found that the aneurysm had two perforating arteries originating from its body. With the intention of sacrificing one perforator, clipping was attempted with an angled ring clip. However, on releasing the clip the blades did not close completely because of the atheromatous wall of the aneurysm. A thin cotton sheet (Bemsheet) was used to keep the clip from slipping out; two strings tied at both ends were used to ligate the wrapped Bemsheet.

Removal of Brain Section to Provide Space for Clip Head

Case Study 12

This 71-year-old woman (Fig. 26-20) suffered an SAH 2 days before the operation. A moderate-size aneurysm was found on the lateral side of the internal carotid artery.

Operation

The internal carotid artery was extremely sclerotic and protruded laterally. The aneurysm was projecting inferiolaterally under the tentorium, to which it was tightly adherent. The posterior communicating

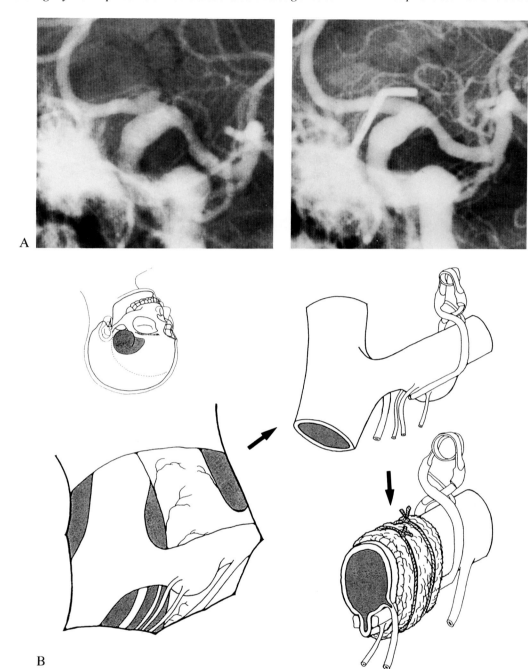

Figure 26-19. (**A**) Pre- and postoperative anteroposterior angiograms of an aneurysm at the A_1 segment of the anterior cerebral artery in Case Study 11 patient. (**B**) Schema of the operation in Case Study 11. Clipping is attempted with a ring clip, but when the clip is released, the blades do not close completely because of the atheromatous wall of the aneurysm. A thin cotton sheet (Bemsheet) is used to keep the clip from slipping out; two strings tied at both ends are used to ligate the wrapped Bemsheet.

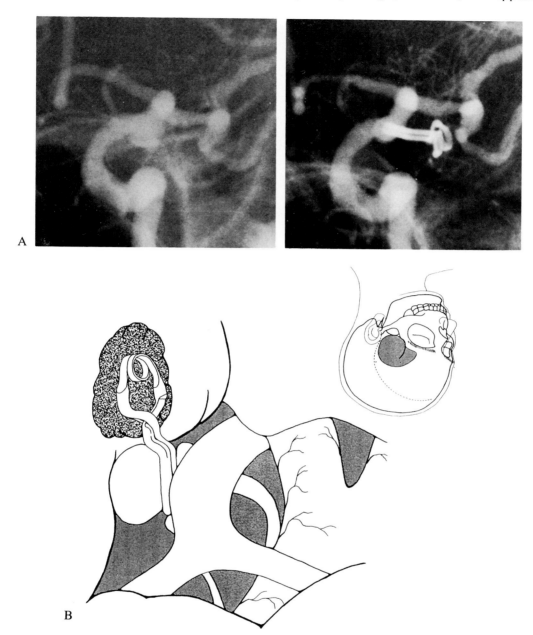

Figure 26-20. (**A**) Pre- and postoperative anteroposterior angiograms of an internal carotid artery aneurysm in Case Study 12 patient. (**B**) Schema of the operation in Case Study 12. A bayonet clip is applied to the aneurysm. Because the clip is applied laterally from the temporal lobe side, the clip head tends to tilt when the retraction is released; therefore, a tiny portion of the temporal lobe of the brain is removed to provide a space for the clip head.

artery was identified in the opticocarotid space, and the anterior choroidal artery was found just proximal to the distal neck, which was dangerously red owing to bleb formation. The tentorium had to be sectioned at its origin from the anterior clinoid process to provide space for the clip blades. A bayonet clip was successfully applied after temporary clipping of the proximal internal carotid artery. The aneurysm ruptured while the clip was being closed. Because the bayonet clip was applied laterally from the temporal lobe side, the head of the clip tended to tilt when the retraction was released; therefore, a tiny portion of the temporal lobe pia mater and brain was removed to provide space for the head.

Placement of Cushion between Clip Head and Neural Structures

To avoid injury to neural structures by the clip, placement of pieces of muscle or Gelfoam between the clip head and surrounding neural structures is recommended.

CONCLUSIONS

In conclusion, we have listed complications associated with aneurysm clipping operations and described various methods to prevent them. Experienced neurosurgeons may have become aware of all these methods through difficult cases,[2,3,12,14,15] but systematic prior knowledge would be more helpful in successfully clipping a given aneurysm than trying to find a suitable method when difficulty is encountered intraoperatively. The following rules represent our basic philosophy when performing clipping operations:

1. Remember that each aneurysm is different.
2. Have all kinds of clips, including special clips, available at surgery.
3. Be prepared for premature rupture at any stage of the operation.
4. Have as many technical options available as possible.
5. Ordinarily, tentative clipping of the aneurysm is preferable to prolonged temporary clipping of the parent artery.

ACKNOWLEDGMENT

We would like to thank Dr. Michael Apuzzo for language correction and valuable suggestions in preparing the text. We also thank Drs. Kazuhiko Kyoshima, Masaki Miyatake, and Tadaetsu Nagasaki for their editorial and technical assistance.

REFERENCES

1. Drake CG: On the surgical treatment of ruptured intracranial aneurysms. Clin Neurosurg 13:122, 1966
2. Drake CG: Giant intracranial aneurysms: Experience with surgical treatment in 174 patients. Clin Neurosurg 26:12, 1979
3. Hongo K, Kobayashi S, Yokoh A et al: Monitoring retraction pressure on the brain. An experimental and clinical study. J Neurosurg 66:270, 1987
4. Kobayashi S, Kyoshima K, Gibo H et al: Carotid cave aneurysms of the internal carotid artery. J Neurosurg 70:216, 1989
5. Nakagawa F, Kobayashi S, Takemae T et al: Aneurysms protruding from the dorsal wall of the internal carotid artery. J Neurosurg 65:303, 1986
6. Sugita K: Microneurosurgical Atlas. Springer-Verlag, Berlin, 1985
7. Sugita K, Hirota T, Mizutani T et al: A newly designed multipurpose microneurosurgical head frame. Technical note. J Neurosurg 48:656, 1978
8. Sugita K, Hirota T, Tsugane R: Application of nasopharyngeal mirror for aneurysm operation. Technical note. J Neurosurg 43:244, 1975
9. Sugita K, Kobayashi S, Inoue T et al: New angled fenestrated clips for fusiform vertebral artery aneurysms. J Neurosurg 54:346, 1981
10. Sugita K, Kobayashi S, Inoue T et al: Characteristics and use of ultralong aneurysm clips. J Neurosurg 60:145, 1984
11. Sugita K, Kobayashi S, Kyoshima K et al: Fenestrated clips for unusual aneurysms of the carotid artery. J Neurosurg 57:240, 1982
12. Sugita K, Kobayashi S, Takemae T et al: Direct retraction method in aneurysm surgery. J Neurosurg 53:417, 1980
13. Sundt TM Jr: Surgical Techniques for Saccular and Giant Aneurysms. Williams & Wilkins, Baltimore, 1990
14. Sundt TM Jr, Piepgras DG, Marsh WR: Booster clips for giant and thick-based aneurysms. J Neurosurg 60:751, 1984
15. Yasargil MG: Microneurosurgery. Vol. 2. Clinical Considerations, Surgery of the Intracranial Aneurysms and Results. Georg Thieme Verlag, Stuttgart, 1984
16. Yokoh A, Sugita K, Kobayashi S: Intermittent versus continuous brain retraction. J Neurosurg 58:918, 1983

27 Cerebral Vasospasm Following Aneurysmal Subarachnoid Hemorrhage

Neal F. Kassell
Mark E. Shaffrey
Christopher I. Shaffrey

Since its recognition in the early 1950s, cerebral vasospasm has been the bête noire of neurosurgeons caring for patients with ruptured intracranial aneurysms. A 40-year investigation into the pathogenesis and pathophysiology of vasospasm has yielded results that form the basis of current management and that promise to make the avoidance of vasospasm a reality within the next several years.

Angiographic vasospasm occurs in 70 to 90 percent of patients at some time during the first 14 days following aneurysm rupture.[3,37,52,111] Ischemic neurologic deficits from clinical vasospasm, usually occurring at the beginning of the second week following the ictus, are found in approximately half of patients demonstrating angiographic vasospasm.[19,51,52,91,111] While rebleeding is the most dramatic and feared complication of aneurysm rupture, vasospasm is still the leading treatable cause of death and disability in patients admitted to tertiary care centers with the diagnosis of aneurysmal subarachnoid hemorrhage (SAH).[52] It has been encouraging that clinical vasospasm is on the wane, having decreased as a cause of mortality from over 40 percent in the 1960s to 15 percent in the early 1980s to 8 percent or less currently.[34,65,89,103]

DIAGNOSIS

The diagnosis of vasospasm rests on a multifaceted clinical syndrome, which may consist of the insidious alteration in level of consciousness and focal neurological deficits (most often occurring 5 to 12 days following SAH) and usually accompanied by gradually increasing blood pressure, headache, fever, and a tendency toward hyponatremia.[30,53,73,99,106,121,126] Occasionally, ischemic deficits may rapidly appear or abruptly worsen as a result of intra-arterial platelet aggregation, local thrombus formation, or microthromboembolism.[43,68,105] In addition, surgery may precipitate deficits, either by exacerbating arterial narrowing or by exhausting compromised cerebrovascular reserve.[3,15]

In diagnosing clinical vasospasm, it is necessary to exclude other causes for neurological deterioration, such as subdural, epidural, or intraparenchymal hematomas, hydrocephalus, or metabolic disturbances. Additionally, to be absolutely certain of the diagnosis, angiography must be performed to confirm that a high degree of arterial narrowing exists in the appropriate vascular territory. Neurological deterioration is quite common in patients with ruptured aneurysms, and frequently, these deficits are multifactorial. When neurological deterioration occurs, however, vasospasm must be suspected because it is the most common and serious contributing factor.

While angiography remains the gold standard for diagnosing vasospasm, the necessity for its use has greatly diminished with the advent of transcranial Doppler ultrasonography.[1,59,75,97] This new noninvasive technique has proved to be a robust surrogate for angiographic demonstration of arterial narrowing and has greatly facilitated the management of vasospasm. The procedure can be performed as often as necessary to diagnose the arterial narrowing in advance of the development of ischemic symptoms.[59,75] Patients with a mean middle cerebral artery velocity greater than or equal to 200 cm/s are generally considered at risk for developing the clinical symptomatology of vasospasm.[36,96] Criticisms that the sensitivity of transcranial Doppler ultrasonography would be adversely affected by a high incidence of distal vasospasm appear unfounded.[75] Advances in local cerebral blood flow measurements using xenon computed tomography and single-photon emission computed tomography (SPECT) make these techniques attractive diagnostic prospects for the future.[17,40,41,62,101]

PATHOGENESIS

The pathogenesis of the arterial narrowing that occurs following SAH is not fully understood. On the basis of studies in animals and humans, it is clear that the arterial luminal narrowing is not an architectural thickening in the vessel wall such as a proliferative vasculopathy.[51,58] While intimal proliferation does occur as a generalized vascular injury reaction, it rarely if ever results in a significant compromise of the arterial lumen.[16,58,98,99,118] Evidence exists, however, that these normal but narrowed arterial walls may become stiffer after SAH.[16,58] Most likely, the cause of cerebral vasospasm is multifactorial, profound vasoconstriction in response to vasoactive substances in the subarachnoid space being the most prominent factor. There is a long list of putative spasmogens, which includes epinephrine,[4,76] norepinephrine,[4,76,114,131] serotonin,[4,14,44,76,107,125,131] angiotensin,[4,44] thrombin or plasmin,[124] fibrin degradation products,[23,39] prostaglandins,[14,25,29,46,69,119,130] thromboxane,[20,43,107,113,117,119] hydroperoxides,[5,6,92,94] and potassium.[112,128] Currently, the most likely etiologic spasmogens under investigation are endothelin[57,86,104] and hemoglobin.[63,66,81,83,110,122] Additional contributing factors probably include inflammation and immunoreactive processes,[61,82,87] endothelial injury and

disturbance of the blood–arterial wall barrier,[51,70,93] loss of vasodilator influences,[10,24,31,35,42,55,64,70] and exposure of smooth muscle cells to vasoactive substances in the plasma.[51] The notion that vasospasm is multifactorial in nature implies that no single pharmacological agent can be identified for blocking or inactivating the spasmogenic substances. The difficulty in finding specific agents for preventing or reversing the SAH-induced arterial narrowing supports this notion.

PATHOPHYSIOLOGY

In order to plan, implement, and evaluate therapeutic approaches to vasospasm, it is essential to have a firm understanding of the pathophysiology. Aneurysmal SAH causes a time-dependent arterial narrowing, which peaks between days 7 and 10 postbleed and leads to increased cerebrovascular resistance.[9,51,100,121] Cerebral blood flow initially is maintained at constant levels by autoregulation, but as the arterial narrowing progresses in severity, autoregulation is exceeded and cerebral blood flow decreases.[9,51] However, the patient's clinical condition still remains constant because in normal situations the brain is supplied with approximately twice as much blood flow as necessary to maintain normal function.[51] As arterial narrowing increases further, the cerebral vascular reserve is exceeded, blood flow falls into the ischemic zone, and patients develop ischemic deficits, which at this level are reversible.[51] If the arterial narrowing progresses even further and blood flow falls below the critical threshold for infarction, the brain dies and permanent deficits develop.[51]

Although the classical presentation of vasospasm is gradual neurological deterioration, occasionally, as previously mentioned, neurological deficits develop or worsen abruptly, as a result of thrombus formation or thromboembolism.[43,68,105] Following SAH there is platelet adhesion to the luminal surface of the arterial walls, which are surrounded by subarachnoid clot; this situation has the potential for platelet aggregation, thrombus formation, and embolism.[43,45]

MANAGEMENT

Theoretical Approaches

There are five potential approaches to the management of vasospasm:

1. Prevention of the arterial narrowing
2. Reversal of the arterial narrowing

3. Prevention of the ischemic consequences of the arterial narrowing
4. Reversal of the ischemic consequences of the arterial narrowing
5. Protection of the brain from infarction if all the above approaches fail

Aneurysmal SAH accounts for approximately 8 percent of all strokes in North America.[48] A fundamental requirement for effective management of patients with vasospasm is maintenance of a high degree of vigilance for early detection of arterial narrowing and/or its ischemic consequences and prompt intervention before permanent changes in the brain can occur.

Prevention of Arterial Narrowing

Theoretically, arterial narrowing can be prevented by inactivating or blocking the spasmogenic substances, by removing blood and spasmogenic substances from the basal cisterns, or by using potent specific or nonspecific cerebral vasodilating agents. A variety of agents have been tried, in both experimental animals and humans, for blocking or inactivating spasmogenic substances, including vitamin E,[54,78,115] ticlopidine,[79] cyclosporine A,[88] thromboxane synthetase inhibitors,[13,56,95,109] and the new 21-aminosteroids.[102,116,133] The use of cyclosporine A, whose protective benefits could be derived either from its role as an immunosuppressant or from its role as a calmodulin antagonist, is an intriguing option, which requires further clinical investigation.[88] Of the agents listed above, the most promising appears to be the 21-aminosteroid Tirilizad, because this agent has the potential to prevent narrowing as well as cytoprotective effects in focal ischemia.[26,27,133] Thus far, preclinical safety studies have failed to disclose any serious pharmacological side effects, and clinical trials of Tirilizad are currently underway.[26,27]

Removal of blood and spasmogenic substances from the subarachnoid spaces can be accomplished at the time of craniotomy for aneurysm obliteration by aspirating and irrigating away the clot.[7,28,67,77,108,130] Not unexpectedly, this results in only partial removal of the subarachnoid hematoma while incurring a significant risk of bruising pial banks and damaging small vessels.[51] Despite successful experimental studies in primates, recent clinical studies cast some doubt on the significance of clot removal in the amelioration of vasospasm.[38,77]

A novel approach for facilitating subarachnoid clot removal is thrombolytic therapy, which consists of irrigating the subarachnoid space with recombinant tissue plasminogen activator (rTPA) or urokinase at the time of surgery or postoperatively.[21,22,72,84] Thrombolytic therapy holds considerable promise, and clinical trials of this modality have been initiated. Preclinical data have demonstrated dramatic clearing of thick clots from the subarachnoid space and have strongly suggested prevention of arterial narrowing and ischemic neurological deficits.[21,22] The major concern about the use of thrombolytic therapy is the possibility of precipitating intracranial bleeding. While initial reports suggest that this approach is safe, results of rigorous clinical trials are necessary to prove safety and effectiveness.

Recently it has been shown that high-dose, continuous intravenous infusions of the calcium antagonist nicardipine can prevent arterial narrowing. Nicardipine at a dose of 0.15 mg/kg/h decreases the incidence of moderate or severe angiographic vasospasm during the peak period (days 7 to 11) by approximately 40 percent and decreases the incidence of clinical vasospasm by approximately 30 percent.[47]

Reversal of Arterial Narrowing

In theory arterial narrowing can be reversed by inactivating or blocking spasmogenic substances, by use of potent cerebral vasodilating agents, or by mechanically dilating the lumina of narrowed arteries by balloon angioplasty. However, once arterial narrowing has been established, no agent identified to date can specifically inactivate or block the spasmogenic substances. Furthermore, intravenous administration of potent vasodilators has failed to reverse arterial narrowing.[127] However, in some but clearly not all patients, intra-arterial and intracisternal administration of papaverine is capable of dilating profoundly narrowed arteries and reversing clinical vasospasm.[32] The use of intra-arterial papaverine is in the earliest stages of evaluation.

Transluminal balloon angioplasty is a relatively new approach for the treatment of vasospasm. In certain patients it has been dramatically effective in reversing the arterial narrowing and the accompanying neurological deficits.[11,18,33,74,132] Complications of this treatment include delayed arterial occlusion, rupture of vessels, conversion of bland to hemorrhagic infarction, and displacement of surgical clips from aneurysm necks.[18,33,74] At this time the safety and efficacy of transluminal balloon angioplasty have not been rigorously proved, although preliminary results indicate that a subgroup of patients who demonstrate progressive clinical deterioration from vasospasm may benefit from this procedure.[74]

Prevention and Reversal of Ischemic Deficits

Ischemic deficits can be theoretically prevented or reversed by optimizing the patient's hemodynamic and rheologic status. This is often referred to as *hypervolemic, hypertensive, hemodilution* (or *triple H*) therapy. Cerebral perfusion pressure can be elevated by increasing mean arterial pressure or by decreasing intracranial pressure. Cardiac output can be increased through the use of cardiac stimulants such as dopamine and dobutamine and/or by increasing the intravascular volume. Likewise, pulse pressure can be increased by increasing intravascular volume. Collateral circulation to the ischemic or potentially ischemic zones can be improved by dilating leptomeningeal collaterals. Blood viscosity can be lowered by decreasing hematocrit by either iso- or hypervolemic hemodilution or by the disaggregating properties of colloid solutions, thus reducing cerebrovascular resistance and increasing cerebral blood flow. Removal of red blood cells is not necessary in patients with aneurysmal SAH.

Treating the ischemic consequences of vasospasm with triple H therapy is a poor second choice to definitive measures for preventing or reversing arterial narrowing. Although triple H therapy has been reported to reverse ischemic neurological deficits in as many as 70 percent of patients, its effectiveness has never been stringently established.[50] However, dramatic clearing of severe neurological deficits in certain patients when mean arterial pressure is raised, followed by reappearance of these deficits when the blood pressure is lowered, has been sufficiently convincing to result in widespread adoption of this approach.

There are a number of serious drawbacks to triple H therapy. This approach is expensive, requiring numerous days in an intensive care unit with costly medications and intravenous fluids, high levels of specialized nursing care, and invasive monitoring by Swan-Ganz catheters and arterial lines with their associated morbidity, which includes sepsis and thromboembolism. Increasing arterial pressure can result in rebleeding of previously unruptured aneurysms, new bleeding from incidental but unsecured aneurysms, intracerebral hemorrhage from ruptured small vessels, conversion of bland to hemorrhagic infarctions, exacerbation of cerebral edema and increased intracranial pressure, and a high incidence of pulmonary edema.[50,80] Nonetheless, for the foreseeable future triple H therapy will be an essential component in the armamentarium of techniques used against cerebral vasospasm.

Prevention of Cerebral Infarction

The final common pathway in vasospasm-related neurological deficits is neuronal ischemia. Because there is no completely reliable method of preventing or reversing vasospasm, cytoprotective agents are currently needed to reduce the impact of neuronal hypoxia. Although they are controversial, cytoprotective agents, including nimodipine, naloxone, and monosialoganglioside, have been reported to be effective in some clinical trials.[8,86,111] Monosialoganglioside, a natural component of neuronal membranes, is reported to improve level of consciousness when compared with placebo over short time periods, but longer studies are necessary to determine the possibility of long-term benefits.[86]

The role of oral nimodipine in preventing or treating delayed ischemic events has recently been reviewed.[111] In all studies the incidence of severe neurological deficits is reduced despite evidence that the incidence and severity of angiographic vasospasm is not diminished.[89] It is suggested that the nonvascular, anti-ischemic effects of nimodipine and nicardipine may be exerted directly on neurons,[47,89,111] possibly because these agents limit excess calcium entry into the neurons, thus reducing ischemia-caused cell damage. Nimodipine and nicardipine are pharmacologically equivalent dihydropyridines, but the equivalent intravenous dose of nicardipine, 10 mg/h, has approximately 10 times the biological equivalency of a 60-mg oral dose of nimodipine given every 4 hours.[47]

University of Virginia Approach for Management of Vasospasm

The above-described theoretical approaches have been translated into the following practical approach used at the University of Virginia. The management of vasospasm and prevention of its potential complications is based on five elements: (1) diagnosis; (2) subarachnoid clot removal; (3) triple H therapy; (4) calcium channel blocking agents; and (5) ischemic protection and rescue.

Diagnosis

Arterial Narrowing

Diagnosis of arterial narrowing is based primarily upon the transcranial Doppler examination. Patients have Doppler examinations at least every other day through the first 14 days following SAH. If the patient's neurological condition changes or if the Doppler signals progressively increase in frequency, the evaluations are performed on a daily basis. In addition, most patients have routine postoperative angiography scheduled between days 7 and 10 following SAH (the period most likely to demonstrate angiographic vasospasm). Angiography is also used if a discrepancy develops between the patient's clinical condition and the Doppler results (e.g., if the patient develops the clinical syndrome of vasospasm and the transcranial Doppler remains normal).

Clinical Vasospasm

Patients are observed in the neurological intensive care unit or the acute care stroke unit for signs and symptoms of clinical vasospasm. During the period of maximum risk for the development of vasospasm, neurological evaluations are performed more frequently—at least every 2 hours. If the Doppler frequencies increase into the vasospasm range or if vasospasm is detected angiographically, the neurological evaluations are performed with greater frequency and the patients are usually transferred to the intensive care unit, where they can be observed on a continuous basis.

Clot Removal at the Time of Surgery

All patients undergo surgery at the earliest convenient time following admission. An attempt is made to open the basal cisterns widely and to gently remove as much of the subarachnoid blood as possible with suction and irrigation. It is our impression, unsubstantiated by rigorous scientific proof, that clot removal may be enormously facilitated in those patients with thick subarachnoid hematomas by installation of rTPA in the subarachnoid space at the time of surgery. This approach is most likely to prevent development of vasospasm in those patients at maximal risk but must be used in the first 2 to 3 days following bleeding to be effective.[22] The obvious concern with this therapy is precipitation of postoperative intracranial bleeding, and the use of intrathecal fibrinolytic therapy will probably require restriction in those patients with significant cortical disruption due either to primary hemorrhage or to surgery.[21]

Hypertensive, Hypervolemic Hemodilution Therapy

In asymptomatic patients, intravascular volume is maintained with fluid intake of approximately 3,000 ml/day, of which approximately one-third is colloid, such as albumin, and two-thirds is crystalloid. Induced hypertension is not used at this stage. We see no indication for raising arterial pressure in asymptomatic patients unless they are significantly hypotensive and their aneurysms have been obliterated.

In asymptomatic patients with vasospasm diagnosed by transcranial Doppler examination or angiography, a fluid intake of approximately 3,000 ml/day is maintained but the ratio of colloid to crystalloid is changed, so that approximately two-thirds of the volume is colloid and one-third is crystalloid. At this point hemodilution consists of maintaining a hematocrit of approximately 35 to 40. While induced hypertension is not used, antihypertensive medications are discontinued.

In clinically symptomatic patients, hypervolemia is induced, to whatever level results in optimal cardiac output as determined by Swan-Ganz catheter, by infusion of large volumes of colloid, crystalloid, and red blood cells in whatever proportions are necessary to maintain normal plasma electrolytes and a hematocrit between 30 and 35. Pulmonary function, as indicated by oxygen saturation, arterial blood gas levels, and chest roentgenograms, is closely monitored. Mannitol is infused at the rate of 50 ml/h for its rheological effect on the microcirculation (prevention of rouleau formation, etc.), as well as its antioxidant properties. Hypertension is induced with dopamine and supplemented by neosynephrine as necessary for additional vasopressor effect. Arterial pressure is titrated to the neurological deficit and heart rate is targeted for 100 to 120 beats per minute. In certain patients it may be necessary to modify the dosage of calcium antagonists in order to induce the appropriate level of hypertension. This is easier to achieve with nicardipine, which is administered in an easily titratable, intravenous formulation with a short half-life. If there is no improvement after 1 hour of hypertensive therapy, the patient is taken to angioplasty.

Calcium Channel Blocking Agents

Calcium channel blocking agents are used in all aneurysmal SAH patients. Nimodipine in a dosage of 60 mg orally every 4 hours has no effect on angiographic vasospasm but does appear to reduce clinical vasospasm. Nicardipine in a dose of approximately 10 mg/h by continuous intravenous infusion reduces angiographic and clinical vasospasm. An intravenous formulation of nimodipine will be unavailable in the United States for the foreseeable future, and intravenous nicardipine should be available following final Food and Drug Administration (FDA) approval.

Ischemic Protection and Rescue

Last, when all the above approaches fail, measures can be undertaken to prevent infarction from developing until the arterial narrowing resolves spontaneously and an adequate blood flow has been restored. In addition to use of potentially cytoprotective agents such as the calcium antagonists and mannitol, other measures include maintaining normal body temperature, maintaining blood glucose below 100 mg/dl, and prevention of seizures. Barbiturate coma has been tried with unsatisfactory results in patients who are desperately ill from vasospasm; this modality should be abandoned.[49]

SUMMARY

Cerebral vasospasm appears to be on the wane. While it is still the leading treatable cause of death and disability secondary to aneurysmal SAH, new therapeutic modalities are on the horizon that promise to significantly attenuate this problem by the mid-1990s. These approaches are based on a new understanding of the pathogenesis and pathophysiology of the arterial narrowing; the arterial narrowing is largely multifactorial but mostly involves profound vasoconstriction. Architectural changes in the arterial wall may play only a minor role, if any. Early diagnosis and referral of patients with ruptured aneurysms, a high level of vigilance, and immediate intervention are essential to capitalize fully on these new therapeutic approaches.

REFERENCES

1. Aaslid R, Huber P, Nornes H: Evaluation of cerebrovascular spasm with transcranial Doppler ultrasound. J Neurosurg 60:37, 1984
2. Adams HP: Calcium antagonists in the management of patients with aneurysmal subarachnoid hemorrhage: A review. Angiology 41:1010, 1990
3. Adams HP, Kassell NF, Torner JC et al: Predicting cerebral ischemia after aneurysmal subarachnoid hemorrhage: Influences of clinical condition, CT results, and antifibrinolytic therapy. A report of the Cooperative Aneurysm Study. Neurology 37:1586, 1987
4. Allen GS, Henderson LM, Chou SN: Cerebral arterial spasm. Part 1: In vitro contraction of vasoactive agents on canine basilar and middle cerebral arteries. J Neurosurg 40:433, 1974
5. Asano T: Relevance of oxygen free radicals, lipid peroxidation, and lipoxygenase products to the pathogenesis of vasospasm. p. 86. In Sano K, Asano T, Tamura K (eds): Acute Aneurysm Surgery. Springer-Verlag, Vienna, 1987
6. Asano T, Tanishima T, Sasaki T et al: Possible participation of free radical reactions initiated by clot lysis in the pathogenesis of vasospasm after subarachnoid

hemorrhage. p. 190. In Williams & Wilkins, Baltimore, 1980
7. Auer LM: Acute operation and preventive nimodipine improve outcome in patients with ruptured cerebral aneurysms. Neurosurgery 15:57, 1984
8. Bell BA, Miller JD, Neto NGF et al: Effect of naloxone on deficits after aneurysmal subarachnoid hemorrhage. Neurosurgery 16:498, 1985
9. Biller J, Godersky JC, Adams HP: Management of aneurysmal subarachnoid hemorrhage. Stroke 19:1300, 1988
10. Brandt L, Ljuggren B, Andersson KE et al: Prostaglandin metabolism and prostacyclin in cerebral vasospasm. Gen Pharmacol 14:151, 1983
11. Brothers MF, Holgate RC: Intracranial angioplasty for treatment of vasospasm after subarachnoid hemorrhage: Technique and modifications to improve branch access. AJNR 11:239, 1990
12. Buchheit F, Boyer P: Review of treatment of symptomatic cerebral vasospasm with nimodipine. Acta Neurochir Suppl (Wien) 45:51, 1988
13. Chan RC, Durity FA, Thompson GB et al: The role of the prostacyclin-thromboxane system in cerebral vasospasm following induced subarachnoid hemorrhage in the rabbit. J Neurosurg 61:1120, 1984
14. Chehrazi BB, Giri S, Joy RM: Prostaglandins and vasoactive amines in cerebral vasospasm after aneurysmal subarachnoid hemorrhage. Stroke 20:217, 1989
15. Chyatte D, Fode NC, Sundt TM: Early versus late intracranial aneurysm surgery in subarachnoid hemorrhage. J Neurosurg 69:326, 1988
16. Clower BR, Haining JL, Smith RR: Pathophysiological changes in the cerebral artery after subarachnoid hemorrhage. p. 124. In Wilkins RH (ed): Cerebral Arterial Vasospasm. Williams & Wilkins, Baltimore, 1980
17. Davis S, Andrews J, Lichtenstein M et al: A single-photon emission computed tomography study of hypoperfusion after subarachnoid hemorrhage. Stroke 21:252, 1990
18. Dion JE, Duckwiler GR, Vinuela F et al: Pre-operative microangioplasty of refractory vasospasm secondary to subarachnoid hemorrhage. Neuroradiology 32:232, 1990
19. Ebeling U, Reulen HJ: Cerebral vasospasm and aneurysm surgery. p. 411. In Auer LM (ed): Timing of Aneurysm Surgery. Walter de Gruyter, New York, 1985
20. Ellis EF, Nies AS, Oates JA: Cerebral arterial smooth muscle contraction by thromboxane A_2. Stroke 8:480, 1977
21. Findlay JM, Weir BKA, Kanamaru K et al: Intrathecal fibrinolytic therapy after subarachnoid hemorrhage: Dosage study in a primate model and review of the literature. Can J Neurol Sci 16:28, 1989
22. Findlay JM, Weir BKA, Kanamaru K et al: The effect of timing of intrathecal fibrinolytic therapy on cerebral vasospasm in a primate model of subarachnoid hemorrhage. Neuorsurgery 26:201, 1990

23. Forster C, Mohan J, Whalley ET: Interaction of fibrin degradation products and 5-hydroxytryptamine on various smooth muscle preparations: Possible role in cerebral vasospasm. p. 186. In Wilkins RH (ed): Cerebral Arterial Spasm. Williams & Wilkins, Baltimore, 1980

24. Fujiwara S, Kassell NF, Sasaki T et al: Selective hemoglobin inhibition of endothelium-dependent vasodilation of rabbit basilar artery. J Neurosurg 64:445, 1986

25. Gaetani P, Marzatico F, Baena RR et al: Arachidonic acid metabolism and pathophysiologic aspects of subarachnoid hemorrhage in rats. Stroke 21:328, 1990

26. Hall AD, Travis MA: Effects of the nonglucocorticoid U740006F on progressive brain hypoperfusion following experimental subarachnoid hemorrhage. Exp Neurol 102:244, 1988

27. Hall AD, Travis MA: Inhibition of arachidonic acid-induced brain edema by the nonglucocorticoid 21-aminosteroid U74006F. Brain Res 451:350, 1988

28. Handa Y, Weir BKA, Nosko M et al: The effect of timing of clot removal on chronic vasospasm in a primate model. J Neurosurg 67:558, 1987

29. Handa J, Yoneda S, Matsuda M et al: Effects of prostaglandins A, E_1, E_2, F_2-alpha on the basilar artery of cats. Surg Neurol 2:173, 1976

30. Hasan D, Wijdicks EFM, Vermeulen M: Hyponatremia is associated with cerebral ischemia in patients with aneurysmal subarachnoid hemorrhage. Ann Neurol 27:106, 1990

31. Hassler W, Chioffi F: CO_2 reactivity of cerebral vasospasm after aneurysmal subarachnoid hemorrhage. Acta Neurochir (Wien) 98:167, 1989

32. Helm GA, Kassell NF: Intra-arterial papaverine for the treatment of cerebral vasospasm, abstracted. Congress of Neurological Surgeons Annual meeting, Orlando, October 1991

33. Higashida RT, Halbach VV, Dormandy et al: New microballoon device for transluminal angioplasty of intracranial arterial vasospasm. AJNR 11:233, 1990

34. Hijdra AH, Braakman R, van Gijn J et al: Aneurysmal subarachnoid hemorrhage. Stroke 18:1061, 1987

35. Hongo K, Kassell NF, Nakagomi T et al: Subarachnoid hemorrhage inhibition of endothelium-derived relaxing factor in rabbit basilar artery. J Neurosurg 69:247, 1988

36. Hutchison K, Weir B: Transcranial Doppler studies in aneurysm patients. Can J Neurol Sci 16:411, 1989

37. Inagawa T: Effect of early operation on cerebral vasospasm. Surg Neurol 33:239, 1990

38. Inagawa T, Yamamoto M, Kazuko K et al: Effect of clot removal on cerebral vasospasm. J Neuorsurg 72:224, 1990

39. Ito M: Experimental vasospasms—significance of oxyhemoglobin, fibrin degradation products and breakdown products of white ghost in the pathogenesis of cerebral vasospasms. Treatment of vasospasms with gabexate mesilate and diphenhydramine. Neurol Med Chir (Tokyo) 20:225, 1980

40. Jakobsen M, Enevoldsen E, Dalager T: Spasm index in subarachnoid hemorrhage: Consequences of vasospasm upon cerebral blood flow and oxygen extraction. Acta Neurol Scand 82:311, 1990

41. Jakobsen M, Overgaard J, Marcusen E et al: Relation between angiographic cerebral vasospasm and regional CBF in patients with SAH. Acta Neurol Scand 82:109, 1990

42. Juul R, Edvinsson L, Gisvold SE et al: Calcitonin gene-related peptide-LI in subarachnoid hemorrhage in man. Signs of activation of the trigemino-cerebrovascular system? Br J Neurosurg 4:171, 1990

43. Juvela S, Hillbom M, Kaste M: Platelet thromboxane release and delayed cerebral ischemia in patients with subarachnoid hemorrhage. J Neurosurg 74:386, 1991

44. Kapp J, Mahaley MS, Odom GL: Cerebral artery spasm. Part 2: Experimental evaluation of mechanical and humoral factors in pathogenesis. J Neurosurg 29:339, 1968

45. Kapp JP, Neill WR, Neill CL et al: The three phases of vasospasm. Surg Neurol 18:40, 1982

46. Kapp JP, Robertson JR, White RP: Spasmogenic qualities of prostaglandin F_2-alpha in the cat. J Neurosurg 44:173, 1976

47. Kassell NF: Nicardipine and angiographic vasospasm. 59th Annual Meeting of the Am Assoc Neurol Surg, New Orleans, April 1991

48. Kassell NF, Drake CG: Timing of aneurysm surgery. Neurosurgery 10:514, 1982

49. Kassell NF, Peerless SJ, Drake CG et al: Treatment of ischemic deficits from cerebral vasospasm with high dose barbiturate therapy. Neurosurgery 7:593, 1980

50. Kassell NF, Peerless SJ, Durward QJ et al: Treatment of ischemic deficits from vasospasm with intravascular volume expansion and induced arterial hypertension. Neurosurgery 11:337, 1982

51. Kassell NF, Sasaki T, Colohan ART et al: Cerebral vasospasm following aneurysmal subarachnoid hemorrhage. Stroke 16:562, 1985

52. Kassell NF, Shaffrey CI, Shaffrey ME: Timing of aneurysm surgery. p. 95. In Wilkins RH, Rengachary SS (eds): Neurosurgery Update. Vol. 2. McGraw-Hill, New York, 1990

53. Kassell NF, Torner JC: The International Cooperative Study on the Timing of Aneurysm Surgery—an update. Stroke 15:566, 1984

54. Kato Y, Sano H, Katada T et al: Experimental and clinical study in the use of intrathecal alpha-tocopherol in vasospasm, abstracted. p. 179. In Proc 2nd Int Symp on Cerebral Aneurysm Surgery in the Acute Stage. Graz, Austria, Sept 1984

55. Kim P, Vanhoutte PM: Endothelium-dependent relaxations and chronic vasospasm after subarachnoid hemorrhage. Blood Vessels 27:263, 1990

56. Komatsu H, Takehana Y, Hamano S et al: Beneficial effect of OKY-046, a selective thromboxane A_2 synthetase inhibitor, on experimental cerebral vasospasm. Nippon Yakurigaku Zasshi 41:381, 1986

57. Kraus GE, Bucholz RD, Yoon KW et al: Cerebro-

spinal fluid endothelin-1 and endothelin-3 levels in normal and neurosurgical patients: A clinical study and literature review. Surg Neurol 35:20, 1991

58. Lehman RM, Kassell NF, Nazar G et al: Morphometric methods in the study of vasospasm. p. 367. In Wilkins RH (ed): Cerebral Vasospasm. Raven Press, New York, 1988

59. Lindegaard KF, Nornes H, Bakke SJ et al: Cerebral vasospasm diagnosis by means of angiography and blood velocity measurements. Acta Neurochir (Wien) 100:12, 1989

60. Masaoka H, Suzuki R, Hirata Y et al: Raised plasma endothelin in aneurysmal subarachnoid hemorrhage. Lancet 2:1402, 1990

61. Mathiesen T, Fuchs D, Wachter H et al: Increased CSF neopterin levels in subarachnoid hemorrhage. J Neurosurg 73:69, 1990

62. Matsuda A, Shiino A, Handa J: Sequential changes of cerebral blood flow after aneurysmal subarachnoid haemorrhage. Acta Neurochir (Wien) 105:98, 1990

63. Mayberg MR, Okada T, Bark DH: The role of subarachnoid hemorrhage in arterial narrowing after subarachnoid hemorrhage. J Neurosurg 72:634, 1990

64. McCulloch J, Uddman R, Kingman TA et al: Calcitonin gene-related peptide. Functional role in cerebrovascular regulation. Proc Natl Acad Sci USA 83:5731, 1986

65. Mee E, Dorrance D, Lowe D et al: Controlled study of nimodipine in aneurysm patients treated early after subarachnoid hemorrhage. Neurosurgery 22:484, 1988

66. Miyaoka M, Nonaka T, Watanabe H et al: Etiology and treatment of prolonged vasospasm: Experimental and clinical studies. Neurol Med Chir (Tokyo) 16:103, 1976

67. Mizukami M, Kawase T, Usami T et al: Prevention of vasospasm by early operation with removal of subarachnoid blood. Neurosurgery 10:301, 1982

68. Moncada S, Vane JR: Arachidonic acid metabolites and the interactions between platelets and bloodvessel walls. N Engl J Med 300:1142, 1979

69. Morgan H, White RP, Pennick M et al: Prostaglandins and experimental cerebral vasospasm. Surg Forum 23:447, 1972

70. Nakagomi T, Kassell NF, Sasaki T et al: Impairment of endothelium-dependent vasodilation induced by acetylcholine and adenosine triphosphate following experimental subarachnoid hemorrhage. Stroke 18:482, 1987

71. Nakagomi T, Kassell NF, Sasaki T et al: Etiology of the disruption in blood arterial wall barrier following experimental subarachnoid hemorrhage. Surg Neurol 34:16, 1990

72. Narayan RK, Narayan TM, Katz DA et al: Lysis of intracranial hematomas with urokinase in a rabbit model. J Neurosurg 62:580, 1985

73. Nelson PB, Seif SM, Maroon JC et al: Hyponatremia in intracranial disease: Perhaps not the syndrome of inappropriate secretion of antidiuretic hormone (SIADH). J Neurosurg 55:938, 1981

74. Newell DW, Eskridge JM, Mayberg MR et al: Angioplasty for the treatment of symptomatic vasospasm following subarachnoid hemorrhage. J Neurosurg 71:654, 1989

75. Newell DW, Grady MS, Eskridge JM et al: Distribution of angiographic vasospasm after subarachnoid hemorrhage: Implications for diagnosis by transcranial Doppler ultrasound. Neurosurgery 27:574, 1990

76. Nielsen KC, Owman C: Contractile response and amine receptor mechanisms in isolated middle cerebral artery of the cat. Brain Res 27:33, 1971

77. Nosko M, Weir BKA, Lunt A et al: Effect of clot removal at 24 hours on chronic vasospasm after SAH in the primate model. J Neurosurg 66:416, 1987

78. Oba M, Mizoi K, Fujimoto S et al: Effect of postischemic administration of mannitol, vitamin E, dexamethasone and perfluorochemicals on cerebral ischemia. An experimental study. p. 267. In Spetzler RF, Carter LP, Selman WR, Martin NA (eds): Cerebral Revascularization for Stroke. Thieme-Stratton, New York, 1985

79. Ono H, Mizukami M, Kitamura K et al: Preventive effect of ticlopidine on cerebral ischemia due to cerebral vasospasm following ruptured aneurysm: A double-blind cooperative study. American Association of Neurological Surgeons, Scientific Programme, Paper 38, 1983

80. Origitano TC, Wascher TM, Reichman OH et al: Sustained increased cerebral blood flow with prophylactic hypertensive hypervolemic hemodilution ("triple-H" therapy) after subarachnoid hemorrhage. Neurosurgery 27:729, 1990

81. Osaka K: Prolonged vasospasm produced by the breakdown products of erythrocytes. J Neurosurg 47:403, 1977

82. Ostergaard JR, Kristensen BO, Svehag SE et al: Immune complexes and complement activation following rupture of intracranial saccular aneurysms. J Neurosurg 66:891, 1987

83. Ozaki N, Mullan S: Possible role of the erythrocyte in causing prolonged cerebral vasospasm. J Neurosurg 51:773, 1979

84. Pang D, Sclabassi RJ, Horton JA: Lysis of intraventricular blood clot with urokinase in a canine model. Part 3. Effects of intraventricular urokinase on clot lysis and post hemorrhagic hydrocephalus. Neurosurgery 19:553, 1986

85. Papadopoulos SM, Gilbert LL, Clinton Webb R et al: Characterization of contractile responses to endothelin in human cerebral arteries: Implications for cerebral vasospasm. Neurosurgery 26:810, 1990

86. Papo I, Benedetti A, Carteri A et al: Monosialoganglioside in subarachnoid hemorrhage. Stroke 22:22, 1991

87. Pelletieri L, Nilsson B, Carlsson CA et al: Serum immunocomplexes in patients with subarachnoid hemorrhage. Neurosurgery 19:767, 1986

88. Peterson JW, Nishizawa S, Hackett JD et al: Cyclosporine A reduces cerebral vasospasm after subarachnoid hemorrhage in dogs. Stroke 21:133, 1990

89. Pickard JD, Murray GD, Illingworth R: Effect of oral nimodipine on cerebral infarction and outcome after subarachnoid hemorrhage: British aneurysm nimodipine trial. Br Med J 298:636, 1989

90. Romner B, Ljunggren B, Brandt L et al: Correlation of transcranial Doppler sonography findings with timing of aneurysm surgery. J Neurosurg 73:72, 1990

91. Ropper AH, Zervas NT: Outcome 1 year after SAH from cerebral aneurysm. J Neurosurg 60:909, 1984

92. Sano K: Cerebral vasospasm and aneurysm surgery. Clin Neurosurg 30:13, 1983

93. Sasaki T, Kassell NF, Zuccarello M et al: Barrier disruption in the major cerebral arteries in the acute stage after subarachnoid hemorrhage. Neurosurgery 19:177, 1986

94. Sasaki T, Wakai S, Asano T et al: The effect of a lipid hydroperoxide of arachidonic acid on the canine basilar artery. An experimental study on cerebral vasospasm. J Neurosurg 54:357, 1981

95. Sasaki T, Wakai S, Asano T et al: Prevention of cerebral vasospasm after SAH with a thromboxane synthetase inhibitor OKY-1581. J Neurosurg 57:74, 1982

96. Sekhar LN, Wechsler LR, Yonas H et al: Value of transcranial Doppler examination in the diagnosis of cerebral vasospasm after subarachnoid hemorrhage. Neurosurgery 22:813, 1988

97. Sloan MA, Haley EC, Kassell NF et al: Sensitivity and specificity of transcranial Doppler ultrasonography in the diagnosis of vasospasm following subarachnoid hemorrhage. Neurology 39:1514, 1989

98. Smith RR, Clower BR, Grotendorst GM et al: Arterial wall changes in early human vasospasm. Neurosurgery 16:171, 1985

99. Smith RR, Yoshioka J: Intracranial arterial spasm. p. 1355. In Wilkins RH, Rengachary SS (eds): Neurosurgery. McGraw-Hill, New York, 1985

100. Solomon RA, Fink ME: Current strategies for the management of aneurysmal subarachnoid hemorrhage. Arch Neurol 44:769, 1987

101. Soucy JP, McNamara D, Mohr G et al: Evaluation of vasospasm secondary to subarachnoid hemorrhage with technetium-99m-hexamethyl-propylenamine oxime (HM-PAO) tomoscintigraphy. J Nucl Med 31:972, 1990

102. Steinke DE, Weir BK, Findlay JM et al: A trial of the 21-aminosteroid U74006F in a primate model of chronic cerebral vasospasm. Neurosurgery 24:179, 1989

103. Stornelli SA, French JD: Subarachnoid hemorrhage—factors in prognosis and management. J Neurosurg 21:769, 1964

104. Suzuki S, Kimura M, Souma M et al: Cerebral microthrombosis in symptomatic cerebral vasospasm—a quantitative histological study in autopsy cases. Neurol Med Chir 30:309, 1990

105. Suzuki H, Sato S, Suzuki Y et al: Endothelium immunoreactivity in cerebrospinal fluid of patients with subarachnoid hemorrhage. Ann Med 22:233, 1990

106. Takaku A, Shindo K, Tanaka S et al: Fluid and electrolyte disturbances in patients with intracranial aneurysms. Surg Neurol 11:349, 1979

107. Tanaka Y, Kassell NF, Torner JC: Effects of subarachnoid hemorrhage on platelet-derived vasoconstriction of rabbit basilar artery. Surg Neurol 32:439, 1989

108. Taneda M: Effect of early operation for ruptured aneurysms on prevention of delayed ischemic symptoms. J Neurosurg 57:622, 1982

109. Tani E, Maeda Y, Fukumori T et al: Effect of selective inhibitor of thromboxane A_2 synthetase on cerebral vasospasm after early surgery. J Neurosurg 61:24, 1984

110. Tanishima T: Cerebral vasospasm: Contractile activity of hemoglobin in isolated canine basilar arteries. J Neurosurg 53:787, 1980

111. Tettenborn D, Dycka J: Prevention and treatment of delayed ischemic dysfunction in patients with aneurysmal subarachnoid hemorrhage. Stroke, suppl IV. 21:IV85, 1990

112. Toda N: Responsiveness to potassium and calcium ions of isolated cerebral arteries. Am J Physiol 227:1206, 1974

113. Toda N: Mechanism of action of carbocyclic thromboxane A_2 and its interaction with prostaglandin I_2 and verapamil in isolated arteries. Circ Res 51:675, 1982

114. Toda N: Alpha adrenergic receptor subtype in human, monkey and dog cerebral arteries. J Pharmacol Exp Ther 226:861, 1983

115. Travis MA, Hall ED: The effect of chronic two-fold dietary vitamin E supplementation on subarachnoid hemorrhage-induced brain hypoperfusion. Brain Res 418:366, 1987

116. Vollmer DG, Kassell NF, Hongo K et al: Effect of the nonglucocorticoid 21-aminosteroid U74006F on experimental cerebral vasospasm. Surg Neurol 31:190, 1989

117. Von Holst H, Granstrom E, Hammarstrom S et al: Effect of leucotriene C_4, D_4, prostacyclin and thromboxane A_2 on isolated human cerebral arteries. Acta Neurochir (Wien) 62:177, 1982

118. Von Mecklenburg C, Chang JY, Delgado T et al: Ultrastructural cerebrovascular changes in a model of subarachnoid hemorrhage in baboon based on triple cisternal blood injection. Surg Neurol 33:195, 1990

119. Walker V, Pickard JD, Smythe et al: Effects of subarachnoid hemorrhage on intracranial prostaglandins. J Neurol Neurosurg Psychiatry 46:119, 1983

120. Weir B: Medical aspects of the preoperative management of aneurysms: A review. Can J Neurol Sci 6:441, 1979

121. Weir B, Grace M, Hansen J et al: Time course of cerebral vasospasm. J Neurosurg 48:173, 1978

122. Wellum GR, Irvine TW, Zervas NT: Cerebral vasoactivity of heme proteins in vitro: Some mechanistic considerations. J Neurosurg 53:777, 1982

123. White RP, Chapleau CE, Dugdale M et al: Cerebral arterial contractions induced by human and bovine thrombin. Stroke 11:363, 1980

124. White RP, Hagen AA, Morgan H et al: Experimental study on the genesis of cerebral vasospasm. Stroke 6:52, 1975

125. White RP, Heaton JA, Denton IC: Pharmacological comparison of prostaglandin F-2 alpha, serotonin and norepinephrine on cerebrovascular tone of monkey. Eur J Pharmacol 15:300, 1971

126. Wijdicks EFM, Vermeulen M, van Gijn J: Hyponatremia and volume status in aneurysmal subarachnoid hemorrhage. Acta Neurochir Suppl (Wien) 47:111, 1990

127. Wilkins RH: Attempted prevention or treatment of intracranial arterial spasm: A survey. Neurosurgery 6:198, 1980

128. Wilkins RH, Levitt P: Potassium and the pathogenesis of cerebral arterial spasm in dog and man. J Neurosurg 35:45, 1971

129. Yamamoto YL, Feindel W, Wolfe LS et al: Experimental vasoconstriction of cerebral arteries by prostaglandins. J Neurosurg 37:385, 1972

130. Yamamoto I, Hara M, Ogura K et al: Early operation for ruptured intracranial aneurysms: Comparative study with computed tomography. Neurosurgery 12:169, 1983

131. Zervas NT, Lavyne MH, Negoro M: Neurotransmitters and the normal and ischemic circulation. N Engl J Med 293:812, 1975

132. Zubkov YN, Nikiforov BM, Shustin VA: Balloon catheter technique for dilatation of constricted cerebral arteries after aneurysmal SAH. Acta Neurochir (Wien) 70:665, 1984

133. Zuccarello M, Marsch JT, Schmitt G et al: Effect of the 21-aminosteroid U-74006F on cerebral vasospasm following subarachnoid hemorrhage. J Neurosurg 71:98, 1989

28 Protection of the Neuronal Pool

Michael L. Levy

Craig Rabb

William T. Couldwell

Vladimir Zelman

Michael L.J. Apuzzo

In any treatise concerning future advances in the management of patients with neurological illness, one can only assume that the current avenues of basic and clinical research are in pursuit of realistic goals. The concept of neuronal protection is inherent to all neurologically based illnesses. Only in being able to understand the pathogenesis of traumatic and ischemic injury can we improve outcome in the neurological surgery patient population. This chapter will specifically deal with current research regarding neuronal protection, including mechanisms of action and pathophysiology. The understanding of this substrate will allow us to progress to a discussion of the most potentially rewarding avenues of therapeutic intervention. We will then discuss the clinical data most related to these avenues and consider the implications of future treatment modalities.

With regard to the management of neurosurgical patients, the tenets of neuronal protection are all-encompassing. Advances in this field will not only have vast implications in our future care of ischemic, traumatic, and surgical disorders but also change the manner in which the neurosurgical community views these disease processes.

Cerebral protection and rescue following anoxic/ischemic insults is not unique to the modern era of medicine.[126,176,299,302] However, the potential for reversibility of injury involving the neuronal pool may be expanded further by using modalities initiated prior to the ischemic event (cerebral protection) and treatments rendered after the event (i.e., rescue).

PATHOPHYSIOLOGICAL MECHANISMS IN ISCHEMIA/HYPOXIA

To address the topic of cerebral protection in the context of neurosurgical procedures, one must have a thorough understanding of the pathophysiological processes that lead to ischemic injury. Once this background is established, one may design strategies for cerebral protection that attempt to interrupt the process of neuronal cell death at multiple steps. Although a detailed discussion of the pathophysiological parameters that lead to neuronal death is beyond the scope of this chapter, a brief review is requisite before proceeding.

Cellular Events

In the absence of oxygen delivery or blood flow to cerebral tissue, oxidative phosphorylation ceases in approximately 15 seconds. This depletion of oxygen results in the inception of anaerobic metabolism, with the production of lactic acid from pyruvate. Anaerobic metabolism continues until depletion of intracellular glucose and glycogen stores (which takes approximately 5 minutes in complete anoxia) occurs, resulting in lactate accumulation (up to a fourfold increase) and a significant decrease in intra- and extracellular pH.[4,160] Concomitant with this lactic acidosis is depletion of adenosine triphosphate (ATP) stores. The resultant tissue acidosis is exacerbated by the presence of preischemic hyperglycemia, leading to increased neuronal cell loss.[134,196,197] Ensuing cellular events are complex and interrelated; the lactic acidosis produces a myriad of effects, including aberrant enzyme function, denaturation of structural proteins, and increased free fatty acid (FFA) liberation,[30] all of which ultimately exacerbate the acidosis.

With depletion of ATP stores there is failure of Na-K ATP-dependent pumps, with resultant increased extracellular K^+ ion, causing membrane depolarization. Membrane depolarization is opening of voltage-dependent calcium channels; this, combined with failure of ATP-dependent Na^+-Ca^{++} pumps and inadequacy of the endoplasmic reticulum as a calcium sequestrum, results in a large rise in intracellular Ca^{++} ion levels.[178] Elevated intracellular Ca^{++} has several functional catabolic consequences, the most significant of which is activation of phospholipases A and C, with subsequent dissolution of membranes (including mitochondrial) and liberation of FFAs. As all cells are susceptible to ischemia-induced intracellular Ca^{++} release (including vascular smooth muscle and glia), neuronal dysfunction is exacerbated by vascular constriction, which further limits blood delivery and causes glial swelling. The ultimate functional results of intracellular Ca^{++} release are vasoconstriction, platelet aggregation, and uncoupled oxidative phosphorylation.

The arachidonic acid liberated is the precursor of thromboxanes, prostacyclin (PGI_2), and the leukotrienes via cyclooxygenase and lipoxygenase pathways. Thromboxanes are potent vasoconstrictor agents; unfortunately, in the postischemic brain prostacyclin, which is vasodilating, is less preferentially synthesized. Leukotrienes are mild vasoconstrictors but also alter membrane permeability. Subsequent to arachidonic acid release is the production of free radicals, which are hypothetical species characterized by an unpaired electron in the outer orbit (e.g., superoxide anion O_2^-, hydroxyl radical OH^-) and are postulated in their transient existence to catalyze destructive reactions in cell membranes,[247] thus

increasing permeability and perpetuating the catabolic process. They have been especially implicated in membrane dissolution following reperfusion.

Finally, cell death may be mediated by voltage-dependent and N-methyl-D-aspartate (NMDA) receptor-dependent calcium channels. The subsequent increase in intracellular Ca^{++} ions may trigger activation of xanthine oxidase, lipases, and proteases,[137,237] which could lead to cell death.

In view of the aforementioned multiple cellular events, it is apparent that there exist several potential areas of therapeutic intervention; we shall proceed with a discussion of these modalities in relation to their mechanism of action.

Patterns of Cerebral Blood Flow during Ischemia

Normal cerebral blood flow (CBF) ranges from 50 to 55 ml per gram of tissue per minute. This range of values is maintained at a fairly constant level by autoregulation, which results from changes in the vasculature in response to changes in systemic blood pressure. Within normal ranges of blood pressure (mean arterial blood pressure >60 mmHg or <140 mmHg), when blood pressure increases, the vessels constrict, and when blood pressure drops, the vessels dilate,[275] so as to maintain a constant level of CBF. Autoregulation may be altered by metabolic factors such as carbon dioxide pressure (PCO_2), oxygen pressure (PO_2), H^+ ions, K^+ ions, and trauma.[245] Nevertheless, it is important to realize that at the regional level those normal values of regional cerebral blood flow (rCBF) reflect primarily the flow in the highly active cortical regions, and the cortical activity in turn relates to regional differences in brain function.

Ischemia results when the supply of oxygen and nutrients does not meet the demands of the tissue supplied. Symptoms of ischemia result when rCBF falls below 30 ml/100 g/min. This may be reflected by changes in the electroencephalogram (EEG) or in somatosensory evoked potential (SSEP). Flattening of the EEG occurs when the rCBF falls to 20 ml/100 g/min,[262] whereas reductions in SSEP amplitudes occur when the rCBF falls below 15 ml/100 g/min.[105] This threshold appears to reflect failure of synaptic transmission. The threshold for metabolic failure of neurons appears to be approximately 10 ml/100 g/min,[20] and if sustained will result in cellular death.[189] Thus, there appears to be a group of neurons that may be salvaged, the so-called ischemic penumbra.[18]

Consequences of Reperfusion of Ischemic Regions

When the brain suffers an ischemic insult, this may become manifest in the vasculature in either of two ways, permanent vessel occlusion[119] or occlusion with subsequent reperfusion. In the latter, secondary phenomena may occur in the form of the so-called no-reflow phenomenon[11] or delayed postischemic hypoperfusion. After occlusion of a vessel, reperfusion may not take place as a result of swelling of vascular elements, changes in blood viscosity, or changes in local perfusion pressure.[80,81] Thus, a potentially reversible event becomes irreversible, the no-reflow phenomenon. Alternatively, if the vasculature experiences a reactive hyperemia subsequent to reversible or irreversible ischemia, this may be followed by increased vascular tone, resulting in decreased flow (delayed postischemic hypoperfusion).[127]

Ischemic Cerebral Edema

Classically, the concept of cerebral edema entails two distinct entities, vasogenic edema and cytotoxic edema.[143] A third type of cerebral edema that may occur is a combination of the two, ischemic cerebral edema. The initial cytotoxic swelling is followed by breakdown of the blood-brain barrier, which by increasing intracranial pressure (ICP) results in further ischemia and thus in a vicious cycle.[207]

PREOPERATIVE MANAGEMENT OF PATIENTS AT RISK FOR BRAIN INJURY

Medical Management: Intravenous Fluids

Fluid Restriction

Fluid management in the neurosurgical patient will obviously vary depending on the clinical scenario. In the presence of presumptive or documented increases in intracranial pressure, fluid restriction to 75 ml/h of isotonic solution in adults and 1,000 to 1,200 ml/m²/day in children is indicated. In the elective surgery setting, patients can remain euvolemic. Most salient to our discussion of fluid management in the attempt to preserve neuronal function and integrity is the concept of cerebral perfusion and its determinants. With this in mind we will now discuss isch-

emic compromise of the neuronal pool and alterations in perfusion resulting from vasospasm.

Hypervolemia and Hemodilution

Rationale

Intravascular volume expansion has become an accepted modality in the prevention and subsequent treatment of cerebral ischemia from vasospasm or, more frequently, acute stroke. However, the guidelines for hypervolemic therapy in terms of the volume and timing of intravenous fluid administration and the target cardiac performance parameters are generally based on anecdotal information. Hence we will explore the rationale for hypervolemic preload enhancement and its effects on cardiac performance and protection of the neuronal pool. In order to minimize complications related to volume expansion, including cardiac, hematologic, and pulmonary sequelae, and to maximize cardiac performance during therapy for cerebral vasospasm, we have used a flow-direct balloon-tipped catheter with cardiac output and hemodynamic monitoring.

Increasing Cerebral Blood Flow by Increasing Cardiac Output

The reversal of ischemic deficits through the use of induced arterial hypertension via volume expansion and vasopressors was initially described in 1951 by Denny Brown.[64] Farhat and Schneider[77] theorized that elevations in the mean arterial pressure resulted in increased rCBF. Using induced hypertension and volume expansion, Kosnik and Hunt[149] documented reversal of postoperative ischemic deficits resulting from vasospasm in six of seven patients. They concluded that cerebrovascular autoregulation was disrupted in ischemic areas of the brain and that perfusion to these regions could be enhanced with increases in mean arterial pressure.[141,250,290]

Relative hypovolemia as a concomitant of subarachnoid hemorrhage (SAH) was first suggested by Kosnik and Hunt[149] in 1976 and is well documented in the literature.[150,168] Such studies suggested that hypovolemia following SAH may play a critical role in delayed ischemia and thus explained why hypervolemic therapy may be an appropriate treatment modality. Solomon et al.[252] confirmed the relationship between hypovolemia and symptomatic vasospasm and suggested that hyperactivity of the sympathetic nervous system due to hypothalamic dysfunction following SAH was an important factor in inducing hypovolemia.

Improving Cerebral Blood Flow By Optimizing Blood Viscosity

Giannotta et al.[95] noted the success of low molecular weight dextran in inducing hypervolemia and improving neurological function, which they ascribed to its putative ability to improve flow through the microcirculation by reducing both cellular aggregation and arteriovenous shunting.

This body of work led some to investigate the possibility that SAH may result in hemorrheological alterations that could contribute to the pathogenesis of cerebral vasospasm. Fisher et al.[82] followed serial determinations of hematocrit, whole blood and plasma viscosity, red cell aggregation, fibrinogen levels, and zeta sedimentation rates in 12 patients with ruptured intracranial aneurysms. On day 4 to day 7 following SAH fibrinogen, plasma viscosity, and zeta sedimentation levels reached their maxima, which were statistically significantly elevated as compared with controls. Thus, hemorrheological alterations may play a role in ischemic complications from ruptured aneurysms, and secondary improvement in such abnormalities with hemodilutional or volume expansion therapies may be of theoretical benefit.

Hypervolemia with Hemodilution

Brown et al.[44] report favorable results in the treatment of cerebral vasospasm due to SAH in four patients following volume expansion, pressure support with dopamine, and a continuous infusion of mannitol. Favorable results have also been documented with the use of isoproterenol or isoproterenol and aminophylline combination therapy.[84–86,261,266] It is likely that the operant factors were increases in cardiac output secondary to the cardiac stimulant effect of these agents and the copious volume of intravenous fluid administered to maintain steady-state levels.

Davis and Sundt[60] demonstrated a critical link between cardiac function and augmentation in blood flow in ischemic areas of brain. Keller et al.[140] supported this concept, demonstrating that increased cardiac output could improve microcirculatory flow without changes in mean arterial pressure or blood viscosity.

Kassell et al.[136] in 1982 reported on one of the largest series of patients with neurological deterioration following cerebral vasospasm secondary to SAH who were treated with volume expansion, vasoblockade, and pressor agents. Reversal of neurological deficits occurred in 43 of 58 patients studied. They relied on hemodynamic monitoring via Swan-Ganz catheterization. Kassell et al. observed that

neurological improvement could occur in the early stages of fluid replacement before mean arterial pressure became elevated. This lent further credence to previous investigators who believed that rheologic phenomena or improved cardiodynamics could contribute to improved CBF. Pritz et al.[227] documented reversal of ischemic neurologic deficits in two patients with SAH-induced vasospasm by maximizing cardiac output. Pritz[226] has further described in detail the use of Swan-Ganz catheterization in monitoring patients treated for cerebral vasospasm following SAH to maximize cardiac output and avoid complications associated with hypervolemic therapy or increased ICP.

It has been subsequently documented by many that CBF progressively decreases in poor-grade patients or those with vasospasm.[33,47,152,177,181,218,221,252] Reductions in CBF occur in the face of increased cerebral blood volume.[102] Rosenstein et al.[232] documented reversal of neurologic deficits associated with increases in CBF following hypervolemic therapy. The seemingly rational basis for such treatment of vasospasm and the immediate and complete improvement seen in many patients treated in this manner supports further studies regarding hypervolemic hypertension as an effective treatment in reversing neurologic deficits secondary to SAH-induced vasospasm.

The contribution of blood viscosity to blood flow has also been analyzed. Wood et al.,[304] using an animal stroke model, documented that nondilutional hypervolemia with autologous whole blood transfusions did not increase perfusion in ischemic regions or reduce the volume of infarcted tissue.

Hypervolemia without Hemodilution

McGillicuddy et al.[172] in a primate model of cerebral vasospasm found a significant increase in CBF with elevations in central venous pressure in the face of stable systemic arterial pressures. CBF increased only in regions of ischemia and remained unchanged in the nonischemic regions, where autoregulation was presumably intact.

Wood et al.[303] subsequently reported that hypervolemic hemodilution with expansion of peripheral vascular volume increased cardiac output more than CBF in nonischemic brain. Increases in ICP and cardiac output (up to 71 percent without attendant change in mean arterial blood pressure) were noted in their animal model. Muizelaar and Becker[193] suggested that autoregulatory adjustments in vascular diameter were present in response both to changes in cardiovascular function and to alterations in serum viscosity.

Isovolemic Hemodilution

Tu et al.[283,284] in 1988 proposed that isovolemic as opposed to hypervolemic hemodilution might circumvent potential adverse effects associated with volume expansion. Isovolemic hemodilution led to a significant reduction in viscosity, which correlated linearly with reduction in hematocrit and with improved neurological outcome following occlusion of the carotid and middle cerebral arteries.

Management of Subarachnoid Hemorrhage-Induced Vasospasm

Management in the Intensive Care Unit

The majority of the patients in the better grades (1 to 3) undergo early operative management with clip ligation of the ruptured aneurysm. Thus, the majority of cases of ischemic complications that we experience are in the postoperative period. The new onset of lethargy with or without a focal neurological deficit is presumed evidence of the onset of cerebral vasospasm until proven otherwise. In rapid succession a computed tomography (CT) scan is obtained to rule out other forms of intracranial pathology, intravenous fluid volumes are increased, and a flow-directed balloon-tipped right heart catheter is placed. Complications of Swan-Ganz catheterization, including infection, pneumothorax, hemothorax, pulmonary infarct, and arrhythmias, can all be avoided with meticulous technique and sterility in conjunction with catheter changes every 3 days. All catheter tips are cultured when removed. An initial bolus of 300 ml of albumisol or hetastarch is given, and the measurement and recording of cardiac parameters is commenced.

Fluid Management

Patients with suspected SAH are immediately admitted to the neurosurgical intensive care unit. Steps are immediately taken to document the cause of the SAH with CT scanning and cerebral angiography. Patients with ruptured intracranial aneurysms are maintained on bed rest with the head elevated to 30 degrees unless significant hypotension intervenes. Vital sign and neurological evaluations are carried out and recorded on an hourly basis. Arterial blood pressure is monitored with automated cuffs or arterial catheters. Young patients or those with no preexisting cardiac history are given 5 percent dextrose in lactated Ringer's solution at rates approximating 150 ml/h. Fluid boluses of up to 300 ml are given preparatory to and following cerebral angiography because

of the significant osmotic diuresis related to the contrast load. A short course of high-dose dexamethasone intravenously (10 mg q3h) is given to patients with poor neurological grades and those awaiting surgery.

Management of Blood Pressure. An attempt is made to determine the preexisting blood pressure. No effort is made to reduce the blood pressure below 15 to 20 mmHg above the premorbid level. For those subarachnoid hemorrhage patients with blood pressure more than 20 mmHg above their normal levels or with systolic pressures above 185 mmHg, sedative medications, including analgesics and phenobarbitol, are initiated. Refractory elevations in blood pressure are managed with intravenous sodium nitroprusside because of its ability to be easily and rapidly titrated. Hypertensive patients with preexisting coronary vascular disease are managed with intravenous nitroglycerin. All patients who require intravenous antihypertensive agents are managed also with Swan-Ganz catheterization. Very rarely is there a place for the use of diuretics in the acute aftermath of a ruptured intracranial aneurysm.

Optimization of Intravascular Volume. Measured parameters include cardiac output, cardiac index, left ventricular stroke work index, systemic vascular resistance, pulmonary artery wedge pressure, pulmonary artery pressure, stroke volume index, and pulmonary artery diastolic pressure. Central venous pressures may also be monitored but are not used as indices of cardiac function.

We have found a poor correlation between pulmonary artery wedge pressure and central venous pressure. However, increases in pulmonary artery wedge pressure up to 14 mmHg did correlate in a statistically significant manner with increases in cardiac index, stroke volume index, and left ventricular stroke work index; there was no statistical correlation between increases in pulmonary wedge pressure above 14 mmHg and improvement in cardiac performance as evidenced by these parameters. Thus, in previously healthy individuals we enhanced fluid volume status until a pulmonary artery wedge pressure of approximately 14 mmHg was maintained. Additional checks on cardiac index will reduce complications such as cerebral edema, congestive heart failure, and pulmonary edema to a minimum.[159]

Management of Vasospasm Refractory to Volume Expansion. In patients who fail to respond to measures for maximizing cardiac performance or in those whose compromised cardiac status results in reduction in cardiac index at the target level of pulmonary wedge pressure, augmentation of cardiac function is accomplished with pressor agents to achieve the desired clinical response. Dobutamine is usually initiated at 10 μg/kg/min. Blood pressure responses are blunted and cardiac parameters enhanced with the simultaneous use of sodium nitroprusside at 0.5 to 8 μg/kg/min. With this regimen pulmonary artery wedge pressures are no longer reliable in assessing cardiac function directly because pulmonary artery wedge pressure is reduced up to 56 percent with initiation of dobutamine and nitroprusside. Thus, we rely solely on cardiac index and stroke volume index, which can increase up to 120 percent following initiation of dobutamine and nitroprusside. This regimen is particularly valuable in patients with ruptured but unsecured aneurysms in the preoperative state. Postoperatively, in cases in which significant elevations of blood pressure are desired and not contraindicated, dopamine is used and blood pressure is titrated up to 200 mmHg systolic until the desired clinical effect is realized.

Management of Failure to Sustain Hypervolemic Treatment. In healthy individuals it may be difficult to maintain a pulmonary wedge pressure in the desired range. As long as the clinical condition is satisfactory, no further measures are taken, but if the desired clinical effect is not obtained, hypertensive therapy is instituted. We have had only limited experience with the use of vasopressin or the mineralocorticoids in attempting to maximize fluid retention. Kassell et al.[136] have recommended this as an effective measure.

Management of Failure to Achieve Hemodilution. In those few patients who have high hematocrits following maximization of hypervolemia and hypertensive therapy and who fail to respond clinically, we have resorted to reducing the hematocrit by therapeutic venesection and removal of 1 to 2 units of packed cells with replacement of plasma. This has been necessary in two patients over the past 5 years.

Failure to Respond to Enhanced Cardiac Output and Hypervolemic Hemodilution. When further neurological deterioration occurs in the face of maximal volume expansion and critical increase in mean arterial blood pressure, ventricular catheterization is carried out, with subsequent intraventricular pressure monitoring and reduction of ICP to maximize cerebral perfusion pressure. Brief periods of hyperventilation are used to acutely reduce ICP spikes. Removal of cerebrospinal fluid (CSF) for cerebral perfusion pressures that fall below 70 mmHg is the next preferred maneuver. Intravenous mannitol,

which also temporarily improves the hemorrheology in the microcirculation, is used for refractory elevations in ICP or reduction in cerebral perfusion pressure. With such a comprehensive program the majority of episodes of cerebral vasospasm can be modified or for the most part ameliorated. There are, however, ischemic sequelae of cerebral vasospasm that are refractory in all forms of treatment. These generally occur in the face of massive SAH, as documented by early CT scanning, and the inability to operatively remove large amounts of the hemorrhagic material in a timely fashion. Multiple SAHs in our experience have also been responsible for the most malignant forms of cerebrovasospasm.

Timing of Discontinuance of Therapy. Hypervolemic and hypertensive therapy is continued until such time as tapering of the vasopressor and/or volume load is not met with a decrease in neurological function. This has been known to take up to 2 weeks in a few cases. In general, following the critical period for vasospasm, namely, day 5 to day 12 following the SAH, most therapeutic maneuvers can be reduced.

Summary of Management in Patients with Aneurysmally Induced Vasospasm

A basic understanding of cardiac physiology with appropriate monitoring and implementation of methods to increase cardiac performance can measurably improve the outcome of patients with cerebral ischemia from vasospasm. Success is predicated on early recognition of the evolving syndrome, with rapid introduction of measures to improve cerebral perfusion pressure and hemorrheology.

Use of Hypervolemia and Hemodilution in Acute Stroke

Clinical trials in ischemic stroke have also shown promising results with hemodilution.[2,101] This should be considered with the admonition, however, that hemorrhagic stroke, suspected increased ICP following head trauma, and large infarction are contraindications to hypertensive therapy. There is also a potential for detrimental effects associated with prolonged hypertension in the face of a disrupted blood-brain barrier; extravasation of osmotically active serum components may be followed by extravasation of fluid, with exacerbation of local edema and increased ICP. Previous studies have demonstrated increased ischemia with hypertension.[274]

In summary, hypertensive hemodilution is efficacious in SAH and potentially useful in focal ischemia, although optimal duration of treatment has yet to be defined, but is of no demonstrable benefit at this time in global ischemia.

Hyperventilation and Hypocarbia in the Management of Intracranial Hypertension

Hyperventilation and associated hypocarbia result in cerebrovascular vasoconstriction, and secondary decreases in cerebral perfusion lead to reduction in ICP. In addition, decreases in arterial carbon dioxide pressure ($PaCO_2$) diminish cerebral CO_2 and increase pH. Jennet and Teasdale[133] initially questioned the usefulness of controlled hyperventilation in 1981. Despite the recommendations of many that controlled hyperventilation may reduce ICP and counteract cerebral lactic acidosis following head trauma and thereby improve outcome, no randomized studies have been performed to date.[31,65,167,169] It is likely that these effects of hyperventilation are only transient and may actually compromise outcome in some cases. Muizelaar[194] have shown that whereas blood pH remains elevated following prolonged hyperventilation, the pH of the CSF returns to baseline within 24 hours. In addition, Muizelaar and associates[195] reported that cerebral arteriolar diameter actually increased following 24 hours of hyperventilation and became hypersensitive to changes in $PaCO_2$, presumably reflecting the loss of bicarbonate buffer from the CSF.

Gordon and Rossanda,[99] in a series of 251 head trauma patients, reported reduction of mortality in 51 patients hyperventilated to a $PaCO_2$ of 25 to 30 mmHg for periods ranging from 6 hours to 41 days. Hyperventilation has not been found to improve outcome following stroke.[51]

In 1991 Muizelaar et al.[194] suggested that hyperventilation may exacerbate existing cerebral ischemia following head injury and result in neuronal death. They evaluated the effects of normal ventilation, hyperventilation, and hyperventilation plus the buffer tromethamine in a randomized study of 113 patients with severe head injury. Tromethamine may overcome the loss of bicarbonate buffer from the CSF following prolonged hyperventilation and thus improve outcome. These results suggest that prophylactic hyperventilation is deleterious in head-injured patients with motor scores of 4 to 5 and that when sustained hyperventilation becomes necessary for ICP control, its deleterious side effects may be overcome with tromethamine.[194] It is known that in cases of fluid percussion injury, oxygen radicals prevent

arteriolar vasoconstriction in response to hyperventilation. Ellis et al.[71] evaluated the effect of the oxygen radical scavenger N-acetylcysteine on restoration of arteriolar response to hyperventilation following fluid percussion injury. They concluded that N-acetylcysteine given pre- or postinjury led to normal reactivity and thus may be useful for treatment of oxygen radical-mediated cerebral injury.

The benefits of hyperventilation in the acute reduction of ICP following head injury and in the intraoperative setting are well documented. However, current research raises questions about the efficacy of prolonged hyperventilation in this scenario and suggests that outcome may even be compromised with such protocols. Agents that restore the buffering effect of the CSF or the arteriolar response to hyperventilation may represent the means by which the benefits of hyperventilation can overcome their potential deleterious effects on outcome following head injury.

Medical Management: Management of Diabetes in the Surgical Patient

The metabolic abnormalities most often associated with diabetes mellitus (DM) can be exacerbated in the face of stressors such as infection and surgery.[145] Plasma glucose concentrations, which are usually 15 percent higher than whole blood glucose concentrations, should be used in the management of DM in the perioperative period.

The treatment of DM in the perioperative period is centered around preventing hyperglycemia and glycosuria and maintaining tight control of plasma glucose concentrations and serum electrolytes throughout the day. Experimental work has correlated the degree of hyperglycemia with neuronal damage in incomplete ischemia.[180,257] Rapid control of normoglycemia following the insult is advocated; this is cogent advice in view of the well-known detrimental effects of hypoglycemia. One must also be cognizant of the possibility of hypovolemia secondary to the osmotic diuresis that accompanies severe hyperglycemia. This can be controlled with frequent monitoring of glucose levels and administration of insulin as indicated. Plasma glucose should remain between 150 and 250 mg/dl; regular insulin should be administered if glucose concentrations exceed 300 mg/dl. Such tight control can prevent episodes of hypoglycemia and ketoacidosis. In addition, the nutritional supplementation of patients with DM should be closely monitored in the perioperative period. Dietary supplementation should include carbohydrate (50 percent of caloric intake) and protein (15 percent of caloric intake).

Should marked alterations in plasma glucose concentrations be evident preoperatively, elective procedures should be postponed until good control is attained. Sliding-scale methods of insulin administration are most effective when bedside determination of serum glucose is possible. Sliding-scale methods based upon urine tests have no place in the management of surgical patients.

Emergent neurosurgical procedures in the face of diabetic ketoacidosis require aggressive perioperative management aimed at replacing fluid, electrolyte, and insulin deficits. If possible, such procedures should be delayed until volume depletion and metabolic acidosis can be reversed. In nonemergent procedures, intravenous fluids should contain 5 percent dextrose solution, and one-half of the patient's normal morning dose of NPH insulin should be given subcutaneously as an intermediate-acting preparation. The patient's glucose concentrations should then be closely monitored and NPH insulin continued with regular insulin supplementation in the event that serum glucose concentrations exceed 300 mg/dl.

Pharmacologic Intervention

Substrate Manipulation

As previously described, subsequent to the onset of ischemia there is rapid depletion of glucose stores and intracellular ATP and a preferential shift of metabolism to the anaerobic mode with production of lactate from pyruvate. In cases of incomplete ischemia with continued delivery of glucose to cerebral tissue, lactate production proceeds with further reduction of intracellular pH, thus increasing cellular toxicity and exacerbating neurological deficit. Therefore, "a little blood flow is worse than no flow at all, if followed by reperfusion."[119] This has been experimentally supported by work in dogs following cardiac arrest; animals resuscitated after 30 minutes of cardiopulmonary resuscitation (CPR) showed significantly worse neurological outcomes than those in which no intervening CPR was performed prior to resuscitation. The clinical implications of this are profound, especially in instances of traumatically induced ischemia, in which there is a significant occurrence of stress-related hyperglycemia, which may be exacerbated by the concurrent use of steroids.[145]

Methodologies have been proposed to circumvent the above-described detrimental anaerobic glucose metabolism. One of these is administration to the brain in the face of ischemia of an alternate substrate that is readily metabolized to nontoxic products. Substrates such as gamma-hydroxybutyrate (GHB) and 1,3-butanediol cross the blood-brain barrier and are readily metabolized by neurons to nontoxic metabolites. Gamma-butyrolactone (GBL) is hydrolyzed in the peripheral circulation to GHB, which crosses the blood-brain barrier and is dehydrogenated to succinic semialdehyde, which is further oxidized to succinate, a tricarboxylic acid cycle intermediate. GBL has been demonstrated to significantly decrease glucose utilization in rat brain (32 percent in gray and 58 percent in white matter).[17] In a hypoxic mouse model, GHB increased survival time significantly (85 percent), but to a lesser extent than that observed with barbiturates or hypoxia in the same model. The predominant factor limiting use of GHB is the major reduction of CBF and cardiac output associated with its clinical use. 1,3-Butanediol is an ethanol dimer, which following administration is rapidly converted by ethanol and aldehyde dehydrogenase to beta-hydroxybutyrate, which is lipophilic, readily crosses the blood-brain barrier, and is metabolized by neuronal tissue. In the Levine rat ischemic-hypoxic model (unilateral carotid ligation and conscious hypoxic exposure), 1,3-butanediol has decreased neurological deficit. It has also been shown to increase hypoxic survival time in mice and rats. Interestingly, while the presumed mechanism for this protective effect has been the provision of a nontoxic substrate, blood levels of beta-hydroxybutyrate did not correlate with increased survival time; as such the precise mode of action of 1,3-butanediol has yet to be determined.[163] Data, however, do support a significant cerebral protective effect of 1,3-butanediol.[164]

Corticosteroids

Mechanisms of Action in Stroke

High-potency glucocorticoids have long been used before neurosurgical procedures in the belief that they can mitigate against edema and provide neuronal protection at a time of anticipated neuronal insult. Experimentally they have been shown to stabilize membranes and decrease arachidonic acid release following ischemia. This protective effect is probably multifactorial. Glucocorticoids have been demonstrated to increase blood flow to injured central nervous system tissue by several postulated mechanisms, including direct vasodilatation, decreased thromboxane A_2 (TXA$_2$) release, and decreased lipid peroxidation. In addition, they have been shown to enhance Na-K ATPase activity (presumably by decreasing lipid peroxidation), thus decreasing ion flux accordingly. Intrinsic antioxidant properties of glucocorticoids also function in free-radical scavenging (see below). In consideration of the above properties, glucocorticoids have been widely touted for their ability to protect against neuronal ischemic damage. One cautionary proviso, however, is the need to be aware that hyperglycemia can be potentiated by their use (see below). In animal studies dexamethasone did not confer any significant cerebral protection in a model of hypoxic-ischemic brain injury.[10]

Head Injury

Clinical trials of glucocorticoids have failed to consistently show a favorable effect on outcome following head trauma. There do exist potential subsets of patients (most notably younger ones) with severe head trauma in whom use of high-dose methylprednisolone may improve outcome.[96] One inherent problem with the use of glucocorticoids in head trauma is the decreased uptake of steroids by contused brain, which thus limits their efficacy. Moderate tissue levels may be attained within 1 hour after the insult; therefore optimal postfacto results would dictate glucocorticoid administration in the field. At the present time the deleterious catabolic side effects of glucocorticoids (in addition to the risk of infection and gastrointestinal blood loss) outweigh their proven benefit in the majority of head trauma cases; however side effects of short-course high-potency glucocorticoids are minimal, and clinical trials of early, large-dose therapy with careful monitoring of serum glucose levels are certainly warranted.

Spinal Cord Injury

Some of the most compelling evidence regarding the use of steroids is the emergent use of glucocorticoids following spinal cord injury. It has been suggested that high-dose glucocorticoids improve posttraumatic spinal cord blood flow, microvascular perfusion, and clinical neurological recovery.[12,13,109,307] A 1990 report of a large randomized controlled clinical trial using high-dose methylprednisolone immediately following traumatic spinal cord injury concluded that methylprednisolone improved neurological functional outcome.[42] It has also been reported that the 21-aminosteroid U74006F improved neurologic functional outcome following traumatic spinal cord injury in cats.[11] Thus, the use of steroids in the treatment of spinal cord injury appears promising. Further studies will be required to elucidate not only the mechanisms of these actions but also the extent of potential recovery possible through their use.

21-Aminosteroids

Current investigative interest in a steroid subgroup, the 21-aminosteroids, has led to a good deal of research regarding cerebral protective effects and potential mechanisms of action. Monyer et al.[187] studied the protective efficacy of novel 21-aminosteroids against several forms of neuronal injury in murine cortical cell cultures. 21-Aminosteroids were found to partially attenuate the damage induced by glucose deprivation, combined oxygen-glucose deprivation, or exposure to NMDA. The maximal protection afforded by 21-aminosteroids was less than that produced by NMDA antagonists, but their combination produced synergistic benefits. 21-Aminosteroid addition had a protective action consistent with inhibition of free radical-mediated lipid peroxidation.

Human leukocytes are known to be recruited to ischemic regions of the brain. The production of hydrogen peroxide and free radicals by leukocytes in these ischemic regions may result in lipid peroxidation and resultant tissue injury. Fisher et al.,[83] in a model of chemiluminescence in stimulated human leukocytes, suggested that the 21-aminosteroid U74500A may reduce lipid peroxidation by reducing the concentration of oxygen metabolites; thus, U74500A may play a significant role in reducing ischemic injury and vasogenic edema. The 21-aminosteroid U74006F has also been reported to inhibit postischemic lipid peroxidation as assessed by the preservation of brain vitamin E and thereby to provide for a membrane protective effect. Such an effect could potentially reverse the influx of calcium into the cell following ischemic insult and allow for a recuperative effect at the cellular level.[108] In a model of global ischemia in cats, U74006F significantly increased cortical blood flow 15 minutes following the ischemic insult as compared with controls. U74006F also significantly improved postischemic maintenance of blood pressure and recovery of SSEPs in addition to reducing postischemic acidosis. These results suggest that U74006F may be a useful adjunct in the early treatment of global ischemia.[110]

Recent animal models of forebrain ischemia suggest that U74006F is of benefit in ameliorating ischemic injury, although such injury may vary in differing regions of the brain, possibly because of a regional variability in lipid peroxidation following ischemic insult.[157] Pretreatment with two 1.5 mg/kg boluses in dogs who subsequently received a global ischemic insult also conferred a protective effect and improved outcome.[214]

21-Aminosteroids have also been documented to have certain protective effects in models of regional ischemia and SAH. Young et al. found that U74006F reduced cerebral edema following middle cerebral artery (MCA) occlusion in the rat. This effect was limited to regions with adequate collateral blood flow.[308] Zuccarello reported that U74006F protected the blood-brain barrier against the effects of SAH by preventing lipid peroxidation and other lipolytic processes that irreversibly damage cell membranes.[311]

It is evident that the protective effect of the 21-aminosteroids in reducing lipid peroxidation can reduce injury resulting from ischemia and potentiate recovery. This protective effect has been described in models of global ischemia, regional ischemia, and SAH. Further research is ongoing with regard to the potential benefit of these drugs in humans following stroke and aneurysmally induced SAH.

Calcium Channel Blockers

The use of calcium channel blockers in neurosurgery was initiated in an attempt to provide a treatment for delayed cerebral vasospasm secondary to SAH. It has been theorized that their mechanism of action involves relaxation of the smooth muscle of the cerebral vasculature. Recent interest in calcium ion activity relates to the fact that Ca^{++} shifts are central in the production of leukotrienes, prostanoids, thromboxanes, and oxidative free radicals and are heavily implicated in the postischemic hypoperfusion syndrome; as described previously, all these factors interrelate and contribute to neuronal injury. Calcium entry blockers have been postulated to decrease ionic calcium shifts, thereby obviating this catabolic cascade. Pretreatment with calcium entry blockers has been reported to provide protection from global cerebral ischemia; recent experimental studies have indicated positive results with administration after global ischemia, both in the short term (24 hours after aortic arch occlusion in dogs[258]) and in the longer follow-up term (96 hours after neck tourniquet placement of 17 minutes in primates.[256] At present there is an ongoing trial of lidoflazine administration following human cardiac arrest. Calcium entry blockers are also potentially applicable in focal as well as global ischemia; they have been demonstrated to decrease the depletion of ATP following focal arterial occlusion.

There has been great enthusiasm about the use of these agents following SAH-induced vasospasm. Nimodipine is a dihydropyridine derivative, which readily crosses the blood-brain barrier. It is a potent voltage-sensitive calcium channel blocker, offers some cerebrovascular specificity, and has been studied in relation to modification of post-SAH vasospasm with encouraging results. Its effectiveness is supported by a 1985 clinical report of improvement of neurological deficit following SAH.[39,148] During multicenter trials in patients with aneurysmal SAH, nimodipine was found to indeed improve outcome.[8,216,217] These results indicated, however, that nimodipine did not improve angiographically visible vasospasm and thus suggested that the drug's mode of action is on the neuron itself. In animal models of cerebral ischemia with reperfusion[112,153,154,192,285] and in models of permanent vessel occlusion,[32,34,90,104,122,236] nimodipine was found to have a protective effect. Nimodipine has also been shown to be effective in excitotoxin-induced injury.[91] Although the drug was not shown to ameliorate angiographic vasospasm, it has been shown in vitro to improve local cerebral blood flow,[166,235,302] which provides a possible mechanism for reduction of postischemic hypoperfusion. This has been corroborated by human studies using positron emission tomography (PET) to quantitate rCBF and regional cerebral oxygen metabolism rate (rCMRO$_2$).[107,116,123,279] Nevertheless, not all investigators agree about nimodipine's protective effects.[165,278,287]

A number of multicenter trials were initiated to assess the efficacy of nimodipine in acute stroke. Gelmers et al.[93] reported improvement in neurological deficits and improvement in survival, the latter being noted only in men. Improved survival and neurological outcome were also noted by Paci et al.[209] and Martinez et al.[170] However, the Trust Study Group found no benefit in acute stroke in either survival or neurological outcome.[282] In 1990, Gelmers and Jennerici[94] reviewed the results of several multicenter trials and found a general trend toward improvement in outcome in patients given the drug.

Nicardipine is a recently developed cerebrospecific congener, which can be administered intravenously; its efficacy awaits appropriate clinical trials.

Calcium channel blockers, however, represent a large and heterogeneous group, encompassing different classes of agents with some specificity of occlusion of different calcium channel subtypes. In addition, they appear to demonstrate some species specificity in their beneficial effects. In general all calcium channel blockers carry risk of hypotension and negative cardiac inotropic effects; however, if this is kept in mind, if the agents are carefully titrated in relation to their side effects, and if cerebroselective blockers are used, calcium channel blockers remain promising for future use in both the pre- and posttreatment of focal and global ischemia.[26]

While the above discussion provides encouragement for the use of these agents, there has been experimental evidence, supported by sporadic case reports, of delayed onset of seizures and progressive neurological deterioration at 72 to 96 hours following their administration. At our institution all patients with aneurysmal SAH, patients undergoing elective clipping of unruptured aneurysms, and all patients having surgery for skull base lesions receive perioperative nimodipine.

Diphenylhydantoin

Most neurosurgeons use diphenylhydantoin in patients with supratentorial lesions that are potentially epileptogenic. Aside from its anticonvulsant properties, this drug has been shown to have direct cytoprotective effects in neurons. Reduction of the ischemic inhibition of Na-K ATPase has been demonstrated in animals.[16] Other mechanisms postulated include reduction of ATP utilization,[52,103] inhibition of calcium-mediated processes,[41,142] and reduction in synaptic activity.

Diphenylhydantoin has been demonstrated to decrease membrane-associated ion flux during both hypoxia and normoxia. It has no significant effect on $CMRO_2$ and produces an overall decrease in CBF. It has been shown to decrease K^+ ion concentration in CSF following cardiac arrest in dogs, and this phenomenon has been presumptively linked to its protective effect[16] under the premise that increased extracellular K^+ concentration precipitates contraction of vascular smooth muscle and astroglial water content, thereby increasing cytotoxic edema. Its anticonvulsive properties, though important in control of postischemic seizure activity, are secondary in its neuronal protection effects. The K^+ increase in CSF most certainly reflects liberation from hypoxic cells; diphenylhydantoin attenuates this K^+ efflux by enhancing ATP-dependent Na-K pump activity or by a direct membrane-stabilizing effect. It decreases this posthypoxic K^+ efflux more effectively than either barbiturates or hypothermia in a canine model.[16] It was previously demonstrated that diphenylhydantoin administered prior to the onset of hypoxia in rats and mice delayed the onset of clinical signs of hypoxia, and similar treatment in cats increased survival. The neuronal protective effects of diphenylhydantoin have been demonstrated whether it is given before or after the ischemic insult[15] although Boxer et al.[41] demonstrated no beneficial effect if it is given more than 2 hours after the insult. Immediate administration following global ischemia in cats decreased histopathologically associated anoxic changes.[15] Maximal benefits are gleaned from anticonvulsant dosages; large doses produce well-known toxic side effects and provide no additional ischemic protection. Future clinical use awaits definitive human trials. We currently administer diphenylhydantoin pre- and postoperatively to patients with supratentorial lesions that involve the cortex.

Inhibitors of Arachidonic Acid Metabolism

During ischemia, arachidonic acid is released from cell membranes. In reference to our original discussion of the pathophysiological consequences of ischemia, the arachidonic acid liberated from phospholipase activity is a precursor via the cyclooxygenase pathway of prostacyclin and thromboxanes. During reperfusion, the arachidonic acid is metabolized through the cyclooxygenase and lipoxygenase pathways, which results in accumulation of prostaglandins, prostacyclin, thromboxanes, and leukotrienes.[230]

In ischemia the desired result of manipulation of this system would be inhibition of thromboxane A_2 synthesis and facilitation of synthesis of prostacyclin, which promote vasodilatation and inhibit platelet aggregation. The use of prostacyclin as a nonspecific vasodilator has been proposed in this circumstance; in particular, it has been advocated as being more efficacious when administered in combination with a cyclooxygenase inhibitor to promote vasodilatation while actively precluding thromboxane synthesis.

Indomethacin is a potent cyclooxygenase inhibitor and has been documented to improve recovery following global ischemia in rabbits.[40] In combination with prostaglandin I_2 it has been documented to decrease focal cerebral ischemia.[22] In fact, indomethacin has been demonstrated to enhance the protective effects of nimodipine and mannitol in a rat model of cerebral ischemia.[267] Eicosapentanoic acid has been shown to inhibit the conversion of arachadonic acid to both prostaglandins and thromboxane A_2, while allowing formation of prostacyclin.[58] In a gerbil model this has been shown to abolish postischemic hypoperfusion.[36] To date no controlled trials in humans have been performed.

The above concept is similarly exploited by use of eicosapentanoic acid, which as a substrate for cyclooxygenase is metabolized via a single-step reaction to yield prostacyclin; this serves to augment the total available supply of vasodilator and also competes with arachidonic acid for cyclooxygenase, thereby decreasing thromboxane production. Human clinical trials are lacking but are enthusiastically anticipated.

Agents That Reduce Blood Viscosity

The current standard of care for patients with aneurysmal SAH and delayed cerebral vasospasm provides for them to receive volume expansion. This acts to improve cardiac output as well as to reduce hematocrit. Pentoxyfylline is an agent that improves the rheology by increasing the deformability of red blood cells, but unfortunately it has not proved effective in human trials of acute stroke.[213]

Xanthine Oxidase Inhibitors

As stated previously, the enzyme xanthine oxidase has been implicated as a key determinant of neuronal cell death. Allopurinol, an inhibitor of this enzyme, is a drug widely used in the treatment of gout. Several animal studies have found allopurinol to be effective in reducing the effects of cerebral ischemia.[132,171,183] Propentofylline, also a xanthine oxidase inhibitor, has also been shown to be effective in ameliorating cerebral ischemia in an animal model.[63] These encouraging results may lead to human trials.

PREOPERATIVE ASSESSMENT OF CEREBRAL BLOOD FLOW

Angiography

Although invasive, angiography is the gold standard in the preoperative evaluation of the cerebral vasculature. Aside from its obvious necessity in vascular neurosurgery, angiography is helpful in evaluating the patency of venous sinuses and the displacement of other major vascular structures by neoplasms. It is particularly helpful for evaluating the patency of sinuses prior to performing complex skull base surgery when a venous sinus may be sacrificed or for identifying the junction between the vein of Labbé and the transverse sinus. We currently have abandoned routine angiography in favor of magnetic resonance imaging (MRI) in the preoperative localization of the carotid arteries for pituitary surgery, and in the future MRI angiography will likely replace conventional angiography in the preoperative assessment of the cerebral vasculature.

MRI Angiography

At present time MRI angiography can provide satisfactory visualization of the extracranial and large intracranial vessels. We have used it with success in selected patients in whom iodinated contrast agents could not be used, but at present it lacks appropriate resolution to warrant routine use in lieu of conventional angiography.

Transcranial Doppler Ultrasonography

Clinical use of transcranial Doppler ultrasonography (TCD) is most frequently detailed in the evaluation and management of patients with aneurysmally induced SAH and resulting vasospasm. Because of the severity of the sequelae associated with vasospasm, it is essential that we establish the time course of vasospasm in each patient to maximize management and outcome. Until recently cerebral angiography was the sole modality by which we could clinically stage the progression of vasospasm. Unfortunately, angiography is an invasive procedure and cannot be performed at the bedside. Currently, TCD provides promise in evaluating the progression of vasospasm in a simple and noninvasive fashion.[1,113,241,242,298]

In evaluating the progression of vasospasm with TCD, blood flow velocity (namely mean flow velocity) is the parameter that has been correlated most closely with severity of vasospasm, in addition to flow velocity and diameter of the middle cerebral artery as determined by angiography.[1,113] TCD blood flow velocities have also been correlated with neurologic deficit.[54,113,129] Flow velocities of 120 cm/s are present in all patients with angiographic evidence of vasospasm.[1,241]

In view of the variability of intracranial flow patterns based upon such factors as ICP, PCO_2, and hematocrit, Klingelhofer et al.[144] evaluated the interdependence of clinical grade, degree of vasospasm, ICP, and TCD parameters by determining mean flow velocity and the index of cerebral circulatory resistance (measure of peripheral vascular flow) in 76 patients with SAH. They concluded that (1) in patients with a resistance index less than 0.5, changes in mean flow velocity reflected the severity of vasospasm; (2) during vasospasm, values of the resistance index above 0.6 with a simultaneously decreased mean flow velocity indicated a rise in ICP; and (3) with marked elevations in ICP, evaluation of vasospasm with TCD based upon mean flow velocity may be unreliable.

The intraoperative benefits of TCD during carotid endarterectomy have also been reported. Steiger et al.[259] reviewed 100 consecutive microsurgical carotid endarterectomies in 93 patients. Cerebral perfusion and activity were monitored with simultaneous TCD and EEG. No perioperative strokes occurred in this series. During the mean follow-up of 15 months, one patient died from stroke ipsilateral to the treated carotid artery; another patient had a minor contralateral stroke; two patients suffered a single reversible neurologic deficit in the distribution of the treated vessel; and four other patients had a single contralateral hemispheric or retinal reversible ischemic attack. Pokrovskii et al. used TCD to study the linear blood flow rate in the MCA during carotid endarterectomy in 25 patients.[222] They documented that changes in linear blood flow rate in the MCA correlate with alterations in blood pressure. Most notably, this flow rate was most reduced during compression of the common carotid artery in patients with marked involvement of the contralateral carotid artery. After the blood flow in the common carotid artery was restored, the linear blood flow rate in the MCA could be determined by the degree of stenosis of the artery undergoing operative intervention and the degree of collateral circulation. Thus it was possible to determine the need for additional measures to protect the brain from ischemia.

The potential benefits of TCD in the management of patients with vasospasm are obvious. Only through aggressive clinical studies can the benefits of TCD in the care of these patients be maximized. At present the use of TCD in carotid endarterectomy remains to be defined.

Positron Emission Tomography/ Single-Photon Emission CT/ Xenon CT

In the preoperative planning of an intracranial procedure, it is often valuable to know the parameters of rCBF in the area of interest. This is particularly true when considering revascularization procedures. The most widely available technique is single-photon emission computed tomography (SPECT), but it unfortunately suffers from poor spatial resolution and inaccuracies resulting from binding of the isotope to tissue receptors.

In xenon-enhanced CT scanning, xenon gas is inhaled by the patient. This technique provides good spatial resolution and reasonably accurate measurements of rCBF. Its main disadvantage is that it does not provide measurements of metabolic activity, and the gas is not infrequently associated with intoxicating effects upon the patient.

The most versatile tool, providing information about rCBF, rCMRO$_2$, and regional glucose utilization, is PET. Although technical difficulties have limited its availability, an increased number of centers are building PET facilities.

INTRAOPERATIVE MANAGEMENT

Principles of Neuroanesthetic Technique

The tenets of neuroanesthetic technique require that cerebral perfusion pressure be optimized while autoregulatory function remains intact. Anesthetics have varying effects on cerebral perfusion, cerebral oxygen demand, and cerebrovascular resistance. The inhalational anesthetics tend to act as vasodilators, thereby increasing intracranial blood volume, which can thus increase ICP. Such increases can be balanced via hyperventilation and associated hypocarbia.[7] The anesthetic agents most commonly used in neuroanesthesia and their effects on cerebrovascular dynamics are discussed below.

Anesthetic Agents

Isoflurane

Neuroprotective agents may exert their effect by reducing CMRO$_2$, increasing cerebral oxygen delivery, or altering ongoing pathological processes. Barbiturates provide neuroprotection by reducing the CMRO$_2$ necessary for synaptic transmission in a dose-related fashion while leaving the component necessary for cellular metabolism intact. Isoflurane may exert a neuroprotective effect by a similar mechanism, but its efficacy is probably less than that of barbiturates owing to adverse effects on CBF.[111] It is unique among volatile anesthetics in that it may potentially produce an isoelectric EGG at clinically relevant concentrations. As with barbiturates, the primary metabolic depressant effect preferentially alters synaptic activity while the metabolism maintaining cellular integrity is unaffected. In contrast to barbiturates, isoflurane exhibits no myocardial depression, has no influence on ICP, and does not allay free fatty acid (FFA) liberation. In addition to metabolic demand reduction, it is believed to improve CBF and to decrease potassium flux with all its attendant catabolic consequences.

Warner et al.[293] evaluated reversible focal ischemia in rats subjected to reversible MCA occlusion while receiving deep methohexital or isoflurane anesthesia. During ischemia, although a regional reduction in flow was noted in both anesthetic groups, mean flow remained greater in the isoflurane group. A study by Newberg and Michenfelder[199] concluded that the predominant protective effect is attributable to reduction of metabolic demand and is effective only at decreasing conductive electrical activity in areas of incomplete ischemia with some element of residual synaptic activity. Other studies have demonstrated protection during hemorrhagic hypotension and carotid endarterectomy.

Enflurane

Enflurane increases CBF and can increase ICP to an extent that may not be countered by hyperventilation and associated hypocarbia. In addition, enflurane has a negative inotropic effect on the heart. Thus, increased ICP in the face of decreased cardiac function can result in decreased cerebral perfusion pressure.[246]

Halothane

Halothane produces a vasodilatory response, which results in increases in CBF. It also results in a decrease in $CMRO_2$ and in hypotension. It has been reported that transient increases in ICP resulting from induction of anesthesia with this agent can be difficult to manage even with the use of hyperventilation.[251]

Nitrous Oxide

Nitrous oxide can lead to a marked increase in ICP, which is refractory to hypocarbia. In combination with other agents it may severely exacerbate intracranial hypertension when a mass lesion is already compromising cerebral dynamics.[5]

Lidocaine

Lidocaine, while similarly preferentially suppressing synaptic transmission has also been invoked in membrane stabilization during ischemia. Evidence for neuronal protection in experimental animal models is promising but has yet to be substantiated in human trials.

Muscle Relaxants

Muscle relaxants increase cerebral blood flow. They also result in differing levels of histamine release with the most marked response following the administration of D-tubocurarine. These properties are most directly involved in their effect on cerebrovascular dynamics.[260] It should be noted that depolarizing agents (i.e. succinylcholine) used directly without being preceded by the use of a nondepolarizing agent, can severely exacerbate intracranial hypertension.

Hypothermia

History

It has long been suspected clinically and supported by anecdotal reports that hypothermia increases neuronal resistance to hypoxic insults; cold water drowning victims with normal functional recovery after 40 minutes of submersion have been documented. Pioneer work of Bigelow and associates in 1950 demonstrated experimental survival in dogs undergoing deep hypothermia. Subsequently Rosamoff[233] demonstrated a reduction in canine MCA infarct size following lowering of core temperature to 22° to 24°C.

Mechanism of Neuroprotective Effect

Cellular Mechanisms

A 1986 study by O'Connor et al.[204] demonstrated normal neurological function in dogs following 1 hour of circulatory arrest with simultaneous cerebral temperature of 13°C, with no resultant discernible neuropathological changes following sacrifice of the animals 7 days postanoxia. The presumptive mechanism in hypothermic neuronal protection is the reduction of metabolic demands (decreased $CMRO_2$); from 37° to 22°C, $CMRO_2$ decreases linearly to 25 percent of normal. Difficulties with the practical applicability of hypothermia have been its limiting side effects, most notably myocardial depression, subsequent pulmonary infections, and gastric ulcers. In addition, the optimal duration of hypothermia for maximal protective effect has not been defined; prolonged hypothermia may indeed be detrimental, with increased blood viscosity and sludging of flow. However, hypothermia with circulatory arrest has been an important adjunct in cardiac surgery (especially in the repair of congenital lesions) and repair of the aortic arch.[204]

Thresholds of Ischemia during Hypothermia

Cerebral protection during surgical procedures necessitating circulatory arrest or low flow remains the factor that most limits the critical time for repair of lesions. Swain et al.[271] reported on the use of in vivo phosphorus 31 nuclear magnetic resonance spectroscopy to assess cerebral metabolism during circulatory arrest in sheep. A flow of 10 ml/kg/min preserved high-energy phosphates and intracellular pH. Therefore deep hypothermia with cardiopulmonary bypass flows as low as 10 ml/kg/min can maintain brain high-energy phosphate concentrations and intracellular pH for 2 hours in sheep, whereas flows of

5 ml/kg/min or intermittent full-flow systemic perfusion between periods of circulatory arrest offer less protection.

Protective Effects of Hypothermia during Hyperglycemia

The effect of hypothermia on the presence or absence of substrate is also being currently evaluated. Lundgren et al.[162] have documented that preischemic hyperglycemia aggravates brain damage following transient ischemia and results in postischemic seizure activity and cellular edema. Their experiments confirmed previous findings that mild hypothermia protects normoglycemic animals against the insult. The results also showed that hypothermia prevented most of the exaggeration of damage caused by hyperglycemia. This suggests that hypothermia has less of a protective effect on mechanisms causing such damage than on neuronal damage in the classic selectively vulnerable regions, particularly the caudoputamen.

Protective Effects of Hypothermia on N-Methyl-D-Aspartate Receptor Activity

Some of the most interesting current work concerns the neuroprotective effects of the noncompetitive NMDA antagonist MK 801. Baker et al.[27] suggest that the neuroprotective properties of hypothermia may reside in part in its ability to prevent increase in the extracellular concentrations of amino acids that enhance the activity of the NMDA receptor complex. This suggestion is based on findings in rabbits subjected to 10 minutes of global ischemia under normothermic (37°C) or hypothermic (29°C) conditions. Corbett et al.[55] have reported that the protective actions of MK 801 may be due entirely to drug-induced hypothermia. Both systemic injection of MK 801 and profound cerebral hypothermia protect vulnerable CA1 neurons from degeneration. Buchan and Pulsinelli[46] have also concluded that the neuroprotective activity of MK 801 against transient global ischemia appears to be largely a consequence of postischemic hypothermia rather than a direct action on NMDA receptor channels. Mohler and Gordon[185] have reported that the thermoregulatory responses of the rabbit to central neural injections of sulfolane also cannot be attributed to direct action of the parent compound but rather is due to attendant hypothermia. Duhaime and Ross[70] have found that degeneration of hippocampal CA1 neurons occurs following transient complete ischemia produced by raised ICP.

Gill and Woodruff[98] have reported that the combination of the excitatory amino acid antagonist kynurenic acid with MK 801 had a synergistic neuroprotective effect in a transient forebrain ischemia model in gerbils. Maintenance of the body temperature of the gerbils at 37°C for 24 hours did not affect the neuroprotective action of MK 801 or kynurenic acid. Ikonomidou et al.[130] have shown that reducing the body temperature of the infant rat also confers partial protection against cerebral ischemia and that mild hypothermia plus MK 801 treatment provides total protection against such damage.

Prediction of Response to Hypothermia

Mathematical relationships have also been developed relating cerebral protection to hypothermia. Michenfelder and Milde[179] have evaluated the relationship between brain temperature and $CMRO_2$ in a canine model during cooling from 37° to 14°C while EEG was continuously monitored. For each temperature interval, the temperature coefficient (Q10) for $CMRO_2$ was calculated by the formula

$$Q10 = CMRO_2 \text{ (at } x°C)/CMRO_2 \text{ (at } 10x°C)$$

Between 37 and 27°C, the Q10 was 2.23, but between 27 and 14°C the mean Q10 was doubled to 4.53. With rewarming to 37°C, CBF and $CMRO_2$ returned to control levels, and brain biopsies revealed a normal brain energy state. Greeley et al.,[100] in a review of hypothermic cardiopulmonary bypass in 46 neonates, infants, and children, suggested that cerebral metabolism is exponentially related to temperature during hypothermic bypass, with a temperature coefficient of 3.65. They formulated a mathematical model, which expresses a numerical hypothermic metabolic index to quantitate the duration of brain protection provided by reduction of cerebral metabolism owing to hypothermic bypass over any temperature range. This index predicts that patients cooled to 28°C have an ischemic tolerance of 11 to 19 minutes and that patients cooled to 18°C have a predicted ischemic tolerance of 39 to 65 minutes.

Clinical Use of Hypothermia

Use during Cardiothoracic Surgery

Most of the literature on cerebral protection resulting from hypothermia concerns its use during cardiovascular procedures with concomitant bypass. Kazui et al.[139] reviewed 21 consecutive patients undergoing surgical correction of aneurysms of the transverse aortic arch, in whom the mean cerebral arrest time was 35.2 ± 3.4 minutes. They reported no cerebral complications. Bachet et al.[24] propose that the technique of "cold cerebroplegia" provides excellent cerebral protection during operations on the aortic arch. The carotid arteries are cannulated and perfused with blood cooled at 6° to 12°C while the core temperature is maintained at moderate hypothermia (25° to 28°C). In a 5-year series of 54 patients they reported no intraoperative mortality. Overall mortality was 13 percent, with only one death related to neurological compromise. Transient postoperative neurological deficit was present in 4.3 percent of their patients.

Watanabe et al.[294] concluded that perfusion flow rate will decide the safe period and that pulsatile assistance will promote brain protection at any flow rate in profoundly hypothermic cardiopulmonary bypass. Hypothermic circulatory arrest also provides for adequate protection during quadruple coronary artery bypass grafting and may eliminate cerebral embolization.

Newman et al.[201] reported on the neuropsychological consequences of prolonged circulatory arrest with hypothermia and barbiturate "protection." Measurements performed during surgery showed a prolonged absence of EEG recording. Postoperative neuropsychological assessment revealed good preservation of function, with the exception of delayed verbal memory and performance on the trial making test. Natale and D'Alecy[198] have also documented that selective brain cooling before and during 10 minutes of cardiac arrest was associated with significantly improved neurological function and 100 percent survival, whereas normothermic cardiac arrest produced marked neurological dysfunction and 100 percent mortality in a canine model.

Mizrahi et al.[184] measured peripheral body temperatures at the onset of hypothermia-induced electrocerebral silence in the intraoperative EEG of 56 adults undergoing cardiovascular procedures. Using EEG-guided hypothermia, they found low morbidity and mortality. These data suggested that electrocerebral silence is a safe and reliable guide for determining the appropriate level of hypothermia during cardiovascular procedures.

Use during Neurological Surgery

Profound hypothermia and thiopentone were used to provide cerebral protection during circulatory arrest in the management of a patient with a giant cerebral aneurysm.[281] Baker et al.[28] have suggested that hypothermia to 24°C may reduce cerebral infarction and edema formation following permanent middle cerebral artery occlusion in the rat. Welsh and Harris[300]

found histological indications that hippocampal injury was not diminished by postischemic hypothermia during the first 2 hours of reperfusion in a gerbil model; maximal histological injury was present in the CA1 neuron subfield in all animals. Crittenden et al.[56] concluded that both antegrade infusion of cerebroplegia and external cranial cooling confer distinct cerebral protective effects after a protracted period of hypothermic circulatory arrest in sheep when compared with systemic hypothermia alone, systemic hypothermia combined with external cranial cooling, or retrograde cerebroplegia. It has also been demonstrated by Welsh et al.[301] that a decrease in head temperature of only 2°C will reduce the degree of CA1 neuron injury in gerbils subjected to 5 minutes of bilateral ischemia.

With regard to any potential role in the protection against radiation injury, ketamine and hypothermia combination therapy has not been found to confer a protective effect against acute radiation-induced mortality.[206]

While the experimental data and clinical results summarized above are encouraging, sight must not be lost of the fact that cerebral lesions have been reported in children following thoracic surgery during hypothermia.[19] In the future the adverse limiting side effects may be moderated by using hypothermia in combination with other modalities (such as hemodilution (considered below). In addition, moderate hypothermia 28° to 30°C may have substantial beneficial effects on cerebral oxygen metabolism with few concomitant adverse side effects. Hypothermia in combination with barbiturates has been demonstrated to reduce $CMRO_2$ by 85 percent.[202] Despite all its proven efficacy, it has yet to be clinically tested in a cardiac arrest outcome model, but it remains potentially important in the future if methods of combating problems associated with its use are developed.

Pharmacologic Intervention

Agents That Reduce Cerebral Oxygen Demand

Barbiturates

As an anesthetic and depressant of cerebral metabolism, pentobarbital induces its effects on the central nervous system by stimulating the binding of gamma-aminobutyric acid (GABA) to its receptor and by inhibiting postsynaptic excitatory amino acid activity.[206] The potential neuronal protective effects of barbiturates have long been recognized. Barbiturates produce a dose-dependent diminution of $CMRO_2$ until EEG silence (up to 50 percent in humans and animals,[257] after which additional doses have no effect; housekeeping functions of the cell are not depressed. This is most assuredly the major protective mechanism; however, barbiturates are responsible for a host of other beneficial cellular effects, including lysosomal membrane stabilization, decreased FFA liberation, and decreasing edema formation, and they also exhibit free-radical scavenging ability. Barbiturates decrease CBF in nonischemic brain, which may actually improve flow in focal ischemia by producing a "reversible steal" phenomenon. The protective effect of barbiturates correlates with their anesthetic properties, while their anticonvulsive properties account for a much smaller percentage of their beneficial effect (diazepam is less effective at increasing survival in posthypoxic mice, although it is superior to barbiturates in preventing seizure activity in this model.[259]

The efficacy of barbiturates in focal ischemia is well documented in both pretreatment and early posttreatment (within 60 minutes) models of middle cerebral artery occlusion; this effect is most applicable in the context of anticipated occlusion of blood flow during a neurovascular procedure. There is some evidence of potential benefit even if the barbiturates are administered in conditions of focal ischemia with restoration of flow within 6 hours.[244] Evidence also exists for their advantage if administered before or shortly following incomplete global ischemia, for example when used following severe hypotension or intraoperatively. Their efficacy before or after complete global ischemia is controversial; different animal models have yielded opposite results. At this time the routine use of barbiturates following cardiac arrest has shown no consistent clinical benefit, although if given within minutes of the reestablishment of normotension they are well tolerated.[234] This is important in consideration of the deleterious side effects of most barbiturates—namely, cardioplegic effects that are dose-dependent and require initiation of pressure support in a significant percentage of patients receiving burst-suppressive doses, the increased risk of infection attributable to barbiturates, and depression of mental status that obscures neurological evaluation. Protection from acute radiation-induced mortality by pentobarbital in the rat model has been shown to be a reproducible phenomenon and is associated with the GABA agonistic activity of the compound. This agonistic property may offer the potential for a novel approach to the enhancement and efficacy of radiation therapy in the treatment of brain tumors.[206]

Current research evaluating the potential protective effects of ultrashort-acting barbiturates also show promise. Kuroiwa et al.[151] demonstrated that the pathological processes leading to delayed neuronal injury in the CA1 sector are induced during the initial 40 minutes of recirculation and that ultrashort-acting barbiturates (e.g., methohexital) infused into the left carotid artery are able to reverse these processes if given during this period.

The efficacy of these agents in severe head trauma is also controversial; studies have failed to demonstrate unequivocal improved outcome following their use. A randomized trial in severe head injury reported in 1985 failed to demonstrate improvement in outcome or ICP control.[292] The questionable benefit and severe potential side effects of these agents preclude their use in the majority of trauma cases. Clinical trials have yet to define potential subgroups (e.g., younger patients who tolerate cardiovascular side effects) in whom use of these agents may be of benefit.

Etomidate

The barbiturate Althesin had been increasingly used during the early 1980s as a first-line agent in controlling increased ICP following severe head injury,[191] but its use has been discontinued owing to induction of histamine release and resultant anaphylaxis. Dearden and McDowall[61] have shown that the decreases in CBF are not simply a result of decreased arterial pressure. They have suggested that etomidate may provide an effective alternative to Althesin in treating increases in ICP following severe head injury and have recommended an initial infusion rate of 50 μg/kg/min for 10 minutes (loading dose) and then 20 to 40 μg/kg/min. They have also suggested that steroid supplements be used to prevent problems with adrenocortical suppression.

Etomidate is a potent, short-acting anesthetic induction agent, which also produces a dose-related decrease in $CMRO_2$. Its protective effects have been substantiated both in functional outcome following ischemia and hypoxia and in cerebral histology in experimental animal models. In canine oligemic hypoxia, higher survival rates are reported with etomidate than with equivalent burst-suppressant doses of thiopental or pentobarbital. At these dose levels there was decreased lactate production and better maintenance of ATP stores than in control animals. The improved efficacy of etomidate as compared with barbiturates has been in part attributed to its lack of cardiodepressant side effects and its short duration of action. Also implicated in its protective effect are decreased ICP and a preferential neocortical electrical suppressant effect via a GABA-mimetic action.[200]

Etomidate secondarily suppresses adrenocortical synthesis, with restoration of normal adrenal function after infusion is finished.[9,79,188,295] With the concurrent administration of corticosteroids during etomidate infusion in critically ill patients, no increased mortality has been observed.[156,173,240,295,306]

Etomidate's effects on cerebral activity have been extensively studied. These progressive changes can readily be seen on the EEG, which serves as a continuous sensitive indicator of cerebral effects during anesthesia.[53,67,68,138,182,190,220,223,249,286,296,306] The EEG progression seen with etomidate is analogous to that described for thiopental.[175] The end point of clinical anesthesia corresponds to the stage 3 end point, which is characterized by the absence of EEG signs of arousal after noxious stimuli are given at stage 3; therefore stage 3 is the EEG equivalent of surgical anesthesia. It is described a having increased-amplitude slow waves interspersed with 1- to 2-second periods of high-frequency, low-amplitude waves. This is similar to the burst pattern seen with thiopental, except that intervals between high-amplitude slow waves (i.e., burst suppression) were seen with etomidate in a dose of only 1 mg/kg in an elderly patient population.[239] Furthermore, aside from a significant decrease in dosage required to reach the stage 3 end point, the initial volume of distribution and the renal clearance of etomidate were significantly reduced in elderly patients; EEG monitoring to titrate etomidate infusions for anesthesia to the clinical response end point is very important, especially with increasing age of the patient. The average plasma concentration of etomidate averaged 310 nmol/L at therapeutic effect (0.3 to 1.0 μg/ml in other studies), or 1.22 μg/ml at a 30 μg/kg/min infusion rate.

Etomidate's effects on cerebral activity can be described in six progressive levels.[53] Level 1 changes possess constant voltage, without partial or total suppression. Level 2 changes have less than one second total/subtotal suppression, separated by 100 to 300 μV bursts of activity. Level 3 has a duration of 1 to 3 seconds, with total (occasionally subtotal) suppression, separated by 100 to 300 μV bursts. Level 4 has total suppression for longer than 3 seconds, separated by bursts of 50 to 100 μV. Level 5 has a longer than 3-second total suppression, with brief bursts less than 50 μV. At level 6, no activity is seen, even with sensitive monitoring.[14]

Using 14 patients with supratentorial tumors, Cold et al.[53] in 1986 measured cerebral blood flow and the CMRO$_2$ with simultaneous serum samples, brain biopsy, and EEG monitoring. The results showed that increasing serum levels correlated with increasing brain levels. High serum etomidate has been associated with suppressed median EEG activity and a decrease in CMRO$_2$. EEG was felt to be only a rough estimate of actual CMRO$_2$, with a wide range of CMRO$_2$ values possible at therapeutic plasma and/or EEG readings. Meinck et al.[175] and Schwilden et al.[240] have concluded that the median EEG was more sensitive than the EEG spectral edge in indicating clinical anesthesia and coma. A blood etomidate concentration of 0.05 μg/ml yielded a median frequency below 5 Hz, well within the desired range of this group's study.[239] A maintenance dose of 0.88 mg/min and a loading dose of 82 mg were calculated, and correlated with their earlier reports showing that a maintenance dose of 0.8 mg/min and a loading dose of 80 mg provided a safe hypnotic effect.

Etomidate infusion has been associated with myoclonus.[14,62,291] Many studies have used muscle relaxants (e.g., pancuronium) to suppress this effect.[14,53,174,188] Studies on cats indicate that etomidate has a disinhibitory effect at the spinal level.[25]

Etomidate infusion with hydrocortisone replacement has also been successfully used to treat refractory status epilepticus when administered at a rate of 20 μg/kg/min, with maintenance to 5 μV on the EEG, absence of burst suppression, and no seizure activity. Hypotension was readily corrected with fluid replacement.[306] Interestingly, clinical seizure activity did not always correlate with activity documented by EEG. This study emphasized the importance of continuous EEG monitoring. With concurrent corticosteroid administration, no increased mortality was reported and all patients recovered.

The major detrimental side effect of etomidate is related to its vasoconstrictive properties (both cerebral and systemic); this may be alleviated by administration of the agent in combination with a vasodilator. However, this vasoconstrictive property may be potentially beneficial in the management of intracranial hypertension and may aid in the redistribution of blood flow to relatively ischemic regions. Experimental data are forthcoming. Currently we are using etomidate infusions during complex skull base surgery and during surgery for intracranial aneurysms in which the possibility of temporary clipping is entertained.

Midazolam

Midazolam is a short-acting benzodiazepine, which has recently gained favor among anesthesiologists as an induction agent.[238] It has been shown to reduce CMRO$_2$ by 55 percent, with a corresponding reduction in CBF of 40 to 45 percent.[121] As a potential protective agent, it has the additional advantage of being reversible by a specific antagonist, RO-15-1788. This antagonist has not been found to have adverse effects on CBF[88] or upon ICP in patients in whom ICP had previously been controlled.[50] At present further work is needed before using midazolam as a protective agent.

Free-Radical Scavengers— Superoxide Dismutase

As the enzyme superoxide dismutase (SOD) is known to catalyze the degradation of the superoxide ($O_2^\cdot$) free radical, some investigators have examined its potential to reduce neuronal injury. In a study of cardiac arrest with reperfusion, intra-arterial SOD was demonstrated to reduce postischemic CBF changes,[48] possibly through inactivation of endothelium-derived relaxing factor.[309] In a rat model of fluid percussion brain injury, SOD improved outcome.[158] Another possible mechanism of cerebral protection is the reduction of cerebral edema, as illustrated in a cold lesion model in cats.[49] One obstacle still to be overcome, however, is the lack of an effective vehicle for intravenous administration.[114]

Iron Chelators

Another mechanism by which the action of free radicals may be attenuated is by administration of deferoxamine. Ferrous ion, released from mitochondrial cytochromes and iron-containing enzymes during ischemia, chelates with ADP following reperfusion; the active complex thereby formed has been postulated to catalyze free-radical formation and thus to contribute to lipid peroxidation.[23] Deferoxamine has been shown to improve outcome in rats following cardiac arrest,[147] although a canine study did not corroborate these findings.[87] Thus, more studies need to be completed before clinical trials may be undertaken.

Reduction of Excitotoxic Injury—N-Methyl-ᴅ-Aspartate Receptor Antagonists

Several studies in animals have examined the efficacy of NMDA receptor antagonists in the attenuation of ischemic injury. Thus, 2-amino-7-phosphonoheptanoic acid (AP-7) was demonstrated to have protective effects in a rat model of global ischemia[248] and in carotid occlusion.[38] Other NMDA antagonists such as MK-801[97] and 3,3 (2-carboxypiperazin-4-yl)propyl-1-phosphonic acid[272] have also proved ef-

fective in animal models. Recently, CPP, a new NMDA receptor antagonist, has been shown to be highly potent in binding to receptor sites and may also prove useful in animal studies.[59] Hopefully, the near future will yield encouraging results with these or similar agents in human studies of cerebral ischemia.

Membrane Stabilization—GM₁ Ganglioside

GM_1 ganglioside, a glycosphingolipid, is a ubiquitous molecule, which is frequently a cell membrane receptor constituent. It has been demonstrated in vitro to enhance outgrowth of dendrites and improve survival and maintenance of neurons.[155] In an animal model of MCA occlusion, GM_1 ganglioside was shown to improve outcome and resulted in improvement of EEG in the recovery period.[146] Its mode of action presumably involves reduction of membrane-bound ATPases[135] or reduction of $CMRO_2$,[277] but definitive data regarding these mechanisms are lacking. Preliminary results in humans have unfortunately not shown a benefit in acute stroke.[120]

Improvement in Oxygen-Carrying Capacity—Perfluorocarbons

Perfluorocarbons have a high affinity for oxygen and a low viscosity. For the latter reason initial efforts have been directed toward their use in cerebral vasospasm. In acute stroke improved outcome has been noted with the use of Fluosol-DA.[212] The use of these agents has also been investigated via CSF injection[208] in cases in which rCBF is insufficient. Protection from air embolism has also been demonstrated with perfluorocarbons.[255] The primary limitation of perfluorocarbons is the theoretical possibility that free radicals may be generated as a result of increased oxygen delivery.

Opiate Antagonists

Since the discovery of the first pentapeptide enkephalins in 1975, much research has been directed toward uncovering the possible physiologic roles of endogenous opioid peptides. Often the potential functions of endogenous opioid peptides have been inferred from studies examining the effects of selective opiate receptor antagonists. Based upon these studies, opiate antagonists have been suggested as potential agents in the treatment of central nervous system trauma and ischemia. There are four distinct groups of opiate receptors, each of which is specific for a group of endogenous opioid peptides; these are the mu, delta, kappa, and epsilon receptors.

The pathophysiology of traumatic and ischemic injuries has led many investigators to evaluate the use of opiate antagonists in this type of injury. It is known that the similarity between traumatic and ischemic injury lies in the reversible secondary decrease in blood flow to the involved region. Ischemia leads to a loss of autoregulation, and thus perfusion becomes dependent on systemic blood pressure. Endorphins released following injury result in hypotension and thereby diminish perfusion to areas with alterations in autoregulation, which leads to exacerbation of the secondary injury. The nonselective opiate antagonist naloxone has been reported to increase cardiovascular function and survival following shock. These effects are dose-related, with dosages greater than 1 mg/kg required. Naloxone works at the mu receptor in low dosages and at the kappa and delta receptors in higher doses.

The use of opiate antagonists for cerebral protection is based upon earlier results supporting their use in the treatment of spinal cord injury. The nonselective opiate antagonist naloxone was documented by Faden et al.[74,75] to increase posttraumatic hypotension, spinal cord blood flow, and neurologic recovery following compression injury in an animal model. Faden et al.[73,76] also showed that thyrotropin-releasing hormone (TRH) was effective in increasing neurologic recovery following compression injury in an animal model. He concluded that TRH may act in vivo as a partial physiologic opiate antagonist that spares analgesic systems. Other investigators have been unable to replicate these findings using varied animal models of spinal cord injury.[106,288,289] More recently (1985), Faden and Jacobs's[72] more specific investigations into kappa receptor antagonists has suggested their potential efficacy in spinal cord injury. Kappa-specific antagonists are more effective in the treatment of shock than mu- or delta-specific antagonists. In addition, kappa-selective agonists lead to hypotension and impair cardiovascular function following injection into the anterolateral hypothalamus.

Faden et al.[73] confirmed the therapeutic benefit of naloxone in improving cortical SSEPs and local cerebral perfusion following an air embolization model of experimental stroke in dogs. Baskin and Hosobuchi[29] reported in 1991 that the levorotatory form of the selective kappa antagonist WIN 44,441-3 acutely improved neurologic function following MCA occlusion. Ogawa et al.[205] also documented increased survival in an animal model of stroke following administration of naloxone and coenzyme Q. Further

results should not only explain the pathogenicity of endogenous opioid peptides in ischemic injury but should also define the role of opiate antagonists as cerebral protectants.

Structural Intervention

Use of Bypass Grafts

In planned occlusion or resection of portions of the intracranial vasculature, bypass grafts have been used to replace the sacrificed segment. Before undertaking such a technically difficult procedure, the necessity for such a graft may be determined by a carotid balloon occlusion test which may yield changes in the clinical examination or in parameters of rCBF as determined by xenon CT. Thus, one may preoperatively evaluate the risk of resecting a major vessel.

If the need to sacrifice a vessel is determined, one may choose three routes: superficial temporal artery (STA)-MCA bypass, EC-IC saphenous vein graft,[262] or petrous-supraclinoid saphenous vein graft.[254] The advantage of the saphenous vein graft procedures is that they provide significantly more flow than the STA-MCA bypass. The petrous-supraclinoid bypass has the additional advantage that torquing of the shunt with head movements is avoided. To avoid ischemic complications from the extended length of the procedure, use of a temporary intraluminal shunt was reported by Hori et al.[124] in 1991.

Techniques of Brain Retraction

Studies in animals have demonstrated that the histologic changes in cortex are observed in normotensive animals after 1 hour of retraction at a retractor pressure of 20 mmHg.[7] During a long surgical procedure the surgeon's focus is upon the operative field, and the consideration of retractor pressure and perfusion of the retracted brain is often neglected. In fact, temporal lobe retraction during surgery for unruptured aneurysms has been correlated with an increased risk of postoperative seizures.[228] To minimize these sequelae, we recommend covering the cortex with Surgicel and then using cottonoid to interface between the Surgicel and the retractor blade, as recommended by Sundt et al.[265] This will provide stability to the retractor blade and reduce ischemic changes at the edges of the blade. Finally, whenever possible periodic loosening of the tension on self-retaining retractor arms will allow reperfusion of any ischemic cortex.

Management of Intraoperative Aneurysm Rupture

Mortality from intraoperative rupture of an intracranial aneurysm may be as high as 70 percent, especially if parent vessel occlusion occurs.[210] An approach to the management of this problem that is based on sound surgical principles and vascular physiological tenets should minimize morbidity and mortality.

A number of authors favor temporary clipping of the parent vessel and/or use of deep hypotension.[7,21,23,43,69,78,89,92,117,125,128,161,211,224,229,253,264,268–270,305] Pertuiset and coworkers[215] have recommended deep hypotension in conjunction with bipolar coagulation of the rent in the aneurysm. Fox,[89] on the other hand, has recommended simple tamponade by pressure of the suction against a cottonoid pad, on the aneurysm dome. For anything other than a very minor hemorrhage that stops rapidly with tamponade, we prefer to use temporary clips in an unhurried, preplanned, careful fashion after having dissected the parent vessels in such manner that temporary clips can be placed without harming small perforating arteries.

Are There Indications for Use of Hypotension?

The use of hypotension as an adjunct for either dissection of the aneurysm or management of the intraoperative rupture has been advocated by many as a means to reduce the incidence of premature rupture and to improve the outcome if a rupture does occur.[3,43,69,78,92,128,229,243] However, there are theoretical disadvantages to its use. Hypotension could exacerbate ischemia-related deficits in the acute aftermath of an SAH and thus would be expected to be associated with altered cerebrovascular reactivity and metabolic activity.[102,115,131,203,219,224,273,280]

Temporary Clipping of Parent Vessel

Symon and Vajda[276] have developed guidelines for the use of temporary vascular occlusion based upon threshold relationships between neuronal electrical function and rCBF. Clips with closing force no greater than 80 g are acceptable. Control of afferent and efferent circulation should be secured to avoid exsanguination of the collateral circulation and subsequent ischemia distal to the aneurysm. Repetitive short occlusions seem to provide no particular advantage over a single prolonged occlusion. Elevation of systemic pressure can improve collateral flow during occlusion and may provide a margin of safety.

We have been unable to ascribe specific neurological deficits to complications related to the use of temporary clips alone. The impact of temporary MCA occlusion in experimental conditions is known. Primates subjected to 2 hours of occlusion suffer minor deficits with small infarcts; 3 hours of occlusion produces variable effects; and 4 hours produces severe edema and death.[57,189,263]

To elucidate the appropriate steps in the management of intraoperative aneurysm rupture, we retrospectively analyzed 276 operative procedures for the management of 317 intracranial aneurysms. There were 36 cases of perioperative or intraoperative rupture. Three management modalities were evaluated, namely, use of tamponade as the primary hemostatic maneuver, use of temporary clips, and use of pharmacologically induced hypotension. There was no statistically significant difference in outcome between those cases in which tamponade was used to control hemorrhage and those in which temporary clipping was used. However, those patients in whom hypotension was used did less well than those in whom it was not used. Thus, we conclude that hypotension may not be a necessary adjunct in the management of intraoperative aneurysm rupture.

Extracorporeal Circulation and Oxygenation

Cardiac arrest is the classic clinical correlate of experimental global ischemia. No therapy has been identifiable to date that consistently reverses normothermic cardiac arrest of longer than 5 minutes with complete neurological recovery. The extension of CPR to CPCR (cardiopulmonary and cerebral resuscitation) commenced in the early 1970s with the realization of the need for cerebral-oriented cardiac resuscitation protocols.[234] External CPR produces marginal cerebral perfusion pressures at best, but if initiated immediately following cardiac arrest, it may maintain heart and cerebral viability for as long as 1 hour.[186] If it is started longer than 3 to 5 minutes after arrest, however, neurological recovery declines exponentially, presumably because of intravascular sludging of the bloodstream. In contrast, open chest CPR and cardiopulmonary bypass provide remarkably improved perfusion pressures. Emergency cardiopulmonary bypass using a membrane oxygenator, heparin infusion, hemodilution with colloid infusion to a hematocrit of 20 to 25 percent, and moderate hypertension produced improved cardiac resuscibility and increased the proportion of awake survivors in a recent protocol using primates.[225] This technique is within present technical feasibility for use in major emergency room or trauma centers; emergency vascular access and competent personnel would be the factors limiting rapid application of extracorporeal circulation in the emergency room. In addition to superior cerebral perfusion pressures, the use of bypass would preclude many of the limiting risks of other potential or concurrently used modalities (e.g., calcium channel blockers or hypothermia). In the neurosurgical operating theater, cardiopulmonary bypass prior to the onset of planned ischemia would allow administration of cardioplegic doses of barbiturates or hypothermia with impunity. At present this technique remains an exploitable resource whose full potential has yet to be realized.

Ancillary Aids

Intraoperative Angiography

Intraoperative angiography has been used in the recent past to determine the completeness of resection of arteriovenous malformations. Recently we have begun using this technology to assess the patency and extent of aneurysm clipping during surgery of giant aneurysms of the carotid and vertebral arteries. In several of our cases this has resulted in repositioning of aneurysm clips, which would have otherwise resulted in insufficient clipping, and in one case use of the technique has prevented clip-induced internal carotid artery occlusion.

Intraoperative Electrocardiography and Somatosensory Evoked Potentials

As noted previously, EEG and SSEPs provide excellent data regarding CBF. During aneurysm surgery we use SSEP monitoring during temporary clipping to provide an added measure of security.

POSTOPERATIVE MANAGEMENT

Revascularization

Angioplasty

Angioplasty has recently been used for treatment of vasospasm secondary to SAH with improvement in neurological symptoms.[118] It is conceivable that stenosis of a vessel anastomosis may be amenable to angioplastic techniques.

Emergency Bypass

Some have advocated emergency bypass surgery in the immediate postoperative period for acute occlusion of the internal carotid artery or MCA. A 1985 review article illustrated 27 cases of improvement among 65 such procedures performed.[66] Although the use of the procedure in this setting is controversial, further consideration and investigation must be undertaken before discounting this indication.

Decompressive Procedures

In the event that the patient sustains a massive hemispheric or cerebellar infarction with severe mass effect, one must consider a decompressive craniectomy.[231] It may still be possible to salvage some remaining neurons in spite of the risk of venous stasis and further ischemia due to incarceration of the involved cortex. If there is any remaining viable brain, the craniectomy may improve the perfusion pressure of the ischemic tissue. Before performing such a procedure, the surgeon must take into consideration the patient's age and hemispheric dominance, complicating illnesses, and the wishes of the family.

Phlebotomy

Rheologically, microcirculatory flow is enhanced with a moderate reduction of hematocrit (decreasing viscosity) to the range of 30 to 35 percent. This may be achieved by colloid/crystalloid infusion (hypervolemic hemodilution) or phlebotomy as necessary.

Antiplatelet/Anticoagulation

Along with disrupted vascular endothelium with ischemia, platelet activation is an additional result of elevated intracellular calcium, causing the liberation of thromboxanes and leukotrienes. The rationale for the use of antiplatelet and anticoagulant agents is that during ischemia the above factors enhance thrombogenesis and increase particulate flow. These agents have been used successfully in patients with known sources of emboli (e.g., carotid ulceration or cardiac sources) and intraoperatively during neurovascular surgery to prevent emboli and thrombosis. At present there have been insufficient studies to demonstrate efficacy for the routine use of antiplatelet agents in focal ischemia; it remains for future trials to determine the clinical circumstances in which they may be of benefit. Likewise the question of heparin use after ischemia is unresolved, as there have been no consistent results following its experimental use.[37,186] Similarly, in head trauma the use of anticoagulants or antiplatelet agents has yet to be defined, but it is likely that the increased risk of hemorrhagic complications in head-injured patients will preclude their use.

Thrombolysis

As the systemic administration of fibrinolytic agents is fraught with hemorrhagic complications, streptokinase has been administered intra-arterially to patients with acute basilar occlusion, with moderate success.[45] This may also provide a nonsurgical method of reestablishing patency of thrombosed bypass grafts. Tissue plasminogen activator catalyzes the conversion of plasminogen to plasmin and thus initiates the dissolution of fresh thrombus. It has previously been demonstrated to produce positive results when used following acute coronary thrombosis; experimental use in cerebral vasculature has yielded controversial results. A 1985 study revealed decreased neurological deficit in rabbits when tissue plasminogen activator was administered after experimental induction of cerebral emboli,[310] and this agent is said to lyse experimental emboli without the concordant risk of hemorrhagic complications. High expectations are held for its future use in the medical management of acute embolic or thrombotic stroke.

CONCLUSION

As more knowledge about the pathophysiological mechanisms of neuronal injury is acquired, more individualized methods of preventing neuronal injury will arise and replace the current standard treatments. They will likely take the form of multimodality regimens that are administered perioperatively. Table 28-1 is a summary of potential therapeutic modalities.

Table 28-1. Potential Therapeutic Modalities

Decrease metabolic demand
  Hypothermia
  Barbiturates
  Anesthetics
    Isoflurane
    Etomidate
    Althesin
    Lidocaine
  Excitatory neurotransmitter antagonists
    2-amino-7 phosphoheptanoic acid
Increase supply
  Perfluorocarbons
Vascular factors
  Hypertension/hemodiluton
  Vasodilators
    Prostacylin (PGl_2)
    Indomethacin
    Eicosapentanoic acid
    Thromboxane (TXA_2)
  Cardiopulmonary bypass
  Rheological factors
    Heparin
    Mannitol
    Antiplatelet
    Tissue plasminogen activator
    Streptokinase/urokinase
  Surgical revascularization
    Carotid endarterectomy
    EC/IC bypass
    Omental transfer

Methods to inhibit ion flux
  Calcium
    Ca^{++} channel blockers
      Nimodipine
      Nicardipine
    Deferoxamoine
    Potassium
    Diphenylhydantoin
    Isoflurane
Membrane stabilization
  Corticosteroids
  Lidocaine
  Free radical scavengers
    Barbiturates
    Vitamin C
    Vitamin E
    Corticosteroids
Substrate manipulation
  Glucose
  Ketones
    1,3-Butanediol
    Gamma-hydroxybutyrate
Modalities of unknown mechanism
  Dimethyl sulfoxide

REFERENCES

1. Aaslid R, Huber P, Nornes H: A transcranial Doppler method in the evaluation of cerebrovascular spasm. Neuroradiology 28:11, 1986

2. Aberg E, Adielson G, Almqvist A et al: Multicenter trial of hemodilution in ischemic stroke—background and study protocol. Stroke 16:885, 1985

3. Aitken RR, Drake CG: A technique of anesthesia with induced hypotension for surgical correction of intracranial aneurysms. Clin Neurosurg 21:107, 1974

4. Aitkenhead A: Cerebral protection. Br J Hosp Med 35:290, 1986

5. Albin MS: Neuroanesthesia. p. 903. In Youmans JR (ed): Neurological Surgery. WB Saunders, Philadelphia, 1990

6. Albin MS, Bunegin L, Gelineau J: ICP and CBF reacting to isoflurane and nitrous oxide during normocarbia, hypocarbia, and intracranial hypertension. p. 719. In Miller JD, Teasdale GM, Rowan JO et al: (eds): Intracranial Pressure. Vol. 6. Springer-Verlag, Berlin, 1986

7. Albin MS, Bunegin L, Helsel P et al: Intracranial pressure and regional cerebral blood flow responses to experimental brain retraction pressure. p. 131. In Shulman K, Marmarou A, Miller JD et al. (eds): Intracranial Pressure. Vol. 4. Springer-Verlag, Heidelberg, 1980

8. Allen GS, Ahn HS, Preziosi TJ et al: Cerebral arterial spasm—a controlled trial of nimodipine in patients with subarachnoid hemorrhage. N Engl J Med 308:619, 1983

9. Allolco B, Stuttmann R, Fischer H et al: Long-term etomidate and adrenocortical suppression. Lancet 2:626, 1983

10. Altman DI, Young RS, Yagel SK: Effects of dexamethasone in hypoxic-ischemic brain injury in the neonatal rat. Biol Neonate 46:149, 1984

11. Ames A III, Wright RL, Kowada M et al: Cerebral ischemia. II. The no-reflow phenomenon. Am J Pathol 52:437, 1968

12. Anderson DK, Means ED, Waters TR et al: Microvascular perfusion and metabolism in injured spinal cord after methylprednisolone treatment. J Neurosurg 56:106, 1982

13. Anderson DK, Saunders RD, Demediuk P et al: Lipid hydrolysis and peroxidation in injured spinal cord: Partial protection with methylprednisolone or vitamin E and selenium. Cent Nerv Syst Trauma 2:257, 1985

14. Arden JR, Holley FO, Stanski DR: Increased sensitivity to etomidate in the elderly: Initial distribution versus altered brain response. Anesthesiology 65:19, 1986

15. Artru AA, Michenfelder JD: Cerebral protective metabolic, and vascular, and protective effects. Stroke 11:377, 1980

16. Artru AA, Michenfelder JD: Anoxic cerebral accumulation reduced by phenytoin: Mechanism of cerebral protection? Anesth Analg 60:41, 1981

17. Artru AA, Steen P, Michenfelder JD: Gamma-hydroxybutyrate: Cerebral metabolic, vascular and protective effects. J Neurochem 35:1114, 1980

18. Astrup J, Siesjo BK, Symon L: The state of "penumbra" in the ischemic brain: Viable and lethal thresholds in cerebral ischemia. Stroke 12:723, 1981

19. Astrup J, Siesjo BK, Symon L: Thresholds in cerebral ischemia: the ischemic penumbra, editorial. Stroke 12:723, 1981

20. Astrup J, Symon L, Branston NM et al: Cortical evoked potentials and extracellular K^+ and H^+ at critical levels of brain ischemia. Stroke 8:51, 1977

21. Ausman J, Diaz F: Comment. Neurosurgery 18:706, 1986

22. Awad I, Little JR, Lucas F et al: Modification of focal cerebral ischemia by prostacyclin and indomethacin. J Neurosurg 58:714, 1983

23. Babbs CF: Role of iron ions in the genesis of reperfusion injury following successful cardiopulmonary resuscitation: Preliminary data and a biochemical hypothesis. Ann Emerg Med 14:777, 1985

24. Bachet J, Guilmet D, Goudot B et al: Cold cerebroplegia. A new technique of cerebral protection during operations on the transverse aortic arch. J Thorac Cardiovasc Surg 102:85, 1991

25. Baiker-Heberlein M, Kenins P, Kikillus H et al: Investigations into the site of central nervous action of the short-acting hypnotic agent R-(+)-ethyl-1-(alpha-methyl-benzyl) imidazole-5-carboxylate (etomidate) in cats. Anaesthesia 28:78, 1979

26. Baethman A, Jansen M: Possible role of calcium entry blockers in brain protection. Eur Neurol 25 (suppl. 1):102, 1986

27. Baker AJ, Zornow MH, Grafe MR et al: Hypothermia prevents ischemia induced increases in hippocampal glycine concentrations in rabbits. Stroke 22:666, 1991

28. Baker CJ, Onesti ST, Barth KN et al: Hypothermic protection following middle cerebral artery occlusion in the rat. Surg Neurol 36:175, 1991

29. Baskin DS, Hosobuchi Y: Treatment of experimental stroke with the opiate antagonist WIN 44,441-3—effects on neurologic function, infarct size, and survival. NIDA Res Monogr 75:531, 1986

30. Bazan NG: Effects of ischemia and electroconvulsive shock on the free fatty acid pool in the brain. Biochim Biophys Acta 218:1, 1970

31. Becker DP, Gardner S: Intensive management of head injury, p. 1593. In Wilkins RH, Rengachary SS (eds): Neurosurgery. McGraw-Hill, New York, 1985

32. Berger L, Hakim AM: Calcium channel blockers correct acidosis in ischemic rat brain without altering cerebral blood flow. Stroke 19:1257, 1988

33. Bergvall U, Steiner L, Forster DMC: Early pattern of cerebral circulatory disturbances following subarachnoid haemorrhage. Neuroradiology 5:24, 1973

34. Bielenberg GW, Burniol M, Roesen R, Klaus W: Effects of nimodipine on infarct size and cerebral acidosis after middle cerebral artery occlusion in the rat. Stroke 21 (suppl. IV):90, 1990

35. Bigelow WG, Lindsay WK, Greenwood WF: Hypothermia: Its possible role in cardiac surgery: Investigation of factors governing survival in dogs at low temperatures. Ann Surg 132:531, 1950

36. Black KL, Hoff JT, Radin NS et al: Eicosapentaenoic acid: Effect on brain prostaglandins, cerebral blood flow and edema in ischemic gerbils. Stroke 15:65, 1984

37. Bleyaert A, Nemoto P: Effect of postcirculatory arrest life support on neurological recovery in monkeys. Crit Care Med 8:153, 1980

38. Boast CA, Gerhardt SC, Janak P: Systemic AP-7 reduces ischemic brain damage in gerbils. p. 249. In Hicks TP, Lodge D, McLennan H (eds): Excitatory Amino Acid Transmission. Alan R. Liss, New York, 1987

39. Boker D, Solymosi L, Wassman H: Immediate postangiographic intracarotid treatment of cerebral vasospasm after subarachnoid hemorrhage with nimodipine. Neurochirurgia (Stuttg) 28:118, 1985

40. Boulu RG, Gueniau C, Plotkine M et al: Recovery of global cerebral ischemia in rabbits: Influence of indomethacin. Eur Neurol 20:230, 1981

41. Boxer PA, Cordon JJ, Mann MD et al: Comparison of phenytoin with noncompetitive N-methyl-D-aspartate antagonists in a model of focal brain ischemia in rat. Stroke 21 (suppl. III):47, 1990

42. Bracken MB, Shepard MJ, Collins WF et al: A randomized, controlled trial of methylprednisolone or naloxone in the treatment of acute spinal-cord injury. Results of the Second National Acute Spinal-Cord Injury Study. N Engl J Med 322:1405, 1990

43. Brown AS, Horton JM: Elective hypotension with intracardiac pacemaking in the operative management of ruptured intracranial aneurysms. Acta Anaesthesiol Scand Suppl 23:665, 1966

44. Brown FD, Hanlon K, Mullen S: Treatment of aneurysmal hemiplegia with dopamine and mannitol. J Neurosurg 49:525, 1978

45. Bruckmann H, Ferbert H, Zeumer H: The acute basilar thrombosis. Angiological, clinical comparison, and therapeutic implications. Presented at 13th Symposium Neuroradiologicum, Stockholm, 1986

46. Buchan A, Pulsinelli WA: Hypothermia but not the N-methyl-D-aspartate antagonist, MK 801, attenuates neuronal damage in gerbils subjected to transient global ischemia. J Neurosci 10:311, 1990

47. Burke AM, Chien S, McMurtry JG III et al: Effects of low molecular weight dextran on blood viscosity after craniotomy for intracranial aneurysms. Surg Gynecol Obstet 148:9, 1979

48. Cerchiari EL, Hoel TM, Safar P, Sclabassi RJ: Protective effects of combined superoxide dismutase and deferoxamine on recovery of cerebral blood flow and function after cardiac arrest in dogs. Stroke 18:869, 1987

49. Chan PH, Longar S, Fishman RA: Protective effects of liposome-entrapped superoxide dismutase on post traumatic brain edema. Ann Neurol 21:450, 1987

50. Chiolero RL, Ravussin P, Anderes JP et al: The effects of midazolam reversal by RO 15-1788 on cerebral perfusion pressure in patients with severe head injury. Intensive Care Med 14:196, 1988

51. Christensen MS: Prolonged artificial hyperventilation in cerebral apoplexy. Acta Anaesthesiol Scand Suppl 62:7, 1976

52. Clifton GL, Taft WC, Blair RE et al: Conditions for pharmacologic evaluation in the gerbil model of forebrain ischemia. Stroke 20:1545, 1989

53. Cold GE, Eskeson V, Eriksen H et al: Changes in $CMRO_2$, EEG and concentration of etomidate in serum and brain tissue during craniotomy with continuous etomidate supplemented with N_2O and fentanyl. Acta Anaesthesiol Scand 30:159, 1986

54. Compton JS, Redmond S, Symon L: Cerebral blood velocity in subarachnoid hemorrhage. A transcranial Doppler study. J Neurol Neurosurg Psychiatry 50:1499, 1987

55. Corbett D, Evans S, Thomas C et al: MK 801 reduced cerebral ischemic injury by inducing hypothermia. Brain Res 514:300, 1990

56. Crittenden MD, Roberts CS, Rosa L et al: Brain protection during circulatory arrest. Ann Thorac Surg 51:942, 1991

57. Crowell RM, Olsson Y, Klatzo I, Ommaya A: Temporary occlusion of this middle cerebral artery in the monkey: Clinical and pathological observations. Stroke 1:439, 1970

58. Culp BR, Titus BG, Lands WEM: Inhibition of prostaglandin biosynthesis by eicosapentaenoic acid. Prostaglandins Med 3:269, 1979

59. Davies J, Evans RH, Herrling PL et al: CPP, a new potent and selective NMDA antagonist. Depression of central neuron responses, affinity for [3H]D-AP5 binding sites on brain membranes and anticonvulsant activity. Brain Res 382:169, 1986

60. Davis DH, Sundt TM Jr: Relationship of cerebral blood flow to cardiac output, mean arterial pressure, blood volume, and alpha and beta blockade in cats. J Neurosurg 52:745, 1980

61. Dearden NM, McDowall DG: Comparison of etomidate and Althesin in the reduction of increased intracranial pressure after head injury. Br J Anaesth 57:361, 1985

62. De Grood PM, Mitsukuri S, Van Egmond J et al: Comparison of etomidate and propofol for anaesthesia in microlaryngeal surgery. Anaesthesia 42:366, 1987

63. DeLeo J, Schubert P, Kreutzbrg GW: Protection against ischemic brain damage using propentofylline in gerbils. Stroke 19:1535, 1988

64. Denny-Brown D: Treatment of recurrent cardiovascular symptoms and the questions of vasospasm. Med Clin North Am 35:1457, 1951

65. DeSalles AAF, Muizelaar JP, Young HF: Hyperglycemia, cerebrospinal fluid lactic acidosis and cerebral blood flow in severely head-injured patients. Neurosurgery 21:45, 1987

66. Diaz FG, Ausman JI, Mehta B: Acute cerebral revascularization. J Neurosurg 63:200, 1985

67. Doenicke A, Loffler B, Kugler J et al: Plasma concentration and EEG after various regimens of etomidate. Br J Anesth 54:393, 1982

68. Doenicke A, Lorenz W, Beigl R et al: Histamine release after intravenous application of short-acting hypnotics: A comparison of etomidate, Althesin (CT 1341), and propanediol. Br J Anaesth 45:1097, 1973

69. Drake CG: Giant intracranial aneurysms: Experience with surgical treatment in 174 patients. Clin Neurosurg 26:12, 1979

70. Duhaime AC, Ross DT: Degeneration of hippocampal CA1 neurons following transient ischemia due to raised intracranial pressure: Evidence for a temperature dependent excitotoxic process. Brain Res 512:169, 1990

71. Ellis EF, Dodson LY, Police RJ: Restoration of cerebrovascular response to hyperventilation by the oxygen radical scavenger *N*-acetylcysteine following experimental traumatic brain injury. J Neurosurg 75:774, 1991

72. Faden AI, Jacobs TP: Effect of TRH analogs on neurologic recovery after experimental spinal trauma. Neurology 35:1331, 1985

73. Faden AI, Hallenbeck JM, Brown CQ: Treatment of experimental stroke: Comparison of naloxone and thyrotropin releasing hormone. Neurology 32:1083, 1982

74. Faden AI, Jacobs TP, Holaday JW: Comparisons of early and late naloxone treatment in experimental spinal injury. Neurology 32:677, 1982

75. Faden AI, Jacobs TP, Mougey E et al: Endorphins in experimental spinal-cord injury: Therapeutic effect of naloxone. Ann Neurol 10:326, 1981

76. Faden AI, Jacobs TP, Smith MT, Holaday JW: Comparison of thyrotropin releasing hormone, naloxone, and dexamethasone treatments in experimental spinal injury. Neurology 33:673, 1983

77. Farhat SM, Schneider RC: Observations on the effect of systemic blood pressure on intracranial circulation in patients with cerebrovascular insufficiency. J Neurosurg 27:441, 1967

78. Farrar JK, Gamache FW, Ferguson GG et al: Effects of profound hypotension on cerebral blood flow during surgery for intracranial aneurysms. J Neurosurg 55:857, 1981

79. Fellows W, Byrne AJ, Allison SP: Adrenocortical suppression with etomidate. Lancet 2:54, 1983

80. Fischer EG, Ames A III, Hedley-Whyte ET et al: Reassessment of cerebral capillary changes in acute global ischemia and their relationship to the "no-reflow phenomenon." Stroke 8:36, 1977

81. Fischer EG, Ames A III, Lorenzo AV: Cerebral blood flow immediately following brief circulatory stasis. Stroke 10:423, 1979

82. Fisher M, Giannotta SL, Meiselman HJ: Hemorheological alterations in patients with subarachnoid hemorrhage. Clinical Hemorheol 7:611, 1987

83. Fisher M, Levine PH, Cohen RA: A 21-aminosteroid reduces hydrogen peroxide generation by and production of chemiluminescence of stimulated human leukocytes. Stroke 21:1435, 1990

84. Flamm ES, Ransohoff J: Treatment of cerebral vasospasm by control of cyclic adenosine monophosphate. Surg Neurol 6:223, 1976

85. Fleischer AS, Raggio JF, Tindall GT: Aminophylline and isoproterenol in the treatment of cerebral vasospasm. Surg Neurol 8:117, 1977

86. Fleischer AS, Tindall GT: Cerebral vasospasm following aneurysm rupture: A protocol for therapy and prophylaxis. J Neurosurg 52:149, 1980

87. Fleischer J, Lanier W, Milde J et al: Failure of deferoxamine, an iron chelator, to improve neurological outcome following complete cerebral ischemia in dogs. Stroke 18:124, 1987

88. Forster A, Juge O, Louis M, Nahory A: Effects of a specific benzodiazepine antagonist (RO 15-1788) on cerebral blood flow. Anesth Analg 66:309, 1987

89. Fox JL: Intracranial Aneurysms. Vol. 1. Springer-Verlag, New York, 1983

90. Fujisawa A, Matsumoto M, Matsuyama T et al: The effect of the calcium antagonist nimodipine on the gerbil model of experimental cerebral ischemia. Stroke 17:748, 1986

91. Gardiner IM, De Belleroche J: Reversal of neurotoxin-induced ornithine decarboxylase activity in rat cerebral cortex by nimodipine. A potential neuroprotective mechanism. Stroke 21 (suppl. IV):93, 1990

92. Gardner WJ: The control of bleeding during operation by induced hypotension. JAMA 132:572, 1946

93. Gelmers HJ, Gorter K, deWeerdt CJ, Wiezer JH: A controlled trial of nimodipine in acute ischemic stroke. N Engl J Med 318:203, 1988

94. Gelmers HJ, Jennerici M: Effect of nimodipine on acute ischemic stroke. Pooled results from five randomized trials. Stroke 21 (suppl. IV):81, 1990

95. Giannotta SL, McGillicuddy JE, Kindt GW: Diagnosis and treatment of postoperative cerebral vasospasm. Surg Neurol 18:286, 1977

96. Giannotta SL, Weiss MH, Apuzzo MLJ, Martin E: High dose glucocorticoids in the management of severe head injury. Neurosurgery 15:97, 1984

97. Gill R, Foster AC, Woodruff GN: MK-1 is neuroprotective in gerbils during the post-ischemic period. Neuroscience 25:847, 1988

98. Gill R, Woodruff GN: The neuroprotective actions of kynurenic acid and MK 801 in gerbils are synergistic and not related to hypothermia. Eur J Pharmacol 176:143, 1990

99. Gordon E, Rossanda M: Further studies on cerebrospinal fluid acid-base status in patients with brain lesions. Acta Anaesthesiol Scand 14:97, 1970

100. Greeley WJ, Kern FH, Ungerleider RM et al: The effect of hypothermic cardiopulmonary bypass and total circulatory arrest on cerebral metabolism in neonates, infants, and children. J Thorac Cardiovasc Surg 101:783, 1991

101. Grotta JC, Pettigrew LC, Allen S et al: Baseline hemodynamic state and response to hemodilution in patients with acute cerebral edema. Stroke 16:790, 1985

102. Grubb RL Jr, Raichle ME, Eichling JO, Mokhtar HG: Effects of subarachnoid hemorrhage in cerebral blood volume, blood flow, and oxygen utilization in humans. J Neurosurg 46:446, 1977

103. Gueldry S, Rochette L, Bralet J: Comparison of the effects of valproate, ethosuximide, phenytoin, and pentobarbital on cerebral energy metabolism in the rat. Epilepsia 28:160, 1987

104. Hadley MS, Abramski JM, Spetzler RF et al: The efficacy of intravenous nimodipine in the treatment of focal cerebral ischemia in a primate model. Neurosurgery 25:63, 1989

105. Hagardine JR, Branston NM, Symon L: Central conduction time in primate brain ischemia—a study in baboons. Stroke 11:637, 1980

106. Haghighi SS, Chehrazi B: Effect of naloxone in experimental acute spinal cord injury. Neurosurgery 20:385, 1987

107. Hakim AM, Evans AC, Berger L et al: The effect of nimodipine on the evolution of human cerebral infarction studied by PET. J Cereb Blood Flow Metab 9:523, 1989

108. Hall ED, Pazara KE, Braughler JM: Effects of tirilazed mesylate on postischemic brain lipid peroxidation and recovery of extracellular calcium in gerbils. Stroke 22:361, 1991

109. Hall ED, Wolf DL, Braughler JM: Effects of a single large dose of methylprednisolone sodium succinate on experimental posttraumatic spinal cord injury. Dose-response and time action analysis. J Neurosurg 61:125, 1984

110. Hall ED, Yonkers PA: Attenuation of postischemic cerebral hypoperfusion by the 21-aminosteroid U74006F. Stroke 19:340, 1988

111. Hall R, Murdoch J: Brain protection: Physiological and pharmacological considerations. Part II: The pharmacology of brain protection. Can J Anaesth 37:762, 1990

112. Hara J, Nagasawa H, Kogure K: Nimodipine prevents postischemic brain damage in the early phase of focal cerebral ischemia. Stroke 21 (suppl. IV):102, 1990

113. Harders AG, Gilsbach JM: Time course of blood velocity changes related to vasospasm in the circle of Willis measured by transcranial Doppler ultrasound. J Neurosurg 66:718, 1987

114. Haun SE, Kirsch JR, Helfaer MA et al: Polyethylene glycol conjugated superoxide dismutase fails to augment brain superoxide dismutase activity in piglets. Stroke 22:655, 1991

115. Heilbrun MP, Olesen J, Lassen NA: Regional cerebral blood flow studies in subarachnoid hemorrhage. J Neurosurg 37:36, 1972

116. Heiss WD, Holthoff V, Pawlik G, Neveling M: Effect of nimodipine on regional cerebral glucose metabolism in patients with acute ischemic stroke as measured by positron emission tomography. J Cereb Blood Flow Metab 10:127, 1990

117. Heros RC, Nelson PB, Ojemann RG et al: Large and giant paraclinoid aneurysms: Surgical techniques, complications, and results. Neurosurgery 12:153, 1983

118. Higashida RT, Halbach VV, Cahan LC: Transluminal angioplasty of intracerebral vessels for treatment of intracranial arterial vasospasm. J Neurosurg 71:648, 1989

119. Hoff JT: (Editorial comment.) J Trauma 23:794, 1983

120. Hoffbrand BI, Bingley PJ, Oppenheimer SM, Sheldon CD: Trial of ganglioside GM1 in acute stroke. J Neurol Neurosurg Psychiatry 51:1213, 1988

121. Hoffman WE, Miletich DJ, Albrecht RF: The effects of midazolam on cerebral blood flow and oxygen consumption and its interaction with nitrous oxide. Anesth Analg 65:729, 1986

122. Hogan M, Ghedde A, Hakim AM: Nimodipine binding in focal cerebral ischemia. Stroke 21 (suppl. IV):78, 1990

123. Holthoff B, Beil C, Hartmann-Klosterkoetter U et al: Effect of nimodipine on glucose metabolism in the course of ischemic stroke. Stroke 21 (suppl. IV):95, 1990

124. Hori T, Ikawa E, Takenobu A et al: The use of an intraluminal shunt for bypass grafts of the cavernous internal carotid artery. J Neurosurg 75:661, 1991

125. Hosobuchi Y: Direct surgical treatment of giant intracranial aneurysms. J Neurosurg 51:743, 1979

126. Hossman KA, Kleihues P: Reversibility of ischemic brain damage. Arch Neurol 29:375, 1973

127. Hossmann KA, Lechtape-Gruter H, Hossmann V: The role of cerebral blood flow for the recovery of the brain after prolonged ischemia. Z Neurol 202:281, 1973

128. Hugosson R, Hogstrom S: Factors disposing to morbidity in surgery of intracranial aneurysms with special regard to deep controlled hypotension. J Neurosurg 38:561, 1973

129. Hunt WE, Hess RM: Surgical risk as related to time of intervention in the repair of intracranial aneurysms. J Neurosurg 28:14, 1968

130. Ikonomidou C, Mosinger JL, Olney JW: Hypothermia enhances protective effect of MK 801 against hypoxic/ischemic brain damage in infant rats. Brain Res 487:184, 1989

131. Ishii R: Regional cerebral blood flow in patients with ruptured intracranial aneurysms. J Neurosurg 50:587, 1979

132. Itoh T, Kawakami M, Yamaguchi Y et al: Effect of

allopurinol on ischemia and reperfusion-induced cerebral injury in spontaneously hypertensive rats. Stroke 17:1284, 1986

133. Jennet B, Teasdale G: Management of Head Injuries. FA Davis, Philadelphia, 1981, p. 255

134. Kalimo J, Rehncrona S, Soderfeldt B et al: Brain lactic acidosis and ischemic cell damage: 2. Histopathology. J Cereb Blood Flow Metab 1:313, 1981

135. Karpiak SE, Li YS, Mahadik SP: Gangliosides (GM1 and AGF2) reduce mortality due to ischemia: Protection of membrane function. Stroke 18:184, 1987

136. Kassell NF, Peerless SJ, Durward QJ et al: Treatment of ischemic deficits from vasospasm with intravascular volume expansion and induced arterial hypertension. Neurosurgery 11:337, 1982

137. Katz AM, Messineo FC: Lipid membrane interactions and the pathogenesis of ischemic damage in the myocardium. Circ Res 48:1, 1981

138. Kay B: A dose-response relationship for etomidate, with some observations on correlation. Br J Anaesth 48:213, 1976

139. Kazui T, Inoue N, Ito T et al: Clinical study on surgical treatment of aortic arch aneurysm using selective cerebral perfusion or hypothermic circulatory arrest. Nippon Kyobu Geka Gakkai Zasshi 37:44, 1989

140. Keller TS, McGillicuddy JE, LaBond VA et al: Volume expansion in focal cerebral ischemia: The effect of cardiac output on local cerebral blood flow. Clin Neurosurg 29:40, 1982

141. Kindt G, Youmans J, Albrand O: Factors influencing the autoregulation of the cerebral blood flow during hypo and hypertension. J Neurosurg 36:299, 1967

142. Kinuchi H, Imaizumi S, Yoshimoto T, Motomiya M: Phenytoin affects metabolism of free fatty acids and nucleotides in rat cerebral ischemia. Stroke 21:1326, 1990

143. Klatzo I: Neuropathological aspects of brain edema. J Neuropathol Exp Neurol 26:1, 1967

144. Klingelhofer J, Sander D, Holzgraefe M et al: Cerebral vasospasm evaluated by transcranial Doppler at different intracranial pressures. J Neurosurg 75:752, 1991

145. Kolde T, Weiloch J, Seisjo BK: Chronic dexamethasone pretreatment aggravates ischemic brain damage by inducing hyperglycemia. J Cereb Blood Flow Metab 5 (suppl. 1):S251, 1985

146. Komatsumoto S, Greenberg JH, Hickey WF, Reivich M: Effect of the ganglioside GM1 on neurologic function, electroencephalogram amplitude, and histology in chronic middle cerebral artery occlusion in cats. Stroke 19:1027, 1988

147. Kompala SD, Babbs CF, Blako KE: Effects of deferoxamine in late deaths following CPR in rats. Ann Emerg Med 15:405, 1986

148. Koos WT, Perneczy A, Auer LM et al: Nimodipine treatment of ischemic neurological deficits due to cerebral vasospasm after subarachnoid hemorrhage: Clinical results of a multicenter study. Neurochirurgia (Stuttg) 28:114, 1985

149. Kosnik EJ, Hunt WE: Postoperative hypertension in the management of patients with intracranial arterial aneurysms. J Neurosurg 45:148, 1976

150. Kudo T, Suzuki S, Iwabuchi T: Importance of monitoring the circulating blood volume in patients with cerebral vasospasm after subarachnoid hemorrhage. Neurosurgery 9:514, 1981

151. Kuroiwa T, Bonnekoh P, Hossmann KA: Therapeutic window of CA1 neuronal damage defined by an ultrashort-acting barbiturate after brain ischemia in gerbils. Stroke 21:1489, 1990

152. Kuyama H, Ladds A, Branston NM et al: An experimental study of acute subarachnoid haemorrhage in baboons: Changes in cerebral blood volume, blood flow, electrical activity and water content. J Neurol Neurosurg Psychiatry 47:354, 1984

153. Lazarewicz JW, Pluta R, Puka M, Salinska E: Diverse mechanisms of neuronal protection by nimodipine in experimental rabbit brain ischemia. Stroke 21 (suppl. IV):108, 1990

154. Lazarewicz JW, Pluta R, Salinska E, Puka M: Beneficial effect of nimodipine on metabolic and functional disturbances in rabbit hippocampus following complete cerebral ischemia. Stroke 20:70, 1989

155. Ledeen RW: Biology of gangliosides: Neuritogenic and neuronotrophic properties. J Neurosci Res 12:147, 1984

156. Ledingham IM, Watt I: Influence of sedation on mortality in critically ill multiple trauma patients. Lancet 1:1270, 1983

157. Lesiuk H, Sutherland G, Peeling J et al: Effect of U74006F on forebrain ischemia in rats. Stroke 22:896, 1991

158. Levasseur JE, Patterson JL, Ghatak NR et al: Combined effect of respirator-induced ventilation and superoxide dismutase in experimental brain injury. J Neurosurg 71:573, 1989

159. Levy ML, Giannotta SL: Cardiac performance indices during hypervolemic therapy for cerebral vasospasm. J Neurosurg 75:27, 1991

160. Ljunggren B, Norberg K, Siesjo BK: Influence of tissue acidosis upon restitution of brain energy metabolism following total ischemia. Brain Res 77:173, 1974

161. Ljunggren B, Saveland H, Brandt L et al: Temporary clipping during early operation for ruptured aneurysm. Preliminary report. Neurosurgery 12:525, 1983

162. Lundgren J, Smith ML, Siesjo BK: Influence of moderate hypothermia on ischemic brain damage incurred under hyperglycemic conditions. Exp Brain Res 84:91, 1991

163. Lundy EF, Klima LD, Huber TS et al: Elevated blood ketone and glucagon levels cannot account for 1,3-butanediol induced cerebral protection in the Levine rat. Stroke 18:217, 1987

164. Lundy EF, Luyckx BA, Combs DJ et al: Butanediol induced cerebral protection from ischemic-hypoxia in the instrumented Levine rat. Stroke 15:547, 1984

165. Lyden PD, Zivin JA, Kochar A, Mazzarella V: Effects of calcium channel blockers on neurologic out-

come after focal ischemia in rabbits. Stroke 19:1030, 1988

166. Mabe J, Nagai J, Takagi T et al: Effect of nimodipine on cerebral functional and metabolic recovery following ischemia in the rat brain. Stroke 17:501, 1986

167. Marmarou A, Anderson R, Ward JD et al: The traumatic coma data bank: monitoring of ICP. p. 549. In Hoff JT, Betz AL (eds): Intracranial pressure VII. Springer-Verlag, Berlin, 1989

168. Maroon JC, Nelson PB: Hypovolemia in patients with subarachnoid hemorrhage: Therapeutic implications. Neurosurgery 4:223, 1979

169. Marshall LF, Marshall SB: Medical management of intracranial pressure. p. 177. In Cooper PR (ed): Head Injury. 2nd Ed. Williams & Wilkins, Baltimore, 1987

170. Martinez-Vila VE, Guillen F, Villanueva JA, Matias GJ et al: Placebo-controlled trial of nimodipine in the treatment of acute ischemic cerebral infarction. Stroke 21:1023, 1990

171. Martz D, Rayos G, Schielke GP, Betz AL: Allopurinol and dimethylthiourea reduce brain infarction following middle cerebral artery occlusion in rats. Stroke 20:488, 1989

172. McGillicuddy J, Kindt G, Giannotta SL et al: Focal cerebral blood flow in cerebral vasospasm: The effect of intravascular volume expansion. Acta Neurol Scand Suppl 72:490, 1979

173. McKee JI, Finlay WEI: Cortisol replacement in severely stressed patients. Lancet 1:484, 1983

174. Mehta MP, Dillman JB, Sherman NM et al: Etomidate anaesthesia inhibits the cortical response to surgical stress. Acta Anaesthesiol Scand 29:486, 1985

175. Meinck HM, Moehlenhof O, Keller D: Neurophysiological effects of etomidate, a new short-acting hypnotic. Electroencephologr Clin Neurophysiol 50:512, 1980

176. Mettler CC: History of Medicine. Blackstrom, Philadelphia, 1947, p. 1215

177. Meyer CHA, Lowe D, Meyer M et al: Progressive change in cerebral blood flow during the first three weeks after subarachnoid hemorrhage. Neurosurgery 12:58, 1983

178. Meyer FB, Sundt TM, Yanagihara T et al: Focal cerebral ischemia: Pathophysiologic mechanisms and rationale for future avenues of treatment. Mayo Clin Proc 62:35, 1987

179. Michenfelder JD, Milde JH: The relationship among canine brain temperature, metabolism, and function during hypothermia. Anesthesiology 75:130, 1991

180. Michenfelder JD, Milde JH, Sundt TM: Cerebral protection with barbiturate anesthesia. Arch Neurol 33:345, 1976

181. Mickey B, Vorstrup S, Voldby B et al: Serial measurement of regional cerebral blood flow in patients with SAH using 133 Xe inhalation and emission computerized tomography. J Neurosurg 60:916, 1984

182. Milde LN, Milde JH: Preservation of cerebral metabolites by etomidate during incomplete cerebral ischemia in dogs. Anesthesiology 65:272, 1986

183. Mink RB, Dutka AJ, Hallenbeck JM: Allopurinol pretreatment improves evoked response recovery following global cerebral ischemia in dogs. Stroke 22:660, 1991

184. Mizrahi EM, Patel VM, Crawford ES et al: Hypothermic induced electrocerebral silence, prolonged circulatory arrest, and cerebral protection during cardiovascular surgery. Electroencephalogr Clin Neurophysiol 72:81, 1989

185. Mohler FS, Gordon CJ: Thermoregulatory responses of the rabbit to central neural injections of sulfolane. Neurotoxicology 10:53, 1989

186. Montgomery W, Donegan J, McIntyre K (eds): American Heart Association: Standards and Guidelines for Cardiopulmonary Resuscitation and Emergency Cardiac Care. JAMA 255:2905, 1986

187. Monyer H, Hartley DM, Choi DW: 21-Aminosteroids attenuate excitotoxic neuronal injury in cortical cell cultures. Neuron 5:121, 1990

188. Moore RA, Allen MC, Wood PJ et al: Peri-operative endocrine effects of etomidate. Anaesthesia 40:124, 1985

189. Morawetz RB, Jones TH, Ojemann RG et al: Regional cerebral blood flow during temporary middle cerebral artery occlusion in waking monkeys. Acta Neurol Scand Suppl 64:114, 1977

190. Morgan M, Lumley J, Whitwam JG: Respiratory effects of etomidate. Br J Anaesth 49:233, 1977

191. Moss E, Gibson JS, McDowall DG, Gibson RM: Intensive management of severe head injuries. Anesthesia 38:214, 1983

192. Mossakowski MG, Gadamski R: Nimodipine prevents delayed neuronal death of sector CA1 pyramidal cells in short-term forebrain ischemia in Mongolian gerbils. Stroke 21 (suppl. IV):120, 1990

193. Muizelaar JP, Becker DP: Induced hypertension for the treatment of cerebral ischemia after subarachnoid hemorrhage. Direct effect on cerebral blood flow. Surg Neurol 25:317, 1986

194. Muizelaar JP, Marmarou A, Ward JD et al: Adverse effects of prolonged hyperventilation in patients with severe head injury: A randomized clinical trial. J Neurosurg 75:731, 1991

195. Muizelaar JP, van der Poel HG, Li ZC et al: Pial arteriolar vessel diameter and CO_2 reactivity during prolonged hyperventilation in the rabbit. J Neurosurg 69:923, 1988

196. Myers RE: Anoxic brain pathology and blood glucose, abstracted. Neurology 26:345, 1976

197. Myers RE, Yamaguchi S: Effects of serum glucose concentration on brain response to circulatory arrest, abstracted. J Neuropathol Exp Neurol 35:301, 1976

198. Natale JA, D'Alecy LG: Protection from cerebral ischemia by brain cooling without reduced lactate accumulation in dogs. Stroke 20:770, 1989

199. Newberg LA, Michenfelder JD: Cerebral protection by isoflurane during hypoxemia or ischemia. Anesthesiology 59:29, 1983

200. Newberg LA, Milde L, Milde J: Preservation of cere-

bral metabolites by etomidate during incomplete cerebral ischemia in dogs. Anesthesiology 65:272, 1986

201. Newman S, Pugsley W, Klinger L et al: Neuropsychological consequences of circulatory arrest with hypothermia. A case report. J Clin Exp Neuropsychol 11:529, 1989

202. Nordstrom CH, Rehncrow S: Reduction of cerebral blood flow and oxygen consumption with a combination of barbiturate anesthesia and induced hypothermia in the rat. Acta Anaesthesiol Scand 22:7, 1978

203. Nornes H, Knutzen HB, Wikeby PL: Cerebral arterial blood flow and aneurysm surgery. Part 2: Induced hypotension and autoregulatory capacity. J Neurosurg 47:819, 1977

204. O'Connor JV, Wilding T, Farmer P et al: The protective effect of profound hypothermia on the canine central nervous system during one hour of circulatory arrest. Ann Thorac Surg 41:255, 1986

205. Ogawa N, Tsukamoto S, Hirose Y, Kuroda H: Survival effect of coenzyme Q10 and naloxone on experimental stroke in gerbils. Pharmacol Biochem Behav 24:315, 1986

206. Olson JJ, Friedman R, Orr K et al: Cerebral radioprotection by pentobarbital: Dose response characteristics and association with GABA agonist activity. J Neurosurg 72:749, 1990

207. Olsson Y, Crowell RM, Klatzo I: The blood-brain barrier to protein tracers in focal cerebral ischemia and infarction caused by occlusion of the middle cerebral artery. Acta Neuropathol (Berl) 18:89, 1971

208. Osterholm JL, Adelman JP, Triolo AJ et al: Severe cerebral ischemia treated by ventriculo-subarachnoid perfusion with an oxygenated fluorocarbon emulsion. Neurosurgery 13:381, 1983

209. Paci A, Ottaviano P, Trenta A et al: Nimodipine in acute ischemic stroke: A double-blind, controlled study. Acta Neurol Scand 80:282, 1989

210. Paul RL, Arnold JG Jr: Operative factors influencing mortality in intracranial aneurysm surgery: Analysis of 186 consecutive cases. J Neurosurg 32:289, 1970

211. Peerless SJ, Drake CG: Treatment of giant cerebral aneurysms of the anterior circulation. Neurosurg Rev 5:149, 1982

212. Peerless SJ, Ishikawa R, Hunter IG et al: Protective effect of Fluosol-DA in acute cerebral ischemia. Stroke 12:558, 1981

213. Pentoxyfylline Study Group: Pentoxifylline in acute ischemic stroke, abstracted. Stroke 18:298, 1987

214. Perkins WJ, Milde LN, Milde JH, Michenfelder JD: Pretreatment with U74006F improves neurologic outcome following complete cerebral ischemia in dogs. Stroke 22:902, 1991

215. Pertuiset B, van Effenterre R, Goutorbe J, Yoshimasu N: Management of aneurysmal rupture during surgery, using bipolar coagulation, deep hypotension, and the operating microscope. Acta Neurochir (Wien) 30:195, 1974

216. Petruk KC, West M, Mohr G et al: Nimodipine treatment in poor-grade patients. Results of a multicenter double-blind placebo-controlled study. J Neurosurg 68:505, 1988

217. Phillipon J, Grob R, Dagreou F et al: Prevention of vasospasm in subarachnoid haemorrhage. A controlled study with nimodipine. Acta Neurochir (Wien) 82:110, 1986

218. Pickard JD, Boisvert DPJ, Graham DI et al: Late effects of subarachnoid haemorrhage on the response of the primate cerebral circulation to drug-induced changes in arterial blood pressure. J Neurol Neurosurg Psychiatry 42:899, 1979

219. Pickard JD, Matheson M, Patterson J, Wyper D: Prediction of late ischemic complications after cerebral aneurysm surgery by the intraoperative measurement of cerebral blood flow. J Neurosurg 53:305, 1980

220. Pickerodt VWA, McDowall DG, Coroneos JJ, Keaney NP: Effect of Althesin on cerebral perfusion pressure, cerebral metabolism, and intracranial pressure in the anaesthetized baboon. Br J Anaesth 44:751, 1972

221. Pitts LH, Macpherson P, Wyper DJ et al: Cerebral blood flow, angiographic cerebral vasospasm and subarachnoid hemorrhage. Acta Neurol Scand Suppl 64:334, 1977

222. Pokrovskii AV, Ermoliuk RS, Kuntsevich GI et al: Evaluation of cerebral hemodynamics by transcranial Doppler ultrasonography in carotid endarterectomy. Khirurgiia (Mosk) 1:16, 1991

223. Popescu DT: Clinical study of Althesin and hypomidate. Acta Anaesthesiol Belg 27 (suppl.):196, 1976

224. Poppen JL: Aneurysm of the middle cerebral artery. p. 160. In Poppen JL: An Atlas of Neurosurgical Techniques. WB Saunders, Philadelphia, 1960

225. Pretto E, Safar P: Emergency cardiopulmonary bypass after 12½ minutes cardiac arrest improves recovery in dogs. Crit Care Med 14:432, 1986

226. Pritz MB: Treatment of cerebral vasospasm: Usefulness of Swan-Ganz catheter monitoring of volume expansion. Surg Neurol 21:239, 1984

227. Pritz MB, Giannotta SL, Kindt GW et al: Treatment of patients with neurological deficits associated with cerebral vasospasm by intravascular volume expansion. Neurosurgery 3:364, 1978

228. Rabinowicz AL, Ginsburg DL, DeGiorgio CM, Giannotta SL: Unruptured intracranial aneurysms: Seizures and antiepileptic drug treatment following surgery. J Neurosurg 75:371, 1991

229. Ransohoff J, Guy HH, Mazzia VDB, Battista A: Deliberate hypotension in surgery of cerebral aneurysms and correlative animal studies. N Y State J Med 69:913, 1969

230. Rehncrona S, Westerberg E, Akesson B et al: Brain cortical fatty acids and phospholipids during and following complete and severe incomplete ischemia. J Neurochem 38:84, 1982

231. Rengachary SS, Batnitzky S, Morantz RA et al: Hemicraniectomy for acute massive cerebral infarction. Neurosurgery 8:321, 1981

232. Rosenstein J, Suzuki M, Symon L et al: Clinical rise

of a portable bedside cerebral blood flow machine in the management of aneurysmal subarachnoid hemorrhage. Neurosurgery 15:519, 1984

233. Rosomoff HL: Hypothermia and cerebral vascular lesions II. Experimental middle cerebral artery interruption followed by induction of hypothermia. Arch Neurol 78:454, 1957

234. Safar P: Cerebral resuscitation after cardiac arrest: A review. Circulation 74 (suppl. IV):138, 1986

235. Salgado AV, Jones SC, Furlan AJ et al: Bimodal treatment with nimodipine and low molecular weight dextran for focal cerebral ischemia in the rat. Ann Neurol 26:5621, 1989

236. Sauter A, Rudin M: Calcium antagonists reduce the extent of infarction in rat middle cerebral artery occlusion model as determined by quantitative magnetic resonance imaging. Stroke 17:1228, 1986

237. Schlaepfer WW: Neurofilaments: Structure, metabolism and implication in disease. J Neuropathol Exp Neurol 11:117, 1987

238. Schulteam-Esch J, Kochs E: Midazolam and flumezenil in neuroanesthesia. Acta Anaesthesiol Scand Suppl 92:96, 1990

239. Schuttler J, Schwilden H, Stoeckel H: Infusion strategies to investigate the pharmacokinetics and pharmacodynamics of hypnotic drugs: Etomidate as an example. Eur J Anaesthesiol 2:133, 1983

240. Schwilden H, Schuttler J, Stoeckel H: Quantitation of the EEG and pharmacodynamic modelling of hypnotic drugs: Etomidate as an example. Eur J Anaesthesiol 2:121, 1983

241. Seiler RW, Grolimund P, Aaslid R: Cerebral vasospasm evaluated by transcranial ultrasound correlated with clinical grade and CT-visualized subarachnoid hemorrhage. J Neurosurg 64:594, 1986

242. Sekhar LN, Wechsler LR, Yonas H: Value of transcranial Doppler examination in the diagnosis of cerebral vasospasm after subarachnoid hemorrhage. Neurosurgery 22:813, 1988

243. Sellery GR, Aitken RR, Drake CG: Anaesthesia for intracranial aneurysms with hypotension and spontaneous respiration. Can Anaesth Soc J 20:468, 1973

244. Selman WR, Spetzler RF, Roessman UR et al: Barbiturate-induced coma therapy for focal cerebral ischemia. Effect after temporary and permanent occlusion. J Neurosurg 55:220, 1981

245. Shaknovich AR, Serbinenko FA, Razumovsky AE: Functional reactivity of cerebral blood flow in patients with cerebrovascular pathology. Acta Neurol Scand Suppl 64:258, 1977

246. Shapiro H: Intracranial hypertension: Therapeutic and anesthetic considerations. Anesthesiology 43:445, 1975

247. Siesjo BK: Cell damage in the brain: A speculative synthesis. J Cereb Blood Flow Metab 1:155, 1981

248. Simon RP, Swan JH, Griffiths T et al: Blockade of N-methyl-D-aspartate receptors may protect against ischemic damage in the brain. Science 226:850, 1984

249. Simpson ME: Pharmakokinetics of Althesin: Comparison with lignocaine. Br J Anaesth 50:1231, 1978

250. Skunhojie E, Hoeot-Rasmussen K, Paulsen D et al: Regional cerebral blood flow and its autoregulation in patients with transient focal cerebral ischemic attacks. Neurology 20:465, 1970

251. Smith AL, Marque JJ: Anesthetics and cerebral edema. Anesthesiology 45:64, 1976

252. Solomon RA, Post KD, McMurtry JG III: Depression of circulating blood volume in patients after subarachnoid hemorrhage: Implications for the management of symptomatic vasospasm. Neurosurgery 15:354, 1984

253. Sonntag VKH, Yuan RH, Stein BM: Giant intracranial aneurysms: A review of 13 cases. Surg Neurol 8:81, 1977

254. Spetzler RF, Fukushima T, Martin N, Zabramski JM: Petrous carotid to intradural carotid saphenous vein graft for intracavernous giant aneurysm, tumor, and occlusive cerebrovascular disease. J Neurosurg 73:496, 1990

255. Spiess BD, Braverman B, Woronowicz AW, Ivankovich AD: Protection from cerebral air emboli with perfluorocarbons in rabbits. Stroke 17:1146, 1986

256. Steen PA, Grisvold SE, Milde JH et al: Nimodipine improves outcome when given after complete cerebral ischemia in primates. Anesthesiology 62:406, 1985

257. Steen PA, Michenfelder JD: Cerebral protection with barbiturates. Relation to anesthetic effect. Stroke 9:140, 1978

258. Steen PA, Newberg LA, Milde JH et al: Cerebral blood flow and neurological outcome when nimodipine is given after complete cerebral ischemia in the dog. J Cereb Blood Flow Metab 4:82, 1984

259. Steiger HJ, Schaeffler L, Boll J, Liechti S: Results of microsurgical carotid endarterectomy. A prospective study with transcranial Doppler and EEG monitoring, and elective surgery. Acta Neurochir (Wien) 100:31, 1989

260. Stoelting RK: Allergic reactions during anesthesia. Anesth Analg 62:341, 1983

261. Sundt TM Jr: Management of ischemic complications after subarachnoid hemorrhage. J Neurosurg 43:418, 1975

262. Sundt TM Jr: Surgical Techniques for Saccular and Giant Intracranial Aneurysms. Williams & Wilkins, Baltimore, 1990

263. Sundt TM Jr, Michenfelder JD: Focal transient cerebral ischemia in the squirrel monkey: Effect on brain adenosine triphosphate and lactate levels with electrocorticographic and pathologic correlation. Circ Res 30:703, 1972

264. Sundt TM Jr, Piepgras DG: Surgical approach to giant intracranial aneurysms. Operative experience with 80 cases. J Neurosurg 51:731, 1979

265. Sundt TM Jr, Sharbrough FW, Anderson RE et al: Cerebral blood flow measurements and electroencephalograms during carotid endarterectomy. J Neurosurg 41:310, 1974

266. Sundt TM Jr, Szurszewski J, Sharbrough FW: Physiological considerations important for the management of vasospasm. Surg Neurol 7:259, 1977

267. Sutherland G, Lesiuk H, Bose R, Sima AA: Effect of mannitol, nimodipine, and indomethacin singly or in combination on cerebral ischemia in rats. Stroke 19:571, 1988

268. Suzuki J, Kwak R, Okudairo Y: The safe time limit of temporary clamping of cerebral arteries in the direct surgical treatment of intracranial aneurysm under moderate hypothermia. Tohoku J Exp Med 127:1, 1979

269. Suzuki J, Yoshimoto T: The effect of mannitol in prolongation of permissible occlusion time of cerebral artery—clinical data of aneurysm surgery. Neurosurg Rev 1:13, 1979

270. Suzuki J, Yoshimoto T, Kayama T: Surgical treatment of middle cerebral artery aneurysms. J Neurosurg 61:17, 1984

271. Swain JA, McDonald TJ Jr, Griffith PK et al: Low flow hypothermic cardiopulmonary bypass protects the brain. J Thorac Cardiovasc Surg 102:76, 1991

272. Swan JH, Evans MC, Meldrum BS: Long-term development of selective neuronal loss and the mechanism of protection by 2-amino-7-phosphoheptanoate in a rat model. J Cereb Blood Flow Metab 8:64, 1988

273. Symon L: Disordered cerebro-vascular physiology in aneurysmal subarachnoid haemorrhage. Acta Neurochir (Wien) 41:7, 1978

274. Symon L, Branston NM, Strong AJ et al: Autoregulation in acute focal ischemia. An experimental study. Stroke 7:547, 1976

275. Symon L, Pasztor E, Dorsch NWC: Physiological responses of local areas of the cerebral circulation in experimental primates determined by the method of hydrogen clearance. Stroke 4:632, 1973

276. Symon L, Vajda J: Management of giant intracranial aneurysms. Clin Neurosurg 36:21, 1989

277. Tanaka K, Dora E, Urbanics R et al: Effect of the ganglioside GM1 on cerebral metabolism, microcirculation, recovery kinetics of ECoG and histology, during the recovery period following focal ischemia in cats. Stroke 17:1170, 1986

278. Tateishi A, Fleischer JE, Drummond JC et al: Nimodipine does not improve neurologic outcome after 14 minutes of cardiac arrest in cats. Stroke 20:1044, 1989

279. Teasdale G, Mendelow AD, Graham DI et al: Efficacy of nimodipine in cerebral ischemia or hemorrhage. Stroke 21 (suppl. IV):123, 1990

280. Tempelhoff R, Modica PA, Rich KM, Grubb RL: Use of computerized electroencephalographic monitoring during aneurysm surgery. J Neurosurg 71:24, 1989

281. Thomas AN, Anderton JM, Harper NJ: Anaesthesia for the treatment of a giant cerebral aneurysm under hypothermic circulatory arrest. Anaesthesia 45:383, 1990

282. Trust Study Group: Randomised, double blind, placebo-controlled trial of nimodipine in acute stroke. Lancet 336:1025, 1990

283. Tu YK, Heros RC, Karacostas O et al: Isovolemic hemodilution in experimental focal cerebral ischemia. Part 1: Effects on hemodynamics, hemorheology, and intracranial pressure. J Neurosurg 69:72, 1988

284. Tu YK, Heros RC, Karacostas O et al: Isovolemic hemodilution in experimental focal cerebral ischemia. Part 2: Effects on regional cerebral blood flow and size of infarction. J Neurosurg 69:82, 1988

285. Uematsu D, Greenberg JH, Hickey WF, Reivich M: Nimodipine attenuates both increase in cytosolic free calcium and histologic damage following focal cerebral ischemia and reperfusion in cats. Stroke 20:1531, 1989

286. Van Aken J, Rolly G: Influence of etomidate, a new short-acting anaesthetic agent, on cerebral blood flow in man. Acta Anaesthesiol Belg 27 (suppl.):175, 1976

287. Vibulsresth S, Dietrich WD, Busto R, Ginsberg MD: Failure of nimodipine to prevent ischemic neuronal damage in rats. Stroke 18:210, 1987

288. Wallace MC, Tator CH: Failure of naloxone to improve spinal cord blood flow and cardiac output after spinal cord injury. Neurosurgery 18:428, 1986

289. Wallace MC, Tator CH: Failure of blood transfusion or naloxone to improve clinical recovery after experimental spinal cord injury. Neurosurgery 19:489, 1986

290. Waltz A: Effect of blood pressure on blood flow in ischemic and non-ischemic cerebral cortex. The phenomena of autoregulation and luxury perfusion. Neurology 18:613, 1968

291. Wanscher M, Tonnesen E, Huttel M, Larsen K: Etomidate infusion and adrenocortical function. A study in elective surgery. Acta Anaesthesiol Scand 29:483, 1985

292. Ward JD, Becker DP, Miller JD et al: Failure of prophylactic barbiturate coma in the treatment of severe head injury. J Neurosurg 62:383, 1985

293. Warner DS, Zhou JG, Ramani R, Todd MM: Reversible focal ischemia in the rat: Effects of halothane, isoflurane, and methohexital anesthesia. J Cereb Blood Flow Metab 11:794, 1991

294. Watanabe T, Miura M, Orita H et al: Brain tissue pH, oxygen tension, and carbon dioxide tension in profoundly hypothermic cardiopulmonary bypass. Pulsatile assistance for circulatory arrest, low flow perfusion, and moderate flow perfusion. J Thorac Cardiovasc Surg 100:274, 1990

295. Watt I, Ledingham M: Mortality amongst multiple trauma patients admitted to an intensive therapy unit. Anaesthesia 39:973, 1984

296. Wauquier A: Brain protective properties of etomidate and flunurizine. J Cereb Blood Flow Metab 2 (suppl. 1):53, 1982

297. Wauquier A: A profile of etomidate. A hypnotic, anticonvulsant, and brain protective compound. Anesthesia 38 (suppl.):26, 1983

298. Wechsler LR, Ropper AH, Kistler JP: Transcranial Doppler in cerebrovascular disease. Stroke 17:905, 1986

299. Weiss MH: The current status of cerebral protection. Neurol Neurosurg Update Ser 6:2, 1985

300. Welsh FA, Harris VA: Postischemic hypothermia fails to reduce ischemic injury in gerbil hippocampus. J Cereb Blood Flow Metab 11:617, 1991

301. Welsh FA, Sims RE, Harris VA: Mild hypothermia prevents ischemic injury in gerbil hippocampus. J Cereb Blood Flow Metab 10:557, 1990

302. White BC, Winegar CD, Wilson RF, Krause GS: Calcium blockers in cerebral resuscitation. J Trauma 23:788, 1983

303. Wood JH, Simeone FA, Kron RE et al: Experimental hypervolemic hemodilution. Physiological correlations of cortical blood flow, cardiac output, and intracranial pressure with fresh blood viscosity and plasma volume. Neurosurgery 14:709, 1984

304. Wood JH, Snyder LL, Simeone FA: Failure of intravascular volume expansion without hemodilution to elevate cortical blood flow in region of experimental focal ischemia. J Neurosurg 56:80, 1982

305. Yasargil MG: Special operative problems. p. 269. In Yasargil MG (ed): Microneurosurgery. Vol. 1. Thieme, Stuttgart, 1984

306. Yeoman P, Hutchinson A, Byrne A et al: Etomidate infusions for the control of refractory status epilepticus. Intensive Care Med 15:255, 1989

307. Young W, Flamm ES: Effect of high-dose corticosteroid therapy on blood flow, evoked potentials, and extracellular calcium in experimental spinal injury. J Neurosurg 57:667, 1982

308. Young W, Wojak JC, DeCrescito V: 21-Aminosteroid reduces ion shifts and edema in the rat middle cerebral artery occlusion model of regional ischemia. Stroke 19:1013, 1988

309. Zhang XM, Ellis EF: Superoxide dismutase decreases mortality, blood pressure, and cerebral blood flow responses induced by acute hypertension in rats. Stroke 22:489, 1991

310. Zivin JA, Fisher ML: Tissue plasminogen activator reduces neurological damage after cerebral embolism. Science 230:1289, 1985

311. Zuccarello M, Anderson DK: Protective effect of a 21-aminosteroid on the blood-brain barrier following subarachnoid hemorrhage in rats. Stroke 20:367, 1989

29 Vascular Occlusive Diseases

Carotid Endarterectomy

James T. Robertson

The efficacy and appropriateness of carotid endarterectomy has been subject to severe criticism by neurologists and other physicians.[1,3,9,10,27,40–42] In 1984 carotid endarterectomy was the most common arterial vascular procedure. Approximately 107,000 operations were performed in 1985, but severe criticism reduced the number of cases to approximately 78,000 in 1989. Whisnant et al.[43] estimated that approximately 35,000 new patients each year with carotid transient ischemic attack (TIA) or recovered stroke with stenosis would be candidates for carotid endarterectomy. If this estimate was correct, the number of carotid endarterectomies each year far exceeded the indications for the procedure in symptomatic patients. Approximately half of the carotid endarterectomies were performed on asymptomatic patients.[3,16,19] In addition to the projected excess number of procedures, the critics afforded evidence that the surgical risk was too high to justify the procedure and that antiplatelet therapy probably had a better outcome than surgical treatment.[1,5,10,14,18,29,39,40] The American College of Physicians statement concerning the indications for carotid endarterectomy concluded that surgical mortality rates of less than 1 percent and stroke-related morbidity of less than 3 percent for patients with TIAs and stroke mortality plus stroke-related morbidity of less than 2 percent for patients with asymptomatic carotid artery disease were the values that must be matched to compete with available medical therapy.[29]

The numerous articles criticizing carotid endarterectomy have provoked a nihilistic attitude toward the surgical management of stroke prevention.[1,3,10,36] This is ironic, particularly since at the same time the National Institutes of Health have funded two large, multicenter, controlled clinical trials to determine the optimal medical versus surgical management of patients with TIAs and small strokes with carotid stenosis or ulceration and patients with asymptomatic carotid stenosis of 60 percent or more.[26,38] As a result, recruitment in these trials has been impaired. A recent consensus of a selected committee of neurologists, neurological surgeons, and vascular surgeons, recognizing the confusion and the nihilistic attitude concerning indications for carotid endarterectomy, recommended that the clinical trials be supported but in the interim, sustained the performance of carotid endarterectomy with low morbidity and mortality in selected patients with appropriate symptoms and a hemodynamic carotid lesion.[4] The limits were categorized by clinical presentation. The combined morbidity and mortality of the procedure should not exceed 3 percent for asymptomatic lesions, 5 percent for TIAs, 7 percent for ischemic stroke, and 10 percent for recurrent carotid stenosis. In addition, the 30-day mortality rate from all causes related to endarterectomy should not exceed 2 percent. Concomitantly, ongoing quality audits should be performed in institutions where endarterectomy is being performed to ensure surgical adherence to these current suggested figures. The committee exhorted until the results of the clinical trials are available that carotid endarterectomy continue to be an established operative procedure for the care of patients with carotid atherosclerotic disease.

An exciting scientific landmark was announced on February 21, 1991 at the International Stroke Conference of the American Heart Association in San Francisco by H. J. M. Barnett, the principal investigator of the North American Symptomatic Carotid Endarterectomy Trial.[6] The interim analysis of approximately 600 patients who had been randomly assigned to either medical or surgical therapy for TIA or mild, nondisabling stroke ipsilateral to a 70 to 90 percent narrowing of the internal carotid artery (ICA) were unequivocally shown to be treated best by surgical therapy. The interim analysis showed that among these symptomatic patients with high-grade carotid stenosis (70 to 99 percent), carotid endarterectomy did indeed reduce the overall risk of fatal and nonfatal ipsilateral carotid stroke, despite any perioperative risk of any type of stroke or of death from any cause. Including perioperative morbidity and mortality or its 32-day equivalent time in the medical group, over 24 percent of the medical group but only 7 percent of the surgical patients had experienced fatal or nonfatal ipsilateral carotid stroke at 18 months. This represents an absolute stroke risk reduction in favor of surgery of 17 percent. An exciting finding was that carotid endarterectomy was beneficial in the prevention of any stroke of any severity in any territory. Of great and supporting interest was the announcement by the British study group headed by Charles Wardlow of a clear benefit for carotid endarterectomy in the same group of patients. The answer is not available for the patients with 30 to 69 percent stenoses who present with ipsilateral TIAs or mild, nondisabling strokes. Further accrual and follow-up will be necessary to decide how best to treat these patients. However, the interim secondary analysis did show that degree of stenosis correlated extremely well with risk reduction after surgery in symptomatic patients. This interim analysis points out the major scientific advantage of a prospective randomized clinical study for obtaining a definitive uncontestable result. This was accomplished with slightly fewer than 600 patients properly allocated to medical versus surgical treatment.

The second study, the Asymptomatic Carotid Artery Study, directed by James F. Toole as principal investigator, now includes 34 centers that contribute patients.[38] All these patients have at least 60 percent blockage of the carotid artery by atherosclerosis but are asymptomatic regarding the ipsilateral artery at the time of randomization. Since many centers operate on asymptomatic high-grade carotid artery stenosis patients, hopefully this study will enjoy more rapid recruitment and completion of its target of 1,500 patients randomly allocated equally to medical and surgical therapy. Presently the study has enrolled 715 patients.

The combined morbidity and mortality resulting from endarterectomy in the United States has been estimated to be 10 percent per year.[1] A recent review of operations performed at large or academic institutions revealed a 2.2 percent stroke rate and a mortality rate of 1.4 percent, for a combined morbidity and mortality of 3.6 percent.[19] For asymptomatic patients, carotid endarterectomy is safer, carrying a combined morbidity and mortality of 2 percent or less.[38] There is little doubt that patient selection for endarterectomy plays an important role in surgical results. In this context Sundt et al.'s[34] grading of preoperative risk according to neurological, medical, and angiographic status serves as an excellent example of the importance of patient selection.[19] Clearly, the clinical presentation, the patient's comorbidity and native stroke risk, and the angiographic findings are critical in patient selection and resulting morbidity and mortality. In Sundt's experience, the neurologically stable patients without other risk in grade 1 had a combined morbidity and mortality of less than 1 percent, whereas, patients without associated medical or angiographically determined risk had a combined morbidity and mortality of 8.5 percent.

The clinical settings in which carotid endarterectomy is indicated are at least a 50 percent carotid stenosis or a large ulcerated plaque with ipsilateral TIAs, a reversible ischemic neurological deficit, a small stroke, or, in selected cases, recurrent symptomatic carotid stenosis.[4,15,19,24,25,27,28,30,32] Individual patients may require surgery for progressing stroke, progressive retinal ischemia, acute carotid occlusion, symptomatic carotid stump syndrome, global cerebral ischemia due to multiple large vessel occlusive disease, selected tandem lesions in which the proximal stenosis is greater than the distal, and, in certain cases, symptomatic carotid dissection and true or false aneurysm. The procedure is not indicated in patients presenting with vertebral basilar distribution TIAs, multi-infarct dementia, severe neurological deficits, evidence of intracranial hemorrhage, or large infarcts. Medical contraindications include congestive heart failure, a recent myocardial infarction, active angina, dementia, advanced malignancy, and uncertain diagnosis.[27,28,32]

PREOPERATIVE MANAGEMENT AND EVALUATION

The physician must take whatever measures are necessary to make sure that the carotid lesion is the cause of the patient's symptoms. The best surgical results are obtained in those patients operated on for true TIAs or amaurosis fugax. Since evidence from postmortem and stroke registries indicates that 15 to 25 percent of ischemic events can be attributed to a cardiac embolic or dysrhythmic source, cardiac evaluation is essential.[1] Patients with active angina pectoris, a myocardial infarction, or congestive failure should be treated medically if at all possible. Since postoperative myocardial infarction is a leading cause of death after carotid endarterectomy, patients must have adequate oxygenation and intravascular volume expansion before surgery. Immediate preoperative use of aspirin for platelet inhibition is recommended, even though, rarely, it will be necessary to administer platelet transfusion because of bleeding aggravated by aspirin therapy at surgery.[32] If the patient is having active TIAs, continuous intravenous heparin therapy, with the partial thromboplastin time kept at one and one-half times control, is recommended.[28] Platelet counts should be performed every third day, and if a thrombopenia occurs, heparin must be stopped to avoid a hypercoagulability syndrome. With short-term (less than 3-day) heparin therapy, this syndrome is rare.

Contraindications for heparin therapy must be followed. If the patient is severely hypertensive, every effort at control of the hypertension prior to surgery or heparin is mandated because of the increased risk of surgery in patients with uncontrolled blood pressures in excess of 180/110 mmHg. Severe chronic obstructive pulmonary disease may be a contraindication to surgery. Preoperative management of pulmonary toilet in an effort to improve function is recommended. Uncontrolled diabetes mellitus must be regulated. Attention should be given to indications of renal insufficiency. If the patient is anemic and surgery is felt to be urgent, after appropriate anemia studies the anemia should be corrected prior to induction of general anesthesia. Careful attention to patient medication is indicated to be certain that appropriate drugs are not discontinued inadvertently.

OPERATIVE PROCEDURE AND COMPLICATION AVOIDANCE

When the brain is presented with an ischemic insult, cerebrovascular reactivity or cerebral autoregulation is impaired or lost. Thus the perfusion pressure of the brain depends upon the systemic mean arterial pressure, and at the same time, because of the loss of autoregulation, the brain is extremely vulnerable to sudden changes in systemic arterial pressure. The anesthesiologist must be aware of this liability in patients presenting for operation with ischemia and choose either Ethrane or Forane for general anesthesia or regional local anesthesia.[7,17,32] The operating table should be horizontal without head elevation and the head should be turned partially to the opposite side with modest elevation of the ipsilateral shoulder. Gentle preparation of the operative site avoids the possibility of dislodging emboli from a fragile carotid plaque. A reverse S-shaped incision is preferred in order to minimize postoperative wound contracture with its associated discomfort and to afford wide exposure (Fig. 29-1). The incision characteristically begins at the level of the mastoid and extends anteriorly along the anteromedial border of the sternocleidomastoid muscle to about one to two fingerbreadths above the sternal notch in the midline. Sharp dissection is essential; use of a Shaw cutting cautery knife blade is preferred by many. After sectioning the platysma muscle vertically, the plane of dissection is anteromedial to the sternocleidomastoid muscle, beginning inferiorly and proceeding superiorly. In the upper midportion of the incision, the transverse cervical nerve, which is responsible for the skin innervation medial to the incision and along the lower jaw, is divided. The external jugular vein is lateral to this incision and is preserved. The approach to the carotid sheath begins inferiorly along the anterior medial border of the sternocleidomastoid muscle and proceeds superiorly. The carotid sheath is a fascial sheath formed by extensions of the deep cervical fascia and the prevertebral fascia. The sheath contains the carotid artery, the jugular vein, and the vagus nerve. Inferiorly, along the common carotid artery (CCA), the carotid sheath is very well deformed; the thickened sheath overlying the CCA is best opened vertically, and this excision is extended superiorly up to the carotid bifurcation. The sheath is less well defined superiorly because of vascular branches. The sheath is preserved and tacked up with small sutures attached to the platysma, which allows subsequent closure of the sheath and also tends to elevate the carotid artery. The CCA should be exposed inferiorly, if possible, to the point of a normal arterial wall. This may involve sectioning the omohyoid muscle. At the point at which dissection of the CCA begins, the patient is given intravenous heparin in a dose of 5,000 to 7,000 units. After 2 to 3 minutes, the patient is considered heparinized, and the vascular surgical procedure can proceed.

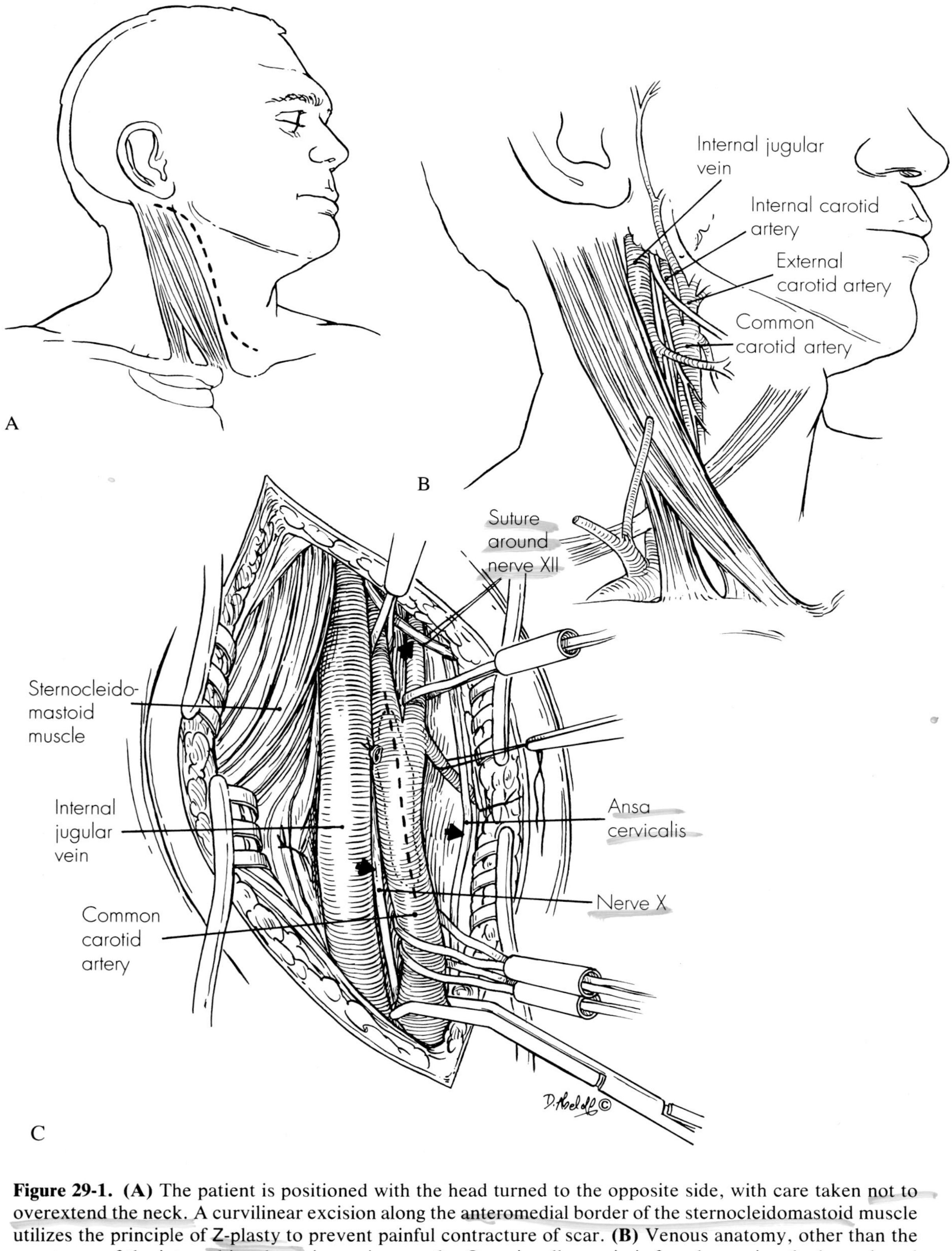

Figure 29-1. (A) The patient is positioned with the head turned to the opposite side, with care taken not to overextend the neck. A curvilinear excision along the anteromedial border of the sternocleidomastoid muscle utilizes the principle of Z-plasty to prevent painful contracture of scar. (B) Venous anatomy, other than the constancy of the internal jugular vein, varies greatly. Occasionally a vein is found covering the hypoglossal nerve, which may result in division of the nerve as the vein is being ligated and divided. Meticulous sharp

The major danger through this portion of the operation is embolization produced by excessive manipulation of the carotid bifurcation.[28,32] The surgeon must be intensely aware of the fragile nature of an atherosclerotic plaque, particularly if ulcerated and/or intraluminal clot. Intraoperative embolization is a major cause of minor or major stroke resulting from the operation. Meticulously the CCA, external carotid artery (ECA), and the ICA are exposed. The external jugular vein may require ligation superiorly as the posterosuperior lobe of the parotid gland is exposed. The common fascial vein enters the jugular vein usually at the level of the bifurcation of the CCA, and routinely requires ligation and division. There may be numerous other branches that must be ligated and divided in order to adequately expose the targeted artery. The available evidence strongly supports monitoring with electroencephalography (EEG) to determine intraoperative episodes of ischemia produced by emboli or shunt occlusion and the necessity of a shunt.[27,31,32] During operation if a major unexpected EEG change occurs, an embolus to the main trunk of the middle cerebral artery (MCA) must be suspected. If this is a minor embolic episode, the change will frequently reverse, but if major, it may persist. If it does, the routine recommended by Sundt includes ensuring that heparinization is present by augmenting the original heparin dose if necessary and immediately giving intravenously 3 mg/kg of thiopental or more if necessary to reach burst suppression of the EEG.[32] Subsequently, the endarterectomy should be completed as quickly as possible, and if the EEG change disappears or is minor subsequently, the patient is allowed to awaken from anesthesia. If not, arteriography on the table is recommended, and if an embolus is found in the MCA, either an MCA embolectomy or extracranial-intracranial (EC-IC) bypass surgery should be done. Another option, which has been used clinically but on which there is a paucity of clinical published results, is administration of intravenous thromboplastin activator or another more common fibrinolytic drug such as streptokinase or urokinase. Spetzler[30] has reported the use of thromboplastin activator to reopen an ICA occluded at the carotid bifurcation intracranially, with subsequent restoration of cerebral flow. This will require repeat arteriography. If these intra-arterial agents are used

to dissolve the embolic clot, the surgeon must be prepared to ensure hemostasis and prevent postoperative arterial bleeding.

If EEG monitoring is not performed, some surgeons routinely introduce an intra-arterial shunt[28,33] (Fig. 29-2), which may be a straight CCA to ICA shunt or else an externally looped shunt. Embolus as a result of shunt use may be produced by intimal injury to the proximal CCA or distal ICA or even dissection of the intima. The shunt may undergo occlusion during the procedure, or emboli may be introduced into the shunt at the time of placement. Sundt[32] emphasizes the unusual but recommended placement of the shunt first into the CCA artery, making certain that any embolic material has been irrigated from this artery, and then after being allowed to bleed slightly, into the ICA. Most surgeons place the shunt into the ICA first and subsequently into the CCA. The shunt should be presoaked in saline treated with heparin in a dose of 50 units/ml. In addition to preventing clotting, the wetting of the shunt prevents air bubbles from forming in the shunt at the time of placement.

At the time of the exposure of the CCA, two Rummel tourniquets are placed around the proximal CCA, and on exposure of the ECA, a Rummel tourniquet is placed around the proximal ECA; a vascular loop is placed around the distal ICA, and the superior thyroid artery is usually occluded by looping an 0-silk suture around it and applying modest tension with a hemostat. This minor tension on the superior thyroid artery and ECA tends to displace the bifurcation inferiorly and elevate the carotid artery from the wound. The ICA may be occluded with a Scoville aneurysm clip or with an 0-silk suture looped around the artery, with a 4-0 suture through the loop to allow the loop to be loosened. Some surgeons use a small elastic vascular loop around the vessel, which is tightened by placing a vascular clip to complete the loop. This is frequently done at the time a shunt is inserted and helps to secure the shunt distally. Whether or not a proximal vascular clamp or the two Rummel tourniquets are used on the CCA, every effort should be made to reach a position proximal to the carotid plaque so as to apply these constricting devices on normal artery. The techniques used to occlude the distal ICA and ECA also emphasize the need to get

dissection is essential to prevent dislodgement of plaque debris. **(C)** During dissection the lymph nodes should be dissected from medial to lateral, remembering that the lymph nodes go with the vein. The ansa cervicalis is usually divided after it is dissected from below up to the hypoglossal nerve to identify the hypoglossal nerve and to prevent sectioning an abnormally located vagus nerve. Arterial structures are isolated between Ramal tourniquets.

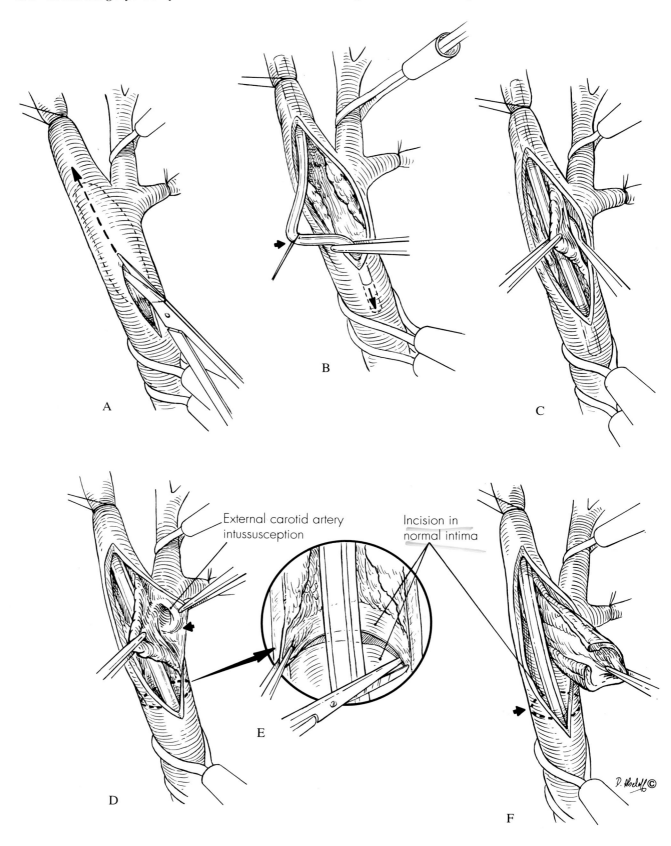

External carotid artery
intussusception

Incision in
normal intima

A

B

C

D

E

F

distal to the atherosclerotic plaque and to minimize damage to the intima. Sundt[32] is a strong advocate of the use of the soft shoe Fogarty occlusive vascular clamp on the CCA. All these efforts are designed not only to prevent damage of normal intima but to prevent fracturing of atherosclerotic plaque with subsequent stenosis or subintimal dissection and to avoid providing a site for thrombus formation with distal embolization postoperatively.

The arteriotomy begins in the proximal CCA and extends into the ICA. A No. 11 blade is used to open the CCA at the site below the plaque, and then Potts scissors are used to incise the artery through the plaque into normal distal ICA. Obviously, the occluding clamps and/or loops are tightened prior to the arteriotomy. Some surgeons insist on removing the plaque from the ICA distally as the initial step. Others will immediately place a shunt in the ICA and subsequently in the CCA or vice versa as described. Then the plaque is carefully dissected from the arterial wall with a blunt dissector (e.g., a Penfield No. 4), and once normal intima is reached in the CCA, the intima is sharply dissected so as to allow no loose flap. The plaque is peeled from below upward to the ECA, where it is carefully dissected from the ECA by intussusception. As this process proceeds up the ECA, it is wise to release the occluding Rummel tourniquet temporarily to allow the plaque to be carefully removed and to ascertain the backflow from the ECA. It is important to make certain that the ECA is left patent.[32]

Subsequently, the plaque is peeled out of the ICA; it usually will peel out quite smoothly distally (Fig. 29-3). If the distal plaque is removed prior to insertion of a shunt, less distal artery need be exposed. On the other hand, if normal intima was exposed distal to the plaque prior to insertion of the shunt, the plaque can quite easily be removed even with the shunt in place. If the plaque peels out easily and leaves a distal smooth surface, no tacking sutures are necessary. If the distal intima remains quite thickened and infiltrated with plaque, it is necessary to remove this to the point of normal intima. The technique of nicking the more available thickened intima with the Potts scissors and peeling out the distal thickened intima circumferentially is recommended.[32] If there is any question about the distal intima being loose, it should be tacked down with 6-0 double-arm Prolene sutures proceeding from within the artery to the outer wall, where the suture is tied. The suture should be placed vertically rather than horizontally to avoid constricting the lumen. During the dissection of the plaque, the endarterectomy bed is frequently irrigated with heparin-containing saline. This irrigation allows identification of loose pieces of debris and plaque, which must be meticulously removed from the endarterectomy site to prevent postoperative clotting. If a shunt has been used, it is helpful to place a 5-0 or 4-0 Prolene suture around the shunt to provide subsequent ease in removal of the shunt through the small remaining arteriotomy at the time of arterial closure (Fig. 29-3). Other surgeons, to minimize migration of the shunt, place 5-0 or 6-0 double-arm Prolene sutures around the shunt and through the arterial wall with a loose tie externally and remove this suture prior to shunt removal.

Once the vessel has been meticulously cleaned, primary closure or closure with a fabric or vein patch ensues. The available evidence in the literature supports the use of a patch over primary closure.[16,19,20,32] There are clearly fewer postoperative carotid occlusions or ischemic events with the use of a patch. In addition, the incidence of restenosis is minimized as compared with primary arterial closure.[8,11,19] Patching, whether fabric or vein is used, and meticulous placement of the suture to ensure a smooth patch or are essential. A 6-0 Prolene suture is recommended as a running suture. Primary closure of the artery should also be effected with 6-0 Prolene suture. Just prior to closure the shunt is removed, all vessels are allowed to flush, and subsequent primary closure is completed. Then the ECA and CCA are opened and subsequently the ICA is opened to minimize air or particulate embolization into the ICA system.

If a fabric patch has been used and properly preclotted, bleeding is easily controlled by application of

Figure 29-2. **(A)** The incision should be made proximal to the plaque in the common carotid artery and then sectioned from normal intima below to normal intima above. **(B)** After flushing the vessels, the shunt is inserted first into the internal carotid artery beyond the plaque and subsequently into the common carotid artery and held in place with occlusive tourniquets. **(C)** The plaque is sharply dissected proximally to normal intima and then sectioned sharply. Plaque is then dissected from below upward, with care taken to remove it from the external carotid artery by intussusception and subsequently from the internal carotid artery under direct view. **(D)** Careful removal of the plaque from the external carotid artery ensures patency. **(E&F)** The plaque will usually peel out from the distal intima very smoothly, however, often additional plaque needs to be peeled off the normal intima to ensure a smooth lining of the artery.

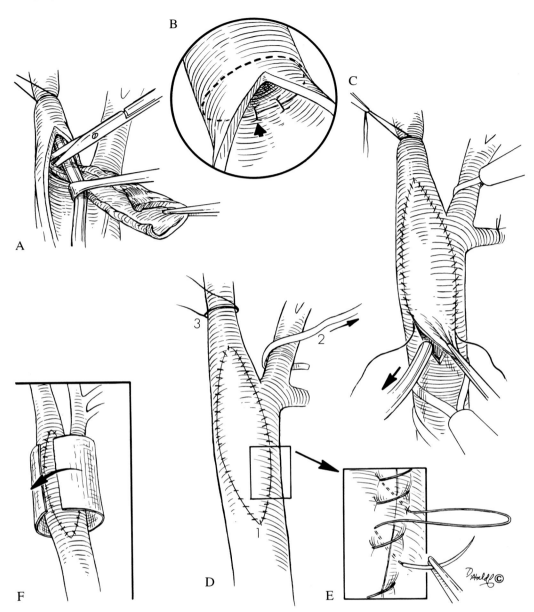

Figure 29-3. (A&B) Distal plaque peeled off normal intima. It is most unusual to require tacking sutures on the intima. They are shown for completeness only. **(C–E)** Patch is sutured with running 5-0 or 6-0 Prolene suture after preclotting. It is important to insert the needle at an exact right angle and suture the patch to the arterial wall. **(F)** Reenforcement of endarterectomy site with Teflon film (optional).

Gelfoam and thrombin wrapped in a sheet of Surgicel to form a good compressive pack. Additional arterial sutures may be needed if the initial suture technique did not ensure close and regular placement of the suture, allowing for site bleeding. Meticulous attention is necessary to avoid damage to the running suture with placement of the additional sutures. Every effort is made to avoid reversing the heparin for at least 20 minutes. Endarterectomy with and without heparinization in animals has shown that after 10 minutes the use of heparin has usually protected the endarterectomy site, allowing a platelet coating without thrombus formation.[32] Longer use of heparin is probably more beneficial, and therefore every effort is made not to reverse the heparin. If bleeding is a problem after the first 10 to 20 minutes, the heparin may be reversed in stages. The half-life of operative heparin is approximately 60 minutes, and this should be taken into account at the time of heparin reversal with protamine hydrochloride. Generally, the heparin is reversed with 1 mg of protamine for every 500 units of heparin. Palpation of the arterial wall is then carried out to determine the presence or absence of a thrill, which would indicate a loose intimal flap or some obstructive intraluminal mass. If a thrill is present, an arteriogram should be performed to determine the characteristics of the endarterectomy. If clot or debris if found inside the lumen, the vessel must be reoccluded and reopened and all debris re-

moved and closure reeffected. If there is any question about the patency of the arterial system, an arteriogram should be performed. Operative ultrasound may be used providing institutional expertise is available. Palpation of the superficial temporal artery should be reconfirmed, if that pulse is diminished or absent, the external carotid artery must be assumed to be partially or completely occluded (Fig. 29-4A&B). A clamp on the proximal ECA should be placed and

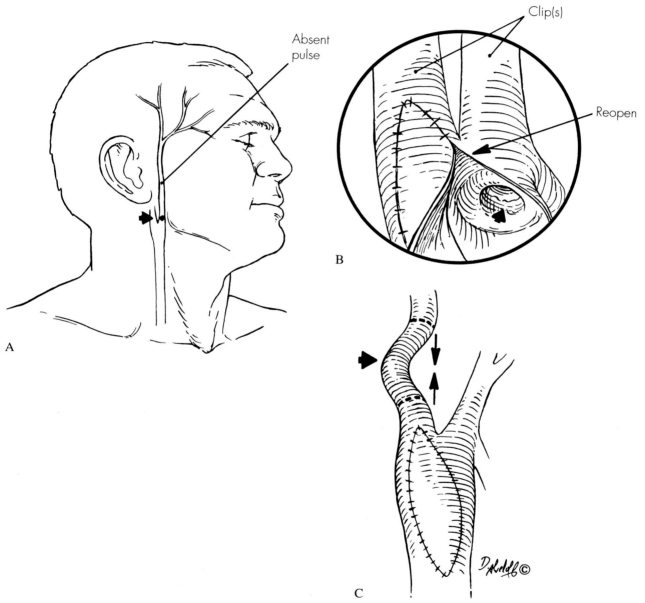

Figure 29-4. (A&B) Absent superficial temporal pulse. Postoperatively it is imperative to palpate the superficial temporal artery pulse. If it is absent, carotid occlusion, or more often external carotid artery occlusion, is suspected and should be confirmed; if present, the vessel must be reopened to remove the source of emboli. **(C)** It is imperative to meticulously reconstruct the vessel. If there is an extensive circuitous curve in the vessel, this should be straightened out by dissection and suture placement in the arterial wall or by resection of the anterior wall with shortening of the vessel.

distal occlusion of the ICA achieved by the placement of Rummel tourniquets or vascular occluding clips or clamps, and then the ECA is opened; almost invariably a dissected intima will be found, which should be removed and flow restored in the ECA. At times it is necessary to patch the ECA to ensure an adequate lumen. This dissection of intima distal to the blind intussusception of the ECA plaque is not unexpected. Patency of the ECA is important to prevent an occluded stump from being a source of emboli postoperatively and also to ensure adequate collateral circulation.

Prior to surgery the surgeon should have determined whether or not the vessel had kinks or loops in it. After the endarterectomy it is essential to remove any significant kinks or loops in the ICA system that are proximate to or part of the operative field (Fig. 29-4C). These can be removed by resection and anastomosis with 6-0 Prolene suture and subsequent vein or fabric patching or plication of a short segment of the endarterectomized vessel.

The overriding surgical principle must be reconstruction of the artery to ensure optimal unimpaired, well-directed arterial flow. The overriding goal is to operate safely and not produce the stroke to prevent which this prophylactic operation has been performed. Hertzer's comment,[19] "few major operations are conceptually so simple, yet technically so unforgiving, as a carotid endarterectomy," must be remembered. Rather than using confirmatory intraoperative arteriography, many surgeons are now using operative ultrasonography to determine the patency and quality of the reconstructed artery. This noninvasive procedure deserves widespread consideration.

Subsequent to meticulous hemostasis, the wound is reconstructed, and if feasible, the fascial sheath of the CCA is resutured. Sundt[32] uses a Teflon sheath around the distal CCA and bifurcation after vein patching to prevent subsequent aneurysmal formation. A Gortex stint may be used around the ICA, either to serve as an external support or to allow distal kinks to be lessened. Subsequent to absolute hemostasis, the wound is closed.

From the viewpoint of flow restoration, it is critical that the blood pressure be maintained at approximately 150 mmHg systolic as a maximum. This may require intravenous use of nitroprusside or nitroglycerin. The sudden restoration of high flow, particularly after the removal of a very tight stenosis and in the presence of heparin and/or aspirin, may produce intracerebral hemorrhage. The meticulous control of blood pressure is the major way of minimizing the hyperperfusion that often occurs following removal of a high-grade stenosis. Sundt[32] has shown flows to increase by over 100 percent after a successful endarterectomy, particularly in patients presenting with a slow stroke syndrome, generalized cerebral ischemia, or multiple, TIAs. Postoperative hypertension is a major treatable and preventable event. Smith has popularized transcranial Doppler ultrasonography to monitor perioperatively for adequate collateral blood flow and hyperperfusion. The therapy of postoperative hypertension should begin at the point of restoration of flow and be maintained throughout the patient's hospital stay. Fortunately, the postoperative instability of blood pressure usually disappears within 12 to 24 hours.

Postoperative hypotension, on the other hand, may be equally disastrous. This instability occurs in at least 50 percent of patients operated on under general anesthesia but is quite unusual on patients operated on under regional anesthesia.[7,17] The instability of blood pressure is due to carotid sinus malfunction.[2] The carotid sinus is a major baroreceptor in normal individuals; elevation in peripheral perfusion pressure stimulates this receptor, and its afferent nerve, the glossopharyngeal nerve, conducts the impulse to the medulla, which, through activation of the sympathetic or parasympathetic system (usually the latter) produces a lowering of peripheral vascular tone and blood pressure and a slowing of pulse rate. If the patient's peripheral blood pressure falls, the reverse occurs on activation of the sympathetic system. Patients with atherosclerosis of the carotid body often lose effective baroreceptor action. Following endarterectomy, the carotid bulb may again distend and the carotid sinus reflex be strongly reactivated, producing postoperative hypotension. On the other hand as a result of the surgical procedure, the reflex may be abolished and postoperative hypotension occur. The latter situation is more common than the former. Significant postoperative hypotension may produce cerebral ischemic complications and can best be treated by placing the patient in a Trendelenburg position, making certain that volume replacement is adequate, because often these patients do not respond well to vasopressors. In an effort to avoid postoperative hypotension, many surgeons routinely section the innervation of the carotid sinus at surgery. Others consider restoration of carotid sinus activity as a bonus to aid in the subsequent management of previously hypertensive patients.

OPERATIVE DAMAGE TO NERVES

The sensory branches of the cervical plexus (namely, the transverse cervical nerve the greater auricular nerve) and the cranial nerves (mandibular branch of the facial nerve, the vagus and its branches, the superior laryngeal and recurrent laryngeal nerves, the spinal accessory nerve, and the hypoglossal nerves) may be damaged at the time of carotid endarterectomy.[21,23,32] In addition damage to the cervical sympathetic chain may produce a complete Horner syndrome, or in cases of high dissection of the ICA, an incomplete Horner syndrome. The Cleveland Clinic has reported a complication rate for injury to the marginal mandibular nerve of 2 percent, to the recurrent laryngeal nerve of 6 percent, to the superior laryngeal nerve of 2 percent, and to the hypoglossal nerve of 5 percent. Some degree of minor injury is probably more common. The sensory losses occurring with damage to the transverse cervical or greater auricular nerves, although annoying, do not produce the significant morbidity of the other cranial nerve injuries. Meticulous surgical technique and knowledge of the anatomy, with application of sharp dissection and routine use of bipolar cautery, will prevent all these complications, with the exception of the routine loss of the transverse cervical nerve in the preferred carotid exposure. Advocates of the transverse cervical incision argue that the transverse cervical nerve can be spared and a more cosmetic postoperative wound produced, but the limits of exposure by this approach are a liability.

Facial Nerve Injury

Total facial nerve paralysis is rare and only occurs when very high exposure of the carotid artery is required. In order to expose the ICA at C2 and above, it is necessary to bring the incision anterior to the tragus of the ear, reflect the superficial lobe of the parotid superiorly and anteriorly, and at times dislocate the jaw to allow access. In the process of this extensive dissection, traction on the main facial nerve trunk may produce complete facial nerve paralysis. Otherwise the most common damage to the facial nerve is to the mandibular branch, which usually occurs secondary to traction. Placing the major vertical traction on the posterior belly of the digastric muscle or incising the deep fascia posteriorly along the sternocleidomastoid muscle will allow higher exposure and minimize traction on the mandibular and parotid aspects of the wound. Injury to the mandibular branch produces asymmetry of the mouth secondary to paralysis of the depressor of the lip. This is annoying to the patient in speech, and in eating the patient may bite the lower lip. Because it is usually a stretch injury and/or because the facial nerve has numerous arborizations, the deficit usually clears within 3 months. In the rare annoying permanent cases of paralysis, plastic surgery may be required.

Vagal Nerve Injury

Vagus nerve injury[12,21,32] can occur in carotid endarterectomy, but injury to the main trunk of the vagus nerve is rare. The nerve usually runs posterior to the carotid artery between it and the jugular vein and is covered by a separate fascia sheath. It may be injured in high exposure and by careless use of the cautery. Injury can be minimized by meticulous attention to anatomical detail and by use of the bipolar cautery. On occasion the vagus nerve may course anterior to the carotid artery on the right. In this circumstance the recurrent branch of the laryngeal nerve arises at the level of the carotid bifurcation, and obviously either the vagus or the recurrent nerve may easily be sectioned. This complication must be avoided by being aware of its occurrence and not sectioning any nerve until its origin has been determined. Therefore the routine should be observed of always identifying the ansa cervicalis and following the nerve proximally to its origin from the hypoglossal nerve prior to section. When an anterior vagus nerve is present, the nerve and its recurrent branch must be dissected and mobilized anteriorly and medially prior to the endarterectomy.

The recurrent branch of the laryngeal nerve is usually damaged by placing a self-retaining retractor deep to the level of the trachea. The nerve arises at the root of the neck at about the C7-T1 level and runs in front of the right subclavian artery. It courses below and behind the artery and then superiorly and medially behind the CCA into the groove between the trachea and the esophagus, where it ascends to the lower border of the cricoid cartilage. It becomes the inferior laryngeal nerve and supplies intrinsic muscles of the larynx that control the vocal cords. Damage results in unilateral vocal cord paralysis. This nerve is rarely, if ever, exposed during carotid endarterectomy, and damage is usually due to traction.

The superior laryngeal nerve is a branch of the vagus nerve at the lower margin of the first cervical vertebra and runs posteriorly and medially to the ICA and ECA. The nerve divides into an internal and an external branch. The internal branch is responsible for the sensory supply of the epiglottis and the larynx above the vocal cords. The external branch is responsible for the motor supply to the cricothyroid muscle and the inferior pharyngeal constrictor. The nerve is covered by loose fascia posterior and medial to the carotid arteries and can best be seen just medial and deep to the carotid bifurcation. It is usually damaged by careless use of cautery or direct posterior compression medial to the carodtid bifurcation. Meticulous technique and use of bipolar cautery will minimize damage to this nerve. It also maybe damaged by high exposure of the ICA at and above C1, so that in high dissection the medial aspect of the vagus nerve must always be respected. Damage to the superior laryngeal nerve is very disabling because the patient not only has difficulty in swallowing but suffers loss of sensation in the right epiglottis and larynx which allows food to migrate into the larynx, producing aspiration and annoying coughing. This is particularly true at night.

Spinal Accessory Nerve Injury

The spinal accessory nerve, a motor nerve, is rarely injured during carotid endarterectomy. In exiting the jugular foramen, the nerve lies superficial to the internal jugular vein and courses into the sternocleidomastoid muscle. The nerve is usually injured by misdirected exposure of the carotid artery into the posterior triangle of the neck or by traction or cautery injury in superior exposures of the ICA. Damage results in complete paralysis of the sternocleidomastoid and trapezius muscles, which causes a dropped shoulder and discomfort in the neck and shoulder. If the nerve is sectioned and recognized, primary suture should be effected.

Hypoglossal Nerve Injury

The hypoglossal nerve is totally responsible for the innervation of the tongue. Paralysis of the nerve produces slight impairment of speech and deviation of the tongue to the side of the paralysis, with subsequent ipsilateral tongue atrophy. The descendens hypoglossi leaves the nerve usually at its inferior curve and runs anterior and medial to the jugular vein and anterior to the carotid artery. The section of the descendens hypoglossi above the cervical branch that forms the ansa cervicalis produces no clinical syndrome. This branch, along with the cervical branch, is responsible for the motor supply of the deep strap muscles of the neck. As an external landmark the hypoglossal nerve usually runs at the level of the occipital artery. It is invariably crossed superiorly by the branch of the occipital artery to the sternocleidomastoid muscle. Occasionally, the nerve is crossed by an aberrant vein, and this vein may be closely adherent to the nerve. The nerve may be injured by direct traction or by use of means other than bipolar cautery in removing a plexus of veins from around it, particularly superiorly. With an overlying vein, the nerve may be ligated and divided with the vein unless the nerve is meticulously and routinely exposed. In order to avoid use of the cautery or unnecessary traction or clamping, the branch to the sternocleidomastoid muscle must be routinely exposed, ligated and divided. The nerve can then be displaced superiorly. If the hypoglossal nerve is sectioned, it should be sutured primarily. Otherwise recovery of function can be anticipated within 3 months.

POSTOPERATIVE COMPLICATIONS

Stroke or Transient Neurological Deficit

If the patient awakens with a postoperative neurological deficit, the surgeon is faced with the major catastrophe of the operation.[28,32] If the patient has a profound hemiplegia and aphasia and eye deviation to the side of the lesion, the prognosis is grave but not hopeless. Usually a much less severe neurological deficit is present. In the presence of a major deficit, the most likely cause is thrombosis of the ICA with or without distal embolization (Fig. 29-5). The next most common cause is a distal ICA or MCA embolus and, rarely, an intracerebral hemorrhage. In the face of an immediate significant deficit that is greater than a preoperative deficit, the patient should be given additional heparin to ensure heparinization and the blood pressure should be elevated with vasopressors. Preparations are made to immediately return the patient to the operating suite. Over the next few minutes if the deficit is improving, therapy should be continued and arteriography planned. If the deficit is unimproved, the patient should be returned to the operating suite and the wound reopened. If an excellent pulse is present in the carotid artery, an on-the-table arteriogram is obtained; if this reveals an arterial flap or partial clot thrombosis in the ICA, appropriate vessel isolation and reopening of the vessel are indicated. If the thrombus is immediately available, it is removed and back bleeding is allowed. At this point the mechanical cause of the thrombosis is usually identified as an intimal flap, and this is repaired.

Before restoration of flow, an internal arteriogram is obtained by placing a 14-gauge intracatheter into the distal internal carotid artery and injecting 4 to 5 ml of contrast medium to ensure that the distal ICA is patent and to determine whether there is an embolus in the MCA. If the vessel is patent with or without an MCA embolus, flow can be restored after reconstruction of the vessel. If an embolus exists in the intracranial carotid artery, the patient's blood pressure may be raised and back bleeding allowed in the hope that

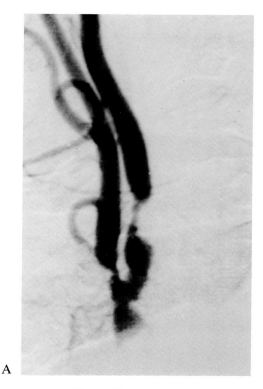 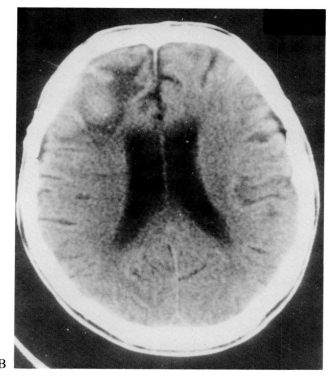

Figure 29-5. **(A)** Irregular carotid stenosis with **(B)** postoperative embolic infarction.

the embolus will flush down the open artery. The arteriogram is repeated, and if the distal ICA occlusion persists, flow should not be restored but preparation for a craniotomy and embolectomy should be considered. Another consideration would be the use of intra-arterial thrombolytic agents and repeat arteriography to determine patency (Fig. 29-6). If arterial patency can be achieved, the vessel is reconstructed and flow restored. If an MCA artery embolus is present, flow should be restored by reconstruction of the artery and subsequent use of thrombolytic agents, or craniotomy and embolectomy EC-IC or bypass surgery should be considered. If on opening the artery, no local thrombus is present and no back flow occurs, a Fogarty catheter should be passed distally to the level of the carotid canal and distended gently to remove any distal thrombus. A distal thrombus without a local operative thrombus would indicate distal intimal damage to the ICA, probably from dissection produced by shunting, or intimal damage produced by forceful clamping. Not infrequently, on returning the patient to the operating room, the artery and arteriogram are found to be normal. In this circumstance it is presumed that either operative ischemia occurred despite monitoring or shunting or that an embolus had occurred and dissolved. A distal branch or branches of the MCA may

be found to contain an embolus. Craniotomy with embolectomy, thrombolytic agents, or medical therapy may be the most satisfactory treatment. Generally, the prognosis with a distal embolus into the cortical arteries mitigates against surgical therapy.

Prevention of postoperative ICA occlusion is best handled by the routine use of a vein or fabric patch. In Sundt's experience,[32] 4 percent of the patients in whom the vessel had been closed primarily suffered a postoperative occlusion. The literature reveals the incidence of postoperative occlusion in primary closure to range from 2 to 5 percent. A literature review and personal experience indicate that a reconstructed, primarily closed artery is more apt to have points of narrowing than an artery reconstructed by the patch technique. Almost invariably, an ICA occlusion is secondary to technical factors, which must be prevented by meticulous surgical technique.

Heparin-induced hypercoagulability may be responsible for postoperative thrombosis. This complication should be prevented by routine monitoring of platelet counts every third day in patients who are receiving a constant heparin therapy and by attempting to limit the heparinization to 3 to 4 days. Once this hypercoagulable state occurs, there is no definitive therapy. Other factors in the prevention of postoperative occlusion at the operative site include rou-

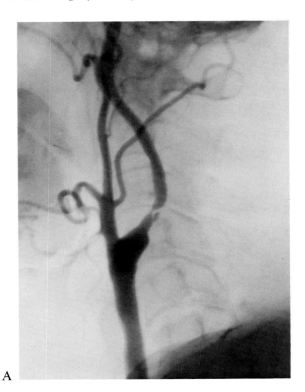

A

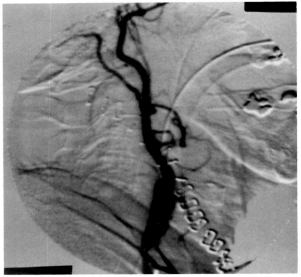

B

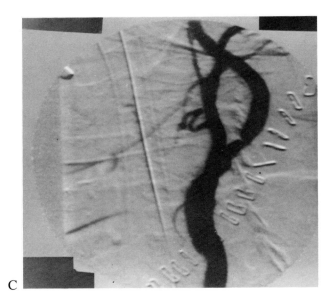

C

Figure 29-6. (A) Severe carotid stenosis. **(B)** Postoperative carotid thrombosis. **(C)** Restoration of flow after local urokinase infusion. Note stenosis at distal suture line, which produced the postoperative thrombosis.

tine use of aspirin and care not to completely reverse the heparinization after restoration of vessel flow. Also, operative and postoperative hypertension must be avoided.

If angiography demonstrates no cause for the neurological deficit but evidence of a mass lesion, an intracerebral hemorrhage is present. If the arteriogram is normal, a postoperative computed tomog-

raphy (CT) or magnetic resonance imaging (MRI) scan is indicated to determine the presence of an intracerebral clot or infarction. If an intracerebral hemorrhage is seen, the patient's blood pressure should be maintained at a normal level. The heparinization must be reversed with protamine hydrochloride. If the patient has received aspirin, giving platelet buttons to reverse the aspirin effect is essential. Subsequently, surgical evacuation may be life-saving. Unfortunately, when intracerebral hemorrhage occurs, bleeding is often massive. If the hemorrhage is extensive and in the major hemisphere, no therapy is probably the most humane course in view of the patient's dismal prognosis.

If arteriography confirms an ECA occlusion, and an embolus is seen in the ICA system or the arteriogram is otherwise normal, the probability is that an embolus arose from the ECA. This patient's ECA should be isolated from cerebral flow end opened, and a thrombectomy should be performed and flow reconstituted, or the patient should be heparinized for 1 week to 10 days to prevent additional embolization. If a CCA occlusion is found, one can suspect an intimal lesion, with dissection as the cause. This will necessitate extending the arteriotomy inferiorly to the clamp site and appropriate repair.

Hematoma and Carotid Suture Line Rupture

Postoperative hematoma with tracheal deviation, pain and discomfort, and an airway embarrassment is best treated by immediately opening the wound. In an emergent situation the wound must be opened in the bed, but if possible, the patient should be returned to the operating room. If the hematoma is quite large and the patient is maintaining the airway, the wound should be opened under local anesthesia after local preparation and draping and before intubation. Often, the hematoma can be evacuated without the necessity of general anesthesia. If possible, rapid induction of general endotracheal anesthesia with respiratory paralysis and an attempt at intubation should be avoided because of major difficulty in placing an endotracheal tube without prior wound opening and partial clot evacuation. If intubation is required, the endotracheal tube probably should be left in place for 2 to 3 days to ensure that the airway is maintained.

On reopening the wound, the patient is frequently found to have either oozing from raw surfaces, associated with aspirin therapy, or an arterial or venous bleeder that requires ligation. The hematoma may also present with interference with swallowing and speech due to posterior dissection. The hematoma may extend into the mediastinum.

Rarely, rupture of the suture line or graft used to close the carotid artery occurs. This is an extreme emergency—the patient's death is imminent unless the airway can be maintained, the bleeding stopped, and shock treated. It may be necessary from a life-saving standpoint to open the wound in the bed and occlude the carotid artery manually or with an available hemostat. If possible, the patient should be intubated and returned to surgery, where the appropriate exposure and isolation of the carotid artery can be achieved. On rare occasions the running suture will have been found to be broken; on other occasions the patch graft may have torn. Whatever the cause, it must be repaired and the artery reconstituted. A ruptured carotid suture line can be avoided by inspecting the arterial suture for areas of thinning and not nicking or knotting the suture in the process of wound closure. In addition, if Prolene is used, sutures should be tied with at least six or seven knots and cut long.

Prevention of hematoma requires meticulous attention to hemostasis during wound closure and awareness of the potential danger of using aspirin or not reversing the heparinization at closure of the artery. In addition, meticulous control of blood pressure in the hypertensive patient is essential.

Unusual Wound and Artery Complications

Postoperative wound infection is rare. Even when a patch graft has been used, provided that the patient is neurologically intact the wound should be opened and drained, the causative organism identified, and appropriate antibiotics given. The great danger is wound disruption secondary to infection or rejection of the graft used for angioplasty. The literature contains very little direction in the management of the wound with a patch graft that becomes infected. My one patient was healed without problem by use of drainage and antibiotics.

On rare occasions a false aneurysm will occur. This is most unusual with primary wound closure and usually occurs with angioplasty. It may be secondary to delayed incompetency of the vein graft, to a low-grade infection of the fabric graft, or to partial delayed rupture of either one. The aneurysm usually presents with a mass in the neck or with episodes of transient ischemia or stroke. Rarely, a twelfth nerve palsy and mass are present. Surgical repair involves wide exposure with excision of the aneurysm and reconstruction of the artery, either by patching or by resection and grafting. If a graft is required, we prefer Gortex tubing with end-to-end anastomosis between the CCA and the ICA, and implantation of the ECA in an end-to-side anastomosis. If the CCA origin is uninvolved in the aneurysmal process, end-to-end anastomosis between the ICA and CCA may be possible.

Ischemic Attacks

Dirrenberger[8b] and Deen[8a] have delineated the healing process after endarterectomy in a superb fashion. They conclusively illustrate the benefit of operative heparinization and not reversing the heparinization after arterial closure. The thrombogenicity of the endarteromized surface is fortunately short-lived. Immediately postsurgery, the operative surface is quite thrombogenic, but after the first 20 minutes it is less, and with heparin it is significantly less. The raw surface is covered by adhering platelets and fibrin. The period of thrombus formation does not exceed 6 to 8 hours, as the protective platelet fibrin coat or the depletion of thromboplastin causes the surface to lose thrombogenicity. Providing that flow has been restored appropriately, postoperative embolization or occlusion of the carotid artery is usually an event of the first few hours after surgical repair. However, ischemic events, whether they are TIAs or reversible ischemic neurological deficits, may occur up to the point of reendothelization of the arterial wall. This requires approximately 1 month. Other causes for delayed ischemic events include unrecognized arterial dissection or damage to the arterial wall secondary to vigorous clamping. An occluded ECA may be the source of emboli producing TIAs. Postoperative ischemic attacks or neurological deficits are best managed by performing a CT scan of the head to exclude hemorrhage or infarction followed by an arteriogram. The status of the arterial tree will then determine whether operative or medical management is recommended.

Hyperperfusion Syndromes

Hyperfusion syndromes[32] occur in surgical patients who have a high risk for carotid endarterectomy and who after endarterectomy have a marked increase in cerebral blood flow (CBF). These patients often have paralysis of autoregulation ipsilatral to the surgery. There is a profound increase in intracranial flow postoperatively, which can be determined by blood flow measurement or by serial transcranial Doppler measurements, preoperatively and postoperatively. When this syndrome occurs, the patient's blood pressure should be meticulously controlled in a low range of 120 to 130 mmHg systolic for several days. The tremendous increase in CBF frequently causes ipsilateral vascular headaches; in fact, ipsilateral headache is not uncommon following endarterectomy owing to increased CBF. Headache may also be produced by carotid artery occlusion; if the patient's headache is better in the sitting position, it is most likely secondary to increased CBF, whereas if it is worse in the sitting position, this may indicate carotid artery occlusion. The headaches are usually treated by analgesics. Aspirin and continued heparin should be avoided in patients with the hyperperfusion syndrome.

Occasionally patients will have migraine-like attacks; these usually are patients with documented increases in CBF. The attacks usually involve visual scotomas in a visual field quadrant. No specific therapy is indicated. Postoperative seizures may occur in patients with the hyperperfusion syndrome, usually occur about 1 week to 10 days following operation. The seizures are treated with Dilantin and are usually short-lived, although they may be difficult to control. A permanent seizure disorder is rare.

The most catastrophic complication occurring from hyperperfusion is intracerebral hemorrhage (Fig. 29-7). Several authors have recorded the risk factors that contribute to the hyperperfusion syndrome; these include advanced age, hypertensive disease, an unstable preoperative neurological condition, a recent cerebral infarction, and routine use of aspirin and heparin. The hemorrhage may be massive and fatal. It should be managed medically, if possible, by reversing the aspirin effect with platelet transfusions, discontinuing heparin, and controlling the blood pressure to low normal.

Myocardial Infarction, Arrhythmia, and Congestive Heart Failure

The leading cause of death after endarterectomy is myocardial infarction, either immediate or, more often, delayed.[1,10,37] In view of the close association between arteriosclerotic heart disease and carotid atherosclerosis, every patient must be assumed to have coronary artery disease. Unstable angina, congestive heart failure, and significant cardiac arrhythmias are relative contraindications for carotid endarterectomy. These conditions should be corrected or ameliorated as much as possible prior to surgery. All patients undergoing endarterectomy need adequate oxygenation and postoperative cardiac monitoring.

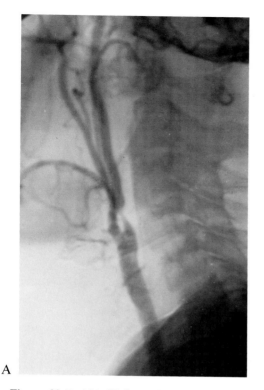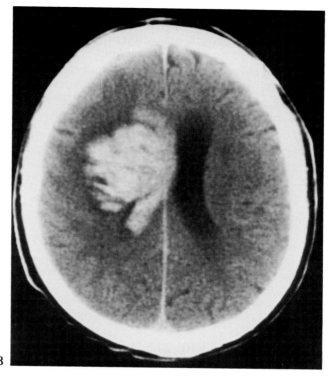

A   B

Figure 29-7. (A) High-grade carotid stenosis with frequent transient ischemic attacks. **(B)** Intracerebral hematoma after endarterectomy on third postoperative day.

Meticulous attention to avoid fluid overload or congestive heart failure is indicated. Maintenance of the patient's preoperative medication is frequently overlooked and may produce postoperative congestive heart failure or arrhythmia.

There will be rare cases in which multiple TIAs are associated with a significant carotid lesion and unstable angina or the development of unstable angina in the postoperative period. With this preoperative situation, simultaneous operation on the carotid artery and coronary arteries may be necessary; however, this invariably carries a higher morbidity than if the operations can be staged. The operations should be staged even if it means having the coronary artery team on call at the time of the endarterectomy. If the heart symptoms are critical, the coronary bypass procedure is performed first.

Recurrent Carotid Stenosis

Late recurrent stenosis is secondary to myointimal hyperplasia or atherosclerosis, usually the former. Recurrent stenosis occurs in 15 to 20 percent of surgical cases, but it is symptomatic in only 2 to 3 percent. Reoperation is feasible but carries a significantly greater risk than primary surgery. Recurrent stenosis may be prevented by routine patching of the arteriotomy.[8,11,32] or by carotid eversion.[22]

SUMMARY

Criticism has appropriately focused on a serious review of the indications for carotid endarterectomy. The prophylactic benefit of this operation depends on very low surgical morbidity and mortality. With symptomatic carotid stenosis (70 to 90 percent of cases) surgery is over three times as effective in reducing stroke as medical therapy. This result was present within 3 months in the recent Symptomatic Carotid Therapy Trial.[26a] Recent literature would confirm the ever-increasing safety of the operation, which is due to meticulous selection of patients and improved perioperative and operative management of those undergoing surgery. The qualifications of the surgeons have improved.

The increasing use of institutional audit may contribute to lower morbidity. The average surgeons do not record or review their surgical results. According to Hertzer,[19] "the stakes are so high and the margin for error is so low that carotid endarterectomy simply must be audited and reaudited at every hospital in which it is performed." Evidence exists that audit has improved the surgical results, either through limiting the unqualified surgeon or forcing the qualified surgeon to understand the treacherous, unforgiving nature of poor surgical care and technique. With the cataloging of complications, evidence now exists as to their incidence, prevention, and management. Surgeons must continue to maintain combined morbidity and mortality for this procedure in the 3 percent range or lower in the good-risk symptomatic or asymptomatic patient.

New angioplastic techniques are being employed with immediately apparent successful radiographic results.[37] Their future will require careful evaluation of risks and long-term benefits.[13]

Cerebral Revascularization

Arthur L. Day
Howard N. Chandler

LITERATURE REVIEW

After extensive investigations of cerebral ischemia and infarction, C. Miller Fisher suggested in 1951 that "anastomosis of the external carotid artery or one of its branches with the internal carotid artery above the area of narrowing should be feasible" and that "someday, vascular surgery will find a way to bypass the portion of the artery during the period of ominous fleeting symptoms."[66] More than 15 years later Yasargil[94] and associates performed the first superficial temporal artery (STA) to MCA microsurgical arterial anastomosis for cerebral ischemia.[61,94,95] Since that time the procedure has been used with increasing frequency to treat a variety of intracranial lesions.

Most earlier clinical series were nonrandomized and poorly controlled and primarily emphasized the radiographic and hemodynamic alterations produced by the procedure. The International Cooperative Study of Extracranial-Intracranial Arterial Anastomosis (the Study), published in 1985, reported on the 5-year outcomes of nearly 1,400 patients who were randomly assigned to surgical and medical limbs.[48,49,62,63,80] This study found that cerebral revascularization was no more effective than aspirin therapy in reducing stroke or stroke-related deaths for all categories studied. Criticisms of the Study's conclusions have been numerous and have been based primarily on the patient groupings used and the substantial number (more than 2,500) of surgical exclusions from the series.[45,47,57,68,72,83,87,88] Since the Study's publication, however, use of the procedure has been greatly reduced.

Data from the Study have clearly indicated that perioperative complications substantially counteract the protective benefits of the procedure for many patients. Table 29-1 lists the types of complications and their incidence as reported in the larger literature series.[52,53,62,64,67,69,81,82,90,96]

Many experienced cerebrovascular neurosurgeons still feel that a significant patient subgroup exists in whom revascularization risks are overcome by the beneficial effects of the procedure. Selection of patients whose risks without surgical treatment appear high, along with careful attention to perioperative details to minimize complications, can magnify these advantages.[51,55,58,93]

PREOPERATIVE, INTRAOPERATIVE, AND POSTOPERATIVE MANAGEMENT

Preoperative Assessment and Management

Table 29-2 lists the pathological lesions potentially amenable to EC-IC bypass.[53,56,82,92,96] The remainder of this chapter deals primarily with problems associated with bypass for arteriosclerotic disease. Such bypass surgery is quite controversial, and surgical indications must be carefully considered in the light of clinical, radiographic, and CBF findings.[50,72]

Table 29-1. Central Nervous System Complications—Types and Incidence (Within 30 Days of Surgery)

| Author, Year | No. of Cases/ No. of Patients | Patency Rate | Deaths (%) | Morbidity | | | | | | |
| | | | | Ischemic | | | Hemorrhage | | Wound | |
				CS	TIA/RIND	Sz	ICH	Other	Inf	Flap
Chater,[52] 1983	400/400	96%	10 (2.5%)	9	?	?	0	7	1	5
Collice et al.,[53] 1985	105/100	90%	1(1%)	1	11	?	0	0	?	?
EC/IC Study,[62] 1985	663/663	96%	4 (0.6%)	20	?	?	?	?	?	?
Eguchi,[64] 1985	113/113	95%	2 (1.7%)	2	3	7	2	1	0	5
Gagliardi,[67] 1985	90/90	94%	1 (1.1%)	1	4	?	0	8	0	2
Gratzl & Roun,[69] 1985	213/200	94%	4(2%)	6	2	?	1	1	1	6
Reale et al.,[81] 1984	100/100	100%	0(0%)	1	6	3	0	2	1	0
Reichman,[82] 1976	68/68	?	3 (4.4%)	3	1	5	1	3	0	5
Sundt et al.,[90] 1985	415/403	99%	5 (1.2%)	15	54	?	2	27	2	?
Yasargil & Yonekawa,[96] 1977	86/84	87%	3 (3.4%)	2	?	5	2	3	5	5
Total/Avg	2253	(94.5%)	(1.5%)	60 (2.7%)	81 (7.3%)	20 (5.4%)	8 (0.9%)	52 (3.5%)	10 (0.8%)	28 (2.9%)

Abbreviations: CS, completed stroke; TIA, transient ischemic attack; RIND, reversible ischemic neurological deficit; ICH, intracerebral hematoma; Other includes subdural and epidural hematomas and hygromas; Inf, infection; Flap, flap ischemia or necrosis; Sz, seizure; ?, information not available from text of article.

Inclusion criteria: Arterial bypasses only (no veins); ischemic disease only (arteriosclerosis, moyamoya, fibromuscular dysplasia, etc.); bypass to MCA only.

Clinical Selection

Symptoms should be localized to the carotid distribution, generally to the region of the middle cerebral artery (MCA). The more common indications include TIAs, reversible ischemic neurological deficits (RINDs), and mild completed strokes with subsequent fluctuations in neurological function. Overall, patients should not be subjected to EC-IC bypass (in spite of "proper" arteriographic indications) when the identified lesion is static and currently asymptomatic, when the sympatomatic lesion has not had a prior trial of medical therapy, or when the lesion is amenable to an extracranial procedure.[47,57,62]

Preoperative evaluation should include routine laboratory work, chest roentgenography, electrocardiography, and a history and physical examination. Any suggestion of cardiac, vascular, or pulmonary disease should be further evaluated by appropriate consultants and tests. Patients with severe disease are not considered, as their expected longevity and systemic operative risks are poor. Patients with long-standing major neurological deficits are also excluded, as revascularization cannot revitalize infarcted brain tissue.

Table 29-2. Pathology Potentially Amenable to Extracranial-Intracranial Bypass

Atherosclerosis
    ICA occlusion
    CCA occlusion
    ICA siphon stenosis, occlusion
    MCA stenosis, occlusion
Planned occlusion
    Aneurysm
    Tumor
Moyamoya disease

Arteriographic Selection

The lesions outlined in Table 29-2 do not represent homogeneous pathological or clinical entities, and EC-IC bypass is not appropriate for all such lesions. Many types of pathology exhibit different mechanisms of symptom production, natural histories, and responses to medical management. For instance, carotid dissections, despite the seeming production of severe stenosis indicated by arteriography, usually cause symptoms due to embolization. Intracranial stenoses often reflect severe systemic arteriosclerotic disease, and the hazards of converting a stenotic lesion to an occlusion following bypass are high. Most stenotic lesions should receive a trial of major anticoagulant therapy (heparin or coumadin) prior to bypass and should undergo surgery only if refractory to *best* medical therapy.[56]

Prior to the final management decision, the radiographic and clinical features of the ipsilateral carotid bifurcation must be carefully assessed. For example, a patient with a single ischemic episode and an ICA occlusion quite likely experienced the episode in close temporal proximity with the occlusion, and surgical treatment should be withheld. Certain other lesions would benefit from an extracranial procedure only. Arteriosclerotic "pseudoocclusion" is not infrequently encountered in this group of patients. An ICA occlusion may go unnoticed, but continued arteriosclerotic progression causing stenosis or ulceration near the ECA origin may lead to later cerebral symptoms. The stump of an occluded ICA can become a source of embolisms into the ECA and the retina or brain.

Donor Vessel Selection

Scalp vessels with angiographic lumina smaller than 1 mm make poor donors (Fig. 29-8). Patency rates are lower, the difficulty of anastomosis is greater, and the amount of irrigation provided by the vessel is reduced. Generally, the larger of the two STA branches (anterior versus posterior) is chosen. The anterior branch is more ideally positioned to facilitate anastomosis to proximal sylvian MCA branches. If no satisfactory arterial channel is available or if immediate high flows are required, a saphenous vein graft is used.[76,77,84,86,89]

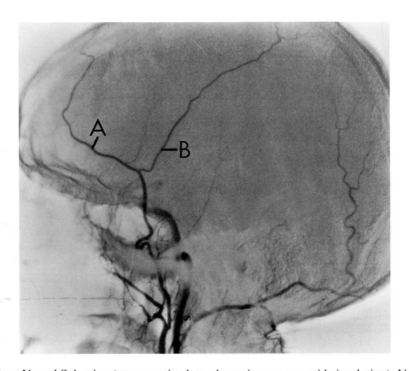

Figure 29-8. Donor Vessel Selection (preoperative lateral arteriogram, carotid circulation): Note anterior (*A*) and posterior (*P*) STA branches; anterior branch is preferable donor because of slightly larger size and more optimal position (vein use preferable for hemispheric revascularization when STA branches are smaller); ICA bifurcation must be carefully investigated for lesion amenable to extracranial procedure.

Surgical Procedure

Anesthesia and Monitoring

Blood pressure is monitored with an intra-arterial line, and wide swings are carefully avoided. A Swan-Ganz catheter is placed whenever cardiac or pulmonary instability or barbiturate loading is anticipated. Hyperventilation is generally not recommended, as its vasoconstrictive effects might further reduce CBF.

Cortical activity is monitored intraoperatively with evoked potentials and EEG. Barbiturates are instituted in many cases, especially when a vein graft is used (because of longer occlusion times) or a major MCA trunk is temporarily clipped. These medications are administered to burst suppression, and continued until flow is restored.

Systemic heparinization is used for vein graft procedures to minimize the risk of graft thrombosis. The heparin is initiated after all preliminary dissection is completed and reversed with protamine after flow has been reestablished. Preoperative heparin therapy should be discontinued early on the morning of surgery; aspirin or dipyridamole can be maintained throughout the operative period.

Operative Position

The patient is placed in the supine position with the head elevated above the heart to reduce venous congestion in the brain. Both STA branches are identified by palpation and Doppler ultrasonography and then externally marked. The head is fixed in skull tongs, with the face rotated 20 degrees up from a pure lateral position. If simultaneous carotid ligation and/or vein graft use is contemplated, the cervical carotid bifurcation is also included in the operative field. The lower leg is prepared and draped when a long saphenous vein is required.

Scalp and Donor Preparation

Under most circumstances STA exposure is best accomplished by a linear incision directly over the donor vessel (Figs. 29-9 and 29-10). While a flap provides better cortical exposure, the donor vessel is more difficult to dissect, and the incidence of scalp necrosis is greater. Scalp infiltration with anesthetic or vasoconstricting agents is not recommended. The incision is begun distally on the STA so that if an injury occurs during its identification, the entire vessel need not be sacrificed. After the initial cut (approximately 2 cm long) passes through the skin and dermal fat, the two edges are retracted and elevated with skin hooks. The external STA surface is identified, and the incision is extended until the entire vessel is visualized down to the zygoma.

A bipolar or carbon dioxide laser is used to prepare a 1-cm pedicle of supporting tissue, with care taken to avoid injury to the main STA trunk. The frontalis branch of the facial nerve, which often accompanies the anterior branch of the STA, is swept anteriorly away from the vessel and preserved. The pedicle is elevated from the temporalis fascia, leaving its connections at its proximal and distal ends to allow continued flow. The artery is bathed in 3 percent papaverine solution and covered with moistened cotton strips until used for anastomosis.

Saphenous Vein Harvesting and Preparation

Generally, the lower leg segment is harvested, as this portion is smaller in diameter and thus the size discrepancy between it and the MCA is minimal. A linear incision is begun distally, just anterior to the medial malleolus, and extended proximally once the vein has been identified. All branches are ligated with 6-0 silk ties, which are carefully placed so as to avoid compromise of the main venous channel. A mark is placed on the external saphenous surface with either an indelible pen or a small-caliber nylon suture, so that future rotation can be easily seen and corrected. The dissected segment is then harvested between two ligatures, the direction of flow being carefully marked. The saphenous nerve is dissected free from the vein and preserved, as injury may cause a painful neuralgia.

After the vessel is irrigated with heparinized saline, a temporary clip is placed over the proximal end, and the vein is gently inflated. A Shiley vein distender is used to calibrate this pressure, as overinflation may damage the endothelium and promote graft thrombosis.[79,91] The vessel is placed into a basin filled with cold heparinized saline until needed.

When a vein is used, the intracranial anastomosis is performed first. The technique for anastomosis is similar to that for an arterial-to-arterial bypass, but since the venous wall is thicker, a slightly larger suture (8-0) is preferable. Once the intracranial anastomosis has been completed, a wide tunnel is carefully prepared to allow atraumatic subcutaneous passage of the vein into the cervical incision site while carefully avoiding rotation of the graft. The cervical anastomosis is then performed with 6-0 Prolene suture. When it is completed, both ends of the graft are flushed and the heparin is reversed.

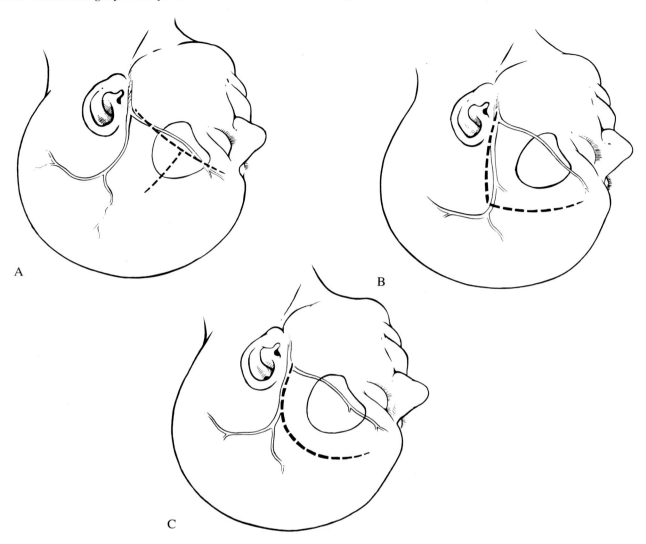

Figure 29-9. Scalp Incision Variations, designed to provide frontotemporal exposure while incorporating course of STA. **(A)** Linear incision over anterior STA branch, T incision posteriorly. **(B)** Linear incision over posterior STA branch, extension anteriorly. **(C)** Traditional frontotemporal flap, with preservation of both STA branches for use if needed.

Intracranial Exposure

Since the revascularization procedure is generally aimed at replenishing the entire MCA territory rather than an isolated branch, we prefer to make the anastomosis in the sylvian fissure near the main MCA trunks[60] (Fig. 29-11). A flap of temporalis muscle and fascia is turned (often divided into anterior and posterior leaflets) and a free bone flap 5 to 6 cm in diameter is elevated.

The proximal sylvian fissure is opened to expose the MCA and its M_2 segments several centimeters below the brain surface. An accessible 1 to 1.5 cm MCA segment that is free of branches is isolated above a latex dam, leaving room for the anastomosis and temporary clips at each end.

Distal STA Preparation

A temporary clip is placed over the proximal STA pedicle, and the distal end is sectioned. The entire pedicle is rotated into the operative field, and an estimate is made about the appropriate length required to reach the recipient MCA site. As cerebrospinal fluid (CSF) drains from the sylvian fissure, the depth of the operative field may become progressively greater, so an extra 1 cm length of STA is allowed.

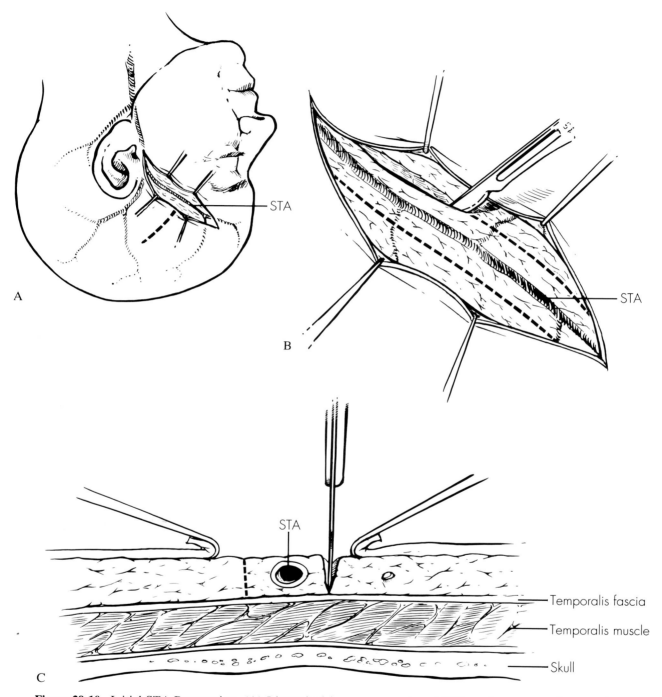

Figure 29-10. Initial STA Preparation. **(A)** Linear incision exposes external STA surface over entire vessel length. **(B)** Skin edges retracted, 1 cm wide vascular pedicle isolated (dotted lines). **(C)** Cross-sectional view of scalp containing donor artery (*STA*); skin retracted with hooks, knife cut parallel to vessel through dermis to deep temporalis fascia.

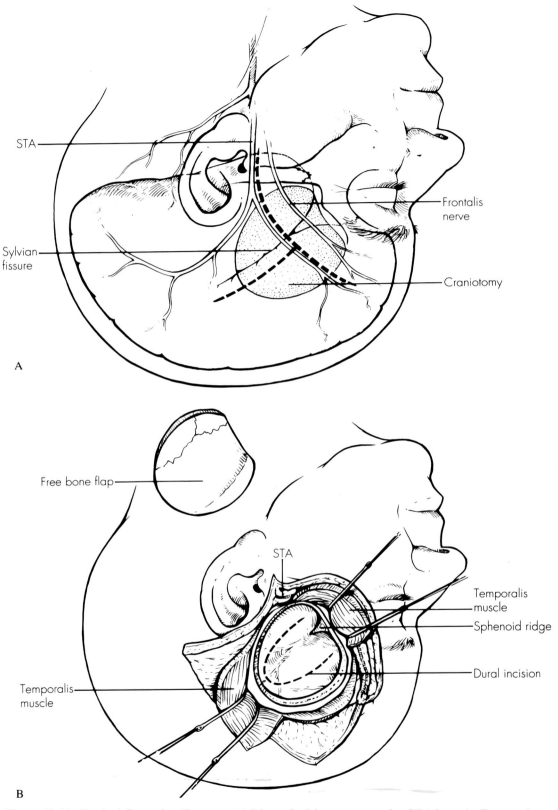

Figure 29-11. Typical Operative Format. **(A)** Linear incision over anterior STA branch, T extension posteriorly (*dotted lines*). Note position of adjacent frontalis nerve, craniotomy (*Cran*), sylvian fissure. **(B)** Temporalis muscle (*T*), fascia divided into anterior and posterior leaflets and retracted with hooks to expose frontotemporal region; anterior STA branch with pedicle swept forward; dural incision (*dotted line*) to expose anterior sylvian fissure. (*Figure continues.*)

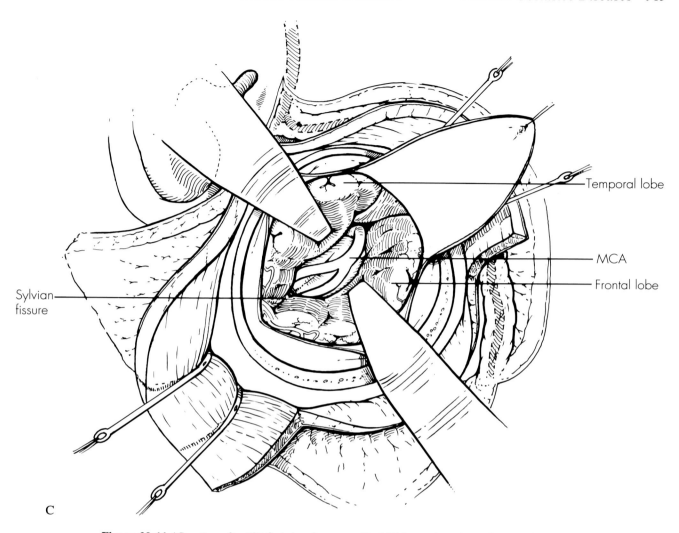

Figure 29-11 (*Continued*). **(C)** Sylvian fissure split, MCA trunk or large branch isolated.

The free end of the STA is dissected of all supporting structures, and a fresh cut is made across the end of the vessel. The proximal clip is temporarily released to verify patency. If no flow appears, the pedicle is checked for causes of obstruction, including graft torsion, thrombosis, or inadvertent injury. If good flow cannot be established, the arterial pedicle should be abandoned for a vein graft. After irrigation with heparinized saline, a fishmouth incision of a length approximately twice the diameter of the vessel is made into the artery. The exact position of the incision is chosen as the STA rests alongside the MCA so as to ensure comfortable access to both sides of the anastomosis.

Anastomosis

Figure 29-12 shows the anastomosis procedure. The MCA segment is isolated between two temporary clips. A linear arteriotomy (two to three times the STA diameter) is made, and a small Silastic stent is placed in the lumen to separate the arterial edges. Microsutures (10-0 nylon on a BV-6 needle) are placed in the STA both at the base of the fishmouth incision and on the side opposite to approximate the two vessels. The most difficult side of the anastomosis is then completed by placing a series of six to eight independent sutures. After placement of all sutures, each is tied with four knots.

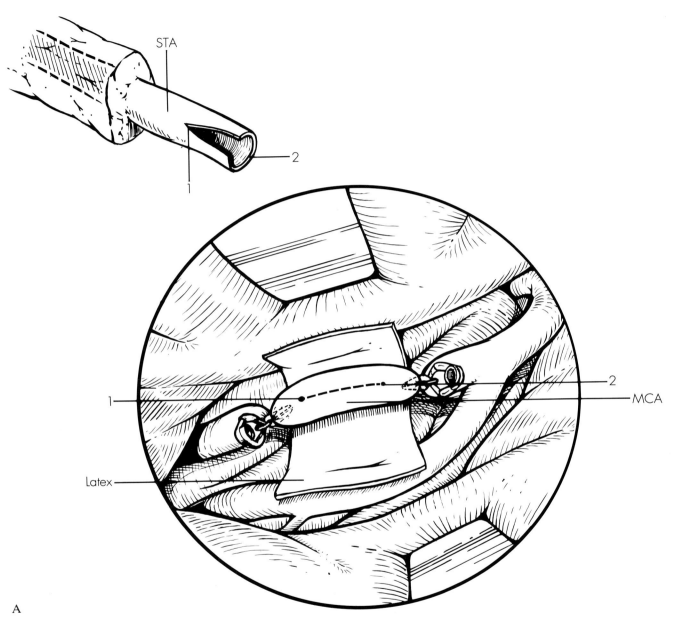

A

Figure 29-12. Anastomosis. **(A)** Distal end of STA has been prepared for anastomosis; fishmouth incision made along length of STA is approximately twice the diameter of the vessel; MCA trunk has been isolated between two temporary clips and elevated over latex platform; length of MCA incision approximately three times STA diameter. To provide retrograde flow into more proximal MCA, point 1 on STA (base of fishmouth incision) is sewn to distal end of MCA incision. (*Figure continues.*)

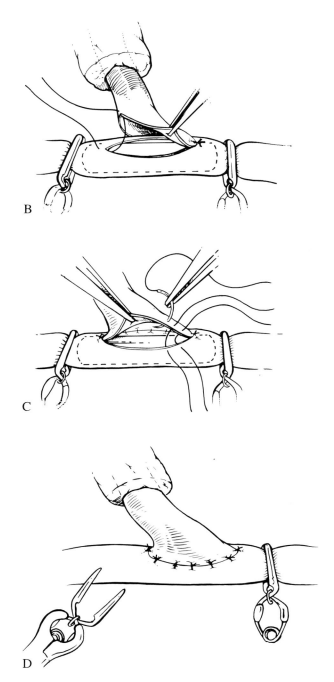

B

C

D

Figure 29-12 (*Continued*). **(B)** After stent (*dotted lines*) is positioned in MCA, two end sutures are placed. **(C)** Back wall of anastomosis has been completed, suture line inspected from interior view, sutures placed in frontal wall of anastomosis, and then stent removed before tying. **(D)** Completed anastomosis: clips removed individually to allow back bleeding of each end into anastomosis site. (*Figure continues.*)

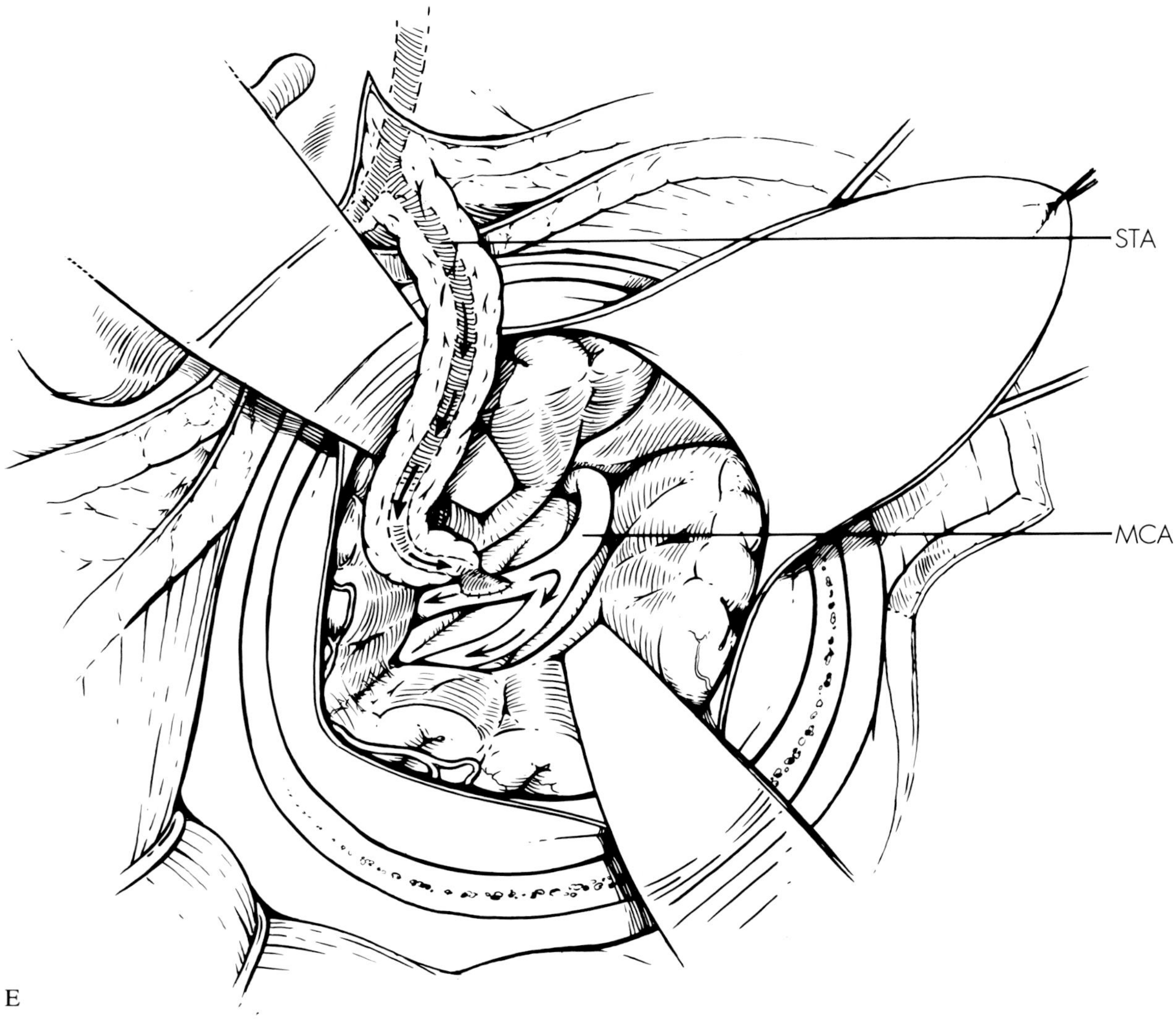

Figure 29-12 (*Continued*). (**E**) Completed anastomosis: flow reestablished, directed toward proximal portions of MCA.

After the completed portion of the anastomosis is internally inspected, sutures are placed in the remaining side. Before the final two are tied, the stent is removed, and the lumen of the anastomosis is gently irrigated. The last two sutures are closed over a vessel full of heparinized saline.

The STA clip is transiently released, which allows any residual debris to be dislodged through gaps in the anastomosis. A similar flush is then done with each end of the MCA. All clips are removed so that free communication is allowed in all directions. Significant gaps are closed with isolated microsuture. Bleeding will often be easily controlled with small Gelfoam pledgets.

If there is any question about patency, the temporary clips should be replaced and several sutures removed from the "easier" side of the anastomosis for direct inspection and back-bleeding from all sources. Obstruction may be corrected by irrigation, replacement of faulty sutures, or elimination of graft compression.

Closure

Once hemostasis is complete, all cottonoids and residual blood products are removed. The dura is loosely reapproximated, leaving a wide channel for donor vessel passage. The residual dural defect is covered with a large sheet of Gelfoam to minimize CSF egress into the subcutaneous tissues (Fig. 29-13A). The base of the bone flap is removed, and the bone edge on the skull is beveled to prevent compression of the donor vessel. The bone flap is secured, and the temporalis fascia is approximated around the periphery of the field (Fig. 29-13B). Only the temporalis muscle is closed centrally, to provide a soft yet firm investment around the STA. The skin is closed in a single layer with interrupted 3-0 nylon mattress sutures.

Postoperative Care

Blood pressure is maintained in the range of 120 to 140 mmHg with parenteral medications until oral intake becomes possible. Prophylactic antibiotics, initiated just prior to the initial skin incision, are used for 24 hours and are generally aimed at skin contaminants. Phenytoin is added for seizure prophylaxis.

Perioperative steroids are administered but quickly tapered in the absence of cerebral edema. One enteric-coated aspirin is administered daily as soon as the patient can tolerate oral intake. Vigorous pulmonary treatments are implemented as needed.

Patients are allowed out of bed the following day and are usually discharged within 7 to 10 days. Skin sutures are removed in 10 days. Tight dressings, oxygen masks, or eyeglasses that might compress the donor vessel are avoided throughout hospitalization.

POSTOPERATIVE COMPLICATIONS

Many complications that may accompany or follow EC-IC bypass are systemic disorders, including such conditions as gastrointestinal hemorrhage or

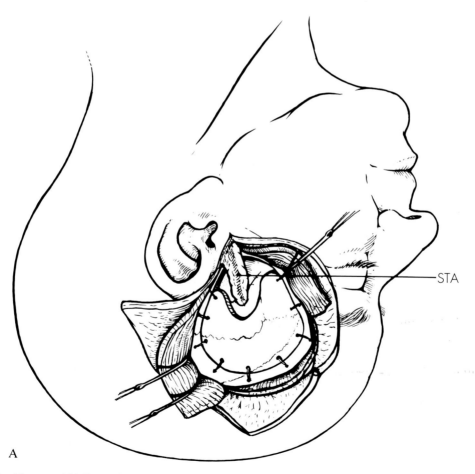

A

Figure 29-13. Closure. **(A)** Dura closed loosely around STA; dura then covered with large sheet of Gelfoam; bone flap replaced, with craniectomy inferiorly to allow STA passage. (*Figure continues.*)

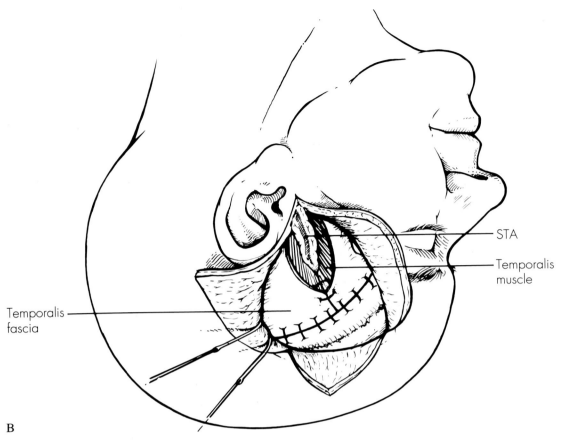

Figure 29-13 (*Continued*). **(B)** Temporalis fascia sutured peripherally to adjacent similar layer, temporalis muscle centrally, and loosely closed around STA to minimize CSF escape.

perforation, myocardial infarction, and pneumonia, such as may accompany any major surgical procedure. Sequential compression stockings are used routinely for prophylaxis of deep venous thrombosis and pulmonary embolism. If thrombosis or embolism should develop beyond the immediate postoperative period (3 to 4 days), the patient can be treated with an anticoagulant (heparin) if indicated. Prior to that time, a vena cava filter may be preferable.

Central nervous system (CNS) complications (Table 29-1) may occur early or late following the procedure, and each must receive prompt attention. Most can be avoided by careful patient selection, hydration and blood pressure maintenance, and meticulous attention to detail in the operating room.

Ischemia

Neurological deterioration in the postoperative period should be evaluated with an emergent CT scan to rule out hemorrhage. If none is identified, arteriog- raphy should be considered to assess graft patency, especially if the deficit is persistent. Poor perfusion secondary to graft thrombosis or insufficiency that does not respond to further hydration and blood pressure elevation may require emergent graft revision.

Conversion of an intracranial stenosis to occlusion may also precipitate acute neurological decline.[46,71,85] The incidence of this phenomenon can be greatly reduced by treating these patients medically for 3 to 6 months with major anticoagulants (heparin and coumadin) *prior* to surgical consideration.[56] Many "high-grade" lesions will resolve in that interval and can thereafter be treated with antiplatelet drugs without need for surgical intervention. Persistent high-grade obstructions may be less prone to embolize or clot off following medical treatment, which makes any subsequent surgical procedure safer. The more proximal placement of the anastomosis nearer the lenticulostriate origins appears to maximize perfusion to greater numbers of vessels and to minimize stagnation in the vessel segment just beyond the stenosis. If a deficit does develop secondary to proximal intracranial occlusion and the graft is patent, the patient is managed with hydration and blood pressure elevation. Symptoms developing at least 3 to 4 days after surgery may be treated with anticoagulants if necessary to minimize further thrombosis risks.

Most early postoperative deficits are transient and may be caused by seizures, dysautoregulation, or cerebral edema.[74,75] These problems are presumably precipitated by the redistribution of flow surrounding the anastomotic bed. Anticonvulsant levels and an EEG should be checked in questionable cases. Steroids are maintained at higher levels until the neurological deficit has largely resolved.

Late complications are mostly ischemic in nature. Continued control of systemic risk factors, particularly blood pressure control and avoidance of smoking, is necessary. Delayed cerebral infarction may be caused by graft thrombosis or compromise, conversion of an intracranial stenosis to an occlusion, progression of disease in the cervical carotid region, or embolization via the graft.[46,54,70,71,85] Patients are maintained on daily antiplatelet drugs indefinitely to minimize these possibilities.

Hemorrhage

Strict control of blood pressure is essential to prevent early postoperative hemorrhagic complications.[59,73] The incidence of bleeding is further lessened if placement of the anastomosis in a region of cystic encephalomalacia is avoided and if the procedure is delayed after a recent stroke. Reestablishment of higher flows to an ischemic (and poorly regulated) vascular bed can lead to perfusion pressure breakthrough bleeding, a phenomenon that occurs more commonly with high-flow vein grafts.[59,77,84,89]

Early bleeding may arise from the anastomosis site and is obviously best handled by prevention. Sutures should be placed close enough to make this problem exceedingly uncommon. The incidence of epidural or subdural hemorrhage can be reduced by meticulous intraoperative hemostasis, the use of epidural tack-up sutures, and reversal of heparin (when used) with protamine prior to closure. Surgical evacuation should be reserved for those hematomas causing a significant mass effect. Repeat bleeding may indicate a pseudoaneurysm at the anastomosis site and may prompt arteriography and revision.

Late bleeding may arise from anastomotic aneurysm formation and rupture or from other unidentified sources.[65,78] This occurrence requires arteriographic investigation, with subsequent intervention based on radiographic and clinical findings.

Fluid Collections

Fluid may accumulate in the subdural space or beneath the scalp and temporalis muscle, especially early after surgery. These collections generally contain both CSF and blood and will usually resolve with time. A tight wound may be tapped with a spinal needle aimed away from the vascular pedicle and directed in a plane superficial to the bone. Excessive decompression via a lumbar puncture may allow the brain to sag away from the inner table and jeopardize the integrity of the anastomotic line. Fluid collections are more common when heparin or a vein graft been used intraoperatively. In those instances, a subdural drain is left in for several days. A subdural shunt may be required for persistent cases.

Wound Healing Problems

Problems with wound healing include scalp necrosis, wound infection, and meningitis. The incidence of scalp necrosis is greatly reduced by using linear incisions directly over the STA, thereby avoiding a large flap whose principal blood supply has been removed.[82] The scalp is handled quite gently to avoid undue trauma to the relatively devascularized edges. The skin is closed with a single layer of mattress nylon suture, interrupted so as to avoid strangulating the edges between sutures and to allow individual suture removal if necessary to drain an infection. If scalp necrosis does develop, a vascularized scalp pedicle may need to be mobilized over the defect.

Meningitis may be sterile (hemogenic) or infectious and is managed with appropriate antibiotics. With superficial suppurations or meningitis, the bone flap is not removed unless the infection fails to respond to extended medical treatment.

REFERENCES

Carotid Endarterectomy

1. Barnett HPM, Plumb F, Walton JN: Carotid endarterectomy—an expression of concern. Stroke 15:941, 1984
2. Bove EL, Fry WJ, Gross WS, Stanley JC: Hypotension and hypertension as consequences of baroreceptor dysfunction following carotid endarterectomy. Surgery 85:663, 1979

3. Brott TG et al: Changes patterns in the practice of carotid endarterectomy in a large metropolitan area. JAMA 255:2609, 1986

4. Callow AD, Kaplan LR, Correll JW et al: Carotid endarterectomy: What is its current status? Am J Med 85:835, 1988

5. Canadian Cooperative Study Group: A randomized trial of aspirin and sulfinpyrazone and threatened stroke. N Engl J Med 299:53, 1978

6. Clinical Alert: Benefit of endarterectomy for patients with high-grade stenosis of the internal carotid artery. Ninds News Release, Feb. 27, 1991

7. Corson JD, Chang BB et al: The influence of anesthetic choice on carotid endarterectomy outcome. Arch Surg 122:807, 1987

8. Das MB, Hertzer NR, Ratliff NB et al: Recurrent carotid stenosis. A five-year series of 65 re-operations. Ann Surg 202:2875, 1985

8a. Deen HG, Sundt TM Jr: The effect of combined aspirin and dipyridamole therapy on thrombus formation in an arterial thrombogenic lesion in the dog. Stroke 13:179, 1982

8b. Dirrenberger RA, Sundt TM Jr: Carotid endarterectomy: temporal profile of the healing process and effects of anticoagulation therapy. J Neurosurg 48:201, 1978

9. Dyken ML: Carotid endarterectomy studies: A glimmering of science. Stroke 17:355, 1986

10. Dyken ML, Pokras R: The performance of endarterectomy for disease of the extracranial arteries of the head. Stroke 15:948, 1984

11. Edwards WH Jr et al: Recurrent carotid artery stenosis. Ann Surg 209:662, 1989

12. Evans WE, Mendelowitz DS, Liapisc et al: Motor speech deficit following carotid endarterectomy. Ann Surg 196:461, 1982

13. Ferguson R: Getting it right the first time. AJNR 1:875, 1990

14. Fields WS, Lemak NA, Frankowski RF: Control trial of aspirin and cerebral ischemia. Stroke 8:301, 1977

15. Fields WS, Masleni K, Myer JS et al: Joint Study of Extracranial Arterial Occlusion: V. Progress report of prognosis following surgery or non-surgical treatment for transient cerebral ischemic attacks and cervical carotid artery lesions. JAMA 211:1993, 1970

16. Fode NC, Sundt TM, Robertson JT et al: Multicenter retrospective review of results in complications of carotid endarterectomy in 1981. Stroke 17:370, 1986

17. Gabelman CG, Gann DS, Ashworth CJ, Carney WI: 100 consecutive carotid reconstructions: Local versus general anesthesia. Am J Surg 145:477, 1983

18. Hass WK, Eastin JD, Adams HP et al: A randomized trial comparing ticlopidine hydrochloride with aspirin for the prevention of stroke in high-risk patients. N Engl J Med 321:501, 1989

19. Hertzer NR: Presidential Address: Carotid endarterectomy—A crisis in confidence. J Vasc Surg 7:611, 1988

20. Hertzer NR et al: A prospective study of vein patch angioplasty during carotid endarterectomy. 3 yr. results for 801 patients in 917 operations. Ann Surg 206:628, 1987

21. Hertzer NR, Feldman BJ, Beven EG, Tucker HM: A prospective study of the incidence of injury to the cranial nerves during carotid endarterectomy. Surg Gynecol Obstet 151:781, 1980

22. Jones CE: Carotid eversion endarterectomy revisited. Am J Surg 157:323, 1989

23. Lusby RJ, Wylie EJ: Complications of carotid endarterectomy. Surg Clin North Am 63:1293, 1983

24. Merrick NJ, Fink A, Park RE, Brook RH: Derivation of clinical indications for carotid endarterectomy by an expert panel. Am J Public Health 77:187, 1987

25. Meyer FB, Sundt TM Jr, Piepgras DG et al: Emergency carotid endarterectomy for patients with acute carotid occlusion and profound neurologic deficits. Ann Surg 203:A2, 1986

26. North American Symptomatic Carotid Endarterectomy Study Group: Carotid endarterectomy: Three critical evaluations. Stroke 18:987, 1987

26a. North American Symptomatic Carotid Endarterectomy Trial Collaborators: Beneficial effect of carotid endarterectomy in symptomatic patients with high-grade carotid stenosis. N Engl J Med 325:711, 1991

27. Ojemann RG, Crowell RM: Cerebral Management of Cerebral Vascular Disease. Williams & Wilkins, Baltimore, 1983

28. Robertson JT, Auer NJ: Extracranial occlusive disease with carotid artery. p. 1559. In Youmans JR (ed): Neurological Surgery. Vol. 3. WB Saunders, Philadelphia, 1982

29. Sebul RD, Whisnant JP: Indications for carotid endarterectomy. Ann Intern Med 111:675, 1989

30. Spetzler RF: Internal carotid artery occlusion. (in preparation)

31. Spetzler RF et al: Microsurgical endarterectomy under barbiturate protection: A prospective study. J Neurosurg 65:63, 1986

32. Sundt TM Jr: Occlusive Cerebral Vascular Disease: Diagnosis and Surgical Management. WB Saunders, Philadelphia, 1987

33. Sundt TM Jr et al: The risk-benefit ratio of intraoperative shunting during carotid endarterectomy. Relevancy to operative and post-operative results in complications. Ann Surg 203:196, 1986

34. Sundt TM Jr, Sandok BA, Whisnant JP: Carotid endarterectomy complications and pre-operative assessment of risk. Mayo Clin Proc 50:301, 1975

35. The EC/IC Bypass Study Group: Failure of extracranial-intracranial bypass to reduce the risk of ischemic stroke. N Engl J Med 313:1191, 1985

36. Theron J et al: New triple coaxial catheter system for carotid angioplasty with cerebral protection. AJNR 11:869, 1990

37. Till JS, Toole F et al: Declining morbidity and mortality carotid endarterectomy. Stroke 18:823, 1987

38. Toole JF: The Asymptomatic Carotid Atherosclerosis Study. U.S. Public Health Service Grant, NINCDS-NS 22611, 1987

39. United Kingdom Transient Ischemic Attack Study Group. United Kingdom Transient Ischemic Attack Aspirin Trial: Interim results. Br Med J 296:316, 1988

40. Wardlow C: Carotid endarterectomy: Does it work? Stroke 15:1068, 1984

41. Whisnant JP, Fisher L, Robertson JT, Scheinberg P: Carotid endarterectomy decreased stroke and death in patients with transient ischemic attacks. Ann Neurol 22:72, 1987

42. Whisnant JP, Sandok BA, Sundt TM Jr: Carotid endarterectomy for unilateral carotid system transient cerebral ischemia. Mayo Clin Proc 58:171, 1983

43. Winslow CM et al: The appropriateness of carotid endarterectomy. N Engl J Med 318:721, 1988

44. Winslow CM, Solomon DH, Chassin MR et al: The appropriateness of carotid endarterectomy. N Engl J Med 318:721, 1988

Cerebral Revascularization

45. Ausman JI, Diaz FG: Critique of the extracranial-intracranial bypass study. Surg Neurol 26:218, 1986

46. Awad IA, Furlan AJ, Little JR: Changes in intracranial stenotic lesions after extracranial-intracranial bypass surgery. J Neurosurg 60:614, 1985

47. Awad IA, Spetzler RF: Extracranial bypass surgery: A critical analysis in light of the International Cooperative Study. Neurosurgery 19:655, 1986

48. Barnett HJM, Fox A, Hachinski V et al: Further conclusions from the extracranial-intracranial bypass trial. Surg Neurol 26:227, 1986

49. Barnett HJM, Sackett D, Taylor DW et al: Are the results of the extracranial-intracranial bypass trial generalizable? N Engl J Med 316:820, 1987

50. Batjer HH, Devous MD Sr, Purdy PD et al: Improvement in regional cerebral blood flow and cerebral vasoreactivity after extracranial-intracranial arterial bypass. Neurosurgery 22:913, 1988

51. Batjer H, Mickey B, Samson D: Potential roles for early revascularization in patients with acute cerebral ischemia. Neurosurgery 18:283, 1986

52. Chater NL: Neurosurgical extracranial-intracranial bypass for stroke: With 400 case. Neurol Res 5:1, 1983

53. Collice M, Arena O, Erminio F, Riva M: Surgical and long-term results in 100 consecutive patients with ICA occlusion. p. 445. In Spetzler RF, Carter LP, Selman WR, Martin N (eds): Cerebral Revascularization for Stroke. Thieme-Stratton, New York, 1985

54. Conley FK: Embolization of a superficial temporal artery to middle cerebral artery bypass: Case report. Neurosurgery 12:342, 1983

55. Crowell RM: Emergency cerebral revascularization. Clin Neurosurg 33:281, 1986

56. Day AL: Indications for surgical intervention in middle cerebral artery obstruction. J Neurosurg 60:296, 1984

57. Day AL, Rhoton AL, Little JR: The extracranial-intracranial bypass study. Surg Neurol 26:222, 1986

58. Diaz FG, Ausman JI, Mehta B et al: Acute cerebral revascularization. J Neurosurg 63:200, 1985

59. Diaz FG, Pearce J, Ausman JI: Complications of cerebral revascularization with autogenous vein grafts. Neurosurgery 17:271, 1985

60. Diaz FG, Umansky F, Mehta B, Montoya S: Cerebral revascularization to a main limb of the middle cerebral artery in the sylvian fissure. An alternative approach to conventional anastomosis. J Neurosurg 63:21, 1985

61. Donaghy RMP: Patch and by-pass in microangeional surgery. p. 75. In Donaghy RMP, Yasargil MG (eds): Microvascular Surgery. CV Mosby, St. Louis, 1967

62. EC-IC Bypass Study Group: Failure of extracranial-intracranial arterial bypass to reduce the risk of ischemic stroke. N Engl J Med 313:1191, 1985

63. EC-IC Bypass Study Group: The international cooperative study of extracranial-intracranial arterial anastomosis (EC-IC bypass study): Methodology and entry characteristics. Stroke 16:397, 1985

64. Eguchi T: Results of EC-IC bypass with and without long vein graft. p. 584. In Spetzler RF, Carter LP, Selman WR, Martin N (eds): Cerebral Revascularization for Stroke. Thieme-Stratton, New York, 1985

65. Fein JM: Bypass induced cerebral aneurysm. Neurol Res 7:46, 1985

66. Fisher CM: Occlusion of the internal carotid artery. Arch Neurol Psychiatry 65:340, 1951

67. Gagliardi R, Benvenuti L, Onesti S: Seven years experience with extracranial-intracranial arterial bypass for cerebral ischemia. p. 413. In Spetzler NF, Carter LP, Selman WR, Martin N (eds): Cerebral Revascularization for Stroke. Thieme-Stratton, New York, 1985

68. Goldring S, Zervas N, Langfitt T: The extracranial-intracranial bypass study. A report of the committee appointed by the American Association of Neurological Surgeons to examine the study. N Engl J Med 316:817, 1987

69. Gratzl O, Roun J: Quality grading of bypass surgery. Operative combined risks less than 4 percent. p. 467. In Spetzler RF, Carter LP, Selman WR, Martin N (eds): Cerebral Revascularization for Stroke. Thieme-Stratton, New York, 1985

70. Gumerlock MK, Coull BM, Howieson J et al: Late stenosis of a superficial temporal-middle cerebral artery bypass: Angiographic and histologic findings. Neurosurgery 16:650, 1985

71. Gumerlock MK, Ono H, Neuwelt EA: Can a patent extracranial-intracranial bypass provoke the conversion of an intracranial arterial stenosis to a symptomatic occlusion? Neurosurgery 12:391, 1983

72. Gur D, Yonas H: Extracranial-intracranial arterial bypass. N Engl J Med 314:1192, 1986

73. Heros RC, Nelson PB: Intracerebral hemorrhage after microsurgical cerebral revascularization. Neurosurgery 6:371, 1980

74. Heros RC, Scott RM, Kistler JP et al: Temporary neurologic deterioration after extracranial-intracranial bypass. Neurosurgery 15:178, 1984

75. Kanter SL, Day AL, Heilman KM, Gonzalez-Rothi LJ: Pure word deafness: A possible explanation of transient deteriorations after extracranial-intracranial bypass grafting. Neurosurgery 18:186, 1986

76. Little JR, Furlan AJ, Bryerton B: Short vein grafts of cerebral revascularization. J Neurosurg 59:384, 1983

77. Marano SR, Spetzler RF: Vein interposition grafts for

anterior circulation ischemia. p. 591. In Spetzler RF, Carter LP, Selman WR, Martin N (eds): Cerebral Revascularization for Stroke. Thieme-Stratton, New York, 1985

78. Parent AD, Smith RR: Traumatic aneurysm complicating EC-IC bypass: successful surgical clipping. Surg Neurol 15:229, 1981

79. Pearce J, Diaz FG, Ausman JI et al: Saphenous vein grafts in neurovascular surgery: Their value and limitations. p. 372. In Spetzler RF, Carter LP, Selman WR, Martin N (eds): Cerebral Revascularization for Stroke. Thieme-Stratton, New York, 1985

80. Peerless SJ: Indications for extracranial-intracranial arterial bypass in light of the EC/IC bypass study. Clin Neurosurg 33:307, 1986

81. Reale F, Benericetti E, Benvenuti L et al: Extracranial-intracranial arterial bypass in typical carotid reversible ischemic deficits: Long-term follow-up in 100 patients. Neurol Res 6:113, 1984

82. Reichman OH: Complications of cerebral revascularization. Clin Neurosurg 23:318, 1976

83. Relman AS: The extracranial-intracranial arterial bypass study. What have we learned? editorial N Engl J Med 316:809, 1987

84. Samson DS, Gewertz BL, Beyer CW, Hodosh RM: Saphenous vein interposition grafts in the microsurgical treatment of cerebral ischemia. Arch Surg 116:1578, 1981

85. Scott RM, Pessin MS, Wolpert SM: Intracranial internal carotid artery stenosis: Occlusion following cerebral bypass surgery. p. 514. In Spetzler RF, Carter LP, Selman WR, Martin N (eds): Cerebral Revascularization for Stroke. Thieme-Stratton, New York, 1985

86. Spetzler RF, Marano SR: Vein interposition grafts for anterior circulation ischemia. p. 201. In Erickson DL (ed): Cerebral Revascularization. Futura, Mt. Kisco, NY, 1988

87. Sundt TM Jr: Was the international randomized trial of extracranial-intracranial arterial bypass representative of the population at risk? N Engl J Med 316:814, 1987

88. Sundt TM Jr, Fode NC, Jack CR Jr: The past, present and future of extracranial to intracranial bypass surgery. Clin Neurosurg 34:134, 1988

89. Sundt TM Jr, Piepgras DG, Marsh WR, Fode NC: Saphenous vein bypass grafts for giant aneurysms and intracranial occlusive disease. J Neurosurg 65:439, 1986

90. Sundt TM Jr, Whisnant JP, Fode NC et al: Results, complications and follow-up of 415 bypass operations for occlusive disease of the carotid system. Mayo Clin Proc 60:230, 1985

91. Sundt TM III, Sundt TM Jr: Principles of preparation of vein bypass grafts to maximize patency. J Neurosurg 66:172, 1987

92. Weinstein PR, Baena RY, Chater NL: Outcome after extracranial-intracranial arterial bypass for internal carotid artery stenosis. p. 440. In Spetzler RF, Carter LP, Selman WR, Martin N (eds): Cerebral Revascularization for Stroke. Thieme-Stratton, New York, 1985

93. Whisnant JP, Sundt TM Jr, Fode NC: Long-term mortality and stroke morbidity after superficial temporal artery–middle cerebral artery bypass operation. Mayo Clin Proc 60:241, 1985

94. Yasargil MG: Diagnosis and indications for operations in cerebrovascular occlusive diseases. p. 95. In Yasargil MG (ed): Microsurgery Applied to Neurosurgery. Thieme, Stuttgart, 1969

95. Yasargil MG, Krayenbuhl HA, Jacobson JH II: Microsurgical arterial reconstruction. Surgery 67:221, 1970

96. Yasargil MG, Yonekawa Y: Results of microsurgical extra-intracranial arterial bypass in the treatment of cerebral ischemia. Neurosurgery 1:22, 1977

30 Aneurysmal Lesions

Anterior Circle of Willis

Intracavernous Carotid Artery Aneurysms

Takanori Fukushima

John Day

Howard Tung

For many years, direct operative attack on lesions within the cavernous sinus has been regarded as extremely risky with little likelihood of success. Uncontrollable, excessive bleeding, postoperative cranial nerve deficits, and potential damage to the intracavernous carotid artery have been effective deterrents to widespread attempts at entering what has been considered the last "no man's land" in neurological surgery. References are abundant in the literature of the first half of the twentieth century regarding surgical strategies for dealing with carotid-cavernous fistulas.[4,5,21,23,24] In a 1937 article, Walter E. Dandy[5] wrote about various techniques of carotid ligation and trapping procedures for the treatment of "carotid-cavernous aneurysms" clinically demonstrated by pulsating exophthalmos. We now know that he was referring to carotid-cavernous fistulas and not the saccular aneurysms discussed in the following pages. In that same year, Browder[4] was the first to report the successful direct approach to the cavernous sinus. He obliterated a carotid-cavernous fistula by packing muscle through an incision in the roof of the cavernous sinus. Before 1960, several authors published their methods of dealing with vascular lesions of the cavernous sinus, none of which included a direct surgical approach to the intracavernous carotid artery.[21,23,24]

The neurosurgical literature was devoid of reference to a successful direct approach to the region until 1965. In that year, Parkinson[33] reported his successful direct repair of a traumatic carotid-cavernous fistula under the anesthetic conditions of hypothermia and cardiac arrest. In the 1970s, development of newer invasive radiological techniques, including detachable balloon catheters, quieted wide enthusiasm for direct operative attack of intracavernous vascular lesions. Later in the same decade and into the 1980s, renewed interest in the definition of the microsurgical anatomy of the region provided the necessary knowledge for several individuals to approach lesions of the cavernous sinus successfully under conventional anesthetic conditions, without hypothermia and cardiac arrest.[8–10,14,16,19,20,22,27,28,32,33,41–43,52] In particular, Dolenc[8,9] should be recognized for his important development of a combined epidural and subdural approach to the cavernous sinus and his success with clipping intracavernous carotid artery aneurysms.

Following Dolenc, other neurosurgeons, including the senior author, have reported their favorable results for various vascular and neoplastic cavernous sinus lesions.[1,6,7,29,30,44] This chapter presents an overview of direct operative attack on aneurysms of the cavernous sinus, including the senior author's personal series of cavernous carotid vascular lesions. Throughout this discussion, special attention is paid to the avoidance of complications.

OPERATIVE SERIES TO DATE

Aside from an isolated case report in 1979 by Johnston[25] of direct attack on bilateral intracavernous aneurysms using Parkinson's approach, Dolenc[8] in 1983 published the first series of intracavernous aneurysms obliterated directly through an intracavernous approach. Several other authors' experiences using Dolenc's technique have been published since his landmark article.[6,7,19,30,50] These series are outlined in Table 30-1, with emphasis on the major complications encountered.

Between 1984 and 1991, the senior author has accumulated an experience in intracavernous aneurysm surgery encompassing 79 cases. Table 30-2 outlines the complications encountered. In 70 percent of the cases, temporary third, fourth, and sixth cranial nerve deficits, singly or in combination, were observed. The temporary palsies resolved in the following 3 to 6 months, similar to cases reported by Hakuba et al.[19] In three cases of direct clipping, unpleasant trigeminal distribution dysesthesias were noted postoperatively. In three cases, permanent diplopia resulted from third nerve damage in two patients and from sixth nerve damage in one patient.

Early in this experience, exposure of the petrous internal carotid resulted in total deafness in two patients secondary to cochlear damage from drilling through the overlying bone. Blindness resulted in two cases of siphon-C_4 aneurysms and in one case utilizing a saphenous vein bypass. The precise cause of optic nerve impairment remains undetermined. Two cases suffered cerebrospinal fluid (CSF) leaks through the sphenoid sinus, necessitating transsphe-

Table 30-2. Permanent Complications of Direct Surgery of Cavernous Sinus Vascular Lesions (79 Cases)

Complication	No. of Cases
Trigeminal facial dysesthesia	3
Diplopia (III, VI)	3
Deafness	2
Blindness	3
Visual field defect	2
Hemiplegia	1
Hemiparesis	2
CSF leak	2
Epidural hematoma	1
Contralateral cerebellar hemorrhage	1
Mortality	0

noidal packing. Two patients who were treated with the Fukushima saphenous vein bypass procedure suffered moderate postoperative hemiparesis, the first from unknown etiology and the second due to acute graft occlusion. One patient who underwent direct clip ligation of a C_4 aneurysm suffered a temporary hemiparesis of unknown cause, probably an embolic event. Another patient who suffered a mild hemiparesis, probably secondary to an embolic event, had a carotid-cavernous fistula of the dural arteriovenous malformation (AVM) type that was successfully eliminated via direct obliteration. The postoperative use of heparin contributed to a contralateral cerebellar hemorrhage in one patient, and another patient suffered an ipsilateral epidural hematoma.

Table 30-1. Reported Complications of Directly Approached Intracavernous Vascular Lesions

Author	Year	No. of Cases	Complications
Dolenc[8]	1983	7 (3 aneurysms, 4 carotid-cavernous fistulas)	Persistent hemiparesis and dysphasia Death secondary to sepsis Death secondary to pulmonary embolus at 10 days Hemiparesis 1 week postoperative, improved at 1 year follow-up
Hakuba et al.[20]	1989	3 (1 giant aneurysm, 2 carotid-cavernous fistulas)	Third nerve palsy in all patients that resolved in 3 to 4 months
Diaz[7]	1989	15 (all aneurysms)	Death secondary to intraoperative IVH Optic nerve infarct in two cases Sepsis
Sundt[50]	1990	2 (both aneurysms)	No new deficits
Linskey et al.[30]	1991	8 (all aneurysms)[a]	Visual deficit, partial third nerve palsy Field cut, Horner's syndrome Partial third nerve palsy, putamen infarct Partial third and fifth palsies, decreased lacrimation, watershed zone cerebral infarcts Partial third nerve palsy, small frontal infarct

[a] Of these eight cases, four were ligated by clipping, two underwent aneurysmorrhaphy, and two were bypassed.

PREOPERATIVE MANAGEMENT

Indications

The pioneering work of the abovenamed individuals and various technical advances have allowed the development of a management strategy for intracavernous aneurysms that encompasses several options. Indirect surgical therapies have traditionally played a primary role in the approach to these lesions.[3,11,15,21,23,46] Technological development of endovascular techniques with precision-directed catheters and detachable balloons have further expanded the surgical armamentarium.[2,13] In the 1990s, with proper preparation of the patient, surgeon, and operating room team, direct surgical attack on intracavernous vascular lesions is a viable option. The indications for direct approaches to asymptomatic intracavernous aneurysms have been a matter of controversy.[29,30] Clearly, in the case of observed enlargement of such a lesion radiographically, delay in treatment is not justified considering current abilities. Many aneurysms can lie quiescent for years and then suddenly begin enlarging with a resultant hemorrhage. It is our opinion that asymptomatic intracavernous aneurysms should be considered the equivalent of their intradural counterparts and be obliterated if the intricate maneuvers later outlined can be performed.

Preoperative Preparation

All patients should undergo a routine general medical examination, including routine preoperative laboratory studies to identify intercurrent systemic illness. A careful neurological examination, accurately documented, is very important to allow precise determination of postoperative improvement or morbidity. A full radiological work-up is imperative to image the offending lesion adequately and to develop surgical strategy.

Angiography remains the "gold standard" for complete definition of the vascular anatomy involved. At the time of angiography, the adequacy of collateral circulation should be ascertained utilizing various compression studies or a balloon occlusion test. A management strategy has been proposed by several authors based on the results of angiographic studies.[30,44] It is obviously important to determine the adequacy of collateral flow prior to the use of temporary clips or to performing any bypass procedure. Magnetic resonance imaging (MRI) with selective views of the cavernous sinus area is an important adjunct in preoperative observation of the alterations in normal cavernous sinus anatomy induced by the lesion. It is possible that the development of techniques using MRI will replace conventional angiography, obviating the need for an invasive radiological procedure.

Medications that are given prior to surgery include anticonvulsants, corticosteroids, and calcium channel blockers in the event of subarachnoid hemorrhage. All patients are started on dilantin, with the goal in mind of attaining a therapeutic level prior to the procedure. This is not critical, however, and patients may be started just prior to induction of general anesthesia with an intravenous loading dose of 15 mg/kg. Patients suffering a subarachnoid hemorrhage are given nimodipine (60 mg PO q4h) from the time of diagnosis until a 21 day course is complete. Subarachnoid hemorrhage patients as well are started on high-dose corticosteroids at the time of diagnosis as a protective measure against ischemia secondary to re-rupture or vasospasm. Elective surgery patients typically receive their initial dose of steroids in the operating suite prior to anesthetic induction. Perioperative antibiotics are routinely utilized. Prophylaxis against the gastrointestinal complications of steroids is strictly practiced with the use of H_2 blockers and antacids. Sequential pneumatic compression boots are applied and their function initiated in the operating room.

OPERATIVE MANAGEMENT

Microsurgical Anatomy

In reducing surgical morbidity, the importance of the individual surgeon's grasp of the detailed surgical anatomy of this region cannot be overemphasized. To operate in this area, conventional anatomical description and dissection are not enough. A clear understanding of the multiple entry points into the cavernous sinus, as outlined below, is fundamental to any successful direct approach.

The cavernous sinus (Fig. 30-1) is located on either side of the sella turcica at the convergence of the anterior base, middle fossa, sphenoid ridge, and petroclival ridge (the "four corners" of cranial base surgery). It is a small, tetrahedron-shaped space, occupying approximately 1 cm³ that is bounded by the leaves of the dura mater on all sides. The floor and most of the medial wall are covered by the periosteal layer, while the roof, lateral wall, and upper medial wall are covered by the dural layer. The space contains a heavy venous plexus with communications to

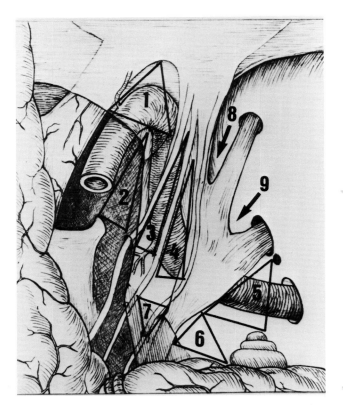

Figure 30-1. The cavernous sinus microsurgical anatomical triangles (triangles 1 through 9).

the ophthalmic veins, the pterygoid plexus, the superior and inferior petrosal sinuses, the central retinal vein, and the middle and inferior cerebral veins. The internal carotid artery and cranial nerves III, IV, V, and VI in their individual courses make their way through the cavernous sinus. The reader is referred to several excellent detailed discussions on the anatomy of the cavernous sinus.[1,16,22,33,43,52,53,54] Through the course of this discussion we will refer to the segments of the internal carotid artery as described by Fischer.[12]

Safe entry into the cavernous sinus may be achieved through 11 triangular-shaped corridors. Figure 30-1 illustrates these areas as viewed from the cranial base.

Anterior (Triangle 1)

The anterior triangle area is defined by the lateral border of the extradural optic nerve, the medial wall of the superior orbital fissure dura, and the dural ring surrounding the internal carotid artery as it courses intradurally.[8–10] This is an epidural space that contains the distal genu of the internal carotid artery (C_3

segment). There is a thin, fibrous membrane over the C_3 carotid, which is the true anteromedial cavernous membrane. Most of the proximal internal carotid, paraclinoid, infraclinoid, and ophthalmic aneurysms can be clipped safely by opening this triangular space alone.

Medial (Triangle 2)

The siphon angle, lateral wall of the intradural internal carotid, posterior clinoid process, and porus oculomotorius delineate the medial triangular space.[10,20] By incising the dura of this triangle, the proximal siphon and horizontal segment of the cavernous carotid artery (C_4) can be well exposed. Most aneurysms of the C_4 segment, carotid-cavernous fistulas, and intracavernous tumors can be exposed through this route.

Superior (Triangle 3)   *oculomotor*

The superior triangle is bounded by the third and fourth cranial nerves laterally, with its posterior margin being the crest of dura at the transition from middle to posterior fossa.[14] This triangle is most suitable for exposure of the C_4-C_5 junction, the usual location of the origin of the meningohypophyseal trunk.

Lateral (Triangle 4)

The lateral (Parkinson's) triangle is a very narrow space bounded by the fourth cranial nerve and the ophthalmic division of the trigeminal nerve. This is the original triangle described by Parkinson[33,34] for entry into the cavernous sinus, and the area is most suitable for access to the ascending C_5 segment of the internal carotid artery.

Posterolateral (Triangle 5)   *Glasscock*

The posterolateral triangle is defined by the posterior rim of the foramen ovale, foramen spinosum, the posterior border of the mandibular division of the trigeminal nerve, and the cochlear apex.[10,17,18] Removal of the bone in this triangle, drilling from the area of the foramen spinosum and continuing medially along the posterior border of the trigeminal mandibular branch, exposes the proximal C_5 segment or the horizontal intrapetrous internal carotid artery. This exposure is for obtaining proximal control of the internal carotid with temporary occlusion in the repair of intracavernous carotid lesions. This segment of the internal carotid is also exposed for the cavernous carotid bypass procedure originally developed by the senior author in 1986.[14]

Posteromedial (Triangle 6) Kawase

The porus trigeminus, cochlea, and posterior border of the mandibular division of the fifth cranial nerve to the posterior apex of the posterolateral triangle define the posteromedial triangle.[26] This triangle was initially described by Kawase et al.[26] and exactly corresponds to the free petrous apex. This portion of the petrous bone contains neither neural nor vascular structures and therefore may be safely drilled away for access to the upper brainstem and root of the trigeminal nerve.

Posteroinferior (Triangle 7)

The posteroinferior triangle is bounded by the fourth cranial nerve, the posterior clinoid process, and the medial porus trigeminus. An incision in this area carried down from the petroclival ligament to the petrosphenoidal ligament (Gruber's ligament) will expose the sixth cranial nerve in Dorello's canal and the distal C_5 segment.

Anterolateral (Triangle 8)

The anterolateral triangle is the area between the ophthalmic and maxillary divisions of the fifth cranial nerve extending anteriorly to a line from the superior orbital fissure to the foramen rotundum.[32] This triangle is used for exposing the superior orbital vein. It is also opened to expose the anterolateral extension of tumors within the cavernous sinus.

Lateralmost (Triangle 9)

Between the foramen rotundum and the foramen ovale a triangle can be defined that is bounded by the second and third divisions of the trigeminal nerve. This is also an area opened for exposure of lateral extensions of cavernous sinus tumors.

Anterior Tip of the Cavernous Sinus

Through the anterior transbasal approach, the apical portion of the cavernous sinus may be exposed. This approach allows bilateral access to the genu of the carotid siphon and the C_4 segment, obtaining a different angle of view compared with approaches through other triangles.

Backside of the Cavernous Sinus

An extended transsphenoidal approach will gain access to the posteroinferior aspect of the cavernous sinus from the underside. Wide removal of the sellar floor toward the carotid eminence will bilaterally expose the C_4 segment from the medial side. Control of cavernous bleeding will be accomplished with careful packing with Surgicel. This exposure is useful in cases of pituitary adenomatous invasion of the cavernous sinus.

Summary

A detailed knowledge of conventional cavernous sinus anatomy, although useful, is inadequate as a basis for attempting a direct attack on intracavernous lesions. Full understanding of the microsurgical anatomy outlined above, as well as precise incision and dissection of these anatomical triangles are crucial to the success of intracavernous microsurgery. Additionally, meticulous attention to hemostasis using monopolar and bipolar coagulation and packing with Surgicel must be maintained. Although Surgicel is very useful, care must be taken to avoid excess packing, which can cause vascular and neural compression with their attendant consequences. The S-shaped course of the intracavernous carotid must be carefully dissected and followed without damage to the vessel wall. All cranial nerves must be meticulously dissected and preserved with a minimum of traction. Because of the complicated anatomy involved and the difficulty with hemostasis, the extremes in microsurgical technique and anatomical knowledge are integral to approaching this delicate area with minimal resultant morbidity.

Operative Procedure

Routine general endotracheal anesthesia is used for all patients, and all patients should be pretreated with anticonvulsant medication and receive dexamethasone pre- and intraoperatively. For adequate intraoperative brain relaxation a lumbar drain may be placed for CSF drainage. Hyperventilation and osmotic agents are also routinely used. In selected patients with preoperative angiographic demonstration of poor collateral circulation, barbiturates are employed for cerebral protection.[47,48] We recommend the routine use of intraoperative electrophysiological monitoring. Cortical cerebral blood flow, electroencephalography (EEG), somatosensory evoked potentials, visual evoked potentials, and brainstem auditory evoked potentials may all be used to provide intraoperative warning of impending cerebral injury. A system monitoring brain retractor pressure is also advocated to reduce retractor-induced cortical injury. A portable C-arm should also be readily available for the occasional use of intraoperative digital subtraction angiography (DSA).

The patient is placed on the operating table in the supine position with the head elevated from 15 to 30 degrees. The head is fixed by three-point fixation in the Mayfield headrest and is rotated away from the side of the lesion 15 to 20 degrees (Fig. 30-2). In addition to the routine preparation for a frontotemporal craniotomy, the neck may be prepared in the same operative field in case proximal control of the cervical internal carotid artery is required. The scalp and temporalis muscle are elevated in a single flap and are retracted anteriorly with the use of several large blunt scalp hooks. Usually, two small pediatric burr holes are placed, one over the pterion and the second posteriorly (Fig. 30-2). The overlying pericranium and a posterior section of the temporalis muscle is harvested for later use in dural closure and packing of the skull base. In principle, the combined epi- and subdural exposure of the frontotemporal region, as described originally by Dolenc,[8,9] is performed.

An extradural approach to the anterior clinoid is first made, identifying the foramen rotundum and foramen ovale in the process. This initial extradural approach is made except in the cases of internal carotid (IC) ophthalmic, infraclinoidal, and paraclinoidal aneurysms. In these aneurysms it is often only necessary to open the anterior or the medial triangle. Therefore, immediate intradural exposure of the cavernous sinus is adequate for visualization and clip ligation of these aneurysms.

The most important anatomical triangle is Dolenc's anterior cavernous triangle. By removing the anterior clinoid process widely and reducing the optic strut, the anterior cavernous triangle is easily exposed. Exposure of this triangle is adequate for handling the majority of proximal internal carotid, ophthalmic, and siphon aneurysms. Clipping of these aneurysms will often require the slight mobilization of the optic nerve that is compressing the dome of the aneurysm. This is accomplished by complete skeletonization of the optic canal with the use of a high-speed drill cooled by constant irrigation. Various sizes of diamond burrs will be required for precise drilling in this area. Extremely secure and gentle drilling is required to avoid damage to any neural or vascular structures. An important technical point, which should be generally practiced, is to drill only until a thin shell of cortical bone remains and then complete the removal with a fine dissector. When reducing the optic strut, it is possible to enter the posterior ethmoid sinus or the sphenoid sinus medially if adequate care is not exercised. If this occurs, it is important to take the necessary steps to avoid a postoperative CSF leak by proper obliteration of the opening with muscle and fibrin glue. A further surgical maneuver that is important in this approach to the anterior triangle is the incision of Pernezky's fibrous ring.[41,42] This fibrous structure should be fully incised from its dorsal to inferior extent, which will allow mobilization of the proximal internal carotid segment, thus facilitating dissection of the ophthalmic artery and the aneurysm.

After completing the extradural dissection, including removal of the lesser sphenoid wing and anterior clinoid process, the surgeon is ready for the intradural approach. The dura is incised in a sort of inverted T, based anteriorly, which creates two flaps that are retracted forward. The incision is much the same as that done in any routine frontotemporal approach with an extension directed along the dura covering the lesser sphenoid ring. The sylvian fissure is dissected to open approximately the anterior 2 to 3 cm. The consequences of interrupting venous drainage through the large sylvian veins can be devastating.

Once the sylvian fissure dissection is completed the lumbar drain is opened to facilitate gentle retraction of the brain. A self-retaining retractor system is utilized to retract the temporal lobe gently inferior

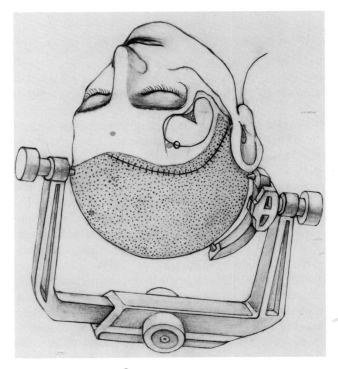

Figure 30-2. The points of pin fixation, incision, and bone flap used for direct access to intracavernous vascular lesions.

and laterally. The frontal lobe is gently retracted superomedially. Some authors have advocated the use of a temporal tip lobectomy to broaden the operative corridor without excess temporal lobe retraction.[44] The senior author, however, has not found this to be necessary in his extensive experience with these lesions. The olfactory tract can easily be identified medially and followed posteriorly to the optic nerve. In the region of the optic nerve and the ophthalmic segment of the internal carotid, the arachnoid is incised. Dissection proceeds posteriorly to the tentorial edge, where the third and fourth cranial nerves are identified. Identification of the dural penetration points of these two nerves is key to proper recognition of the triangles that are dissected to expose the intracavernous carotid artery. The medial, superior, and lateral triangles are all recognizable with identification of these two nerves. By incising the outer dural membrane the third and fourth cranial nerves may be exposed from their dural entrance points to the superior orbital fissure. The nerves are mobilized, maintaining their positions in the inner dural membrane, and are protected by cottonoids. It is preferable to use a thinner and softer composition of cottonoid than that generally commercially available. We favor a special soft cottonoid developed especially for protecting such delicate anatomical structures (Fukushima cottonoids, Kawamota Corp., Japan; American Silk Sutures, Lynn, MA). With accurate dissection of these triangles, aneurysms of the C_4 segment, as well as carotid-cavernous fistulas, can be approached.

One of the fundamental tenets of cerebral aneurysm surgery is the acquisition of proximal and distal control of the involved segment. In most intracavernous aneurysm surgeries involving the siphon, C_4, or C_5 segments, this may be attained with exposure of the intrapetrous internal carotid artery. Unroofing of the carotid canal is accomplished by drilling away the posterolateral (Glasscock's) triangle through an extradural approach.[8,10] Great care must be taken to preserve the cochlea, tensor tympani muscle, and eustachian tube in this exposure.[14] Additionally, one will observe that as the carotid is exposed, moving laterally, the investment of a thick periosteal adventitia thins to a more usual density of adventitial covering. It is important to maintain this thick covering, as its removal will compromise the postoperative integrity of the vessel. Furthermore, in all manipulations of the carotid, it is imperative that extraordinary care be exercised. Reports of postoperative fusiform aneurysms of the carotid developing secondary to surgical manipulation are not unknown to the literature.[52] With completion of this maneuver, the carotid is available for application of temporary clips and

for anastomosis of a saphenous vein graft in the Fukushima bypass procedure.[14,49] In cases of proximal internal carotid, ophthalmic, paraclinoidal, and supraclinoidal aneurysms, proximal control may be obtained by exposure of the extradural internal carotid siphon in the anterior triangle. A temporary clip may be applied here if necessary. If aneurysmal rupture occurs prior to or during the exposure of the proximal artery, compression of the cervical carotid artery will in most cases prove adequate.

With the acquisition of proximal and distal control and completed dissection of the aneurysm, clip ligation of the aneurysm is performed. The basic principles of circumferential definition of the aneurysm neck, visual identification of all perforators, and maintenance of parent vessel patency should be strictly applied. All manner of clip shapes and sizes should be readily available. The surgeon must be prepared to maximize his creative faculties in devising an optimal clip configuration. It is not uncommon in the senior author's experience that multiple clips and booster clips are necessary for adequate ligation. When temporary clips are applied, and in the bypass procedure, brain protection through the use of barbiturates should be practiced. The proper sequential release of temporary clips will avoid complications secondary to air and clot emboli. Intraoperative digital subtraction angiography should be available at this juncture for confirmation of carotid and/or graft patency.

In the case of a giant aneurysm of the intracavernous carotid, specifically the C_4 segment, anticipated technical difficulties with clip ligation are an indication for performance of a C_5 to C_3 segment saphenous vein interposition graft procedure. First developed by the senior author, it has since been successfully utilized to exclude these hazardous lesions from the circulation.[14,49] For this procedure, the leg should be prepped for saphenous vein harvest. Proper technique of graft preparation should be strictly observed. The reader is referred to an excellent review of these principles by Sundt and Sundt.[51] The internal carotid artery is exposed in the anterior and posterolateral triangles. One author has proposed the use of a shunt during the anastomosis of the interposition graft.[1] The efficacy of reduction of ischemic complications related to temporary occlusion of the internal carotid by use of such an intraoperative shunt remains to be determined at this time.

As in all skull base operations, direct surgical approaches to the cavernous sinus tend to be somewhat bloody operations. The surgeon must endeavor to maintain a hemostatic, clean operative field in order to assist navigation through this treacherous region of human anatomy. It is also important to help minimize the necessity of blood transfusion with its well known attendant complications. Utilizing the specially designed Fukushima monopolar malleable coagulator, skull base bone bleeding and dural oozing are readily controlled. Bipolar coagulation is also frequently used for the dura and intradural structures. Bone wax and, most importantly, Surgicel packing are crucial for cavernous hemostasis. With appropriate packing, any bulk of venous bleeding from the cavernous sinus can be managed. A spectrum of shapes and sizes of Surgicel should be readily available on the operating overtable. When three to four pieces have been packed, they should stay in place several minutes, after which one or two pieces are removed. This will prevent excessive packing, which results in nerve damage secondary to compression and occlusion of major blood vessels.

It is imperative that the surgeon be familiar with the areas that are amenable to packing with Surgicel to reduce compression-induced morbidity. In the anterior triangle small pieces of Surgicel may be inserted between the internal carotid and optic nerve, at the mouth of the intracavernous sinus, between the internal carotid siphon tip and the sphenoid bone, and against the medial wall of the superior orbital fissure dura (the true cavernous membrane). In the lateral aspect of the anterior triangle, Surgicel must be modestly used to avoid pressure on the oculomotor nerve that is running here, concealed by the medial aspect of the superior orbital fissure dura. Opening the medial triangle toward the posterior clinoid produces a large amount of bleeding. Packing inferiorly can be performed with impunity, as this space only communicates with the clival basilar venous plexus and contains no neural or arterial structures. Laterally directed packing, however, must be modest, as the third, fourth, and sixth cranial nerves are in close proximity. Consideration of the above guidelines will be helpful in achieving hemostasis in this area and avoiding complications.

At the completion of the intradural portion of the procedure, hemostasis should be complete. The neurovascular structures are finally inspected for evidence of correctible compression or damage. The dura is closed in a watertight fashion with the use of 4-0 nylon suture, usually utilizing a running interlocked method. If complete primary closure is not possible, a dural patch graft with temporalis fascia or pericranium should be utilized. The extradural bony dissection is then inspected for any communication between the intracranial contents and bacterial-flora-bearing structures. It is important to inspect the area of the eustachian tube, and, if it has been violated,

occlude its orifice with a fat or muscle graft covered with fascia. When the exposure has necessitated extension to possible involvement of the aerodigestive tract contents, it is advisable to consider coverage with a vascularized free flap. This will not only reduce the chances of infection but also satisfy functional and cosmetic considerations. The bone flap is replaced and secured, usually with wire. The scalp flap is then closed in layers. Routinely, the patient does not leave the operating suite until satisfactorily free of the effects of general anesthesia, allowing examination of the general neurological condition.

Postoperative Care

Initially patients are managed in the neurosurgical intensive care unit, with routine neurological examinations and vital sign monitoring by the nursing staff. We advocate the routine use of postoperative electrophysiological monitoring for 48 to 72 hours. All patients are treated with corticosteroids for protection against possible ischemia. The use of corticosteroids necessitates the use of H_2 blockers and antacids as prophylactic measures against gastrointestinal complications. Patients are also maintained on therapeutic levels of anticonvulsant medication. A postoperative seizure, with its attendant complications, can cause an otherwise uneventful recovery to sour. Patients who remain seizure free for 6 months have their anticonvulsants withdrawn. Sequential pneumatic compression stockings are maintained on patients while recumbent until they are ready to be discharged from intensive care. These are then replaced by compression stockings. It is important to mobilize all patients as quickly as possible to hasten their recovery.

ILLUSTRATIVE CASES

During the past 8 years, from 1984 to 1991, a total of 79 cases with various cavernous vascular lesions have been operated upon by the senior author. The variety and number of these cases are summarized in Table 30-3.

Proximal Internal Carotid Paraclinoid Giant Aneurysms

Seventeen cases in the proximal internal carotid have been directly approached through the anterior triangle. Seven cases presented with subarachnoid

Table 30-3. Direct Cavernous Surgery for Cavernous Carotid Vascular Lesions (1984–1991)

Lesion	No. of Cases
Aneurysms	
C_3 siphon	13
Ophthalmic	11
IC proximal-paraclinoid giant	17
C_4 horizontal	5
Primitive trigeminal	1
Intracavernous giant	20
Carotid-cavernous fistula	
Spontaneous	8
Traumatic	3
Siphon stenosis	
Bypass	1
Total	79

hemorrhage, the other 10 presenting with visual symptoms. An innovative technique was used for obliteration of the aneurysm prior to clipping, employing temporary occlusion of the cervical carotid and continuous suction of the aneurysm dome with an 18-gauge butterfly needle. This maneuver greatly facilitates proper clipping of these giant aneurysms. Occasionally, the back flow from the distal carotid artery was significant enough to require temporary clipping distally. Great care should be taken to preserve the posterior communicating artery and Dawson's perforators when placing this temporary clip.

All cases required the use of multiple clips for ligation, ranging from four to seven clips, with various combinations of angled and fenestrated clips (Figs. 30-3 to 30-6). We developed a special clip with a long window that was particularly suitable for these lesions (long window locking clips, designed by Fukushima, manufactured by the Mizuho Co., Tokyo). This clip has an 8- to 9-mm aperature that can be applied over the initial fenestrated clip to achieve double tandem clipping (Fig. 30-7). Figure 30-8 illustrates a representative case using four regular fenestrated clips in concert with three long window locking clips.

Ophthalmic Artery Aneurysms

Of the 11 aneurysms in the ophthalmic artery, five presented with subarachnoid hemorrhage, three with visual symptoms, and three as incidental findings. Figure 30-9 demonstrates the case of a 67-year-old woman who presented with grade II subarachnoid hemorrhage. On day 7 posthemorrhage, she underwent a direct approach that utilized five clips to ligate

the aneurysm. The result was excellent, with no postoperative neurological deficit. Another case was complicated postoperatively by a small visual field defect and transient diabetes insipidus. The diabetes was presumably secondary to obliteration of proximal internal carotid or superior hypophyseal (Dawson's) perforators. Only one aneurysm in this location was directed into the cavernous sinus proper. This patient presented with subarachnoid hemorrhage and underwent direct clipping utilizing just one angled Sugita clip. The clip was shown in a postoperative angiogram to be slipping halfway from the aneurysm neck. It is important to consider that some clips have a relatively weak closing tension, necessitating the use of a double or triple tandem clipping technique for adequate closure strength.

Carotid Siphon Aneurysms

Of the 13 cases in this group, 10 were asymptomatic and detected incidentally. Two presented with subarachnoid hemorrhage, and one patient suffered visual symptoms. Figure 30-10 illustrates the case of an incidentally diagnosed aneurysm in a 44-year-old man. Through a direct approach exposing only the anterior triangle a small, right-angled clip was used to ligate the aneurysm with no resultant morbidity. The case of a 62-year-old woman presenting with subarachnoid hemorrhage is demonstrated in Figure 30-11. The aneurysm bled intrathecally through the dura over the medial siphon angle. The aneurysm was clipped uneventfully with a small, right-angled aperature clip. Figure 30-12 shows a large, irregularly shaped siphon aneurysm with a daughter dome protruding into the right optic nerve. This 52-year-old woman presented with chronic headache and a field cut. Three fenestrated clips and one straight clip were required to ligate the aneurysm successfully. This case was an excellent candidate for intraoperative DSA to confirm adequate clip placement and arterial patency (Fig. 30-12C).

C_4 Segment Aneurysms

Aneurysms in the C_4 segment are particularly difficult to obliterate by clip ligation. The surgeon will typically be faced with a broad-necked aneurysm, additionally complicated by a variably thick, irregular, or fragile wall. A medial triangle exposure is used under most circumstances. It is important to expose an adequate length of the third cranial nerve and to retract it laterally with its dural sleeve intact. A key

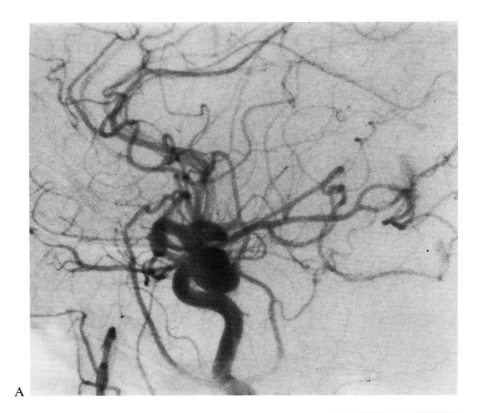

A

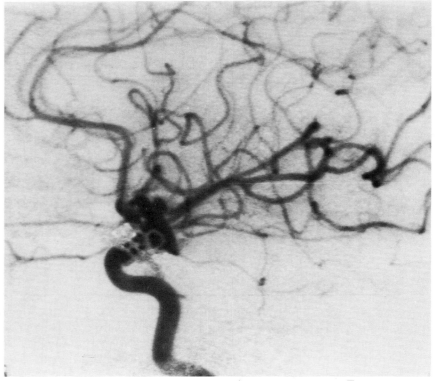

B

Figure 30-3. Pre- and postoperative angiograms of a 52-year-old woman presenting with subarachnoid hemorrhage. **(A)** On the left lateral carotid angiogram a large infraclinoidal aneurysm was detected. **(B)** The postoperative angiogram demonstrates clip ligation of the aneurysm.

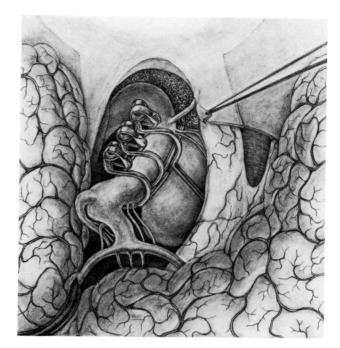

Figure 30-4. The clip configuration utilized in Fig. 30-3.

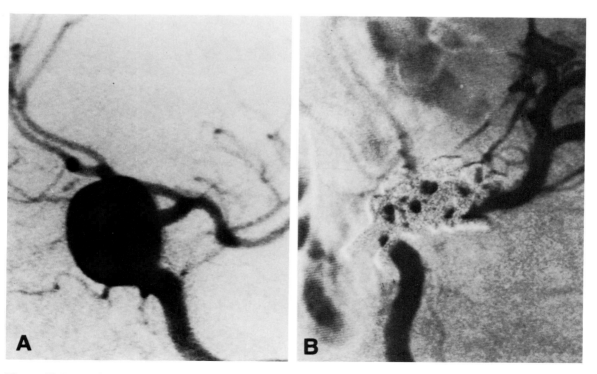

Figure 30-5. Angiographic demonstration of a paraclinoidal aneurysm in a 46-year-old woman presenting with subarachnoid hemorrhage. **(A)** Preoperative left carotid angiogram reveals a giant paraclinoidal aneurysm. **(B)** Intraoperative digital subtraction angiography showing successful clip ligation utilizing seven clips.

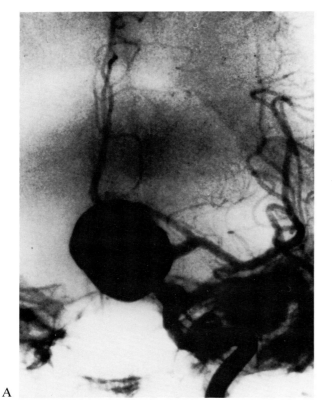
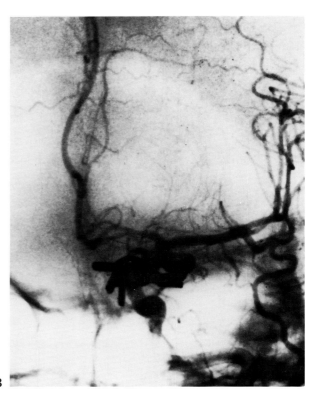

A   B

Figure 30-6. A 69-year-old woman presented with decreased visual acuity and a bitemporal hemianopsia. Angiography revealed this giant paraclinoidal aneurysm. **(A)** Preoperative left AP carotid angiogram. **(B)** A quadruple clip configuration was required for ligation and is shown postoperatively.

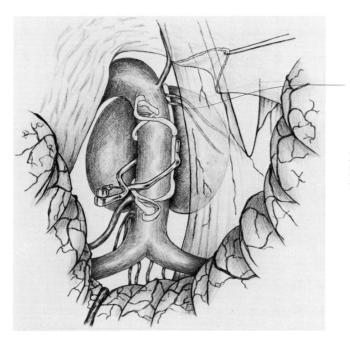

Dawson's perforators.

Figure 30-7. Fukushima's long window locking clip. The locking clip is placed over the primary aperture clip in tandem fashion.

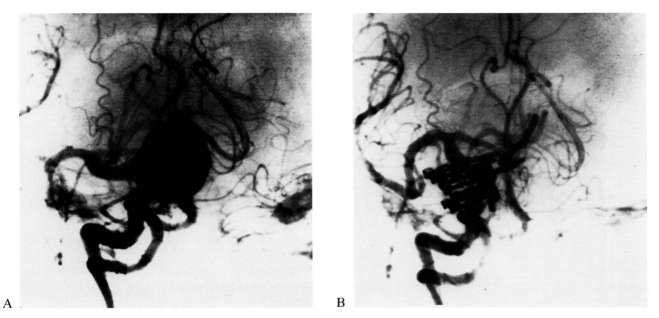

Figure 30-8. A 60-year-old woman presented with a visual deficit on the right. **(A)** Preoperative right retrograde brachial angiography demonstrates a giant paraclinoidal aneurysm. **(B)** Successful clip ligation of the aneurysm with seven clips is shown.

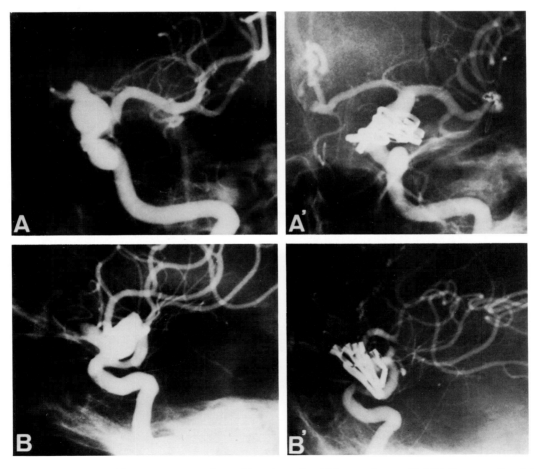

Figure 30-9. A 67-year-old woman presenting with subarachnoid hemorrhage. **(A&B)** Preoperative lateral and AP angiograms outline a multilobulated large ophthalmic segment aneurysm. **(A'&B')** Postoperative angiogram demonstrates successful clip ligation utilizing five clips.

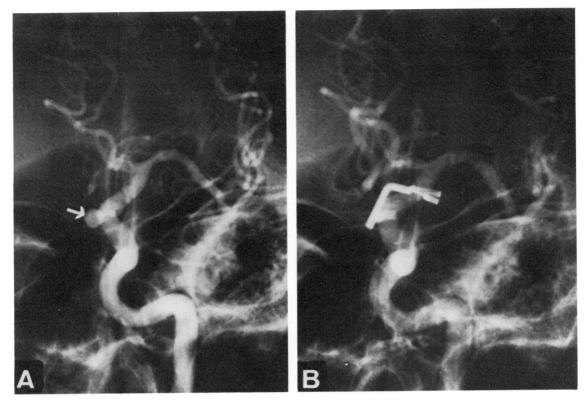

Figure 30-10. A 44-year-old man with a small carotid siphon aneurysm that was discovered incidentally. **(A)** Preoperative carotid angiogram. The white arrow points to the aneurysm, which is protruding medially. **(B)** Successful clip ligation is demonstrated on the postoperative angiogram.

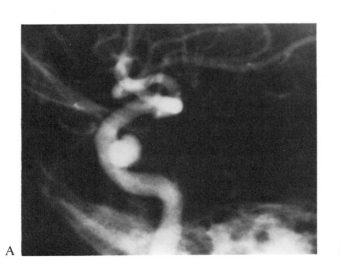

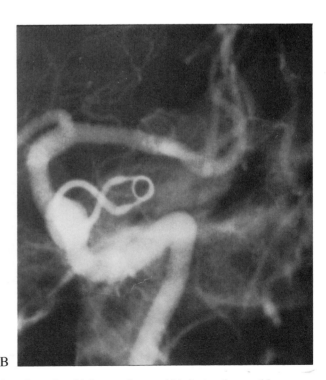

Figure 30-11. A 62-year-old woman who presented with subarachnoid hemorrhage. **(A)** Lateral carotid angiogram revealed a carotid siphon aneurysm with a bleb, which was the likely point of rupture. **(B)** Postoperative angiogram showing successful clipping with a right-angled, fenestrated clip.

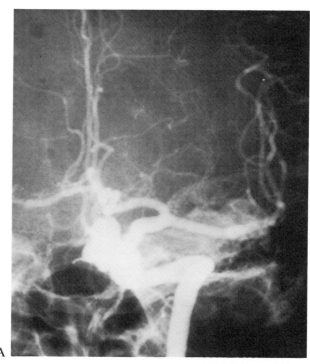

Figure 30-12. This 52-year-old woman presented with the complaints of a chronic headache accompanied by a visual field defect. **(A&B)** Preoperative AP and lateral carotid angiogram shows an irregular, multilobulated carotid siphon aneurysm. **(C)** Intraoperative digital subtraction angiography demonstrated satisfactory clip ligation.

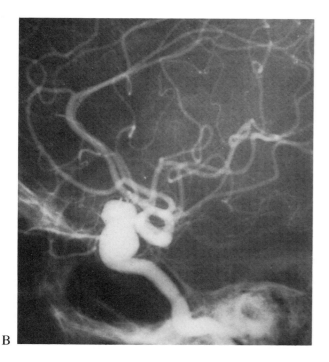

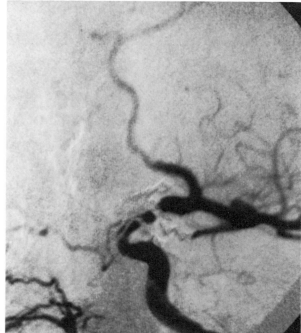

issue here is adequate hemostasis of the cavernous bleeding, which will be most challengingly encountered in this situation. Intraoperative DSA is indispensible in these cases to confirm proper clip placement. When technical difficulty is anticipated preoperatively, the patient's leg or thigh should be included in the surgical preparation for possible saphenous vein harvesting if a bypass procedure becomes necessary. Figure 30-13 demonstrates a case of a directly clipped C_4 segment aneurysm.

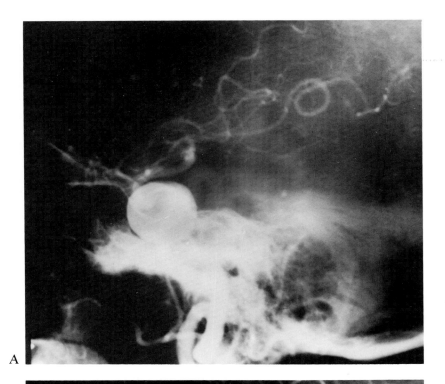

A

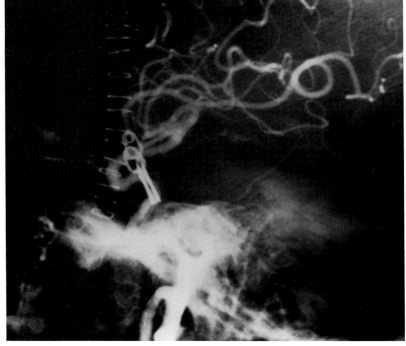

B

Figure 30-13. A 50-year-old woman with a sixth nerve palsy and diplopia was found to have this C4 segment aneurysm. **(A)** Preoperative angiogram demonstrated a giant C_4 aneurysm. **(B)** The aneurysm was clipped through a direct intracavernous approach, with the result demonstrated in this postoperative angiogram.

Intracavernous Giant Aneurysms

The management of intracavernous giant aneurysms remains one of the most controversial issues in neurosurgery. Simple carotid ligation or trapping of the aneurysm, with or without external carotid–internal carotid bypass has been the standard surgical treatment.[15,46,50] More recently the development of endovascular techniques has allowed attempts to obliterate these aneurysms utilizing detachable balloons.[2,13] Additionally, artificial thrombosis produced by running an electrical current through fine copper wires introduced into the aneurysm through a needle has been tried.[32] For asymptomatic aneurysms a rather conservative attitude has been advocated, based on the belief that the natural history of these lesions does not support the need for urgent therapy.[29,30] Attempts at direct surgical repair were first reported by Dolenc et al.[10] Their experience is notable for rather significant technical difficulty in reconstructing the cavernous carotid lumen. Three cases were complicated by internal carotid artery occlusion and significant cranial nerve morbidity (Table 30-1).

In 1986, inspired by the lack of a satisfactory approach to these lesions, the senior author developed a new bypass procedure, utilizing a petrous carotid-to-carotid siphon saphenous vein interposition graft to eliminate the aneurysm while preserving distal blood supply.[14] Additionally, bypass procedures involving interpositional grafts between the high cervical and petrous carotid, and the high cervical carotid and carotid siphon have been developed (Fig. 30-14).[31] To date, 25 bypass procedures have been performed, the majority with favorable results (Table 30-4). Acute postoperative graft occlusion developed in only one case, with an asymptomatic delayed occlusion discovered on follow-up study in another, resulting in a 92 percent patency rate. Figure 30-15 details an artist's conception of Fukushima's cavernous bypass. The procedure requires no manipulation of the aneurysm. The proximal C_5 petrous carotid and the C_3 siphon segments are exposed, followed by end-to-side anastomosis of a 5- to 7-cm-long saphenous vein interposition graft. This completely eliminates the cavernous giant aneurysm from the circulation. Figures 30-16 to 30-18 illustrate several clinical cases.

Carotid-Cavernous Fistulas

Surgical treatment of these lesions has likewise been controversial. Traditionally, conventional therapy involved various trapping procedures combined

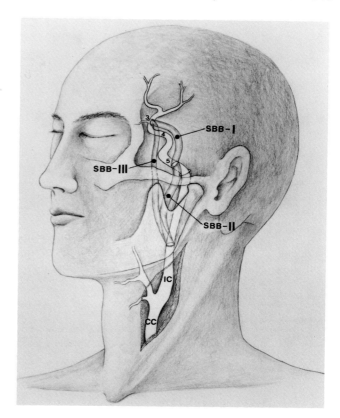

Figure 30-14. The three types of Fukushima skull base bypass (SBB). *SBB-I*, The so-called skull base cavernous bypass, which connects the proximal C_5 segment to the distal C_3 siphon segment. *SBB-II*, Links the high cervical internal carotid artery to the C_5 intrapetrous segment. *SBB-III*, The high cervical carotid artery is connected to the C_3 siphon segment through a submandibular pterygoid fossa route.

by various methods of embolization with muscle.[5,21,23] Direct surgical repair was first reported in 1965 by Parkinson[33] in his landmark paper and more recently by Dolenc.[8–10] Presently, the procedure of first choice is endovascular balloon occlusion, which

Table 30-4. Skull Base Cavernous Bypass (1986–1991)

Lesion	No. of Cases
C_5–C_3	
Cavernous giant aneurysm	17
C_4 fusiform aneurysm	1
Meningioma	2
Siphon stenosis	1
	21
High cervical–C_5 tumor	3
High cervical–C_3 cavernous giant aneurysm	1
Total	25

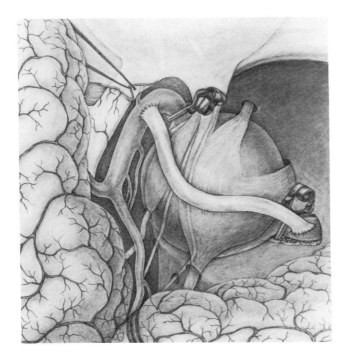

Figure 30-15. An artist's illustration of the skull base cavernous bypass. A short, saphenous vein interposition graft is placed over a giant cavernous carotid artery aneurysm from C_3 to C_5 utilizing an end-to-side anastomosis.

has thus far resulted in an acceptable success rate of occlusion of these lesions, despite a moderate risk of carotid artery occlusion.[2,13] The senior author's series includes 11 cases of carotid-cavernous fistulas that were directly approached. Three were of trau-

matic etiology, two secondary to aneurysm rupture, and six were of the dural AVM type. In all cases, the CCF disappeared after microsurgical reconstruction of the offending segment. Complications encountered consisted of one case of postoperative mild

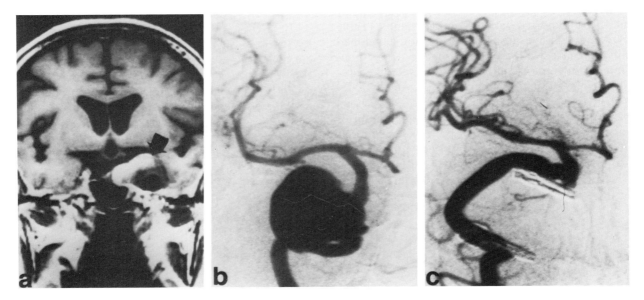

Figure 30-16. A 66-year-old woman who presented with a left Garcin's syndrome. **(a)** MRI clearly demonstrates the giant intracavernous aneurysm and its resultant mass effect. **(b)** Preoperative AP angiogram showing this giant aneurysm. **(c)** The aneurysm was successfully excluded from the circulation utilizing the skull base cavernous bypass.

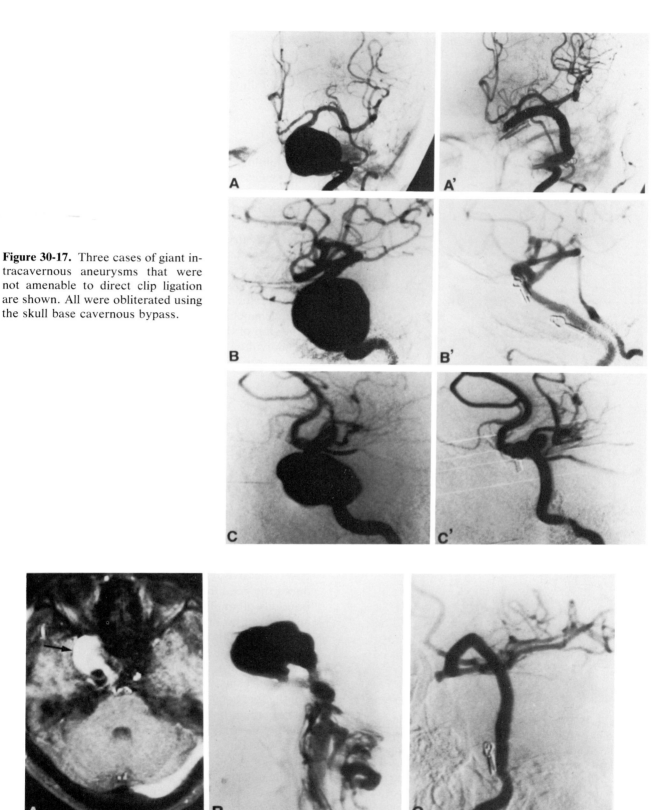

Figure 30-17. Three cases of giant intracavernous aneurysms that were not amenable to direct clip ligation are shown. All were obliterated using the skull base cavernous bypass.

Figure 30-18. This 46-year-old man presented with a left sixth cranial nerve palsy accompanied by retro-orbital pain. **(A)** MRI appearance of the lesion. **(B)** The preoperative lateral carotid angiogram shows a giant cavernous aneurysm with an associated carotid-cavernous fistula formed by rupture of the aneurysm. **(C)** The postoperative angiogram demonstrates the complete elimination of the aneurysm and the carotid-cavernous fistula after performance of a saphenous vein interposition bypass graft procedure.

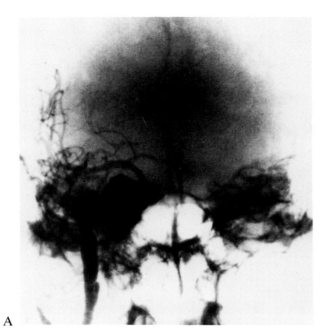

A

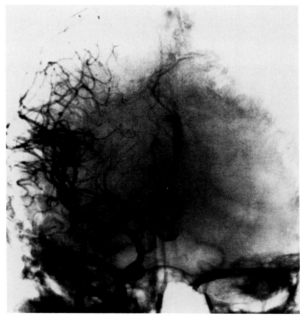

B

Figure 30-19. This figure demonstrates the obliteration of a carotid-cavernous fistula by a direct intracavernous approach. **(A)** The preoperative angiographic appearance of the carotid-cavernous fistula is demonstrated. **(B)** After a direct cavernous approach, the carotid-cavernous fistula is shown to be completely eliminated in this postoperative angiogram.

hemiparesis and one case of permanent diplopia. Figure 30-19 illustrates one case.

SUMMARY

Technological developments have pushed back many neurosurgical frontiers in the past quarter century. In no area have certain advances contributed more to an ability to attack surgically previously inaccessible lesions than in the case of intracavernous aneurysm surgery. The above discussion outlines a complex and intricate procedure with innumerable pitfalls before, during, and after its performance. A thorough knowledge of the microanatomy and ample surgical experience are crucial to the individual surgeon's chances of success. Consideration and implementation of the above outlined principles will serve the individual surgeon well who endeavors to face these hazardous lesions.

Carotid Ophthalmic Aneurysms
Steven L. Giannotta
Michael L. Levy

Certain anatomical and physiological characteristics of carotid ophthalmic artery aneurysms present the cerebrovascular surgeon with a unique set of management-related challenges. Situated at the skull base, the overlying anterior clinoid process introduces the need for a powerful high-speed drill within fractions of a millimeter of a large pulsating sac. The adjacent optic nerve, frequently compressed to the point of functional compromise, needs to be manipulated—but at the same time protected—throughout the surgical procedure. Unlike other anterior circulation aneurysms, between 25 and 50 percent of carotid ophthalmic aneurysms may be large or giant, and up to 50 percent of cases may present in the absence of subarachnoid hemorrhage with minimal symptoms, thereby making surgical decision making even more difficult.[56,58–61,64,66] The occasional necessity of obtaining control of various sources of collateral flow to the area, along with the everpresent spectre of the need for a trapping procedure with or without hemispheric revascularization, adds to the complexity of the decision making. Furthermore, the high likelihood of the presence of calcium in the aneurysmal wall, the need for occasional surgical excursions into the cavernous sinus, and the requirement of specialized equipment such as angled fenestrated clips round out a group of circumstances that are fraught with the potential for complications.

CLASSIFICATION

Most intracranial aneurysms are named according to associated or adjacent branches of the aneurysm's parent vessel.[65] Carotid ophthalmic aneurysms, however, have been categorized by a number of other criteria. Although the term *carotid ophthalmic* endures, it implies a constant relationship to the ophthalmic artery, which is too restrictive. Thus we prefer the classification of Day,[58] who refers to these lesions as *ophthalmic segment* aneurysms and divides them into ophthalmic and superior hypophyseal depending on the location of the neck in relation to either perforating branches or the ophthalmic artery itself.[58] Further description of each aneurysm is related to important characteristics that govern case selection and surgical technique and includes size and direction of the dome, as well as location of the neck. For the purpose of this discussion, we will address those aneurysms that arise distal to the carotid dural ring and proximal to the origin of the posterior communicating artery.

IMAGING

Aside from establishing the diagnosis, various imaging modalities can be instrumental in treatment planning and, as a result, in complication avoidance. With respect to cerebral angiography, a number of prerequisites must be understood in order to maximize information relative to complication avoidance and patient selection. Occasionally, carotid ophthalmic aneurysms are small enough to escape detection on cursory examination. Given the fact that up to 25 percent of carotid ophthalmic aneurysms are associated with multiple aneurysms, careful scrutiny of this area as well as the possible need for optional views such as obliques and submental vertex must be kept in mind.[56,58–61,64,66] Cross-compression studies imaging the anterior communicating artery will be helpful to rule out associated aneurysms as well as to arm the surgeon with valuable information regarding potential sources of collateral circulation. The presence and size of the superficial temporal artery, should the need arise for revascularization, is also a helpful adjunct. Finally, the direction of the dome, one of the most critical features and strategies related to clip ligation, must be assessed early and reassessed at the

beginning of the operative procedure, since dorsally projecting aneurysms can be embedded in the inferior aspect of the frontal lobe and are subject to rupture upon retraction.

Computed tomographic (CT) scanning can be of immeasurable aid in patient selection and complication avoidance. In the instance of multiple aneurysms, the location or thickness of adjacent cisternal clots can give evidence as to which aneurysm is the source of hemorrhage. Both calcium in the aneurysm wall, and laminated clots within the dome of the aneurysm, usually well seen on CT scans, are two hazards that must be planned for in the surgical setting. Pneumatization of the anterior clinoid process, a frequently unrecognized phenomenon, can lead to postoperative cerebrospinal fluid (CSF) rhinorrhea—a complication best avoided by recognition and appropriate surgical preplanning.

SURGICAL MANAGEMENT

Case Selection

A discussion on surgical management implies that a number of critical decisions have already been made. The most obvious decision relates to the patient's chances of successfully meeting the operative risks. Once this has been determined, the overall management strategy for the patient must be planned. Important decisions relate to whether a direct approach to the aneurysm is advisable as opposed to carotid ligation in the neck versus an endovascular approach. Key factors in this decision relate to the expertise of the surgeon in using the specialized techniques necessary for management of carotid ophthalmic aneurysms. The breadth and depth of experience of the endovascular team will determine whether an endovascular approach is a satisfactory alternative. It may be best to delay use of the direct approach to large or complex carotid ophthalmic lesions until experience with small or less technically demanding lesions and comfort with exposure of the cavernous sinus, decompression and deflection of the optic nerve, use of fenestrated clips, and temporary occlusion techniques are gained.

Craniotomy and Initial Exposure

The classical pterional craniotomy as described elsewhere in this text is used for all carotid ophthalmic lesions (Fig. 30-20A). Little modification of the original description by Yasargil is necessary.[69] How-

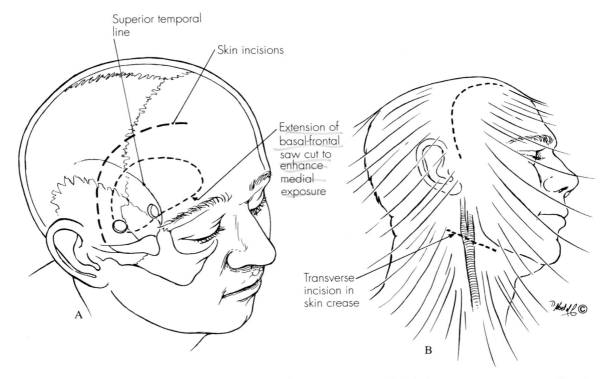

Figure 30-20. (A) Typical pterional craniotomy for approach to ophthalmic segment aneurysms. Basal-frontal saw cut is extended a variable distance, depending on whether a contralateral aneurysm will also be approached. **(B)** Typical skin crease incision for exposure of the internal carotid artery when proximal control is desired.

ever, if carotid exposure for proximal carotid control is necessary, the draping and preparation of the patient can be preplanned to include both incisions in one surgical field (Fig. 30-20B). It is important to extend the basal frontal cut with the craniotomy saw an extra 2 to 4 cm to enhance exposure to allow for the free movement of retractors in the event that bilateral aneurysms are to be attacked through one surgical exposure. After removal of the sphenoid wing and opening of the dura, it is expedient to split the proximal sylvian fissure for 1 to 2 cm. This will dramatically improve the ability to manipulate clips and clip appliers—especially when dealing with large or globular aneurysms. This will also facilitate temporary occlusion of the A_1 and M_1 segment should such a maneuver be necessary. Liberal opening of the sylvian fissure also lowers retractor pressure, thereby reducing the possibility of ischemic injury to the frontal and temporal lobes (Fig. 30-21).

Before exposure of the proximal carotid artery and anterior clinoid, a quick check of the imaging studies should be carried out to determine if a dorsally placed aneurysm may be vulnerable to disruption with deep placement of retractors or retraction of the frontal lobe. Once the sylvian fissure is split and re-

tractors are deepened, the lumbar subarachnoid drain is opened to allow further relaxation, enhancing the reduction of intracranial pressure obtained through the use of osmotic diuretics. Arachnoid investments of the proximal carotid artery and optic nerve are opened widely to enhance further exposure and retractability of the frontal lobe. Ultimately, the carotid and chiasmatic cisterns will be maximally exposed. Care should be taken to preserve, if possible, the olfactory tract. This again is obviated by wide opening of the sylvian fissure.

Removal of Anterior Clinoid

Removal of the anterior clinoid is one of the most critical procedures to the successful management of ophthalmic segment aneurysms. A few words regarding equipment may be helpful. The drill to be used for removing the clinoid must fulfill several requirements. The device must come with an array of steel cutting and diamond-tipped burrs of appropriate size. The drill should be reversible and preferably controlled by a foot pedal as opposed to a device on the drill handpiece itself. The drill should fit comfortably

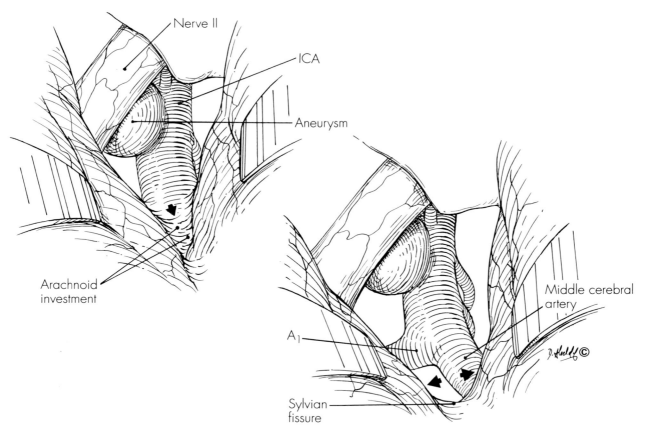

Figure 30-21. Medially protruding aneurysm under the optic nerve. The sylvian fissure is opened and the frontal and temporal lobes gently retracted for maximal flexibility in dealing with the lesion.

in one hand, should have excellent balance, and should not be encumbered by a heavy air hose so as to require the expenditure of extra energy to hold the drill steady. A ready and precise supply of cooling irrigation fluid is mandatory. This can be accomplished in several ways. Suction irrigation tips held in the surgeon's nondominant hand are most ideal for this procedure. Alternatively, a precise irrigating device wielded by the surgical assistant looking through the operating microscope observer arm can be used. A third option involves a drip system through a strategically placed needle above the surgical field directed over the area of the clinoid.

Drilling of the clinoid is preceded by opening the dura. A semicircular dural flap based over the entire anterior clinoid process, as well as the optic canal, must be outlined with either bipolar or, more efficiently, unipolar cautery. Careful palpation over the optic canal is necessary to identify that portion that may be covered only by dura and therefore may allow inadvertent thermal or compression injury to the optic nerve (Fig. 30-22A). A dural flap can be reflected over the proximal carotid artery, optic nerve,

and aneurysm to serve as a further protective barrier (Fig. 30-22B&C). For large clinoid processes in experienced hands, a steel 2-mm cutting burr can be utilized to begin clinoid removal. In general, the largest burr one can use is the most efficient and safe choice. As one approaches the aneurysm, the dura, or the optic nerve, diamond-tipped drill bits are most appropriate. It is advantageous to remove the entire clinoid process so as to expose the proximal cavernous sinus and the most distal carotid-dural ring. It is also important to unroof the optic nerve completely, especially the bone on the medial border, so as to be able to deflect the optic nerve from lateral to medial gently and without undue counterpressure. Clinoid removal will predictably result in bleeding from the cavernous sinus, which should be controlled using judicious packing of Surgicel and bipolar electrocautery. In excessively pneumatized anterior clinoid processes, packing with bone wax will obviate postoperative CSF rhinorrhea. In certain circumstances, the sphenoid sinus may be inadvertently opened, especially when decompressing the medial aspect of the optic canal. If the mucosa is intact, simple occlusion of the

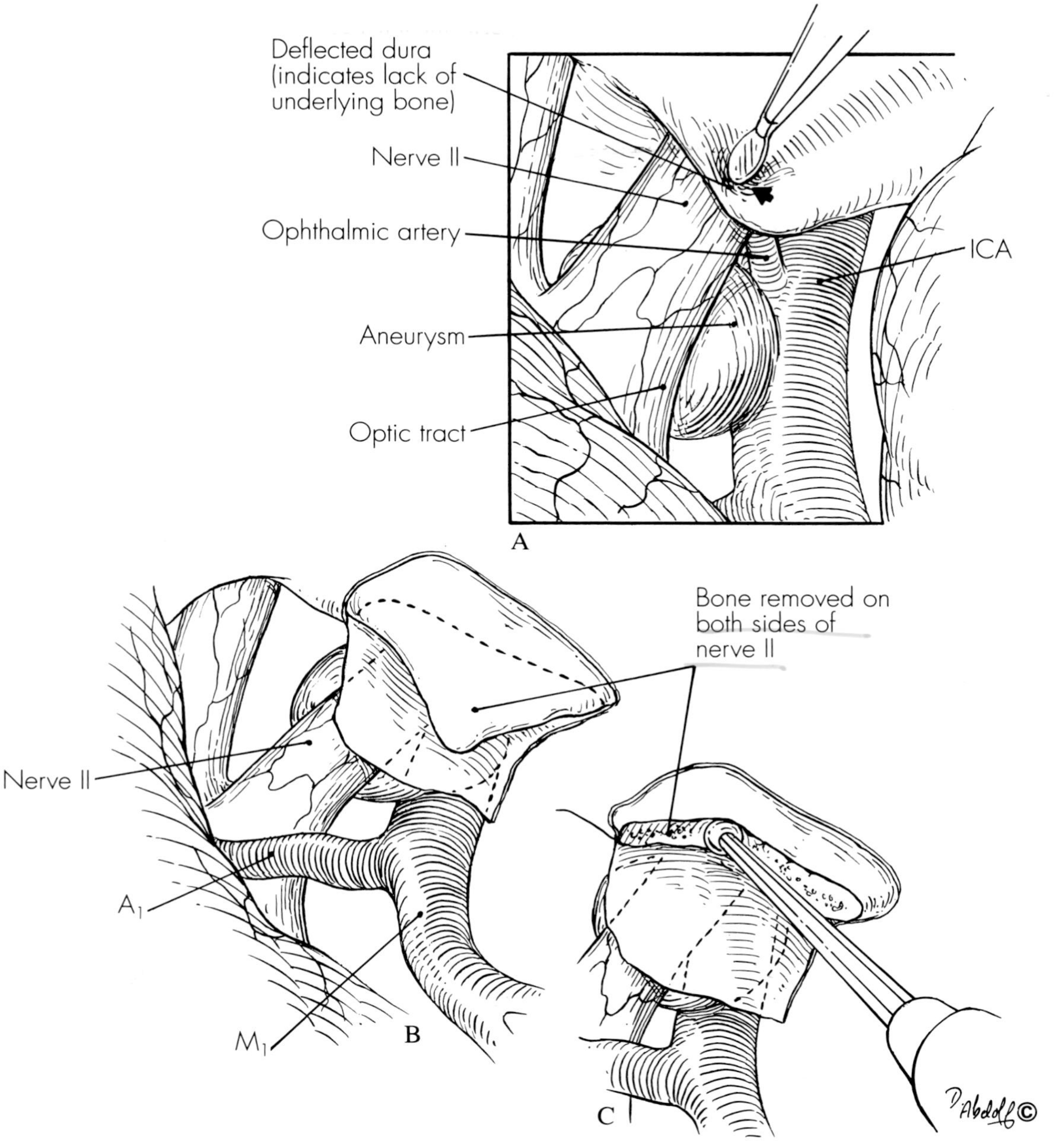

Deflected dura
(indicates lack of
underlying bone)

Nerve II

Ophthalmic artery

ICA

Aneurysm

Optic tract

A

Bone removed on
both sides of
nerve II

Nerve II

A₁

M₁   B

C

Figure 30-22. **(A)** Palpation of the dura over the anterior clinoid to determine the extent of bony covering of the optic nerve prior to coagulation and incision of the dura. **(B&C)** Following dural incision, the clinoid is removed with a drill. Note the dural flap protecting the carotid artery, optic nerve, and aneurysm during this maneuver.

bony aperture with bone wax will suffice. If the mucosa is opened, obliteration of the sinus may be necessary. Packing with autologous fat and exenteration of all mucosa should be accomplished to obviate CSF rhinorrhea and the possibility of a craniotomy infection.

Dissection of the Aneurysm

A word regarding instrumentation is appropriate prior to discussing dissection techniques. Small spatulas, probes, and scissors designed specifically for aneurysm surgery should be used. Spatulas and scissors should be sharp, without burrs that could inadvertently tear the aneurysm sac. Suction tips that have been used for for removal of the clinoid should be exchanged for those that have not been injured by inadvertent touching of the drill tip. Sharp dissection instruments should be used to their maximal advantage, as intraoperative aneurysm rupture is more commonly associated with maneuvers utilizing blunt instrumentation.[57]

To complete the exposure of the carotid segment that the aneurysm occupies, opening of the inner layer of dura (dura propria) along the lateral aspect of the optic nerve is necessary. This exposes the carotid artery more proximally and also allows exposure of the origin of the ophthalmic artery. If the neck of the aneurysm extends further proximal to this, then opening of the carotid ring with dissection of the su-

periormost aspect of the cavernous sinus will be necessary. Once the appropriate segment of carotid artery has been exposed, the extent of the aneurysm neck should be identified and dissection begun. Arachnoid investments should be taken down sharply, using fine arachnoid scissors and intermittent dissection with fine spatulas and probes commenced in order to identify completely and to dissect superior hypophyseal perforators as well as perforators to the optic chiasm. The ophthalmic artery should be dissected free of the neck of the aneurysm so as to preserve its origin at the time of clip application. Ultimately the aneurysm will, unless it is quite small, need to be deflected in various directions in order to be able to identify all arachnoid investments and free the neck from perforating branches (Fig. 30-23A). This can be done with the barrel of a smooth

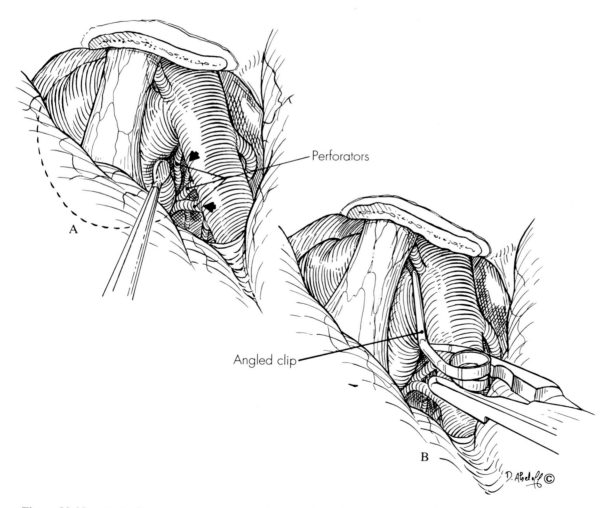

Figure 30-23. (A) Deflection of aneurysm sac to identify perforators to the optic chiasm and hypophysis. **(B)** Use of angled clip to avoid perforators.

sucker tip or spatula dissectors. Intermittent deflection of the optic nerve may also be necessary. We recommend intermittent retraction of the optic nerve and have not had experience with continuous mechanical retraction as advocated by others.[68] Depending on the size of the aneurysm, the origin of posterior communicating artery and anterior choroidal artery may need to be dissected free of either the dome or the neck of the aneurysm. At some point prior to clip application, an instrument should be passed completely behind the neck of the aneurysm to ensure an unobstructed passage to both aneurysm clip blades. This may require the passage of either an angled or a curved dissector or probe. Any apparent resistance to this maneuver should be immediately followed by further dissection techniques and deflection of the aneurysm in order to site and properly dissect any obstructing perforator or arachnoid investment. Since faulty or aborted attempts to place aneurysm clips prior to proper complete dissection of the aneurysm is one of the most common causes for intraoperative rupture, thought should be given to temporary occlusion of the carotid artery and deflation of the aneurysm so that proper exposure can be obtained prior to clip placement (Fig. 30-23B).

Carotid Control

For globular or large ophthalmic segment aneurysms, strong consideration should be given to proximal carotid control for the purposes both of managing inadvertent intraoperative rupture and as a definitive maneuver to deflate the aneurysm prior to clip placement. Distally, the most appropriate place for temporary occlusion would be between the aneurysm and the posterior communicating artery. If this is not feasible, a site just distal to the posterior communicating artery should be selected. If necessary, temporary occlusion of both M_1 and A_1 segments of the carotid bifurcation must be considered.

Proximal control, however, can be accomplished at three potential sites. Perhaps the most easily accomplished is that of carotid control in the neck. A 5 cm transverse incision is made in a skin crease below the angle of the jaw. The sternocleidomastoid muscle is retracted and the carotid sheath identified and opened longitudinally. Tapes are placed around both internal and external carotid arteries. A second option involves the extradural exposure and temporary clip occlusion of the petrous portion (C_5) of the carotid artery. The dura is elevated from the floor of the middle fossa and secured with one blade of the self-retaining retractor. The middle meningeal artery is followed to the foramen spinosum, where it is coagulated and divided. Medially and anteriorly to the foramen spinosum will be found the foramen ovale. Directly posterior to the foramen ovale and medial to the foramen spinosum, the carotid can be exposed by drilling away the floor of the middle fossa. Occasionally the carotid can be exposed without removal of much bone, as there may be incomplete coverage of the carotid in this area. The eustachian tube lies lateral to the C_5 portion of the internal carotid artery and should be left intact. Approximately 10 to 12 mm of carotid artery can be exposed with judicious drilling. A venous plexus frequently surrounds the carotid and must be carefully controlled with bipolar electrocautery. A temporary aneurysm clip can be placed across this portion of the carotid artery at the appropriate time for proximal carotid control. A third and more distal site for carotid control is the short distance of carotid between the two dural carotid rings. The first carotid ring is almost invariably identified during removal of the anterior clinoid process. With further dissection toward the anterior cavernous bend of the internal carotid artery, a second dural ring is identified. Between these two rings is provided a space for temporary placement of a clip to obtain proximal control of carotid flow. This site also provides for an alternative should the need for carotid control arise in an unplanned situation.

Clip Application

Following complete mobilization and dissection of the aneurysm, the decision is made regarding clip selection. Considerations here include the orientation of the longest dimension of the neck in relation to the long axis of the parent vessel. Except in aneurysms with very narrow necks, the clip should be placed parallel with the long axis of the parent vessel so as not to kink it. Other considerations include preservation of perforators, the orientation of the overlying optic nerve, and whether a fenestrated clip must be used to incorporate the carotid artery, the optic nerve, or both (Fig. 30-24A).[67] Not infrequently the need to remove and reposition the clip will arise. Our philosophy is that there is no substitute for perfect clip application. Several sizes or configurations of clips may need to be applied in an effort to obtain complete aneurysm obliteration while maintaining the appropriate lumen dimension of the carotid artery. Care should be taken so as not to place the clip too close to the base of the aneurysm, thus unwittingly narrowing the internal diameter of the parent vessel. In this regard, intraoperative angiography and

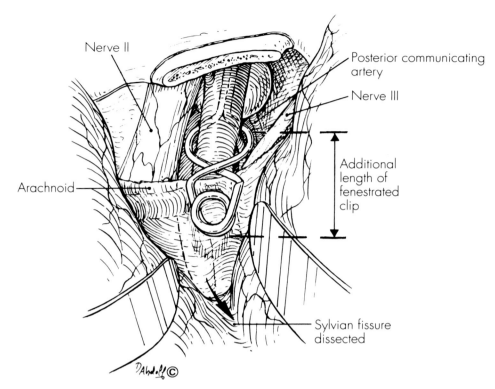

Nerve II

Posterior communicating artery

Nerve III

Additional length of fenestrated clip

Arachnoid

Sylvian fissure dissected

Figure 30-24. Fenestrated clip encompassing the carotid artery within its aperture.

the judicious use of intraoperative Doppler ultra-sonography will be helpful in ensuring satisfactory flow through the parent vessel.

For globular or large aneurysms, almost invariably temporary occlusion with deflation of the aneurysm will be necessary—or at least advisable—prior to clip placement (Fig. 30-25B&C). We have not used hypotension for this maneuver, as frequently hypo-tension alone will not sufficiently slacken the aneu-rysm for appropriate clip placement. The aneurysm will tend to "pulsate off" a poorly placed clip. It is much more efficient to obtain definitive proximal and distal control with or without the use of cerebral pro-tective agents so as to deflate the aneurysm for proper appropriate clip placement. Hypotension is contraindicated during this maneuver. Invariably, angled fenestrated clips will be necessary for globular aneurysms to "reconstruct" the lumen of the parent vessel. Frequently, tandem clips will be used on those aneurysms in which the neck is excessively long or the aneurysm unusually large. Various com-binations of straight clips and aperture clips can be positioned so as to obliterate even the largest of ca-rotid aneurysms. It is important here to leave a small amount of aneurysm neck between the clip blade and the parent vessel so as not to constrict flow through the carotid too much.

We have instituted the use of evoked potential monitoring during those cases in which temporary carotid occlusion is anticipated. Preservation of the responses accurately predicts cerebral tolerance to this maneuver, whereas attenuation of responses usually heralds the need for cerebral protective agents before reocclusion is attempted.

For large aneurysms with intralumenal clot or for those that are partially calcified, complete carotid control with opening of the sac is advisable. An en-darterectomy or complete removal of laminated clot can then be accomplished with complete irrigation of the lumen using heparinized saline. Following this maneuver, appropriate clip placement can be accom-plished without risk of embolization of either orga-nized clotted material or calcific debris.

Occasionally after clip application the optic nerve may be slightly deflected from its normal course due to the presence of the clip. In most circumstances, this is easily tolerated, especially if the optic canal has been decompressed with removal of the anterior clinoid process. Only in undue angulation of the optic nerve should clip application be altered. Obviously, if the optic canal has not been properly decom-pressed, lesser degrees of optic nerve deflection due to the presence of the clip will be tolerated.

Prior to dural closure, the area of the clinoid re-

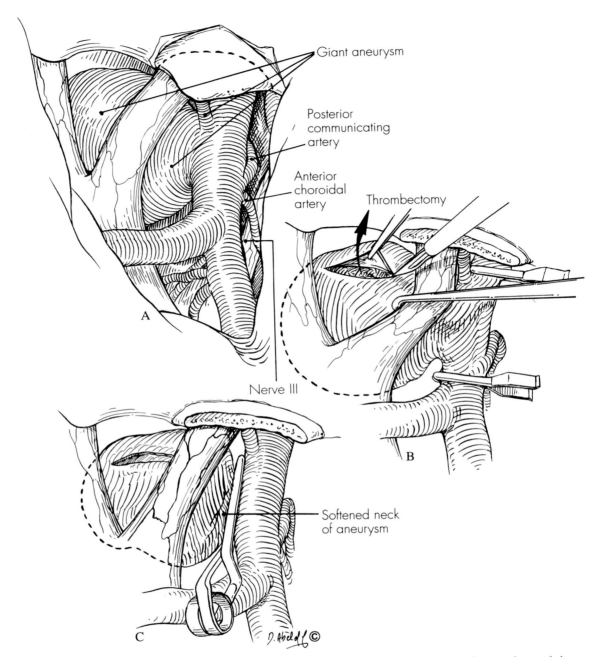

Figure 30-25. (A) Large ophthalmic segment aneurysm under both optic nerves. **(B)** Evacuation and thrombectomy following temporary occlusion of the internal carotid and ophthalmic arteries. **(C)** Clip ligation of the aneurysm neck following evacuation of the sac.

moval as well as the area of the tuberculum should be reinspected for possible sites of CSF leakage and appropriate packing and/or waxing be accomplished. Postoperatively, fluid losses are replaced prior to leaving the operating theater so as to maintain adequate circulatory volume and to avoid the possibility of postoperative hypotension.

Contralateral Clip Application

In cases of bilateral carotid ophthalmic aneurysms, consideration may be given to approaching the contralateral aneurysm through the ipsilateral craniotomy (Fig. 30-26).[62,63] This is most feasible in cases in which the contralateral aneurysm is reasonably small

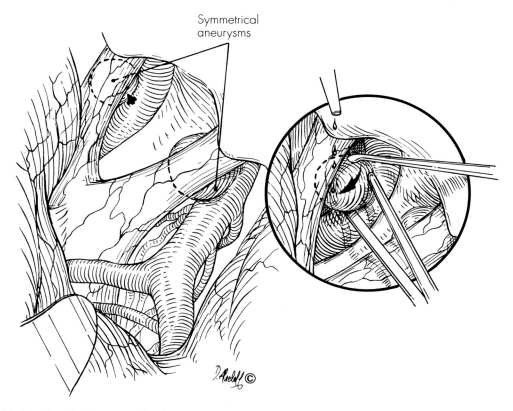

Figure 30-26. The ideal presentation in a patient with bilateral ophthalmic segment aneurysms. In approaching one aneurysm in this manner the contralateral internal carotid artery can be easily evaluated.

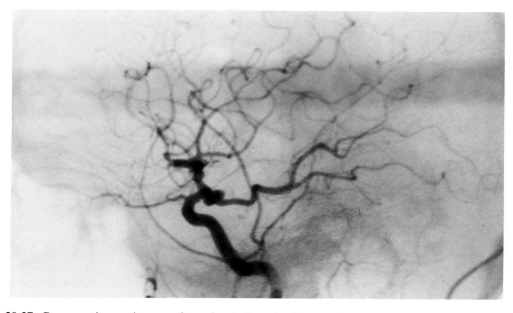

Figure 30-27. Preoperative angiogram of a patient believed to have an internal carotid-posterior communicating artery aneurysm. The lesion was actually an ophthalmic segment-superior hypophyseal (ventral carotid) aneurysm.

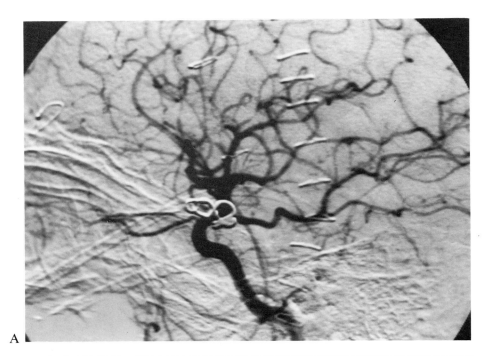

A

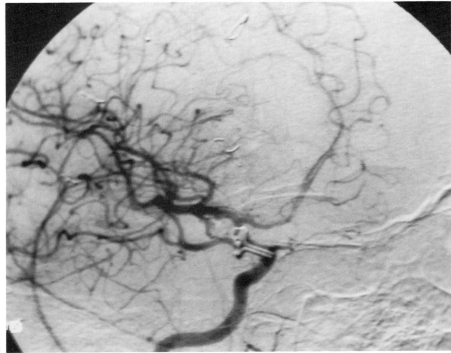

B

Figure 30-28. Postoperative angiograms of a patient with an ophthalmic segment-superior hypophyseal (ventral carotid) aneurysm. Note the use of a fenestrated clip, which encompasses the carotid artery within its aperture.

and projects either medially from the carotid artery or dorsally. Following secure clip application of the ipsilateral aneurysm, the retractor blade can be redirected contralaterally across the midline. The ipsilateral olfactory tract may be injured if overly vigorous retraction is used. Wide opening of the carotid and chiasmatic cisterns so as to expose the opposite optic nerve and carotid artery lying inferiorly to the optic nerve is necessary. Intermittent elevation of the contralateral optic nerve will frequently expose the aneurysm or aneurysm neck. The origin of the ophthalmic artery is identified, and arachnoid investments are dissected with probes or scissors. In left-sided approaches to right-sided aneurysms, it is frequently advisable to place the clip with the left hand. The surgeon should feel reasonably comfortable with this maneuver prior to embarking on contralateral clip application. Occasionally, the overhanging tuberculum sella will impede the appropriate placement of the clip. This will necessitate a removal of the tuberculum via appropriate drilling techniques. Again, if the mucosa of the sphenoid sinus is violated, appropriate steps to exenterate the sinus and to pack it must be carried out to avoid either CSF leakage or infectious complications (Figs. 30-27 to 30-31).

RESULTS

Tables 30-5 to 30-7 summarize our statistics related to the direct approach in 43 patients who harbored ophthalmic segment aneurysms. Over one-half of the cases presented in the absence of subarachnoid hemorrhage. Typically, there were 29 associated vascular lesions, mostly other aneurysms. In five cases bilateral ophthalmic segment lesions were present.

Of 43 cases, there was one death due to inadvertent carotid occlusion prior to our institution of intraoperative angiography and evoked potential monitoring. There was only one case of postoperative

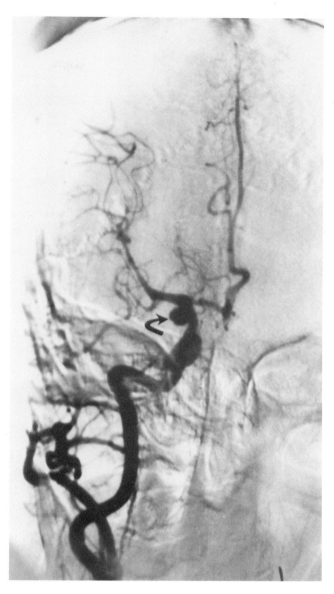

Figure 30-29. Preoperative angiogram of a patient with a right internal carotid artery aneurysm (*curved arrow*).

Table 30-5. Ophthalmic Segment Aneurysm Presentations

Presentation	No. of Cases
SAH	16
Incidental to another aneurysm	10
Visual loss	5
Headache	5
Incidental to nonvascular condition	5
Embolic stroke	2
	43

Table 30-6. Ophthalmic Segment Aneurysms and Associated Vascular Lesions

Lesion	No. of Cases
Aneurysms	
Posterior communicating artery	13
Contralateral ophthalmic artery	5
Middle cerebral artery	4
Basilar artery	2
Pericallosal artery	2
Anterior communicating artery	1
Carotid bifurcation	1
Arteriovenous malformation	1

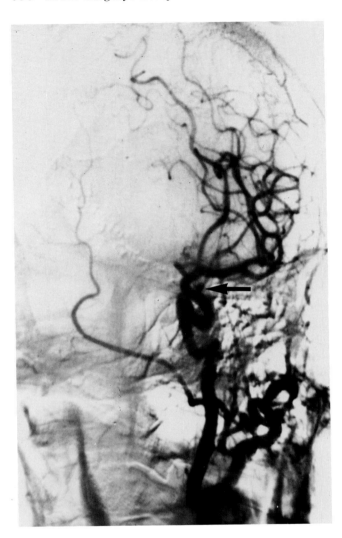

Figure 30-30. Preoperative angiogram of the same patient documenting a small left ophthalmic segment aneurysm (*straight arrow*).

visual loss, which was temporary. No patient with preexisting visual loss suffered visual deterioration, and two cases were dramatically improved.

Surgical complications and their avoidance and management are summarized in Table 30-8.

Table 30-7.   Ophthalmic Segment Aneurysm Complications

Complication	No. of Cases
Vasospasm	4
Carotid occlusion	1
Visual loss	1
Subdural hematoma	1
Cerebral edema	1
Myocardial infarction	1

CONCLUSIONS

Proper management of ophthalmic segment aneurysms requires meticulous attention to details, impeccable surgical judgement, and facility with techniques not used with other anterior circulation aneurysms. It is suggested that the following steps will help to minimize complications in managing ophthalmic segment aneurysms:

1. Tackle smaller lesions before attempting larger ones.
2. Become comfortable with drilling techniques at the skull base.
3. Review the use of aperture clips.
4. Develop a protocol for temporary carotid occlusion, including cerebral protection.

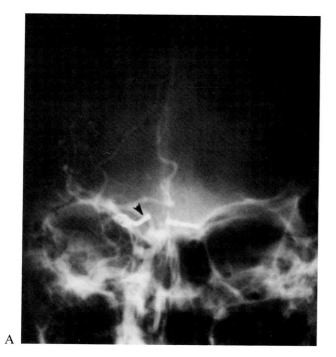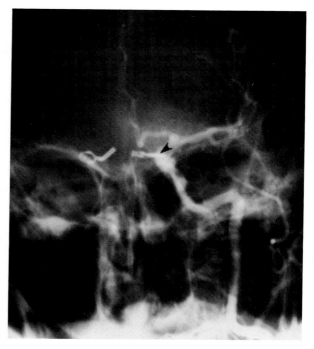

A   B

Figure 30-31. Postoperative angiograms demonstrating successful obliteration of the right internal carotid artery aneurysm and the left ophthalmic segment aneurysm through a right-sided approach.

Table 30-8.   Avoidance and Management of Complications in Carotid Ophthalmic Aneurysm Surgery

Complication	Avoidance	Management
Aneurysm exposed not responsible for hemorrhage	Exhaustive preoperative imaging	Repeat studies
		Urgent reoperation
Postoperative CSF rhinorrhea	Wax pneumatized anterior clinoid and pack sphenoid	Lumbar drainage
		Reoperation
Early intraoperative aneurysmal rupture	Early proximal control for large dorsal aneurysms	Tamponade
		Carotid compression
Frontal lobe retractor injury	Lumbar drainage and opening of the sylvian fissure	Steroids
		Normotension
Optic nerve injury	Proper drilling technique and equipment. Adequate irrigation. Decompression of the optic canal with intermittant gentle nerve retraction.	Steroids
		Volume expansion
		Reoperation if progressive
Delayed intraoperative rupture	Sharp technique with complete dissection prior to clipping	Tamponade
		Proximal control
		Temporary clips
Carotid artery narrowed or occluded	Clip blades should be parallel to the long axis of the aneurysm neck. Use of fenestrated clips and intraoperative angiography.	Consider reoperation
Aneurysm fills on postoperative angiogram	Use of tandem and/or booster clips with evacuation of the aneurysm after clipping	Reoperation

Midcarotid Artery (Posterior Communicating and Anterior Choroidal Artery) Aneurysms

Eugene S. Flamm

This chapter is focused on aneurysms of the middle portion of the supraclinoid carotid artery. In spite of the high frequency of aneurysms at the posterior communicating (PCoA) and anterior choroidal (AChA) artery, there has been little written that specifically addresses the complications of surgery for these aneurysms (Table 30-9). Since both of these aneurysms arise in the same vicinity of the carotid artery, the complications associated with their management are often quite similar. Most significant is the occurrence of an ischemic event related to their surgical correction. While occlusion of the carotid artery is rare, flow alteration with resultant ischemia due to compromise of the specific arteries and their branches is probably the most frequent cause of postoperative complications following surgery.

DIAGNOSIS

With the exception of a third nerve palsy, the well-known signs and symptoms of an subarachnoid hemorrhage (SAH) are usually no different following rupture of a PCoA or AChA aneurysm. The third nerve palsy associated with these aneurysms almost always involves the pupil. There have been a few instances in which pupillary sparing has been noted.[72,74,76] At this time we still recommend angiography to rule out an aneurysm as the cause of a third nerve palsy with pupillary involvement. Without pupillary involvement, myasthenia gravis and diabetes mellitus must be considered. Ultimately one must be certain that an aneurysm is not the cause of a third nerve palsy even

Table 30-9. Distribution of Aneurysms in Author's Series

Location	No. of Cases	Percent
Ophthalmic	114	11.2
Posterior communicating	244	24.0
Anterior choroidal	49	4.8
Carotid bifurcation	40	3.9
Anterior communicating	194	19.1
Distal anterior cerebral	32	3.1
Middle cerebral	209	20.6
Vertebrobasilar	135	13.3
Totals	1,017	100.0

if the pupil is spared. In the foreseeable future, magnetic resonance angiography (MRA) may be utilized to exclude an aneurysm, thus avoiding the need for a formal arteriogram. At the present time this remains an innovational and not fully established technique with which to rule out an intracranial aneurysm.[78-80] When an aneurysm is discovered with MRA, the surgeon must decide if sufficient information is provided to avoid performing a standard angiogram (Fig. 30-32). At the present time, we do not operate on the basis of MRA alone.

In addition to the general complications that can occur with major craniotomies, specific problems related to aneurysms at these two locations will be addressed. The discussion will begin with a general approach used by the author and then cover several intraoperative and perioperative problems that can affect the outcome.

OPERATIVE TECHNIQUES

Anesthetic Techniques— Aids to Exposure

To maximize the exposure of the circle of Willis and to reduce the amount of retraction required, several adjuncts are utilized. An infusion of 20 percent mannitol (0.5 to 1.0 g/kg) is begun at the time of the skin incision. Another important adjunct is spinal drainage. A catheter introduced through a Touhey needle is inserted into the lumbar subarachnoid space after induction of anesthesia. The drainage is not opened at this time. When the dura has been exposed and tented, the spinal drainage is opened. This delay prevents stripping away of the dura, which may cause epidural bleeding that is difficult to control. Furthermore, it is easier to open the leaves of the arachnoid in the sylvian fissure if some cerebrospinal fluid (CSF) is present. In addition to the relaxation of the brain, this method facilitates the microdissection since the surgeon can work in a drier field. Spinal drainage is avoided in patients with moderate amounts of atrophy, since intracranial access to CSF is easy. The risk of excessive removal with subsequent collapse of the brain is thus avoided. The final step to achieve a slack brain is to maintain the $PaCO_2$ in the range of 25 to 30 mmHg before the dura is opened; thereafter PCO_2 is kept between 30 and 35 mmHg. Exposure of carotid artery aneurysms is the single most important step for successful surgery of these lesions. Failure to achieve this with a relaxed brain sets the stage for laceration of the brain because of excessive retraction, poor microdissection, and an increased risk of intraoperative rupture.

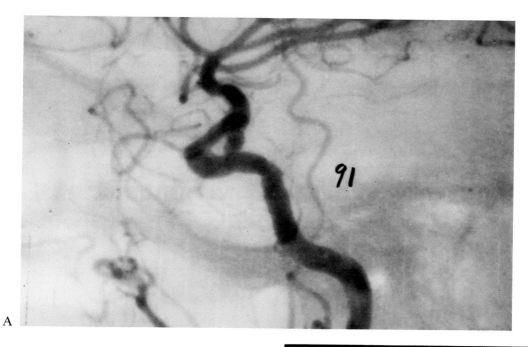

Figure 30-32. Imaging of a PCoA aneurysm. **(A)** Lateral conventional carotid arteriogram showing aneurysms at the origin of the PCoA. **(B)** Same patient as in Fig. A. Magnetic resonance arteriogram (MRA). Segmented view of internal carotid artery showing PCoA aneurysm.

Positioning the Patient

The patient is positioned with the head secured in a pin headholder. The use of the Sugita headholder has eliminated the occasional problem of penetration of the skull by the spring-loaded pins. Since the pins used with the Sugita headholder are tightened by hand, the risk of producing an epidural hematoma is virtually eliminated. The pin sites are infiltrated with a local anesthetic to avoid any rise in blood pressure because of pain. All intracranial microsurgery should be performed with the head secured by skull fixation. This is necessary to reduce any movement of the head that will interfere with the microdissection that is carried out at ×16 to 20 magnification. A system that permits this as well as the attachment of self-retaining retractors and other adjuncts is particularly helpful.

The head is turned to a full lateral position, and the vertex is dropped slightly toward the floor. The zygoma is almost parallel with the floor. This permits better direct visualization of the region of the optic nerve and carotid artery and reduces any obstruction to vision by the temporalis muscle or floor of the skull. A folded sheet or shoulder roll should be placed beneath the ipsilateral shoulder to reduce the amount of stretch placed on the carotid artery and jugular vein. As in all craniotomies, the head should be slightly above the level of the heart to permit gravitational venous drainage (Fig. 30-33).

Techniques of Craniotomy

Skin Incision

As shown in Figure 30-34, a curvilinear incision just behind the hairline is used. It extends from the level of the zygoma, 1 cm in front of the tragus, to a

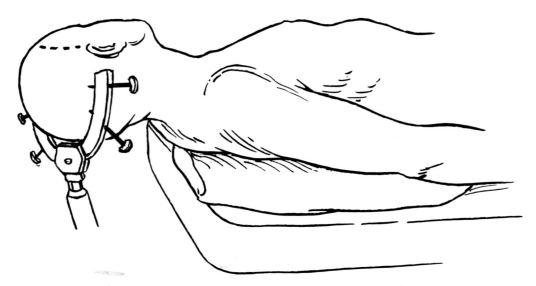

Figure 30-33. Position of patient for pterional craniotomy.

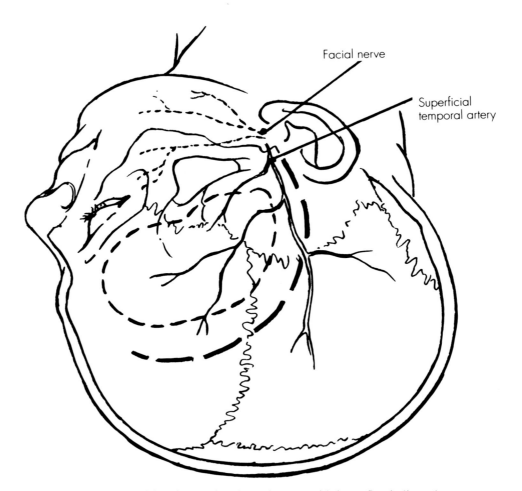

Figure 30-34. Incision for pterional craniotomy with bone flap indicated.

point between the midline and pupillary line. To avoid injuring the frontal branch of the facial nerve, the incision should not extend too low or be made too anterior to the tragus. The incision line may be infiltrated with local anesthetic, but epinephrine is not used because of the chance of sudden elevation in the blood pressure. Care is taken to preserve the superficial temporal artery. The craniotomy is the same for virtually all aneurysms of the carotid circulation and upper basilar artery.

Scalp Flap

The temporalis fascia is incised with a scalpel; this permits closure as a separate layer that reduces postoperative swelling in the area. The scalp flap is reflected inferiorly in a single layer with the cutting cautery to separate the temporalis muscle from the skull. By reflecting the scalp flap in a single layer, injury to the frontal branch of the facial nerve is avoided. The bony landmarks that are utilized are the zygomatic process of the frontal bone, the lateral margin of the supraorbital ridge, and the zygoma. The muscle is reflected downward until these structures are visualized or, in the case of the zygoma, easily palpated (Fig. 30-35).

Bone Flap

A single burr hole is placed in the temporal region where it can be covered by the temporalis muscle. From this hole a free bone flap measuring 4 × 5 cm is created with a craniotome. An initial cut is made from the burr hole to sphenoid wing as far as is possible. The craniotome is then returned to the burr hole and the remainder of the flap created. It is usually necessary to crack the bone at the sphenoid wing by elevating the flap. It is essential that the bony opening be flush with the floor of the frontal fossa. Care must be taken, however, not to enter the orbit with the craniotome in an attempt to make the flap too low. A minor variation is made when a left- or right-sided exposure is used. For a right-handed surgeon, a left-sided craniotomy should have 1 to 2 cm more

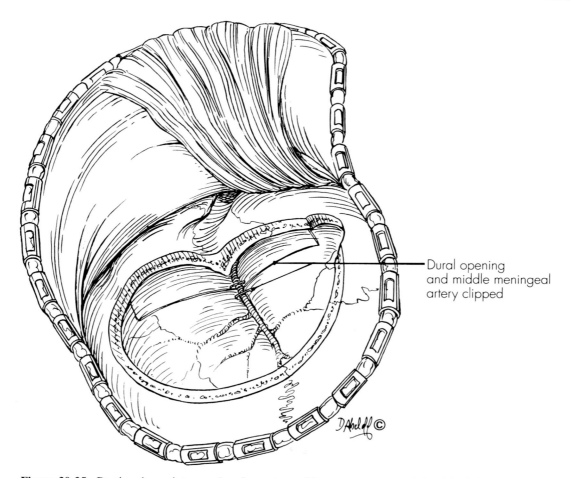

Dural opening
and middle meningeal
artery clipped

Figure 30-35. Pterional craniotomy showing extent of bony exposure and dural incision indicated.

frontal exposure to permit the free introduction of instruments without coming into contact with the margin of the flap. This is less of a problem when the exposure is on the right side, since instruments in the surgeon's right hand will cross the temporal lobe. Care should be taken to avoid entering the frontal sinus. If this occurs special attention must be given to the closure to prevent a CSF rhinorrhea (see below).

The lateral aspect of the sphenoid wing is then rongeured so that it will offer no obstruction to the line of vision. It is not necessary to drill this away, since 1.5 cm of the wing can easily be removed with rongeurs. After dural tenting sutures have been placed, the spinal drainage is opened. A linear dural incision is made along the base of the exposure, 2 cm from the craniotomy margin. Care is taken not to coagulate the dura so that a good dural closure can be performed. If necessary, the middle meningeal artery is secured with small titanium clips.

Cosmetics

The pterional approach provides good access through a relatively small opening. It heals well, leaving an almost unnoticeable operative site. Attention to several details will improve the cosmetic results. When possible, bone overlying the temporal lobe should be included in the bone flap removed with the craniotome. This reduces the bony defect that may produce a poor cosmetic result after the incision has healed. Another source of a poor appearance of the wound site is atrophy of the temporalis muscle. Since the innervation of the muscle comes from nerve branches deep to the muscle, they should not be coagulated when the muscle is elevated from the bone.

At the time of the closure several other steps are helpful to ensure a cosmetically acceptable incision. I prefer to use silk sutures rather than wire to secure the bone flap. This is well tolerated and will not protrude through the scalp. It is important to insert the sutures to minimize any noticeable subcutaneous lump. They can be placed beneath muscle, behind the hairline, or countersunk. When reattaching the free bone flap, the anterior, medial margin should be seated first. This will minimize any irregularities of the bone flap in visible areas of the scalp.

Intraoperative Techniques

It is difficult to describe all the nuances of the dissection techniques used in aneurysm surgery. The first step, after elevating the frontal lobe, is to identify the optic nerve. Once this has been done, the exposure is maintained with a self-retaining retractor. The landmarks for identifying the optic nerve are the olfactory tract and the sphenoid wing. The nerve is found at the point of intersection of these two structures. Retraction of the medial border of the temporal lobe is usually necessary for clipping of PCoA and AChA aneurysms. It is important, however, not to disturb the relationship between the dome of the aneurysm and the temporal lobe before good visualization of any adhesions can be achieved.

The operating microscope is now brought into use, and the dissection proceeds at increasing magnifications as the carotid artery and aneurysm are exposed. The first step of the microdissection is to divide various arachnoid connections. This frees the aneurysm from any undue traction and increases the room in which to operate within the subarachnoid space. The arachnoid between the frontal lobe and optic nerve is first divided. This plane is extended laterally into the sylvian fissure and medially to the interhemispheric fissure. As the arachnoid is divided additional retraction increases the exposure of the carotid artery. Once this arachnoid is opened the dissection can proceed along the carotid toward the point of origin of the aneurysm.

Intraoperative Rupture

One of the most serious intraoperative complications of all aneurysm surgeries is the occurrence of intraoperative rupture. This is particularly difficult to manage when it occurs during the initial exposure, prior to definition of the anatomy of the aneurysm. Aneurysms of the PCoA may be particularly susceptible to this when they are adherent to the temporal lobe. In this situation rupture of the aneurysm may occur when the temporal lobe is retracted to gain the initial exposure. One should be alert to this possibility in those patients with aneurysms of the PCoA who do not have a third nerve palsy. This may indicate that the aneurysm is adherent to the temporal lobe rather than in the usual close relationship with the third nerve. This should also be suspected when the angiogram shows the aneurysm projecting lateral to the carotid artery. In these situations special attention to the placement of the temporal retractor is necessary. This should be delayed until good visualization of the aneurysm is available through the microscope. Since retraction of the temporal lobe may still be necessary, it should be done under direct visualization of the aneurysm to avoid tearing an adhesion that can safely be dissected and divided.

Even before the planes around the aneurysm are well established, the surgeon should develop a mental picture of the location of the neck. Should rupture occur before the dissection has been completed, it is helpful to have a good idea of where the neck is located so that a rapid and accurate dissection and application of the clip can be carried out while bleeding is controlled by the suction. Should rupture occur, the first step is to maintain visualization of the operative field. This can often be accomplished with the accurate placement of a suction over the dome. Clip application should be attempted only after adequate dissection has been done. A temporary clip may be helpful if additional time is needed to complete the final delineation of the neck of the aneurysm as well as the branches of the carotid artery.

Proximal Control

In aneurysms of the carotid artery at the PCoA and AChA, one can usually obtain proximal control of the intracranial carotid artery. In some situations the PCoA aneurysm may be quite proximal or the aneurysm may be partially covered by the anterior clinoid process. In these situations control of the carotid artery can only be obtained by exposure of the carotid artery in the neck. While this is not often necessary, it should not be overlooked as a means of facilitating the clipping or increasing the safety of the procedure. With the widespread use of subtracted films, the relationship between the aneurysm and the anterior clinoid process and base of the skull may be overlooked. Proximal control of the carotid artery should also be utilized in cases of large aneurysms (see below).

Clip Application

Selection of appropriate clips should begin early in the course of the dissection so that the surgeon has a good idea which clips and clip appliers will be best suited for the particular aneurysm. It is important to remember that the neck of an aneurysm becomes wider than the initial diameter when it is compressed. It is important to have a clip long enough to account for this increase. *It is necessary to add about one-third of the diameter of the neck to the length of the blades of the clip to encompass the entire neck when it is flattened out. This can be expressed by the formula: $L = \pi d/2$, where L is the length of the clip and d is the diameter of the neck of the aneurysm.*

Although smaller carotid aneurysms (<8 mm) can be safely clipped by placing the clip at right angles with the parent vessel, it is advisable to apply the clip so that the blades are parallel with the parent vessels (Fig. 30-36). This is particularly important when dealing with large, thick-walled aneurysms. Failure to do this increases the chances of compromising the lumen of the vessel or producing a kink in the parent vessel and its branches.

If more than one clip is required because of the presence of two aneurysms, it is better to complete the dissection of both aneurysms prior to applying the first clip. If one clip must be applied before the second aneurysm is completely dissected, it should be positioned so that it will not interfere with the application of the second clip.

In almost all cases, the aneurysm should be punctured and opened after it has been clipped. Only in this way can the surgeon be certain that the goal of

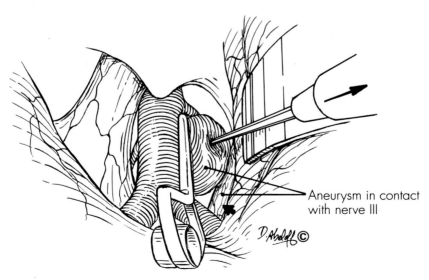

Aneurysm in contact with nerve III

Figure 30-36. Clip application parallel to the parent vessel.

obliterating the aneurysm has been achieved. It is surprising how often an aneurysm can bleed when this is done after a seemingly perfect clip application. The only exception is when no further adjustment of the clip is safe or possible. While this occurs with some of the larger ophthalmic region aneurysms, it should not pose a problem for the more distal carotid aneurysms. In those cases in which the aneurysm is not punctured, a postoperative angiogram is used to ensure complete closure of the aneurysm.

One final point to be emphasized is the need for patience and the willingness to readjust the clip until a satisfactory application has been achieved. This is important for complete obliteration of the aneurysm as well as preservation of flow in the parent vessels.

If modern clips that are MR compatible are used, there is little if any chance of slippage. With older clip designs this was a problem that was occasionally encountered. It should be considered in patients who are being followed many years after the original surgery.

Techniques of Closure

A watertight closure of the dura should be attempted. If the frontal sinus has been opened, care must be taken to prevent a CSF leak from developing. In addition to a careful dural closure, a pericranial flap should be developed to cover the opening of the frontal sinus. The sinus is filled with gelatin foam and the pericranial flap sutured to the dura. Glue or acrylic is not used. The bone flap must be securely fastened to provide a good cosmetic result. The temporalis muscle and fascia are closed in separate layers. A drain with a closed vacuum system is placed beneath the scalp flap for 24 hours. This reduces the periorbital swelling that may develop.

SPECIFIC SOURCES OF INTRAOPERATIVE COMPLICATIONS

Vascular Considerations

Two major vessels must be considered when one operates upon midcarotid artery aneurysms. The branches of the carotid artery have important territories of supply that demand their preservation.

Posterior Communicating Artery

In most cases the PCoA itself can be separated from the neck of the aneurysm and thereby preserved. In a review of 200 cases of PCoA aneurysms in the author's series, the position of the PCoA in relation to the aneurysm could be determined. In 75 percent of these cases the artery arose on the proximal side of the aneurysm neck.[75] In 12 percent of the cases a direct origin of the posterior cerebral artery from the carotid artery was encountered. In the remaining 13 percent the PCoA was visualized on the distal side of the aneurysm neck. When a direct origin of the PCoA is encountered, this vessel must be preserved to avoid a significant infarct in the posterior temporal and occipital lobes. It is important to remember that the PCoA is not a straight conduit. There are often two to four branches from the PCoA that supply the optic chiasm, optic tract, pituitary stalk, and hypothalamus.[77] In addition to the possible loss of visual fields, excessive manipulation or occlusion of these branches may produce diabetes insipidus.

Anterior Choroidal Artery

There is no specific clinical presentation of aneurysms arising from the region of the AChA. They are relatively uncommon, comprising only 5 percent of the present series. In the author's series, the presentation was SAH in 29 of 50 cases, temporal lobe seizures in 2, and a partial third nerve palsy in 2. They were found in association with another aneurysm in 12 cases, the most common association being with an adjacent PCoA aneurysm. Because of the important territory of the brain supplied by the AChA, every effort should be made to identify the origin of the artery itself.[77] Failure to do this will frequently cause the vessel to be included in the clip. This is poorly tolerated and results in an infarction in the internal capsule that produces a severe hemiparesis from which recovery is incomplete at best.

The dissection and clipping of aneurysms in this location is quite similar to PCoA aneurysms. The major difference is the need to identify the AChA with certainty. An important aid to visualize the AChA is to obtain adequate room to work at the distal end of the carotid artery. This is facilitated by widely opening the sylvian fissure. Although this is generally done as part of the initial approach to carotid aneurysms and certainly for aneurysms of the carotid bifurcation, an extra effort should be made in cases of anterior choroidal aneurysms, because there is often a tendency to regard them as PCoA aneurysms that do not require the same amount of exposure (Fig. 30-37). The AChA may course medial to the aneurysm. In this situation it is necessary to separate the vessel from the aneurysm neck to prevent its inclusion in the clip. Sometimes this can be done by working from the medial side of the carotid artery between the vessel and the optic nerve. In rare instances the AChA may arise from the carotid artery proximal to

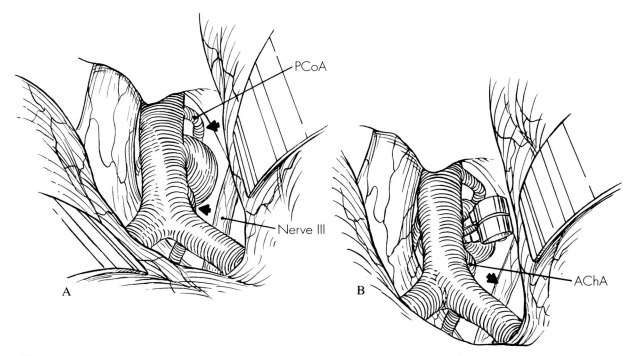

Figure 30-37. **(A)** Distal fissure opened for adequate exposure. **(B)** Clip applied at right angle to the parent vessel when aneurysm is small.

the PCA (Fig. 30-38). This anomaly must be recognized to avoid inadvertent sacrifice of the AChA.

Bridging Veins

The decision to coagulate and divide the bridging veins along the temporal lobe has been discussed many times. Some surgeons do not divide these veins routinely. In most instances I have preferred to do this prior to the placement of retractors. This should obviate the need to interrupt the dissection of the aneurysm if these veins tear later during the procedure. Collateral venous drainage of the anterior temporal lobe is adequate to permit this without producing swelling.

Figure 30-38. Angiogram showing anomalous origin of both branches. The AChA is seen arising from the carotid artery proximal to the origin of the PCoA.

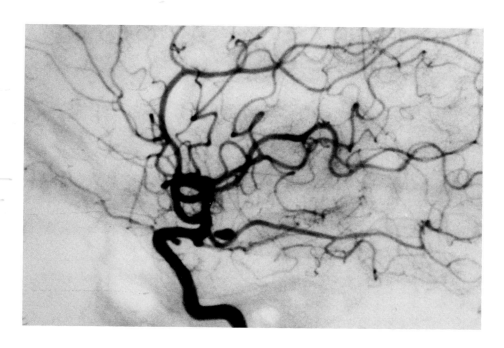

Cranial Nerves

An additional source of problems with aneurysms arising from the midportion of the carotid artery are the cranial nerves in this area. They may be injured during the initial exposure through a pterional approach or at some specific point of the dissection.

Olfactory Tract

The olfactory tract is subject to damage during any standard pterional approach. This occurs during the initial elevation of the frontal lobe to expose the optic nerve and carotid artery. Another point of the procedure at which the olfactory tract may be damaged is the placement of the frontal retractor. Care must be taken to prevent small venous hemorrhages along the olfactory tract, because attempts to coagulate these bleeding points may lead to disruption of the nerve.

Prevention of these problems can be achieved by careful attention to retractor placement and to the degree of traction placed on the tract. To limit the amount of bleeding along the tract and to reduce the need for coagulation, Gelfoam should be placed in the region of the cribriform plate. This is done as soon as the frontal retractor is placed. The undersurface of the frontal lobe including the olfactory tract should be covered with cottonoids before the retractor is placed. In spite of these precautions the loss of smell and thus the loss of special taste can be expected in about 10 percent of patients undergoing a pterional craniotomy. A considerably higher incidence has recently been reported.[70] Bilateral damage to the olfactory tracts may occur during a unilateral craniotomy. All too often the olfactory tracts are regarded as expendable. Loss of olfaction and taste are significant problems that affect patients' daily activities; for this reason care should always be taken to prevent this occurrence.

Optic Nerve

The optic nerves and chiasm are not usually injured during exposure or dissection of PCoA or AChA aneurysms. To reduce any damage to these structures, I do not cover the optic nerve or chiasm with cottonoid so that they remain in view during all of the dissection along the carotid artery. Should visualization of these structures be lost during the procedure when hemorrhage occurs, great care must be taken as all instruments are moved in and out of the field.

Oculomotor Nerve

The oculomotor nerve is another structure that is particularly vulnerable during operations on aneurysms of the midcarotid artery. Although the association of aneurysms of the PCA with the third nerve is well known, it should be remembered that the anterior choroidal artery and aneurysms arising at its origin may also have a close relationship with this nerve. Injury may come from stretching during retraction, direct injury, or during the course of mobilizing an aneurysm in this vicinity. Traction injury can be prevented by widely opening the arachnoid around the nerve to isolate it from any transmitted traction. Sharp, careful opening of the arachnoid along the course of the nerve is far less traumatic than indiscreet traction to the temporal lobe.

Another potential source of injury to the third nerve during surgery is through compression of the nerve by a self-retaining retractor. The surgeon may inadvertently rest his hand on the arm or blade of the temporal self-retaining retractor, causing it to slip and to compress the third nerve along the edge of the tentorium (Fig. 30-39).

Although it is advisable to puncture any aneurysm that is compressing the third nerve after it has been clipped, a more extensive decompression of the nerve through dissecting the entire aneurysm from the nerve is not advisable. This is more likely to damage the nerve further rather than to improve the chances of recovery.

Other Cranial Nerves

While other cranial nerves may be injured during procedures on aneurysms of the PCoA or AChA, this is unusual. The sixth nerve and the first two divisions of the trigeminal nerve may be injured if there is need to coagulate the dura over the cavernous sinus. Coagulation in this area should be done only with bipolar cautery to prevent any current spread that might injure adjacent nerves.

GIANT ANEURYSMS

Approximately 14 percent of giant aneurysms in my series arose in the vicinity of the PCoA or AChA (Table 30-10). Often these produced no specific symptoms, but in 10 percent subarachnoid hemorrhage was associated with visual complaints or pituitary dysfunction due to the location of the SAH. Great attention must be paid to these lesions to avoid

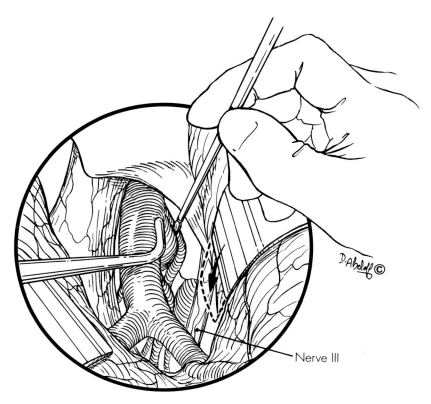

Figure 30-39. Slipped retractor against the third nerve. Also shown is the relative distal origin of the AChA.

a number of intraoperative and postoperative complications. These include intraoperative rupture, distal embolization, and delayed occlusion of the carotid artery or its branches.

Proximal Control

As mentioned above, proximal control can be accomplished in the neck with temporary occlusion of the internal carotid artery or intracranially with the

Table 30-10. Giant[a] Cerebral Aneurysms in Author's Series

Location	Total	Giant	Percent
Ophthalmic	114	49	42.9
Posterior communicating	244	17	7.0
Anterior choroidal	49	6	12.2
Carotid bifurcation	40	10	25.0
Anterior communicating	194	19	9.8
Distal anterior cerebral	32	2	6.6
Middle cerebral	209	33	15.8
Vertebrobasilar	135	32	23.7
	1,017	168	16.5

[a] Size, 2.0–6.0 cm; mean, 3.1 cm.

use of a temporary clip on the supraclinoid artery. I currently use the carotid occlusion clamp designed by Heifiez.[73] In both situations I utilize monitoring of somatosensory evoked potentials to provide some indication of impending cerebral ischemia.

An additional problem encountered with carotid aneurysms, especially larger ones, is the tension within the aneurysm itself. This often prevents a clip from closing completely; there is also an increased chance of rupture if the clip does not completely obliterate the aneurysm when it is applied. Several techniques are available to reduce the tension within the aneurysm. Temporary occlusion of the internal carotid artery in the neck dramatically reduces the pressure in the supraclinoid carotid artery and within the aneurysm. This is utilized for large aneurysms arising from the proximal supraclinoid carotid artery. Although temporary clips can be applied directly to the supraclinoid carotid artery for more distal carotid aneurysms, they must be positioned so that the working space necessary to clip the aneurysm is not compromised.

We prefer to utilize intermittent periods of occlusion ranging from 3 to 5 minutes. This is carried out with normal to slightly elevated blood pressure. No putative cerebral protective agents are used at the time of occlusion or in the postoperative period. The goals of temporary occlusion for management of giant aneurysm are twofold. First, the risk of intraoperative rupture is reduced. Second, the tension within the aneurysm at the time of clip application is reduced. This improves the accuracy of the clip placement. It also allows the clip to close completely and to remain in proper alignment with the carotid artery.

Trapping and Decompression

In some situations temporary occlusion of the proximal carotid artery is not sufficient to slacken a giant aneurysm. Prior to clip application it may be necessary to trap the aneurysm and/or to carry out suction decompression. The decision to perform this maneuver should be made before multiple clip applications are attempted. This is important in large and giant aneurysms that may contain thrombus. Excessive manipulation of such an aneurysm increases the risk of distal embolization from the lumen of the aneurysm. With trapping or intravascular decompression, this risk is reduced.

Another technique that has been helpful with large, thick-walled aneurysms is suction decompression.[11] A 19-gauge scalp vein needle with the flanges removed is connected to the operating room suction. By puncturing the dome of the aneurysm where it is thick, blood can be suctioned through the aneurysm and the intraluminal tension reduced. Although this may not cause the thick-walled aneurysm to collapse, the aneurysm will become softer and more pliable. The clip can then be closed down easily and more safely. Blood loss has not been more than 100 ml when this technique is employed. More recently, Samson and Batjer (personal communication) have utilized a suction technique through the lumen of the cervical carotid artery to achieve decompression of the aneurysm. A catheter is introduced into the exposed carotid artery in the neck. The aneurysm is trapped by placing a clip distal to the aneurysm, and the aneurysm is decompressed by suction through the catheter.

Aneurysmorrhaphy

Giant aneurysms of the midcarotid artery may contain organized thrombus and calcified plaque along the neck where the clip is to be applied. This can be dealt with by removing this material from the lumen of the aneurysm. This will improve the chance of accurate clip placement and reduce the risk of tearing the neck at its junction with the carotid artery.

The area of the aneurysm must be trapped. The clips used for this should be positioned carefully so that they do not interfere with subsequent dissection (Fig. 30-40A&B). The opening into the dome of the aneurysm must be far enough removed from the carotid artery to preserve sufficient tissue for closure and reconstruction of the vessel. Microdissectors, ring forceps, suction, and, occasionally, the ultrasonic aspirator can be used to remove the contents and thin the wall.

Before attempting to clip the base of the aneurysm, it is essential to allow some bleeding through the carotid artery. Failure to "back bleed" the system sets the stage for distal embolization of clot or air that is in the opened carotid artery.

Arterial Reconstruction

With giant aneurysms of the midcarotid artery, the goal is often more than achieving occlusion of the aneurysm. With larger aneurysms, the wall of the carotid artery is shared with the dome of the aneurysm (Fig. 30-40C). Closure of the aneurysm requires reconstruction of the carotid artery itself. The portion of the artery that has been incorporated into the dome of the aneurysm must be returned to its cylindrical configuration. Temporary occlusion, trapping, or suction decompression all are helpful to accomplish this.

A variety of clips are useful. They should be selected and loaded prior to beginning the dissection. The major principle to remember is preservation of the lumen of the carotid artery as well as the PCoA and AChA (Fig. 30-40D). Except when there is a fetal origin of the posterior cerebral artery from the carotid artery, the PCoA may sometimes have to be sacrificed to occlude a large midcarotid artery successfully.

These ends are accomplished by the use of fenestrated clips or long, angled straight clips that can be applied with the blades parallel to the course of the carotid artery. Multiple clips should be used when needed.

POSTOPERATIVE MANAGEMENT AND COMPLICATIONS

The goals of postoperative care are to maintain adequate cerebral perfusion, to reduce any postoperative cerebral swelling and increase in intracranial

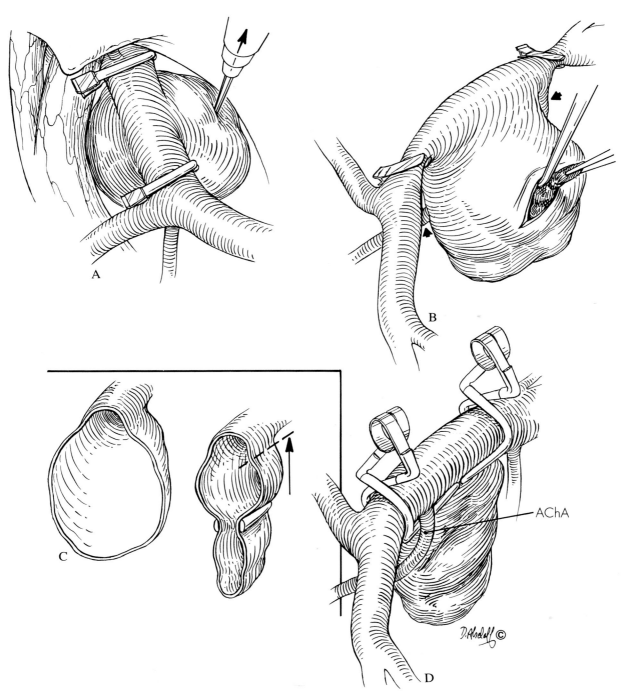

Figure 30-40. Aneurysmorrhaphy of giant midcarotid artery aneurysm. **(A)** Aneurysm is trapped, and suction decompression is performed. **(B)** Trapped aneurysm is opened and contents removed. **(C)** Shared wall of the carotid artery with the aneurysm is shown. A segment of the aneurysm is utilized to reconstruct the carotid artery into a cylinder. **(D)** Reconstruction of the carotid artery and obliteration of the aneurysm with fenestrated clips.

pressure, and to prevent seizures. These aims can be accomplished by continuing the preoperative medical regimen of corticosteroids, anticonvulsants, and fluids.

Upon transfer of the recovery room, blood pressure is maintained at normal to slightly elevated levels. Central venous pressure is maintained at 6 to 8 cmH$_2$O by administering colloid. Corticosteroids, in our practice methylprednisolone 250 mg every 6 hours, are maintained at this level for 3 days and then tapered over the next 5 days. Levels of anticonvulsants are determined initially after surgery and during the postoperative period.

Since most aneurysms have been opened intraoperatively, we do not routinely perform postoperative angiography. If there is any change in the patient's neurological condition or if the aneurysm was not opened at surgery, angiography is carried out.

Most patients are now operated on within 3 days of SAH. It is therefore important to maintain an expectant attitude with regard to the development of delayed ischemia. At present all patients are being managed with a dihydropyridine calcium channel blocker to reduce the incidence of cerebral vasospasm and delayed ischemia. The efficacy of this regimen is monitored with transcranial Doppler measurements and follow-up angiography when indicated by neurological deterioration. We prefer to document vasospasm rather than presume that it is the cause of any neurological deterioration.

Finally, it is important to remain vigilant when dealing with midcarotid aneurysms. All too often one hears an inexperienced surgeon say that this case is *"just* a PCoA aneurysm." An experienced surgeon is never so blithe. The pitfalls are many, but can be avoided with attention to these details.

Carotid Bifurcation Aneurysms

Christopher S. Ogilvy
Robert M. Crowell

Representing about 15 percent of all internal carotid artery (ICA) aneurysms, carotid bifurcation aneurysms manifest a distinct clinical presentation, anatomical configuration, and surgical challenge. Review of relevant literature and of our own experience shows that characteristic surgical complications in this group of aneurysms come from injury to associated arterial perforating branches and to intraoperative aneurysmal rupture.

We believe that perforator injury and aneurysmal rupture are best prevented by (1) specific *microsurgical approach* dictated by the projection of the aneurysm, (2) wide *sylvian exposure* of parent and perforator vessels near the aneurysm, and (3) *temporary clipping,* which greatly assists in precise dissection and aneurysm obliteration without rupture.

In this report we examine details of the specialized surgical approach to carotid bifurcation aneurysms. We also review the many complications from ICA bifurcation aneurysms that are similar to those from other aneurysms.

LITERATURE REVIEW

In the premicrosurgical era, the clipping of ICA bifurcation aneurysms carried with it significant morbidity and mortality rates.[99] Af Bjorkesten[81] reported seven bifurcation aneurysms treated surgically. One lesion was clipped directly, three were suture ligated, and three were wrapped. The results of these procedures are difficult to separate from those in all the patients reported in this early series of ICA lesions. McKissock et al.[90] reported a 41 percent mortality rate in 44 patients with bifurcation aneurysms treated surgically. In 10 lesions approached with direct surgery, David and Sachs[85] had one death. Perria et al.[94] reviewed bifurcation lesions reported in the literature prior to 1965; they identified 35 cases treated with carotid ligation and 50 cases treated with direct wrapping or clipping. Of the patients treated with carotid ligation, there was a 14 percent postoperative mortality rate. Ischemic complications and ineffectiveness have led to disuse of carotid ligation for ICA bifurcation aneurysms whenever direct surgery is possible. In the Perria et al. series of patients treated with direct surgery, a 34 percent postoperative morbidity rate was recorded. In an exceptional series of nine patients, Sengupta[97] was able to clip eight lesions with no operative deaths and a single neurological worsening.

The results of the series of carotid bifurcation aneurysms operated on with an operating microscope are presented in Table 30-11. As can be seen, the use of the operating microscope and microsurgical techniques has significantly reduced the morbidity and mortality rates to a total of 5 to 15 percent.[99] DaPain et al.[84] stress that a wide opening of the sylvian fissure is important in order to avoid the complication of unnecessary retraction of brain to expose these lesions. In addition, for anteriorly projecting lesions they caution approach via the sylvian fissure instead of following the ICA in order to avoid rupture of the

Table 30-11. Results of a Series of Carotid Bifurcation Aneurysms Operated on with an Operating Microscope

Author	Year	No. of Cases	Mortality	Morbidity
DaPain et al.[84]	1979	21	1	0
Yarsargil[100]	1984	55	2	4
Ojemann et al.[93]	1988	14	1	1
Laranjeira et al.[88]	1990	18	0	1
Total		108	4	6
Percent			4	6

dome of the aneurysm, which is often adherent to the ICA. Intraoperative rupture is known to triple the incidence of complications of aneurysm surgery.[82] Posteriorly projecting aneurysms are particularly prone to adherence to important deep perforating arteries on the dome of the lesion. In a review of 18 patients by Laranjeira et al.,[88] emphasis was placed on detailed definition of the perforating vessels. The only complication in this series was due to compromise of the perforating arteries during clipping of a giant ICA bifurcation aneurysm.

COMPLICATION AVOIDANCE AND MANAGEMENT

Major complications from ICA bifurcation aneurysms are listed in Table 30-12. While many complications may occur without operative intervention, for example, vasospasm or hydrocephalus, because of the current practice of early surgery these problems often emerge in the postoperative period. Medical problems can arise with or without surgery. Note that most of these complications may also be encoun-

Table 30-12. Major Complications of ICA Bifurcation Aneurysm Surgery: Avoidance and Management

Manifestation	Complication	Diagnostic Technique	Treatment	Avoidance
Immediate postoperative deficit	Arterial (intraoperative perforator) occlusion	Clinical examination	Adjust clip	Perfect clipping, intraoperative angiography
Delayed postoperative deficit	Subdural, epidural, or intracerebral hemorrhage	CT	Surgical evacuation	Precise hemostasis intraoperative blood pressure check
	Hydrocephalus	CT	?Ventriculostomy ?VP shunt	Avoid Amicar
	Vasospasm	CT + transcranial Doppler (angiography)	BP, CVP, mannitol, ?angioplasty	Avoid Amicar, nimodipine
	Meningitis	Lumbar puncture	Antibiotics	Careful asepsis, prophylatic antibiotics
	Seizures	EEG	Anticonvulsants	Prophylatic anticonvulsants
	Electrolyte imbalance	Serum electrolytes	Appropriate fluid management	Careful fluid treatment
Medical problems	Myocardial infarction	ECG, enzymes	Medical	Avoid hypotension
	Deep vein thrombosis	Colorflow Doppler venogram	Umbrella (or anticoagulation 6 days postoperative)	Thigh-high air boots, avoid steroids
	Pulmonary embolus	PA angiography	Umbrella (or anticoagulation 6 days postoperative)	Thigh-high air boots, avoid steroids
	Respiratory failure	Arterial blood gasses	Intubation, etc.	Preoperative pulmonary function tests

tered in relation to balloon catheter treatment of aneurysms.

In the following presentation of a treatment program for ICA bifurcation aneurysms, we emphasize prevention of these complications, both intraoperatively and perioperatively. Methods of managing complications are presented as well.

The most important *intraoperative complications* are rupture and perforator occlusion. Obviously intraoperative precautions are crucial to prevent these catastrophes. The major strategy to prevent rupture is temporary clipping. The major strategy to prevent perforator occlusion is wide sylvian exposure. Details are described below.

The most important *perioperative complications* are recurrent SAH, vasospasm, and hydrocephalus. These are prevented by measures applicable to intracranial aneurysms generally.

PREOPERATIVE MANAGEMENT

The most common presentation of carotid bifurcation aneurysms is subarachnoid hemorrhage (SAH). The computed tomographic (CT) scan will often show extensive hemorrhage in the basal subarachnoid cisterns, especially prominent in the anterior cisterns on the side of rupture. In some instances, the hemorrhage may cause focal symptoms and CT appearance of deep basal ganglionic hemorrhage, owing to protrusion of the aneurysmal sac into the frontal lobe. Occasionally when a carotid bifurcation aneurysm reaches giant size, it may present with local symptoms and signs of compression, such as visual disturbance or hemiparesis. Occasionally when thrombus builds up in a carotid bifurcation aneurysm, distal embolization may cause hemispheric ischemia or infarction.

Though the presence of an ICA aneurysm may be suspected from the CT scan, angiography provides confirmation, and oblique or base views may also be helpful (Fig. 30-41). The angiogram is crucial in discerning the projection of the aneurysm and thus in surgical planning to avoid intraoperative rupture or perforator damage.

Before surgery, we manage ICA bifurcation aneurysms the same as other aneurysms. For patients with subarachnoid hemorrhage, immediate CT documents SAH, and angiography pinpoints the lesion. Blood pressure is controlled as soon as possible. Nimodipine, phenytoin, and hypervolemic hemodilution are begun. Early surgery is undertaken as soon as possible in all good-grade (1 to 3) and some poor-grade (4 and 5) patients. Early obliteration is the best way to avert catastrophic recurrent SAH.

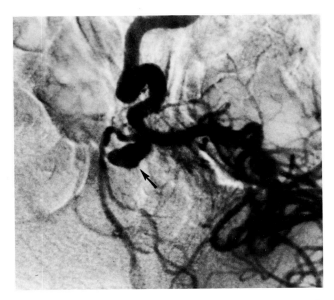

Figure 30-41. Oblique angiogram shows superiorly directed ICA aneurysm (*arrow*) from surgeon's point of view. Same case as in Figs. 30-43 to 30-45.

OPERATIVE TECHNIQUE

Induction

Every effort is made to avoid a hypertensive episode, which might cause recurrent aneurysmal rupture. Preanesthetic medication is given on call to the operating room. In preparation for intraoperative angiography the patient is placed supine on an Amsco radiolucent operating table. A 14- or 16-gauge cannula is inserted into an arm vein for satisfactory venous access. An arterial line is inserted into the radial artery for continuous blood pressure monitoring. In some patients who are especially anxious or in whom venous and arterial access are difficult, it is better to proceed with induction of anesthesia using only an intravenous access placed in an appropriate limb vein.

After venous and arterial access are obtained, preoxygenation is carried out. Then the patient is given isoflurane (0.5 to 2.0 percent). Once the patient is deeply drowsy, thiopental is given intravenously (150 to 300 mg, in increments) to a full sleep dose. With the patient asleep, gentle laryngoscopy is carried out, and the vocal cords are sprayed with topical lidocaine. No effort at intubation is made at this moment. The patient is ventilated with mask technique for several minutes to obtain vocal cord anesthesia. Then laryngoscopy and gentle intubation are carried out. All of these maneuvers are designed to minimize the hypertensive response during intubation. Blood pressure is monitored continuously, and should there be an undue elevation intubation is aborted until a satisfactory preparation is achieved.

During the entire procedure, end-tidal PCO_2 is monitored in an effort to maintain a level of approximately 30 mmHg. Arterial blood gases (ABG) are checked intermittently to ensure this level of hypocarbia, in an effort to promote brain relaxation. Concomitantly, esophageal core temperature is monitored with a standard flexible probe. A nasogastric tube is placed in order to provide for emptying of the stomach during and after surgery to avoid aspiration. Standard electrocardiographic (ECG) monitoring is carried out with both limb and precordial leads. A Foley catheter is placed in sterile fashion for continuous drainage of urine and monitoring of urine output.

In selected cases with cardiac pathology, a pulmonary arterial (PA) line is placed for continuous monitoring of PA pressures and intermittent determination of cardiac output (CO). A central venous pressure (CVP) catheter is placed for monitoring of CVP to guide fluid management and provide access for fluid administration both intra- and postoperatively. After placement of CVP or PA lines, a chest film is required to ensure proper positioning of the catheter and to exclude the possibility of a pneumothorax. Prophylactic preoperative antibiotics are given intravenously before the skin excision (Ancef 1 g IV). In the absence of symptomatic brain swelling, we do not routinely give corticosteroids because of the increased incidence of deep venous thrombosis and pulmonary embolism. In patients who have been screened preoperatively with noninvasive Doppler methods to exclude deep venous occlusive disease, thigh-high pneumatic compression air boots are utilized to minimize the chance of deep venous thrombosis during surgery. In patients with large or giant carotid bifurcation aneurysms, a lumbar spinal catheter is inserted for drainage of spinal fluid to assist in the exposure of the intracranial aneurysm. No CSF is purposely removed at this time.

Positioning

A limited frontotemporal shave is accomplished. Then the patient is placed in the radiolucent three-point skeletal head rest device. Prior to placement of the pins, the anesthesiologist gives an additional increment of thiopental to avoid a hypertensive reaction to the painful pin insertion.

The general principles of head positioning hold for these aneurysms: The head is placed above the heart by flexion of the neck. To avoid venous obstruction, the clavicle and mandible should be at least 2 cm

apart. To permit the brain to fall away from the skull base, the vertex is placed 10 to 15 degrees below the horizontal. For obliteration of an ICA bifurcation aneurysm and preservation of crucial perforator arteries, generous exposure of the ICA, middle cerebral artery (MCA), and anterior cerebral artery (ACA) must be provided, especially for large and giant lesions. This exposure is obtained by rotation of the head 30 to 60 degrees off the vertical (Fig. 30-42). The ideal angle of attack upon most aneurysms is perpendicular to the neck. Thus in order to place the visual axis vertical, it is best to position the neck of the aneurysm in the horizontal plane. With these princi-

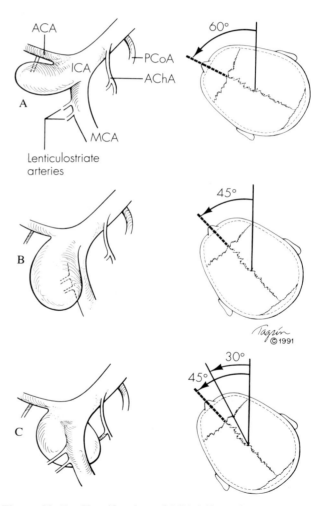

Figure 30-42. Classification of ICA bifurcation aneurysm with operative positioning. Anatomy as seen at right pterional craniotomy. **(A)** Superiorly (medially) directed aneurysm requires 60 degree head turn. **(B)** Posteriorly directed aneurysm requires 45 degree head turn. **(C)** Inferiorly directed aneurysm requires 30 to 45 degree head turn.

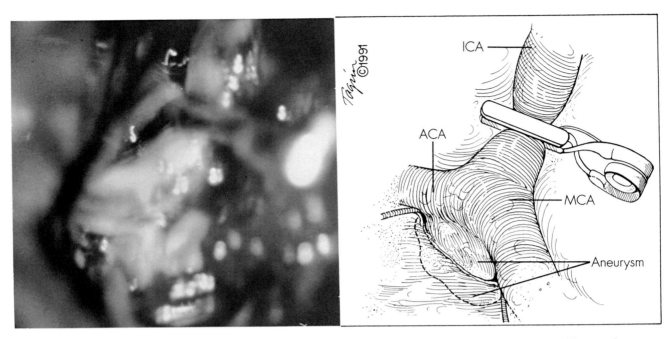

Figure 30-43. At right pterional craniotomy, wide sylvian exposure and temporary ICA clip facilitate safe dissection of aneurysm.

ples in mind, one can estimate the optimum head rotation by reference to the aneurysmal configuration as depicted in the cerebral angiograms.

It is important to note that carotid bifurcation aneurysms typically point in one of three directions:

superiorly (medially), posteriorly, or inferiorly.[100] *Superiorly* directed carotid bifurcation aneurysms impinge on the orbital frontal gyrus or olfactory tract. This is the most common configuration. The aneurysm projects along the A_1 segment of the ACA. Ex-

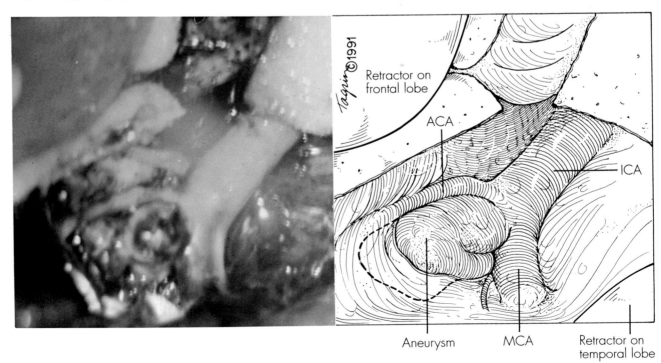

Figure 30-44. Final preparation of aneurysm. A_1 and M_1 perforating branches beneath aneurysm have been separated.

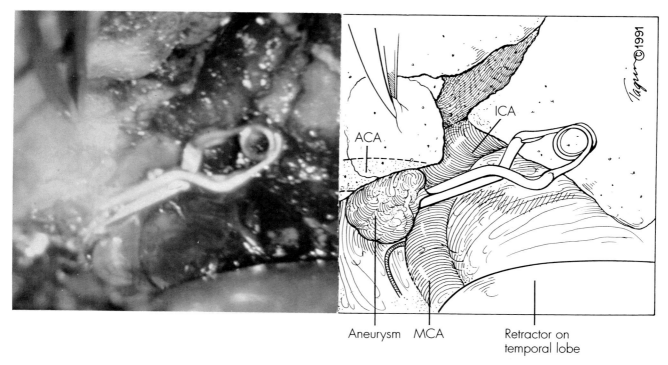

Aneurysm MCA   Retractor on
                 temporal lobe

Figure 30-45. Clip obliteration of aneurysm with straight Sugita clip.

posure of such a lesion is similar to exposure of an anterior communicating aneurysm, and the head is best turned 60 degrees off the vertical (Figs. 30-41 and 30-43 to 30-45). *Posteriorly* directed aneurysms generally occupy the sylvian cistern and accompany the MCA. These lesions are best approached with the head turned approximately 45 degrees. *Inferiorly* directed aneurysms generally drape down over the posteromesial aspect of the internal carotid and may enter the interpeduncular cistern (Fig. 30-46). A precisely perpendicular approach to such an aneurysm would require access through the brain and is thus not strictly possible. The best practical approach is rotation of the head 30 to 45 degrees, with wide splitting of the sylvian fissure for extensive exposure of the carotid bifurcation area. This is also the best exposure for a giant aneurysm in this area.

Incision

The scalp flap is essentially a frontotemporal flap, similar to a pterional flap but providing a bit more temporal exposure by swinging slightly posteriorly (Fig. 30-47A). This type of exposure provides satisfactory access to the ICA, ACA, and MCA. The incision begins at the widow's peak in the midline and curves posteriorly above the ear and then down to the zygoma just in front of the tragus. The incision is taken to the midline to avoid an incision on the forehead but to provide access to the key hole just behind

the zygomatic process of frontal bone. The incision is taken down to the zygoma to permit access to the temporal lobe, with the incision just in front of the tragus to avoid injury to the frontalis branch of the facial nerve. In this area, the posterior branch of the superficial temporal artery is dissected free and divided between 3-0 silk ligatures, with careful preservation of the trunk and anterior branch in case of need for extracranial-intracranial bypass. Next the

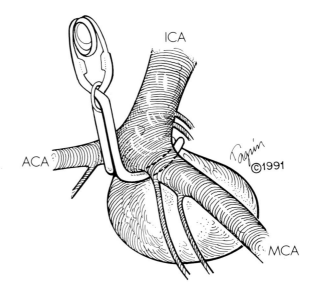

Figure 30-46. Large inferiorly directed aneurysm obliterated with curved Sugita clip.

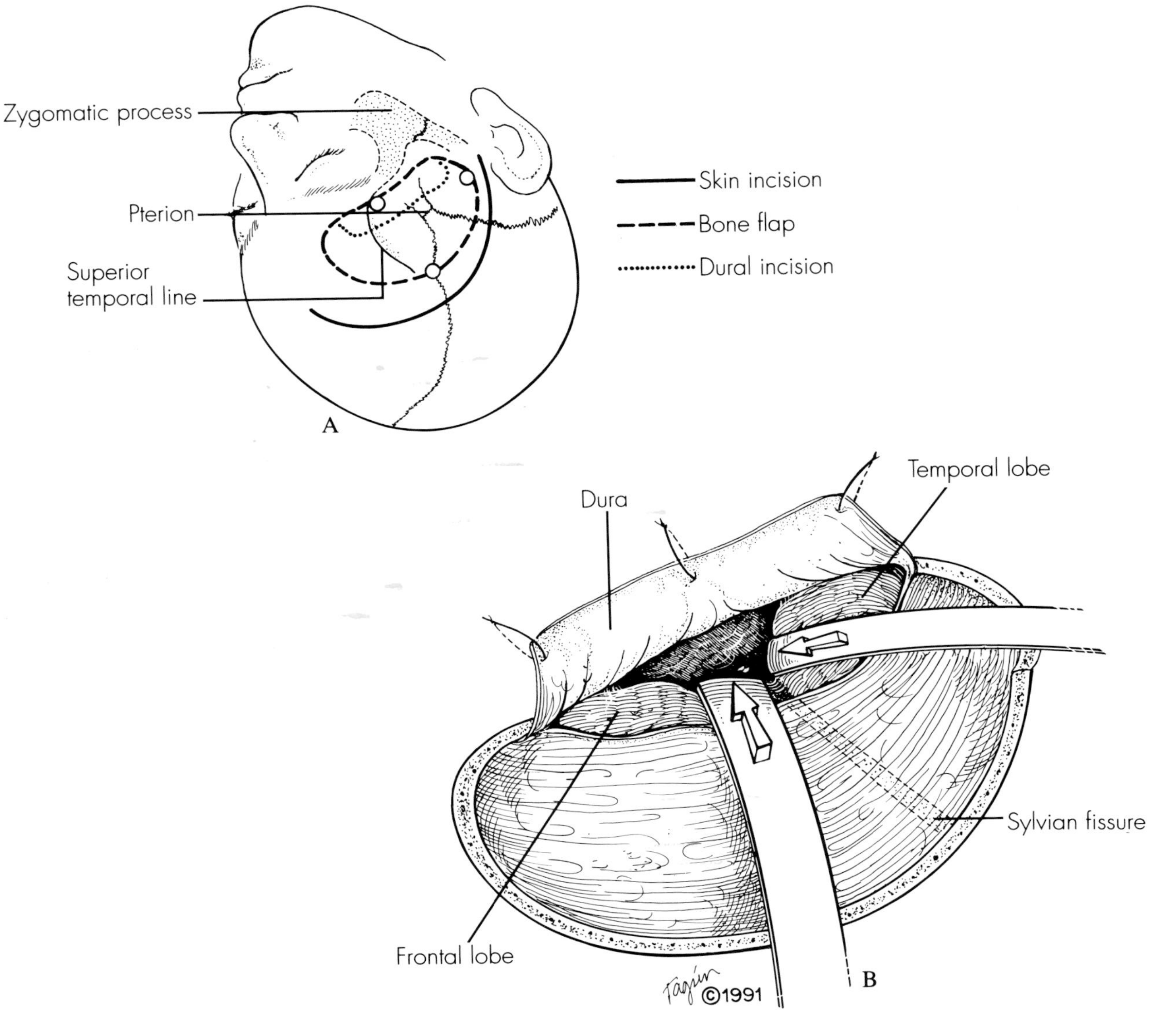

Figure 30-47. (A) Incision and bone flap. Modified pterional craniotomy provides substantial frontal and temporal exposure. **(B)** Initial exposure corridors. The temporal corridor is used for superiorly directed aneurysms, and the frontal for posteriorly directed aneurysms.

temporalis fascia is incised sharply, and the muscle is opened with the cutting cautery down to the skull. The temporalis muscle is reflected with the cutting cautery down to the frontozygomatic process, and the soft tissues are pulled back with 3-0 silk retraction sutures.

Bone Flap

As the bone flap is being turned, mannitol 100 g and furosemide 10 mg are given to promote diuresis and brain relaxation. This is done to provide satisfac-

tory deep exposure without retractor injury. The bone flap is prepared with burr holes just behind the zygomatic process of the frontal bone, in the low temporal area, and on the superior temporal line posteriorly (Fig. 30-47A). After the dura is separated from the bone with a Penfield 3 instrument, the bone flap is cut with the Midas Rex craniotome. The anterior portion swings low for 2.5 cm over the anterior cranial fossa, like the bone flap for an anterior communicating artery aneurysm. The posterior portion swings posteriorly like the bone flap for a middle cerebral aneurysm. In essence this is an expanded pterional bone flap.

After waxing of the bony edges and control of any dural bleeders such as the middle meningeal artery, the lateral one-third of the sphenoid ridge is removed for improved exposure. This is done with separation of the dura on both the temporal and frontal sides down to the lateral edge of the superior orbital fissure. The orbitomeningeal artery is coagulated and cross cut. The Leksell ronguer and angled up-biting Kerrison instrument are used in most cases to flatten the sphenoid ridge. In some cases, the high-speed drill may be used instead. Bony edges are waxed, and dural to pericranial stitches are placed.

Initial Exposure Corridors

Loupes (2.5×) and headlight illumination are used for initial exposure in order to take advantage of the ease of variable-angled visualization at adequate magnification. The dura is opened along the skull base about 2 cm above the bone edge for convenience of later closure. The ends of this straight incision are curved inferiorly in the frontal and temporal zone to promote a smooth, nonbuckled surface to the tented dura. The tenting sutures of 4-0 Nurolon are placed around the periphery of the dura, angling the corner stitches on the dural flap outwards to flatten this surface (Fig. 30-47B).

Next, the brain is elevated for initial approach to the ICA. At this juncture, it is wise to ensure that PCO_2 and diuresis have been optimal to promote brain relaxation. In the case of a giant aneurysm, withdrawal of subarachnoid fluid is accomplished at this point, usually 50 to 100 ml.

The *strategy of retraction* depends on which way the aneurysm points: If it points along the ACA (superiorly), temporal retraction only is used until the lesion is in view. If it points along the MCA (posteriorly), then frontal retraction alone is used to start. If it points back down the mesial ICA, then both frontal and temporal retraction may be used from early on.

When the aneurysm is *posteriorly or inferiorly* directed, one begins with a subfrontal exposure to avoid encounter with the aneurysm (Figs. 30-42, 30-46, and 30-48). A cottonoid is advanced along the

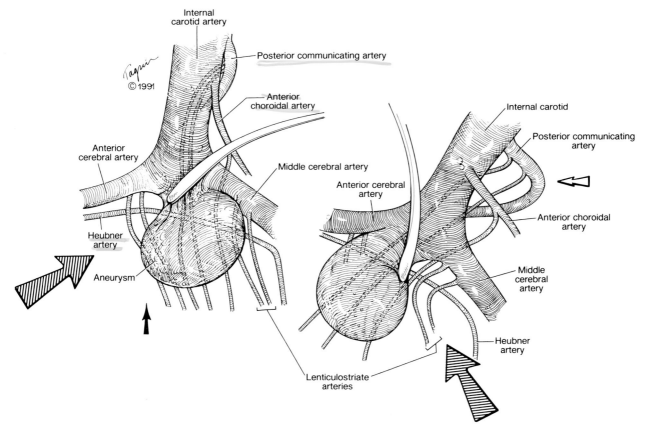

Figure 30-48. Vascular anatomy and microexposure. Large striped arrows indicate principal frontal and temporal accesses. Small open arrow shows lateral and medial carotid accesses. Small black arrow shows sylvian access.

sylvian fissure on the inferior aspect of the frontal lobe. The olfactory tract is identified and followed posteriorly to the optic nerve. The cistern around the optic nerve is opened, permitting flow of CSF for additional brain relaxation. The arachnoid is opened more laterally over the ICA. At this point the cottonoid is replaced with Bicol, and a 0.5×3 inch cottonoid is placed on the Bicol and gently retracted with a self-retaining Greenberg retractor. Retraction lifts the frontal lobe off the optic nerve and simultaneously tends to open the sylvian fissure. The fissure is carefully opened microsurgically. After the aneurysm is visualized, the temporal lobe is gently retracted with the cottonoid to permit coagulation and division of temporal tip draining veins. Then a strip of Bicol is placed over the temporal lobe, which is covered with a cottonoid and gently retracted with a Greenberg retractor. The two retractor blades are approximately perpendicular to each other with minimal pull on the temporal lobe.

For the common aneurysms directed *superiorly* (Figs. 30-41 to 30-45), frontal retraction is avoided initially and a temporal approach is favored to avoid the aneurysm initially. Aggressive frontal retraction could lead to rupture, and therefore minimal frontal retraction is utilized. Safer temporal retraction is favored instead to permit exposure and control of the internal carotid artery with CSF drainage. Only after the aneurysm is visualized do we begin frontal retraction. The final retractor array is as described above, with minimal retraction on the frontal lobe.

Critical Anatomy and Microexposure

Safe exposure of ICA bifurcation aneurysms is difficult because the anatomical location is deep and a host of critical perforating arterial branches is intimately related to the aneurysmal sac. The ICA gives off critical deep branches via the posterior communicating artery and anterior choroidal artery. The A_2 segment of the ACA gives off Heubner's artery, which runs recurrently to the deep distribution of the lenticulostriate territory. The MCA gives off medial lenticulostriate perforating arteries to the internal capsule. In addition, aneurysms of the internal carotid bifurcation are related to important veins. The superficial sylvian vein should be preserved with the temporal lobe, but occlusion of this vessel probably does not cause important consequences. On the other hand, the basal vein of Rosenthal and its tributary, the medial sylvian vein, both of which may be found in relation to ICA bifurcation aneurysms, are crucial and must be preserved to avoid significant neurological deficit.

To expose the lesion, the *sylvian fissure is opened widely* under the microscope, beginning deeply in most cases and working toward the surface. First ICA, then MCA and ACA are dissected free, with great care to preserve all perforating branches (Figs. 30-42 and 30-48). Intraoperative review of the angiogram often helps to identify important branches.

Next the *aneurysm neck is prepared*. Once the ICA, ACA, and MCA are controlled, the surgeon has the opportunity for temporary trapping of the lesion, should rupture occur. The final, most difficult, and most dangerous portion of the dissection involves separation of the perforating vessels from the aneurysmal neck prior to clipping. Often this is quite difficult because the perforators may be deep to the bifurcation and the aneurysmal neck. If the neck is expanded, the perforators may actually be incorporated into the neck. With a larger or giant aneurysm, the perforators may be substantially hidden from the surgeon's view. Generally speaking, the strategy is to angle the microscope in from the frontal side to visualize MCA branches and from the temporal side to visualize ACA branches, with a combination of angles of attack for the ICA branches (Fig. 30-48).

Temporary Clips

Intraoperative rupture triples the number of complications of intracranial aneurysm surgery.[82] For small aneurysms, modest hypotension (systolic blood pressure 90 mmHg) may suffice to prevent rupture during dissection and clipping of the lesion. Most often, however, especially with large or giant aneurysms, the safer strategy is the use of temporary clips to make the aneurysm slack and to prevent catastrophic rupture. Elective utilization of temporary clips when rupture seems likely prevents intraoperative rupture.[83,86] Mannitol has been used to prevent ischemic infarction during temporary clipping,[83,87] and pentobarbital has also been shown to be effective as cerebral protection.[86] When barbiturate protection is used, Durity[86] suggests dosage to burst suppression on electroencephalography (EEG) or loading with 10 mg per kg, followed by 5 mg per kg every 10 minutes during cross-clamping. We have generally preferred a regimen of mannitol and induced hypertension to permit prompt awakening of the patient after surgery. For elective temporary clipping, mannitol 100 g is given intravenously 15 minutes prior to cross-clipping of the parent arteries. When mannitol cannot be used because of medical problems (renal, cardiac, or hyperosmolarity) or in the case of precipitous rupture demanding temporary clips, then barbiturate protection is preferred.

For ICA bifurcation aneurysms, a 10-mm temporary Sugita straight clip is placed on the ICA proximal to the anterior choroidal artery. In some cases, we add 7-mm Sugita straight clips on the MCA and ACA, clear of perforating branches. As these clips are being placed, the blood pressure is carefully raised to the 150 to 160 mmHg systolic level in patients whose cardiac reserve can tolerate such a measure.

Temporary clips prevent rupture and make the aneurysm soft. This markedly enhances the complete dissection of the neck and careful preservation of perforating branches. However, there is limited time available (1 hour maximum), and the surgeon must move quickly with the dissection. The Rhoton 6 instrument is helpful, and sweeping or spreading movements with the bipolar fine cautery are often effective. A small cotton ball helps to maintain the dissection plane between the aneurysm neck and the perforating blood vessels. It is worthwhile to free a generous length of perforating vessels from the aneurysm neck to avoid kinking or tearing as the obliterating clip is placed. A 360-degree dissection of the neck must be performed in order to permit safe clipping. The surgeon approaches the lesion from the frontal and temporal avenues and as needed below the A_1 and M_1 segments on either side of the ICA (Fig. 30-48). Full neck dissection is necessary to ensure that all perforant vessels are spared and the aneurysm neck is completely prepared. Ordinarily these measures do not require complete dissection of the dome.

Another adjunct that may be helpful is the use continuous aspiration of the aneurysm immediately prior to clipping the lesion. This is accomplished with a 19-gauge butterfly needle attached to a suction device and held with a Kelly clamp by the assistant. This maneuver may collapse the aneurysm to allow final dissection and obliteration.

Lesion Obliteration

The best method of aneurysm obliteration is a perfectly placed *clip across the neck,* sparing all native vessels. This is in fact the most usual method and may require several reapplications to get the clip just right. Very commonly a straight clip of the proper length can be worked across the neck (Fig. 30-49A). It is important to avoid an excessively long clip, which may occlude a perforating vessel or the A_1 segment. Rarely, when it cannot be dissected off the aneurysmal neck, it is justified to obliterate the A_1 segment purposefully in that the anterior cerebral circulation may be carried by the anterior communicating artery. However, this maneuver should only be

utilized if cross-circulation was documented at the time of angiography. As the clip is placed one must see the tip as it goes beyond the neck. By gentle, slight axial wiggling, the surgeon may minimize friction between the clip and the aneurysmal neck. Whenever there is significant resistance to the advance of the clip, careful inspection should be done to avoid tearing of a perforator or the neck of the aneurysm.

In a number of cases, the neck will be broad enough that application of a straight clip may produce crimping of the parent vessels, a dogear of the aneurysm, or both. To avoid these problems, *a clip in the axis of the A_1 and M_1 vessels* is preferred, usually with a gentle curve just to match the bifurcation (Fig. 30-49B). In a selected minority of cases, a fenestrated clip may be helpful. The fenestration may be placed around the middle cerebral artery (Fig. 30-49C) or the ICA (Fig. 30-49D). The clip format may be either straight (Fig. 30-49A) or curved (Fig. 30-49B), the latter especially if the lesion is inferiorly directed (Fig. 30-46). In all cases, careful inspection before, during, and after clipping must be done to ensure that all perforating vessels have been spared with obliteration of the aneurysmal neck. The Sano double-jointed clip applier is particularly useful for application of such specialized clips.

In some cases, *bipolar cauterization* of the neck of the aneurysm may be the key maneuver for obliteration, with or without an additional clip, depending on the vascular anatomy. In applying coagulation, caution must be used to avoid current spread to perforator vessels. It is best to start with a very low cautery current and short durations of current application, with continuous irrigation, gradually increasing the current and duration, in order to obtain a progressive thickening and whitening of the neck of the aneurysm. There is a potential for aneurysmal neck rupture, and this method must be cautiously utilized. Risk is minimizes by placing the blades of the forceps all the way across the neck to avoid hot spots of current, with a very light squeeze-release maneuver to minimize the possibility of sticking. We prefer the standard Malis bipolar cautery unit over the Biceps unit for this maneuver because of the problem of popping encountered with the Biceps.

Occasionally a *ligature* is helpful. Doubled, waxed 3-0 silk suture can usually be passed with a forceps down one margin of the neck to be retrieved on the other margin of the neck. The suture is then tied with a surgeon's knot by the use of two hemostats. If there is worry of possible avulsion, the surgeon then accepts less than total occlusion with the suture, and the job is completed with a clip.

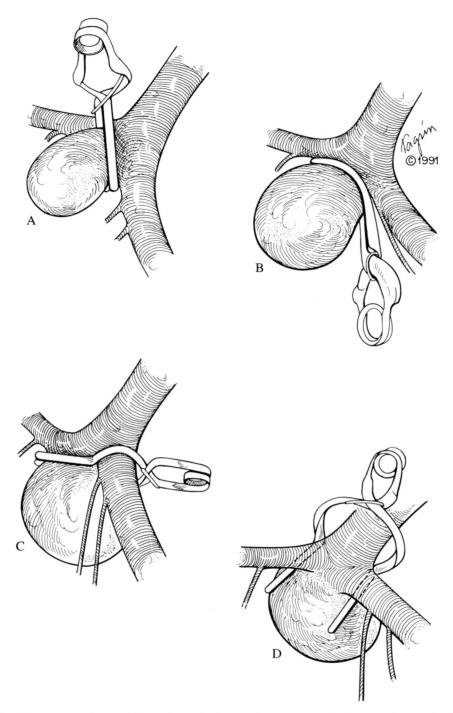

Figure 30-49. Clipping techniques. **(A)** Straight clip for small aneurysm. **(B)** Curved clip in axis of A_1 and M_1 segments. **(C)** Fenestrated clip encircles MCA. **(D)** Fenestrated clip encircles ICA to occlude neck of inferiorly directed aneurysm.

When the lesion cannot be safely obliterated by any of these techniques, *muslin* is the best answer. This agent is known to cause an intense local scar to re-enforce the wall of the aneurysm without vascular thrombosis. It is important to keep the muslin away from sensitive neural structures such as the optic chiasm and optic nerves. Reinforcement of this sort appears to be somewhat effective over time,[91] and the approach appears to be safer and more effective than the cyanoacrylate adhesives.[96]

It should also be kept in mind that the surgeon can retreat if the risk of attack seems too great. There is now the option of transvascular balloon or coil obliteration or even no surgery at all, particularly in an unruptured lesion.

After the lesion has been obliterated, by whatever technique, the surgeon must inspect the blades carefully for potential perforators caught in the clip. If this is the case, the clip must be adjusted to preserve these crucial little vessels. Moreover, one should inspect the parent vessels—the ICA, ACA and MCA. If there is any question of their patency, then testing is in order. This can be done with the application of a miniaturized Doppler flow probe to indicate the direction of flow. In the absence of this device, a two-forceps test can be applied, in which two forceps are applied to the vessel in question and gently moved apart while maintaining occlusion. Release of the proximal forceps should then permit prompt refilling of the proximal segment, thus proving the presence of antegrade flow.

Another important check, appropriate in many cases, is the aspiration of the lesion with a 25-gauge spinal needle. If the lesion is collapsed by this maneuver and does not fill, then complete obliteration of the distal lesion is proved.

We have just begun to utilize *intraoperative angiography* at the end of the case. In this situation, the patient is on the outset placed on a radiolucent table with the head in a radiolucent headrest. The groin is prepared when the scalp is prepared. At the conclusion of the procedure, with the open cranial wound covered, the neuroradiology team proceeds with transfemoral catheterization of the ICA. Digital videotape is exposed in appropriate planes and recorded on the OEC digital system. Review of the videotape ensures appropriate obliteration of the aneurysm and preservation of normal structures. If there is a problem, we readjust the clip and repeat the angiographic study to confirm appropriate clip placement. Precise indications for intraoperative angiography have yet to be established.

Closure

Once the aneurysm has been secured, it is then appropriate to inspect the area and to remove any hematoma, by careful suction or forceps extraction. Then hemostasis is carefully confirmed, eventually with the blood pressure raised (systolic 150 to 160 for 5 minutes). We then place pledgets of Gelfoam soaked in papaverine on the parent vessels to minimize the chance of subsequent vasospasm. Surgical strips are placed on the retracted surfaces of the frontal and temporal lobes as well as any area of cortisectomy. The wound is routinely closed with 4-0 running Nurolon to the dura. The bone flap is sutured in place with 0 silk. The temporalis muscle is then closed, followed by the fascia. The galea is closed with interrupted sutures and the skin with 3-0 running nylon. Bacitracin irrigation is carried out between layers. An appropriate dry sterile dressing is placed. Only rarely is a drain left in place.

Giant Aneurysms

Direct clip obliteration is the most effective treatment for giant aneurysms. However, giant aneurysms of the ICA bifurcation pose special problems in that the important perforating arteries are often draped over the neck and dome. Wide exposure with temporary clipping for precise definition of the parent arteries and perforators, as described above, may permit safe separation of critical vessels from the aneurysm. Even if this can be accomplished, the neck of such a lesion is often broad and thick walled, incorporating the take-offs of both anterior and middle cerebral arteries. In some cases, the A_1 and M_1 origins of the cerebral arteries can be safely reconstructed with aneurysm clips. Care must be taken to ensure that dysplastic, thin aneurysm wall is not left behind, for this often leads to recurrence and SAH. On the other hand, the surgeon must place the clips far enough off the vessel origins to avoid occlusion (often 1.5 to 2 arterial widths). In some cases, satisfactory clip obliteration may be achieved with good results.[98]

If there is a well-defined neck on angiography, particularly in a younger patient, it is probably worthwhile to explore the aneurysm, but if the surgeon finds an unclippable or high-risk aneurysm, then indirect treatment should be considered. In some cases, an immediate bypass procedure may be performed under the same anesthetic.

Hunterian ligation has been performed for ICA bifurcation aneurysms. Unfortunately, proximal ICA occlusion is often ineffective for aneurysms above the ophthalmic take-off and most especially for bifurcation lesions. In some cases, aneurysm trapping has been combined with distal bypass to the MCA. This approach, however, runs the risk of cerebral ischemia, and intraoperative monitoring to identify such a problem is as yet imperfect.

An alternative approach combines a generous revascularization of MCA with subsequent balloon trapping of the aneurysm with the patient awake. We prefer external carotid artery–saphenous vein–middle cerebral branch bypass. Aneurysmal rupture can occur if there is a waiting period prior to ICA occlusion. Intraoperative angiography can suggest the magnitude of graft flow and thus the likelihood of aneurysm blow-out. If this seems small, we take the patient to the intensive care unit and maintain the blood pressure in the low normal range for 1 week. At that point, balloon trapping of the aneurysm is carried out, with the patient awake with EEG monitoring, under full heparinization. After 3 days, we switch to coumadin, aiming at a prothrombin time of 1.5 × control for 6 weeks.

Balloon obliteration of a giant ICA bifurcation with parent vessel sparing is possible ("reconstructive" procedure). We have done one such ICA bifurcation aneurysm with success and angiographic confirmation. This approach has not been verified yet by long-term clinical and angiographic follow-up. However, we consider this method preferable to trapping in the setting of a narrow neck (where dysplastic wall can likely be obliterated) and acute SAH (where trapping would require delay and heparinization, both threatening recurrent SAH).

Postoperative Management

The patient is awakened in the operating room as promptly as possible. This maneuver is timed carefully by the anesthesiologist. If the clinical examination demonstrates an *immediate marked hemiparesis or hemiplegia,* the most likely cause is often an occluded perforating vessel, probably caught in the clip. If there is any reasonable likelihood of this circumstance, it is probably warranted to reopen the wound and readjust the clip position to restore normal perforator flow and avert hemiplegia. We have twice done this, with gratifying restoration of flow and function.

If the patient is neurologically intact upon awakening and then later develops a *delayed neurological deficit,* the differential diagnosis is substantially more complex (see Table 30-12). An accumulating sub-

dural, epidural, or intracerebral hemorrhage is best detected by prompt CT scan. Treatment is immediate re-exploration of the wound to remove the hematoma, except in cases of insignificantly small hematomas. The best prevention is meticulous hemostasis at the conclusion of the original procedure. Advancing hydrocephalus can also cause deterioration and is confirmed on CT scan. When hydrocephalus is mild, careful follow-up may be warranted, but severe hydrocephalus may require ventriculostomy and even eventual ventriculoperitoneal shunt placement. Prevention of hydrocephalus includes avoidance of ε-aminocaproic acid and careful attention to the basal cisterns with removal of all possible clot at the initial procedure. Symptomatic cerebrovascular vasospasm is strongly suspected when the CT shows neither hematoma nor hydrocephalus, and the transcranial Doppler studies disclose increasingly high flow velocities in the anterior circulation. Direct confirmation requires angiography. When vasospasm is moderate, we institute medical therapy including blood pressure elevation as high as 200 systolic, with hypervolemia (CVP 8 to 10 mmHg). Mannitol 100 g every 8 hours by continuous infusion is given for support of microcirculation. When vasospasm is severe by neurological examination and transcranial Doppler testing, we favor immediate angiography and angioplasty.[92] Prevention of symptomatic vasospasm is probably enhanced by hypervolemia, hemodilution, and nimodipine.[95] Other causes of delayed deterioration must sometimes be sought: meningitis is detected by lumbar puncture, antibiotics are used for treatment, and aseptic technique is the best prevention. Seizures may not be clinically obvious, and an EEG may be required for diagnosis (even repeated examinations may be needed). Anticonvulsants will be required for therapy, and avoidance of cortical manipulation and incision may limit the likelihood of this complication. Electrolyte imbalances, including diabetes insipidus and cerebral salt wasting, may be detected by serial electrolyte determinations. Adjustment of fluid therapy with fluid restriction or administration of hypertonic saline may be required for correction.

Various *medical problems* may also supervene. Unexplained changes in vital signs may suggest myocardial infarction, which is confirmed by ECG and serial creatine phosphokinase determination. Therapy may involve trinitroglycerine utilization and avoidance of hypertension. Avoidance of hypertension may also be an important preventive measure, and all patients should have a 12-lead ECG in the recovery room to investigate covert myocardial infarction. Deep venous thrombosis may be disclosed by Doppler studies or venography of the lower extremities. Transvenous placement of an inferior vena cava filter is usually the appropriate treatment early in the postoperative period, and after 5 days heparin and coumadin could be used instead. Avoidance of steroid therapy and utilization of thigh-high compression stockings decrease the incidence of this complication. Subsequent pulmonary embolus from deep venous thrombosis may be suspected by ECG criteria and deteriorating ABG, but a pulmonary angiogram is required to confirm the diagnosis. Inferior vena cava filter placement and heparinization are the treatments of choice.

Middle Cerebral Artery Aneurysms

Bryce K. Weir
J. Max Findlay
Lew Disney

ANATOMY

The complications specific to middle cerebral artery (MCA) aneurysm surgery are related to the anatomy of the MCA and to the regions of brain it supplies. Grand,[110] Gibo et al.,[109] Umansky et al.,[125,126] Rosner et al.,[118] and Yasargil[130] have undertaken and reported elegant microanatomical studies of the MCA and its branches, thus providing the precise understanding of these vessels necessary for successful microsurgical procedures.

Beginning as the largest of the two terminal branches of the internal carotid artery, the MCA passes laterally to immediately enter the deep part of the sylvian fissure. The more superficial part of the sylvian fissure narrows superiorly as temporal and frontal lobes approach each other. The proximal part of the fronto-orbital gyrus and the superior temporal gyrus often indent each other and interlock inside the fissure, which conceals the deeper portion of the sylvian fissure and complicates its surgical opening. The sylvian fissure also contains the superficial and deep middle cerebral or sylvian veins, which receive branches draining the temporal and frontal lobes. The superficial sylvian vein, which may be duplicated, often lies on the temporal side of the fissure and empties into the sphenoparietal and cavernous sinuses. This vein is often anastomosed with the transverse sinus via the vein of Labbé. The deeper vein receives lenticulostriate venous branches and courses medially to join the basal vein of Rosenthal.

The sylvian fissure is preferably opened on the medial or frontal lobe side of the veins. Coagulation and division of small veins passing between the two lobes or bridging from the temporal lobe to the sphenoparietal sinus is acceptable and generally safe, but great care must be taken to preserve the large venous trunks travelling down the fissure.

The deeper part of the fissure, also known as the sylvian cistern, transmits the MCA. The sylvian cistern communicates medially with the carotid cistern and is divided into an anteromedial "sphenoidal compartment" and a posterolateral "operculoinsular compartment." Frequently overlying the artery along this course is a web of tough arachnoid fibers connecting temporal and frontal lobes. When exposing the MCA these dense condensations of arachnoid are best divided sharply. The floor of the sphenoidal compartment of the sylvian cistern and the region over which the proximal MCA travels is the middle and lateral zone of the anterior perforated substance. The anterior perforated substance is bounded anteriorly by lateral and medial olfactory striae; posteriorly by optic tract and temporal lobe; laterally by limen insulae; and medially it extends above optic chiasm to the interhemispheric fissure. The anterior perforated substance is the site of penetration of the anterior perforating arteries, which will be considered shortly. Because the sylvian cistern is completely enclosed by brain, MCA aneurysms often become embedded in brain substance as they enlarge; consequently, when they rupture they frequently present with intracerebral in addition to subarachnoid hemorrhage.[117] The incidence of intracerebral hematomas in patients with MCA aneurysms was found to be as high as 50 percent in one large series.[113] The particular propensity of MCA aneurysms to cause focal signs such as hemiparesis or partial epilepsy is due to this tendency to bleed at least partially into brain substance. The intracerebral hematomas tend to track into the temporal and frontal lobes and less commonly into the basal ganglia.

The main trunk of the MCA, also referred to as the "sphenoidal," "horizontal," or "M_1" segment, lies posterior and parallel to the sphenoid ridge, coursing laterally beneath the anterior perforated substance within the sphenoidal compartment of the sylvian cistern. The main division of M_1 may occur at any point along this path, but it usually is near the anterior edge of the island of Reil (limen insulae), giving M_1 an average length of 15 mm. The outer diameter of 70 unfixed M_1 arteries hand injected with polyester resin was found to be 3 ± 0.1 mm.[126] In most cases the main division of the M_1 segment is a bifurcation. Gibo et al.[109] found a true bifurcation in 78 percent, a trifurcation in 12 percent, and a division into four or more trunks in 10 percent of 50 hemispheres studied. Umansky et al.[126] analyzed 70 hemispheres and found the MCAs divided in four ways: bifurcation, 64 percent; trifurcation, 29 percent; quadrification, 1 percent; and a single-trunk type of MCA with no major division, 6 percent. The secondary trunks arising from the main division of M_1 are the M_2 segments, and they overlie the insula within the operculoinsular compartment of the sylvian cistern. They consist of inferior and superior divisions when M_1 bifurcates, and a middle division is also found in the event of an M_1 trifurcation. Gibo et al.[109] found that the MCAs that bifurcated could be divided into three groups: equal bifurcation (23 percent), inferior trunk dominant (36 percent), or superior trunk dominant (41 percent). The M_2 segment length is approximately 11 mm, and outer diameter after resin injection as described above approximated 2 mm.[126] Gibo et al.[109] referred to those segments coursing over the fronto-parietal and temporal opercula as M_3 or opercular segments and those branches that spread out over the cortical surface as the M_4 segments.

The branches of the MCA are either perforating or cortical. The early cortical branches originate from the temporal side of M_1, which different authors refer to as either the *lateral* or *anterior* surface of the artery. These can include the uncal artery, the polar and anterior temporal arteries, and occasionally an orbitofrontal artery. Frequently the uncal artery originates from the distal internal carotid artery. The polar and anterior temporal arteries can arise from a single stem off M_1. Yasargil[130] has pointed out that a common temporal arterial branch, if large enough, can be mistaken as an early M_1 bifurcation. These early cortical branches are not always present.

The perforating branches of the MCA are commonly referred to as the *lenticulostriate vessels*. They generally originate on the frontal side of the M_1 and proximal M_2 segments, referred to as either the *posterior*[118,125] or *medial*[130] surface of the artery, depending on whether one considers the MCA to travel directly laterally or posterolaterally within the fissure. The origin of these branches can be situated on either the superior or inferior aspect of the artery, and in the latter case the surgeon separating the sylvian fissure from above must retract the MCA slightly in order to observe their sites of origin. In one study of 34 hemispheres the number of perforating branches per MCA varied from 5 to 29 (mean 14.9 ± 0.7 vessels.[125] However, 50 percent of the perforators counted had originated from common stems, which could give rise to as many as 13 individual branches. Yasargil[130] observed that all of the len-

ticulostriate vessels arose from one single large stem artery 40 percent of the time. The outer diameter of single vessels ranges from 0.1 to 1.1 mm (mean 0.39 ± 0.02 mm), whereas the common stems range from 0.6 to 1.8 mm (mean 0.87 ± 0.04 mm).[125] Both Rosner et al.[118] and Umansky et al.[125] found that 80 percent of lenticulostriate vessels arose from the M_1 segment, and most of the remainder arose from proximal parts of the M_2 segments. It was found that the earlier the bifurcation, the greater the number of postbifurcation perforating branches. The angle of origin is variable for the more medially originating lenticulostriates but usually acute for the longer lateral vessels, which follow a recurrent course to reach the anterior perforated space.

Rosner et al.[118] divided the lenticulostriate arteries into medial, intermediate, and lateral groups. The medial were the least constant and pursued a direct path to the midzone of the anterior perforated substance. The intermediate frequently included a common stem that arborized extensively while passing to a more lateral zone of the anterior perforated substance. The lateral group frequently included one or more vessels that arose directly from the M_1 bifurcation. Anterior perforating vessels also arise from the internal carotid artery, the anterior choroidal artery, the anterior cerebral artery, and the recurrent artery of Heubner. The anterior perforating vessels supply those deep cerebral structures located above the anterior perforated substance, including the internal and external capsules, the globus pallidus, putamen, and caudate nucleus.

Although considerable variation exists among individuals, the distal cortical branches frequently emanating from the superior M_2 trunk include the orbito-frontal, fronto-opercular, prefrontal, precentral, central, and anterior and posterior parietal arteries. The cortical branches that frequently stem from the inferior M_2 trunk include the middle and posterior temporal arteries and the angular artery. More unusual variations and anomalies of the MCA have recently been reviewed.[124] These include fenestration of the M_1 segment or complete duplication of M_1 beginning at or near the terminal internal carotid artery. An "accessory MCA" is a vessel originating from the anterior cerebral artery that follows a recurrent path to reach the sylvian cistern, where it then parallels the course of M_1, providing early cortical and lenticulostriate branches.

Bearing in mind the many variations that can occur in the MCA branching pattern, perhaps the best mental picture of the MCA for the surgeon to retain is that shown in Figure 30-50, which is a schematic representation of the MCA from above after the sylvian fissure has been opened widely. Fox[108] has compiled a superb set of intraoperative photographs that demonstrate this perspective of the MCA during microsurgical opening of the sylvian fissure. When dealing with aneurysms of the MCA, the surgeon must be particularly familiar with the pattern of division of the M_1 segment, since this is the location of the majority (up to 85 percent) of MCA aneurysms.[132] At this location aneurysms usually point laterally in the direction of the long axis of the prebifurcation segment of the main trunk (the direction of maximal hemodynamic thrust in the preaneurysmal segment of the parent artery). The lateral and intermediate lenticulostriate arteries may arise on or near this bifurcation and the neck of the aneurysm. The origin of the branches may be hidden on the posterior wall near the neck of the aneurysm, and vessels that might appear to be arising from the fundus of the aneurysm are usually only closely applied and adherent to the fundus and actually originate from the bifurcation region. Aneurysms can also occur near the origins of large lenticulostriate arteries on the M_1 segment, and these frequently point superiorly. Aneurysms are occasionally found in relation to the origin of early cortical branches of M_1 or at main branch points of the M_2 segments. More peripheral aneurysms are quite rare and generally have an inflammatory etiology.

The variations in MCA anatomy have been emphasized; however, in a given individual the right and left MCAs are often quite symmetrical in pattern. Perhaps related to this is the higher than expected incidence (by chance alone) of mirror MCA aneurysms among patients with multiple aneurysms.[119]

The MCA supplies most of the lateral surfaces of the cerebral hemispheres and the deep structures of the frontal and parietal lobes. It nourishes the motor and premotor areas, the sensory and auditory projection areas, and higher receptive association regions. Accidental or spontaneous occlusion at its origin is usually fatal. MCA occlusion can cause weakness owing to involvement of the corticospinal tract at its origin in the central gyrus or deeper within the internal capsule, sucking and grasping reflex owing to involvement of the premotor area, personality changes from involvement of the prefrontal area, visual field defects from damage to the geniculocalcarine tract and the temporoparietal occipital lobes, reduction in discrimination ability and spatial neglect from parietal lobe involvement, Gerstmann's syndrome (finger agnosia, right-left disorientation, dyscalculia, and dysgraphia) owing to involvement of the parietooccipital junctional area (angular gyrus) in the dominant hemisphere, or receptive (Wernicke's) dysphasia from disturbance of the dominant temporoparietal

area. One or two orbital branches run forward and laterally to the inferior surface of the frontal lobe and the inferior frontal gyrus. Occlusion of one of these vessels in the dominant hemisphere can result in a motor (Broca's) dysphasia.

SURGICAL MANAGEMENT

Early surgical experience with MCA aneurysms, which included direct aneurysm obliteration as well as carotid ligation and aneurysm investment with muscle or gauze, have been reviewed.[127] The high incidence of mortality and morbidity associated with treatment in the premicrosurgical era of neurosurgery was in part related to (1) excessive brain manipulation during dissection of the sylvian fissure and aneurysm; (2) inadvertent kinking, occlusion, and damage to the major trunks or lenticulostriate branches with aneurysm clipping; and (3) the inadequate protection from rebleeding conferred by aneurysm wrapping or proximal vessel ligation. Lougheed and Marshall[113] provided an unprecedented type of analysis of their management results for anterior circulation aneurysms, which included a total of 156 patients with MCA aneurysms, treated between 1954 and 1970 at the Toronto General Hospital. In this series 54 percent were operated in the first week, and all angiographically proven aneurysms were recorded and followed, whether operated on or not, so that the total effectiveness of management (management morbidity and mortality) as well as the results of surgery (operative morbidity and mortality) could be assessed.

Seventeen grade V patients, eight of whom were treated surgically, died. For the remainder of patients, grades I to IV, the management mortality rate within 3 months of admission to the hospital was 23.5 percent. The operative mortality rate for 115 cases of single and multiple ruptured aneurysms, grades I to IV, was 13.9 percent for the same time period. Three operated patients died within several years from repeat hemorrhages from either wrapped or inadequately clipped aneurysms, and another patient died within 1 year of surgery from infarction due to MCA occlusion at surgery. As expected, younger, alert patients fared much better with surgery, and although excellent surgical results could be obtained by delaying surgery several weeks from the hemorrhage, the authors concluded that alert patients may be operated upon within 1 week, providing no technical difficulties in obliterating the aneurysm are anticipated and no spasm is present. The authors also found that operative morbidity and mortality rates dropped im-

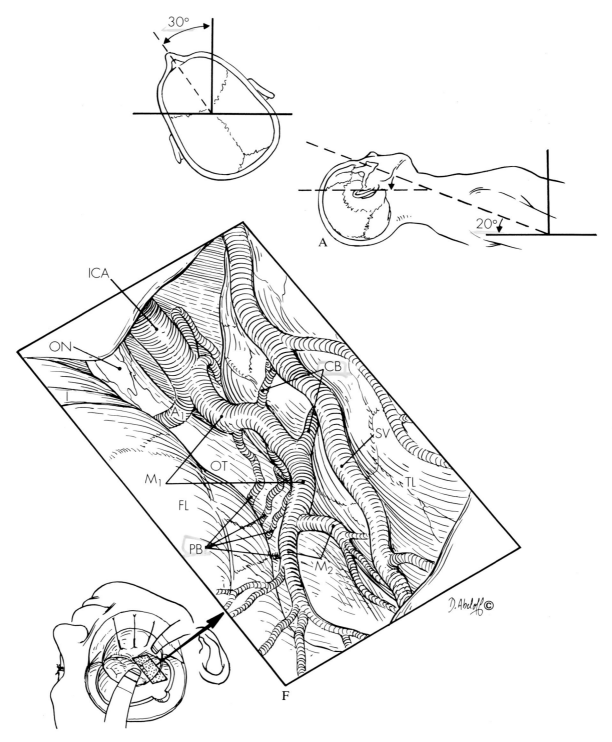

Figure 30-50.   (A&F).

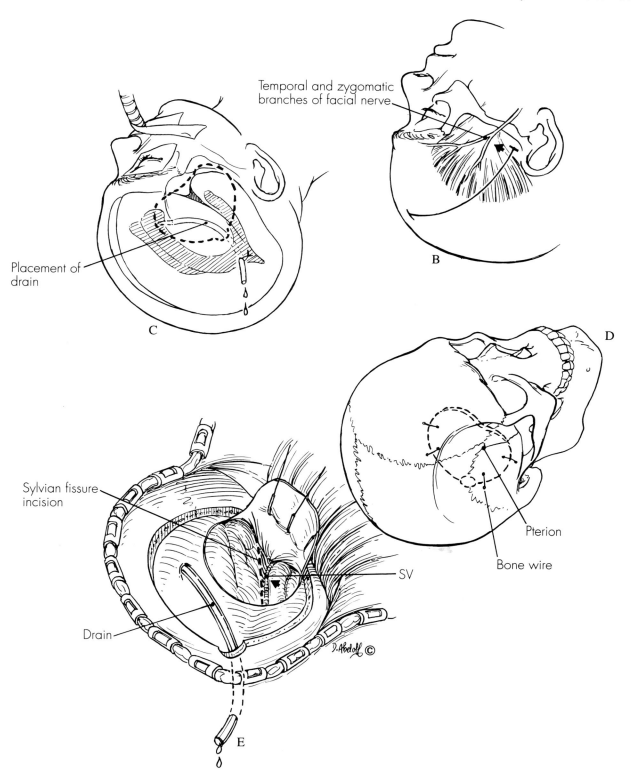

Figure 30-50. (B–E).

pressively toward the end of the series with the introduction of the operating diploscope; of 18 patients undergoing microsurgery not one patient died or was made worse with operation. Since this series, most relevant reports on MCA aneurysm surgery have concerned the employment of microsurgical exposure for definitive aneurysm clipping. These have often been personal series of experienced aneurysm surgeons in which patients are selected to some extent; consequently surgical results are generally good, and overall management mortality statistics are not given. In addition, it is rarely possible when analyzing the overall results of aneurysm surgery to distinguish adverse effects of aneurysm rupture and cerebral vasospasm from direct complications of surgery. The following is a review of an MCA aneurysm surgical series that includes mention of technical aspects favored by the individual author/surgeon.

Fox[107] recommended positioning patients with MCA aneurysms with the head considerably extended during a frontotemporal exposure, which allows for a view of the MCA somewhat perpendicular to its main axis, and a more comfortable opening of the sylvian fissure. To gain proximal control of the MCA in the event of premature rupture, Fox prefers to begin the M_1 dissection at the ICA bifurcation. He cautions that if one elects to descend directly to the aneurysm through a fissure distended by clot a sudden release of pressure on the aneurysm may result in intraoperative rupture. Between 1975 and 1981, using the operating microscope, Fox operated on 35 MCA aneurysms, with a zero percent mortality rate. Most patients underwent surgery 10 to 14 days after subarachnoid hemorrhage. Surgical morbidity and complications were not detailed.

In 1984, Suzuki et al.[122] reported their surgical technique and results for MCA aneurysms. A total of 265 cases of single MCA aneurysms, including patients of all clinical grades, was divided into 174 patients operated on prior to 1975 and 91 patients operated on after this time, when a standard approach had been developed. In both groups surgery was performed using binocular loupes or the naked eye. The Suzuki et al. technique is to put the head in a neutral position with the chin elevated 5 to 10 degrees. A small frontotemporal craniotomy is performed and the internal carotid artery and proximal M_1 exposed. After the administration of 500 ml of 20 percent man-

Figure 30-50. **(A)** The head is rotated approximately 30 degrees away from the side of the aneurysm in MCA aneurysm surgery. **(B)** The skin incision is behind the hairline if possible, beginning from within less than 1 cm from the ear and above the zygomatic arch to reduce the risk of damage to the frontalis branch of the facial nerve. The skin, galea, and temporalis muscle can be turned in one layer. The bone flap is cut flush with the floor of the anterior fossa in the lateral supraorbital area to reduce the amount of brain retraction. With MCA aneurysms more bone is removed over the temporal lobe than with anterior communicating artery aneurysms. **(C)** A sufficient bone opening (burr hole size) is made posteriorly for the ventricular drain to pass through. Extensive rongeuring of bone under the temporalis muscle is avoided as much as possible to avoid late, unsightly depressions. **(D)** Four wires are used to reduce the chance of late bone tilting or settling with resultant cosmetic deformity. **(E)** The dural incision is shown. Rarely a straight cut backwards over the sylvian fissure is required for greater exposure. The dural flap is held back with fish hooks. The placement of the ventricular drain is shown. **(F)** Once the ipsilateral optic nerve and internal carotid artery are identified and exposed, the frontal lobe is elevated and temporal lobe is retracted posteriorly using self-retaining retractors, and the sylvian fissure is opened or ''split'' in a proximal to distal fashion using sharp dissection. A ''wide-open'' sylvian fissure after arachnoid dissection is shown. The typical MCA and sylvian fissure anatomy is shown from the surgeon's perspective. Deep and superficial sylvian veins (*SV*) run parallel to, and have a variable relationship with, the MCA. Some veins may have to be coagulated as they bridge the sylvian fissure in order to permit proper exposure of the M_1 trunk and of the aneurysm dome. The deep part of the sylvian fissure, or the sylvian cistern, transmits the main trunk of the MCA, or the M_1 segment, which has an average length of 15 mm. In about two-thirds to three-fourths of cases, the M_1 segment terminates as a bifurcation. Most of the remainder end as trifurcations. The early cortical branches (*CB*) of the M_1 segment originate from the temporal side of the M_1 segment. These can include the uncal artery, the polar and anterior temporal arteries, and occasionally an orbitofrontal artery. The perforating branches (*PB*) of the MCA are usually referred to as the lenticulostriate vessels. They originate on the frontal side of the M_1 and proximal M_2 segments. They must be carefully protected during MCA aneurysm surgery. In the common situation of the M_1 segment bifurcating, two M_2 segments result, a superior division that sends cortical branches to the opercular, frontal, and parietal regions, and an inferior division that sends cortical branches to the posterior temporal and parietal regions (*I*, olfactory tract; *ON*, optic nerve; *OT*, optic tract; *FL*, frontal lobe; *TL*, temporal lobe; *ICA*, internal carotid artery; A_1, first segment of ACA; M_1, first segment of MCA; M_2, second segments of MCA; *PB*, perforating branches of MCA; *CB*, cortical branches of MCA; and *SV*, sylvian veins).

nitol for cerebral protection, a temporary clip is moved distally along the M_1 trunk as it becomes exposed during opening of the sylvian fissure. When the aneurysm and M_2 branches are identified, temporary clips are also placed on the latter, thus trapping the aneurysm and facilitating its dissection and clipping, ligation, or wrapping. In this surgical series, after 6 months 80 percent of patients operated on before 1975 were in either good or excellent condition, whereas in the group who underwent surgery after 1975, 94 percent were in good or excellent condition at follow-up. Suzuki et al. feel that the most important principle for aneurysm surgery is to secure the afferent artery prior to aneurysm exposure and repair. They use temporary clips in almost all cases, and in their hands the MCA has been safely occluded after the administration of mannitol for up to 40 minutes. Most patients in this series had occlusion times between 10 and 20 minutes, and average occlusion times did not differ among those patients with excellent, good, fair, poor or fatal results. Suzuki et al.[122] feel that aggressive removal of subarachnoid clot reduces the risk of postoperative vasospasm, and surgery within 48 hours is optimal for this purpose.

Volume II of Yasargil's four volume series[129] on microneurosurgery, which contains descriptions of his operative approaches for intracranial aneurysms and surgical results, was published in 1984. One hundred eighty-four patients who underwent operation for aneurysms of the MCA were presented, which represented 18.2 percent of his entire aneurysm series. Yasargil noted the variability in width, length, and depth of the sylvian cistern, which correlated with the difficulty of surgical dissection. As well, the course of the MCA is variable. In Yasargil's series, MCA aneurysms were located in one of five principal locations: (1) anterior temporal (4 percent), (2) lenticulostriate (8 percent), (3) bifurcation (83 percent), (4) second or M_2 bifurcation (3 percent), and (5) distal (2 percent). Fifty-three percent of the aneurysms were unilobular, 25 percent were bilobular, 14 percent trilobular, and 4 percent truly multilobular. Yasargil employs a standard pterional craniotomy. In his opinion the decision as to where to enter the sylvian cistern and begin dissection of the MCA depends on the radiographic anatomy of the aneurysm and associated hematoma, on the fullness of the brain at the time of exposure, on the course of the MCA, and, to some extent, on the experience and confidence of the operating surgeon. The area of dissection is divided into three parts: area I, at the base of the sylvian fissure, where the sylvian cistern communicates with the basal cisterns; area II, over the MCA proximal to the bifurcation; and area III, over the peripheral branches of the MCA beyond the bifurcation.

Yasargil prefers to begin in area I in order to gain proximal control of the MCA, although if hematoma is present in either the temporal or frontal lobe he advises that a portion of it be removed through an incision in the superior temporal or inferior frontal gyrus, leaving some hematoma around the aneurysm. After relaxing the brain in this fashion he then proceeds to either area I or area II proximal to the ruptured aneurysm. Yasargil stresses the importance of identifying lenticulostriate arteries arising from the bifurcation, often beneath the neck of the aneurysm. It is important to exclude these, as well as any frontal or temporal cortical branches adherent to the aneurysm fundus, from the clip blades. The dissection of these vessels from the aneurysm can be tedious. A temporary clip on M_1 can be used to soften the aneurysm and make aneurysm dissection safer, and temporary clips are placed on the M_2 vessels if the aneurysm is to be intentionally opened. In this series temporary clipping was employed in 11.4 percent of patients without any apparent deleterious consequences. Yasargil uses bipolar coagulation on the aneurysm and resects the fundus, removing and adjusting aneurysm clips until he is satisfied that every part of the aneurysm is excluded. In Yasargil's series of 184 MCA aneurysms, 69 percent were neurologically normal or grades I or II. Eighty-four percent had a good result, 11 percent were fair to poor, and 5 percent died. Only nine patients were operated in grade IV condition. Almost one-half of the semicomatose patients with large hematomas were able to return to a normal life and to their previous occupations. Eight patients who underwent operation with fixed dilated pupils and absent respirations (grade V) died. In this series, 100 percent of grade IV and V patients had significant hematomas, which was considered to indicate that depression of consciousness in these patients is due to mass effect and herniation rather than direct brainstem injury from the hemorrhage. Yasargil felt that only three patients in the 184 (1.6 percent) who developed postoperative infarction were actually made worse by operation. Hydrocephalus requiring shunting occurred in 5 percent of patients and epilepsy in 6 percent.

Except for instances of an unusually short M_1 segment, Fein and Flamm[104] prefer to approach MCA aneurysms through a purely sylvian exposure beginning laterally and proceeding in a proximal direction. They point out that rupture of the aneurysm may make exposure of the proximal vessel difficult, but, with careful control of the patient's blood pressure and good microsurgical technique, this problem can usually be avoided. To minimize the amount of retraction required, these authors routinely employ mannitol, furosemide, and lumbar drainage. They point out that adequate exposure of MCA aneurysms dictates that the neck of the aneurysm is visible from all directions, sometimes requiring that the entire aneurysm be mobilized from surrounding brain. The structure of MCA aneurysms and their relationship to the afferent and often multiple efferent vessels is often complex, and in these situations a combination of clips may be necessary to safely obliterate the sac. The authors consider it necessary, at times, to sacrifice a small MCA branch to achieve complete repair of the aneurysm, although in several cases a divided distal branch has been reimplanted into the proximal artery with an end-to-side anastomosis. These authors do not favor temporary clipping of the M_1 segment for MCA aneurysm repair, and in some instances elect to puncture the aneurysm dome with a 21-gauge scalp vein needle connected to suction in order to soften the aneurysm and facilitate dissection and clipping. In their series of 114 patients there were 87 (76.3 percent) excellent, 12 (10.5 percent) good, and 8 (7.0 percent) poor results, and 7 (6.2 percent) patients died. One death was related to traumatic injury to lenticulostriate vessels complicated further by a postoperative acute subdural hematoma. A subdural hematoma was the cause of death in another patient, and poor results were attributed to a postoperative MCA thrombosis in one patient and a subdural empyema in a second.

Heros[111] has outlined the three basic approaches to MCA aneurysms, which are the medial or subfrontal transsylvian approach, the lateral transsylvian approach (both of which have been described in preceding sections), and the approach that he himself prefers for the majority of MCA aneurysms, the superior temporal gyrus or transtemporal approach. With the patient in the supine position, the head is turned about 60 degrees to the contralateral side, which is a greater angle than for the usual pterional approach. As soon as dura is opened the microscope is brought into the field and a 2 to 3 cm incision is made in the superior temporal gyrus beginning about 1 cm behind the front of the sylvian fissure and continuing posteriorly in a direction parallel to the fissure. With suction and bipolar coagulation, the incision is extended medially into the vertical segment of the sylvian fissure over the insula. The sylvian veins are not disturbed. The branches of the MCA are then identified and followed proximally toward the aneurysm without disturbing the dome. This is done by following the division on the side away from the aneurysm until

the distal portion of the MCA M_1 trunk can be seen. Once the distal M_1 and the main divisions have been identified, he then proceeds with dissection of the entire aneurysmal complex, taking the precaution of leaving adherent brain and clot on the dome in the area of likely rupture. In the event of intraoperative rupture Heros prefers to raise the blood pressure and to apply a temporary clip on M_1 if necessary, but temporary clips are not used routinely. Heros does not feel that the transtemporal approach is suited to aneurysms that arise on the M_1 trunk proximal to the main division, to those that occur at an early M_1 bifurcation, or those uncommon aneurysms that project backward over the insula, obstructing a distal approach. In such instances he prefers a medial transsylvian approach. Heros believes that in the remainder of MCA aneurysms the transtemporal approach requires less brain retraction, minimal disturbance of the sylvian veins and MCA perforators, and better visualization of the more complex posterior aspect of the aneurysmal complex and hence safer clip application. The primary disadvantage is that the aneurysm is exposed before afferent vessel control is assured. Despite this, he believes that it is particularly useful in patients with a temporal lobe hematoma, in patients operated on early when considerable brain swelling hinders medial to lateral opening of the sylvian fissure, and in patients with large aneurysms that project laterally, anteriorly, or inferiorly. Of 68 consecutive operations for MCA aneurysms, including 49 patients operated on through the superior temporal gyrus, there were 50 good, 11 fair, and 3 poor results, and 4 patients died, all of whom were grade IV or V. Late surgery was preferred, with day 14 the median day of operation. Heros listed the following specific operative complications experienced with MCA aneurysm surgery (a single patient with each of the following): (1) intracerebral hemorrhage after induced hypertension; (2) massive brain swelling and death after excision of a giant aneurysm; (3) hemiplegia as a result of occlusion of the MCA after attempted repair of a giant ruptured aneurysm; (4) Broca's aphasia from excessive frontal retraction; and (5) hemiparesis resulting from inadvertent occlusion of a large cortical branch.

Sengupta and McAllister[120] point out that branches of the MCA invest primary division aneurysms like a candelabra, and the sac is cushioned between the frontal and temporal lobes. These branches may grip the aneurysm during the process of growth, and preoperative angiographic studies cannot distinguish between vessels that actually originate from the aneurysm wall and those that originate from normal vessel proximal to it and have the artery adherent to the aneurysm wall (which is almost always the case). Sengupta and McAllister[120] favor the more lateral transsylvian approach. Of 99 cases of MCA aneurysm 64 patients were in grades I or II, 27 in grade III, and 8 in grade IV at the time of operation. Seventeen percent had postoperative neurological complications. At the time of discharge 71 patients had made a good outcome and 6 had died.

MCA aneurysms accounted for just over 20 percent of supratentorial aneurysms seen by Lindsay Symon[123] at the National Hospital in London, England. Most of these cases were operated on late after SAH. He approaches those aneurysms arising at an early bifurcation or from the M_1 segment along the medial sylvian fissure, but for the common type of MCA aneurysm located at the distal main division of M_1 he resects the anterior 1 1/2 inch of the superior temporal gyrus staying below the pia of the sylvian fissure. The major branches of the MCA are identified on the surface of the insula and deep to the pia with microscopic dissection before the sylvian fissure or the arachnoidal spaces of the insula are opened. The disadvantage of this approach is that the fundus is again reached for the M_1 trunk, but in the event of a massive intraoperative rupture Symon would consider placing a temporary clip on the previously dissected terminal internal carotid artery. When the aneurysm and the efferent artery have been identified, he does not hesitate to occlude the distal M_1 trunk temporarily for periods up to 10 minutes while dissecting the aneurysm neck. Longer periods of occlusion are often tolerated by patients harboring large and giant MCA aneurysms that often have to be opened and emptied of clot before clipping can be carried out. The longest occlusion time of the MCA with an excellent postoperative result was 40 minutes. In an endeavor to increase the safety of temporary arterial occlusion intraoperative somatosensory evoked response monitoring is carried out. Symon's observations would suggest that if the evoked response persists for a period of 3 to 4 minutes after occlusion, even though it may subsequently disappear, occlusion times of 10 to 15 minutes will be safely tolerated. If the response remains constant, then an infinite time is probably available. If, however, the conduction rapidly disappears after temporary occlusion, then less than 10 minutes is safe. For clipping Symon prefers the Scoville clip anchored in place after final adjustments with a drop of acrylic placed on the curved spring shank. Of a total of 95 aneurysms of the MCA, the operative mortality rate was 4.2 percent, and unacceptable morbidity oc-

curred in only one grade IV patient, who was confused and suffering from appreciable hemiparesis preoperatively and was densely hemiplegic postoperatively.

Since 1970 Weir[127] has managed 115 patients with MCA aneurysms. Of these, 81 patients had suffered subarachnoid hemorrhage from the MCA aneurysm, 22 had multiple aneurysms with subarachnoid hemorrhage due to rupture of an aneurysm other than the MCA aneurysm, and 12 had unruptured aneurysms with or without symptoms. Of the 81 patients with subarachnoid hemorrhage from the MCA aneurysm, 16 (20 percent) were grade 1, 27 (33 percent) were grade 2, 20 (25 percent) were grade 3, 12 (15 percent) were grade 4, and 6 (7 percent) were grade 5. Forty (49 percent) of patients had good outcome, 16 (20 percent) were left moderately disabled, 10 (12 percent) were severely disabled, 1 (1 percent) was vegetative, and 14 (17 percent) died. All but 11 of the 81 patients had surgical treatment of their aneurysms; 10 patients died preoperatively, and 1 was transferred to a hospital in another province.

In the group in which the subarachnoid hemorrhage was due to rupture of an aneurysm other than the associated MCA aneurysm, 14 (64 percent) had a good outcome, 3 (14 percent) were moderately disabled, 1 (5 percent) was severely disabled, and 4 (18 percent) died. In this group residual disability was always due to the original subarachnoid hemorrhage, and no specific complications arose from the incidental MCA aneurysm. Of these 22 patients, 5 had the MCA aneurysm clipped at the time of surgery to clip the ruptured aneurysm, 11 underwent separate procedures at a later date to clip the MCA aneurysm, and in 6 no clipping was undertaken. Two of these patients died from their initial subarachnoid hemorrhage, 2 were left severely disabled and were not considered candidates for clipping, and 2 harbored small (3 mm) aneurysms that were thought to represent a low risk of rupture. Of the 12 patients with unruptured aneurysms, 9 (75 percent) had a good outcome, 1 (8 percent) was moderately disabled, 1 (8 percent) was severely disabled, and 1 (8 percent) died. The patient left moderately disabled had a large MCA bifurcation aneurysm that had a major lenticulostriate vessel and three smaller vessels emanating from its dome. After careful dissection it was deemed unclippable and left wrapped. The patient developed a small infarct in the territory of the left MCA postoperatively, with a resultant mild hemiparesis and expressive dysphasia. The patient left severely disabled suffered an intraoperative rupture of the aneurysm during dissection of a lateral lenticulostriate vessel adherent to the dome. Both the vessel and the aneurysm had to be occluded in the clip to control the hemorrhage, but the patient was left with a severe hemiparesis and dysphasia. The patient who died had a large calcified MCA bifurcation aneurysm. At surgery the neck of the aneurysm appeared very atherosclerotic, and it was felt that it would likely fracture if clipping was attempted. It was wrapped in muslin gauze, but the patient presented 8 months later with a massive subarachnoid hemorrhage and subsequently died.

Delayed ischemic deficits secondary to vasospasm occurred in 19 (23 percent) of the patients with a ruptured MCA aneurysm. These followed the usual time course, with most deficits having their onset 6 to 9 days after subarachnoid hemorrhage. Rebleeding occurred in 7 (9 percent) patients. The most common time for rebleeding was within 24 hours of the initial hemorrhage, with three patients rebleeding during this period. Hydrocephalus occurred in 14 (17 percent) patients and required insertion of a shunt in 11 (14 percent).

Operations were carried out on 107 MCA aneurysms in 98 patients. Clipping of the aneurysm was accomplished in 98 of the aneurysms. The aneurysm was wrapped in five cases due to vessels being incorporated in the dome of the aneurysm, precluding clipping. Early in the series a Silverstone clamp was used in two instances to occlude the internal carotid; one of these was explored and found to be unclippable prior to this. In one patient operated on as early grade 4, swelling of the brain prevented visualization of the aneurysm and the patient died of his original hemorrhage before another attempt at clipping could be carried out. One patient with a 10-cm giant aneurysm presented with symptoms due to mass effect from the aneurysm that was debulked but not clipped; he has remained in a much improved condition for the 8 years of follow-up.

Intraoperative rupture of the aneurysm occurred in 8 instances. Temporary clips were used in 12 cases, with occlusion times ranging from 30 seconds to 28 minutes. No specific complications relating to the use of temporary clips occurred.

Documented occlusions of vessels by the aneurysm clip occurred in three patients. One patient presented as a grade 4 subarachnoid hemorrhage but rebled 5 hours later and was taken to the operating room on an urgent basis as grade 5 to evacuate an intracerebral clot and clip a 10 mm aneurysm. Postoperative angiography carried out with the patient still under general anaesthesia revealed occlusion of M_1. The patient was returned to the operating room and the clip repositioned, but M_1 had been occluded

for 2 hours and the patient died of a massive hemispheric infarction. Another patient underwent clipping of an unruptured 15 mm MCA aneurysm shortly after a ruptured anterior communicating aneurysm was clipped. Postoperative angiography with the patient still under anaesthesia revealed the aneurysm continuing to fill while the distal MCA branches were occluded. The clip was therefore repositioned, and the patient awoke without a significant deficit. The third patient was previously described in which a lateral lenticulostriate vessel was known to be occluded while controlling the intraoperative rupture of an unruptured aneurysm. There is a learning curve for each operator at this site as for all aneurysms. As a rule a high price is paid for timidity and the failure to examine in minute detail the anatomical situation following the presumed completion of the clip application.

In the Cooperative Aneurysm Study[112] the mean diameter of the MCA aneurysms proximal to the main division was 10.1 mm, and at the main division it was 9.1 mm. Those MCA aneurysms that are classified as large (10 to 25 mm) or giant (>25 mm) are a particular therapeutic problem. In Fox's world literature review[106] the MCA was the location of 9 percent of all giant cerebral aneurysms. In the process of growth they become structurally complex and tend to carry the origins of both cortical and lenticulostriate branches up onto their walls. Assuming an aneurysm neck can be found, clot partially filling the aneurysm and atheroma within its wall can interfere with clip application. Consequently, incidentally discovered giant MCA aneurysms, or those producing only mild mass effects, transient cerebral ischemia, or epilepsy are often treated medically, especially in older persons. Aneurysms that have bled and otherwise symptomatic aneurysms in young patients mandate more aggressive management. Options include (1) wrapping the aneurysm sac with gauze in the hope of strengthening its wall; (2) proximal vessel ligation with or without extraintracranial bypass in an attempt to promote aneurysm thrombosis without distal infarction; and (3) direct clipping or ligation of the aneurysm neck or sac, with or without excision of the sac (the preferred choice if possible).

Wrapping the aneurysm confers incomplete protection from bleeding and is considered by most to be the last therapeutic resort. MCA aneurysms do not lend themselves to treatment by proximal ligation. Ligation proximal to M_1 does not reliably stimulate thrombosis of MCA sac, and M_1 occlusion, even if preceded by a superficial temporal artery to an MCA cortical branch bypass, can result in MCA distribution infarction due to the absence of an effective col-

Table 30-13. Middle Cerebral Artery Aneurysm Surgery (*Continued*)

Neurosurgical Complications	Avoidance
Failure of clip release mechanism	Rehearse clip application and release just prior to use on aneurysm. Do not panic if the clip applier cannot be withdrawn from clip; strong pressure and removal of the clip and applier usually works. Reclipping is then done
Bleeding	Use bipolar coagulation in a methodical fashion on all sacrificed vessels Do not put bridging veins on the stretch Use hemostatic collagen material on oozing pial banks Avoid provocative elevations of arterial or venous pressure to "check on" hemostasis If unable to catheterize ventricles after three passes, desist
Frontalis branch of facial nerve injury	Retract skin and all soft tissues in one flap following sharp dissection Keep inferior incision about 1 cm or less anterior to the ear
Postoperative Neurological from cerebral infarction	Gentle and complete dissection, definitive clipping, and preservation of normal vasculature Remove intracerebral and subarachnoid clot Avoid deliberate hypotension Maintain circulatory blood volume Avoid intracranial hypertension
Infections	Meticulous operative technique Immediate preoperative antibiotic administration and use of antibiotics in irrigating fluids Use of drains is kept to a minimum Use subcuticular absorbable suture and skin tapes to avoid having to draw contaminated skin suture material through the depths of the wound Avoid aspirating subgaleal collections unless absolutely necessary
Hydrocephalus	Remove as much subarachnoid blood as possible at time of surgery CT scan should be obtained shortly postoperative and at 1 or 2 months thereafter More frequent CT scans should be performed if the ventricles are enlarging or if the patient's condition is abnormal and not improving or deteriorating Early shunt insertion is indicated if hydrocephalus is evident
Seizures	Phenytoin for 1 year in therapeutic dosages if no allergy or contraindication, if the patient had a significant parenchymal clot and/or ischemic infarct, particularly in younger patients
Cosmetic defect	Do not rongeur away frontal or temporal bone, leaving a bone defect. Wire flap down with four wires so it does not sag or tilt
General medical	Maintain a high level of intensive and nursing care Early ambulation Use minidose heparin and intermittent compression stockings in cases with paretic lower extremities

the aneurysm ruptures prematurely. The surgeon himself should check the patient's neurological condition immediately before surgery so that any change postoperatively can be recognized and its etiology appreciated. He should have studied the MCA anatomy and aneurysm thoroughly on the angiogram to develop a working three-dimensional sense of the structures about to be uncovered. In particular, he should acquaint himself with any large MCA M_1 branches that may serve as useful landmarks during the dissection of the sylvian fissure. In patients with multiple aneurysms he should feel confident that the aneurysm being repaired is the culprit that has bled.

It is usually the larger or more lobulated aneurysm, and in cases of ruptured MCA aneurysms there should be a greater concentration of blood in the surrounding sylvian cistern visible either on CT scan or magnetic resonance imaging (MRI).[105]

Intraoperative Patient Positioning and Preparation

Pin fixation of the skull should not be applied until an adequate level of anesthesia has been reached. Otherwise the pain stimulus may precipitate a rise in blood pressure and aneurysm rupture. For anterior circulation aneurysms, including MCA aneurysms, we position the patient supine on the operating table, and, keeping the axis of neck and head at right angles to the shoulder line, the head is turned 30 degrees to the side opposite the aneurysm and tilted about 20 degrees vertex down with the trunk elevated about the same amount (Fig. 30-50). The surgeon's view can be varied considerably by changing the trajectory of the microscope light beam, and this must usually be continually altered during the dissection. When doing this it is wise to check once again the now posted x-rays to ensure that the correct side has been exposed. It is found useful to have an oblique view "upside down" since this gives an approximation of the actual anatomy as viewed at operation. This positioning will bring the ipsilateral sphenoid ridge (over which lies the initial corridor of exposure) into a more vertical position and will allow the frontal lobes to fall away from the orbital roof, facilitating dissection and retraction beneath the brain. We routinely employ a combination of mannitol and furosemide as well as moderate hyperventilation (PCO_2 30 to 35 mmHg) to reduce intracranial pressure prior to dural opening.

Craniotomy

A frontotemporal or "pterional" craniotomy is performed. Great care must be taken particularly in older patients not to tear dura when cutting and elevating the bone flap. We generally create a single burr hole at the junction of the frontal and sphenoid bones anteriorly and then develop an oval flap about 7 × 4 cm with a high-speed drill. Slightly more temporal bone is included for MCA aneurysms than for other anterior circulation aneurysms. When the free bone flap is turned, the key to adequate exposure is to remove bone along the base of the anterior fossa floor anteroinferiorly to the pterion and toward the middle fossa floor in front of the temporal lobe dura inferolaterally to the pterion. Frontal and temporal bone should not be rongeured away, since such defects may become unsightly in the late postoperative period. The greater sphenoid wing is resected laterally to medially, but extensive removals do not greatly facilitate surgery on most MCA aneurysms. Temporalis muscle must be retracted firmly away from the pterional exposure with fishhooks to provide an unobstructed view down the sphenoid ridge and in front of the temporal pole.

Yasargil has described how the frontotemporal branch of the facial nerve, which serves frontalis muscle, can be consistently preserved.[131] This nerve courses anterocephalad over the zygomatic arch approximately 1 cm anterior to the superficial temporal artery, so that the posterior limb of the skin incision should not go below the level of the zygomatic arch and should be no more anterior than 1 cm in front of the auricle. The nerve then travels anteriorly external to the zygomatic process of the frontal bone (overtop of the site of the keyhole) invested in a fascial covered sickle-shaped layer of fat. During surgery, if the galea is being separated from temporalis muscle, this fascial covered fatty layer can be identified on top of the anterior fourth of the temporalis muscle, and at this point dissection should be continued *deep* to this layer until the zygomatic process is reached; in this way the enclosed frontotemporal nerve is lifted up with skin and galea and is protected. A frontalis palsy is a distressing cosmetic and visual problem that may often recover spontaneously. We believe we can reduce the frequency of this problem by turning galea and muscle in one layer with no dissection between them.

Dural Opening

If the dura is found to be rock-hard after mannitol and furosemide infusions and there is assurance of optimal arterial blood gases, and if this situation is inconsistent with the patient's preoperative condition, the possibility exists that the aneurysm has rebled either with induction, pin placement, or craniotomy. In the case of MCA aneurysms one can make a stronger case for pressing on with the operation rather than closing and taking the patient for an urgent CT scan, primarily because of the possibility of an intracerebral hematoma that requires decompression. Prior to opening dura an attempt should be made to catheterize the lateral ventricle for cerebrospinal fluid (CSF) drainage (see below). In desperate circumstances a rapid anterior temporal lobectomy may be required if brain herniates through the dural opening.

For MCA aneurysms we open dura in a flat half-circle based anteriorly with the posterior extreme about 5 cm from the origin of the sylvian fissure. If the brain is quite tight and particularly if preoperative hydrocephalus was evident on CT scan, a ventricular catheter is passed through the exposed frontal lobe toward the frontal horn of the lateral ventricle. We feel that this is preferable to lumbar drainage. Ventricular drains may be placed preoperatively if the patient is in very poor condition. With intraoperative CSF drainage a remarkable degree of brain relaxation can usually be achieved, and a red, angry, swollen brain becomes manageable.

At this point it is useful to apply the bars for the self-retaining retractors and to line the craniotomy exposure with clean, dark-colored surgical towels. Fresh surgical gloves should be donned. Prior to dural opening we select and load several temporary clips and at least one straight permanent clip. In addition the clip applicators should be checked to ensure that they release the clips smoothly and properly. The nurses will have draped and prepared the operating microscope.

Microsurgical Approach

When a large temporal or frontal lobe hematoma and attendant brain swelling preclude access to the base of the brain or easy sylvian dissection, an incision is made where the clot is closest to the surface, usually through the superior temporal gyrus, until hematoma is entered. Rather than try to remove all of the hematoma or work through the hematoma until aneurysm is encountered, we prefer to suck away gently enough of the clot to slacken the brain and then turn to a transsylvian exposure of the aneurysm. If possible, we clip the aneurysm in the usual fashion and then remove the clot.

The next step in these patients and the initial step in the remainder is to elevate the frontal lobe and identify the ipsilateral optic nerve. All exposed parts of brain should be covered with a protective layer of cottonoid, especially beneath retractors, in order to prevent brain laceration. If brain laceration does occur the injury should be covered with Gelfoam and a cottonoid, and a retractor placed overtop. The chiasmatic and carotid arachnoid cisterns are then opened, in that order. It is worthwhile to be patient at this point and allow time for CSF to drain and be aspirated from the basal cisterns, as this provides yet more brain relaxation prior to sylvian dissection.

Whenever possible, we approach MCA aneurysms along M_1, thereby having proximal vessel control in the event of intraoperative rupture. In addition, the ample room for temporary clip application usually available on M_1 facilitates temporary occlusion during particularly difficult aneurysm dissections prior to rupture. M_1 segment MCA aneurysms and aneurysms arising from a proximal bifurcation are approached by following the MCA distally from the internal carotid bifurcation. Beginning at the level of the internal carotid artery the frontal lobe is elevated medially, the temporal lobe is retracted laterally, and, using a sharp arachnoid knife, the tough arachnoid bands connecting the two lobes are divided. Continued opposing traction on the frontal and temporal lobes facilitates splitting of the sylvian fissure. While small veins bridging the fissure can be coagulated and divided, the main venous trunks within the fissure should be preserved.

The more common distal bifurcation aneurysms can be approached after directly exposing the M_1 segment distally in the sylvian fissure rather than working distally from the internal carotid bifurcation. This is easier, particularly in patients with slightly swollen brains due to recent subarachnoid hemorrhage, when deep retraction and dissection is difficult, and in patients with especially high internal carotid bifurcations or long M_1 segments. With retractor pressure parting frontal and temporal lobes, arachnoid is divided just medial to the superficial sylvian veins. Once a cortical artery is identified within the fissure it can be followed down to the MCA, which is often tucked into the medial aspect of the sylvian cistern as one descends through the fissure. Once M_1 is identified, it is followed distally on its superior and lateral surface, thus staying clear of lenticulostriate vessels arising on the opposite side of the artery. Careful study of the angiogram and measurement of the distance along the MCA will give the approximate vicinity of the aneurysm. During this dissection blood clot should be cleared from within the sylvian fissure in an effort to minimize postoperative vasospasm.

Some larger MCA aneurysms project slightly anteriorly from the bifurcation and can almost reach the surface of the sylvian fissure. This should be suspected from the angiogram and looked for intraoperatively prior to fissure dissection. When there is blood within the subarachnoid space the red aneurysm dome can be difficult to see. Large anteriorly directed aneurysms can block proximal M_1 exposure in some cases, and these are times we find we must approach the aneurysm from the distal sylvian fissure. Very rarely an anteriorly directed dome will actually be adherent to dura over the sphenoid ridge or anterior middle fossa.

If during a proximal transsylvian dissection the aneurysm ruptures prior to identification of the aneurysm, a temporary clip should be placed upon M_1 and hypertensive arterial blood pressure measured. Dissection should then proceed quickly but safely up the sylvian fissure to the aneurysm.

Aneurysm Clipping

Once the aneurysm is reached the anatomy of the complex must be unravelled in a methodical fashion. Since most M_1 divisions are bifurcations, the superior and inferior trunk need to be identified as one works around the base of the aneurysm. Sharp dissection is preferred. It is not always possible to predict from the angiogram how many branches emanate from the main division. Very commonly both cortical and lenticulostriate branches loop up and adhere to the aneurysm dome. When these vessels are especially adherent or when the aneurysm dome is very thin walled (one can appreciate the blood cells swirling within it with each pulsation of the heart), M_1 temporary occlusion may be carried out for repeated short intervals as required to facilitate dissection by softening the aneurysm. During dissection the assistant should keep the aneurysm wet with irrigation so that it does not dry out under the microscope lights and become sticky, increasing the risk of rupture when it is handled. When the aneurysm does burst during its final dissection the immediate response should be to place a tiny cottonoid patty on top of the sac and apply suction. In the case of MCA aneurysms this will often control the bleeding and allow continued dissection. Often suction and even the cottonoid (if it is obscuring dissection) can be gently removed under saline after several minutes if the tear is pinpoint. When the rupture is more substantial a proximal M_1 temporary clip, already loaded, should be applied. If the bleeding is still severe (and it usually is not), temporary clips can be placed on the efferent arterial branches, but each additional clip clutters the operative field and obscures further dissection. Their use is preferable, however, to flooding of the operative field by vigorous bleeding.

Where the aneurysm is embedded within brain or densely adherent to arachnoid, this often is the point of previous rupture, and it should be avoided during early dissection. If the aneurysm must be mobilized from this point to identify distal branches then one should leave the confines of the subarachnoid space and leave brain substance, clot, or arachnoid attached to this part of the dome.

When the neck has been adequately exposed and a passage for the clip blades has been tested with a microdissector, an appropriate clip is very slowly slid into place and closed, keeping the aneurysm wet. If rupture occurs at this point it may cease when the blades are fully closed, meaning that the hole was distal to the blades and the blades completely occluded the neck of the aneurysm. If bleeding persists and the rent is distal to the clip, the clip may have incompletely crossed the aneurysm neck. If this is clearly seen, the clip should be reapplied more deeply, or another longer clip may be placed just distal to the first one. Once bleeding ceases the initial clip can be adjusted. If bleeding originates proximal

to the clip, this is a more difficult situation. If a neck remnant still exists on this side of the clip, then a second clip can be slid along proximal to the first clip, covering the tear. Hopefully this will leave the parent vessels patent. If there is no proximal neck then proximal and distal temporary clips should be applied and the tear plicated with multiple small clips.

After clipping, the entire aneurysm and clip should be visualized from all sides, ensuring complete obliteration and the absence of any branches included within clip blades. It is very common that adjustments are necessary at this stage of MCA aneurysm surgery. The consequences of major branch stenosis or occlusion with faulty clip application can be inferred from the previous section on MCA anatomy. On occasion a small remnant of aneurysm needs to be left in order to be certain that a major vessel is left patent. In such cases we use shreds of muslin gauze to invest the proximal aneurysm and adjacent artery.

Closure

We do not artificially elevate blood pressure to "check" aneurysm hemostasis. Many either resect or aspirate the aneurysm dome to ensure that it no longer fills but this is usually unnecessary. Retractors and cottonoids are withdrawn under constant saline irrigation, any brain contusions or lacerations are covered with Gelfoam or Avitene, and dura is closed in a watertight fashion. If time is of the essence staples are used; if not, absorbable sutures in layers and skin tapes are considered the optimal method.

Illustrative Cases

Figures 30-51 to 30-58 illustrate varieties of MCA aneurysms and their CT, angiographic, and operative appearances.

POSTOPERATIVE MANAGEMENT

Patients with raised intracranial pressure are left with a ventricular catheter. An attempt is made to achieve fluid balance at the conclusion of surgery. Intraoperative angiography should be carried out if available when highly complex aneurysms are dealt with. Patients who awaken with an unexpected neurological deficit are considered for immediate postoperative cerebral angiography. If an M_1 or M_2 occlusion is identified, then the surgeon should strongly consider returning the patient to the operating room for clip repositioning.

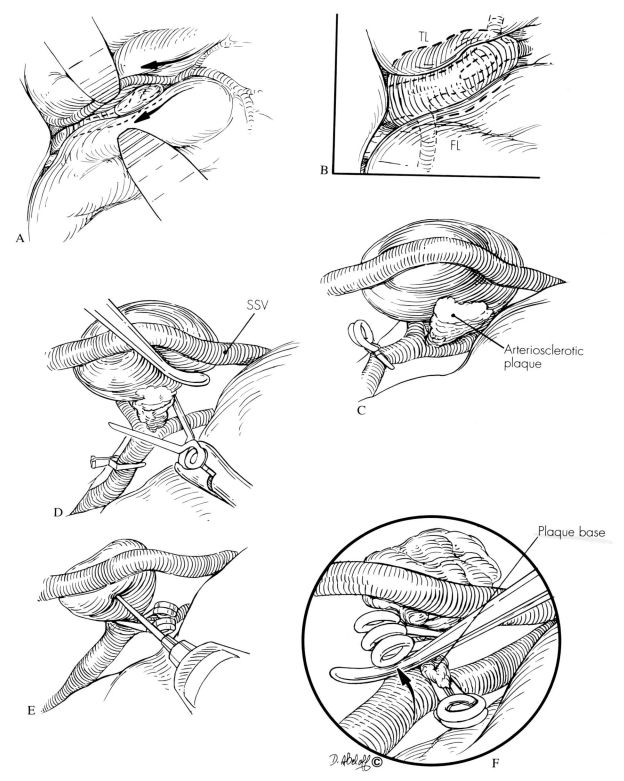

Figure 30-51. (A&B) The aneurysm was immediately visible on dissection of the sylvian fissure, as it arose on the anterolateral aspect of the MCA and lay superficial to the M_1 trunk. **(C)** A superior sylvian vein (*SSV*) was adherent to the aneurysm dome, and the neck of the aneurysm was atherosclerotic. **(D)** A temporary clip was placed on the M_1 segment prior to aneurysm neck clipping. The neck of the aneurysm was clipped with two large Sugita clips, and a neck remnant was left proximal to the clip. **(E)** The aneurysm was punctured with a 22-gauge needle and collapsed with aspiration. **(F)** The residual neck remnant was clipped with a smaller curved clip. The sylvian vein was left intact.

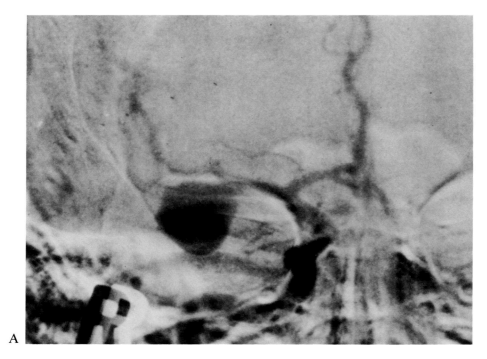

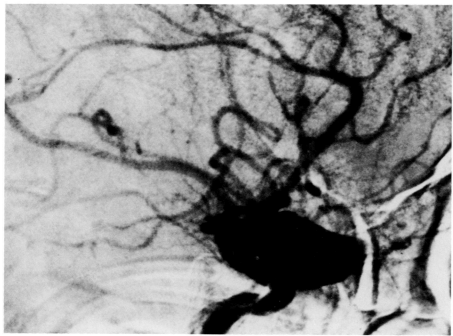

Figure 30-52. (A&B) Preoperative and **(C&D)** postoperative angiograms for the patient illustrated in Fig. 30-51 are shown. (*Figure continues.*)

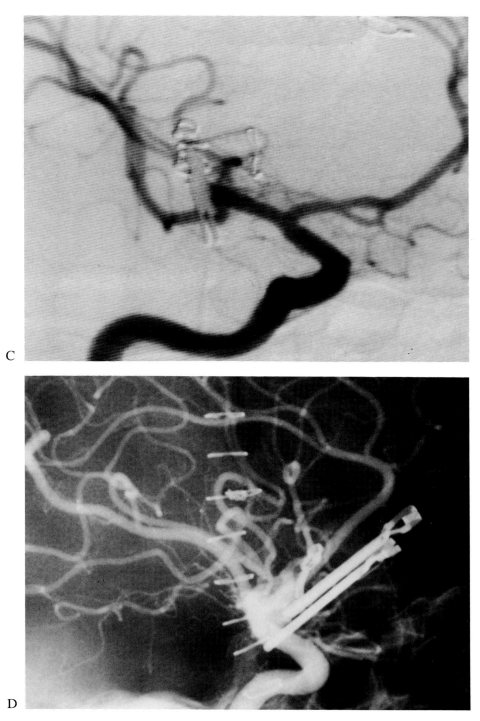

Figure 30-52 (*Continued*).

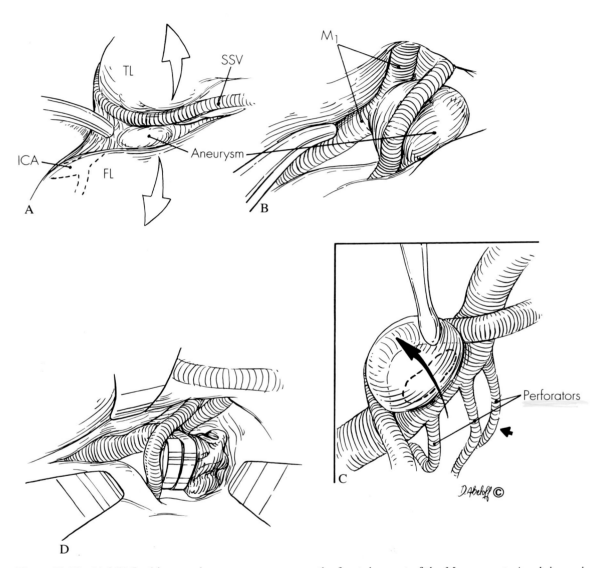

Figure 30-53. **(A&B)** In this case the aneurysm arose on the frontal aspect of the M₁ segment. A sylvian vein (*SSV*) was adherent to the dome. Retracting the aneurysm laterally permitted exposure of the **(C)** medial lenticulostriate vessels, which must be kept absolutely free of the aneurysm clip **(D)**.

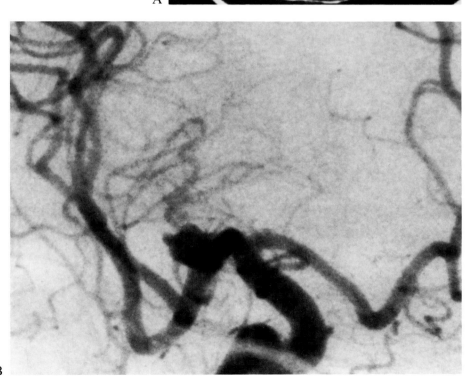

Figure 30-54. **(A)** Preoperative CT scan and **(B)** angiogram and **(C)** postoperative CT scan and **(D)** angiogram for the patient illustrated in Fig. 30-53. (*Figure continues.*)

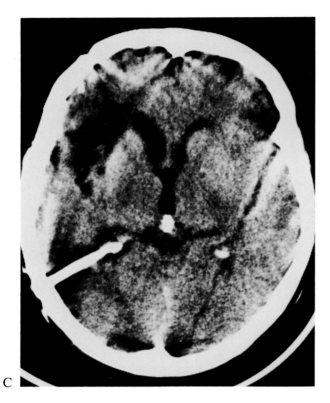

C

Figure 30-54 (*Continued*).

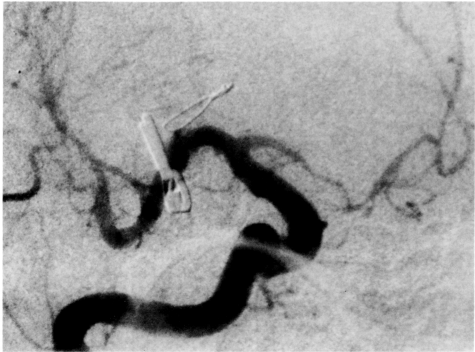

D

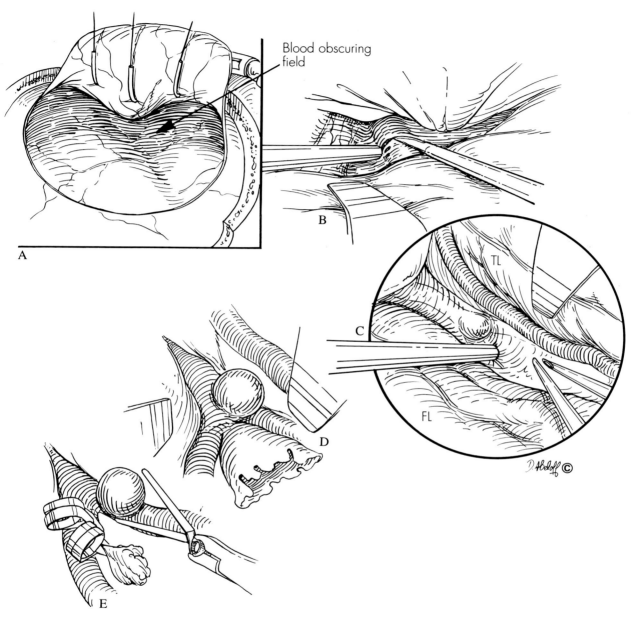

Figure 30-55. (A) The sylvian fissure was distended with blood in this case of a ruptured right MCA aneurysm. **(B)** The arachnoid of the carotid and chiasmatic cisterns was opened and CSF aspirated. **(C)** The sylvian fissure was opened and clot aspirated, and small bridging veins had to be divided. **(D)** The larger aneurysm at the M₁ bifurcation was adherent to organized clot, and the more proximal aneurysm bleb was unruptured. **(E)** An initial clip on the large aneurysm left some residual neck so a second clip was placed flush with the bifurcation. The smaller M₁ aneurysm was then clipped.

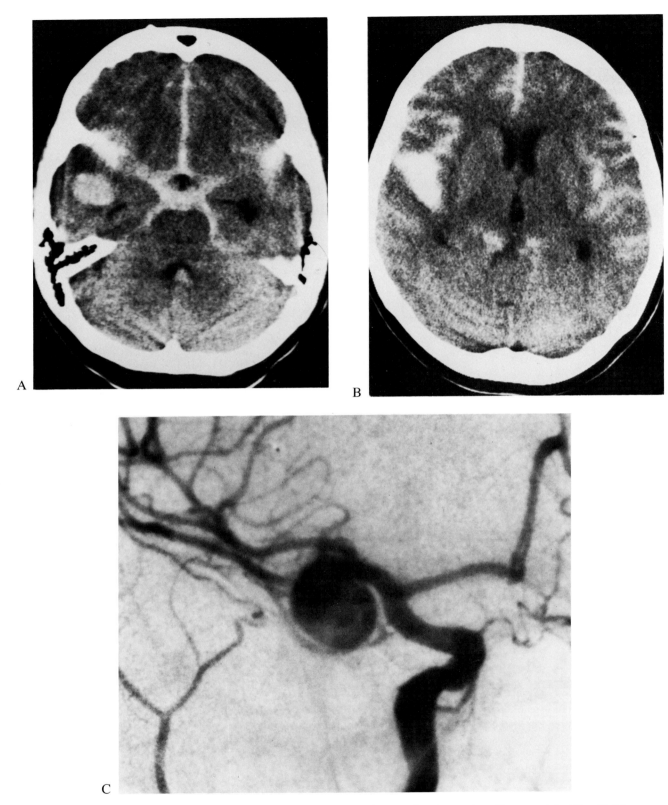

Figure 30-56. (A&B) Preoperative CT scans and **(C)** angiogram for the patient illustrated in Fig. 30-55. **(D&E)** Postoperative CT scans show right MCA distribution infarction due to vasospasm apparent on the postoperative angiogram **(F)**. (*Figure continues.*)

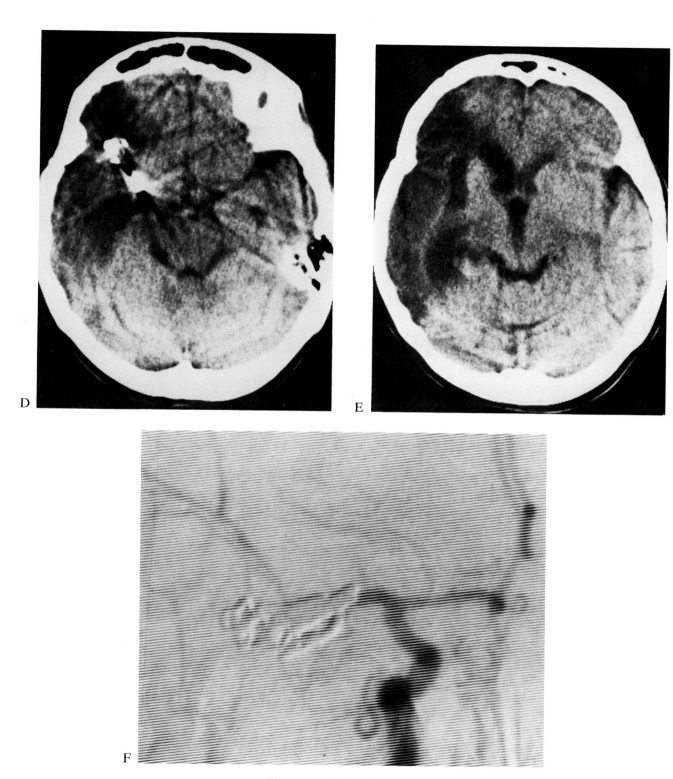

Figure 30-56 (*Continued*).

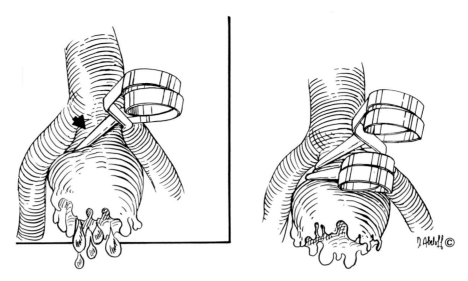

Figure 30-57. If placement of the initial clip across the bleeding aneurysm neck fails to stop hemorrhage, then a more distal deeply placed clip is necessary. The more proximal aneurysm clip should then be placed more deeply, flush with the artery bifurcation, to exclude an aneurysm remnant. The distal side of the aneurysm neck should then be exposed to ensure that the clips are properly placed and do not cross a third MCA division or lenticulostriate vessel.

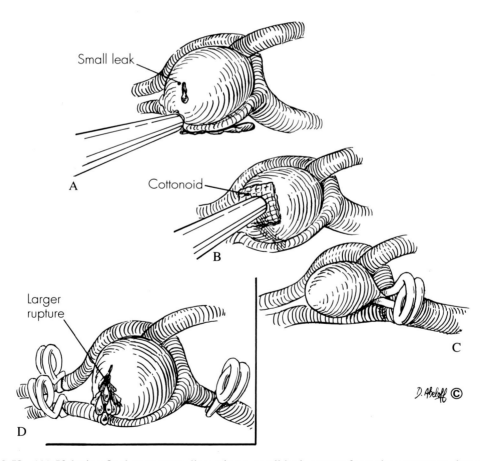

Figure 30-58. **(A)** If during final aneurysm dissection a small leak occurs from the aneurysm dome, this can often be controlled with placement of a small cottonoid and low suction over the rent **(B)**. The aneurysm neck can then be prepared and clipped. Flow from this intraoperative aneurysm rupture is likely to be small if there has been proximal M_1 temporary clipping. **(D)** In a situation of large intraoperative MCA aneurysm rupture, temporary clips should be placed on both the afferent M_1 segment and the large efferent M_2 branches while the aneurysm neck is prepared and clipped. This will stop aneurysm bleeding from the dome and prevent exsanguination of the distal, hypoperfused cerebral cortex.

Anterior Communicating Artery Complex Aneurysms

John L. Fox

R.P. Sengupta

A reputable surgeon does not deliberately set out to create a surgical complication. One can philosophize, therefore, that a surgical complication is an accident. One might hold the opinion that an accident, by definition, cannot be prevented or avoided. But certainly we can do our best to reduce the *incidence* of surgical accidents or complications. One method, not to be taken lightly in some circumstances, is not to operate—or at least not to operate under certain conditions.

The risks of surgical treatment to prevent rupture of an anterior communicating artery (ACoA) aneurysm has lessened since the beginning of the 20th Century. Much of this is due to significant advances in the medical and surgical diagnosis and treatment of intracranial aneurysms. The occurrence of subarachnoid hemorrhage (SAH) and the existence of an intracranial aneurysm have been known since antiquity.[178,261] The clinical syndrome of SAH due to cerebral aneurysm was described in 1923 by Symonds.[270] The method of diagnostic confirmation of an aneurysm and its possible surgical treatment became apparent when Moniz[229] introduced angiography in 1927 and Dott[167] first illustrated an aneurysm by angiography in 1931. The first aneurysm to be treated by direct surgery after preoperative identification with angiography was also by Dott,[167] when he wrapped a carotid bifurcation aneurysm with muscle in 1931. Dandy[164] was the first to obliterate an aneurysm with a clip in 1938, and this is the method that has remained the ideal goal up to the present time.

After the Second World War, neurosurgeons, recognizing the appalling consequences of a ruptured cerebral aneurysm, rushed to obliterate this time bomb. But the results of such surgery itself were dismal, forcing McKissock et al.[226] to report that bedrest was better than surgery. Trying to avoid a direct attack on the aneurysm, some surgeons resorted to proximal ligation of the parent A_1 artery,[216] while others returned to Dott's original technique of wrapping the aneurysm.[172,189]

Norlén and Barnum[233] recognized very early that delaying surgery until after the insult from SAH was over produced better surgical results than early surgery. Botterell et al.[152] introduced a grading system according to the clinical status of the patient, and

they noted improved results in the better grade patient. The same surgeons, who persisted with direct obliteration of the aneurysm, realized that some cerebral protection against anoxia during temporary clipping of the proximal vessels (to avoid premature rupture) could be provided by hypothermia.[219]

Another milestone in safer aneurysm surgery began when Adams and Witt[133] borrowed an operating microscope from their otological colleagues and used it for dissection of the aneurysm. Pool and Colton[245] stressed the advantages of good illumination and magnification of the anatomical details during aneurysm surgery. It was Yasargil[283] who made even the most reluctant surgeon acknowledge the benefit of the operating microscope in reducing the incidence of surgical complications. Simultaneously aneurysm clips were being improved.[181] In parallel with these surgical advances came the invention of computed tomography (the CT scan) in 1973,[198] and this allowed a better understanding of the ongoing pathophysiological processes in the patient. A significant peak to conquer has been cerebral vasospasm.[279] The deleterious consequences of cerebral vasospasm (cerebral ischemia) are reduced by newer methods of promoting cerebral perfusion. With better teamwork and advances in diagnostic facilities, technical aids, aneurysm clips, bipolar coagulation, anesthesia, and rational postoperative care, the ruptured ACoA aneurysm, in good risk patients, can now be obliterated with excellent results in most cases (Table 30-14).

Appreciation of the morphological characteristics associated with ACoA aneurysms can be very instructive.[140,257] Lying buried between the frontal lobes, they are often enclosed and obscured by the parent trunks of the anterior cerebral arteries. Their close proximity to the hypothalamus and other diencephalic structures and their blood supply make surgical obliteration particularly hazardous.[160] Because of this, the surgical approach to the ACoA aneurysm has an interesting history of evolution.[178]

In 1936, Tönnis[274] was the first to operate directly on an ACoA aneurysm. He operated through the midline, by splitting the genu of the corpus callosum (*approach No. 1*). Such an approach through an important area of the brain did not find general acceptance. Dandy[164] described what now is often considered the pterional approach (*approach No. 2*), but he was much ahead of his time. Hamby[191] and Falconer[174] used the unilateral subfrontal approach (*approach No. 3*). In spite of these much thought out approaches, the surgical outcome generally remained unsatisfactory. To lessen the incidence of surgical complications by a direct attack, Logue,[216] a disciple of Dott, employed the indirect method of proximal

Table 30-14.   ACoA Aneurysms[a]: Grade of Surgery Versus Outcome

| Grade | Outcome | | | | |
	Good	Fair	Poor	Dead	Totals
1 & 2	140	20	5	1	166
3, 4, & 5	26	22	0	7	55
Total	166	42	5	8	221

[a] From files of author R.P.S.

anterior cerebral artery (A_1 artery) occlusion to avoid interference with the aneurysm. Hamby[190] resorted to exposure of both carotid arteries in the neck so that they could be temporarily occluded to avoid a premature rupture of the aneurysm. Williamson and Brackett[280] believed that temporary occlusion of the proximal part of both anterior cerebral arteries during exposure of the aneurysm gave improved results. Pool[242–246] popularized the technique of a bifrontal midline approach (*approach No. 4*); he also utilized a temporary occlusion of both A_1 arteries. Further modifications of this technique were advocated by French et al.,[185] who found that premature aneurysm rupture occurred less commonly after removal of the anteromedial part of the frontal lobe. Kempe and coworkers[202,203,277,278] advanced Falconer's concept by describing an approach through the gyrus rectus based on which direction the aneurysm projected. The principle of this approach was to avoid exposing the fundus of the aneurysm. Then came the introduction of the use of the microscope in aneurysm surgery.[133] With the pioneering work by Yasargil[283] in the use of the operating microscope, a new era of surgical aneurysm technique began. The microsurgical approach to the ACoA aneurysm, using a modification of the pterional route with complete exposure of the vascular anatomy,[164,165] was illustrated by Yasargil et al.[284] and Fox.[176,178]

Concerned at the risks of vascular manipulation during the acute stage of SAH, Sengupta[258] and Sengupta and McAllister[261] advocated careful study of the angiograms to assess the circulatory pattern through the circle of Willis, any associated anomalies, and the morphological aspects of the ACoA aneurysm. The neck of the aneurysm and the exact location and relationship of its sac to the surrounding vessels were noted. They advocated using a modified subfrontal, gyrus rectus approach and keeping expo-

sure and manipulation of the vessels to a minimum. A search for newer avenues to these midline aneurysms continued. Hakuba et al.[189] described an orbito-zygomatico-infratemporal approach, which permitted less brain retraction. Finally, Smith and colleagues[264] reported an operative method involving the removal of portions of the orbital rim, orbital roof, and sphenoid bone.

PREOPERATIVE ASSESSMENT

Review of Imaging Studies

In the majority of cases the senior author (J.L.F.) operates on nearly all cases of ACoA aneurysms from the right frontotemporal (pterional) approach to avoid retraction on the dominant hemisphere. Additionally, the right-sided approach is technically easier for a right-handed surgeon. Exceptions occur in cases in which the dome of the aneurysm projects directly to the right, in cases where the left frontal lobe already is damaged by hematoma or infarction (Fig. 30-59), or in cases in which another aneurysm is located on the left carotid circulation. The dominance of the right or the left horizontal segment of the anterior cerebral artery (A_1 artery) or the site of origin of the ACoA aneurysm rarely plays a role in this author's decision regarding side of approach.

Table 30-15 summarizes the factors to be analyzed preoperatively before operating on the ACoA aneurysm. The relevance of the side of the hematoma or infarct, if any, has been mentioned. Cerebral edema is a contraindication to surgery (see Fig. 30-59). Operating under these circumstances will lead to serious postoperative morbidity. The clinical status (alertness) of the patient and the CT scan or magnetic resonance image (MRI) will differentiate between increased intracranial pressure (ICP) due to edema or clot and increased ICP due to hydrocephalus (Fig. 30-60). If hydrocephalus is present, surgery to clip the aneurysm often can be done, but placement of an indwelling cerebrospinal fluid (CSF) needle or catheter should be planned. Additionally one might consider opening the arachnoid membrane of Liliequist (membrane of Key and Retzius) and/or the lamina terminalis at surgery to treat the hydrocephalus.

In analyzing the angiogram preoperatively it is useful to know if the intracranial internal carotid artery (ICA) is short or long. The longer the ICA, the more

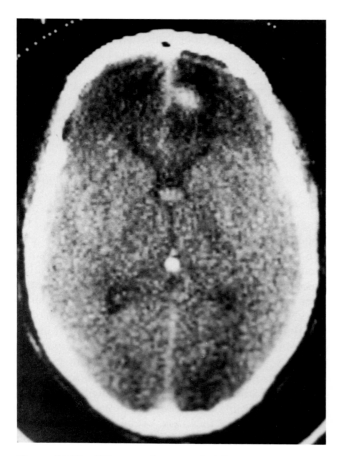

Figure 30-59. CT scan of ruptured ACoA aneurysm with left frontal hematoma and bifrontal edema.

difficult it is at surgery to see the ICA bifurcation and follow the A_1 artery to the ACoA aneurysm. Excess frontal lobe retraction must be avoided in this circumstance, such retraction leading to inadequate cerebral perfusion pressure under the retractor and subsequent cerebral infarction (Fig. 30-61).

Kempe et al.[202,203,277,278] used the gyrus rectus approach (via their pterional craniotomy) for the ACoA aneurysm that projected forward and/or downward. Yasargil et al.[284] removed a small portion of the gyrus rectus routinely in nearly all ACoA aneurysm cases (as do the authors). Kempe used this approach to avoid elevating the frontal lobe and disrupting the forward projecting dome of the aneurysm; that is, go through the gyrus rectus and intercept the neck of the aneurysm before disturbing its dome. But Yasargil found that the frontoorbital artery, arising from the

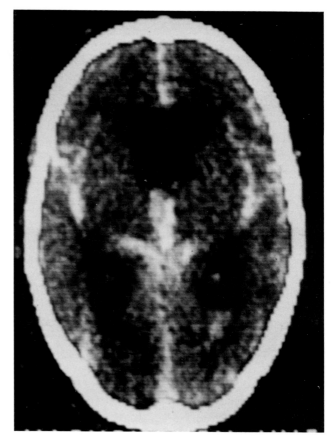

Figure 30-60. CT scan of ruptured ACoA aneurysm with hydrocephalus and blood in interhemispheric fissure, sylvian fissure, ambient cistern, and third ventricle. (From Fox and Nugent,[184] with permission.)

Table 30-15. Factors Concerning Approach to the ACoA Aneurysm

Other aneurysms
Hematoma
Infarction
Edema
Hydrocephalus
Length of internal carotid artery
Direction ACoA aneurysm projects
Shape, size, origin of ACoA aneurysm
Arterial anomalies
Circle of Willis pattern
Frontal sinuses

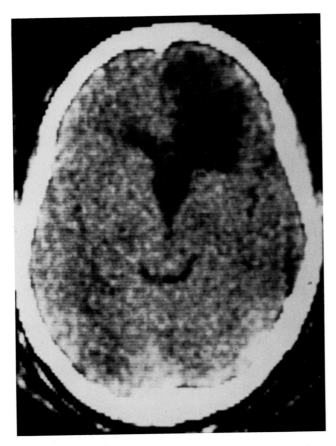

Figure 30-61. CT scan of ACoA aneurysm clipped 3 years earlier. Note hypodensity indicating frontal lobe infarction from brain retraction pressure. (From Fox,[178] with permission.)

A_2 segment of the anterior cerebral artery (A_2 artery), often was adherent to the dome of the ACoA aneurysm, which projected upward between the A_2 arteries. Elevation of the frontal lobe stretches the frontoorbital artery, which then pulls on the dome of the aneurysm. Premature rupture occurs. Thus even in cases in which the ICA is short (permitting the surgeon to see the A_1 artery and follow it), it is prudent in most circumstances to plan to enter the gyrus rectus and expose the ACoA region without any significant retraction on the medial aspect of the frontal lobe.

The shape of the ACoA aneurysm is quite variable: globular, elongated, multilobular. Although these aneurysms can be large, a giant size (2.5 cm or more in diameter) is uncommon among the ACoA aneurysms: rupture generally occurs before a large size is achieved.[178] Optic nerve compression signs are rarely seen in these cases. The angiogram must be analyzed carefully, for what may appear to be a single-domed

ACoA aneurysm at first glance may in fact be a bi- or trilobular aneurysm (or actually two or three separate aneurysms on the ACoA). At surgery one may see the obvious dome projecting toward the surgeon and miss the other dome or second aneurysm projecting deep between and behind the take-offs of the A_2 arteries (Fig. 30-62). Clipping the one dome may leave the second dome unsecured (at best) or tear the origin of the second dome, resulting in hemorrhagic complications.

Of course there is some comfort in knowing the exact site of origin of the ACoA aneurysm: (1) at the left A_2/ACoA junction, (2) at the right A_2/ACoA junction, or (3) along the entirety of the ACoA. The angiogram may, if done with special views and attention to detail, provide this information. Often, however, the exact site of origin is unclear. Even after exposing the ACoA aneurysm at surgery, the surgeon may have difficulty determining which side of the aneurysm is the origin and which side is only tightly adherent to the other A_2/ACoA junction. In general the aneurysm tends to arise from the side of the larger A_1 artery.[284]

The angiogram must be analyzed in terms of the direction to which the fundus of the ACoA aneurysm points. If it points downward and forward (Fig. 30-63A), elevation of the frontal lobe risks tearing the wall of an aneurysm adherent to the optic nerves or tuberculum sellae. In our experience, most ACoA aneurysms point superiorly between the A_2 segments of the anterior cerebral arteries (Fig. 30-63B). Here the dome of the aneurysm may be adherent to one or both A_2 arteries. Uncommonly the fundus points posteriorly (Fig. 30-63C); in this case the dome may be tightly adherent to hypothalamic perforators. Knowing this prior to the surgery allows the surgeon to know ahead of time the possible problems in aneurysm dissection that may occur.

Arterial anomalies are important to recognize on the angiogram. Failure to do so may result in confusion regarding anatomy at operation. And in the case of a loop of a third (accessory) A_2 artery, the loop may be mistaken for an aneurysm on angiography and at surgery. Lie[214] has described many important cerebrovascular anomalies. He has shown examples of carotid-basilar anastomoses, carotid-vertebral anastomoses, aplasia of the internal carotid artery, and carotid-anterior cerebral anastomoses (Fig. 30-64). The latter is an anomalous artery from the ICA (near the ophthalmic artery take-off). It "passes below and medial to the optic nerve and ascends in front of the chiasm to join the anterior communicating artery."[214] The artery perfuses the homolateral anterior cerebral artery (or the entire anterior cere-

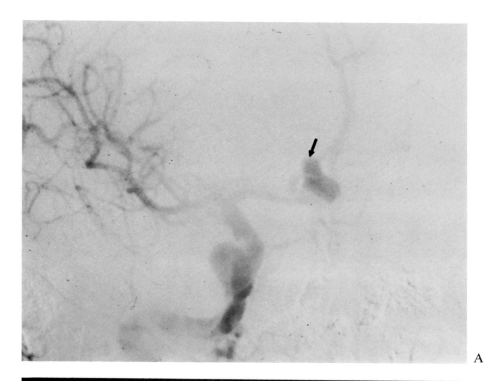

A

Figure 30-62. (A) Angiogram of bilobed ACoA aneurysm. *Arrow:* posterior-superior lobe between frontal lobes (hidden from surgeon). **(B)** Angiogram of two ACoA aneurysms (*arrowheads*). (Fig A from Fox,[178] with permission.)

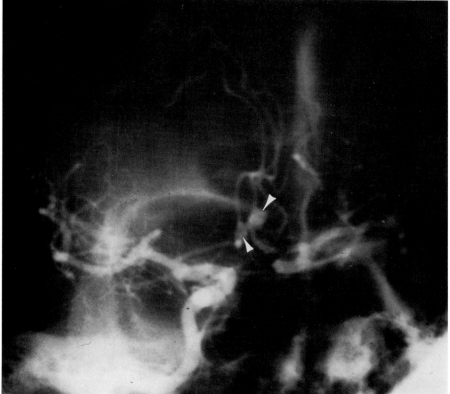

B

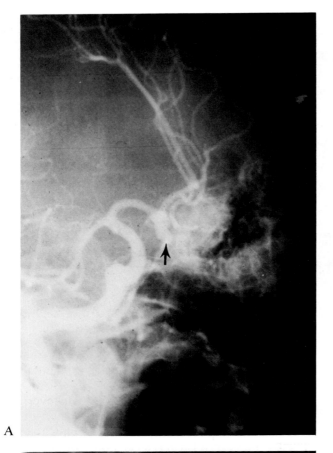

A

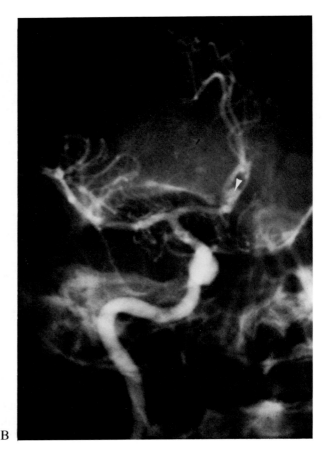

B

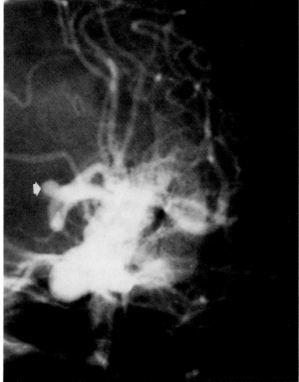

C

Figure 30-63. Angiograms of ACoA aneurysms. **(A)** Projecting downward and forward (*arrow*). **(B)** Pointing superiorly (*arrow*). **(C)** Pointing posteriorly (*arrow*); left carotid angiogram with oblique view through right orbit. (From Fox,[178] with permission.)

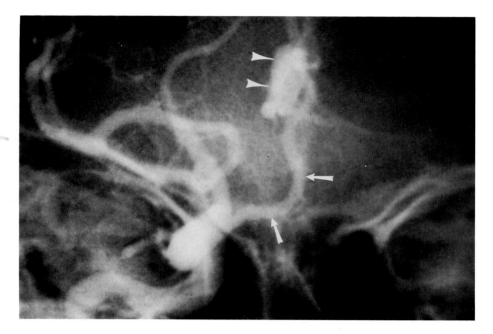

Figure 30-64. Angiogram (frontal view) of ACoA aneurysm (*arrowheads*) and anomalous carotid-anterior cerebral anastomosis (*arrows*). The right internal carotid, middle cerebral, and posterior communicating/ cerebral arteries are shown. At surgery there was a minute right A_1 artery.

bral circulation bilaterally if the contralateral A_1 is hypoplastic or absent).

The anterior communicating artery may be long, short, or nearly absent. Frequently there are two or three ACoA and/or bridging arteries between the ACoA and the A_2 segment (Fig. 30-65). These variations are common without or with the presence of an ACoA aneurysm,[144,174,175,205,240] but they often are not identified on routine cerebral angiography. Heubner's artery usually arises from the A_2 artery just above the ACoA, but it may arise higher up, at the A_1/A_2 communication, or from the A_1 artery. Occasionally, it arises as a common trunk with the fronto-orbital artery (see Fig. 30-65). The frontopolar artery, normally not seen at surgery, may arise from the ascending anterior cerebral artery close to the ACoA.

Variations in the circle of Willis are so common as to almost be the norm. Knowledge of the pattern of this arterial circle should be assessed preoperatively—especially in terms of blood (contrast media) flow through the A_1 arteries. At times the recurrent artery of Heubner[194] will be larger than the hypoplastic A_1 artery. In this case the opposite A_1 artery serves the anterior cerebral circulation. Here one will use the utmost care to prevent an aneurysm clip from compromising the main A_1 artery or the ACoA.

The frontal sinuses vary considerably in extent. If enlarged they may appear to interfere with a basal approach to the aneurysm. We do not hesitate to enter the sinuses and seal them with Gelfoam soaked in an antibiotic. But one must be wary of postoperative rhinorrhea if adequate closing technique is missed.

Murphy's Law is the principle that whatever can possibly go wrong will.[145] The law was named after a statement of frustration by Captain Murphy, a development engineer at Edwards Air Force Base in 1949. This led to simulated crash force testing in a "consistent effort to deny the inevitable."[145] As important as the surgeon's experience is the close attention to the preoperative imaging studies, especially the angiogram. In this way the surgeon can best be alerted to normal and abnormal anatomical variations and improve the chances of avoiding untoward intraoperative surprises.

Timing of Surgery

The issue of patient selection and timing of ACoA aneurysm surgery (as well as surgery for other intracranial aneurysms) following SAH is under continued debate. Reference is made to other reviews on the subject.[178,196,197,261] In general, surgeons tend to operate early (within the first 3 days of the bleed) if the patient is in a grade I or II condition and operate late (10 to 20 days after the bleed) in patients initially in poorer grades. Yet a grade I patient's impending vasospasm may be made considerably worse by manipulation of the cerebral vasculature and the addition of surgical blood to the previous SAH blood in the cisterns. Contrariwise, a secured aneurysm no

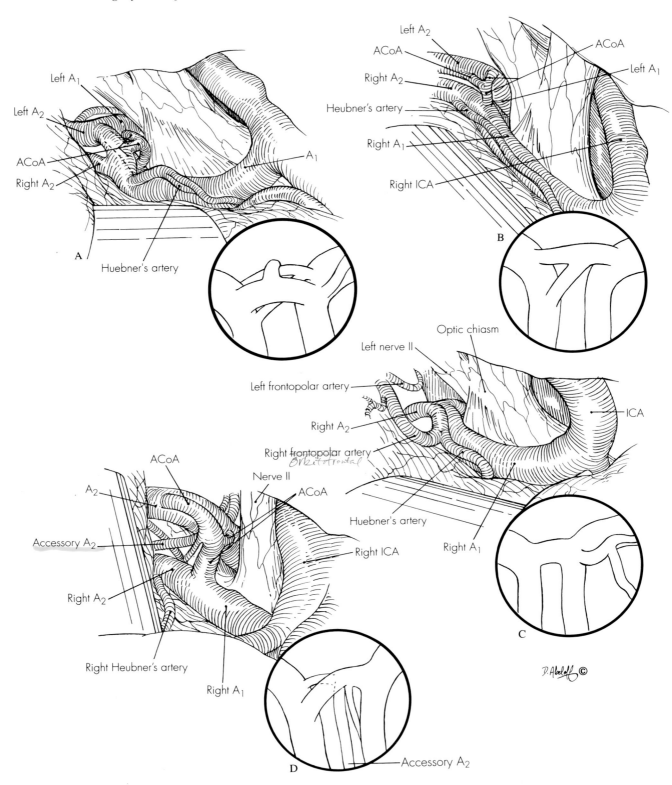

Figure 30-65. Anatomical variations in the ACoA region as viewed by the surgeon through a right frontotemporal craniotomy. **(A)** Triplicate ACoAs with bridging. **(B)** Y-shaped ACoA. **(C)** Common trunk origin of fronto-orbital artery and Heubner's artery. **(D)** Y-shaped ACoA with bridging and origin of a third (accessory) anterior cerebral (A_2) artery. (Fig. A adapted from Fox,[178] with permission; Figs. B–D adapted from Fox,[176] with permission.)

longer threatened by therapeutic institution of vascular hypertension and increased cerebral blood flow raises one's confidence in measures to combat cerebral vasospasm. Since the literature support for early versus late surgery has not resulted in an overwhelming consensus of opinion, we prefer not to make recommendations here but to leave the decision up to the individual surgeon as particular circumstances may dictate.

Gillingham[188] pointed out that in his experience the most important single factor in determining success or failure in the operative treatment of intracranial aneurysms was the conscious level of the patient prior to operation. There is rather universal agreement that the results of intracranial surgery (like the results of nonoperative treatment) are better when the patient is in a good grade.[178] This problem is not unique to ACoA aneurysm cases, but is seen in patients with ruptured aneurysm at all intracranial subarachnoid sites. Additional considerations regarding preoperative assessment of intracranial aneurysm patients are given elsewhere.[170,179,186,187,234]

INTRAOPERATIVE PROBLEMS

Aneurysm Rupture at Surgery

Intraoperative problems with intracranial aneurysm surgery include those of any craniotomy with surgical manipulation about the circle of Willis. The significant exception is intraoperative *rupture* of the aneurysm, an intraoperative problem unique to aneurysm surgery and one of the causes of the postoperative complications discussed later in this chapter.[156,157,159,196,197,238,242] In 1952 Hamby[191] stated "The greatest surgical hazard seems to lie in rupture of the aneurysm during its exposure. This often leads to the clipping of vessels that have not been properly identified." He concluded that the surgeon "was much in the position of the hunter arousing a tiger when stalking a deer." Several authors have discussed intraoperative rupture of the ACoA aneurysm.[173,192,242,244,280] The incidence of intraoperative aneurysm rupture (approaching 50 percent of cases in earlier years) has lessened with the routine use of microsurgical techniques, hypotensive anesthesia, and improved aneurysm clips.[178] Yet aneurysm rupture at surgery is not uncommon, and the wise surgeon will be mentally and emotionally prepared by *assuming* that the aneurysm *will* rupture and by dealing effectively and calmly with the matter should rupture actually occur. Table 30-16 summarizes points

Table 30-16. Prevention of Intraoperative ACoA Aneurysm Rupture

1. Careful induction of anesthesia
2. Patient well anesthetized when skull pins inserted
3. Careful cracking of base of skull flap
4. Good blood pressure control
5. Gentle hematoma release
6. Careful elevation of frontal lobe
7. Careful aneurysm dissection
8. Avoid atherosclerotic plaques when clipping
9. Place wings of clip across entire aneurysm
10. Use strong aneurysm clip of proper size and shape
11. Have a steady surgeon's hand
12. Use appropriate clip applier and withdraw applier slowly
13. Avoid excess early CSF drainage by lumbar puncture
14. Keep wall of aneurysm wet

regarding prevention of premature aneurysm rupture.

There are several critical periods during surgery when intraoperative rupture may occur[178,211,230,236]:

1. Any elevation of blood pressure (BP) or rapid changes in ICP during induction of anesthesia may change the differential transmural pressure of the aneurysm wall sufficient to rupture the aneurysm.
2. During skull fixation with pinions through the scalp, the patient must be well anesthetized so that BP does not suddenly rise.
3. When the bone flap is turned, there may be a sudden reduction in ICP. This, combined with the vibrations (especially if the aneurysm is adherent to the skull base) due to the drilling, sawing, and cracking, may precipitate rupture. Hence, before this point it may be wise to start lowering the BP.
4. Upon opening the dura the tamponading ICP is reduced to near-atmospheric pressure.
5. Upon release of a hematoma surrounding the aneurysm, the aneurysm is no longer tamponaded and may bleed.
6. The aneurysm may be disturbed and rupture during elevation of the frontal lobe.
7. Gentle technique and controlled BP are advisable during dissection of the aneurysm, for this is the point at which most such ruptures occur.
8. Rupture may occur during the use of methods to reduce the diameter of the neck of the aneurysm.
9. During clipping of the aneurysm a weak spot in the neck-artery junction may give way (especially if it is atherosclerotic), the clip may not be fully across the aneurysm neck, the clip may be too weak or defective, the neck may be stretched between a rigid artery and adherent brain tissue, or the surgeon's hand may be too tremorous.
10. The clip applier may fail to be withdrawn smoothly during its removal.
11. The clip may slip off the aneurysm during closure of the wound.

Techniques of controlling intraoperative aneurysm rupture have been discussed by a number of authors.[155,157,178,191,202,204,211,242,247,269,284] Although we rarely do this, temporary clips may be placed on both A_1 arteries. Induced vascular hypotension may be useful (but dangerous if temporary clips are used also). When the aneurysm ruptures during its exposure or dissection, the operating microscope is of great assistance in providing light and visualization so that the dissection can continue while the suction tube clears the field of blood. This procedure is much more easily done if the patient is under controlled hypotension. More often than not, if the aneurysm was exposed before rupture, the surgeon will see the start of the leak before it gets out of control. Pressure of the suction apparatus against a cottonoid on the aneurysm allows effective tamponading while the surgeon isolates the neck for clipping. Bipolar forceps can be used to continue the dissection, close the neck of the aneurysm, and arrest the bleeding by closure and electrocoagulation. Readjustment of the clip or use of a second clip may be effective. Fascial or muscle wrapping, use of encircling clips, and application of tissue adhesives are uncommonly done now. Microsurigcal suture repair of a parent artery is an occasional consideration.

SURGICAL TECHNIQUE

The technique any given surgeon uses is based on experience, training, and observation. One surgeon's technique is not necessarily better than another's. The technique described in this section is that of author J.L.F., which differs in some aspects from that of author R.P.S. Regardless of technique and regardless of which cranial opening (Fig. 30-66) is used, the end result will depend on a rigorous, methodical, systematic, and step-by-step approach to the target, securing it with minimal injury to surrounding structures. The final clipping process is threatened if earlier steps to access the aneurysm have been incorrectly carried out or if needed modifications are recognized too late. It would be rather like trying to take an enemy target in warfare without having all one's troops and armor in proper position at the proper time. Knowing when and where to place these troops and armor takes years of training and experience to achieve and is based on previous mistakes and losses. Such sad and bitter lessons, if learned, will lead to better results and fewer losses in the future. Both the adept student of intracranial aneurysm surgery and the clever student of modern warfare will try to learn much from the mistakes of others in the past, through reading, observing, and assisting.

Frontotemporal Approach

For purposes of clarity and consistency the *right* frontotemporal (pterional) approach will be summarized, with attention to avoidance of possible complications of ACoA aneurysm surgery. This approach is further illustrated in other publications.[176,178–180] Basic concepts stated here can be applied to other approaches that other neurosurgeons may prefer.

Hopefully, the patient has a tranquilized state of mind upon entering the operating room. Good neuroanesthetic methods are critical to a successful outcome.[135] As in other intracranial aneurysm operations the brain must be relaxed and cerebral blood flow sufficient for cerebral metabolism. At times there needs to be a compromise between vascular hypotension to reduce the risk of aneurysm rupture and normotension (or even hypertension during temporary parent artery occlusion) to maintain good cerebral perfusion in the face of vasospasm and brain retraction pressure. Controlled passive hyperventilation, without or with intravascular osmotic drugs such as mannitol, has become routine methodology in controlling ICP.[177,182,193] Since these anesthetic and monitoring issues are not unique to ACoA aneurysm surgery, we will not detail them here. Suffice it to say that if, before or upon opening the dura, the brain is tense and hydrocephalus or hematoma are not a factor, the surgery should be terminated and the patient reassessed for aneurysm clipping at a later date.

The stepwise process leading to successful isolating and clipping of an ACoA aneurysm begins with the construction of a solidly based, four-dimensional pyramid conceptualizing this patient's medical care. The three-dimensional construct is laid down by valuable and continuing contributions from radiology, medicine, surgery, anesthesiology, engineering, nursing, and related fields. Construction continues over time in the operating room. Laying the final brick (clipping the aneurysm) at the peak of the pyramid requires that all of the previous underlying bricks (1) are present, (2) are made from good material, and (3) are well in place at the proper time. For example, if one of the bipolar forceps (Fig. 30-67A) are faulty and a backup set is not readily available or if the microsurgical dissectors (Fig. 30-67B) were missing that day, then one or two of the thousands of bricks are not well laid. Numerous other examples could be given.

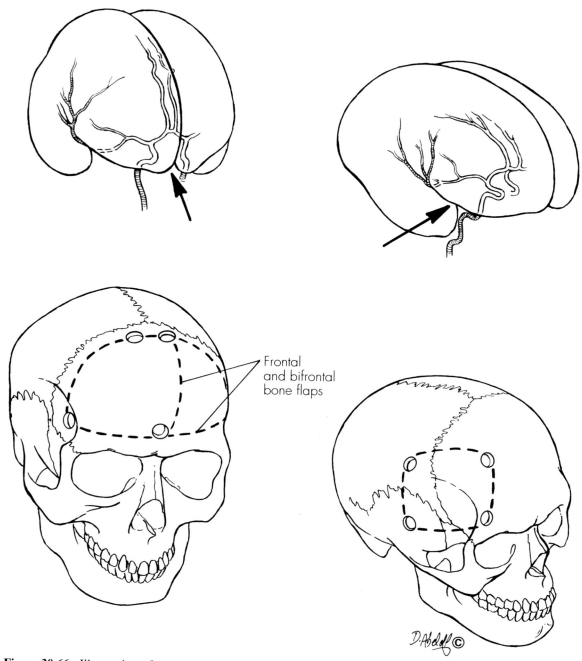

Figure 30-66. Illustration of two commonly used approaches to the ACoA region. **(Left)** frontal or bifrontal approach. **(Right)** frontotemporal (pterional) approach.

As we construct our portion of this allegorical pyramid in the operating room, we can begin with the positioning of the anesthetized patient. Our patient is placed on the American Sterilizer operating room (OR) table so that the patient's head is at the foot-end of the table (Fig. 30-68). This has the following advantages: (1) the table pedals are not in the way of the sitting surgeon's feet; (2) there is more room for the base of the microscope positioned on the surgeon's left; and (3) the normal opening in the OR table lies under the lumbar region of the patient's back, facilitating lumbar CSF drainage without turning the patient.

With the patient's head turned about 40 degrees to the left, tilted about 15 degrees to the left, and dropped back about 15 degrees, we insert the three-

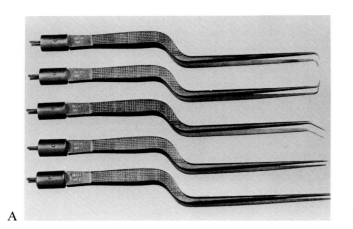
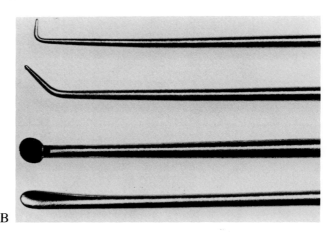

Figure 30-67. Example of **(A)** bipolar forceps and **(B)** microdissectors. (From Fox,[178] with permission.)

point skull fixation apparatus (Mayfield-Kees skull clamp) to immobilize the head. The horizontal part of this headholder should be nearly parallel with the floor (Fig. 30-69). Placed thusly, the head is held firmly without parts of the clamp getting in the way of the Leyla-Aesculap self-retaining retractor to be attached later. The patient must be well anesthetized prior to inserting the skull pins, or a surge in blood pressure may occur. Proper alignment of the head at this stage is very critical: it allows the frontal lobe to fall away from the frontal floor after opening the sylvian fissure, following which a direct path to the aneurysm can be developed. Without aligning the head in this manner for the pterional approach, the sur-

geon later will find an awkward line-of-sight from his eye through the microscope to the target. Details of draping and instrumentation (microscope, surgeon's chair, microinstruments, and so forth) can be found elsewhere.[176,178,179]

The bipolar electrocautery forceps (see Fig. 30-67) is so critical that we summarize its application here. We use the bipolar forceps as the principal dissecting and tissue-separating instrument intracranially. For this reason the blades of the forceps must have proper spreading tension, yet not be so tense as to make tip approximation uncomfortable. They must not rotate inappropriately in the surgeon's hand. In terms of time, its actual application for electrocauter-

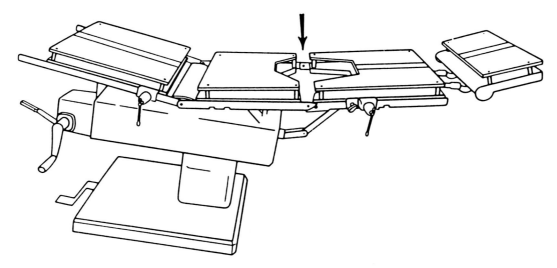

Figure 30-68. Sketch of American Sterilizer operating room table. The usual head-end is to the observer's left. The headrest has been removed from this end and placed at the normal foot-end on the observer's right. The patient's head initially rests on the headrest on the observer's right, with that end elevated 10 to 15 degrees and with the lumbar region of the patient's back resting over the opening (*arrow*) in the table. (From Fox,[178] with permission.)

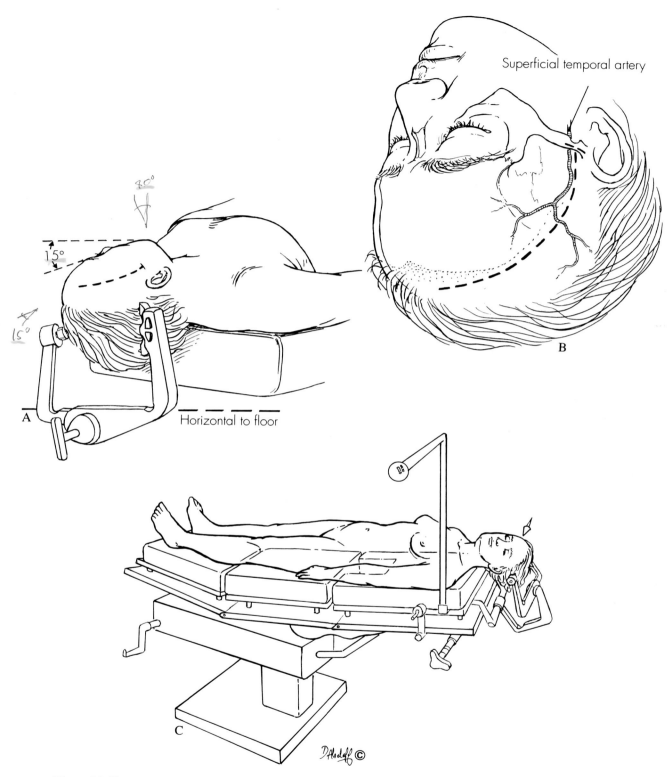

Figure 30-69. **(A)** Illustration of three-point skull fixation apparatus clamped into patient's skull. Dotted line indicates incision for right pterional approach. **(B)** Incision (*dotted line*) is made behind hair line. **(C)** Diagram of patient positioned on operating table. Arrow indicates direction of right pterional approach to ACoA aneurysm.

ization is quite short compared to its use as a tissue dissector, perforator, spreader, separator, and grasper. It is used to place and remove cottonoids, cotton balls, Gelfoam, oxycellulose, and rubber or plastic sheets. For us, the suction tube (in the surgeons' left hand) and the bipolar electrocautery forceps (in the right hand) have become the main microsurgical instruments (in terms of frequency and duration of use) during intracranial aneurysm surgery.

The Cranial Opening

As the head now is positioned, the so-called psychopathic point comes into the center and highest point of the operative field. This is the point where the zygomatic process of the frontal bone, the orbital ridge, and the temporal line meet.[176,178,203,278] The first burr hole will be placed here just above the temporal line (others prefer it below the temporal line at the "keyhole" site, which puts part of the burr hole in the right orbital cavity). At the end of the surgery this hole is covered with bone chips and periosteum, thus preventing any cosmetic indentation. The temporal burr hole is in front of the right ear just above the zygomatic arch. These are interconnected with rongeurs (inferiorly under the temporalis muscle) and craniotome. In older patients two additional burr holes (frontal and parietal) may be drilled and a Gigli saw used. Either way it is important to have the cranial flap large enough to permit gentle retraction of the frontal lobe with the self-retaining retractor. Otherwise the retractor blade will strike against the frontal bone, limiting adequate frontal lobe retraction.

The bone flap is then turned laterally and down while attached to the temporalis muscle. Incising the temporalis muscle (using a free bone flap) and pulling it back leads to excessive future atrophy of the temporalis muscle. Turning the temporalis muscle as a part of the skin flap causes excess soft tissue bulk at the base of the exposure; this leads to the need for more brain retraction in order to visualize the pathway to the ACoA aneurysm.

Figure 30-70 illustrates the need for removal of much of the sphenoid wing prior to opening the dura. If this is not done, the ACoA aneurysm area cannot be directly visualized without excess brain retraction pressure. Such pressure leads to postoperative brain edema and necrosis. Removal of this bone with rongeurs and high-speed drills significantly improves the eventual exposure. The sphenoid bone should be removed down to the base of the anterior clinoid process. The technical details of removal are given elsewhere.[176,178] The dura now is opened. The dura already has been tacked up to the cranial edge to eliminate epidural bleeding. We use 4-0 sutures passed through holes already drilled for future reattachment of the bone flap. The bone flap and galea have been covered with Surgicel (oxycellulose) and retracted away with fishhook retractors and rubberbands.

Transsylvian Exposure

To clip the ACoA aneurysm, we need to expose part or all of the aneurysm. We can do this by pulling hard enough on the brain (frontal lobe) to bring it into view, but this damages brain tissue and perforating vessels. After removal of the sphenoid wing a low basal exposure has opened up the peripheral or craniobasal side of the tunnel leading to the aneurysm. The next step in the pterional approach is to open up the central or cerebral wall of this path under illumination and magnification. It is this step, opening the sylvian fissure, that is either omitted or minimized by many surgeons in the past. It is a step that can be difficult and frustrating until experience is gained, yet this step is as important as sphenoid wing removal in gaining good, direct exposure of the anterior communicating region without excess retraction.

Vital in opening the sylvian fissure is proper placement of the temporal lobe and frontal lobe retractors. We use the Leyla (Yasargil-Aesculap) system, which attaches to the OR table on the left side.[178] The connecting bar is positioned so that the surgeon's left hand can partially rest on it. The cable inside the flexible ball-and-socket arm is tightened to make the arm rigid after the retractor blade is in position. This arm is attached to the end (not the center) of the retractor blade, which is bent in such a manner as to (1) keep the end of the ball-and-socket arm away from the cranial opening, (2) allow the retractor blade to enter the cranial opening without obstructing the surgeon's line of vision, and (3) pull gently on a cottonoid between the blade and the brain. This latter step in effect puts slight traction on the frontal lobe in an anteromedial direction and the temporal lobe in a posterior direction, thus stretching the arachnoid in the sylvian fissure between them. As this arachnoid is cut toward the carotid cistern, the retractor blades are moved deeper to separate more basal portions of the sylvian fissure (Fig. 30-71A). We no longer hesitate to coagulate and sever veins running between these two lobes of the brain. The exposure is carried down on the frontal lobe side of the sylvian veins and the deeper, tougher arachnoid at the base of the syl-

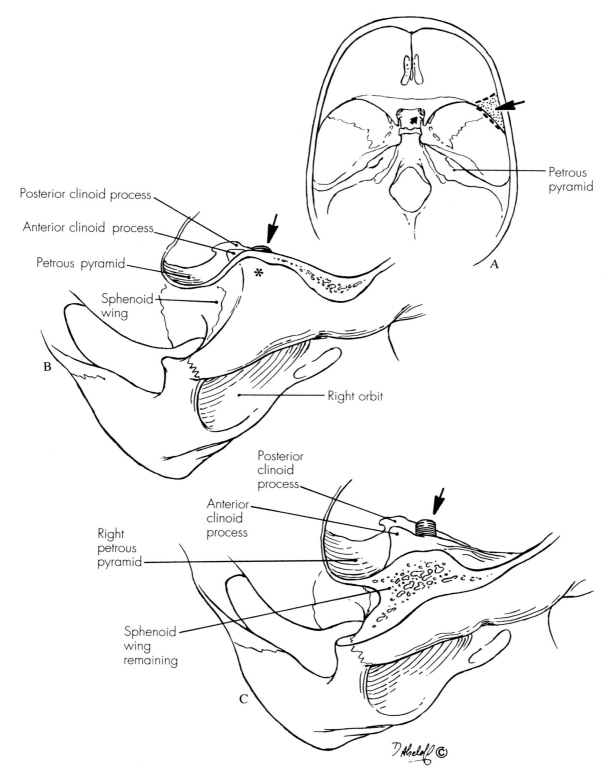

Figure 30-70. Diagram of dry skull. **(A)** Direction of cranial approach (*arrow*) to ACoA area. **(B)** View of ACoA "aneurysm" (*arrow*) blocked by sphenoid wing (*asterisk*). **(C)** View of ACoA "aneurysm" (*arrow*) after much of sphenoid wing has been drilled away. Note: view is with skull held upright.

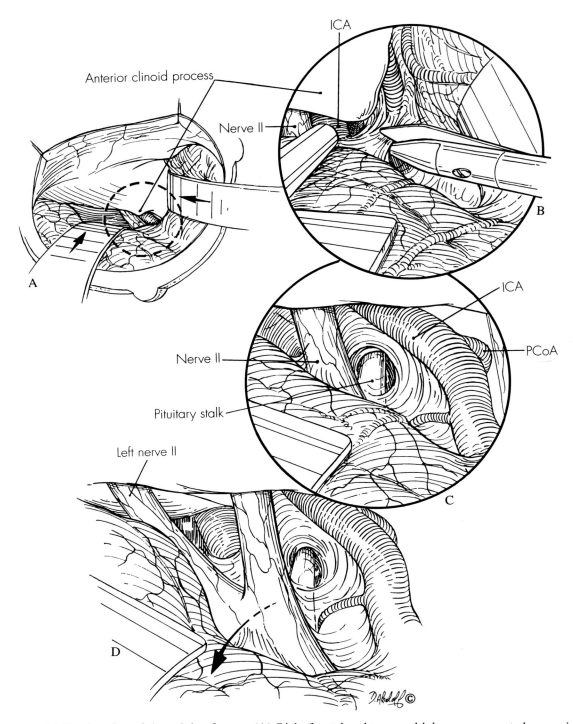

Figure 30-71. Opening of the sylvian fissure. **(A)** Right frontal and temporal lobes are separated, exposing carotid cistern. **(B)** Cutting basal arachnoid in sylvian fissure. **(C)** Elevating frontal lobe. **(D)** As frontal lobe drops back, chiasmatic cistern and cistern of the lamina terminalis are seen.

vian fissure is cut (Fig. 30-71B). Now the frontal lobe can be elevated before detaching the gyrus rectus from the optic nerve; middle cerebral arterial branches come into view. If the intracranial internal carotid artery is short, the optic tract and chiasm will come into direct view immediately. This brings our access to the ACoA aneurysm close with minimal brain retraction pressure. Care is taken to keep the exposed middle cerebral and carotid arteries wet with CSF (stop the lumbar CSF drainage once good brain relaxation is in effect).

Gyrus Rectus Approach

After opening the sylvian fissure great care must be continued to avoid premature rupture of the aneurysm. The surgeon and anesthesiologist must be in continuous communication regarding BP control and fluid balance. In most circumstances the optic tract and the A_1 artery will not be immediately seen after opening the sylvian fissure. More often the surgeon is confronted with structures exposed in the carotid cistern and lateral part of the chiasmatic cistern (Fig. 30-71C).[176] The frontal lobe retractor must not slip unnoticed against Heubner's artery or the optic nerve. The frontal lobe should not be elevated simply to expose the A_1 artery or optic chiasm (these may be seen anyway if the carotid artery is short or there is a prefixed optic chiasm). This may risk unnecessary brain retraction pressure and tension on the wall of the aneurysm.

In the absence of adhesions and edema the frontal lobe may fall away with exposure of the chiasmatic cistern (Fig. 30-71D). If the ICA is short and the optic chiasm is prefixed, the chiasmatic cistern will come into full view (Fig. 30-72A). The ACoA aneurysm and the medial A_1 arteries will lie deeper in the cistern of the lamina terminalis. This cistern lies medial to the arachnoid band seen squeezing the A_1 artery in Figure 30-72. Such arachnoid bands should be cut with microscissors to avoid traction on the A_1 artery and its perforators. But following the A_1 artery (Fig. 30-72B) to the ACoA usually must be avoided. The frontoorbital artery shown in Figure 30-73A often is stuck to the wall of the ACoA aneurysm. Pulling on the frontal lobe stretches this artery and risks rupture of the aneurysm. It is for this reason that Kempe's direct approach through the gyrus rectus is advised in most cases of ACoA aneurysm clipping.[176,178,202,277] Figures 30-73A and 30-74A show the anatomy of the gyrus rectus and the zone through which the surgeon initiates the incision. This is a triangular or quadrangular zone formed by (1) the optic nerve/frontal lobe

junction (Fig. 30-73A) or the A_1/frontal lobe junction (Fig. 30-74A), (2) the olfactory tract and retractor blade, and (3) the fronto-orbital artery as the self-retaining retractor blade first exposes the gyrus rectus medial to the olfactory tract. The initial incision is made in the gyrus rectus within this zone. The pia is cauterized and incised with microscissors or a knife blade. Then with suction, bipolar forceps, and microscissors, a zone of brain tissue 1 cm in length is removed down to the medial pia-arachnoid layer.

The fronto-orbital artery will lead the surgeon directly to the ACoA complex. Extreme care must be taken since this artery often is adherent to the dome of the aneurysm. As the aneurysm is approached, this artery can be electrocoagulated and severed. In this way, any retraction on the frontal lobe with a consequent pulling on the frontoorbital artery will not result in traction on the ACoA aneurysm wall. Once the medial pia-arachnoid layer of the gyrus rectus is reached, fibrin and clot obscuring the aneurysm may be encountered. The pia-arachnoid layer is carefully opened, and any fibrin and clot around the ACoA, its A_1/A_2 branches, and the neck of the aneurysm are removed by suction and forceps. Adhesions are lysed. The dome of the aneurysm initially is avoided and the self-retaining retractors maintained in proper position to permit exposure of the neck without movement of the dome of the aneurysm.

The Aneurysm

Figures 30-73B and 30-74B each demonstrate an ACoA aneurysm projecting superiorly in relation to the patient. The fundi lie between the A_2 arteries and project to the surgeon's left. In the first case there is only a limited exposure of the ACoA complex through the right gyrus rectus opening (Fig. 30-73B). In the second case a more extensive exposure is seen through the gyrus rectus opening (Fig. 30-74B). In dissecting out the neck and fundus of the aneurysm a major risk occurs if the neck of the aneurysm tears at the A_2 artery junction (probe site in Fig. 30-73B). This actually occurred in the second case. In this circumstance pressure is applied on the opening with the suction tube on a small cottonoid. The BP is kept low (about 80 mmHg systolic). Blood is cleared from the field with irrigation and a second suction in the surgeon's right hand. Then dissection is continued to isolate the aneurysm. The clip is applied parallel to the ACoA (Fig. 30-74C), with the tips of its wings advanced enough to occlude the hole yet not so far as to occlude the origin of the A_2 artery. Placing the clip perpendicular to the ACoA often is done but risks

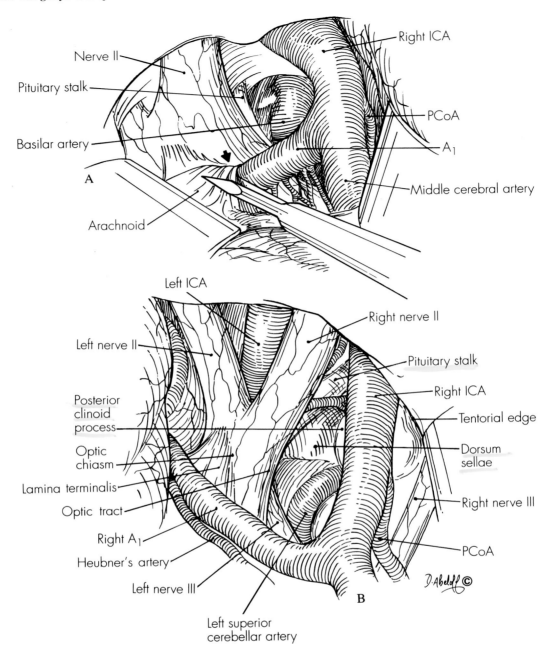

Nerve II

Pituitary stalk

Basilar artery

A

Arachnoid

Right ICA

PCoA

A₁

Middle cerebral artery

Left ICA

Left nerve II

Posterior clinoid process

Optic chiasm

Lamina terminalis

Optic tract

Right A₁

Heubner's artery

Left nerve III

Left superior cerebellar artery

Right nerve II

Pituitary stalk

Right ICA

Tentorial edge

Dorsum sellae

Right nerve III

PCoA

B

D. Abeloff ©

Figure 30-72. Diagrams illustrating the surgeon following the right A₁ artery medially. **(A)** The intracranial carotid artery is short, and there is a prefixed optic chiasm. **(B)** The intracranial carotid artery is long, but the frontal lobe has fallen back with exposure of the A₁ artery, Heubner's artery, and the lamina terminalis.

tearing the aneurysm at its A₂ junction. Here a second clip is placed on the fundus. Depending on circumstances, an encircling clip may be needed to encircle the right A₂ artery and occlude the aneurysm in a direction parallel to the ACoA.

Tears at the neck of the aneurysm during clipping are less likely to occur if the entire aneurysm is isolated (not just the neck). A tear in the dome can be

more easily handled with cottonoid pressure, hypotension, bipolar electrocoagulation (Figs. 30-73C, 30-73D), and/or an initial clip across the waist of the fundus.

Bipolar electrocoagulation of an ACoA aneurysm not only can be used to halt aneurysm bleeding by sealing off the bleeding site but also can be applied to narrow the waist of an aneurysm in order to visualize

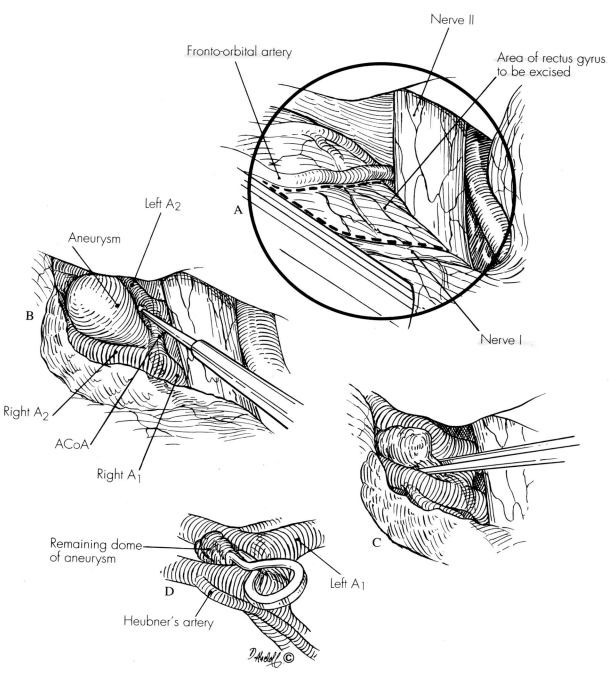

Figure 30-73. Exposure of ACoA aneurysm via the gyrus rectus without following the A$_1$ artery (see text). **(A)** Dotted lines outline area of right gyrus rectus to be incised. **(B)** ACoA aneurysm exposed. **(C)** Bipolar electrocoagulation of aneurysm. **(D)** Aneurysm collapsed after clip applied.

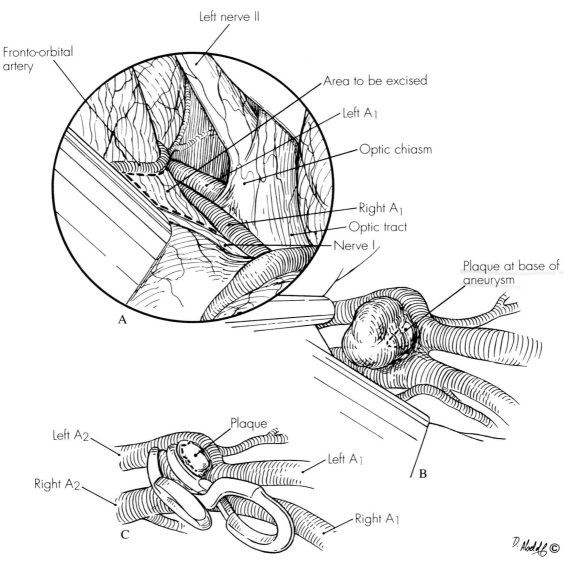

Fronto-orbital artery

Left nerve II

Area to be excised

Left A₁

Optic chiasm

Right A₁

Optic tract

Nerve I

Plaque at base of aneurysm

A

B

Left A₂

Plaque

Left A₁

Right A₂

Right A₁

C

D. Abdd ©

Figure 30-74. Another exposure through the right gyrus rectus (see text). **(A)** Dotted lines outline area of gyrus rectus to be incised. **(B)** Globoid ACoA aneurysm exposed through gyrus rectus incision. **(C)** Two aneurysm clips placed parallel to ACoA with occlusion of aneurysm.

around it better and permit better clip application.[284] The following excerpt from Fox[178] summarizes the technique and critical points:

For large, thick-walled aneurysms use the large-tip forceps. When changing to small-tip diameters (1.0–0.5 mm), lower the electrocautery output (usually use No. 25 on the Malis unit sold by Codman and Shurtleff). The current density increases as the forceps-aneurysm contact surface decreases. Place cotton microsponges between perforators (vessels) and the forceps. Be sure the forceps tips are completely across the aneurysm neck; otherwise the aneurysm may rupture at the point at which the tips touch the aneurysm. Avoid perforators or branches beyond the aneurysm. Close the

forceps blades slowly around the aneurysm neck and keep the blades a short distance from the parent vessel wall. Use intermittent bursts of electricity (a few seconds at a time). Inspect and repeat the process as needed. Stop the current when the wall begins to desiccate, fry, and shrivel. Reinspect and repeat as needed. Keep the field wet as needed to avoid drying and cracking of the aneurysm wall and to avoid sticking of the forceps tips. Knead, or rapidly but minimally open and close, the forceps tips and the coagulation continues. It may help to evacuate some blood in the aneurysm by compressing the dome of the aneurysm with the suction tube against cotton on the aneurysm fundus. If the aneurysm ruptures during the process, insert the forcep blades deeper, close the forceps, and continue the electrocauterization.

We have just demonstrated two examples of ACoA aneurysms pointing superiorly and lying between the A_2 arteries (see Figs. 30-73 and 30-74). Figure 30-75 illustrates aneurysms pointing anteriorly and posteriorly in a case with two ACoA aneurysms (Fig. 30-75A), anteriorly (Fig. 30-75B), and posteriorly (Figs. 30-75C&D). The aneurysm shown in Figure 30-75B was discovered incidently when the frontal lobe was elevated during surgery for another aneurysm. This frontal lobe elevation risked premature rupture of the aneurysm, but the dome had no adhesions of significance. The ACoA aneurysm in Figure 30-75A

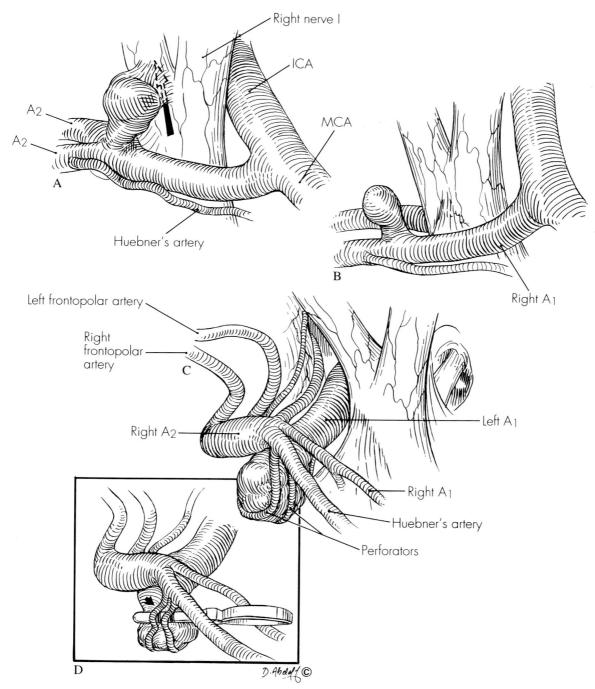

Figure 30-75. Other projections of an ACoA aneurysm (see text). **(A)** Dome of exposed aneurysm stuck to left optic nerve and chiasm by adhesions (a second ACoA aneurysm projecting posteriorly is hidden at this point). **(B)** An ACoA aneurysm projecting forward above optic chiasm and lamina terminalis. **(C)** An ACoA aneurysm projecting backward against lamina terminalis. **(D)** Same aneurysm after clip applied between aneurysm and hypothalamic perforators.

was exposed through the gyrus rectus; it had its anterior dome stuck firmly on the left optic nerve. Adhesions between this dome and nerve were gently lysed with separation by sharp (microscissors) and blunt dissection. In this case a second dome (actually separate aneurysm) pointed posteriorly (downward with respect to the surgeon) and was initially hidden by the right A_1/A_2 junction. The oblique angiographic study had alerted the surgeon to this circumstance. Both aneurysms were isolated and clipped; the deeper aneurysm could be seen only by elevating the right A_2 artery at its junction with A_1 and the ACoA.

The aneurysm shown in Figures 30-75C&D presented a complex situation: (1) the right A_1 artery was hypoplastic, (2) both A_2 arteries were fed by a large left A_1 artery, (3) there was a low take-off of both frontopolar arteries, (4) the aneurysm projected back against the lamina terminalis, (5) the aneurysm had hypothalamic perforators stuck to its dome. Identification of anatomy was difficult. It took a tediously long time to dissect the adherent perforators from the dome before the clip could ligate the neck of the aneurysm (Fig. 30-75D).

The old adage of exposing only the neck of the aneurysm and getting out fast is history.[178] With the aid of microtechnique and modern anesthesia, the surgeon usually can safely dissect out the fundus (or most of it). This allows one to apply the clip without tearing the junction of the neck with its parent artery—for if the dome is not free, the neck of the aneurysm may, in some cases (especially in the presence of atherosclerosis), be stretched between the fixed dome and the parent artery as the clip squeezes down on it. It is easier to deal with a dome ruptured by dissection than with a tear in the neck caused by clipping. Before application of the clip, the surgeon and anesthesiologist must confer regarding blood pressure and any other pertinent assessments. The surgeon should already have selected any clips most likely to be used (in case of a sudden, premature rupture). At this time, the surgeon selects the specific clip to be applied and tests it near the aneurysm without actually applying the clip. Adjustments may have to be made in the length and angle of the clip blade. The surgeon may determine that the clip must be applied with the left hand instead of the dominant right hand. We never use the original type of "encircling" clip around the anterior communicating artery, for it may occlude vital perforators. However, we often use the modern encircling clips to provide a passage for the A_1 or A_2 artery, a perforator, or another aneurysm clip. The clip holder must have the advantage of being bayonet in shape. Final dissections are completed. The surgeon takes the clip-

holder and unlocks it *before* the clip is applied (otherwise the tremor of the unlocking motion may tear and rupture the aneurysm).

The wings of the clip are spread to encircle the aneurysm. They are used to dissect between the neck and adjacent tissues before closure around the aneurysm. Slow, deliberate movements are required. Do not apply the clip as close as possible to the ACoA—especially if one is not applying the clip with its wings parallel to the ACoA. Otherwise, there is a high risk of tearing the A_2/ACoA aneurysm junction. The clip should be about 1 mm from the ACoA to allow the aneurysm wall at that junctional point to bend as it is pulled inward by the clip blade. We often apply a larger clip on the center of the dome first to collapse the aneurysm and then follow with a second, smaller clip about the neck. The wings of the clip must strangle the neck gradually, followed by slow and cautious disengagement and removal of the clip applier. A second clip may be applied on the fundus and parallel to the first clip. We often have applied an extra clip to buttress the first. If any unsecured aneurysm remains and cannot be clipped safely, we cover that part of the aneurysm with cotton fibers followed by Gelfoam (the latter to separate the future cotton foreign body reaction from the optic chiasm and nerves). Table 30-17 summarizes points regarding correct aneurysm clip placement.

Closure

After application of the clip or clips, care is taken to be sure no parent arteries or perforators are trapped in the clip or that part of the aneurysm is not secured. More often than not we have to readjust the clip. Three percent papaverine often is applied topically to take perforators out of local spasm. The

Table 30-17. Concerns Regarding Intracranial Aneurysm Clip Placement

1. Place wings of clip across entire diameter of aneurysm
2. On large aneurysm place initial clip on equator of fundus to collapse aneurysm and avoid clip slipping onto parent artery
3. Do not occlude perforators
4. Do not occlude parent arteries
5. Place clip parallel to parent artery if possible
6. Avoid squeezing plaque or clot into parent artery lumen
7. Leave room on neck of aneurysm for tissue to fold in and form wall of artery
8. Do not leave part of aneurysm unprotected
9. Buttress one clip with another clip as needed
10. Clip second or third loculus or aneurysm at same site (do not miss it)

lamina terminalis may be punctured if hydrocephalus is present.

As in any craniotomy a watertight closure is recommended. We have used subgaleal drains in the past; but they seemed not to have any substantial effect on the postoperative course, and this practice has been discontinued in most cases. Any air sinus opening must be sealed with a periosteum or galeal transplant to avoid CSF leaks. A triangular piece of periosteum is rotated and sutured to the temporalis fascia to cover the frontal burr hole filled with bone chips. Standard galeal and skin closure is effected.

POSTOPERATIVE ASSESSMENT

Perioperative Factors

Postoperative complications after surgical treatment of the ACoA aneurysm may be secondary to the adverse effects of (1) disturbances in the ACoA region,[161] (2) aneurysm surgery,[196,197,227] (3) craniotomy, and (4) the original subarachnoid hemorrhage.[149,163,200,222,256,261,265] Rational postoperative care and management of any likely complication requires a clear appreciation of how problems arise, how to prevent them, and how to treat them.[157,178,196,197,207, 239,271,272,285]

Operative treatment of a ruptured intracranial aneurysm is a preventive therapy against further hemorrhage. The anesthesia, surgical manipulation of the brain and blood vessels, various drugs used, and the patient's anxiety produce an additional insult to the brain already compromised by the SAH. Furthermore, SAH is an ongoing pathological process that may be manifested in the postoperative period. The postoperative condition of the patient will be considerably influenced by the various perioperative factors.[207,218] These include

1. *Clinical condition.* Fewer postoperative complications are seen in patients operated in a better clinical grade.
2. *Age.* With advancing age of the patient, the patient's cardiovascular and respiratory reserves diminish. Such patients are more prone to postoperative complications.[139,260]
3. *Associated medical conditions.* Rupture of an intracranial aneurysm occurs more often in the middle-aged and elderly. These patients may suffer from treated or untreated medical conditions that can complicate postoperative recovery. Patients with chronic hypertension show morphological changes in the blood vessels, which do not tolerate surgical manipulation well. Also these patients do not tolerate hypotensive anesthesia well due to poor cerebral autoregulation. Similarly, those with chronic respiratory or myocardial disease are prone to postoperative complications.[224]

4. *Technical difficulties.* An aneurysm located in a difficult area, a giant aneurysm, or an aneurysm without a clear neck will produce more problems during the postoperative period than those that are technically easier to obliterate.
5. *Vascular anatomy.* Anomalies at the circle of Willis will alter the area of supply of the major cerebral arteries, and this may result in compromising the collateral circulation. In the face of postoperative vasospasm these patients suffer more from delayed ischemic neurological deficits. Anomalies also add to the surgeon's technical difficulties.
6. *Surgical methods.* Obliteration of the aneurysm from the cerebral circulation with intact cerebral vasculature is the ideal surgical treatment. If alternative methods such as proximal ligation, trapping, or wrapping are used, there are other dangers with each method. Elective occlusion of a cerebral vessel may aggravate cerebral dysautoregulation; this patient is prone to a cerebral vascular accident more often than is one with intact cerebral vasculature.[273] Wrapping, even when adequately performed, does not protect the aneurysm from rupture in the immediate postoperative period. In a difficult aneurysm that cannot be clipped the process of effective wrapping may injure small vessels surrounding the aneurysm or cause intraoperative rupture.
7. *Skill and experience.* The postoperative condition is considerably influenced by the skill and experience of the surgeon and the surgical team. The role of anesthesia in aneurysm surgery is well recognized, but the skill and experience of the anesthesiologist are often less well credited. Anesthesia alters the cerebral metabolism and cerebral circulation. Providing an ideal operating condition in a brain that has already been affected by SAH requires unique anesthetic and monitoring technique.
8. *Timing of surgery.* Without careful selection, many patients can be operated soon after the SAH. However, when the brain is still adversely affected by the SAH, surgical manipulation can cause a stormy postoperative course.

Successful obliteration of a ruptured aneurysm is only one facet, although a significant one, in the recovery of the patient. There are so many hazards in the postoperative period that careful management at this stage is no less important than the surgical procedure. If anesthesia is prolonged or a surgical problem causing brain swelling is known to have taken place during surgery, we usually ventilate the patient electively in the intensive care unit. Neurological deterioration in the patient seen immediately after surgery usually is due to injury to small perforators or compromise of a major vessel,[258] prolonged temporary clipping,[136] embolization from the aneurysm itself,[141] or parenchymal injury with hematoma formation or edema from undue retraction.

Intensive Nursing Care

It must be appreciated that a team of skilled nurses is an equal partner of the surgeon and anesthesiologist in the successful recovery of the patient. Observation and assessment of this type of patient by the nurse are much more reliable than the most sophisticated monitoring system. It is routine practice to record pulse, blood pressure, respiratory rate, temperature, fluid intake and output, and drug administration. The neurological assessment sufficient for the nurses to record includes level of consciousness, pupillary size and reaction, limb movements, and other parameters described in the Glasgow Coma Scale. For the recording of intra-arterial blood pressure it is important to confirm the reading of the electronic devices with traditional blood pressure cuff methods to avoid errors.

Routine Laboratory Investigations

Profound changes in the cellular and plasma component of blood from the effect of SAH, craniotomy, and various drug administrations may occur. Kuwayama et al.[212] found a close correlation between the preoperative grade of the ACoA aneurysm patient and the incidence of defective postoperative hypophyseal endocrine function. Landolt et al.[213] analyzed 126 operated aneurysm cases. One ACoA aneurysm patient developed inappropriate secretion of antidiuretic hormone, five (four were ACoA aneurysm cases) had diabetes insipidus, and two ACoA aneurysm patients had disturbance of the hypothalamic thirst center. Forty-two patients developed mild to severe low serum sodium concentrations. Serum sodium depression is common after SAH and aneurysm surgery.[166,183,201,231] Takaku et al.[271,272] discovered only a 2 percent incidence of fluid and electrolyte imbalance in postoperative aneurysm patients, and most of these were ACoA aneurysm patients. The proximity of the ACoA aneurysm to the hypothalamus and its perforators cannot escape notice here. Careful monitoring of full blood count, serum electrolytes, blood urea nitrogen, creatinine, and osmolality is necessary. Arterial blood gases, including PCO_2, PO_2, and pH, can now be performed with a bedside gas analyzer.

Continuous Monitoring Program

With advances in various sophisticated monitoring devices, continuous information about the patient's physiological milieu has complemented clinical observation. Some or all of the following parameters are observed and recorded.

1. Heart rate and electrocardiogram.
2. Arterial blood pressure monitoring. The control of blood pressure is one of the most significant steps in the postoperative management of aneurysm surgery. The intra-arterial catheter used during the anesthesia can easily be connected to one of the transducers in the intensive care unit. Maintenance of systolic blood pressure above the preoperative level with or without blood volume expansion offers protection against ischemic problems.[209,248,249] On the other hand, surgical manipulation of intracranial vessels and postoperative restlessness with rising ICP may raise the blood pressure to excessive levels. However, it may be dangerous to reduce the blood pressure with excess medication in the face of elevated ICP and vasospasm. Sedation, analgesia, fluid control, and head elevation are adequate in most cases to reduce the blood pressure gradually to an acceptable level. To limit cerebral edema total crystalloid fluid intake may have to be limited.[143,158,262,282] When necessary, the blood pressure should be elevated by giving blood and other colloids. Hypertensive medication usually is not necessary. The calcium antagonist nimodipine, which has been in common use, tends to lower the blood pressure.
3. ICP monitoring. In our experience the continuous monitoring of ICP is less useful than clinical assessment and CT. If ICP monitoring is used, the method of Lundberg[221] is helpful; a pressure transducer is connected to an indwelling ventricular catheter, which can be used for draining CSF if necessary. Transducers or rigid fluid-containing conduits implanted intracranially may be preferred by others. With rising ICP one must differentiate one or more causes, including hematoma (intracerebral, subdural, epidural) formation; hydrocephalus; infarction; ischemia from vasospasm; cerebral edema from brain retraction; and meningitis. Treatment will depend on the cause, and this usually is best identified by CT scanning. CSF examination will be needed if septic meningitis is suspected.
4. Right atrial venous pressure monitoring. We monitor the central venous pressure (CVP) when a large fluid intake is necessary, especially during the use of dopamine to improve cerebral perfusion. The CVP usually is increased to about 8 to 12 mmHg, with careful attention to possible cerebral or pulmonary edema or heart failure as adverse effects.

Brain Protective Agents and Other Medication

1. *Calcium antagonists.* In spite of various assertions,[138,142,241] we are not yet convinced that nimodipine is very useful in the prevention and treatment of vasospasm.
2. *Corticosteroids.* The value of dexamethasone or

methylprednisolone in this circumstance has not been proven. Some advocate their use to prevent brain swelling.[239] On the other hand, these steroids can be a cause of upper gastrointestinal tract bleeding.

3. *Antacids*. Antacids may minimize the risk of gastritis.
4. *Barbiturates*. The use of barbiturates such as pentabarbitol to induce coma and exert a protective effect against ischemia and edema has been discussed.[195] We have not used this drug in postoperative aneurysm cases. Its value here remains uncertain.

Prevention of Infection

Intracranial infection is a serious but uncommon occurrence after aneurysm surgery.[157,285] The routine use of prophylactic antibiotics is controversial. A single dose of penicillin with preoperative medication reduced the infection rate in one series.[199] With the addition of various monitoring devices, a patient is more vulnerable to infection from an arterial cannula, an ICP catheter, a urinary catheter, and so forth. In some patients additional antibiotic coverage may be needed.

Prevention of Seizures

The routine use of anticonvulsants is not universally accepted. Anticonvulsants do reduce the incidence of postoperative seizures,[154,252] but allergic or other side effects can be serious. Seizures after SAH have been reported to occur in 10 to 20 percent of patients and are 20 times greater than in the general population.[254,268,281] They are more common in men, in the elderly, in those with intracerebral hemorrhage, after rupture of a middle cerebral artery aneurysm, and with a swollen brain.[207] Although seizures at the onset of SAH do not increase the risk of further seizures, surgical manipulation or cortical incision will increase the risk of a seizure.

Prevention of Thromboembolism

Postoperative phlebothrombosis and pulmonary embolism can occur after craniotomy for obliteration of an aneurysm as in any other major surgery.[200,263,276] Neurosurgical patients in whom fluid restriction may be necessary and in whom operative procedures are long in duration are more vulnerable. Although subcutaneous heparin in low doses (5,000 units every 12 hours) is of proven value, its use after an intracranial operation is rare. We rely on the use of full-length stockings, passive leg exercises, and/or alternating air pressure stockings, as well as clinical detection

and confirmation with a radioisotope scan or phlebogram.

Postoperative Cerebral Angiography

Postoperative angiography is not universally practiced, since many believe that microsurgical techniques and possible opening of the aneurysm sac will ensure satisfactory obliteration of the aneurysm. However, postoperative angiography may be useful for the following reasons:

1. The proximal part of the aneurysm neck may enlarge.[275]
2. A clip may slip.[137,169]
3. A loculus may remain occluded.[171,267]
4. A clip may be incorrectly placed.
5. It can give assurance to the patient and the surgeon.
6. If preoperative angiogram was limited to the area of the bleed, a full study of the cerebral vessels would be necessary.
7. Before operating on a second, remote, incidental aneurysm, it may be necessary to know that satisfactory obliteration of the previously ruptured aneurysm has been accomplished without injuring a major vessel.

PROGRESSIVE NEUROLOGICAL DETERIORATION

Progressive neurological deterioration is one of the most worrying problems after aneurysm surgery. Careful and early management during this period can save the majority of these patients from mortality or severe morbidity. During postoperative management of over 1,000 aneurysm cases by author R.P.S. the following causes of progressive neurological deterioration were encountered:

1. Ischemia from vascular occlusion
2. Ischemia from vasospasm
3. Cerebral edema
4. Hydrocephalus
5. Biochemical disturbances
6. Blood gas disturbances
7. Convulsive seizure
8. Intracranial hematoma
9. Aneurysmal hemorrhage (from operated or other aneurysm)

The diagnosis and treatment of these problems are those of intracranial aneurysm surgery in general. Cerebral infarction may occur from vasospasm, thrombosis, embolic phenomena, encroaching atherosclerotic plaques at clipping site, blood hypercoagulability, excess brain retraction (especially with vascular hypotension), prolonged temporary clip on a vessel, occlusion of venous drainage, trapping procedures, local inflammation, vascular hypotension, and carotid artery atherosclerosis.[132a,168,178,196,197,220,253,259,267] Ischemic signs increase with age (Table 30-18).

Hydrocephalus (acute or chronic) may evolve and be clinically significant in 5 to 10 percent of postoperative aneurysm patients.[157,178,196,208,211,235,250,286] CT scanning confirms the diagnosis. External CSF drainage or CSF shunting may be required.

Postoperative subarachnoid hemorrhage now is less common than in previous years due to advances in microsurgical technique, instrumentation, and imaging studies. In 1965, Lougheed et al.[220] stated that the second most common cause of postoperative death was recurrent bleeding from inadequate aneurysm clipping (brain infarction being the most common cause). Bohm and Hugosson[148] reported a 4 percent incidence of death from rebleed: two from unrecognized aneurysms and three from aneurysms to which a synthetic coat had been applied. In their review of the literature, Horwitz and Rizzoli[196,197] noted cases of rebleeding from the same or another aneurysm.

Postoperative intracranial hematoma is a known complication of any craniotomy procedure. Table 30-19 summarizes causes of this complication in ACoA aneurysm patients.

Recurrent hemorrhage, routine postoperative angiography, repeat surgical exposure, and/or autopsy examinations have documented many incidences of either inadequate clipping where part of the aneurysm remains at risk or actual slippage of the clip from the aneurysm.[134,137,147,148,150,151,162,168,169,171,196,197,220,225,235,237,255,267] Drake and Allcock[169] found a 13 percent incidence of inadequate clip placement in 329 aneurysm patients who underwent postoperative angiography. Paterson[237] reported an 8 percent incidence in 77 case of ICA aneurysm. Sato and Suzuki[255] claimed a 3 percent incidence in 369 cases. Steven[267] reported an 18 percent incidence (especially for ACoA aneurysm cases) in 250 cases stud-

Table 30-19. Causes of Postoperative Intracranial Hematoma

1. Slipped clip
2. Inadequately placed clip
3. Weak clip
4. Aneurysm required another buttressing clip
5. Torn bridging vein
6. Blood clotting defect
7. Excess brain retraction causing hemorrhagic infarct
8. Dura not well tacked up
9. Head not elevated
10. Rupture of another aneurysm
11. Poor cerebral autoregulation with intracerebral hemorrhage as blood pressure rises
12. Hemostasis not sufficient

ied. Bohm and Hugosson[147] had a 22 percent incidence where the aneurysm could not be adequately clipped at surgery, but this statistic is not comparable to those cited above: these authors considered aneurysms that they knew at surgery could not be clipped, whereas the others included only aneurysms that were clipped but which proved at angiography that they were not adequately occluded.

Other postoperative complications may include rhinorrhea or otorrhea if a low frontal or frontotemporal bone flap involved a frontal sinus or temporal bone air cells.[243] Gastrointestinal bleeding from esophageal, gastric, or duodenal ulceration may be a cause of a dropping red blood cell count, especially in ACoA aneurysm cases.[251] As in any surgical case, pulmonary embolism may be a complication.[132a,157,200,266,276] Standard diagnostic evaluation and treatment is used. Other pulmonary complications relate to infection, atelectasis, CVP catheter problems, and pre-existing lung disease. We reported a case of acute fibrinolysis following intraoperative rupture of an ACoA aneurysm.[178] The patient died from disseminated intravascular coagulopathy.

Optic nerve injury is uncommon but may occur secondary to clip pressure, retractor pressure, or nearby dissection with injury to optic nerve vascular supply. The most common cranial nerve injury in ACoA aneurysm operations is to the olfactory nerve with consequent complaints of loss of smell and "taste" if both nerves are injured.[157,196,197,223] Oculomotor or abducent nerve signs would occur from increased ICP.

Several authors have demonstrated psychiatric disturbances (transient and permanent) in patients who had undergone craniotomy for ACoA aneurysms.[146,153,206,213,215,217,228,232,259,271,272,285] Often these patients exhibited the Korsakoff's syndrome (hallucinations, confusion, amnesia, and confabulation).

Table 30-18. Age Versus Ischemic Signs After Craniotomy for Aneurysm[a]

Age (years)	No. of Cases (%) With Ischemia	Total No.
<30	7 (7.8)	89
30–59	87 (16.4)	530
>60	19 (22.6)	84
All groups	113 (16.0)	703

[a] From the files of author R.P.S.

Loss of initiative, personality changes, emotional lability, and memory and intellectual deficits have been described. Many of these had deficits prior to surgery. In 1966 Lindqvist and Norlén[215] reported Korsakoff's syndrome in 17 of 33 cases operated for ACoA aneurysms. More recent evaluations have revealed a considerable reduction in the incidence of this complication.

SUMMARY

We have reviewed our experience in perioperative assessment of patients undergoing cranial surgery to remove the threat of hemorrhage from an ACoA aneurysm. These aneurysms make up about 25 percent of all intracranial aneurysms, usually are found after an SAH and uncommonly are found incidentally, rarely achieve a "giant" size, have a male sex predisposition, and involve vital arteries and perforators to upper brainstem and cerebral functions.[178,261] The incidence of complications in the surgical management of the ACoA aneurysm patient is best reduced not just by training and experience but also by learning from one's own past mistakes and those of others. We are not dogmatic about specific operative approaches or about the timing of surgery. ACoA aneurysm surgery techniques, like other medical procedures, are in a state of continual evolution. Perhaps the greatest enemy of the surgeon is complacency: assuming that the brick was well cemented when in fact it was not.

Distal Anterior Cerebral Artery Aneurysms
William Shucart

Aneurysms arising from the anterior cerebral artery (ACA) distal to the anterior communicating artery (ACoA) are reported to represent from 2 to 7 percent of all intracranial aneurysms. Reviews of this topic stress that there is a high incidence of associated aneurysms in other locations and that the aneurysms can be difficult to treat surgically despite often being relatively small.

The most common location for aneurysms of the distal ACA is at the branching into the pericallosal and callosal marginal arteries (Figs. 30-76 and 30-77). Aneurysms also arise just distal to the ACoA where the orbitofrontal branch arises, at the origin of

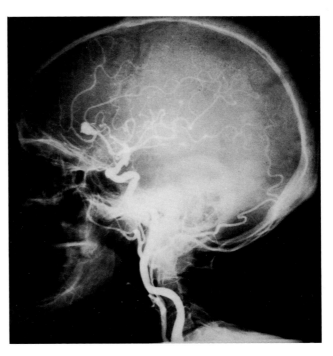

Figure 30-76. Lateral left carotid arteriogram showing typical aneurysm origin at pericallosal-callosal marginal bifurcation.

the frontopolar branch, and at callosal marginal branches. The latter are much less common. The mortality rate with surgery for distal ACA aneurysms remains about 8 percent despite advances in the techniques of surgery and anesthesia. However, most series are small, so variation of one or two cases will markedly affect the percentages. Complications reported following surgical treatment of these aneurysms include difficulty with recent memory, hemiparesis (generally with the leg more severely involved than the arm), and decreased verbal output, which is usually temporary but may last for months.

It is clear that surgical intervention is often much more difficult than one would suspect from either the size or the angiographic appearance of the aneurysm. Particularly for aneurysms occurring from the ACoA to the top of the genu of the corpus callosum, the approach is often awkward, and the difficulty is compounded because this is not an area commonly dealt with surgically. Reasons given for the unusual difficulty in dealing with these aneurysms have been that the space between the hemispheres is quite narrow, which limits exposure; the subarachnoid space between the hemispheres (the callosal cistern) is small so that releasing cerebrospinal fluid (CSF) does not provide the excellent exposure it does in other locations; and there are often dense adhesions between the cingulate gyri which limit retraction.

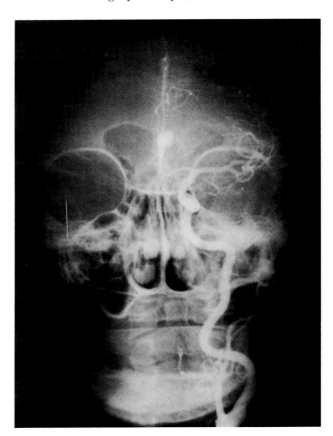

Figure 30-77. AP view of left carotid arteriogram showing dome of aneurysm going to left side.

A broad base of the aneurysm is a very common finding and makes the surgery more difficult. It has been said that these aneurysms tend to bleed when relatively small so that technical problems have been related to the small size of the aneurysm rather than to the usual problems associated with larger aneurysms. Some authors report that these aneurysms rupture very infrequently intraoperatively, whereas others, myself included, have been impressed with how frequently they can rupture intraoperatively. The reason for the latter is that the dome of the aneurysm is often embedded in a frontal lobe and during the course of retraction the dome of the aneurysm can be avulsed.

OPERATIVE TECHNIQUE

My preference is to operate on patients when they are in a good surgical grade. A grade I patient can be operated on at any time. The usual preoperative preparations of making certain that the patient is in good cardiopulmonary status are followed. Anticonvulsants are started at the time the patient is admitted to the hospital, and corticosteroids are given to the patient on the day of surgery. Lumbar spinal drainage is used in all patients to facilitate brain retraction. Intravenous mannitol is given at the time the bone flap is being elevated; the usual dose is 12.5 to 25 g intravenously. Systemic hypotension is not generally used during surgery for distal ACA aneurysms. In dealing with these aneurysms it is best to begin with known anatomy and proceed toward the abnormal site. Attempts to come down directly on the dome of the aneurysm are often very difficult. Confusion has been reported not only in deciding which is the right or left ACA but also in deciding whether the artery being initially exposed is proximal or distal to the aneurysm. It can also be difficult to differentiate the callosal marginal artery from the pericallosal artery.

Aneurysms originating on the ACA from just beyond the ACoA to the top of the genu of the corpus callosum are dealt with in one fashion, and those more distally located, that is, those located on top of the body of the corpus callosum, are dealt with in another fashion. For patients with aneurysms arising on the ACA from the ACoA to the genu of the corpus callosum, the patient is placed in the supine position with the head in neutral position and the neck slightly extended. The head is kept straightforward or turned approximately 5 degrees to the left and fixed in head pins (see Fig. 30-78A). A bicoronal skin incision is made extending slightly further toward the zygomatic process on the right side than the left. The scalp flap is reflected down to the supraorbital ridge. Essentially all distal anterior cerebral aneurysms are approached from the right side unless there are specific reasons to approach them bilaterally or from the left such as multiple aneurysms to be clipped at one operation, or a situation in which the dome of the aneurysm is large and clearly embedded in the right hemisphere such that retraction on the right side would be hazardous. A unilateral right frontal bone flap is made extending from the supraorbital ridge to a point approximately 8 cm above the ridge in the midline (see Fig. 30-78B). If the frontal sinus is small, an attempt is made to place the medial anterior burr hole just above the frontal sinus with the medial edge just to the right of the midline. If the frontal sinus is large it is worth going through the sinus to facilitate exposure. When the sinus is penetrated it is repaired in the usual fashion of stripping the mucosa, packing with fat, and then swinging down a pericranial flap to the dura to exclude the frontal sinus. As the bone flap is

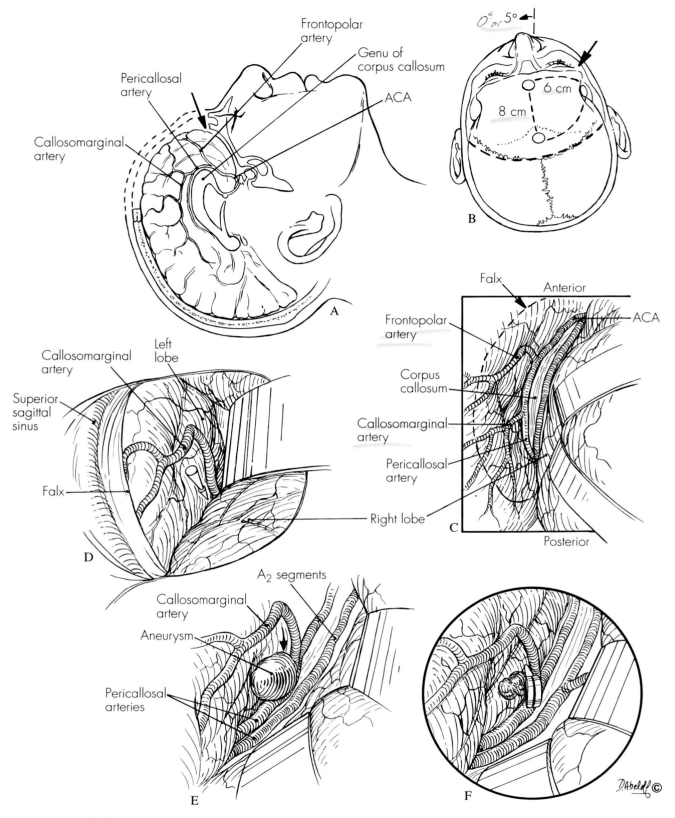

Figure 30-78. (A) Direction of approach, (B) bone flap, and (C) relation of frontopolar and callosomarginal branches to pericallosal artery. (D–F) Technique of following callosomarginal artery back to its origin and locating and clipping aneurysm is shown.

being removed the patient is given 12.5 to 25 g of mannitol intravenously. It is important that the floor of the frontal fossa be reached at some point above the supraorbital ridge and that the lateral aspect of the sagittal sinus be exposed. One need not go across the midline. A dural flap about the same size as the bone flap is then raised, being hinged along the sagittal sinus. As the dura is elevated care is taken not to avulse any of the underlying corticodural veins. One or two small draining veins to the sagittal sinus usually have to be cauterized and divided to provide easy hemispheric retraction.

The least confusing approach to the aneurysm is to begin with normal proximal arterial anatomy. This ensures both proximal vascular control as well as identification of normal vessels before getting close to the area of the aneurysm. The closer the aneurysm is to the ACoA the more imperative it is to begin as inferiorly and proximally as possible (see Fig. 30-79A).

The right cerebral hemisphere is gently retracted away from the falx, which is then followed down to the crista galli. Care is taken to avoid injuring the olfactory tracts. Once the crista is identified, gentle retraction of the right frontal lobe is begun. Adhesions between the frontal lobes will be encountered that should be sharply divided. Retraction is carried back to the top of the chiasm and the ACoA complex just above it. The two pericallosal arteries are then sharply dissected free in the subarachnoid space. This approach is followed, despite the fact that the dissection may be tedious, for it avoids the confusion of identifying the pericallosal arteries and differentiating them from other small arteries (see Fig. 30-79B). One should know from the preoperative studies how far distally on the pericallosal artery dissection has to be carried out, and, if a magnetic resonance image (MRI) has been obtained, whether or not the dome is embedded in the brain.

The further distally on the ACA toward the genu the aneurysm is located the greater the temptation to come directly down on the aneurysm and not do the tedious dissection required when approaching from the ACoA. The problem is that most often the surgeon will wind up exposing the pericallosal arteries distal to the aneurysm and not have proximal control. Identification of the very white corpus callosum, which best identifies the location of the pericallosal arteries, is useful primarily for those aneurysms situated along the body of the corpus callosum and not those below the genu.

As dissection proceeds distally on the pericallosal arteries above the ACoA complex, the pericallosal arteries are situated more anteriorly. When the proximal portion of the neck of the aneurysm is reached careful retraction and dissection are used to identify the distal pericallosal arteries before dealing with the aneurysm neck. It is not always possible to tell before surgery the exact anatomy of the origin of the aneurysm. It is imperative that this be done at the time of surgery, which can require considerable dissection. My preference is to increase the magnification on the microscope progressively as the aneurysm is approached. The aneurysm neck is often broad, in which case the aneurysm clip is best applied along the long axis of the pericallosal arteries. If the aneurysm neck is very atherosclerotic care is taken to avoid fracturing the neck during application of the clip. If the neck of the aneurysm is small, the clipping becomes much easier. Following placement of the aneurysm clip the dome of the aneurysm should be further shrivelled either by aspiration through a small-gauge needle or with bipolar cautery. This allows careful and complete inspection around the clip to make certain that the parent vessel is patent.

Aneurysms more distal on the corpus callosum are much easier to deal with but one should still obtain proximal control. The same coronal skin incision can be used, but the bone flap can be placed 1 to 2 cm higher above the supraorbital ridge and be essentially of the same dimensions. The same general rules of careful, limited retraction of the hemisphere and trying to preserve the larger draining veins still obtain. These are likewise generally approached from the right side unless there is some compelling reason to expose the left side. The exposure to reach the proximal portion of the pericallosal artery as it comes around the curve of the genu of the corpus callosum is much the same as for approaching the corpus callosum itself. The cingulate gyri may be very adherent to one another. The corpus callosum is identified by its very white color, and in the absence of hydrocephalus the two pericallosal arteries are usually fairly close together. Once again, both the proximal and distal portions of the ACAs have to be seen before the clip can be safely applied. These aneurysms are rarely large enough that temporary clipping or aspiration of the aneurysm are required prior to placing the clip.

An alternative approach rather than going to the ACoA and following the pericallosal arteries distally is to separate the frontal lobes very inferiorly and retract posteriorly until either a frontal polar or callosal marginal artery is identified on the medial hemispheral surface (see Fig. 30-78C). The preoperative

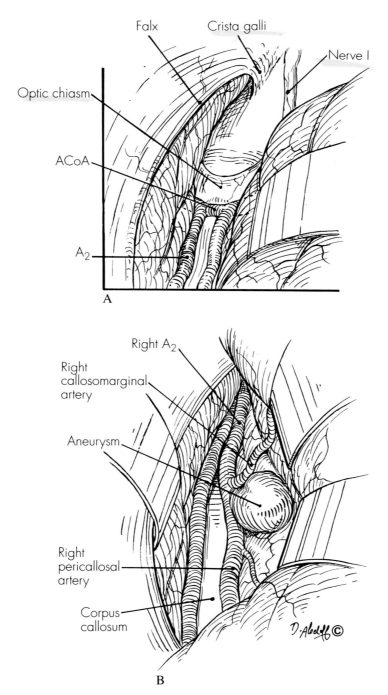

Figure 30-79. **(A)** Interhemispheric approach beginning at ACoA to follow A_2 segments distally. **(B)** Aneurysm at callosomarginal artery origin at about the level of the genu of the corpus callosum.

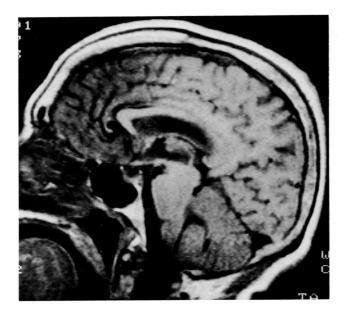

Figure 30-80. Lateral MRI showing relationship of aneurysm to genu of corpus callosum.

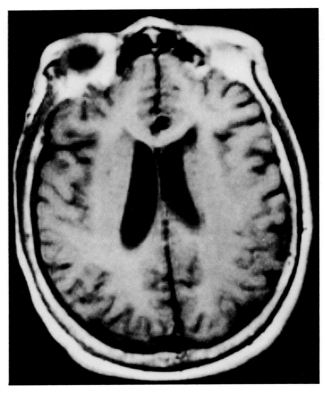

Figure 30-81. Axial MRI showing aneurysm dome imbedded in medial surface of left hemisphere.

arteriogram should make the anatomical relationships of these vessels fairly clear. The appropriate vessel to follow depends on the location of the aneurysm. If either branch is followed back along the medial surface of the hemisphere it will go to the pericallosal artery. The same can be done with a callosal marginal vessel (see Fig. 30-78D–F).

Careful preoperative study of the arteriogram is essential so that correlations can be easily done. Preoperative MRI studies are often helpful for showing the true size and location of the dome of the aneurysm, particularly if the aneurysm is buried in the medial surface of one hemisphere or the other (see Figs. 30-80 and 30-81). If this is seen, retraction can be done primarily against the contralateral hemisphere to decrease the likelihood of rupturing the aneurysm intraoperatively.

COMPLICATIONS

Complications occurring with these aneurysms are much the same as with other intracranial aneurysms. The problem of delayed ischemic deficits can be seen with these aneurysms after they hemorrhage and are treated the same as ischemic deficits with aneurysms in other locations. The interhemispheric exposure creates some of its own problems especially if retrac-

tion is too aggressive and prolonged against the cingulate gyri. This can give rise to a syndrome very similar to akinetic mutism, but is usually transient if it is related to mild retraction. A similar picture can be seen just with the rupture of the aneurysm if there has been significant hemorrhage in or around the cingulate gyri.

The small size of the pericallosal arteries and the fact that the neck is often atherosclerotic make compromise of the lumen of the parent vessel more likely. This can be difficult to evaluate at the time of surgery and is best avoided by paying considerable attention to this possibility during surgery and using meticulous technique. Topical papaverine can be helpful for at least temporarily increasing the size of the pericallosal arteries to help evaluate the adequacy of the clipping and the lack of compromise of the parent vessel. The small hematomas that are often associated with these aneurysms are usually best left alone unless they are more than a few cubic centimeters in volume and/or interfere with the dissection.

Posterior Circle of Willis

Basilar Artery Bifurcation Aneurysms
Charles G. Drake

The aneurysm arising at the bifurcation of the basilar artery has proved to be the most difficult of the posterior aneurysms in terms of achieving results comparable to those on the anterior circulation. With few exceptions, the techniques have not changed significantly from those described in *Clinical Neurosurgery* 1979. This review is concentrated on our experience in the last decade in the avoidance of problems and their management. The problems are related to the approach, the narrow local access, the position, size, and shape of the aneurysm, the perforating vessels, rupture of the aneurysm, and satisfactory clip placement.

APPROACH

The subtemporal approach (Fig. 30-82) has prevailed on this unit. Trials of the transsylvian exposure have not been persuasive, largely because of its narrower confines, the difficulty placing a temporary basilar clip, the inability to do high or low aneurysms, and the difficulty seeing behind the aneurysm, where most of the trouble lies. It is still used occasionally, particularly when an anterior circulation aneurysm is to be done at the same time. Those surgeons who prefer the transsylvian approach and who have difficulty with exposure of an aneurysm should know that it is simple to convert to the subtemporal approach by removing the temporal squama down to the zygoma. When the temporal pole is untethered by large temporosphenoidal veins, it can be retracted after the sylvian fissure is split so as to expose the anterior third or so of the middle fossa for a "half and half" approach.

The right side is used unless the direction or shape of the aneurysm, a left oculomotor palsy, or a right hemiparesis demand an approach under the dominant temporal lobe. Modern neuroanesthesia routinely provides a slack brain, so that light retractor pressure

is used to elevate the base of the temporal pole to expose the incisura. This occurs even early after bleeding, with mannitol and lumbar drainage of the spinal fluid as the dura is being opened.

Removal of the zygomatic arch, either to lessen temporal lobe pressure or to see higher bifurcations, has not seemed necessary; nor has anterior temporal lobe resection. Ipsilateral carotid-ophthalmic and carotid-communicating aneurysms are easily exposed by moving the retractor tip forward under the temporal pole, but carotid bifurcation and anterior communicating aneurysms usually demand the transsylvian exposure. The vein of Labbé is usually well posterior, but must not be injured by the retraction. Small veins to the dura in the middle fossa or at the incisura may be taken without consequence. Mobilization of the temporal pole by dividing large temporal sphenoidal veins can lead to dangerous hemorrhagic venous infarction; large veins should be left intact.

The access to the interpeduncular cistern and fossa is narrow, bounded by the dorsum sellae in front and the peduncle behind, the hippocampus and uncus above, and the tentorial edge below, with the third nerve crossing the field obliquely (Fig. 30-82A&B). As this nerve is usually adherent to the uncus, it can be elevated out of the way by placing the retractor tip at the base of the uncus, which also marks the entrance to the cistern. Only occasionally is it necessary to separate the third nerve from its uncal adherence for a better view of the neck, but some of its arachnoid sheath anteriorly may have to be divided to ease angulating tension on the nerve. The opening into the cistern can also be enlarged by reflecting the edge of the tent firmly downward by a suture tied to the dura of the floor of the middle fossa. Care must be taken to ensure that the suture is placed just lateral to the insertion and course of the trochlear nerve. As much as 1 cm can be added to the vertical exposure. Occasionally, it is necessary to divide the inner third of the tentorium for a low-placed bifurcation region aneurysm, particularly to see enough of the basilar artery for a temporary clip.

The size of the interpeduncular cistern is quite variable. Ordinarily, 1 cm or so of space exists between the crus and the dorsum laterally, although the crus tends to angle forward medially toward the interpeduncular fossa. Occasionally, the brainstem can

1041

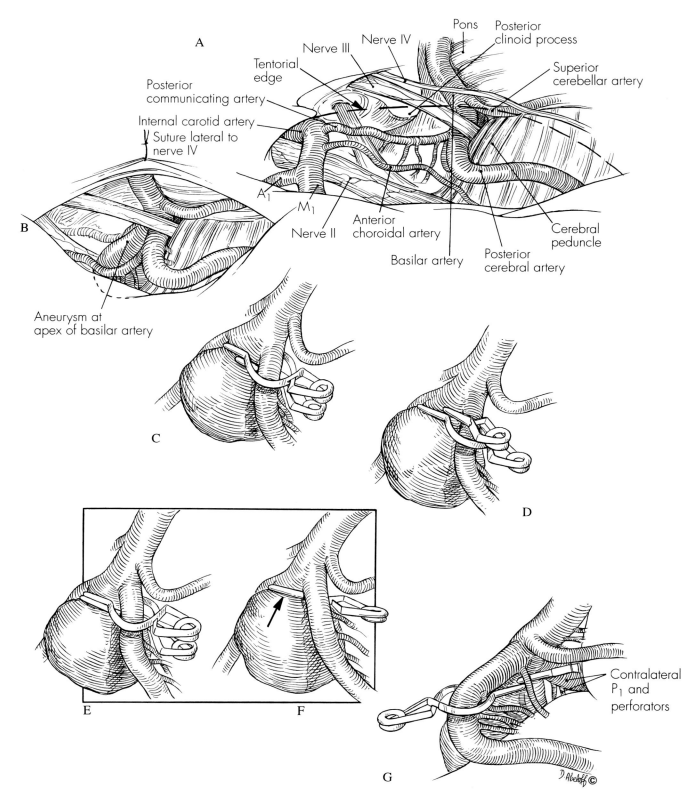

Figure 30-82. **(A)** An expanded schematic view of the anatomy of the incisural and interpeduncular regions relative to the subtemporal approach. **(B)** Typical subtemporal exposure of interpeduncular region and bifurcation aneurysm. The edge of the tentorium has been reflected inferiorly to expand the opening into the cistern. The third nerve is usually adherent to the uncus, and its elevation by the retractor tip on the uncus

be crowded against the clivus, hiding the interpeduncular fossa; however, the crus is remarkably retractable without hemiparesis in order to see the basilar artery and the base of the aneurysm. It has never been necessary to remove the dorsum sellae or to divide the posterior communicating artery (PCoA), which usually gives rise to a host of anterior thalamoperforating arteries.

Usually, the basilar bifurcation is at the level of the dorsum sellae, with the aneurysm projecting upward and a little backward in line with the curve of the artery and half buried in the interpeduncular fossa, hidden by the crus. The waists of large aneurysms abut the clivus anteriorly. After opening Liliequist's membrane widely, carefully to avoid injury to the superior cerebellar artery and PCoA, the cistern variably may be clear or choked with fresh or old clot or, sometimes in delayed cases, a dense arachnoiditis. To lessen retractor pressure that might be needed to follow the posterior cerebral artery, it is practical to follow the superior cerebellar artery medially around the crus, sucking clot in a direction away from the known position of the dome of the aneurysm. This will lead to the basilar artery and the origin of P_1 just above so that the position of the base of the aneurysm is now known.

Aneurysm necks arising from a bifurcation well above the dorsum require more forceful retraction of the parahippocampal region, but only two very high necks could not be seen clearly enough for clipping. It is here that zygoma removal might be helpful, although these necks were buried behind the mammillary bodies. For aneurysm necks below the dorsum, the suture reflection of the tentorial edge inferiorly usually suffices to expose enough of the basilar artery for the temporary clip. The upper edge of the "tic" craniectomy may have to be removed further so that more lateral temporal lobe retraction will give a better line of sight to this region. If the aneurysm neck and enough basilar artery cannot be seen by these measures, then the inner one-third or so of the tentorium should be divided. Even though the pontomesencephalic junction will be crowded against the cli-

vus, it can be retracted enough, on either side of the fourth nerve, to expose enough of the basilar artery for temporary clipping. Because of the angulation, an angled clip applier may have to be used.

At this stage, it is best to free a segment of the basilar artery below the superior cerebellar artery, which is free of perforators, for 2 or 3 mm for the placement of the temporary clip. Of all the measures to solve the technical problems of clipping this aneurysm, temporary basilar clipping has been the most important. Only gentle temporary clips are used and only for 3 or 4 minutes at a time, during which much dissection can be done. Surely any major cerebral artery can be temporarily occluded for such brief periods without ischemic consequences. The circulation is allowed to resume for about 5 minutes in between temporary clippings. Mannitol, 1 to 2 g/kg, has been used as an anti-ischemic measure in case temporary clipping needs to be prolonged. If one or both of the PCoAs are large, one or both can be temporarily occluded too, for trapping. As a consequence, deep systemic hypotension has been largely abandoned on our unit.

As the base of P_1 is exposed, the anterior aspect of the neck of the aneurysm comes into view. It is usually fairly easy to expose the anterior neck, and even to see the opposite P_1 directly or by indenting the neck with the sucker tip or narrow dissector. Angling the retractor forward, more under the temporal pole, may be helpful to see the opposite side of the neck, P_1, and its perforators. Occasionally, the waist of a larger sac needs to be separated from adherence to the dorsum of the clivus very carefully under high magnification and temporary clipping.

P_1 and the superior cerebellar artery can be identified by their relation to the third nerve. P_1 is above, and the PCoA joins it; the superior cerebellar artery is below the nerve. The same relationship can be used to identify these vessels on the opposite side.

It is behind this aneurysm where most of the surgical troubles lie. A few sacs will stand free in the interpeduncular cistern, but most are half buried in the interpeduncular fossa. The exposure of the back

allows most bifurcation aneurysms to be dissected free and clipped beneath it. Here it is shown freed from the uncus for a higher placed aneurysm. **(C&D)** The fenestrated clip is placed first to occlude accurately the opposite side and center of the neck. The second tandem straight clip is usually placed above **(C)** but maybe below **(D)** the fenestrated clip and behind **(C)** or in front of **(D)** the P_1 segment of the posterior cerebral artery. **(E)** A longer straight tandem clip has been applied across the neck beyond the fenestrated clip. **(F)** The fenestrated clip has been removed, and the straight clip has been repositioned down to the base of the neck. **(G)** Schematic view of clipping using successive bilateral subtemporal approaches. The first fenestrated clip application was not or could not be positioned accurately on the far side of the neck. The opposite subtemporal exposure allows easy application of a straight clip on the residual neck either in front of or behind P_1. Bilateral hippocampal retraction has not produced amnestic syndromes.

of the neck begins at the root of P_1 behind or even as low as the superior cerebellar artery if the aneurysm is large. With the temporary clip in place, the peduncle is retracted with a small dissector while using a small sucker tip to expose the root of the neck laterally and behind, even to move the bifurcation slightly and gently forward. Most of the perforators arise at or near the origin of P_1, but not infrequently one or more will arise from the back of the basilar bifurcation. A large perforator has been seen crossing the back and even the front of this aneurysm. The P_1 perforators are usually applied to the side and the posterolateral aspect of the neck, and are usually separable, which must be far enough up the back of the aneurysm so that a clip blade underneath will not kink them. It is necessary to work across the back of the neck, across the interpeduncular cistern, even to see the origin of the opposite third nerve by indenting the waist of the aneurysm even more with the sucker tip and aided with the small dissector. This often reveals the opposite P_1 and its perforators.

Perforators stuck to thin-walled aneurysms are worrisome. Temporary basilar occlusion is most helpful here, for one can be bolder in their separation when the sac is softer with a tiny, narrow dissector or tiny, sharp hook under high magnification, and usually they can be teased away. Laterally placed, adherent perforators can be left open in the aperture of the clip, with the proximal blade closure being just at their position on the neck. Often when the neck is collapsed by such clipping, the perforators can be more boldly freed and the clip reapplied.

It is possible usually to see the opposite P_1, either in front or behind, and its perforators, and even to separate them from the sac. It is important to see the level of take-off of the opposite P_1 to note the angle for applying the clip blades.

CLIP SELECTION AND PLACEMENT

In recent years, with its safety established in hundreds of aneurysm cases, temporary clipping of the basilar artery during dissection of the aneurysm and clip placement is almost routine and has contributed greatly to the safety and the sureness of the procedure.

A straight clip can be used with the subtemporal lateral approach to the aneurysm when the neck arises mostly in front of or behind the rise of the P_1s, which are free or can be freed from the sac. When P_1s are near the front, the tips of the clip can be spread so that the anterior blade goes under P_1 and the poste-

rior blade under the perforators. Both tips have to be watched carefully so that the aneurysm is not punctured and the posterior blade is inside the perforators. For P_1s arising on the back of the aneurysm, the posterior blade must be in front of both the origin of P_1 and the perforators. A sac softened by temporary clipping makes this maneuver much simpler and safer.

More commonly, the P_1s rise up midlaterally, applied to the neck and waist except that with smaller sacs they may stand free. The P_1 adherence can be dense and dangerous to free, even using temporary basilar clipping. The Drake or Drake-Sugita fenestrated clips avoid such a dissection and dangerous clip application by placing P_1 and even its perforators in the aperture, while the blades fall across the neck of the aneurysm. There are three concerns when using this clip. First, the fenestrating ring beyond the applier tips tend to obscure vision in these narrow confines, especially behind the aneurysm. Second, the clip blades must be no longer than the flattened, occluded neck or else the P_1 origin(s) and its perforators may be stenosed or occluded. A flattened neck is about 1.5 times the width of an open, circular neck. If the proper length blades are not available, longer blades may be trimmed with wire cutters and/or a diamond burr and polished with a whetstone. Two common errors are to use blades longer than necessary, which either may occlude the opposite P_1 or its perforators or be placed too far out on the neck. It is remarkable how short the blades need to be when placed down at the very origin of the neck at the P_1 roots. The third concern is that not uncommonly a bit of the neck is left open in the aperture just medial to the ipsilateral P_1 root. This is usually the cause of an aneurysm that still pulsates or bleeds on needling, although it must be certain that the clip tips cross to the far side of the neck. Repositioning of the clip a little lower or with slightly longer blades may suffice to occlude the remaining neck. Otherwise, a straight tandem clip can be used (see below).

While coagulation is occasionally useful to shrink and firm up bulbous or otherwise awkward necks of other aneurysms, it has rarely been used at the basilar bifurcation. It is not only that forceps blades usually cannot be closed across the neck in the lateral approach without including P_1, but the fear that an unseen perforator(s) might be coagulated too. Rarely coagulation has been used cautiously to firm up the neck on either side of a very adherent perforator so that more force can be used in its separation.

If single, fenestrated clip blades cannot be positioned perfectly without concern for the P_1 origins or perforators, then two other methods may be used:

1. Formerly, a fenestrated clip with shorter, fenestrated blades was placed so as to occlude accurately the far three-fourths or so of the neck, leaving a bit of the near neck, P_1, and perforators open in the fenestration. Usually then with the neck collapsed by the blades, it is simple to separate this bit of narrowed but open neck from P_1 and its perforators with a small dissector and place a tandem straight clip in front of or behind P_1 and the perforators to occlude the neck remaining open in the aperture. But this may leave a "dog ear" of neck at P_1, and two clip handles obscure even more of the field for inspection and aspiration.

2. In recent years, and preferred, instead of using short blades for the tandem clip just to occlude the remaining near neck, a longer straight clip is used, and worked across the whole of the neck, just beyond the fenestrated clip, which then can be removed. Then this clip can be repositioned accurately so that the tips just occlude the far side of the neck and dome with the blades placed flush with the upper origins of the P_1s. Kinking of the ipsilateral P_1 by the blades has not been a problem even when P_1 rises midlaterally on a large neck. This method is of particular value if the fenestrated clip has slid down to stenose $p_1(s)$. If the neck is thick at the fulcrum, it may keep the blades of the longer clip open on the far side to allow continued filling of the aneurysm. Then placement of a tandem fenestrated clip next to the partially open clip blades will close the far side of the neck.

Inadvertent rupture of this aneurysm in these narrow confines can be harrowing, although less frequent now with temporary basilar clipping. Panic should be avoided and enough suction used to clear the field to see the position of the rent. Some at or near the dome will stop after the clip is opened or removed, with the re-expansion of the sac and tamponade against the brainstem. Small tears will often stop spontaneously after suction over a pattie. Reapplication of the temporary clip, even trapping if necessary, for larger rents will usually slow the bleeding enough that rapid completion of the dissection of P_1 and the perforators can be done and a clip applied. Tearing just above or at the neck may be controlled by exquisitely accurate clip placement, but the integrity of the perforators and both P_1s must be maintained. A rent at or near the basilar artery bifurcation can sometimes be plugged with Surgicel and shortened fenestrated clip blades applied on top of the Surgicel.

As soon as clipping is completed, the neck and clip blades must be inspected to be certain no perforators are caught, especially behind and on the far side. Rotating the clip handle forward usually exposes the posterior blade, and looking just above the blade will determine whether any perforators are emerging from underneath. It is humbling how often, when surely all the perforators have been seen and separated, one or more will be found caught under the blade. If perforators are or are even suspected to be caught in the blades, the clip must be removed. Clip reapplication should be done as many times as necessary for perfect positioning. However, before removing, a few seconds should be taken with the narrow dissector or small hook to be sure that the perforators are free of the sac above the blades. Blunt or sharp hooks should be used with great caution in these depths, for, with attention diverted, removal may tear the fourth nerve or a small arterial branch. If the perforators are stuck, they can be freed boldly from the slack sac so that with the next application the blade can easily be replaced inside them. It is remarkable that brief perforator occlusion with the strong blades, even for several minutes, has not usually produced infarction.

Although sometimes difficult to see because of the clip handles, an effort should be made to needle and collapse the sac to prove completed clipping. It must be certain that the origin of the opposite superior cerebellar artery is not mistaken for P_1, or else inadvertent occlusion of the basilar bifurcation will occur. In six cases in which it seemed dangerous to complete the occlusion on the far side because of encroachment on P_1 or perforators or in which postoperative angiography revealed that side still to be open, an early second craniotomy was done on the opposite side. In each, the neck remaining was easily occluded with a straight clip, and in none was there any evidence of injury to the memory mechanisms from bilateral hippocampal retraction.

POSITION, SIZE, AND SHAPE OF ANEURYSM

High Basilar Bifurcations

The greater the height above the dorsum sella, the greater must be the retraction of the mesial temporal parahippocampal region. If the neck of the sac reaches the apex of the interpeduncular space, it and the perforators are more effectively hidden by the mamillary bodies in front and the peduncle laterally and behind. However, only in two earlier cases was it necessary to abandon clipping for incomplete gauze packing because of its obscuration by the height of the bifurcation. It is here perhaps that zygoma removal might be helpful. Gentle retraction of the mamillary bodies or crus has not had any known serious consequences.

Low Basilar Bifurcations

At the other extreme, the bifurcation may be quite low, at the level of the floor of the sella or even lower down the clivus. This position of the neck is confining to the surgeon, because the edge of the insertion of the tentorium cannot be reflected downward as much by the "tenting" suture and tends to hide the base of the sac, which is wedged between the pontomesencephalic junction and the clivus. Often with a little more retraction applied under the temporal lobe laterally and with more squamal removal if necessary to increase the angle of vision over the depressed tentorial edge, it may be possible to see and clear the neck for clipping without dividing the tentorium. The waist of a larger sac may have to be separated from adherence to the dorsum or clivus carefully under high magnification and temporary clipping. However, if the neck is obscured or enough of the basilar artery cannot be seen for temporary clipping, the inner third of the tentorium should be divided, beginning behind the insertion of the fourth nerve and the anterior leaflet sewn back into the floor of the middle fossa to give more line of sight down behind the clivus. The fourth nerve should be freed of any arachnoid attachment so that undue tension is not put upon it. For these low aneurysms, it is always wise to have the scalp marked for a posterior temporal flap in case more lateral division of the tentorium is necessary.

The transmastoid-transpetrosal sinus approach, through a completely divided tentorium, has occasionally been used for a difficult, large, low-placed neck. This avoids the danger of division of the sigmoid or lateral sinus by combining a posterior temporal bone flap with a lateral suboccipital craniectomy and removal of the posterior mastoid and petrous apex to expose the upper sigmoid sinus with enough dura in front of it for a tight closure, this uncovers the lateral and sigmoid sinuses with their confluence. After complete division of the tentorium to the superior petrosal sinus and opening the presigmoid dura up to that sinus, the sinus is divided. This mobilizes the confluence so that it and the anterolateral cerebellum can be retracted posteriorly for a wide exposure of the upper (or lower) angle. Care must be taken before division of the sinus that the vein of Labbé enters the lateral sinus behind it.

After the tentorium is divided, the dissection of the neck is usually done medial to the fifth nerve and on either side of the fourth nerve. This slender, fragile nerve is a nuisance in this exposure, for great care must be taken to avoid tearing it with an inadvertent movement with a blunt hook or sucker. This has occurred six times, usually in a trying circumstance, such as bleeding from a large aneurysm. Single suture repair of the nerve has not resulted in reinervation and diplopia on downward gaze has persisted.

Bifurcation aneurysms may project forward or backward or be multilocular. Unfortunately rare, the forward-projecting sac usually presents no problems with perforators. If the dome is adherent to the dorsum sellae, the first clip application should be very accurate, for clip closure may avulse the ruptured dome from its adherence.

However, on backward sacs, the search for perforators must include all sides of the neck. Those on the opposite side may not be seen until the clip blades close. It must be certain, too, that a backward sac is not really a bend in an upward projecting neck, so that a clip only across the bend will leave open neck in front at the bifurcation. There have been three deaths from rebleeding from this mistake when the residual neck "blew out" to form another aneurysm after a few years. Very rarely, this aneurysm may project laterally from a bifurcation that is rotated as much as 90 degrees to one side or the other in the coronal plane; the approach should be on the side of the projection as for superior cerebellar artery aneurysms.

A bilocular sac may have a neck that emerges at right angles in front of and behind the basilar bifurcation. Softened by temporary clipping, it may be possible to make a neck by working the clip blades upward with some pressure to "gather in" enough of the base of each saccule to allow the blades to close above the P_1 origins. If the neck is too large or thick, then each loculus can be clipped separately as backward (first) and forward projecting saccules, with clips lying side by side just behind and in front of the P_1 origins.

Large Aneurysms

Globular aneurysms with thick-walled or yellow atherosclerotic, steeply sloping necks or those with a "beer belly" in front or, worse, behind, can be troublesome. The fenestrated clip blades tend to slip down the steep slopes to occlude the P_1s and even the top of the basilar artery. Similarly, beware of the large aneurysm where the P_1 origins project inferiorly from the neck, rather than laterally, for clip blades across the neck may occlude their orifices. With temporary clipping, even trapping with temporary PCoA occlusion, an attempt may be made to "work" the blades further up on the neck by ''gathering in'' this wider neck between the blades with the hope that with closure they will seat themselves further up on the neck. If the sac can be needled and collapsed, their position will be retained by the arterial pressure below.

Adding clips in parallel beyond the first that occludes P_1 or the basilar bifurcation may finally produce a stable clip so that those proximal can be removed. If a clip can be placed across the waist, it is often possible to add a fenestrated clip below that will hold position. Repeated clip application sometimes softens up the neck so that one will stay. On occasion on thick necks, a very short-bladed Drake-Sugita clip (1 to 2 mm) has been placed to occlude the very termination of the basilar artery, leaving the orifices for P_1 on either side; it must be certain that no perforators arise from the back of the bifurcation. When thrombus extends down around the neck of a larger aneurysm, shortened fenestrated blades can be used to close the open neck centrally and leave the thrombosed near neck in the aperture while the tips close flush with the thrombus on the other side.

The upper basilar artery giving rise to larger aneurysms is usually ectatic, giving the impression of P_1s and even superior cerebellar arteries arising from the neck. However, when clip placement has been achieved just above the origins of P_1, this ectatic segment has not been known to ''blow out'' to form another aneurysm, as may occur when actual neck is left open.

If there is any doubt about the probability of clipping a large or unusual basilar aneurysm, the alternative of proximal basilar artery occlusion should be investigated preoperatively. The size and potential of the PCoA should be known, and Allcock's test will determine if these vessels do not fill spontaneously from the carotid injections. If these vessels are obviously large enough to carry the upper basilar circulation, then the basilar artery can be occluded by a clip. If they seem marginal, then the tourniquet can be placed to test the collateral the next day when the patient is awake.

Giant Aneurysms

The problems with giant bifurcation aneurysms are simply a magnification of those with large aneurysms, although about one in three have necks that can be clipped in one fashion or another. In most, however, proximal basilar artery occlusion is the other choice and is very effective when enough posterior communicating collateral exists to irrigate the upper basilar circulation. However, large posterior cerebral arteries, especially if unilateral, tend to keep the neck and waist of the aneurysm open. Stenosis of the involved P_1 segment with a clip has been tried on several occasions, but with limited effect. Intraluminal thrombosis of residual sac with thrombogenic wire has increased the occlusion, but unfortunately never to include the neck.

Patients with huge aneurysms and severely compressed brainstem are very fragile. Failed attempts at clip application, the application of the Drake microtourniquet, or even mere exploration will tip their

Table 30-20. Basilar Bifurcation Aneurysms—Small (<12.5 mm)

Years and Grades	No. of Cases	Excellent	Good	Poor	Dead
1958–1990					
Grade					
0	60	53	6	1	
I	268	219	26	13	10
II	88	55	20	9	4
III	31	12	10	7	2
IV	6	1	1	4	
Totals	453	340	63	34 (7.5)[a]	16 (3.5)
Good risk (0, I, II)	416	327	52	23 (5.5)	14 (3.4)
1983–1990					
Good risk (0, I, II)	135	113	16	5 (4.4)	1 (0.8)

[a] Values in parentheses are percentages.

Table 30-21.   Basilar Bifurcation Aneurysms—Large (12.5–25 mm)

Years and Grades	No. of Cases	Excellent	Good	Poor	Dead
1958–1990					
Grade					
0	29	22	4	3	
I	119	87	17	9	6
II	57	31	16	9	1
III	21	2	7	10	2
Total	226	142	44	31 (13)	9 (4)
Good risk (0, I, II)	205	140	37	21 (10)	7 (3.4)
1983–1990					
Good risk (0, I, II)	92	68	16	7 (7.6)	1 (1)

a Values in parentheses are percentages.

brainstem function over the brink with varying degrees of postoperative stupor, bulbar paresis, and quadriparesis. This phenomenon has often been associated with remarkable change in the distribution and degree of thrombosis within the sac.

With increasing experience, and particularly the use of temporary basilar artery clipping, the results of treatment of aneurysms at the basilar bifurcation, in recent years, have been more satisfying.

After the results in the whole series were studied, the good risk patients were compared before and after 1983, when temporary basilar clipping became more routine (Tables 30-20 and 30-21). The recent period is characterized by a reduction of the overall surgical morbidity rate, down to 5.2 percent for small and 8.6 percent for large basilar bifurcation aneurysms.

Basilar Apex Aneurysms

H. Hunt Batjer
Duke S. Samson

Aneurysms arising from the distal basilar artery either at the origin of the superior cerebellar artery or from the true basilar apex account for more than one-half of the aneurysms occurring in the vertebrobasilar circulation.[358,359] Despite their relative frequency considering the posterior circulation as a whole, they represent the most recent aneurysms to come under direct surgical attack. Undoubtedly, the relative delay in the arrival of safe and routinely available verte-

bral angiography played some role in this sluggish development, but more important factors relate to the anatomical complexity of the interpeduncular cistern and its central location within the cranial vault. Standard modern surgical approaches must traverse 6 to 7.8 cm of subarachnoid space to arrive at the basilar apex,[353] thus mandating exquisite illumination and magnification for the safe exposure of associated pathological structures.

While many early investigators felt that vertebrobasilar aneurysms posed less threat to patients of initial or subsequent bleeding episodes, evidence to the contrary is now abundant (Table 30-22). Uihlein and Hughes[352] described 14 patients with vertebrobasilar

Table 30-22.   Complications Noted in the Literature

Etiology	Author
Rebleeding	Uihlein and Hughes[352]
	Sachs et al.[333]
	Gillingham[321]
	Troupp[351]
	Richardson[341]
Problems from early operation	Jamieson[323]
Parent vessel sacrifice	Jamieson[323]
	Richardson[341]
Perforator sacrifice	Drake[309]
	Pelz et al.[340]
Incomplete aneurysm occlusion	Drake[311]
	Yasargil[359]
	Batjer et al.[302]
Posterior projection	Yasargil[359]
Large size	Peerless and Drake[339]

aneurysms, eight of whom died of rebleeding.[352] Sachs et al.[343] reviewed 23 cases of nonsurgically treated basilar aneurysms and noted that 65 percent died. Gillingham[321] found 100 percent mortality in 26 nonoperatively treated vertebrobasilar aneurysm cases followed for 3 years. Troupp[351] followed 20 patients who had developed subarachnoid hemorrhage (SAH) from basilar aneurysms and found that 40 percent died of rehemorrhage during follow-up of 4 to 52 months. Similarly, Richardson[341] documented a 50 percent mortality rate in patients with ruptured basilar aneurysm treated with bedrest alone.

The unique features of the neural and vascular anatomy of the interpeduncular cistern are directly linked to the historical reluctance to attempt surgical exposure and with heighted morbidity and mortality rates associated with treatment of aneurysms in this region, and they have provided substantial stimulus for the development of creative and ingenious means of accessing the structures. The subarachnoid space within the interpeduncular cistern is enclosed by the clivus and posterior clinoid processes anteriorly, the mesial aspects of the temporal lobes and tentorial edges laterally, the cerebral peduncles posteriorly, and the mamillary bodies and posterior perforated substance superiorly.[345] The terminal basilar artery has a normal diameter of 2.7 to 4.3 mm and has been found to lie within 15 to 17 mm posterior to the posterior aspect of the internal carotid arteries.[331,347,355] This latter anatomical relationship to the internal carotid has provided a basis for seeking a more anterior, transsylvian route into the interpeduncular cistern. Within this cistern and proximal to its bifurcation, the basilar artery gives origin to the superior cerebellar arteries, which are usually vessels of just over 1 mm diameter but which may be duplicated unilaterally or bilaterally. Frequently, the microsurgical appearance of these vessels is considerably less atheromatous than either the basilar trunk or the posterior cerebral arteries, and they usually appear reddish and thin walled. Blood flow through the superior cerebellar arteries is approximately 50 ml/min, and they form the principle arterial supply for large portions of the cerebellar hemispheres and for the dentate nuclei of the cerebellum.[357] The posterior cerebral arteries arise within 2 to 3 mm of the origin of the superior cerebellar arteries and represent the bifurcation of the basilar artery. These branches are typically 2 to 3 mm in diameter and carry 85 to 125 ml/min in blood volume.[345] The size of the proximal segment of each posterior cerebral artery (P_1 segment) is dependent on the extent to which it replaced the fetal posterior cerebral supply. In patients with a truly persistent fetal pattern, the P_1 may simply be a

vestigial fibrous band. The posterior cerebral arteries via their critical thalamoperforating branches supply the bulk of the mesencephalon and the posterior aspect of the diencephalon.[322] The large cortical branches of the posterior cerebral arteries irrigate the posterior, inferior regions of the temporal lobes and the majority of the occipital lobes. While considerable individual variability exists, the thalamoperforating arteries arise from the posterior aspect of the basilar trunk, the proximal P_1 segments, and the posterior communicating arteries. Two final anatomical structures frequently involved in morbidity in treating interpeduncular aneurysms are the oculomotor nerves. These nerves emerge from the mesencephalon within triangles formed by the basilar, posterior cerebral, and superior cerebellar arteries. They travel anteriorly within the interpeduncular cistern just inferior to the posterior communicating arteries toward their site of entrance into the roof of the cavernous sinus. The anterior confines of the interpeduncular cistern are defined by a thick arachnoidal plane (the membrane of Liliequist) which is anchored superiorly in the region of the mamillary bodies. This membrane extends inferiorly and anteriorly and then folds posteriorly, forming the roof of the prepontine cistern.[333] Its relationship with the posterior communicating arteries and third cranial nerves laterally encases the distal basilar artery and not infrequently confines a minor subarachnoid hemorrhage, preventing generalized spillage.

A number of vertebral-basilar aneurysms were encountered unexpectedly during posterior fossa exploration during the 1930 to 1950 period and occasional triumphs recorded. Most procedures performed during this early era for known or suspected aneurysmal disease were based on the principles of Hunterian ligation extracranially to decrease distension of the sac. Logue[334] may have been the first to report intracranial ligation of the vertebral artery in 1958 in treating two fusiform vertebral aneurysms, and Mount and Taveras[35] are credited with the first deliberate basilar artery ligation in 1962. In reviewing literature prior to 1960, Drake[308] found documentation of six directly treated aneurysms of the basilar bifurcation. Three of these lesions had been packed, and one death was reported. He had treated four basilar bifurcation aneurysms himself, and two patients died.

The 1960s were characterized by substantial interest in distal basilar aneurysms, and this interest was facilitated by technological advances in magnification and illumination. In 1964, Jamieson[323] published his initial experience with 19 patients harboring vertebrobasilar aneurysms and noted an overall postoperative mortality rate of 53 percent. Patients operated on early (within the first week) did less well than those operated on later following their hemorrhage: 64 vs 50 percent mortality rate. Of note, in this series he described trapping the basilar aneurysmal segment in three patients, two of whom expired (Table 30-22). In 1968, Jamieson followed this with a further report of nine additional cases.[324] In the second report, temporary basilar artery occlusion was successfully employed to deal with intraoperative rupture. His mortality rate had decreased to 22 percent in this later experience, but he noted the persistence of poor results in patients with basilar bifurcation aneurysms.

Drake[309] reported further experience with basilar artery aneurysms in 1965 and noted that, while morbidity from basilar trunk lesions appeared to be relatively low, persistently poor results were seen with basilar bifurcation aneurysms; of the first seven patients, only two had a favorable recovery. It was clear to him that the key to progress in this area was in the understanding of the anatomy of the thalamo-perforating arteries with their critical supply to the brainstem and diencephalon (Table 30-22). He pursued operative exposures and techniques that facilitated their dissection from the posterior aspect of the aneurysm sac and avoided blind clip placements that could possibly jeopardize these vessels. It became clear that the subtemporal approach could facilitate the avoidance of these critical structures by clear visualization posterior to the aneurysms. Three years later he reported an additional 12 cases with outstanding results: no deaths and only two poor results (both poor grade preoperatively).[310] The use of deep hypotension during dissection and clipping was thought to add safety to the procedure.

In 1972, Richardson[341] reported a nonrandomized trial of medical versus surgical treatment for patients with ruptured basilar aneurysms. To enter the surgical arm patients had to be in good grade. In Richardson's surgical group, 65 percent of patients ultimately returned to work, and a 50 percent mortality rate was noted in the medically treated patients. Sixty-eight percent of the surgical patients underwent clipping (22 percent mortality), 29 percent underwent wrapping (20 percent mortality), and 3 percent underwent vertebral artery occlusion (100 percent mortality) (Table 30-22).

Hunterian ligation obviously had a primary role in the early pioneering work with basilar artery aneurysms, and, despite the emergence of the microsurgical era and major improvements in clip technology, this technique's usefulness persists. Drake[311,312] and Peerless and Drake[338] dramatically expanded its ap-

plicability by the use of a microsurgically applied tourniquet that could be tightened to occlude the basilar artery after the patient had recovered from surgery. This principle of parent trunk occlusion with awake neurological monitoring represented a major advance in the treatment of giant aneurysms of the upper basilar artery that were not classically treatable by neck occlusion. In a report from London, Ontario, two-thirds of 71 patients treated with vertebral or basilar ligation had favorable outcomes.[340] The dramatic evolution of endovascular technology will undoubtedly facilitate the clinical use of awake monitoring during trial occlusion well into the future.

Intraluminal thrombosis has been championed by Mullan et al.[336] but failed to gain wide acceptance perhaps due to the concurrent introduction of the surgical microscope. This technology was applied with the injection of horse hair in two cases and copper beryllium wire in one case. A small amount of residual neck ultimately expanded, producing death in two of these patients (Table 30-22). The principle of intraluminal thrombosis is currently undergoing a resurgence by the use of endovascularly detached balloons and microcoils. As follow-up accrues in such patients, it will be critical to determine the consequences of subtle imperfections in neck occlusion. Despite the subsequent risk of enlargement and possible rupture, these major advances at the very least provide a means to palliate patients with medical conditions not permitting general anesthesia.

Literature published after the mid-1970s largely concerned microsurgical technology; the use of proximal arterial occlusion, intraluminal thrombosis, wrapping, or trapping procedures was largely reserved for those patients in whom direct neck obliteration was not possible. Chou and Ortiz-Suarez[306] noted that basilar bifurcation aneurysms still carried a higher mortality rate (30 percent) than those elsewhere in the posterior circulation.[306] In 1979, the distal basilar experience of Kodama et al.[329] was published, and 50 percent of patients with basilar bifurcation aneurysms did poorly or died whereas results elsewhere in the posterior circulation were excellent. Major improvement in outcome for patients with basilar aneurysms was reported by Sugita et al.[349] in 1979 using strictly microsurgical principles. Ninety-one percent of their patients were noted to make favorable recoveries. Similar microsurgical results obtained with the transsylvian approach (3 percent mortality) were documented by Yamaura et al.[356]

After elegantly applying the pterional transsylvian exposure with its potential modifications in exposing interpeduncular anatomy, Yasargil[359] reported operative results with basilar bifurcation lesions in 1984.[359] He was able to clip all small aneurysms definitively, greater than one-half of the large aneurysms, and 33 percent of giant aneurysms. The importance of aneurysmal projection was well illustrated, with better results in those aneurysms projecting anteriorly and superiorly (Table 30-22). Of 10 patients treated with coagulation, wrapping, and acrylic coating two died and one had a poor result. In 50 cases of bifurcation aneurysms, 8 percent died and 10 percent had a poor outcome.

In 1985, Peerless and Drake[339] reported personal experience with a massive series of posterior circulation aneurysms in which they achieved a 6 percent mortality rate in lesions of the basilar bifurcation. Their results clearly highlighted the negative impact of large and giant size (Table 30-22). While they did employ the transsylvian exposure in selected cases (multiple aneurysms), the overwhelming majority of their procedures were performed subtemporally. Using this philosophy they had previously reported achieving 11 percent morbidity and mortality in treating aneurysms projecting posteriorly from the basilar bifurcation.[338] The accomplishment in aneurysms projecting posteriorly and typically encased in perforators together with the breadth of this surgical experience in London, Ontario, adds tremendous weight to these surgeons' strong advocacy for the subtemporal approach in preference to the transsylvian route. The unique aspects and potential pitfalls of the two major operative exposures (transsylvian and subtemporal) are discussed in detail below, along with their potential modifications and our general recommendations for employing specific advantages of each in planning surgery for the individual patient.

OPERATIVE TECHNIQUE

After a protracted evolution of thought and creative surgical innovation, two basic surgical exposures have emerged as dominant means of accessing the interpeduncular cistern using microsurgical techniques: the pterional or transsylvian approach and the subtemporal approach. Both of these fundamental approaches have been expanded and modified and in each case became more versatile and adaptable to unique aspects of individual patient anatomy. Each approach has particular strengths, weaknesses, and potential complications that must be carefully considered in the complex thought process of planning an operative attack on a basilar artery aneurysm. In-timate familiarity and considerable experience with each approach and repeated efforts at "pushing the limits" of exposure as seen from both these perspective are, in our opinion, prerequisites for achieving the versatility needed in effectively handling the myriad of anomalies and pathological variations encountered in patients with distal basilar aneurysms. This section will consider in detail each of these operative exposures, including a technical description and illustration of operative technique, and will emphasize points during the procedure that we have found to be critical in preventing surgical injury to the vital tissues in this region.

Pterional (Transsylvian) Approach

The application of the pterional exposure to the treatment of patients with distal basilar aneurysms has been elegantly described and performed by Yasargil et al.[360] This approach expands the standard exposure used by all neurosurgeons in treating more common anterior circulation aneurysms as well as neoplasms in the basal cisterns. In fact, a major strength of this procedure is its familiarity to the majority of neurosurgeons gained from repetitive use. The early observation of Yasargil et al.[360] that the basilar bifurcation resides only 15 to 17 mm posterior to the posterior aspect of the carotid artery and that wide opening of the membrane of Liliequist provides adequate visualization of the upper basilar trunk, the superior cerebellar, as well as posterior cerebral arteries provided early incentive for careful investigation of the applicability of this approach to basilar bifurcation aneurysms. In general, most surgeons recommend approaching appropriate midline basilar apex aneurysms from the right side so that the nondominant frontal and temporal lobes and internal carotid artery are retracted and manipulated. Unique aspects of the aneurysmal anatomy may suggest, however, that a left-sided approach would be safer. An asymmetric tilt of the aneurysm to the left side (Fig. 30-83) implies that the dissection of the left P_1 segment from the neck will be the most critical and demanding and is usually most easily accomplished from the left side. In addition, if the patient has a third cranial nerve palsy it is usually advisable to operate from the side of the cranial nerve deficit to avoid bilateral ptosis postoperatively. Occasionally, the entire distal basilar artery may be widely displaced to the left side, and this configuration is usually very difficult to expose adequately from a right pterional exposure.

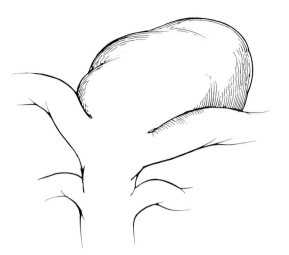

Figure 30-83. While most prefer to perform the pterional exposure from the right side, a significant tilt of the aneurysm to the left side suggests that dissection of the left P₁ from the aneurysmal neck will be the most difficult aspect of the dissection and is often best accomplished from the left side.

Patient Positioning

Due to the confining space available in the interpeduncular cistern and the minimal flexibility in line of sight, precise head positioning is extremely critical in approaching the distal basilar artery by the pterional route. The specific goals of positioning are to minimize the necessary degree of brain retraction and to ensure that all necessary vascular structures are accessible. We have found that placing the Mayfield-Kees skull fixation device so that two pins are anterior on the contralateral side of the frontal bone and the single pin is superior to the mastoid process (Fig. 30-84A) consistently yields a flat surgical field that does not restrict the surgeon's freedom of movement. The head is elevated slightly above the long axis of the body to maximize venous drainage.

The head is then *rotated* away from the operative side by about 20 degrees (Fig. 30-84B). We have frequently found that exposure of uncomplicated and small superiorly and anteriorly projecting basilar bi-

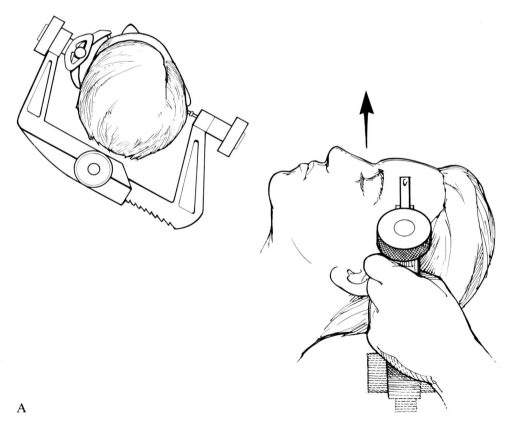

A

Figure 30-84. *Positioning* for a pterional approach to the distal basilar artery. **(A)** The Mayfield-Kees skull fixation device is placed with two pins anteriorly across the midline and the single pin posteriorly to facilitate a flat, unobtrusive surgical field. The head is elevated slightly from the long axis of the body. (*Figure continues.*)

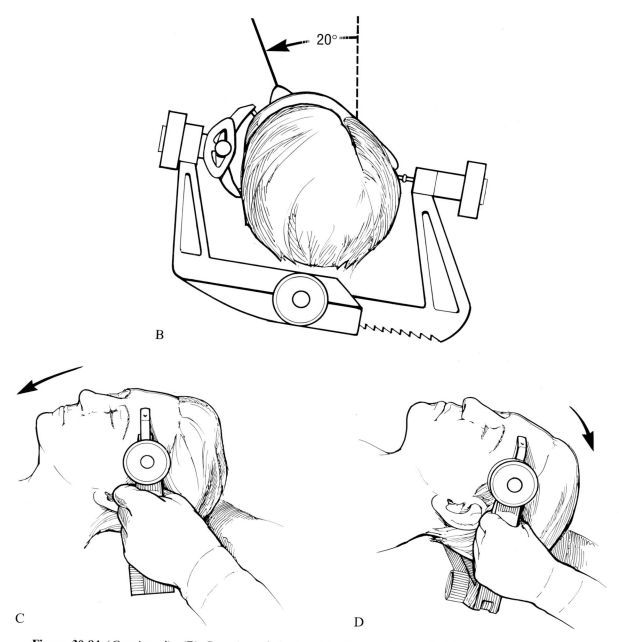

Figure 30-84 (*Continued*). **(B)** *Rotation* of the head to the contralateral side by 20 degrees minimizes subsequent temporal lobe encroachment on the operative field. **(C)** *Flexion* of the neck brings the chin toward the contralateral shoulder and ensures that the plane of the floor of the anterior cranial fossa is perpendicular to the long axis of the body. This maneuver allows maximal surgical comfort and flexibility and prevents encroachment of the surgeon's arms and microscope onto the ipsilateral shoulder. **(D)** *Extension* of the head is then achieved in a somewhat exaggerated degree compared with anterior circulation surgery to minimize subsequent diencephalic retraction. The maxillary eminence is elevated well above the superior orbital ridge.

furcation aneurysms can be obtained without temporal lobe retraction if the sylvian fissure has been widely dissected with the head very minimally rotated. Further rotation produces obstruction of view by the temporal lobe, whose spontaneous gravita-

tional displacement then encroaches on the tentorial incisura instead of widening the exposure laterally by posterior migration. Additionally, rotation by more than 30 degrees restricts exposure medial to the carotid and mandates that the bulk of dissection be done in the retrocarotid planes regardless of individual carotid anatomy or target pathological anatomy.

After the proper rotation is noted, the neck should be gently *flexed* (Fig. 30-84C). This maneuver, which essentially pulls the chin toward the contralateral shoulder, ensures that the floor of the anterior cranial fossa remains perpendicular to the long axis of the body. We have found that this particular aspect of positioning allows the seated surgeon comfortable bimanual access to the depths of the interpeduncular cistern, facilitates instrument exchange, and avoids the tendency of the surgeon to be forced laterally toward the ipsilateral shoulder if appropriate flexion is not achieved.

The final maneuver in head positioning is probably the most important in distal basilar surgery. The head is *extended* on the neck so that the maxillary eminence is well superior to the superior orbital ridge (Fig. 30-84D). This maneuver, common to all pterional craniotomies, is exaggerated when the distal basilar artery is the target. This extension allows maximal gravitational displacement of the frontal and temporal lobes after cerebrospinal fluid (CSF) evacuation and when exaggerated somewhat allows favorable visual access to the interpeduncular cistern without severe mechanical retraction of the optic tracts or diencephalon.[345]

Scalp Incision

Our incision for a pterional exposure of distal basilar lesions differs only slightly from the technique employed for anterior circulation disease. The incision is begun at the zygoma, carried superiorly in a straight line for 8 to 10 cm above the superior temporal line, and curves gently anteriorly to the midline at the level of the normal hairline (Fig. 30-85). The incision is deepened sharply through the galea, preserving at least one major branch of the superficial temporal artery. In addition to maximizing scalp healing potential, preservation of this vessel provides flexibility should unexpected findings or complications necessitate a revascularization procedure. Subsequent dissection exposes adequate temporal squama for a generous craniectomy. While we have found that the interfascial temporalis dissection as described by Yasargil et al.[361] has provided superior exposure of the anterior and inferior aspects of the middle cranial fossa, we have generally been satisfied with reflection of the temporalis in a single layer with the scalp. If care is taken to ensure that the base of the scalp incision is within 1 cm anterior to the tragus, the frontalis branch of the facial nerve can always be preserved. We remain unconvinced that any

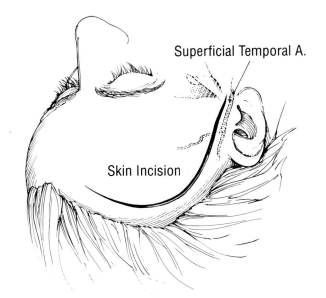

Figure 30-85. The scalp incision for a pterional approach to the basilar bifurcation extends vertically from the zygoma 1 cm anterior to the tragus for 8 to 10 cm and then curves gently anteriorly meeting the hairline in the midline.

technique offers particular superiority in minimizing subsequent cosmetic complications from temporalis muscular atrophy as long as care is taken to avoid coagulation injury to the deep neurovascular bundle that lies in the deepest portion of the muscle belly. Our current preference is to incise the temporalis fascia and muscle with the cutting cautery exposing the root of the zygoma and gently elevate the muscle off the temporal squama (Fig. 30-86). This resultant scalp flap is retracted with fishhook retractors and protected with a folded surgical sponge beneath it to ensure adequate tissue perfusion.

Craniotomy

A three- or four-hole craniotomy is performed, the optional fourth (forehead) burr hole being deleted in young patients and utilized in the elderly with adherent and easily lacerated dura. The first burr hole is placed inferiorly in the temporal squama and the second just inferior to the superior temporal line immediately superior (vertical) from the first hole. The third burr hole is performed at the "anatomical key" superior to the frontozygomatic suture. The optional fourth burr hole is placed medial to the second hole and slightly anterior (Fig. 30-87). A power-driven craniotome is then used to incise the bone along the lines illustrated in Figure 30-87. The incision is carried well anteriorly and inferiorly to the midpoint of the supraorbital ridge, avoiding entering the frontal

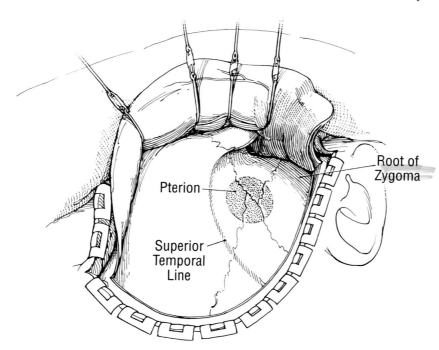

Figure 30-86. The temporalis fascia and muscle are incised with the cutting cautery with care to avoid injury to the deep neurovascular bundle in the muscle. The resultant single layer flap is dissected from the underlying bone and retained with fishhook retractors.

sinus if possible. In patients with very large frontal sinuses, the craniotomy should not be compromised by fear of sinus exposure; rather, adequate bony exposure obtained and prior to closure sinus exenteration and pericranial covering of the sinus performed.

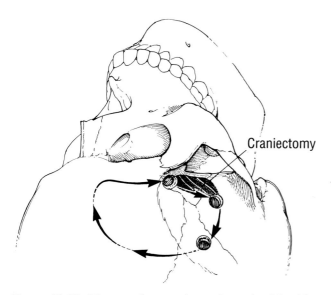

Figure 30-87. The craniotomy is performed with either three or four burr holes connected along the lines indicated. A critical aspect of the craniotomy is a generous anterior temporal craniectomy.

After elevation of the free bone flap, a generous temporal craniectomy is performed, exposing the dura overlying the temporal tip back to the zygomatic root. This degree of temporal exposure is particularly critical in cases in which conversion to "half and half" or true subtemporal exposure is considered possible or likely, as is discussed below.

A critical aspect of bony exposure as relates to interpeduncular exposure concerns the aggressive resection of the sphenoid ridge.[361] After reflection of the dura from the bony sphenoid ridge, rongeurs are used to remove as much of the ridge in conjunction with the temporal squama as possible. A cutting burr on an air-driven drill is then used to resect the lateral one-third to the sphenoid ridge at least to the site of emergence of the orbitomeningeal artery and preferably to the lateral aspect of the superior orbital fissure (Fig. 30-88). In addition, the inner table of the frontal bone is removed for a distance of about 2 cm medial to the burr hole at the anatomical key. This wide bony resection completely exposes the dural coverings of the sphenoidal and opercular-insular portions of the sylvian fissure and flattens all bony encroachment on the floor of the anterior cranial fossa. If the orbit is inadvertently entered, exposing either periorbita or fat, oxidized cellulose may be tucked into the bony defect to restrain the tissue from protruding into the extradural space. Hemostasis must be metic-

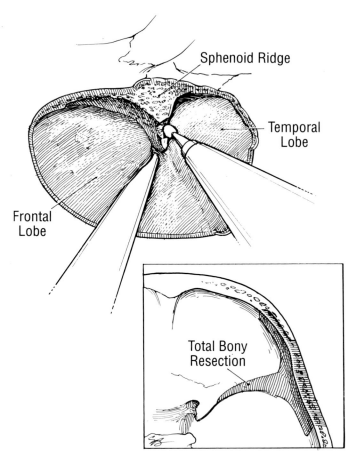

Sphenoid Ridge

Temporal
Lobe

Frontal
Lobe

Total Bony
Resection

Figure 30-88. After removal of the free bone flap and aggressive anterior temporal squama resection, the sphenoid ridge is radically resected with a high-speed drill and cutting burrs. The inner table of the frontal bone is resected in continuity with the sphenoid ridge for about 2 cm.

ulous at this point so that "run down" bleeding will not distract the surgeon in critical parts of the dissection. Bone wax and oxidized cellulose can usually control the bony and extradural venous bleeding routinely seen after sphenoidal resection. Cotton pledgets should not be placed in this space, as the bulk of this material will negate the anatomical advantages of aggressive bony removal.

Next, the dura is incised in a semilunar fashion with the medial limb extending to the frontal bone incision and the lateral limb crossing the sylvian fissure and angling anteriorly to a point 1 cm inferior to the sylvian fissure at the margin of the craniectomy (Fig. 30-89). The dura overlying the remainder of the temporal lobe is stellated, as shown in Figure 30-89, and the dural flaps retracted with stay sutures. This anatomical arrangement minimizes the chances for necessary revision of dural opening or exposure even if a full subtemporal conversion is required.

Due to the fact that basilar bifurcation aneurysms

not infrequently rupture into the ventricular system and our practice of pursuing early surgery for the good grade patient, we often encounter a tight, hydrocephalic brain at this point in the procedure. After becoming chronically frustrated at the frequent failure of spinal drainage in maximizing brain relaxation, Dr. Jonathan Paine from our medical center determined reliable landmarks for frontal ventricular access through a pterional craniotomy.[337] A point on the frontal lobe is defined as follows: The point is the vertex of an isosceles right triangle whose hypotenuse overlies the sylvian fissure and whose sides are 2.5 cm in length (Fig. 30-90). The frontal cortex is punctured perpendicularly with a Silastic catheter, yielding extremely reliable access to the frontal horn of the lateral ventricle. The catheter may then be sutured to the dura posteriorly and left in place during the microsurgical portion of the procedure.[345] The surgical microscope is then brought in and employed for the remainder of the procedure prior to closure.

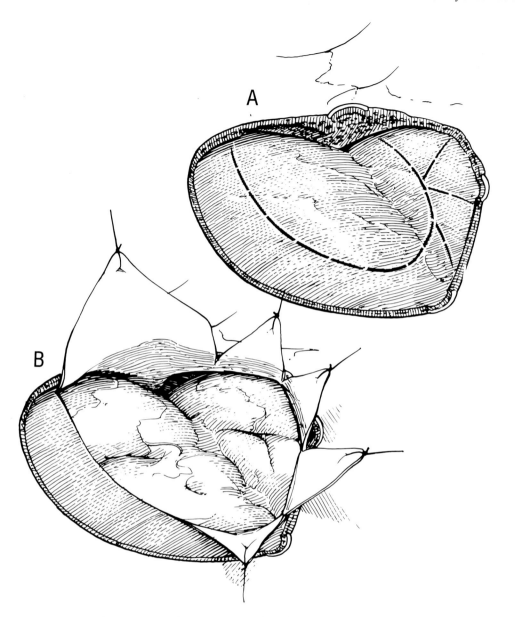

Figure 30-89. Dural incision. **(A)** The frontotemporal dura is opened with the medial limb extending to the margin of the frontal craniotomy and the lateral limb crossing the sylvian fissure. The residual temporal dura is stellated. **(B)** Resultant dural flaps and edges are retracted with stay sutures to maximize exposure and hemostasis.

Initial Subarachnoid Exposure

The early portions of the microsurgical procedure in the patient harboring a basilar bifurcation aneurysm have two specific goals: maximizing brain relaxation by generous arachnoidal opening, allowing egress of CSF, and extensive dissection of the sphenoidal portion at the sylvian fissure. If a ventricular puncture has been performed or a spinal drain placed previously, brain relaxation may already be adequate. More commonly, however, in the fresh post-subarachnoid hemorrhage patient loculated CSF collections still exist in the various basal cisterns, and the evacuation of this CSF further enhances the ultimate exposure. The degree of frontal lobe and potentially temporal lobe retraction necessary to expose aneurysms of the basilar bifurcation adequately can result in kinking of the middle cerebral artery in its initial portion if the dense arachnoidal adhesions of the medial sylvian fissure are not extensively opened

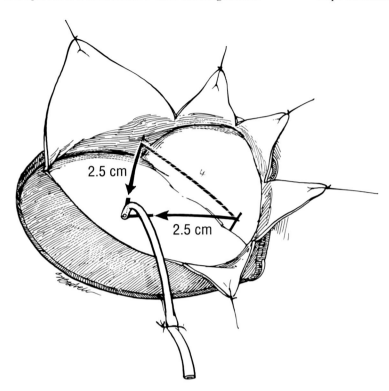

2.5 cm

2.5 cm

Figure 30-90. Reliable access to the frontal horn of the lateral ventricle may be obtained during a pterional craniotomy employing "Payne's point." The landmarks for this point involve the creation of a 2.5 cm isosceles right triangle whose anterior limb abuts on the dura overlying the sphenoid ridge and whose posterior limb touches the sylvian fissure. The hypotenuse overlies the sylvian fissure. A Silastic brain catheter is used to enter the frontal cortex perpendicularly at the vertex of the triangle.

prior to retraction. Due to these concerns, we prefer to initiate the procedure by gently placing a small brain retractor at the posterior inferior aspect of the frontal lobe just anterior to the middle cerebral vein and advance the retractor across the orbital cortex for a distance of about 3 cm along the sphenoid ridge. The orbital surface of the frontal lobe is gently elevated to place the superficial arachnoid of the sylvian fissure on stretch. The microscope is then adjusted so that the lateral aspect of the sphenoidal portion of the fissure may be sharply incised (Fig. 30-91). Initially superficial dissection may be carried medially right down the sylvian fissure, incorporating the carotid cistern into this initial opening. Once that maneuver has been accomplished, we usually place a small T directed laterally and posteriorly in the direction of the insertion of the third cranial nerve into the roof of the cavernous sinus. At that point, the sylvian fissure is entered again laterally, and this dissection with the help of further elevation of the lateral orbital cortex is deepened initially laterally and subsequently medially into the posterior aspect of the carotid cistern. This deep arachnoidal dissection will ultimately en-

counter the dense arachnoidal attachments between the frontal and temporal lobes immediately overlying the carotid bifurcation and the proximal portion of the M_1 segment. In addition, a small bridging vein between the frontal and temporal lobes is frequently encountered in this tissue, and it is usually helpful to cauterize and section this vein. The resultant exposure allows aggressive frontal or temporal retraction (or both) without placing any traction on the internal carotid artery, A_1 segment, or middle cerebral artery (Fig. 30-92). The final step in the initial arachnoidal exposure is to dissect the arachnoid sharply, binding the optic nerve to the gyrus rectus and ultimately yielding wide opening of the prechiasmatic cistern.

With meticulous patient positioning and adequate CSF evacuation, the temporal lobe will spontaneously migrate posteriorly within the middle cranial fossa. The degree of displacement achieved with these initial maneuvers, however, is frequently inadequate for exposure of low-lying basilar bifurcation aneurysms. In addition, not infrequently, a significant portion of the uncus will be found to have actually herniated into the tentorial incisura anteri-

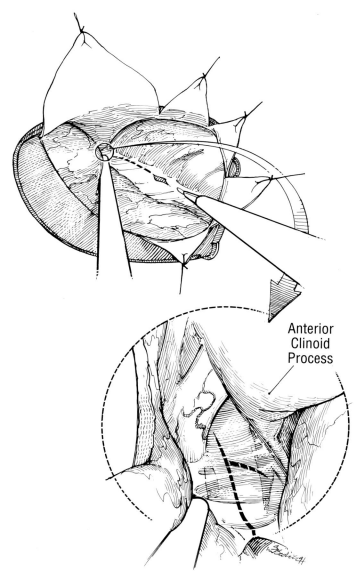

Figure 30-91. The initial microsurgical maneuver is directed at incision of the lateral aspect of the sphenoidal portion of the sylvian fissure. The incision is deepened and carried into the carotid cistern medially. A small T incision is then made posterolaterally directed at the insertion of the third cranial nerve into the cavernous sinus.

orly. While this finding has no real pathological significance, it can greatly obstruct access into the interpeduncular region. While the most traditional option to correct this problem is medial temporal lobe retraction by a stationary retraction device, we have been very impressed that a limited subpial resection of the uncus dramatically opens this space and significantly improves the illumination of the deeper subarachnoid space. When a fixed retractor arm is chosen, it is important to angle the retractor blade 90 degrees so that the retractor tip can be placed on the medial temporal lobe with a vector of force posteriorly, and the superficial aspect of the retractor blade will lay flat against the lateral temporal cortex and not unduly inhibit the surgeon's ability to manipulate instruments bimanually. When the target aneurysm arises below the level of the posterior clinoid and virtually certain temporal lobe retraction is going to be required with or without conversion into a "half and half" approach, it is advisable to detach the anterior veins draining from the temporal pole into the sphenoparietal sinus. Attention to these

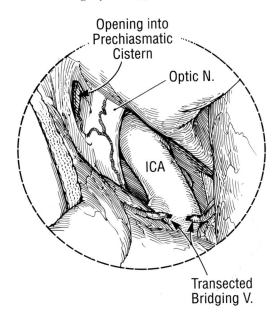

Opening into
Prechiasmatic
Cistern

Optic N.

ICA

Transected
Bridging V.

Figure 30-92. The initial subarachnoid exposure is ended with complete dissection of the medial sylvian fissure, including a frequently encountered bridging vein and wide opening of the prechiasmatic cistern.

veins at this early juncture of the procedure prevents the very unfortunate circumstance of bleeding from anteriorly within the middle cranial fossa due to increased temporal retraction during a period of temporal arterial occlusion. This complication needlessly protracts temporary clipping and serves to fill the interpeduncular cistern with additional blood. Figure 30-93 illustrates the subpial decompression of a medially displaced uncus resulting in a legitimate compromise from the insertion of a temporal retractor in the circumstance of a very favorably located basilar bifurcation aneurysm at the level of or superior to the posterior clinoid process. The resultant exposure with or without stable temporal lobe displacement yields access to the three potential routes into the interpeduncular cistern: (1) through the space between the optic nerve and carotid artery, (2) through the retrocarotid space, and (3) superior to the carotid bifurcation (Fig. 30-94).

Access to the Interpeduncular Cistern

While we have made some distinction between the three general routes of access to the interpeduncular cistern, ideally the fluid progress of the subarachnoid dissection occurs simultaneously in all three spaces. Some unique circumstances obviously prohibit access to one or more of these spaces; namely, a very densely atherosclerotic and calcified carotid artery that resists manipulation or the presence of a poste-

rior carotid wall aneurysm may mandate the selection of a more restricted field of dissection. In most cases, however, patient and complete dissection in the subarachnoid space will allow mobilization both laterally and medially. In initiating the dissection, however, attention should be given to the orientation of the patient's particular anatomy. If the supraclinoid carotid is relatively vertical in orientation and immediately apposed to the optic nerve, the initial dissection should proceed posterior to the carotid artery along the inferior aspect of the posterior communicating artery (Fig. 30-95). If the supraclinoid carotid courses more horizontally, either laterally or posteriorly, a significant triangle opens between the optic nerve and the anterior carotid wall. This anatomical circumstance provides very nice access for the initial dissection to occur through this triangle (Fig. 30-96). This triangle is bordered superiorly by the optic tract and the anterior cerebral artery. The third specific route (superior to the carotid bifurcation) may be very helpful to pursue in patients with a very short supraclinoid internal carotid and in those with a very high basilar bifurcation 1 cm or more above the posterior clinoid processus.

While subsequent dissection should ideally display the anatomy from each of these prospectives (particularly medial to and lateral to the internal carotid) the safest route of access to the interpeduncular cistern is the progressive dissection of the inferior aspect of the posterior communicating artery. Development of this plane protects the anterior thalamoperforating arteries, which emanate from the medial and superior aspect of the vessel, and ensures that the inferior aspect of the P_1-P_2 junction will be identified, preventing inadvertent dissection superior to the P_1 segment that may encounter the aneurysmal fundus prematurely. The posterior communicating artery is followed until it pierces the membrane of Liliequist, and it is frequently helpful to dissect the tenuous arachnoidal attachments between the posterior communicating artery and the third cranial nerve. After delineation of the P_1-P_2 junction, the membrane of Liliequist should be radically divided inferior to that point. This membrane is often thickened by a recent subarachnoid hemorrhage and may encase a thick subarachnoid hemorrhage under pressure. After the membrane is divided significantly both inferiorly and medially, the next stage in the subarachnoid dissection may occur (Fig. 30-97). In routine cases, it is our practice at this point to dissect medial to the internal carotid artery and follow the posterior communicating back to the P_1-P_2 junction by further dissecting the membrane of Liliequist. The extra moment spent in completing this exposure greatly improves the sur-

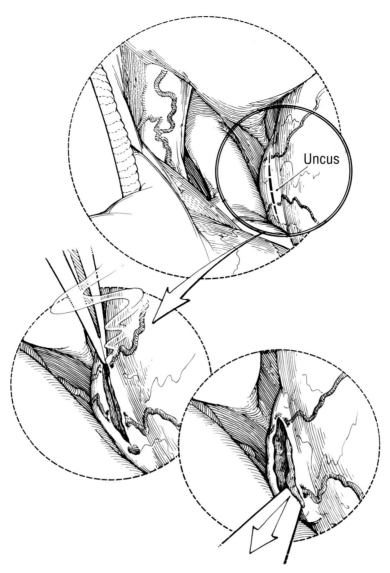

Figure 30-93. When approaching a favorably situated basilar bifurcation aneurysm at the level of or superior to the posterior clinoid process, subpial resection of the uncus may provide an alternative to the placement of a second (temporal lobe) retractor if the uncus appears to encroach upon the tentorial incisura.

geon's three-dimensional appreciation of the anatomy as well as the illumination to the deep vascular structures.

Once the anatomy of the P_1-P_2 junction is widely exposed, the sharp dissection proceeds medially along the inferior aspect of the P_1 segment (Fig. 30-98). This maneuver almost invariably requires some degree of medial displacement of the internal carotid. Confining dissection at this point to the inferior surface of the P_1 prevents inadvertent exposure of the fundus and keeps the surgeon free of the posterior thalmoperforating arteries arising from the superior and posterior aspects of the P_1 segments.

The identification of the origin of the inferior aspect of the P_1 segment from the basilar trunk is a very reassuring moment when the cistern is densely packed with blood. Medial progression of the sharp dissection across the face of the basilar trunk invariably exposes the contralateral superior cerebellar origin and the inferior aspect of the contralateral P_1. At this point, proximal arterial control has been achieved, and an appropriate site for the placement of a temporary clip should be identified (Fig. 30-99). Occasionally, the space between the P_1 and superior cerebellar artery on one or both sides is so confining that a temporary clip site must be prepared inferior to

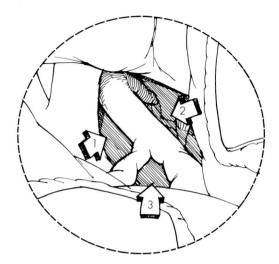

Figure 30-94. Surgical access to the interpeduncular cistern from the pterional exposure may traverse one or all of these three routes: (1) through the space between the optic nerve and carotid artery, (2) retrocarotid along the posterior communicating artery, and (3) superior to the carotid bifurcation.

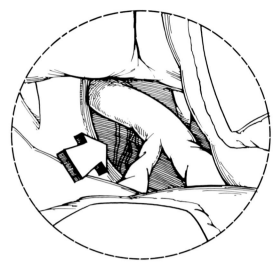

Figure 30-96. If the supraclinoid carotid artery lies more horizontally, the triangle between the optic nerve, carotid artery, and A_1 segments opens, yielding favorable access for the initial dissection.

the superior cerebellar origins. After the establishment of proximal control attention is then focused on the contralateral left P_1 segment. This vessel is initially extensively exposed inferiorly, and ultimately the superior aspect of this vessel is sharply defined from the hematoma, arachnoidal adhesions, and the aneurysmal fundus. Once this exposure is obtained,

the ipsilateral P_1 is thoroughly divested of its arachnoidal attachments, and the superior aspect of this vessel is defined. At this point, while the aneurysm cannot be safely clipped without jeopardizing perforators, complete trapping of the distal basilar complex could be employed should intraoperative hem-

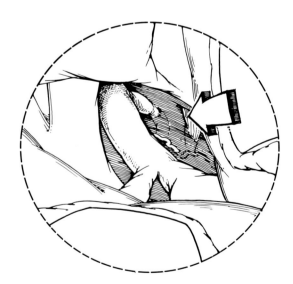

Figure 30-95. If the carotid artery is vertical in orientation and closely apposed to the optic nerve, initial dissection should proceed in the retrocarotid space along the inferior aspect of the posterior communicating artery.

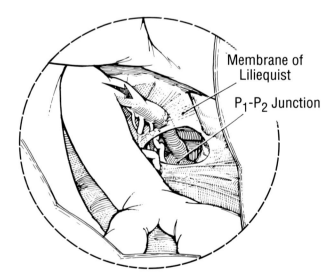

Membrane of
Liliequist

P_1-P_2 Junction

Figure 30-97. Utilizing a retrocarotid approach, the inferior surface of the posterior communicating artery is followed through the membrane of Liliequist to the P_1-P_2 junction. This thick membrane can then be widely opened inferiorly and inferomedially, allowing removal of hematoma.

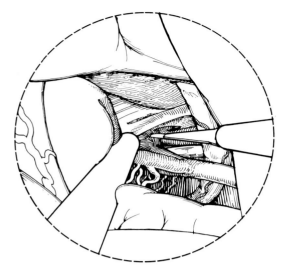

Figure 30-98. Following identification of the anterior aspect of the P_1-P_2 junction, dissection is directed medially along the inferior surface of the P_1 segment.

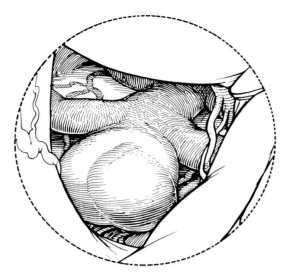

Figure 30-100. Bilateral dissection of the P_1 segments permits definitive temporary trapping of the distal basilar complex, should this become necessary.

orrhage occur (Fig. 30-100). Following the three-dimensional appreciation of these critical anatomical structures, sharp dissection is carried into the neck of the aneurysm by dissecting along the superior aspect of the contralateral P_1 toward its origin. As this dissection plane is deepened and the aneurysm is mobilized superiorly, the medial and posterior P_1 perforating arteries must be sharply and definitively freed from the aneurysmal sac. Following the completion of this dissection, the same maneuvers are employed on the ipsilateral side (Fig. 30-101). Due to the invari-

able presence of perforating arteries arising from the distal basilar trunk and streaming superiorly along the posterior aspect of the fundus, a definitive view from the ipsilateral side of the posterior aspect of the aneurysm is mandatory before safe clipping can be entertained. Occasionally, gentle displacement of the aneurysmal sac with the suction tube will allow sufficient mobilization both superiorly and anteriorly of the deeper aspect of the sac to identify safely a plane

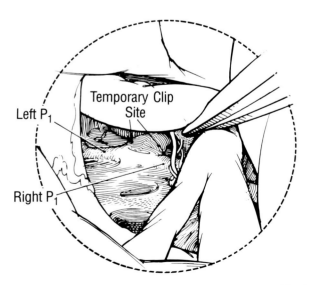

Figure 30-99. After visualizing the inferior aspects of both P_1 segments, bilateral sites for the placement of a proximal temporary basilar clip should be dissected.

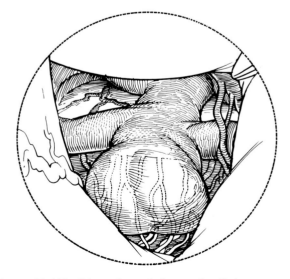

Figure 30-101. Dissection of the neck of the aneurysm from the pterional approach is critically dependent on the mobilization of the thalamoperforating arteries arising from the P_1 segments and the upper basilar trunk streaming superiorly.

for passage of the ipsilateral clip blade. Frequently, this maneuver is much more effectively and safely done with a proximal temporary arterial clip applied (Fig. 30-102). With the use of pharmacological cerebral ischemic protective agents, brief periods of proximal temporary basilar occlusion are very well tolerated (up to approximately 10 to 15 minutes). After adequate visualization of the posterior aspect of the sac, clipping may be performed with the temporary clip still in place.

While the final stages of dissection are similar regardless of the route of access chosen, a brief comment should be made about the use of the approach above the carotid bifurcation. When this exposure becomes necessary, the leash of perforating vessels emanating from the A_1 and M_1 segments can be divested of their arachnoidal attachments, and a surprisingly capacious space may be opened as a result. This space may be further developed by the insertion of a very narrow subfrontal retractor that passes over the carotid bifurcation and abuts the optic tract. The leash of anterior thalamoperforating and hypothalamic vessels that superficially obstructs the view of the interpeduncular cistern from this approach can be gently teased apart with sharp dissection. The progressive cleavage in the inferior to superior direction will ultimately separate these vessels, and the elastic properties of their arachnoidal encasements further display a potential space between them. With patience an adequate exposure can always be obtained.

Clip Application

After clear definition of both aspects of the aneurysm neck, the surgeon is ready for the selection of an appropriate clip and applier. Regrettably, the narrow confines of the interpeduncular cistern when viewed from the anterior aspect frequently become a major problem to the surgeon whose field is further encumbered by a bulky clip applier. As the clip applier is navigated past the internal carotid artery, the surgeon may be able to see the ipsilateral neck and clip blade, but frequently the contralateral anatomy will be completely obscured. One way of dealing with this problem is to insert the ipsilateral clip blade very gently while ensuring that the contralateral blade is widely opened; at this point, the line of sight of the microscope can be subtly adjusted with either mouth control or the surgeon's nondominant hand. The adjustment of the scope must then focus directly on the contralateral neck, allowing placement and advancement of that aspect of the clip. The difficulty of this maneuver may be magnified in aneurysms with very broad necks. We have had particular success with a couple of methods of circumventing this problem. The first maneuver makes use of the previously described extensive exposure both medial and lateral to the carotid artery. It is often possible for the right-handed surgeon in a right pterional craniotomy to achieve good visual access of the entire complex from the retrocarotid approach. The clip applier may

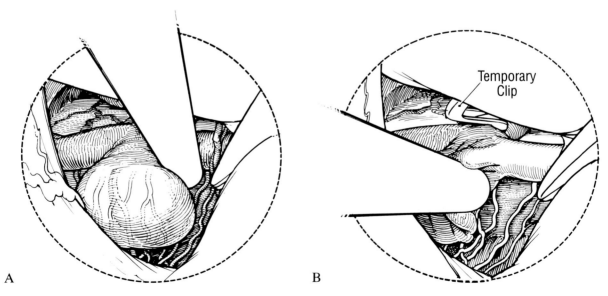

Figure 30-102. Definitive dissection of the aneurysmal neck requires superior and anterior displacement of the sac to clear adherent thalamoperforators posteriorly. **(A)** Commonly the direct injection of blood from the basilar artery into the aneurysm renders it extremely turgid, preventing safe mobilization to the extent necessary. **(B)** Brief proximal arterial occlusion with a temporary clip often softens the sac adequately for mobilization.

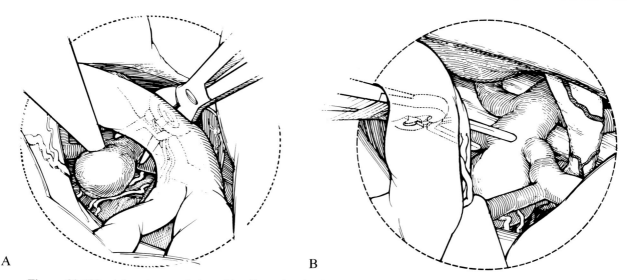

A   B

Figure 30-103. Advantages of the wide dissection both medial and posterior to the carotid artery can be exploited during clip application. **(A)** The right-handed surgeon when operating from the right side may gain visual access of the aneurysm neck through the space medial to the carotid artery and insert the clip applier through the retrocarotid space, thus eliminating loss of vision due to the bulky clip applier. **(B)** Similarly, a left-handed surgeon operating from the right side may focus the microscope through the retrocarotid space and insert the clip applier gently through the triangle medial to the carotid until the blades of the clip come into view.

then be inserted posterior to the carotid artery and the suction device inserted medial to the carotid artery, thereby eliminating one source of visual obstruction, namely, the suction tube. It is also possible to achieve adequate visual access to the aneurysmal neck from the space between the carotid and optic nerve. The right-handed surgeon may then insert the clip applier through the retrocarotid space, thereby eliminating the bulky applier as a source of visual loss. The clip is then inserted gently until the clip blades enter the surgeon's visual field (Fig. 30-103A). Similarly, the left-handed surgeon when operating through a right pterional craniotomy may achieve visual exposure of the complex through a retrocarotid microscope projection. The clip and clip applier can then be inserted medial to the carotid artery in a similar fashion, gently allowing the clip blades to enter the surgeon's field of vision (Fig. 30-103B). A second maneuver that has proven quite useful is the use of an appropriate length bayonetted clip. When the clip is placed upside down in the slightly angled clip applier, the tip of the blades are easily visualized as they encounter the aneurysm neck while the surgeon's view is not encumbered by the rest of the clip and the clip applier apparatus (Fig. 30-104). The exposure is typically too narrow to accommodate what would seem to be a superior solution, that being to use the bayonetted clip right side up.

Occasionally the size of the base of large basilar bifurcation aneurysms mandates the use of an excessively long clip simply to open wide enough to span the neck. Great care must be used in applying long clips from a pterional exposure, as depth perception is difficult and use of excessive length of the clip will almost invariably incorporate perforating arteries or injure the mesencephalon (Fig. 30-105). The surgeon must "feel" the clip pass the posterior aspect of the neck and gently close the clips, partially inspecting both aspects of the neck to see if the aneurysm has been completely spanned and if any critical perforating arteries are jeopardized.

Limitations of Exposure

The pterional approach offers excellent exposure of most aneurysms whose necks arise between the middepth of the sella turcica and a line 1.0 cm superior to the posterior clinoid process (Fig. 30-106). Aneurysms lying inferior to these limits are best approached by a subtemporal exposure or occasionally a "half and half" conversion. Aneurysms arising from extremely high bifurcation are difficult to expose by any route but are probably best exposed transsylvian above the carotid bifurcation. The degree of temporal lobe retraction required to expose these lesions subtemporally is difficult to justify. De-

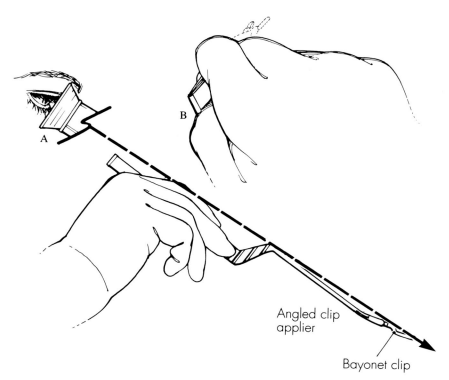

Angled clip
applier

Bayonet clip

Figure 30-104. The narrow confines of the interpeduncular anatomy may be circumvented by the use of a bayonetted clip. **(A)** Using a Yasargil clip applier with slightly angled jaws, the bayonetted clip is grasped upside-down. **(B)** As the clip and applier are deepened, the angle is often very favorable for an unencumbered view of both clip blades.

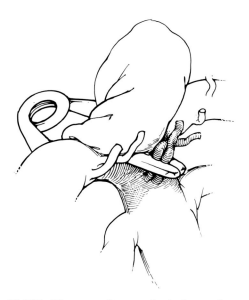

Figure 30-105. The use of excessively long clips may be mandated by the breadth of many large and giant lesions. The surgeon must be very cautious and avoid the temptation to advance the clip "to the hilt." Such a practice will invariably injure perforating arteries.

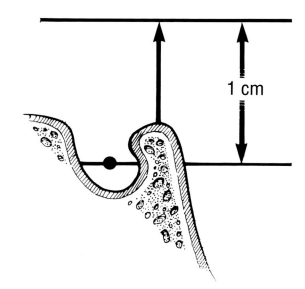

1 cm

Figure 30-106. The pterional exposure yields excellent exposure of the neck of basilar bifurcation aneurysms that originate between the mid-depth of the sella turcica and a line 1.0 cm superior to the posterior clinoid process.

spite the many attractive features of the pterional approach, including its familiarity and the excellent access to the contralateral P_1 segment, variations in bony and vascular anatomy can clearly limit the applicability of this approach. Operative findings of a large bony exostosis or an angiographically unpredictable cartilaginous cap of posterior clinoid process, an extremely atheromatous internal carotid artery, or coexisting carotid wall aneurysms can produce significant impediments to adequate exposure of the interpeduncular cistern. A number of potential solutions to these problems have been developed over the years and will be mentioned.

Yasargil[359] described resection of the posterior clinoid process as a direct solution to inadequate inferior exposure secondary to intervening bone. This maneuver requires reflection of the dural covering of the posterior clinoid process and air drill resection of underlying bone. This is a somewhat difficult technique and carries some risk to the neighboring vascular and neurological anatomy, particularly the internal carotid artery. The use of a drill in this setting is in our opinion considerably safer than the use of rongeurs, whose sudden shifts during bone biting can be catastrophic in this setting.

Yasargil et al.[360] described division of the posterior communicating artery to gain access to aneurysms lying inferiorly in the interpeduncular cistern. Use of this maneuver is predicated on the adequacy of the ipsilateral P_1 segment to supply the posterior cerebral territory and eliminates the potential to include the P_1 segment in the aneurysm clipping in the treatment of giant aneurysms. Prior to employing this maneuver, which by definition sacrifices a component of the circle of Willis that may have negative consequences particularly in the acute subarachnoid hemorrhage patient destined to develop ischemic complications, the surgeon should be certain that the posterior communicating vessel itself is an impediment to his exposure or that the increased mobilization of the carotid artery after section of this vessel will improve his access to the interpeduncular cistern. Fox[318] has used this maneuver routinely and has not noted increased morbidity with its usage. If this measure is to be employed, the vessel should be gently coagulated in a segment that does not contain anterior thalamoperforating vessels.

Similarly, we have found that division of the proximal A_1 segment is occasionally of great value in treating superiorly located basilar aneurysms. The employment of this technique is predicated on the knowledge that a patent anterior communicating artery exists and that the contralateral A_1 is of a size

that would suggest safe preservation of flow to the distal anterior cerebral distribution bilaterally.

As is discussed below, on a number of occasions we have been faced with the realization that the aneurysm under attack could not be adequately exposed from a pterional route due to its inferior location. In this setting conversion to a subtemporal approach is a legitimate alternative, although one that is quite difficult to effectively perform. The patient's head is in an extremely different position from that acquired in the true lateral position that is ideal for the subtemporal approach. After numerous frustrating experiences, we recommend that when this alternative is used, the head should first be repositioned, including rotation as far laterally as is possible while avoiding vascular compromise and then tilting the operating table to provide additional inclination for a lateral exposure. Due to the degree of rotation necessary, it may be necessary for the anesthesiologist to secure the patient's body to the table with tape beneath the surgical drapes prior to the completion of this maneuver.

Drake[312] initially described the "half and half" exposure for the clipping of coincident basilar and carotid aneurysms. This approach with its potential modifications represents an outstanding surgical exposure in and of itself and in many situations represents an attractive middle ground between the pterional and subtemporal dissections. This exposure can be acquired from the pterional exposure very quickly while maintaining continuity of anatomical detail previously dissected. Conversion to this approach usually obviates any need for deep bone resection or division of the posterior communicating artery. The cornerstone for conversion of the pterional approach to the "half and half" is the application of temporal lobe retraction in the posterosuperior direction. A temporal lobe retractor is placed on the most anterior and inferior portion of the temporal tip in the middle cranial fossa. Once the blade has been passed over the temporal tip, it is then elevated to expose the tentoral incisura and uncus (Fig. 30-107). The arachnoidal adhesions binding the uncus to the third cranial nerve can be divided and the uncus completely disengaged. The microscope's line of vision is adjusted posterior and lateral to the carotid, allowing the surgeon access to the vascular anatomy previously obscured by the clivus and posterior clinoid and extreme lateral exposure along the ipsilateral P_2 segment. Perhaps the most valuable aspects of this additional exposure are improved illumination into the wound and the ability to inspect carefully the posterior wall of an aneurysm that hangs somewhat

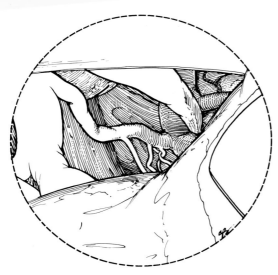

Figure 30-107. The "half and half" modification is achieved by retracting the temporal tip posterosuperiorly, providing elevation of the uncus from the tentorial incisura.

posteriorly into the interpeduncular fossa. In addition, the full use of this conversion can provide even more access to clip maneuvers such as the one illustrated in Figure 30-103.

Subtemporal Approach

It has been our preference to employ the pterional transsylvian exposure to most basilar bifurcation aneurysms due to the specific anatomical advantages discussed previously, including easy access to the contralateral P_1 for definitive temporary trapping if necessary, general familiarity to the majority of neurosurgeons, and the adaptability of this approach to the circumstance of multiple aneurysms. There are a number of circumstances, however, in which we feel that the pterional approach is not indicated. As previously mentioned, aneurysms arising below the mid-depth of the sella turcica are typically not clippable from a pterional view, and in the rare event that the surgeon is able to visualize the neck from this approach there would not be sufficient exposure of the basilar trunk to permit temporary clipping should complications arise. Patients with posteriorly projecting aneurysms similarly are not safely treated from a pterional approach. While the neck of the aneurysm can frequently be clipped by a gently curved clip projecting inferiorly over the bifurcation, the clip blades are placed blindly at their most inferior extent, and the association of the fundus of the aneurysm to thalamoperforating arteries renders prohibitive risk

to the patient. In addition, aneurysms that are large and project anteriorly may be quite difficult to expose from a pterional approach due to the limitation in working space imposed by the mass of the aneurysm itself. Each of these situations is successfully managed by the anterior subtemporal approach. The facts that only 10 to 15 percent of intracranial aneurysms involve the vertebral basilar circulation and that approximately 85 percent of distal basilar aneurysms arise at the level of or above the posterior clinoid process and are therefore, with the exceptions noted above, approachable from a pterional exposure, the subtemporal procedures are used relatively infrequently in our practice.[331,347,359] Nevertheless, this approach, which has been developed and modified by Drake,[312] provides tremendous flexibility with which to manage the gamut of basilar apex aneurysms as well as the ability to manage unexpected findings or complications during surgery. We believe that a detailed familiarity with the subtemporal approach and its potential advantages and limitations is essential whether or not it serves as the basilar aneurysm surgeon's primary route of access.

Positioning

While we prefer to retract the nondominant temporal lobe, certain circumstances we feel justify and occasionally mandate a left-sided procedure. A dense left third nerve palsy or dense right hemiparesis probably contraindicate a right-sided approach due to the risk of injury in any subtemporal approach to the ipsilateral third cranial nerve and cerebral peduncle. In addition, certain anatomical circumstances make a left-sided approach somewhat preferable. Occasionally an unusual tilt of the basilar bifurcation such that the left-sided aspect of the neck and P_1 origin are significantly superior to the right-sided anatomy poses significant risk that an approach from the right side could result in occlusion of the left P_1 segment (Fig. 30-108).

Because of the severity of temporal lobe elevation required, CSF evacuation is mandatory, particularly in the postsubarachnoid hemorrhage patient. While we have tried both polyethylene catheters and indwelling spinal needles, we have frequently been frustrated with the positional lability of the catheters in current use. To avoid the difficulty of manipulating these catheters beneath the drapes should they malfunction, we have more recently relied heavily on indwelling spinal needles connected to extension tubing and drainage bags as the preferred method of CSF drainage.[346] When using indwelling spinal needles, it is extremely important to place a foam rubber donut

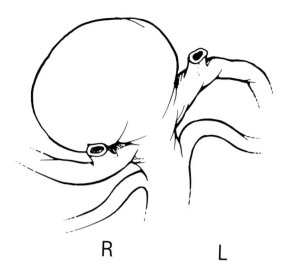

Figure 30-108. A tilt of the basilar bifurcation to the right such that the left P$_1$ origin and the left aspect of the neck lie significantly superior to their right-sided counterparts is probably safer to approach from a left subtemporal exposure as the left P$_1$ may be inadvertently occluded when clipped from the right side.

carefully around the needle and to place a protective cup over the needle so that the scrub nurse will not accidentally contact the needles during manipulation of the Mayo stand. The drain is left closed until the bony removal has been completed.

In particularly difficult cases, it is advisable to place the Mayfield fixation device so that conversion to a frontal temporal incision could be performed without redraping the patient. We have had reasonable success with placing either one or two pins anteriorly on the forehead in achieving this flexibility (Fig. 30-109). Traditionally, we have used an axillary role with a sling attachment for the dependent arm. More recently the use of the now standard gel pads on the operating table have in our opinion obviated the need for axillary roles. Using a large foam sling, the dependent arm and elbow can be very conveniently and anatomically protected within the confines of the Mayfield apparatus (Fig. 30-109). The head position most commonly used is achieved by slightly elevating the head and opening the space between the dependent shoulder and ear and then tilting the vertex of the skull inferiorly 10 to 20 degrees below the horizontal.

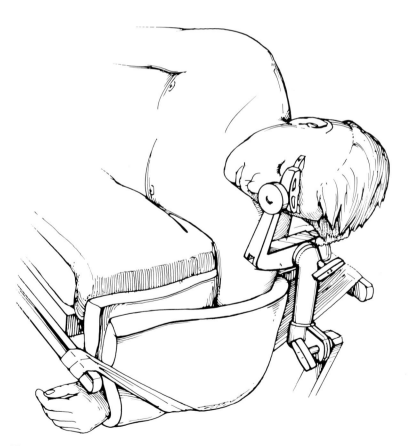

Figure 30-109. Patient positioning for a right subtemporal procedure.

Scalp Incision

Most basilar bifurcation aneurysms can be treated through a linear scalp incision as advocated by Drake.[312] We rarely employ this incision, however, due to the facts that we tend to operate on the subarachnoid hemorrhage patient early and that we employ the subtemporal exposure typically for low-lying basilar bifurcation aneurysms. We have found that a larger craniotomy is beneficial in the early subarachnoid hemorrhage patient in whom brain resection may be performed. A tentorial retraction stitch is quite helpful in exposing aneurysms arising at about the level of the posterior clinoid and just below, but when the neck of the aneurysm lies at the level of the lower aspect of sella turcica or below, it is rarely possible to expose the neck without a full tentorial incision, this maneuver being facilitated by a larger bony opening. Nevertheless, we do use the classically described linear incision and anterior temporal craniectomy for unruptured aneurysms that project posteriorly or aneurysms of a favorable altitude that have hemorrhaged several weeks prior to the operative procedure. The typical incision and craniectomy are illustrated in Figure 30-110. An incision is performed from approximately 1 cm anterior to the tragus and extends directly superiorly over a length of about 10 cm. The subsequent craniectomy is based on the zygoma and root of the zygoma and has a diameter of 3 to 3.5 cm.

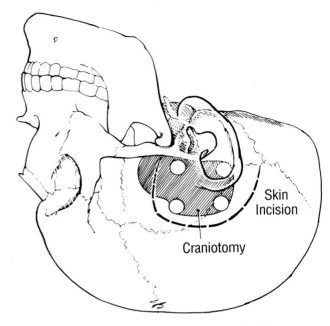

Figure 30-111. For patient with low-lying basilar apex aneurysm in whom tentorial incision is anticipated or for the early postsubarachnoid hemorrhage patient in whom temporal lobe resection may be required, a temporal scalp flap and small craniotomy are performed in addition to an anterior craniectomy.

For particularly low-lying aneurysms (at the level of the lower aspect of the sella turcica), we tend to use a formal temporal scalp flap and small temporal craniotomy in addition to the previously described anterior craniectomy (Fig. 30-111). This wider exposure gives excellent access for temporal lobe resection should this be necessary. A point of major importance in either of these incisions is to maximize the exposure at the inferior aspect of the bony removal to expose the floor of the middle cranial fossa, thus minimizing subsequent brain retraction.

Dural Opening

Regardless of whether a craniectomy or craniotomy is performed, we have found it helpful to perform a cruciate or stellated dural incision such that the inferior dural flap can be secured with a retention suture firmly apposed to the inferior bony edge and the temporalis muscle (Fig. 30-112). This maneuver minimizes extradural bleeding.

Initial Subarachnoid Exposure

The initial approach beneath the temporal lobe is quite dependent on adequate brain relaxation. While CSF drainage, hyperventilation, and patience will

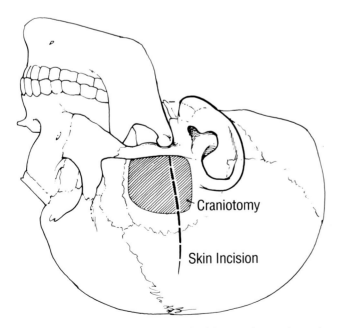

Figure 30-110. Classical linear incision and anterior subtemporal craniectomy. The area of planned bony removal is defined by hatched lines.

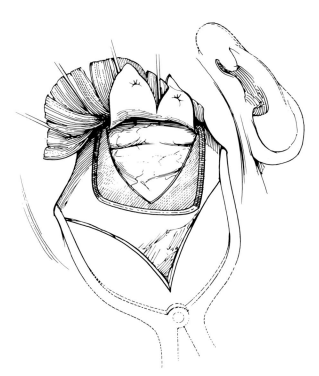

Figure 30-112. After craniotomy or craniectomy, the dura is opened in a cruciate fashion so that it can be secured inferiorly, eliminating extradural run-in bleeding.

usually result in satisfactory brain relaxation, the early subarachnoid hemorrhage patient occasionally cannot be managed by these techniques alone. We have found no evidence of neurological complications associated with resection of the inferior or middle temporal gyrus together with the fusiform and parahippocampal gyri in achieving access to the tentorial incisura. When this resection is done, we have found it extremely beneficial to leave the medial pia-arachnoidal tissue intact so that the retractor blade can rest on this tissue; subsequent elevation of the retractor will then result in superior migration of the third cranial nerve due to its arachnoidal attachments to this tissue. As the uncus is elevated from the tentorial edge, the third cranial nerve will be seen to be slightly elevated with the uncus (Fig. 30-113). While this maneuver does expand the space between the tentorial edge and the third cranial nerve, in general it is extremely helpful to place a tentorial retraction stitch as described by Drake[312] to maximize inferior exposure (Fig. 30-114). This suture is placed by identifying the fourth cranial nerve and placing the stitch just anterior to the site of its insertion and securing it to the dura of the floor of the middle cranial fossa. Should the aneurysm under attack be extremely low lying, we have usually found it necessary to incise the tentorium. This simple maneuver is often compli-

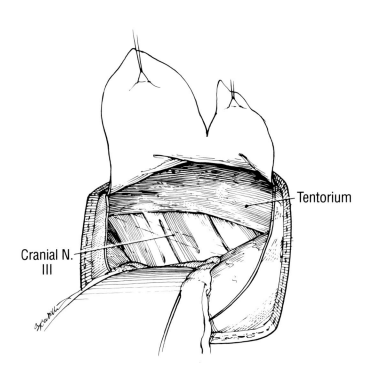

Figure 30-113. As the uncus is elevated by the brain retractor, the third cranial nerve can be seen through the arachnoid to be elevated with the retractor, thus expanding the working space beneath it.

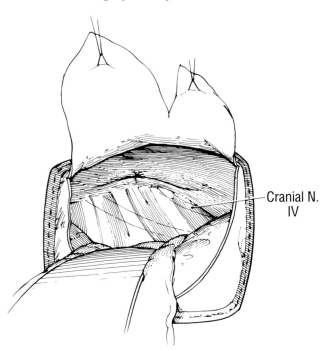

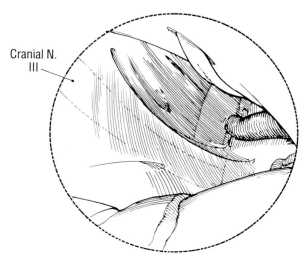

Figure 30-115. The approach to the interpeduncular cistern is begun by incising the arachnoid between the third cranial nerve and tentorial edge and identifying the superior cerebellar artery.

Figure 30-114. Inferior access to the interpeduncular cistern can be maximized by a tentorial retraction stitch placed just anterior to the insertion of the fourth cranial nerve.

cated by aggressive venous bleeding through the folds of the tentorium after they are opened. This hemorrhage is perhaps best controlled by the insertion of small cottonballs placed between these dural leaves with a nerve hook. Care should be exercised to use the minimal amount of bulk possible so as not to eliminate the exposure achieved by the previous tentorial incision. After one or both of these maneuvers are performed, the subarachnoid space may be entered by incising the arachnoid immediately beneath the third cranial nerve. The key landmark to be achieved at this point is the superior cerebellar artery as it begins to angle posteriorly around the cerebral peduncle into the ambiens cistern (Fig. 30-115).

Approach Into the Interpeduncular Cistern

The superior cerebellar artery can be safely followed medially to its origin from the basilar artery. From this perspective, the anterior and posterior margins of the basilar artery can be divested of arachnoid and blood clot and prepared for potential proximal temporary clipping immediately superior to the superior cerebellar artery origin (Fig. 30-116). Under high-power magnification, the dissection is extended superiorly to the point at which the ipsilateral P_1 segment emerges from the basilar artery-aneurysm com-

plex. The most distal portion of the basilar artery will often be noted to begin to expand in the anteroposterior diameter as the region of the neck of the aneurysm is approached. Once the ipsilateral P_1 segment is clearly identified, the contralateral aspect of the basilar artery should be directly inspected. Due to the limitation in early posterior exposure imposed by the cerebral peduncle and the natural anterosuperior initial course of most P_1 segments, dissection across the anterior aspect of the basilar artery with gentle compression of the artery is the most predictable

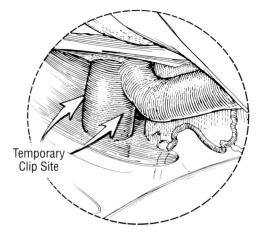

Figure 30-116. The superior cerebellar artery is followed medially to its origin from the basilar artery. A provisional side for temporary arterial occlusion should be prepared immediately distal to the origin of the superior cerebellar artery.

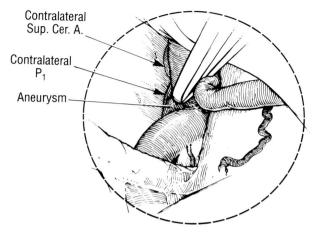

Figure 30-117. With gentle posterior displacement of the distal basilar artery, the proximal P$_1$ segment can be identified as it emerges typically anterosuperiorly from the basilar artery-aneurysm complex.

means of identifying the contralateral P$_1$ (Fig. 30-117). A major potential source or morbidity lies in mistaking the contralateral superior cerebellar artery from the P$_1$ segment. Such an error could result in the placement of a clip occluding the P$_1$ origin with its associated perforators. Several mechanisms are available to help clarify this anatomy. As has been shown in Yasargil's series, the P$_1$ segment is usually the dominant supply of the posterior cerebral artery.[357] Under these circumstances, the P$_1$ is substantially larger than the superior cerebellar artery and usually much more thick walled and atheromatous.

The superior cerebellar by contrast is frequently red in color and apparently thin walled. While anatomical variants, including persistence of the fetal circulation, a hypoplastic P$_1$ segment, and a doubled contralateral superior cerebellar artery, may make these distinctions vague, continuation of the dissection laterally displaying the P$_1$-P$_2$ junction and the contralateral third cranial nerve passing inferior to the P$_1$ segment will prevent any misconception (Fig. 30-118).

Aneurysm Dissection and Clipping

In the typical circumstance of a superior projecting basilar apex aneurysm, the clarification of the contralateral P$_1$ anatomy from anterior to the basilar artery brings into clear perspective the anterior aspect of the aneurysm neck which typically has no associated perforating arteries, and this dissection may be finalized by sharply dissecting the remaining arachnoidal attachments to the clivus and posterior clinoid processes and removal of any hematoma. The more critical aspect of the dissection must then be performed posterior to the arterial complex. This dissection is best initiated immediately posterior to the ipsilateral P$_1$ segment origin. By gentle displacement of the cerebral peduncle as this dissection plane is deepened, the distal basilar artery perforating vessels can be identified and reflected posteriorly off the aneurysm neck. This dissection plane should be carried directly across the interpeduncular cistern until the neck has been spanned (Fig. 30-119). Since the contralateral posterior cerebral artery often cannot be identified in this posterior plane, it is critical to maintain the three-dimensional dynamics of this anatomy by mov-

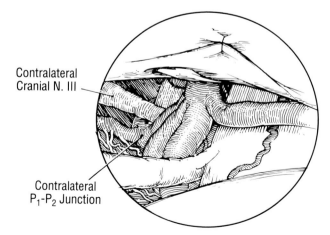

Figure 30-118. Extension of contralateral dissection to display the contralateral P$_1$-P$_2$ junction and third cranial nerve (beneath P$_1$) prevents mistaking a contralateral superior cerebellar artery for a P$_1$ segment.

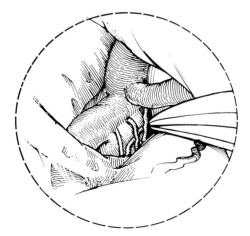

Figure 30-119. The critical posterior dissection plane frequently requires gentle posterior displacement of the cerebral peduncle to mobilize thalamoperforating vessels from the aneurysm neck and fundus.

ing the microscope back into the anterior dissection plane to identify the P_1 segment and frequently look back and forth.

The posterior dissection must guarantee safe passage for the posterior clip blade without incorporation of any perforating arteries. Often the most difficult perforators to spare are not those emanating from the distal basilar artery and streaming superiorly but those arising from the most proximal aspect from the contralateral medial P_1 segment. These vessels may be exceptionally adherent to the aneurysm, and even the ipsilateral ones may be quite difficult to dissect free. Once this has been accomplished, however, an aperture clip can be used to occlude the aneurysm neck accurately, reconstitute the previously bulbous distal basilar artery, and encase the ipsilateral P_1 and its perforators within the aperture (Fig. 30-120). It is critical, however, to ensure that excessive clip length is not used as the contralateral aspect of the neck and P_1 junction is relatively obscured particularly regarding perforators arising from the medial contralateral P_1 segment. Excessive clip length will invariably occlude these vessels (Fig. 30-121).

Anterior projecting aneurysms from the basilar bifurcation, while posing much less perforator risk, frequently obscure the origin of the contralateral of the P_1 segment. Not infrequently, the P_1 can only be visualized during the final aspects of clip closure, and this maneuver requires exquisite control of the microscope by a mouthpiece (Fig. 30-122). Posteriorly projecting aneurysms are optimally exposed by the subtemporal approach but require deliberate and patient dissection of perforating vessels that typically

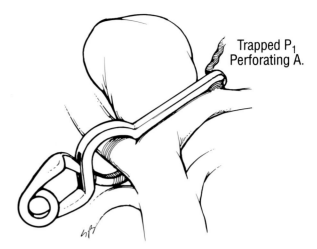

Figure 30-121. Precise clip blade length is critical, as excessive length will invariably occlude contralateral P_1 perforating vessels.

encase the inferior aspect of the aneurysmal sac (Fig. 30-123).

Multiple Aneurysms

The subtemporal approach lends itself extremely well to the treatment of associated posterior carotid wall aneurysms. Simply moving the retractor 1.0 to 1.5 cm anteriorly along the tentorial edge will define

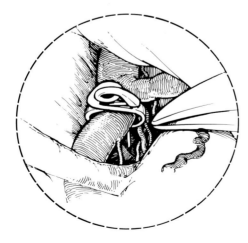

Figure 30-120. Use of fenestrated or aperture clips with short blades has greatly facilitated clipping of basilar apex aneurysms. The ipsilateral P_1 segment is enclosed by the aperture.

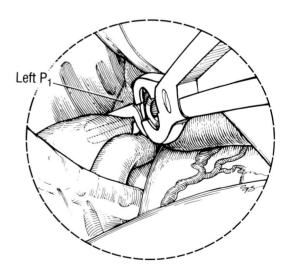

Figure 30-122. Anterior projecting basilar apex aneurysms pose the risk that the contralateral P_1 segment may be caught to the clip as it is obscured by the aneurysm mass. Manipulation of the microscope depth of focus using mouthpiece control can allow visualization of the P_1 as the clip closes.

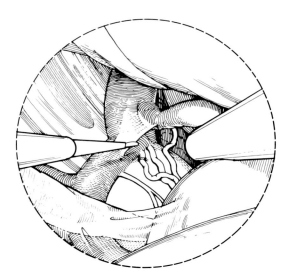

Figure 30-123. Posterior projecting aneurysms must be divested of associated perforating arteries most heavily associated with the inferior aspect of the sac.

the posterior aspect of the carotid cistern. The arachnoid superior to the insertion of the third cranial nerve into the roof of the cavernous sinus is opened, exposing the lateral carotid cistern. The posterior carotid wall is then at a very convenient inclination for definitive dissection of associated aneurysms (Fig. 30-124).

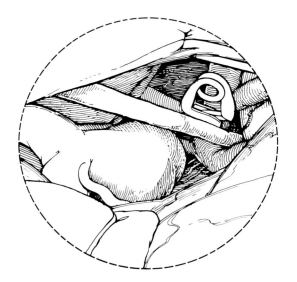

Figure 30-124. The subtemporal approach yields excellent exposure of the posterior carotid wall. By moving the retractor 1.0 to 1.5 cm anteriorly from the interpeduncular cistern, the arachnoid superior to the insertion of the third cranial nerve can be incised and posterior carotid wall aneurysms dissected and clipped.

OPERATIVE COMPLICATIONS

A number of technical advances in recent years have improved the outlook for patients reaching neurosurgical attention who suffer SAH or other symptoms leading to a diagnosis of intracranial aneurysm. Notable contributors to this enhanced level of care include precision in radiological diagnosis, dramatic improvement in neuroanesthetic management leading to a very favorable operative environment, safe temporary clips, brain ischemic protective regimens, and a myriad of safe and effective aneurysm clips. In spite of all these developments, however, the outlook for patients suffering aneurysmal SAH remains guarded.[328] Patients suffering from basilar apex aneurysm are not unique to the general SAH patient in their frequent failure to recover due to brain destruction from the initial hemorrhage, early rebleeding, and development of delayed cerebral ischemia. The unique aspects of the anatomy of the interpeduncular cistern, however, do magnify the toll of surgical and management misadventure in patients suffering from aneurysms in this particular site. In this section are examined the management complications in patients with basilar bifurcation aneurysms, particularly those unique to the distal basilar artery, and some of the preventive and therapeutic measures that have proven of value in our experience are discussed. These arbitrary categories of neurological morbidity are by no means all inclusive but do represent an analysis of our own experience with distal basilar artery aneurysm treated over the past several years in which we noted 8 percent mortality and 11 percent permanent neurological disability.[304] As one might expect, most patients with poor outcome developed neurological complications of more than one type as well as various systemic insults. In our previously published report, we attributed unfavorable outcome to the following specific causes: (1) direct effect of hemorrhage, (2) errors in surgical timing, (3) conceptual errors, (4) technical errors, (5) delayed cerebral ischemia, (6) complications of hypertensive hypervolemic therapy, and (7) "bad luck." For the purposes of the present discussion, we will emphasize management and surgical complications unique to the basilar apex with emphasis on prevention and remedial measures (Table 30-23).

Timing of Operation

The Cooperative Aneurysm Study provided excellent documentation that the peak incidence of aneurysmal rebleeding occurs during the first

Table 30-23. Intraoperative Complications

Etiology	Avoidance/Management
Timing of operation (too early)	Restrict early surgery to those patients in whom TAO will be less than 10 minutes Restrict early surgery to cases accessible by pterional approach Avoid early reoperation to clip unruptured basilar apex aneurysm after SAH from other lesions
Improper choice of operative approach	Avoid pterional approach when neck is inferior to midsellar depth or when aneurysm projects posteriorly
Inadequate treatment	Avoid "wrapping" Eliminate residual neck Document results angiographically
Ischemia from TAO	Restrict to approximately 15 minutes
Perforator injury	Employ TAO to mobilize sac Approach posteriorly projecting aneurysms subtemporally Caution in aggressive decompression of giant, thrombotic sac Always dissect posterior aspect of neck

Intraoperative rupture	Avoidance
	    Sharp dissection
	    Liberal use of TAO
	Management
	    Avoid panic
	    Tamponade
	    Administer brain-protective agents
	    TAO
	    Precise clipping

Abbreviation: TAO, temporary arterial occlusion.

48 hours.[327,328] A large body of information documents that the peak incidence of symptomatic vasospasm occurs between days 7 and 10 following SAH.[332,334,348,354] For a number of years, our impression has been that the good grade patient is best served by an early operation to secure a ruptured aneurysm to minimize the risk of rebleeding and to maximize the efficacy of hypertensive/hypervolemic therapy should ischemic signs develop. Because of this philosophy, early rebleeding prior to surgical therapy has been rare in our basilar apex patients. It is likely that our impression substantially underestimates the actual incidence of death from early rebleeding, as referring physicians and hospitals probably do not initiate transfer of many patients who are mortally ill.

Careful review of our experience has suggested that certain subsets of patients with ruptured basilar bifurcation aneurysms, unlike their counterparts with anterior circulation disease, may not tolerate early procedures well (Table 30-23). Specifically, patients with broad-based large and giant aneurysms, particularly partially thrombotic lesions, are best managed in our experience by the use of temporary arterial occlusion (often complete trapping), pharmacological brain protection, aspiration, and decompression fol-

lowed by clipping (Fig. 30-125).[301,304] Our results have been favorable in patients operated on early in the first week following SAH in whom the duration of temporary occlusion was 10 minutes or less. In cases requiring longer intervals of occlusion, tolerance has been unpredictable. It is often possible to predict a number of features of the targeted aneurysm based on preoperative angiography, CT scanning, and MRI. Truly giant sacs and in particular those with calcified walls or laminated thrombus usually require relatively longer periods of occlusion. In this circumstance, we feel that the patient is probably best served by treatment with antifibrinolytics, which should minimize the risk of rebleeding (0.8 percent per day after day 2)[327] and delaying operation until the second or third week. We still recommend early operation in patients with large aneurysms that are not thrombotic or calcified and in which we would anticipate a relatively brief period of temporary occlusion.

We have noted some relationship between tolerance of early operation and the specific procedure chosen (Table 30-23). As has been previously illustrated, our preference is to use the transsylvian exposure for all aneurysms favorably situated for this approach. In general, we have noted very satisfactory

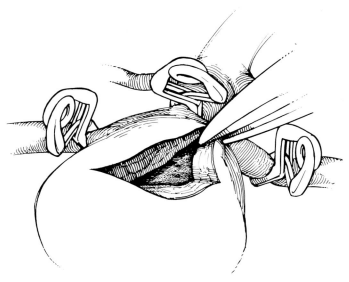

Figure 30-125. Giant partially thrombotic aneurysms are best treated in our experience by temporary trapping, metabolic suppression, aneurysm aspiration or evacuation, and clip reconstruction. In many lesions, the surgeon can predict that this procedure will require substantial intervals of temporary occlusion.

brain relaxation, even in the early days following subarachnoid hemorrhage following pterional craniotomy, ventricular puncture, and anterior temporal lobectomy when necessary. Our experience has not been as favorable in patients with low-lying lesions subjected to subtemporal procedures; we have frequently found that despite adequate CSF evacuation, modest hyperventilation, and inferior temporal resection the exposure remains tight and that the blood-packed interpeduncular cistern does not give adequate room for surgical manipulation in those early days. This impression may be biased in part by the fact that we only use this procedure for those lesions lying inferiorly behind the clivus in which the interpeduncular cistern is likely a much more confining anatomical region than in the more superiorly located aneurysms.

For the past several years, hypertensive/hypervolemic therapy has been the mainstay in our unit for the management of patients with symptomatic delayed cerebral ischemia. Consistent with this management policy, it has been our goal in patients with multiple aneurysms to secure all aneurysms if at all possible prior to the onset of the period of highest risk, particularly in those patients with CT evidence of high risk of vasospasm.[317] This practice has not been associated with significant morbidity when additional anterior circulation aneurysms were clipped at a second sitting; regrettably on a few occasions patients with ruptured anterior circulation aneurysms who were returned to the operating room for clipping of asymptomatic basilar bifurcation aneurysms failed

to regain their preoperative neurological status. While these negative results may relate to poor patient selection (elderly patients) on our part, we nevertheless believe that caution should be exercised in extremely aggressive management of this type, and perhaps consideration should be given to early intervention with angioplasty when carotid circulation vasospasm becomes symptomatic in these situations.

Choice of Operative Approach

Early experience in our unit suggested that the posterior clinoid process posed an inferior limit to the transsylvian exposure.[347] With continued experience and with application of the previously mentioned modifications of the pterional procedure, it has become clear that the inferior limit of this approach in our hands is approximately at the level of the midsellar depth. In the course of defining these limits, a number of procedures were attempted from the transsylvian route that were ultimately unsuccessful in gaining adequate exposure for either definite neck occlusion or for proximal temporary arterial occlusion (Fig. 30-126). As previously mentioned, all approaches to the interpeduncular cistern mandate precise patient positioning to maximize one's ability to work in these narrow confines. In addition to attempted anterior exploration of lesions too inferiorly located, we have incorrectly chosen a subtemporal route to several patients' giant aneurysms due to a posterior-projecting lobe. This approach is based on

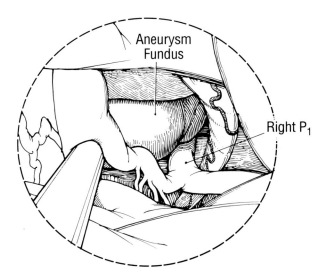

Figure 30-126. Aneurysms arising inferior to the midsellar depth are usually not adequately exposed by the pterional exposure and have required conversion to an alternate approach with less than optimal positioning.

the presumption that adequate aneurysm softening can be achieved with simple proximal basilar artery temporary occlusion. Regrettably in several cases proximal occlusion did not adequately soften the aneurysm sac, and, despite attempts at tandem clipping, crushing of the aneurysm neck, and finally stacking a number of clips on the involved lesion, migration of sequential clips down on to the posterior cerebral arteries occurred. This situation was only remedied by conversion to a transsylvian view, permitting definitive temporary trapping of the distal basilar complex and placement of permanent clips with the aneurysm empty.

The cauliflower-shaped aneurysm deserves mention in this context, because it has been associated with morbidity following inappropriate operative selection. A pterional approach to a cauliflower lesion with anterior and posterior lobes poses an extremely high risk of inclusion of posterior perforating vessels during clip application (Fig. 30-127). This complication can be prevented either by employing a subtemporal approach or by definitive trapping of the basilar artery and both P_1 segments followed by aspiration of the aneurysm and mobilization out of the interpeduncular fossa prior to definitive clipping.

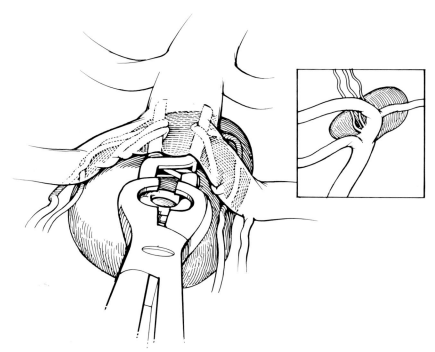

Figure 30-127. The "cauliflower-shaped" aneurysm with lobes projecting both anteriorly and posteriorly poses high risk of perforating artery injury when clipped from a pterional approach. Solutions to this problem include using the subtemporal approach or definitive temporary trapping with aneurysm deflation and mobilization out of the interpeduncular fossa prior to the clipping.

A catastrophic complication during a procedure in which an inappropriate operative approach has been selected is the development of premature rupture. While this complication is discussed in some detail below, having poor visualization of the ruptured site or lack of access for temporary arterial occlusion can convert a relatively modest hemorrhage into a life-threatening situation when the surgeon is not viewing anatomy from the optimal perspective.

Inadequate Treatment

Evidence is accumulating, particularly from surgeons with extensive experience and excellent follow-up, that incompletely treated aneurysms as well as some aneurysms that are by all criteria well clipped do have some tendency to recur over time (Table 30-23).[311,359] In Yasargil's recently reported series, 2 of 10 patients whose basilar aneurysms were wrapped with muscle or acrylic subsequently enlarged or bled fatally.[359] While the problem of the imperfectly placed clip is dealt with below, one could certainly draw parallel conclusions between aneurysms treated with wrapping procedures and those found to have small residual sacs after clipping or endovascular treatments. We have seen one patient who suffered a second subarachnoid hemorrhage 5 years after a basilar bifurcation aneurysm was coated with acrylic. We have also lost a patient following a wrapping procedure of an asymptomatic fusiform basilar aneurysm and carotid occlusion for a giant cavernous aneurysm when hemodynamic changes enlarged and ruptured the basilar aneurysm.[302] The basilar apex is unfortunately not an anatomical site that lends itself well to aneurysm coating or to wrapping with muscle or cotton. It is not possible to encase circumferentially any but the most trivial aneurysms. Occasionally, we are forced to use this maneuver, but endovascular technology probably offers the patient somewhat more protection than these modalities. Nevertheless, the endovascular patients must be followed long term, just as must those with aneurysmal rests to determine if subsequent enlargement is going to occur.

Complications Related to Temporary Occlusion

In our opinion, the development of atraumatic and safe temporary clips and the ample laboratory documentation that various pharmacological approaches successfully depress cerebral metabolism and oxygen consumption during periods of temporary ischemia have made intracranial aneurysm surgery in general a safer undertaking. We have found these surgical principles particularly applicable to surgery of the distal basilar artery with some limitations. The principle goal of applying temporary clipping to basilar apex aneurysms is either to soften the sac adequately for sufficient mobilization and definition of the posterior aspect of the aneurysm or to mobilize a posterior projecting sac from the interpeduncular fossa. Unfortunately, the latter maneuver often requires complete trapping of the distal basilar trunk and both P_1 segments. It has also been our feeling that the application of a proximal basilar temporary clip immediately prior to the application of a permanent clip across the neck has decreased the risk of aneurysmal shearing and intraoperative hemorrhage. Failure to perform temporary arterial occlusion has been felt to result in shearing injuries to aneurysms in at least two patients with basilar bifurcation aneurysms in recent experience. Regrettably adequate softening of the aneurysms is not always achieved by simple proximal occlusion. We have seen a number of circumstances in patients with large and bulbous lesions in which, despite proximal clipping, multiple clip attempts simply would not adhere to the aneurysm neck. In some circumstances, this situation has been complicated by our lack of access to the contralateral P_1 segment by virtue of using a subtemporal approach. This situation mandates the hasty conversion to a more anteriorly directed exposure so that the complete complex can be isolated. We feel that any approach to a large and giant lesion should be undertaken with provision for not only proximal, but, if necessary, distal temporary clipping as well. Inadequate exposure for this maneuver is also encountered in the low-lying basilar apex aneurysms approached from anteriorly in which insufficient inferior exposure precludes clipping of the distal basilar artery if complications arise. The availability of either "half and half" conversion or true subtemporal conversion should prevent this complication.

Regrettably, the amount of time available during temporary arterial occlusion is dependent on a number of variables some of which are not clinically ascertainable. For simple proximal clipping, the presence of one very large posterior communicating artery should provide reassurance that relatively protracted temporary basilar clipping should be tolerated but also that it may be less efficacious in softening the aneurysm. While there are good data that cerebral metabolic activity may be depressed by approximately 50 percent with the use of pharmacological brain-protective agents, it is also clear that this level of suppression does not protect the brain indefinitely. Particularly early after subarachnoid hemorrhage intervals of occlusion in the range of 15 minutes become unpredictable in terms of tolerance. Unfortunately, in our experience, we are not infrequently surprised by the actual duration of occlusion necessary to secure a difficult lesion. Our current regimen employs a normotensive anesthetic with the use of etomidate to achieve electroencephalographic-documented burst suppression and mild induced hypothermia in order to optimize available working time.[301]

Technical Errors

For reasons that have been previously highlighted, the interpeduncular cistern is an unforgiving site in which technical flaw is rarely asymptomatic. The injury to a posterior thalamoperforating vessel by poor dissection technique, inclusion in permanent clipping, or irreversible endothelial injury as a result of transient occlusion in a permanent clip is a catastrophe that highlights the unique aspects of basilar apex aneurysms from other intracranial aneurysms, including those located more inferiorly in the basilar trunk (Table 30-23). Drake's early experience[312] with this problem led him to champion the subtemporal approach as it consistently yielded an optimal view of these important vessels. We have noted a peculiar tendency of patients to develop transient low-density lesions in their diencephalon following procedures in which all perforating vessels were definitively spared. These low-density CT areas typically disappear over the next week and do not appear to be associated with permanent dysfunction. It is possible that the use of temporary occlusion predisposes to these transient lesions. Patients may also develop perforator distribution CT low density as well as focal neurological deficits during episodes of symptomatic vasospasm. Once established with CT lesions, this diencephalic injury due to vasospasm has tended to be permanent and symptomatic. The message is clear from our experinece as well as from that of other surgeons with experience in this anatomical site that efforts to spare these vessels irrigating the midbrain and diencephalon are of paramount importance in planning and carrying out surgical clipping of basilar bifurcation aneurysms. Temporary arterial occlusion with softening of the sac allows improved visualization, particularly when an anterior exposure is being used.

While modern microsurgical technique has allowed excellent visualization of aneurysm anatomy, the complexity of aneurysms of the basilar bifurcation as well as their broad base and frequent atheromatous components in the setting of a very narrow surgical exposure have resulted in numerous patients left with seemingly trivial "dog ears" or small tags of aneurysmal tissue at the base of the clip after the neck is gathered (Fig. 30-128). Whenever possible every attempt should be made to apply a second small clip to this tag of tissue to re-create as normal a parent artery as possible. Admittedly, this task is not always feasible in the narrow confines of the interpeduncular cistern. A mounting body of information clearly shows that this tissue can develop into a new aneurysmal sac in the future and enlarge and hemorrhage.[299,313–315] Diagnosing these lesions is usually straightforward during the primary operation but may be quite difficult on postoperative angiography. Not infrequently, due to local spasm and mild ectasia in the region of the aneurysmal neck, one gets the impression that a millimeter of abnormal tissue has been left behind. This circumstance can be clarified only after all arterial spasm has resolved and usually one will see a healthy-appearing artery on follow-up study. Whether to recommend re-exploration to patients with clear remnant tags of aneurysm tissue is a very difficult decision. Because of some early poor experiences with the re-exploration,[298] we were leaning toward protracted angiographic follow-up on a

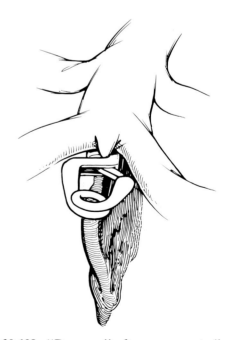

Figure 30-128. "Dog ears" after permanent clip application should be treated with a second small clip whenever possible, as new aneurysms can arise from this tissue even after several years.

yearly or a 5-year basis for patients with this type of pathology and recommending re-exploration only if progression occurs.

It is clear, however, that this type of imperfect clip application should be differentiated from the aneurysm that remains persistently patent after clipping. While occasional giant aneurysms are left with slight filling of the sac when limited space precludes additional clip application, this is a circumstance that we feel is unstable, and it remains the surgeon's burden to prove that thrombosis occurs or to plan a subsequent exploration to clip the aneurysm definitively. In our experience, the aneurysm usually undergoes thrombosis within 2 to 4 days (Table 30-23).

We have included a discussion of intraoperative rupture with technical errors although in some cases the actual cause of bleeding is unknown. Hemorrhage from an aneurysm during the various stages of craniotomy and dissection is not uncommon and in fact was documented in 19 percent of an early series from our medical center in which the majority of patients were undergoing treatment for anterior circulation aneurysms.[303] Despite the fact that aneurysm sites in the anterior circulation are somewhat more accessible for remedial measures should hemorrhage develop, only 62 percent of the patients in our series made favorable neurological recoveries. Obviously this circumstance even in anterior circulation aneurysms is one that carries substantial risk to the patient and should be avoided at all cost. As previously mentioned, the development of hemorrhage from the interpeduncular cistern even of seemingly trivial magnitude immediately obscures perforator anatomy and is a significant technical challenge to manage. While in our opinion gentle tamponade should always be the mainstay of therapy, brain-protective agents should be administered at that time if not previously and preparations made for temporary arterial occlusion if approximately 5 minutes of tamponade does not abate the hemorrhage. Definitive clipping of an actively bleeding carotid, middle cerebral, or anterior communicating aneurysm is possible and not very dangerous. This maneuver is quite hazardous for the patient with a basilar apex aneurysm due to the limited visibility of perforator anatomy. Great emphasis should be placed on prevention of this complication, and in our opinion temporary arterial occlusion together with meticulous sharp dissection techniques probably represent the safest possible alternative for the patient currently available (Table 30-23).

It is our early impression that the endovascular interventional neuroradiologist offers substantial expertise in dealing with aneurysms of the basilar apex.

This region is easily accessible by current catheter technology, and the delivery of platinum microcoils into basilar aneurysms of all sizes is quite feasible. It is our hope that patients thus treated will be followed aggressively to document the long-term results of what must anatomically represent incomplete aneurysm conclusion. In addition to the small areas of residual neck that are often left patent, it is questionable whether re-endothelialization will occur as it does following clip occlusion. With these reservations, this technology offers substantial benefit to patients who are gravely ill neurologically from their hemorrhage as a means to prevent rebleeding during their initial recovery, medically ill patients who are not candidates for general anesthesia, and certain patients with particularly difficult recurrent giant basilar aneurysms in whom re-exploration carries substantial morbidity.

The aggressive temporal lobe retraction necessary during the subtemporal approach can be poorly tolerated in the acute subarachnoid hemorrhage patient. At completion of the procedure, the lobe should be very carefully inspected, and, if significant mottling or edema is noted, an inferior temporal lobe resection or in more severe cases an anterior temporal lobectomy should be seriously contemplated. The trivial morbidity associated with these maneuvers is a small price to pay when considering the potentially lethal complications of an expanding middle cranial fossa mass (Table 30-24).

The vein of Labbé is a structure to be respected in all procedures involving temporal lobe retraction. Protracted occlusions of this structure during temporal lobe elevation or a permanent laceration will frequently give rise to extensive venous infarction and subsequent edema and hemorrhage into the temporal lobe. We suggest placement of moist cotton patties or Gelfoam surrounding the termination of the vein into the transverse or sigmoid sinus prior to retraction to prevent this complication (Table 30-24). We have seen complications in basilar bifurcation giant aneurysms that may have resulted from overaggressive efforts at evacuating thrombus and clot from within the lumen after clipping.[304] This problem may have resulted from perforating vessel compromise as the giant sac collapsed. Perhaps an argument can be made for a more conservative approach to the decompressive aspect of surgery for giant basilar aneurysm particularly in the patient not disabled by mass effect symptoms (Table 30-23). Follow-up of patients with giant carotid aneurysms treated without aneurysm evacuation have shown that many spontaneously lose volume over time.[342]

Table 30-24. Intraoperative Complications

Etiology	Avoidance/Management

Temporal lobe injury	Avoidance
	    Preserve Labbé
	    Willingness to resect inferior temporal gyrus at
	        primary procedure.
	Management
	    Delayed resection if mass lesion develops

Delayed ischemia (vasospasm)	Avoidance
	    Calcium channel blockers?
	    Prophyllactic angioplasty?
	Management
	    Maintain hypervolemia, hemodilution
	    Immediate use of pressors once symptoms
	        appear
	    Angioplasty for medical failures
	    Calcium channel blockers?

Complications from vasospasm therapy
  Progressing edema
	Avoidance
	    Stop hyperdynamic therapy when ICP in-
	        creases or mass effect develops
	Management
	    Diuresis
	    Resection

Recurrent aneurysms	Avoidance
	    Early angioplasty?
	Management
	    Direct repair?
	    Endovascular repair?
	    No therapy?

Symptomatic Vasospasm

Ischemic injury due to vasospasm remains the major cause of death and disability following subarachnoid hemorrhage. Approximately 14 percent of all subarachnoid hemorrhage patients ultimately suffer severe neurological consequences.[326,328] Chui et al.[307] have earlier suggested that vasospasm from vertebrobasilar aneurysms tends to be focal rather than generalized. This has not been our experience, and we have found that patients tend to become symptomatic in cerebral regions predictable from their posthemorrhage CT scan.[317] While the therapeutic keystones of hypertensive/hypervolemic therapy are frequently effective in reversing neurological deficits, failure of this medical therapy has led us to pursue other alternatives, including revascularization.[300] The potential of the endovascular radiologist to access this region rapidly and by quickly performing angioplasty to augment the vascular diameter of the basilar and posterior cerebral arteries offers an attractive alternative to more radical medical therapies, including barbiturate coma. It is our current practice to maintain postoperative patients in a

mildly volume expanded and hemodiluted state, and pressors are initiated at the time ischemic signs develop. If the patient does not immediately respond to hypertension and additional volume, angioplasty is undertaken. This regimen obviously mandates early surgery for securing of the aneurysm and the incorporation of the endovascular radiologist as an integral component of the management team. In our opinion, the endovascular option should be pursued early rather than late in an attempt to augment flow prior to the establishment of cerebral infarction (Table 30-24).

There is good evidence that therapeutic hypertension and hypervolemia offer a substantial chance for salvage of ischemic neurologic tissue in the setting of cerebral vasospasm.[305,316,325,330] Unfortunately, this therapy is not always entirely safe. In addition to the cardiovascular complications and intracranial hemorrhage that have been well described,[320,325,350] our basilar aneurysm series has been complicated by progressive and malignant cerebral edema as well as by the presumed mechanical induction of recurrent aneurysms (Table 30-24). In our opinion, the complication of cerebral edema is due to persistent aggressive hypertension and hypervolemic therapy in the setting of established infarction. CT evidence of mass affect and any increase in ICP must be taken as certain evidence that extracellular fluid is beginning to accumulate and that further hyperdynamic insult to this tissue will result in the conversion of a patient with a focal neurological deficit into one with a life-threatening complication. It is now our standard practice to begin intermittent diuresis and to stop pressor therapy immediately when either of these two signs develop.

The use of hypertensive/hypervolemic therapy over protracted intervals in occasional patients has resulted in angiographically documented recurrent aneurysmal sacs.[298,304] This phenomenon probably represents an iatrogenic acceleration of the evolution of small "dog ears" left at the time of aneurysm clipping. It remains unknown whether years of normotension in the future will result in regression or stabilization of these new sacs. We are currently conservative about offering re-exploration in the early weeks following the development of this complication. We believe that vigilant angiographic follow-up is probably the safest alternative for the patient.

SUMMARY

Perhaps the most obvious evidence that basilar aneurysms pose persistent and unique challenges to the neurosurgeon lies in the relative simplicity with which we currently evaluate patients with anterior circulation pathology. The surgeon's judgment is exercised chiefly in evaluating the issue of surgical timing with consideration of the patient's clinical grade and risk of symptomatic vasospasm by CT criteria. The rupture of a basilar bifurcation aneurysm by contrast also requires careful consideration of the timing of operation, complicated in this situation not only by clinical grade but also by specific anatomical detail and its impact on the operative approach to be offered. The use of temporary arterial occlusion remains a major source of controversy, particularly regarding maximum length of safe occlusion, optimal position of temporary clips, and whether or not brain-protective regimens are of benefit. In addition, controversy exists regarding which aneurysms are not surgically treatable and once that decision is made whether the patient should be referred to the interventional radiologist or whether his future should be left up to the natural history of the disease. This relative complexity requires careful consideration of known natural history data, specific anatomical information relative to the individual patient, and intimate familiarity with the various operative and nonoperative therapeutic techniques available. Only repetitive experience and thoughtful insight into the advantages and limitations of each therapeutic alternative will allow the neurosurgeon to offer the patient the optimal opportunity for a successful neurological outcome.

Posterior Cerebral and Superior Cerebellar Artery Aneurysms
David G. Piepgras

Aneurysms of the posterior cerebral (PCA) and superior cerebellar (SCA) arteries are uncommon vascular lesions, the former contributing 1 to 2 percent of the aneurysms in several major series.[367,381,385,387] Even more rare are aneurysms arising from the SCA proper (those arising from the basilar trunk/SCA junction appropriately being classified as basilar artery aneurysms). Yasargil[387] found only two peripheral SCA aneurysms in his series of greater than 1,000 cases, and in our Mayo series of approximately 1,750 aneurysms there were three SCA trunk aneurysms treated, each of these arising on the proximal or pontomesencephalic segment of the SCA trunk.[385]

This discussion focuses primarily on the unique features of these aneurysms, their surgical management, and an analysis of the problems that have been encountered as reported in the literature and in our own experience. Hopefully this review will allow a better anticipation of management risks and their avoidance.

ANATOMY

Posterior Cerebral Artery

A sound understanding of the vascular anatomy and macrocirculation is of obvious importance in successfully dealing with aneurysms at any site. Several anatomical schemes have been proposed for classification of the segments of the PCA, and its pathology. The descriptions of Krayenbuhl and Yasargil[374] divide the PCA into four segments, designated P_1 through P_4. This system is simple and functional and is utilized in this discussion (Figs. 30-129 and 30-130). For detailed studies on the anatomy of the PCA, the reader should consult the papers of Zeal and

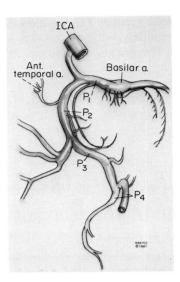

Figure 30-129. Segmental divisions of PCA anatomy according to the system of Krayenbuhl and Yasargil.[374] (By permission of Mayo Foundation.)

Rhoton,[388] Pedroza et al.,[378] and Margolis et al.[375] It should be remembered that there can be considerable variation from the norm, particularly if vascular pathology exists. The first rule toward minimizing complications for a particular surgical case is not only to understand the vascular anatomy as it normally exists but also to have an optimal definition angiographically and to maintain mental flexibility for subtle variations from the norm during the vascular dissection.

Posterior Communicating and P₁ Segments

The PCA takes origin from the basilar artery in the majority of instances although will arise from the internal carotid artery (ICA) in a fetal configuration

unilaterally in approximately 20 percent and bilaterally in approximately 8 percent of cases.[372,386] Whether large or small, the posterior communicating artery gives rise to perforating vessels, notably for this review, those to the mamillary bodies and the retromamillary perforated substance.

The segment of the PCA from its origin from the basilar artery to the posterior communicating artery (PCoA) has been termed the *P₁ segment* by Krayenbuhl and Yasargil[374] and is also referred to as the *proximal peduncular* or *precommunicating segment*. Drake[367] has called attention to the compound curve that this segment of the artery takes as it arises forward and outward to cross the third nerve before turning around the peduncle. Taking origin from the P₁ segments are one or more thalamoperforating branches. These branches typically arise from the posterior or superior aspect of the proximal P₁ segment as one or two trunks. Individual variation may exist, however, with none or multiple trunks being present.[378] These perforators enter the posterior perforated substance and interpeduncular fossa to nourish the anterior and posterior thalamus, the hypothalamus and subthalamus, posterior internal capsule, substantia nigra, red nucleus, and portions of the rostral mesencephalon.[375,388] The critical need for identification and preservation of these branches has been emphasized by Drake[367] and constitutes a major contribution in the progress of vertebrobasilar aneurysm surgery. Their occlusion may produce a variety of neurological deficits oftentimes devastating to the patient, including contralateral hemiplegia, abnormal ocular motility, and major disturbances of consciousness.[388]

Short and long circumflex perforating arteries arise from the P₁ and P₂ segments and encircle the midbrain, medial to the PCA trunk, as they course to the

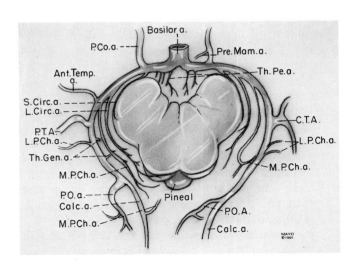

Figure 30-130. Diagrammatic portrayal of PCA anatomy as viewed from inferiorly, showing major segments, circumflex and perforating branches. *PCo a*, posterior communicating artery; *Pre Mama*, premamillary artery; *Ant Temp a*, anterior temporal artery; *Th Pe a*, thalamo perforating arteries; *S Circ a*, short circumflex arteries; *L Circ a*, long circumflex arteries; *PTA*, posterior temporal artery; *CTA*, common temporal artery; *L PCh a*, lateral posterior choroidal arteries; *M PCh a*, medial posterior choroidal arteries; *Th Gen a*, thalamogeniculate arteries; *POA*, parieto occipital artery; *Calc a*, calcarine artery. (By permission of Mayo Foundation, and as modified from Zeal and Rhoton,[388] with permission.)

geniculate and quadrigeminal bodies, respectively. Thrombosis or surgical compromise of these branches could result in visual field defects or, in the case of the quadrigeminal branches, deficits in vertical gaze.[388]

P₂ Segment

Distal to the entrance of the PCoA, the PCA arches laterally and posteriorly between the hippocampal gyrus and midbrain within the ambient cistern. In this course it typically crosses above the tentorial margin to lie below the basal vein of Rosenthal and above the fourth nerve and SCA. This ambient segment of the PCA back to the major inferior temporal trunk has been designated the P₂ segment. Branches from this segment include several thalamogeniculate arteries and direct peduncular branches that directly penetrate the cerebral peduncle to supply the corticospinal and corticobulbar pathways. The former group of arteries perfuse the posterolateral thalamus, the posterior limb of the internal capsule, the geniculate body, and optic tracts. Interruption of these branches results in thalamic infarction which, if extensive, may be accompanied by loss of contralateral sensation and possible hyperpathic pain (Dejerine-Roussy syndrome) as well as hemiplegia, chorioathetosis, and homonymous hemianopsia.[388] Medial and lateral posterior choroidal arteries also typically arise from the P₂ segment, the medial group usually originating from the anterior one-half of the segment while the lateral groups arise more posteriorly. They provide vascular supply to the choroid plexus of the lateral ventricle, but also may send branches to the peduncle, thalamus, and colliculi.

P₃ Segment

Krayenbuhl and Yasargil[374] have designated the P₃ PCA segment as that portion of the vessel distal to the major inferior (posterior) temporal branch extending to the origin of the parieto-occipital and calcarine branches. The P₃ segment therefore typically travels in the posterior ambient cistern to the quadrigeminal cistern. For angiographic reference it should be remembered that the PCAs approach each other in the quadrigeminal cistern and on the frontal projection of the angiogram reach their closest proximity with an average separation of 1 to 2 cm.[375] Typically the PCA trunk then continues posteriorly beneath the splenium of the corpus callosum to terminate in the parieto-occipital and calcarine branches. Variations are not uncommon, and in the study of Zeal and Rhoton[388] the parieto-occipital artery was found to

arise with almost equal frequency from the P₂ and P₃ segments.

P₄ Segments

Cortical P₄ branches include the inferior temporal branches, the parieto-occipital and calcarine arteries, as well as the splenial artery, which most often arises as a branch from the parieto-occipital trunk. The supply of these branches is generally well known and will not be specified in this discussion other than to emphasize that not only the calcarine but also the parieto-occipital arteries contribute supply to the visual cortex. Finally, it is important to remember the extensive leptomeningeal collaterals that exist between the distal cortical branches of the posterior cerebral, anterior, and middle cerebral arteries. In addition, there are anastomoses between choroidal and SCA branches. These anastomoses are notable in providing luxurient collateral flow into the PCA branches and averting infarction in cases of proximal PCA occlusion or thrombosis (Fig. 30-131).[377]

Superior Cerebellar Artery

Aneurysms of the SCA are very rarely encountered, and this discussion of the SCA anatomy will accordingly be capsulized. Following a course inferior to the PCA in the prepontine and perimesencephalic cisterns, the SCA gives rise in its lateral course to a marginal branch and more medially to hemispheric, vermian, and precentral cerebellar arteries. Perforating branches arise from the proximal SCA trunk to supply portions of the pons and midbrain, while perforators off the marginal branch contribute to the dentate nucleus and superior and middle cerebellar peduncles. In the quadrigeminal cistern, fine perforating branches reach to the inferior caliculi. For a more detailed presentation of the gross and radiographic anatomy, the reader is referred to the discussion of Hoffman et al.[371]

CLINICAL FEATURES

Although PCA aneurysms represent only a small fraction of intracranial aneurysms, the literature concerning these lesions indicates that they have particular clinical features as well as a tendency for certain anatomical characteristics that warrant special consideration. The series of cases reported by Drake[367] and Yasargil[387] as well as those collected by Pia and Fontana[381] indicate that the majority of PCA aneu-

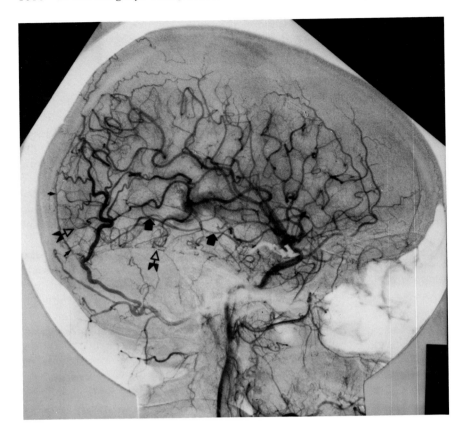

Figure 30-131. Right ICA angiogram (lateral view) following clipping of small right ICA aneurysm and trapping of a giant right P_2 aneurysm. The study shows rapid retrograde filling of the PCA trunk (bold arrows) via leptomeningeal middle cerebral artery collaterals in the occipital and temporal regions (open arrows). The small arrows posteriorly indicate an external carotid dural branch that also contributes collateral flow to the PCA. These collateral channels were well developed in the preoperative angiogram as well, and it was anticipated that the patient would tolerate proximal PCA occlusion if necessary. Aneurysm trapping was carried out with no resultant neurological deficit.

rysms are found on the proximal portion of the PCA, namely, the P_1 and P_2 segments. In our series of 32 cases of PCA aneurysms, if the three mycotic aneurysms (peripherally located on P_4 branches) are excluded, two-thirds of the aneurysms were located along the P_1 and P_2 segments.[385]

As with intracranial aneurysms at other sites, subarachnoid hemorrhage is the most frequent presenting symptom, occurring in 76 percent of the reported cases reviewed by Zeal and Rhoton.[388] With or without hemorrhage, for those aneurysms located on the proximal PCA, there may be associated signs of third nerve palsy and contralateral hemiparesis, owing to the proximity and involvement of the third nerve as well as direct injury to the cerebral peduncle and/or adjacent perforating branches. Symptoms of focal mass effect in the anterolateral tentorial region may also develop and progress related to giant aneurysm formation. Dandy[365] observed the tendencies for aneurysms of the PCA to reach large dimensions and to mimic a neoplasm. Although it has been stated that there may be a predilection for PCA aneurysms to reach giant proportions compared with aneurysms at other sites, this may reflect a bias in case referral and reports rather than fact. In the collected cases of Pia and Fontana[381] 9 of 40 PCA aneurysms (22 percent)

were described as "giant" (larger than 2 cm). In Drake's reports[366,367] of vertebrobasilar system and giant aneurysms compiled in 1978, only 2.4 percent of the combined vertebrobasilar aneurysm series were PCA aneurysms, but almost one-third of these were of giant proportions. Of note is the observation that all of the P_1 giant aneurysms were fusiform, whereas those from P_2 were saccular, characteristics having major implications for their surgical treatment alternatives.[366] In a review of 10 patients with 13 PCA aneurysms, Chang et al.[364] found 6 to be saccular, 5 fusiform, 1 broad based, and 1 giant and fusiform. All but one of these were located along the P_1 and P_2 segments.

Among the 29 nonmycotic PCA aneurysms treated in our series on the cerebrovascular services of the Mayo Clinic, 12 were classed as giant saccular, 2 as fusiform, and 3 as giant/fusiform. Also, one-half of our cases had partial thrombosis of the aneurysm sac[385] (Figs. 30-132 and 30-133).

Finally, the experience with collected cases reveals that the PCA is a relatively common site for aneurysms in young people, and many of these are giant in size.[366,369,376] In summary, while PCA aneurysms are uncommon, when encountered they are usually along the P_1 and P_2 portions of the artery,

Figure 30-132. Contrasted CT scan of a 20-year-old male with a history of progressive headache and numb sensations on the right side of the body; the large enhancing mass arising in the left ambient cistern proved to be a partially thrombosed giant aneurysm.

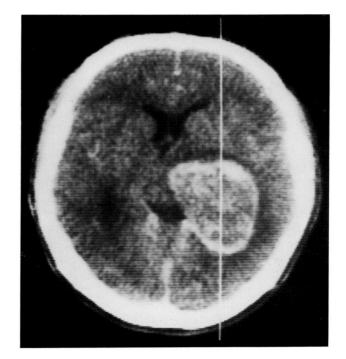

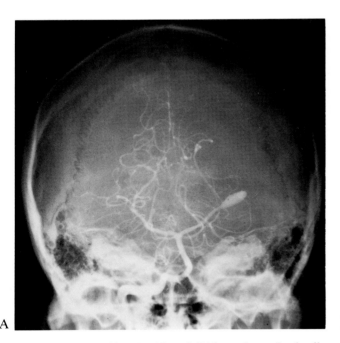

A

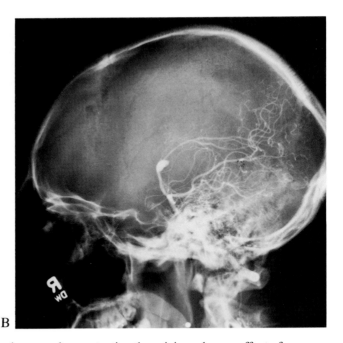

B

Figure 30-133. (A) AP and (B) lateral vertebrobasilar angiograms demonstrating the origin and mass effect of the giant aneurysm shown in Fig. 30-132. The neck was located at the P_2-P_3 junction and the origin of the posterior temporal branch. The aneurysm was exposed through a left subtemporal craniotomy and the P_2 segment temporarily clipped. Thrombectomy of the aneurysm was then accomplished to allow development of an aneurysm neck that could be successfully clipped with preservation of the PCA trunk. The patient had a transient postoperative right hemiparesis that resolved.

have a tendency to be complicated in size and form, and account for a significant proportion of the giant aneurysms that occur in childhood.

PERIOPERATIVE RISKS AND COMPLICATIONS

To minimize operative risks and complications, the neurosurgeon must be well versed in the major difficulties attending the planned treatment. Review of operative series of PCA (and SCA) aneurysms by various authors as well as a detailed analysis of our own experience with 32 cases over the past 10 years provide insight into the problems that can occur. Table 30-25 summarizes the major surgical complications in the order of their magnitude for potential harm to the patient and frequency of occurrence. Also listed are those factors that most likely affect their occurrence.

PCA Perforating Branch Ischemia

Perforating artery injury and resultant diencephalic and mesencephalic focal infarction undoubtedly constitutes the major risk and source of complications in dealing with PCA aneurysms. As indicated in the preliminary discussion of the anatomy of the PCA, the majority of the perforating vessels arise from the P_1 and proximal P_2 segments of the PCA. Sacrifice of one or several perforating branches, as may occur with clipping or, especially, trapping of a P_1 or P_2 PCA aneurysm, may not preclude an excellent outcome for the patient. Review of the published series as well as of our own experience reveals many patients who have early postoperative deficits, such as hemiparesis, confusion, and visual field cut, go on to complete recovery. Although these are usually attributed to "retraction and swelling," late postoperative CT scans in these patients often reveal lacunar-type infarctions in the diencephalon, and a more likely etiology is ischemia secondary to perforator compromise. As already mentioned, however, devastating irreversible infarction may result from compromise of a single dominant thalamoperforating trunk, and the surgeon must make a concerted effort to identify and preserve every perforating vessel along the involved segment.

Considering the fact that there are a large proportion of P_1 and P_2 aneurysms that are of a giant and fusiform nature and not amenable to simple clipping of the neck, and thus often require proximal

Table 30-25.   Major Perioperative Complications and Causative Factors Attending Operative Repair of PCA and SCA Aneurysms[362,364,367,369,380,381,385,387]

Complication	Causation
Ischemia	

Perforating arteries, especially thalamoperforating, thalamogeniculate, direct peduncular, and circumflex perforating arteries	Especially P_1 and P_2 aneurysms
	     Direct occlusion with aneurysm clipping or trapping
	     Propagated thrombus after No. 1
	     Intraoperative temporary occlusion

Cortical arteries, temporal, parieto-occipital, calcarine, splenial PCA branches, hemispheric SCA branches	Especially P_2 and P_3 aneurysms
	     Direct branch occlusion with neck clipping or trapping
	     Inadequate collateral or propagated thrombus after proximal PCA occlusion

Nerve injury	
Oculomotor (III)	Especially P_1 prox. P_2 aneurysm Direct injury—traction, contusion
Trochlear (IV)	Especially P_2, P_3, and SCA Direct injury—traction, laceration, incl. section of tentorium
Temporal lobe injury, edema, and ICH	Excess retraction pressure Failure to achieve "slack brain"; prolonged, fixed retraction; inadequate subtemporal exposure Venous compromise, sacrifice, or retractor pressure Arterial ischemia, branch occlusion, hypotension, retractor pressure
Premature rupture of aneurysm, uncontrolled hemorrhage	Exposure and dissection techniques
Seizures	Lack of perioperative anticonvulsants; temporal lobe injury
Recurrent hemorrhage	Delayed surgery, especially mycotic aneurysm

edema and hemorrhage. Foremost would be those related to retraction of the temporal lobe, which must necessarily be deep to explore the PCA at the tentorial margin. Indeed, more and deeper retraction may be necessary to expose the PCA than the basilar caput, owing to the anatomical fact that the artery in its perimesencephalic course is covered by the hippocampal gyrus. This structure must be elevated to expose the P_2 and P_3 segments, making for a more difficult exposure. Drake[367] and Peerless and Drake[379] have stressed the importance of both operating with a slack brain to minimize retraction pressure on the temporal lobe and combining mannitol-induced diuresis, CSF drainage, and moderate hyperventilation to achieve this. Recent subarachnoid hemorrhage and secondary swelling may work against the ability to achieve good brain relaxation, though this can usually be overcome with the aforementioned measures. Duration of retraction may also be a major factor and must be kept in mind when deciding between surgical alternatives such as the relatively simple proximal PCA occlusion or trapping or the prolonged reconstruction of the PCA.

Venous compromise by either deliberate sacrifice of inferior temporal veins or their avulsion, obstruction, or thrombosis due to retractor blades undoubtedly is a major contributing factor to temporal lobe edema and hemorrhage. Utmost care must be taken to protect and preserve all veins possible, especially the vein of Labbé. Arterial ischemia may also be causative or aggravate temporal lobe edema and hemorrhage. Ischemia may be related to sacrifice or thrombosis of inferior temporal arteries with the aneurysm repair and also with intraoperative hypotension, especially if coupled with strong retractor pressure. A final factor worthy of consideration relates to our impression that the temporal lobe seemingly has poorer tolerance to direct lateral retraction compared with more anterior subtemporal elevation and posterior displacement. The latter is utilized in the modified pterion or "half-and-half" approach applicable to P_1 and anterior P_2 segment aneurysms, whereas the former (direct lateral subtemporal approach) is necessary for P_2 and P_3 segment aneurysms.[384]

Premature Aneurysm Rupture

In aneurysm surgery at all locations, premature aneurysm rupture and uncontrolled hemorrhage is a major contributor to complications, and techniques must be utilized throughout the preparation and exposure to minimize this risk. General principles for aneurysm surgery apply, including exposure and dissection that allow proximal control before the aneurysm itself is approached and utilization of temporary clipping or trapping to allow dissection of a nonturgid aneurysm (Figs. 30-136, 30-138, below). Other dissection techniques aimed at minimizing aneurysm rupture are beyond the scope of this discussion, but the reader is referred to the elegant discussions of Yasargil[386] and Sugita and Kobayashi.[383]

Postoperative Seizures

Usually seizures are not considered a major complication; however, their occurrence in the early postoperative period raises immediate concern regarding the possibility of postoperative clot, and in themselves seizures can be a source for hypoxia and increased intracranial pressure, which may cause or contribute to major morbidity. The risk for postoperative seizures is undoubtedly higher in cases of subtemporal exposure as opposed to transsylvian or subfrontal approaches. For this reason, administration of prophylactic anticonvulsants (usually phenytoin) perioperatively is advocated for patients undergoing surgery for repair of these aneurysms. In our series of 29 cases of PCA aneurysm operated on via the subtemporal approach, four patients had postoperative seizures in spite of anticonvulsant prophylaxis.[385] In none of these cases was the seizures a cause for additional morbidity, and three of the four cases had excellent outcome. In the fourth patient there was a complicating subdural and intracerebral hemorrhage that undoubtedly caused not only the seizure but the poor outcome as well.

Recurrent Hemorrhage

The final complication to be considered with an aim toward avoidance is not usually operative but preoperative, namely, recurrent aneurysmal hemorrhage. Nowadays this dreaded complication is effectively reduced in its frequency by early surgery to repair the aneurysm, which is generally advocated for good grade patients with uncomplicated anterior circulation aneurysms. Such an approach has not been widely utilized for posterior circulation aneurysms, although in experienced hands the morbidity has not been increased.[380] Extra caution must be applied, however, in surgery for complicated and giant aneurysms for which the benefits of early surgery may be outweighed by the increased risks accompanying a swollen brain or an inexperienced surgical team. As we have seen, PCA aneurysms are often complicated in their size, form, and location, and, along with their infrequency of occurrence, these factors necessitate cautious surgical planning.

Mycotic aneurysms would seem to constitute an exception to the foregoing, owing to their truly unpredictable nature for devastating recurrent hemorrhage. In our series of 32 PCA aneurysms, three were mycotic due to bacterial endocarditis.[385] Each arose from a P$_4$ branch and presented with hemorrhage, either subarachnoid or intraventricular, and each suf-

fered a major recurrent intracerebral hemorrhage while being treated with antibiotics and stabilized prior to planned craniotomy. Emergency surgery became necessary to salvage the patient. In each case obliteration of the aneurysm was easily accomplished after evacuation of the clot. The outcome was poor in two cases and good in one. These recurrent hemorrhages have led us to advocate early intervention in cases of mycotic aneurysm that have hemorrhaged.

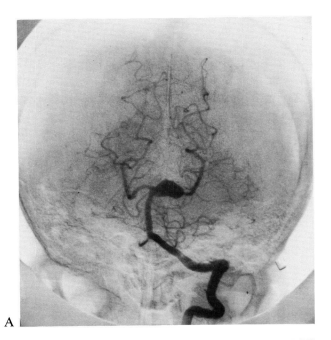

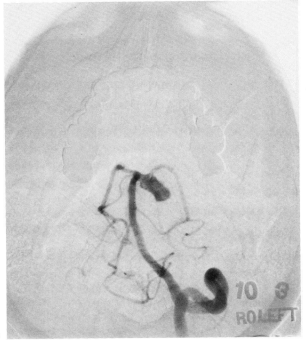

Figure 30-134. AP angiograms of a giant, partially thrombosed, left P$_1$ segment aneurysm. The Towne view **(A)** did not demonstrate the origin of the aneurysm as clearly as the submental-vertex view **(B)**. **(C)** A straight AP view of the aneurysm shows the thrombus filled sac as determined on CT scan and at surgery, outlined in black.

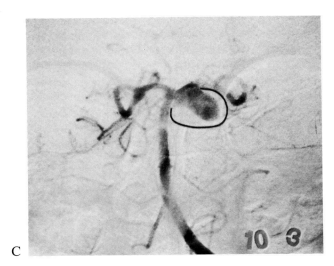

PREOPERATIVE EVALUATION

Because of the tendency for PCA aneurysms to be large and have complicated features, including broad neck, fusiform sac, and intra-aneurysmal thrombosis, optimal preoperative assessment must include noncontrasted and contrasted CT scans or MRI in addition to high-quality selective angiography. Obviously, both carotid and vertebrobasilar systems must be studied, as PCA aneurysms can be perfused by the carotid system, the vertebrobasilar system, or both. Also, because of the tendency for PCA and SCA aneurysms to be superimposed on anteroposterior and lateral views of the angiogram, oblique views and submental vertex views may be necessary to identify the exact site of the neck (Figs. 30-134 and 30-135).[377]

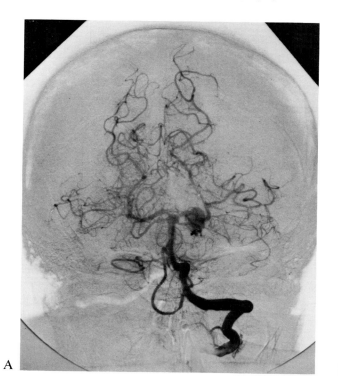

A

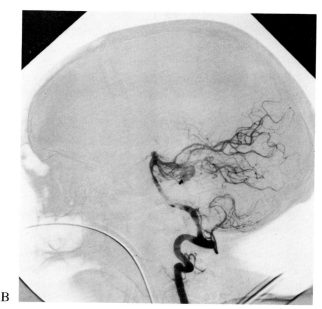

B

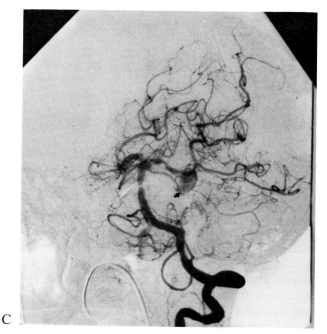

C

Figure 30-135. (A) AP, **(B)** lateral, and **(C)** oblique vertebrobasilar angiograms demonstrating a large left superior cerebellar artery aneurysm. Confusion as to the origin of this aneurysm (PCA vs. SCA) is resolved on the oblique angiogram, which confirms the neck (small arrows) on the ambient segment of the SCA.

It is critical that the location of aneurysms arising from the distal PCA (P_3 and $P3_4$ segments) be correctly identified on preoperative studies, as those aneurysms in the ambient cistern (P_3 segment) will usually be exposed best from a subtemporal approach whereas a posterior interhemispheric approach is necessary for those at the P_3-P_4 junction in the quadrigeminal cistern.

SURGICAL APPROACHES AND TECHNIQUES

Patient preparation for PCA and SCA aneurysm surgery follows those principles for aneurysm surgery at other sites. In cases that have sustained subarachnoid hemorrhage, attention must be paid to optimal blood volume expansion with colloid and crystalloids. As already mentioned, timing for surgery should be individualized, depending on the patient's condition, the complexity of the aneurysm, and the availability of the optimal surgical team. Anticonvulsant prophylaxis is initiated preoperatively for all patients undergoing subtemporal approaches.

Proximal PCA and SCA Aneurysms

For aneurysms located on the proximal and middle segments of the PCA and SCA, the operation is carried out with the patient in the recumbent position with a lumbar drain in place. Our preferred approach to aneurysms located on the proximal segments of the PCA (P_1 and P_1-P_2) and proximal SCA is through a modified pterion craniotomy, whereas those on the middle segments or ambient portions of these vessels (P_2 and P_2-P_3) have been more suitably exposed through a direct subtemporal approach as advocated by Sundt[384] and Drake.[367]

Modified Pterion, Anterior Temporal Approach

The modified pterion, anterior temporal exposure is versatile and has been called the "half-and-half" approach by Drake[367] because of its modification from a pterion transsylvian to an anterior (but not lateral) subtemporal approach. We have preferred it when exposing the region of the anterior tentorial foramen and upper basilar artery because the exposure can be wide and because of the seemingly better tolerance of the anterior temporal lobe to elevation and posterior displacement.[384] The patient is positioned supine, with the head and shoulders elevated

above the heart. The head is secured in a three-point head holder and rotated 30 degrees away from the side of surgery and perhaps slightly flexed to afford a view down the posterior clinoid process and clivus. The skin incision and craniotomy are diagrammed in Fig. 30-136A&B.

In addition to a classical pterion craniotomy with removal of the lateral sphenoid wing, bone removal is extended posteriorly and subtemporally along the floor of the middle fossa to allow optimal exposure beneath the temporal lobe with the least amount of retraction possible. During the craniotomy, mannitol (up to 1 g/kg body weight) diuresis is induced, and, with opening the dura, slow withdrawal of CSF via a lumbar needle is begun to ensure a slack brain as the exposure progresses. The dura is opened and secured to the bone margins to minimize epidural bleeding, and the remainder of the surgery is carried out with the aid of the operating microscope. It is usually helpful to open the sylvian fissure to facilitate elevation of the temporal lobe; however, in cases in which the fissure is poorly developed, it is possible to proceed without this step inasmuch as the "half-and-half" approach will be under the temporal tip rather than through the fissure (Fig. 30-136C&D).

The anterior temporal veins to the sphenoparietal sinus are carefully exposed and each coagulated and divided to ensure that the anterior temporal lobe may be fully elevated. Medial sylvian veins entering the sinus should also be sacrificed rather than retracted under tension and risk their avulsion and profuse hemorrhage at a later time when aneurysm dissection is underway. Veins off the inferior surface of the anterior temporal lobe may also be safely sacrificed, though more posterior veins should be carefully protected.

Temporal retraction must proceed slowly with further removal of CSF through the lumbar needle as necessary to ensure adequate brain relaxation. The brain surface under the retractor is carefully protected with Gelfoam and one layer of cottonoid, the former providing the best "nonstick" protection to the cortex. The anterior clinoid process, internal carotid and posterior communicating arteries, and tentorial margin are identified as the exposure is developed. The arachnoid overlying the third and fourth nerves is carefully opened with sharp dissection with care taken to avoid injury to the underlying vessels and aneurysm. Care must be taken at this time to ensure that the tip of the retractor elevating the temporal lobe and uncus does not compromise the internal carotid, middle cerebral, or posterior communicating arteries or avulse small arterial branches to the temporal lobe.

To facilitate the exposure, it is preferable to elevate the free margin of the tentorium with a suture positioned just anterior but free of the fourth nerve insertion and secured to the adjacent middle fossa dura (Fig. 30-136E&F). This retraction is usually sufficient to allow good exposure of the basilar caput and P_1 and proximal P_2 segments without dividing the tentorium, a maneuver often causing significant bleeding from the vascular channels within the tentorial margin. Dissection of the aneurysm must proceed with caution under moderate hypotension (90 to 100 mmHg systolic), but profound lowering of the blood pressure should be avoided if at all possible. Often the aneurysm anatomy cannot be easily discerned and especially for identification of the perforating branches and exposure of the aneurysm neck it is preferable to carry out temporary proximal occlusion of the PCA or even the distal basilar artery if necessary to facilitate this dissection. If temporary occlusion is planned, especially for the proximal basilar artery, it is advisable first to restore the blood pressure to normal levels. To optimize cerebral protection during the period of temporary occlusion, it is also desirable either to administer barbiturate (thiopental 3 to 5 mg/kg) or, theoretically better, to raise the level of a protective anesthetic agent (isoflurane) during the time of occlusion. Finally, prolonged periods of temporary occlusion (greater than 10 minutes) are generally avoided in favor of intermittent periods of temporary occlusion and reperfusion.

In certain instances, satisfactory exposures of P_1 or P_{1-2} segment aneurysms may be facilitated by ligation and division of a small PCoA. Careful consideration and study of the anatomy and aneurysm must be done before carrying out this maneuver so as to ensure protection of the perforating vessels that arise from the PCoA as well as preserving this vessel as a collateral source to the PCA if P_1 trapping becomes necessary.

It should be kept in mind, particularly with aneurysms at this proximal site on the PCA, that as they enlarge to near giant size they are often fusiform or without a discernible neck so that direct clipping is not possible. In these cases proximal occlusion or trapping is the only alternative and can often be carried out safely, provided critical perforating branches are protected (Fig. 30-136G–I). In cases in which trapping is to be done, the isolated segment should be reduced as much as possible by opening and emptying the sac and then reapplying clips as closely as possible to the aneurysm and ensuring that as many perforating branches as possible are perfused. Especially at this proximal location, attention must be fo-

cused on thalamoperforating and circumflex arteries, which may be difficult to identify when the anatomy is obscured by a large aneurysm and overlying hemorrhage. For giant aneurysms that have been trapped (or successfully clipped) opening and decompression of the aneurysm is also preferable to allow maximal decompression of the adjacent structures. Thrombus must be removed gently so as to avoid traction forces on arterial branches and brain and may be facilated by use of an ultrasonic aspirator. As a rule it is preferable to leave the decompressed aneurysm sac in situ rather than to excise it.

Midposition PCA and SCA Aneurysms

Aneurysms of the middle segments of the PCA (Fig. 30-137) and SCA must be exposed through a lateral subtemporal or "Drake" approach, which is diagrammed in Fig. 30-138A&B. The details of this exposure and subtleties to minimizing trauma to the brain and maximizing visualization of the tentorial aperture have been well described by Drake[367] and by Sundt.[384] Several points aimed at minimizing complications deserve emphasis, the first being proper patient positioning with head and shoulders elevated above the heart to facilitate venous drainage. The head position can be slightly rotated upward for more proximal PCA and SCA exposure but for those more posteriorly (P_3) no rotation is advisable. The sagittal plane of the head is parallel to or angled toward the floor only slightly. A craniotomy under a horseshoe scalp flap carried over the ear is preferable for exposure of the perimesencephalic segments of the PCA and SCA. Care must be taken that the posterior burr hole avoid the top of the sigmoid sinus and also that the exposed mastoid air cells are carefully sealed.

Good brain relaxation with mannitol- or furosemide-induced diuresis and CSF drainage is of paramount importance, as are protection of the temporal lobe and more posterior draining veins, especially the vein of Labbé, as retraction progresses. As already stated, the careful application of Gelfoam over the surface of the brain and around the veins has been most helpful in producing a nonadherent protective covering under cottonoids, though protection of the vein of Labbé also necessitates its being visualized enough to ensure that traction is not excessive. Disruption or thrombosis of this vein, especially in the dominant hemisphere, can lead to hemorrhagic infarction and major neurological deficits, and its protection cannot be stressed enough.

Because of its elevated position above the tentorial margin, exposure of the PCA in its ambient location

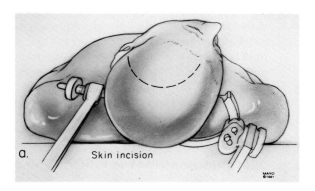

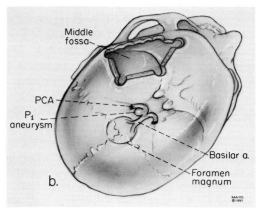

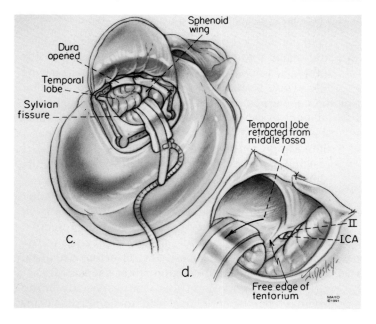

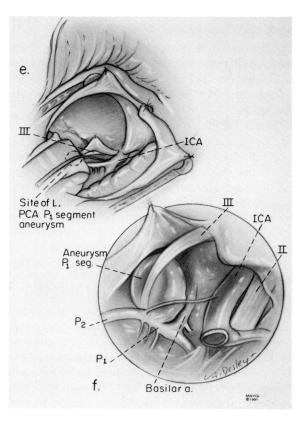

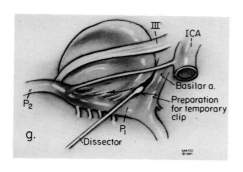

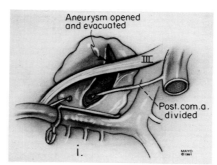

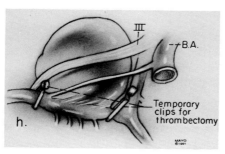

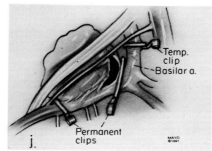

Figure 30-136. (A) Patient positioning and **(B)** modified pterion craniotomy for anterior, subtemporal or "half and half" approach to a proximal PCA trunk aneurysm. The head is rotated approximately 30 degrees and only slightly extended. The standard pterion craniotomy is extended posteriorly and the temporal squama removed to the floor of the middle fossa to allow more subtemporal as opposed to transsylvian exposure. The following sequence demonstrates the surgical approach and management alternatives for the left P_1 aneurysm demonstrated in Figure 30-134. **(C)** The dura has been opened and secured to the craniotomy margins. The sylvian fissure is opened if possible, the dissection being facilitated by gentle frontal retraction to open the plane of dissection. Anterior temporal veins to the sphenoparietal sinus are coagulated and divided. **(D)** The self-retaining retractor is shifted to allow elevation and posterior displacement of the temporal tip exposing the free margin of the tentorium and carotid and crural cisterns. **(E)** The free margin of the tentorium is retracted laterally with a suture secured to the dura of the middle fossa to further expose the crural cistern. The arachnoid is opened with sharp dissection to expose the ICA, posterior communicating, basilar, and PCA arteries. The constant location of the third nerve beneath the PCA, usually the proximal P_2 segment, serves as a landmark for further identification of the PCA, which becomes covered by the uncus and hippocampal gyrus. **(F)** In the case of the P_1 aneurysm shown in Fig. 30-134, the neck arises from the inferior surface of P_1, but the giant aneurysmal sac is filled with thrombus and medially is adherent to the basilar trunk. Preservation of the small PCoA is desirable, but this vessel may be ligated and divided if absolutely necessary, taking care to preserve its perforating branches. The giant partially thrombosed sac and its adherence to the basilar trunk makes management of this aneurysm difficult. Optimal treatment of the aneurysm (i.e., neck clipping) requires reflection of the aneurysm sac away from the basilar trunk **(G)** to allow placement of temporary clips **(H)**, evacuation of the aneurysm, and application of permanent clips **(I)**. This dissection requires great care lest the fragile aneurysm neck tear, necessitating trapping with isolation of the P_1 segment and its perforating branches **(J)**. If aneurysm neck clipping is not possible or is felt to carry high risk of perforator compromise, a single permanent clip on P_1 proximal to the aneurysm is an alternative. (By permission of Mayo Foundation.)

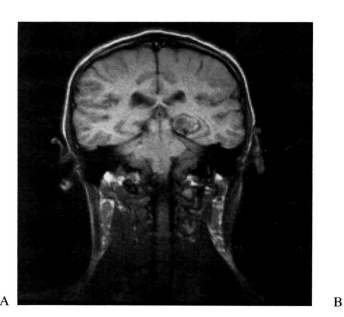

A

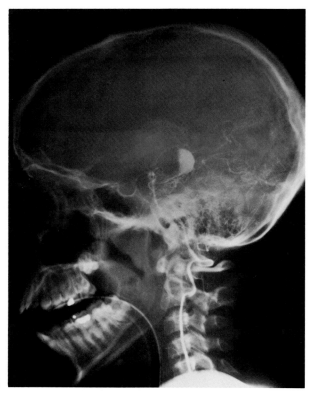

B

Figure 30-137. **(A)** Sagittal T$_1$-weighted MRI showing a large partially thrombosed P$_2$ segment aneurysm in the left ambient cistern. **(B)** Lateral view of the vertebrobasilar angiogram demonstrating the same partially thrombosed aneurysm.

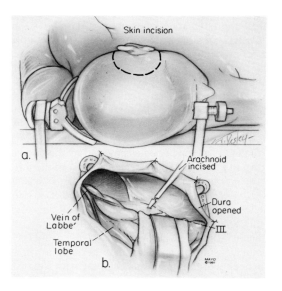

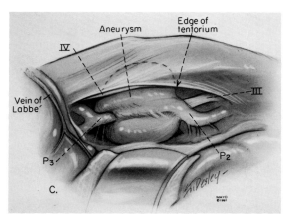

Figure 30-138. **(A)** For the lateral subtemporal approach to the midsegments of the PCA or SCA, the head is positioned laterally or with the brow turned up only slightly. **(B)** The temporal craniectomy has been carried to the floor of the middle fossa. Elevation of the temporal lobe proceeds only after brain relaxation has been achieved with mannitol diuresis and CSF drainage. Special care must be taken to protect the vein of Labbé as the temporal lobe is elevated. Gelfoam pledgets and cottonoid protect the brain surface under the self-retaining retractor. **(C)** The large fusiform aneurysm of the P$_2$-P$_3$ PCA segments (as demonstrated in Figure 30-137) is exposed lateral to the midbrain. (*Figure continues.*)

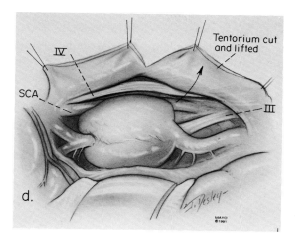

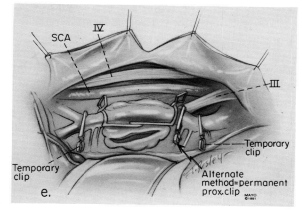

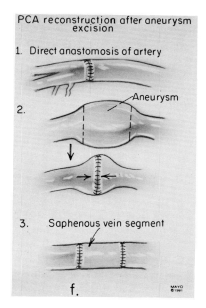

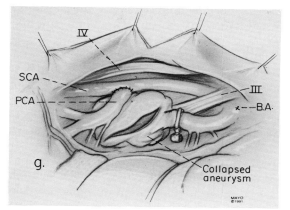

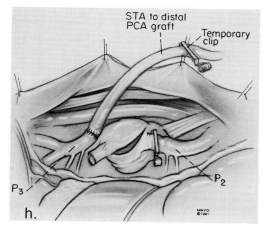

Figure 30-138 (*Continued*). **(D)** The tentorial margin is retracted with a suture or, if necessary, divided just posterior to the entrance of the fourth nerve into the dura. **(E)** Aneurysms along the PCA trunk may not be amenable to simple neck clipping. Temporary trapping and evacuation of the aneurysm may allow a neck to be constructed. Attention must be paid to protect perforating and circumflex branches medial to the aneurysm and PCA. If aneurysm clipping is not possible, reasonable alternative options include proximal PCA clipping as close to the aneurysm as possible or permanent trapping. If collateral flow to the distal PCA is poor, microvascular reconstruction options include **(F)** excision of the aneurysm and end-to-end anastomosis of PCA if adequate length (*1*) or aneurysm wall (*2*) allows; interposed saphenous vein segment (*3*) is a possible but difficult alternative. Restoration of distal PCA flow by end-to-side anastomosis to SCA trunk **(G)**; a superficial temporal artery to distal PCA end-to-end anastomosis **(H)**. (By permission of Mayo Foundation.)

requires more retraction than exposure of the SCA. For the former, the tip of the retractor must elevate the hippocampal gyrus, or on occasion some of this tissue may need to be resected. Large aneurysms often distort the usual course of the artery, and the only reliable method of exposure is to follow the artery from its proximal location over the third nerve to the pathology posteriorly. As has been stated by Rhoton et al.,[382] it is safest to follow the inferior surface of the artery as it is usually devoid of perforators.

For the exposure of the SCA, it is necessary to retract the tentorial margin. In some situations a simple retraction suture may suffice, but more often it is necessary to divide the tentorium for a short distance (Fig. 30-138C–E). This maneuver requires care first to identify and then to preserve the fourth nerve, making the section posterior to its point of entry. Venous bleeding from the tentorial margin is best controlled with bipolar cautery and section in small increments.

Aneurysms of the PCA and SCA are often best dissected and repaired with the use of temporary proximal occlusion. In cases of more complex or larger aneurysms, temporary trapping for dissection, thrombectomy, or neck reduction may be helpful. Care must be taken in application of temporary and permanent clips to avoid compromise of perforating branches, especially those lying medial to the PCA.

We have already discussed the options and attendant risks in treating some of the large and complex PCA aneurysms with permanent proximal occlusion or trapping. Unquestionably this can often be the simplest and safest alternative. The decision to reconstruct or revascularize the PCA distal to the aneurysm must take into account the pathological anatomy, the condition of the patient, the microsurgical skills of the surgeon, the extended time to complete such a repair, and, most importantly, the assessment of distal collateral as judged by the preoperative angiogram and back-bleeding at surgery (Fig. 30-138F–H). More often than not, the decision not to carry out a revascularization process can probably be justified.

Distal PCA and SCA Aneurysms

Because of the rarity of PCA and SCA aneurysms, a detailed discussion regarding their surgical approach and the attendant complications will not be undertaken here. More important is to emphasize the need for careful assessment of the preoperative studies, particularly in the case of the more distal (P_3 segment) aneurysms to determine their exact location (i.e., in the lateral ambient vs. the quadrigeminal cistern). If there is doubt, a standard MRI or MR angiogram may be helpful in determining the site and the best operative approach. Distal PCA aneurysms (P_3-P_4 and P_4) will be best exposed through a parieto-occipital craniotomy and interhemispheric approach to the quadrigeminal cistern as described by Yasargil.[387] Similarly, the distal SCA aneurysms, unlike those on the more proximal trunk, will be best treated through a supracerebellar exposure with the patient in either the sitting or prone position.

POSTOPERATIVE CARE

Care of the patient following surgery for PCA or SCA aneurysms is no different than that for other aneurysms or SAH. Attention must be paid to preservation of normal blood volume, normotension, and cardiac output. Post-SAH delayed cerebral ischemia is treated according to the usual guidelines. Temporal lobe edema is best managed by ensuring optimal ventilation, head elevation, and, if profound, mannitol diuresis. Steroids may also be of benefit. Although uncommon, postoperative temporal lobe hemorrhagic infarction or ICH may be life-threatening and should be treated with aggressive reoperation and resection of hematoma and necrotic tissue. Anticonvulsant drugs should probably be continued for 3 to 6 months.

REFERENCES

Intracavernous Carotid Artery Aneurysms

1. Al-Mefty O, Khalil N, Elwany MN, Smith RR: Shunt for bypass graft of the cavernous carotid artery: an anatomical and technical study. Neurosurgery 27(5):721, 1990
2. Berenstein A, Ransohoff J, Kupersmith M, Flamm E, Graeb D: Transvascular treatment of giant aneurysms of the cavernous carotid arteries. Surg Neurol 21:3, 1984
3. de Morais JV, Lana-Peixoto MA: Bilateral intracavernous carotid aneurysms: treatment of bilateral carotid ligation. Surg Neurol 9:379, 1978.
4. Browder J: Treatment of carotid artery-cavernous sinus fistula. Report of a case. Arch Ophthalmol 18(Supp. 2):95, 1937
5. Dandy WE: Carotid-cavernous aneurysms (pulsating exophthalmos). Zentralb Neurochir 2:77, 1937
6. Diaz FG, Ohaefbulam S, Dujovny M, Ausman JI: Surgical management of aneurysms in the cavernous sinus. Acta Neurochir (Wien) 91:25, 1988
7. Diaz FG, Ohaegvulam S, Dujovny M, Ausman J: Sur-

gical alternatives in the treatment of cavernous sinus aneurysms. J Neurosurg 71:846, 1989

8. Dolenc V: Direct microsurgical repair of intracavernous vascular lesions. J Neurosurg 58:824, 1983

9. Dolenc V: A combined epi- and subdural direct approach to carotid-ophthalmic artery aneurysms. J Neurosurg 62:667, 1985

10. Dolenc V, Kregar T, Ferluga M, Fettich M, Morina A: Treatment of tumors invading the cavernous sinus. p. 377. In Dolenc V (ed): The cavernous sinus. A multidisciplinary approach to tumorous and vascular lesions. Springer-Verlag, 1987

11. Faria MA, Fleischer AS, Spector RH: Bilateral giant intracavernous carotid aneurysms treated by bilateral carotid ligation. Surg Neurol 14:207, 1980

12. Fischer E: Die Lagabweichrugan der vorderen Hirnarterie in Gefassbild. Zentralb Neurochir 3:300, 1938

13. Fox AJ, Vinuela F, Pelz DM et al: Use of detachable balloons for proximal artery occlusion in the treatment of unclippable cerebral aneurysms. J Neurosurg 66:40, 1987

14. Fukushima T: Direct operative approach to the vascular lesions in the cavernous sinus: summary of 27 cases. Mt Fuji Workshop Cerebrovasc Dis 6:169, 1988

15. Gelber BR, Sundt TM: Treatment of intracavernous and giant carotid aneurysms by combined internal carotid ligation and extra-to-intracranial bypass. J Neurosurg 52:1, 1980

16. Gibo H, Lenkey C, Rhoton AL: Microsurgical anatomy of the supraclinoid portion of the internal carotid artery. J Neurosurg 55:560, 1981

17. Glasscock ME: Exposure of the intra-petrous portion of the carotid artery. p. 135. In Hamberger CA, Wersall J (eds): Disorders of the Skull Base Region: Proceedings of the Tenth Nobel Symposium, Stockholm, 1968. Almqvist and Wicksell, Stockholm, 1969

18. Glasscock ME III, Smith PG, Whitaker SR et al: Management of aneurysms of the petrous portion of the internal carotid artery by resection and primary anastomosis. Laryngoscope 93:1445, 1983

19. Hakuba A, Matsuoka Y, Suzuki T et al: Direct approaches to vascular lesions in the cavernous sinus via the medial triangle. p. 272. In Dolenc VV (ed): The Cavernous Sinus. Springer-Verlag, Wien, 1987

20. Hakuba A, Tanaka K, Suzuki T, Nishimura S: A combined orbitozygomatic infratemporal epidural subdural approach for lesions involving the entire cavernous sinus. J Neurosurg 71:699, 1989

21. Hamby WB, Dohn DF: Carotid-cavernous fistulas: report of thirty-six cases and discussion of their management. Clin Neurosurg 11:150, 1964

22. Harris FS, Rhoton AL: Anatomy of the cavernous sinus: a microsurgical study. J Neurosurg 44:169, 1976

23. Hayes GJ: Carotid cavernous fistulas: diagnosis and surgical management. Am Surg 24:839, 1958

24. Jefferson G: On the saccular aneurysms of the internal carotid artery in the cavernous sinus. Br J Surg 26:267, 1938

25. Johnston I: Direct surgical treatment of bilateral intracavernous internal carotid artery aneurysms: case report. J Neurosurg 51:98, 1979

26. Kawase T, Toya S, Shiobara R, Mine T: Transpetrosal approach for aneurysms of the lower basilar artery. J Neurosurg 63:857, 1985

27. Lesoin F, Jomin M, Boucez B et al: Management of cavernous sinus meningiomas. Report of twelve cases and review of the literature. Neurochirurgia 28:195, 1985

28. Lesoin F, Jomin M: Direct microsurgical approach to intracavernous tumors. Surg Neurol 28:17, 1987

29. Linskey ME, Sekhar LN, Hirsch W et al: Aneurysms of the intracavernous carotid artery: clinical presentation, radiographic features, and pathogenesis. Neurosurg 26(1):71, 1990

30. Linskey ME, Sekhar LN, Horton JA et al: Aneurysms of the intracavernous carotid artery: a multidisciplinary approach to treatment. J Neurosurg 75:525, 1991

31. Miyazaki S, Fukushima T, Fujimaki T: Resection of high-cervical paraganglioma with cervical-to-petrous internal carotid artery saphenous vein bypass: report of two cases. J Neurosurg 73:141, 1990

32. Mullan S: Treatment of carotid-cavernous fistulas by cavernous sinus occlusion. J Neurosurg 50:131, 1979

33. Parkinson D: A surgical approach to the cavernous portion of the carotid artery: anatomical studies and case report. J Neurosurg 23:474, 1965

34. Parkinson D: Transcavernous repair of carotid-cavernous fistula: case report. J Neurosurg 26:420, 1967

35. Parkinson D: Carotid cavernous fistula: direct repair with preservation of the carotid artery. Technical note. J Neurosurg 38:99, 1973

36. Parkinson D, Downs AR, Whytehead LL, Syslak WB: Carotid cavernous fistula: direct repair with preservation of carotid. Surgery 76:882, 1974

37. Parkinson D: Aneurysms of the cavernous sinus. p. 79. In Pia HW, Lagmaid C, Zierski J (eds): Cerebral Aneurysms: Advances in Diagnosis and Therapy. Springer-Verlag, Berlin, 1979

38. Parkinson D: Surgical management of internal carotid artery aneurysms within the cavernous sinus. p. 819. In Schmideck HH, Sweet WH (eds): Operative Neurosurgical Techniques: Indications, Methods and Results. Grune & Stratton, Orlando, FL, 1982

39. Parkinson D: Carotic cavernous fistula. History and Anatomy. p. 3. In Dolenc VV (ed): The Cavernous Sinus. Springer-Verlag, Berlin, 1987

40. Parkinson D, West M: Lesions of the cavernous plexus region. p. 3351. In Yeomans J (ed): Neurological Surgery. 3rd Ed. WB Saunders, Philadelphia, PA, 1990

41. Perneczky A, Knosp E, Borkapic P, Czech T: Direct surgical approach to infraclinoidal aneurysms. Acta Neurochir (Wien) 76:36, 1983

42. Perneczky A, Knosp E, Czech T: Para- and infracli-

noidal aneurysms. Anatomy, surgical technique and report on 22 cases. p. 252. In Dolenc VV (ed): The Cavernous Sinus. Springer-Verlag, Berlin, 1987

43. Sekhar LN, Burgess J, Akin O: Anatomical study of the cavernous sinus emphasizing operative approaches and related vascular and neural reconstruction. Neurosurgery 21:806, 1987

44. Sekhar LN, Sen CN, Jho HD: Saphenous vein bypass of the cavernous internal carotid artery. J Neurosurg 72:35, 1990

45. Seltzer J: Bilateral symmetrical aneurysms of internal carotid artery within the cavernous sinus. J Neurosurg 14:448, 1957

46. Silvani V, Rainoldi F, Gaetani P et al: Combined STA/MCA arterial bypass and gradual internal carotid artery occlusion for treatment of intracavernous and giant carotid artery aneurysms. Acta Neurochir 78:142, 1985

47. Spetzler RF, Schuster H, Roski RA: Elective extracranial-intracranial arterial bypass in the treatment of inoperable giant aneurysms of the internal carotid artery. J Neurosurg 53:22, 1980

48. Spetzler RF, Martin N, Hadley MN: Microsurgical endarterectomy under barbiturate protection: a prospective study. J Neurosurg 65:63, 1986

49. Spetzler RF, Fukushima T, Martin N, Zabramski JM: Petrous carotid-to-intradural carotid saphenous vein graft for intracavernous giant aneurysm, tumor, and occlusive cerebrovascular disease. J Neurosurg 73:496, 1990

50. Sundt TM: Surgical Techniques for Saccular and Giant Intracranial Aneurysms. Williams & Wilkins, Baltimore, 1990

51. Sundt TM III, Sundt TM Jr: Principles of preparation of vein bypass grafts to maximize patency. J Neurosurg 66:172, 1987

52. Sutton LN, Gusnard D, Bruce DA: Fusiform dilatations of the carotid artery following radical surgery of childhood craniopharyngiomas. J Neurosurg 74:695, 1991

53. Umansky F, Nathan H: The lateral wall of the cavernous sinus: with special reference to the nerves related to it. J Neurosurg 56:228, 1982

54. Umansky F, Elidan J, Valarezo A: Dorello's canal: a microanatomical study. J Neurosurg 75:294, 1991

55. Van Loveren H, Keller JT, El-Kalliny M et al: The Dolenc technique for cavernous sinus exploration (cadaveric prosection). J Neurosurg 74:837, 1991

Carotid Ophthalmic Aneurysms

56. Almeida GM, Shibata MK, Biaco E: Carotid ophthalmic aneurysms. Surg Neurol 5:41, 1976

57. Batjer HH, Samson D: Intraoperative aneurysm rupture: incidence, outcome, and suggestions for surgical management. Neurosurgery 18:701, 1986

58. Day AL: Aneurysms of the ophthalmic segment. J Neurosurg 72:677, 1990

59. Drake DG, Vanderlinden RG, Amacher AL: Carotid-ophthalmic aneurysms. J Neurosurg 29:24, 1968

60. Ferguson GG, Drake CG: Carotid-ophthalmic aneurysms: Visual abnormalities in 32 patients and the results of treatment. Surg Neurol 16:1, 1981

61. Guidetti B, La Torre E: Management of carotid-ophthalmic aneurysms. J Neurosurg 42:438, 1975

62. Milenkovic Z, Gopic H, Antov P et al: Contralateral pterional approach to a carotid-ophthalmic aneurysm ruptured at surgery. Case report. J Neurosurg 57:823, 1982

63. Nakao S, Kikuchi H, Takahashi N: Successful clipping of carotid-ophthalmic aneurysms through a contralateral pterional approach. Report of two cases. J Neurosurg 54:532, 1981

64. Nutik SL: Ventral paraclinoid carotid aneurysms. J Neurosurg 69:340, 1988

65. Pia HW: Classification of aneurysms of the internal carotid system. Acta Neurochir 40:5, 1978

66. Sengupta RP: Natural history of carotid ophthalmic aneurysms and its influence on surgical management. p. 63. In Kikuchi H, Fukushima T, Watanabe K (eds): Intracranial Aneurysms. Nishimura Co., Niigata, Japan, 1986

67. Sugita K, Kobayashi S, Kyoshima K et al: Fenestrated clips for unusual aneurysms of the carotid artery. J Neurosurg 57:240, 1982

68. Sugita K, Kobayashi S, Takemae et al: Direct retraction method in aneurysm surgery. J Neurosurg 53:417, 1980

69. Yasargil MG, Gasser JC, Hodosh RM et al: Carotid-ophthalmic aneurysms: direct microsurgical approach. Surg Neurol 8:155, 1977

Midcarotid Artery (Posterior Communicating and Anterior Choroidal Artery) Aneurysms

70. Eriksen KD, Bge-Rasmussen T, Kruse-Larsen C: Anosmia following operation for cerebral aneurysms in the anterior circulation. J Neurosurg 72:864, 1990

71. Flamm ES: Suction decompression of aneurysms: technical note. J Neurosurg 54:275, 1981

72. Good EF: Ptosis as the sole manifestation of compression of the oculomotor nerve by an aneurysm of the posterior communicating artery. J Clin Neuro Ophthalmol 10:59, 1990

73. Heifetz MD: Carotid control for intracranial aneurysms. Technical note. J Neurosurg 69:142, 1988

74. Kissel JT, Burde RM, Klingele TG, Zeiger HE: Pupil-sparing oculomotor palsies with internal carotid-posterior communicating artery aneurysms. Ann Neurol 13:149, 1983

75. Krayenbuhl H, Yasargil MG, Flamm ES, Tew JM: Microsurgical treatment of intracranial saccular aneurysms. J Neurosurg 37:678, 1972

76. Kwan ES, Laucella M, Hedges TR 3d, Wolpert SM: A cliniconeuroradiologic approach to third cranial nerve palsies. AJNR 8:459, 1987

77. Rhoton AL, Saeki N, Perlmutter D, Zeal A: Micro-surgical anatomy of common aneurysm sites. Clin Neurosurg 26:248, 1979

78. Ross JS, Masaryk TJ, Modic MT et al: Intracranial aneurysms: evaluation by MR angiography. AJNR 11:449, 455, 1990

79. Sevick RJ, Tsuruda JS, Schmalbrock P: Three-dimensional time-of-flight MR angiography in the evaluation of cerebral aneurysms. J Comput Assist Tomogr 14:874, 1990

80. Trobe JD: Isolated pupil-sparing third nerve palsy. Ophthalmology 92:58, 1985

Carotid Bifurcation Aneurysms

81. af Bjorkesten G: Arterial aneurysms of the internal carotid artery and its bifurcation: an analysis of 69 aneurysms treated mainly by direct surgical attack. J Neurosurg 15:400, 1958

82. Batjer HH, Samson D: Intra-operative aneurysmal rupture: incidence, outcome, and suggestions for surgical management. Neurosurgery 18:701, 1986

83. Crowell RM, Jafar JJ: Temporary clips and mannitol protection for aneurysm surgery (in press)

84. DaPain R, Pasqualin A, Scienza R: Direct microsurgical approach to aneurysms of the internal carotid bifurcation. Surg Neurol 13:27, 1980

85. David M, Sachs M: Les aneurysms de la bifurcation de le carotide interne. Neurochirurgia 10:96, 1967

86. Durity FA: Temporary occlusion and barbiturate protection in cerebral aneurysm surgery. Neurosurgery 25:54, 1989

87. Jafar JJ, Johns LM, Mullan SF: The effect of mannitol on cerebral blood flow. J Neurosurg 64:754, 1986

88. Laranjeira M, Sadasivan B, Ausman JI: Direct surgery for carotid bifurcation artery aneurysms. Surg Neurol 34:250, 1990

89. Lassman LP: Internal carotid artery bifurcation aneurysms. In Pia H et al (eds): Cerebral Aneurysms, Advances in Diagnosis and Therapy. Springer-Verlag, Berlin, 1979

90. McKissock W, Richardson A, Walsh L: Posterior communicating aneurysms: a controlled trial of conservative and surgical treatment of ruptured aneurysms of the internal carotid artery at or near the point of origin of the posterior communicating artery. Lancet 1:1203, 1960

91. Mount LA, Antunes JL: Results of treatment of intracranial aneurysm by wrapping and coating. J Neurosurg 42:189, 1975

92. Newell DW, Eskridge JM, Mayberg MR: Angioplasty for the treatment of symptomatic vasospasm following subarachnoid hemorrhage. J Neurosurg 71:654, 1989

93. Ojemann RG, Heros RC, Crowell RM: Internal carotid artery aneurysms. p. 179. In Surgical management of cerebrovascular disease. Williams & Wilkins, Baltimore, 1988

94. Perria L, Rivano C, Rossi GF, Viale G: Aneurysms of the bifurcation of the internal carotid artery. Acta Neurochir 19:51, 1968

95. Pickard JD, Murray GD, Illingworth R et al: Effect of oral nimodipine on cerebral infarction and outcome after subarachnoid hemorrhage: British aneurysm nimodipine trial. Br Med J 298:636, 1989

96. Samson D, Marshall D: The use of isobutyl-2-cyano-acrylate in embolization. Surg Neurology 28:319, 1987

97. Sengupta RP: internal carotid bifurcation aneurysms and their treatment by direct surgery. J Neurol Neurosurg Psychiatry 38:826, 1975

98. Sundt TM: Surgical Techniques of Saccular and Giant Intracranial Aneurysms. Williams & Wilkins, Baltimore, 1990

99. Weir B: Carotid bifurcation artery aneurysms. p. 456. In Aneurysms Affecting the Nervous System. Williams & Wilkins, Baltimore, 1987

100. Yasargil MG: Microneurosurgery. Vol. 2. Management and Surgical Results for Intracranial Aneurysms. Springer-Verlag, Berlin, 1987

Middle Cerebral Artery Aneurysms

101. Batjer HH, Frankfurt AI, Purty PD et al: Use of etomidate, temporary arterial occlusion, and intraoperative angiography and surgical treatment of large and giant cerebral aneurysms. J Neurosurg 68:234, 1988

102. Brandt L, Sonesson B, Ljunggren B, Saveland H: Ruptured middle cerebral artery aneurysm with intracerebral hemorrhage in younger patients appearing moribund: emergency operation? Neurosurgery 20:925, 1987

103. Drake CG: Giant intracranial aneurysms: experience with surgical treatment in 174 patients. Clin Neurosurg 26:12, 1978

104. Fein JM, Flamm ES: Cerebrovascular Surgery. Vol. III. Springer-Verlag, New York, 1985

105. Findlay JM, Weir BKA: Prevention of aneurysmal subarachnoid hemorrhage. In Norris JW, Hachinski VC (eds): Prevention of Stroke. Springer-Verlag, New York, 1991

106. Fox JL: Intracranial Aneurysms. Vol I. Springer Verlag, New York, 1983

107. Fox JL: Intracranial Aneurysms. Vol. III. Springer-Verlag, New York, 1983

108. Fox JL: Atlas of Neurosurgical Anatomy. The Pterional Perspective. Springer-Verlag, New York, 1989

109. Gibo H, Carver CC, Rhoton AL et al: Microsurgical anatomy of the middle cerebral artery. J Neurosurg 54:151, 1981

110. Grand W: Microsurgical anatomy of the proximal middle cerebral artery and the internal carotid artery bifurcation. Neurosurgery 7:215, 1980

111. Heros RC: Middle cerebral artery aneurysms. p. 1376. In Wilkins RH, Rengachary SS (eds): Neurosurgery. Vol. II. McGraw-Hill, New York, 1985

112. Kassell NF, Torner JC: Size of intracranial aneurysms. Neurosurgery 12:291, 1983

113. Lougheed WM, Marshall BM: Management of aneurysms of the anterior circulation by intracranial procedures. p. 731. In Youmans JR (ed): Neurological Surgery: a Comprehensive Reference Guide to the Diagnosis and Management of Neurosurgical Problems. 1st Ed. WB Saunders, Philadelphia, 1973

114. McDermott MW, Durity FA, Borozny M, Mountain MA: Temporary vessel occlusion and barbiturate protection in cerebral aneurysm surgery. Neurosurgery 25:54, 1989

115. Mooij JJA, Buchthal A, Belopavlovic M: Somatosensory evoked potential monitoring of temporary middle cerebral artery occlusion during aneurysm operation. Neurosurgery 21:492, 1987

116. Peerless SJ, Hamph CR: Extracranial to intracranial bypass in the treatment of aneurysms. Clin Neurosurg 32:114, 1988

117. Reynolds AF, Shaw CM: Bleeding patterns from ruptured intracranial aneurysms: an autopsy series of 205 patients. Surg Neurol 15:232, 1981

118. Rosner SS, Rhoton AL Jr, Ono M, Barry M: Microsurgical anatomy of the anterior perforating arteries. J Neurosurg 61:468, 1984

119. Sahs AL, Perret GE, Locksley HB, Nishioka H: Intracranial Aneurysms and Subarachnoid Hemorrhage: A Cooperative Study. JB Lippincott, Philadelphia, 1969

120. Sengupta RP, McAllister VL: Subarachnoid Hemorrhage. Springer-Verlag, Berlin, 1986

121. Suzuki J, Mizoi K, Yoshimoto T: Bifrontal interhemispheric approach to aneurysms of the anterior communicating artery. J Neurosurg 64:183, 1986

122. Suzuki J, Yoshimoto T, Kayama T: Surgical treatment of middle cerebral artery aneurysms. J Neurosurg 61:17, 1984

123. Symon L: Surgical management of aneurysms of the middle cerebral artery. p. 957. In Schmidek HH, Sweet WH (eds): Operative Neurosurgical Techniques. Grune & Stratton, Orlando, FL, 1988

124. Umansky F, Dujovny M, Ausman JI et al: Anomalies and variations of the middle cerebral artery: a microanatomical study. Neurosurgery 22:1023, 1988

125. Umansky F, Gomes FB, Dujovny M et al: The perforating branches of the middle cerebral artery: a microanatomical study. J Neurosurg 62:261, 1985

126. Umansky F, Juarez SM, Dujovny M et al: Microsurgical anatomy of the proximal segments of the middle cerebral artery. J Neurosurg 61:458, 1984

127. Weir B: Aneurysms Affecting the Nervous System. Williams & Wilkins, Baltimore, 1987

128. Wheelock B, Weir B, Watts R et al: Timing of surgery for intracerebral hematomas due to aneurysm rupture. J Neurosurg 58:476, 1983

129. Yasargil MG: Microneurosurgery. Vol. II. Clinical Considerations, Surgery of Intracranial Aneurysms and Results. Georg-Thieme Verlag, Stuttgart, 1984

130. Yasargil MG: Microneurosurgery. Vol. I. Microsurgical Anatomy of the Basal Cisterns and Vessels of the Brain, Diagnostic Studies, General Operative Techniques and Pathological Considerations of the Intracranial Aneurysms. Thieme-Stratton, New York, 1984

131. Yasargil MG, Reichman MV, Kubik S: Preservation of the frontotemporal branch of the facial nerve using the interfascial temporalis flap for pterional craniotomy. Technical article. J Neurosurg 67:463, 1987

132. Yasargil MG, Smith RD: Management of aneurysms of anterior circulation by intracranial procedures. In Youmans JR (ed): Neurological Surgery. Vol. III. WB Saunders, Philadelphia, 1982

Anterior Communicating Artery Complex Aneurysms

132a. Adams CBT, Louch AB, O'Laoire SA: Intracranial aneurysms: analysis of results of microneurosurgery. Br Med J 2:607, 1976

133. Adams JE, Witt JA: The use of the otological microscope in the surgery of aneurysms. Presented at the 17th Annual Meeting of the Neurosurgical Society of America, Lichfield Park, Arizona, 1964

134. Af Björkesten G, Troupp H: Changes in the size of intracranial arterial aneurysms. J Neurosurg 19:583, 1962

135. Albin MS: Neuroanesthesia and aneurysmal surgery. p. 263. In Hopkins LN, Long DM (eds): Clinical Management of Intracranial Aneurysms. Raven Press, New York, 1982

136. Alexander E Jr, Adams JE, Davis CH Jr: Complications in the use of temporary intracranial arterial clip. J Neurosurg 20:810, 1963

137. Allcock JM, Drake CG: Postoperative angiography in cases of ruptured intracranial aneurysm. J Neurosurg 20:752, 1963

138. Allen GS, Ahn HS, Preziosi TJ et al: Cerebral arterial spasm. A controlled trial of nimodipine in patients with subarachnoid hemorrhage. N Engl J Med 308:619, 1983

139. Amacher AL, Drake CG: Aneurysm surgery in the seventh decade. p. 263. In Fusek I, Kunc A (eds): Present Limits of Neurosurgery. Elsevier, Amsterdam, 1972

140. Andrews RJ, Spiegel PK: Intracranial aneurysms: characteristics of aneurysms by site with special reference to anterior communicating artery aneurysms. Surg Neurol 16:122, 1981

141. Antunes JL, Correll JW: Cerebral emboli from intracranial aneurysms. Surg Neurol 6:7, 1976

142. Auer LM, Brandt L, Ebeling U et al: Nimodipine and early aneurysm operation in good condition SAH patients. Acta Neurochir 82:7, 1986

143. Bakay L, Crawford JD, White JC: The effect of intravenous fluids on cerebrospinal fluid pressure. Surg Gynecol Obstet 99:48, 1954

144. Baptista AG: Studies on the arteries of the brain. II. The anterior cerebral artery: some anatomical fea-

tures and their clinical implications. Neurology 13:825, 1963

145. Bloch A: Murphy's Law. Price/Stern/Sloan, Los Angeles, 1977

146. Bohard F, Saillant C: Syndrome de Korsakoff post-opératoire symptomatique d'un anévrisme de l'artère communicante antérieure (étude clinique et chimiotherapique). Evol Psychiatry (Paris) 34:109, 1969

147. Bohm E, Hugosson R: Experiences of surgical treatment of 400 consecutive ruptured cerebral arterial aneurysms. Acta Neurochir 40:33, 1978

148. Bohm E, Hugosson R: Results of surgical treatment of 200 consecutive cerebral arterial aneurysms. Acta Neurol Scand 46:45, 1970

149. Boisvert DPJ, Pickard JD, Graham DI et al: Delayed effects of subarachnoid hemorrhage on cerebral metabolism and the cerebrovascular response to hypercapnia in the primate. J Neurosurg Psychiat 42:892, 1979

150. Bonnal J, Stevenaert A: Evolution angiographique des anévrysmes artériels du polygone antérieur après intervention directe incomplète. Schweiz Arch Neurol Neurochir Psychiatr 104:11, 1969

151. Bonnal J, Stevenaert A: Thrombosis of intracranial aneurysms of the circle of Willis after incomplete obliteration by clip or ligature across the neck. J Neurosurg 30:158, 1969

152. Botterell EH, Lougheed WM, Scott JW et al: Hypothermia and interruption of carotid or carotid and vertebral circulation, in the surgical management of intracranial aneurysms. J Neurosurg 13:1, 1956

153. Brion S, Derome P, Guiot G et al: Syndrome de Korsakoff par anévrysme de l'artère communicante antérieur; le problème des syndromes de Korsakoff par hémorrhagie méningée. Rev Neurol (Paris) 118:293, 1968

154. Cabral RJ, King TT, Scott DF: Epilepsy after two different neurosurgical approaches to the treatment of ruptured intracranial aneurysm. J Neurol Neurosurg Psychiatry 39:1052, 1976

155. Carton CA, Heifetz MD, Kessler LA: Patching of intracranial internal carotid artery in man using a plastic adhesive (Eastman 910 adhesive). J Neurosurg 19:887, 1962

156. Chou SN, Ortiz-Suarez HJ: Surgical treatment of arterial aneurysms of the vertebrobasilar circulation. J Neurosurg 41:671, 1974

157. Clark K: Complications of aneurysm surgery. Clin Neurosurg 23:342, 1976

158. Collins WF: Neurosurgical complications. Fluid and electrolyte imbalance. Clin Neurosurg 23:417, 1977

159. Connolly RC: Cerebral ischaemia in spontaneous subarachnoid haemorrhage. Ann R Coll Surg Engl 30:102, 1962

160. Critchley M: The anterior cerebral artery and its syndrome. Brain 53:120, 1930

161. Crompton MR: Hypothalamic lesions following the rupture of cerebral berry aneurysms. Brain 86:301, 1963

162. Crompton MR: Recurrent haemorrhage from cerebral aneurysms and its prevention by surgery. J Neurol Neurosurg Psychiatry 29:164, 1966

163. Cruickshank JM, Neil-Dwyer G, Brice J: Electrocardiographic changes and their prognostic significance in subarachnoid haemorrhage. J Neurol Neurosurg Psychiat 37:755, 1974

164. Dandy WE: Intracranial aneurysms of internal carotid artery. Cured by operation. Ann Surg 107:654, 1938

165. Dandy WE: Intracranial Arterial Aneurysms. Comstock, Ithaca, New York, 1944

166. Dóczi T, Bende J, Huszka E et al: The syndrome of inappropriate secretion of ADH after subarachnoid hemorrhage. Neurosurgery 9:394, 1981

167. Dott NM: Intracranial aneurysms: cerebral arterioradiography: surgical treatment. Edinb Med J 40 (section on Trans Med-Chir Soc Edinburgh):219, 1933

168. Drake CG: On the surgical treatment of ruptured intracranial aneurysms. Clin Neurosurg 13:122, 1965

169. Drake CG, Allcock JM: Postoperative angiography and the "slipped" clip. J Neurosurg 39:683, 1973

170. Drake CG, Jory TA: Spontaneous intracranial haemorrhage: "subarachnoid haemorrhage": a review of investigation and treatment in 189 cases. Can J Surg 4:4, 1960

171. Drake CG, Vanderlinden RG: The late consequences of incomplete surgical treatment of cerebral aneurysms. J Neurosurg 27:226, 1967

172. Dutton JEM: Intracranial aneurysm. A new method of surgical treatment. Br Med J 2:585, 1956

173. Elvidge AR, Feindel WH: Surgical treatment of aneurysm in the anterior cerebral and the anterior communicating arteries diagnosed by angiography and electroencephalography. J Neurosurg 7:13, 1950

174. Falconer MA: The surgical treatment of bleeding intracranial aneurysms. J Neurol Neurosurg Psychiatry 14:153, 1951

175. Foltz EL, Ward AA Jr: Communicating hydrocephalus from subarachnoid bleeding. J Neurosurg 13:546, 1956

176. Fox JL: Atlas of Neurosurgical Anatomy. Springer-Verlag, New York, 1989

177. Fox JL: Development of recent thoughts on intracranial pressure and the blood-brain barrier. J Neurosurg 21:909, 1964

178. Fox JL: Intracranial Aneurysms. Springer-Verlag, New York, 1983

179. Fox JL: Management of aneurysms of anterior circulation by intracranial procedures. p. 1689. In Youmans JR (ed): Neurological Surgery. 3rd Ed. WB Saunders, Philadelphia, 1990

180. Fox JL: Microsurgical exposure of intracranial aneurysms. J Microsurg 1:2, 1979

181. Fox JL: Vascular clips for the microsurgical treatment of stroke. Stroke 7:489, 1976

182. Fox JL, Albin MS, Bader DCH et al: Microsurgical treatment of neurovascular disease. Neurosurgery 3:285, 1978

183. Fox JL, Falik JL, Shalboub RJ: Neurosurgical hyponatremia: the role of inappropriate antidiuresis. J Neurosurg 34:506, 1971

184. Fox JL, Nugent GR: Recent advances in intracranial aneurysm surgery. West Virginia Med J 72:104, 1976

185. French LA, Zarling ME, Schultz EA: Management of aneurysms of the anterior communicating artery. J Neurosurg 19:870, 1962

186. Giannotta SL, McGillicuddy JE, Kindt GW: Diagnosis and treatment of postoperative cerebral vasospasm. Surg Neurol 8:286, 1977

187. Gillingham FJ: The management of ruptured intracranial aneurysm. Ann R Coll Surg Engl 23:89, 1958

188. Gillingham FJ: The management of ruptured intracranial aneurysms. Scot Med J 12:377, 1967

189. Hakuba A, Liu S, Nishimura S: The orbitozygomatic infratemporal approach: a new surgical technique. Surg Neurol 26:271, 1986

190. Hamby WB: A method for control of carotid cerebral circulation during operation. J Neurosurg 2:241, 1945

191. Hamby WB: Intracranial Aneurysms. Charles C Thomas, Springfield, IL, 1952

192. Harris P: Aneurysms of the anterior communicating artery. Cincinnati J Med 42:1, 1961

193. Hayes GJ, Slocum HC: The achievement of optimal brain relaxation by hyperventilation technics of anesthesia. J Neurosurg 19:65, 1962

194. Heubner O: Zur Topographie der Ernahrungsgebiete der einzelner Hirnarterien. Zbl Med Wissenschaft 10:817, 1872

195. Hoff JT, Marshall L: Barbiturates in neurosurgery. Clin Neurosurg 26:637, 1979

196. Horwitz NH, Rizzoli HV: Aneurysms and arteriovenous fistulas. p. 83. In Postoperative Complications in Neurosurgical Practice. Recognition, Prevention, and Management. Williams & Wilkins, Baltimore, 1967

197. Horwitz NH, Rizzoli HV: Aneurysms and arteriovenous malformations. p. 182. In Postoperative Complications of Intracranial Neurological Surgery. Williams & Wilkins, Baltimore, 1982

198. Hounsfield GN: Computerised transverse axial scanning (tomography): part 1. Description of system. Br J Radiol 4b:1023, 1973

199. Ingham HI, Kalbag RM, Allcutt D et al: Simple perioperative antimicrobial chemoprophylaxis in elective neurosurgical operations. J Hosp Infect 12:225, 1988

200. Joffe SN: Incidence of postoperative deep vein thrombosis in neurosurgical patients. J Neurosurg 42:201, 1975

201. Joynt RJ, Afifi A, Harbison J: Hyponatremia in subarachnoid hemorrhage. Arch Neurol 13:633, 1965

202. Kempe LG: Operative Neurosurgery. Vol. 1. Cranial, Cerebral and Intracranial Vascular Disease. Springer-Verlag, Berlin, 1968

203. Kempe LG, VanderArk GD: Anterior communicating artery aneurysms. Gyrus rectus approach. Neurochirurgia (Stut) 14:63, 1971

204. Kikuchi H, Furuse S, Karasawa J: Microsurgery of cerebral aneurysm in acute phase (within 1 week after subarachnoid hemorrhage). p. 202. In Koos TH, Böck FW, Spetzler RF (eds): Clinical Microneurosurgery. Georg Thieme Verlag, Stuttgart, 1976

205. Kirgis HD, Fisher WL, Llewellyn RC et al: Aneurysms of the anterior communicating artery and gross anomalies of the circle of Willis. J Neurosurg 25:73, 1966

206. Kodama T, Uemura S, Nonaka N et al: [The quantitative analysis of psychiatric sequelae after direct surgery of anterior communicating aneurysm. Follow-up study.] Neurol Med Chir (Tokyo) 17(p2):227, 1977

207. Kolluri VRS, Sengupta RP: Factors which influence outcome in aneurysm surgery. p. 252. In Sengupta RP, McAllister VL (eds): Subarachnoid Haemorrhage. Springer-Verlag, Berlin, 1986

208. Kolluri VRS, Sengupta RP: Symptomatic hydrocephalus following aneurysmal subarachnoid hemorrhage. Surg Neurol 21:402, 1984

209. Kosnik EJ, Hunt WE: Postoperative hypertension in the management of patients with intracranial aneurysms. J Neurosurg 45:148, 1976

210. Kosteljanetz M: CSF dynamics in patients with subarachnoid and/or intraventricular hemorrhage. J Neurosurg 60:940, 1984

211. Krayenbühl HA, Yasargil MG, Flamm ES et al: Microsurgical treatment of intracranial saccular aneurysms. J Neurosurg 37:678, 1972

212. Kuwayama A, Okada C, Takanohaski M et al: [Endocrine function in postoperative patients with anterior communicating aneurysms.] Neurol Med Chir (Tokyo) 17(pt2):209, 1977

213. Landolt AM, Yasargil MG, Krayenbuhl H: Disturbances of the serum electrolytes after surgery of intracranial arterial aneurysms. J Neurosurg 37:210, 1972

214. Lie TA: Variations in cerebrovascular anatomy. p. 432. In Fox JL (ed): Intracranial Aneurysms. Springer-Verlag, New York, 1983

215. Lindqvist G, Norlén G: Korsakoff's syndrome after operation on ruptured aneurysm of the anterior communicating artery. Acta Psychiatr Scand 42:24, 1966

216. Logue V: Surgery in spontaneous subarachnoid haemorrhage. Operative treatment of aneurysms on the anterior cerebral and anterior communicating artery. Br Med J 1:473, 1956

217. Logue V, Durward M, Pratt RTC et al: The quality of survival after rupture of an anterior cerebral aneurysm. Br J Psychiatry 114:137, 1968

218. Lougheed WM: Selection, timing, and technique of aneurysm surgery of the anterior circle of Willis. Clin Neurosurg 16:95, 1969

219. Lougheed WM, Marshall BM: The place of hypothermia in the treatment of intracranial aneurysms. Prog Neurol Surg 3:115, 1969

220. Lougheed W, Morley T, Tasker R et al: The results of surgical treatment of ruptured berry aneurysms. p. 295. In Fields WS, Sahs AL (eds): Intracranial Aneurysms and Subarachnoid Hemorrhage. Charles C Thomas, Springfield, IL, 1965

221. Lundberg N: Continuous recording and control of

ventricular fluid pressure in neurosurgical practice. Acta Psychiatr Neurol Scand 36:(Suppl 149):1, 1960

222. Maroon JC, Nelson PB: Hypovolemia in patients with subarachnoid hemorrhage: therapeutic implications. Neurosurgery 4:223, 1979

223. Maspes PE, Marini G: Aneurysms of the anterior communicating artery. Result of direct surgical treatment. Acta Neurochir 11:479, 1963

224. Mauney FM Jr, Ebert PA, Sabiston DC Jr: Postoperative myocardial infarction: a study of predisposing factors, diagnosis and mortality in a high risk group of surgical patients. Ann Surg 172:494, 1970

225. McKissock W: Recurrence of an intracranial aneurysm after excision. Report of a case. J Neurosurg 23:547, 1965

226. McKissock W, Richardson A, Walsh L: Anterior communicating aneurysms. A trial of conservative and surgical treatment. Lancet 1:873, 1965

227. Merory J, Thomas DJ, Humphrey PRD et al: Cerebral blood flow after surgery for recent subarachnoid haemorrhage. J Neurol Neurosurg Psychiatry 43:214, 1980

228. Mihara T, Asakura T, Kawamura H et al: [Postoperative psychiatric symptoms and electrocardiographic changes in aneurysm of the anterior communicating artery.] Brain Nerve (Tokyo) 23:1271, 1971

229. Moniz E: L'encéphalographie artérielle, son importance dans la localisation des tumeurs cérébrales. Rev Neurol 2:72, 1927

230. Morgan F: Removal of anterior clinoid process in the surgery of carotid aneurysm. With some notes on recurrent subarachnoid haemorrhage during craniotomy. Schweiz Arch Neurol Neurochir Psychiatry 111:363, 1972

231. Nelson PB, Seif SM, Maroon JL et al: Hyponatremia in patients with subarachnoid hemorrhage: a study of vasopressin and blood volume. p. 654, part B. In Wilkins RH (ed): Cerebral Vasospasm. Williams & Wilkins, Baltimore, 1979

232. Norlén G: Aneurysm of the anterior communicating artery. Prog Brain Res 30:295, 1968

233. Norlén G, Barnum AS: Surgical treatment of aneurysms of the anterior communicating artery. J Neurosurg 10:634, 1953

234. Nornes H, Magnaes B: Intracranial pressure in patients with ruptured saccular aneurysm. J Neurosurg 36:537, 1972

235. Nornes H, Wikeby P: Results of microsurgical management of intracranial aneurysms. J Neurosurg 51:608, 1979

236. Nyström SHM: On factors related to growth and rupture of intracranial aneurysms. Acta Neuropathol (Berl) 16:64, 1970

237. Paterson A: Direct surgery in the treatment of posterior communicating aneurysms. Lancet 2:808, 1968

238. Paul RL, Arnold JG Jr: Operative factors influencing mortality in intracranial aneurysm surgery: analysis of 186 consecutive cases. J Neurosurg 32:289, 1970

239. Peerless SJ: Pre- and post-operative management of cerebral aneurysms. Clin Neurosurg 26:209, 1979

240. Perlmutter D, Rhoton AL: Microsurgical anatomy of the anterior cerebral-anterior communicating-recurrent artery complex. J Neurosurg 45:259, 1976

241. Pickard JD, Murray GD, Illingworth R et al: Effect of oral nimodipine on cerebral infarction and outcome after subarachnoid haemorrhage: British Aneurysm Nimodipine Trial. Br Med J 298:636, 1989

242. Pool JL: Aneurysms of the anterior communicating artery. Bifrontal craniotomy and routine use of temporary clips. J Neurosurg 18:98, 1961

243. Pool JL: Bifrontal craniotomy for anterior communicating artery aneurysms. J Neurosurg 36:212, 1972

244. Pool JL: Timing and techniques in the intracranial surgery of ruptured aneurysms of the anterior communicating artery. J Neurosurg 19:378, 1962

245. Pool JL, Colton RP: The dissecting microscope for intracranial vascular surgery. J Neurosurg 25:315, 1966

246. Pool JL, Potts DS: Aneurysms and Arteriovenous Anomalies of the Brain. Diagnosis and Treatment. Harper & Row, New York, 1965

247. Poppen JL: Discussion. Clin Neurosurg 11:183, 1964

248. Pritz MB, Giannotta SL, Kindt GW et al: Treatment of patients with neurological deficits associated with cerebral vasospasm by intravascular volume expansion. Neurosurgery 3:364, 1978

249. Pritz MB, Giannotta SL, McGillicuddy SE et al: Reversal of neurological deficits due to cerebral vasospasm by controlled increased of intravascular volume. Neurosurgery 2:158, 1978

250. Raimondi AJ, Torres H: Acute hydrocephalus as a complication of subarachnoid hemorrhage. Surg Neurol 1:23, 1973

251. Redondo A, Hanau J, Creissard P et al: Complications gastro-duodénalos des ruptures anévrismales due système communicante antérieur. Neurochirurie 16:471, 1970

252. Richardson AE, Uttley D: Prevention of postoperative epilepsy. Lancet 1:650, 1980

253. Robinson JL, Roberts A: Operative treatment of aneurysms and Coanda effect: a working hypothesis. J Neurol Neurosurg Psychiatry 35:804, 1972

254. Rose FC, Sarner M: Epilepsy after ruptured intracranial aneurysm. Br Med J 1:18, 1965

255. Sato S, Suzuki J: Prognosis in cases of intracranial aneurysm after incomplete direct operations. Acta Neurochir 24:245, 1971

256. Sengupta RP: Anatomical variations in the origin of the posterior cerebral artery demonstrated by carotid angiography and their significance in the direct surgical treatment of posterior communicating aneurysms. Neurochirurgia (Stutt) 18:33, 1975

257. Sengupta RP: Anterior communicating aneurysm: its surgical approach and result. p. 266. In Suzuki J (ed): Advances in Surgery for Cerebral Stroke. Berlin: Springer-Verlag, 1988

258. Sengupta RP: Anterior Communicating Aneurysms and Their Management After Subarachnoid Haemorrhage. (Thesis.) Newcastle University, Newcastle-upon-Tyne, 1978

259. Sengupta RP, Chiu JSP, Brierley H: Quality of survival following direct surgery for anterior communicating artery aneurysms. J Neurosurg 43:58, 1975

260. Sengupta RP, Lassman LP, Hankinson J: The scope of surgery for intracranial aneurysms in the elderly: a preliminary report. Br Med J 2:246, 1978

261. Sengupta RP, McAllister VL: Subarachnoid Haemorrhage. Springer-Verlag, Berlin, 1986

262. Shenkin HA, Bezier HS, Bouzarth WF: Restricted fluid intake. Rational management of the neurosurgical patient. J Neurosurg 45:432, 1976

263. Silver D: Pulmonary embolism: prevention, detection and nonoperative management. Surg Clin North Am 54:1089, 1974

264. Smith RR, Al-Mefty O, Middleton TH: An orbitocranial approach to complex aneurysm of the anterior circulation. Neurosurgery 24:385, 1989

265. Spallone A, Mariani G, Rosa G et al: Disseminated intravascular coagulation as a complication of ruptured intracranial aneurysm. Report of two cases. J Neurosurg 59:142, 1983

266. Stein M, Koota GM, Simon M et al: Pulmonary evaluation of surgical patients. JAMA 181:765, 1962

267. Steven JL: Postoperative angiography in treatment of intracranial aneurysms. Acta Radiol (Diagn) 5:536, 1966

268. Storey FB: Psychiatric sequelae of subarachnoid hemorrhage. Br Med J 1:261, 1967

269. Sundt TM Jr, Nofsinger JD: Clip-grafts for aneurysm and small vessel surgery. Part 1: repair of segmental defects with clip-grafts; laboratory studies and clinical correlations. Part 2: clinical application of clip-grafts to aneurysms; technical considerations. J Neurosurg 27:477, 1967

270. Symonds CP: Contributions to the clinical study of intracranial aneurysms. Guys Hosp Rep 72:139, 1923

271. Takaku A, Shindo K, Tanaka S et al: Fluid and electrolyte disturbance in patients with intracranial aneurysms. Surg Neurol 11:349, 1979

272. Takaku A, Tanaka S, Mori T et al: Postoperative complications in 1,000 cases of intracranial aneurysms. Surg Neurol 12:137, 1979

273. Tindall GT: The treatment of anterior communicating artery aneurysms by proximal anterior cerebral artery ligation. Clin Neurosurg 21:134, 1974

274. Tönnis W: Erfolgreiche Behandlung eines Aneurysma der Art. commun. ant. cerebri. Zbl Neurochir 1:39, 1936

275. Uihlein A, Thomas RL, Cleary J: Aneurysms of the anterior communicating artery complex. Proc Mayo Clin 42:73, 1967

276. Valladares BJ, Hankinson J: Incidence of deep vein thrombosis in neurosurgical patients. Neurosurgery 6:138, 1980

277. VanderArk CD, Kempe LG: Classification of anterior communicating aneurysms as a basis for surgical approach. J Neurosurg 32:300, 1970

278. VanderArk CD, Kempe LG, Smith DR: Anterior communicating aneurysms: the gyrus rectus approach. Clin Neurosurg 21:120, 1974

279. Wilkins RH: Attempted prevention or treatment of intracranial arterial spasm: a survey. Neurosurgery 6:198, 1980

280. Williamson WP, Brackett CE Jr: Management of intracranial aneurysms of the anterior communicating artery. Am Surg 22:100, 1956

281. Winn HR, Richardson AE, Jane JA: Late mortality and morbidity of common carotid ligation for posterior communicating artery aneurysms. A comparison with conservative treatment. J Neurol Neurosurg Psychiatry 38:406, 1975

282. Wise BL: Fluid and Electrolytes in Neurological Surgery. Charles C Thomas, Springfield, IL, 1965

283. Yasargil MG: Microsurgery Applied to Neurosurgery. George Thieme Verlag, Stuttgart, 1969

284. Yasargil MG, Fox JL, Ray MW: The operative approach to aneurysms of the anterior communicating artery. p. 113. In Krayenbuhl H (ed): Advances and Technical Standards in Neurosurgery. Vol. 2. Springer-Verlag, New York, 1975

285. Yasargil MG, Smith RD: Surgery on the carotid system in the treatment of hemorrhagic stroke. Adv Neurol 16:181, 1977

286. Yasargil MG, Yonekawa Y, Zumstein B et al: Hydrocephalus following spontaneous subarachnoid hemorrhage. J Neurosurg 39:474, 1973

Distal Anterior Cerebral Artery Aneurysms

287. Becker GH, Newton TH: Distal anterior cerebral artery aneurysm. Neurosurgery 4:495, 1979

288. Huber P, Braun J, Hirschmann D, Agyeman JF: Incidence of berry aneurysms of the unpaired pericallosal artery: angiographic study. Neuroradiology 19:143, 1980

289. Laitinen L, Snellman A: Aneurysms of the pericallosal artery: a study of 14 cases verified angiographically and treated mainly by direct surgical attack. J Neurosurg 17:447, 1960

290. Mann KS, Yue CP, Wong G: Aneurysms of the pericallosal-callosomarginal junction. Surg Neurol 21:261, 1984

291. Ohno K, Monma S, Suzuki R, Masaoka H, Matsushima Y, Hirakawa K: Saccular aneurysms of the distal anterior cerebral artery. Neurosurgery 27:907, 1990

292. Perlmutter D, Rhoton AL Jr: Microsurgical anatomy of the distal anterior cerebral artery. J Neurosurg 49:204, 1978

293. Sindou M, Pelissou-Guyotat I, Mertens P et al: Pericallosal aneurysms. Surg Neurol 30:434, 1988

294. Snyckers FD, Drake CG: Aneurysms of the distal anterior cerebral artery: a report on 24 verified cases. S Afr Med J 47:1787, 1973

295. Wisoff JH, Flamm ES: Aneurysms of the distal anterior cerebral artery and associated vascular anomalies. Neurosurgery 20:735, 1987

296. Yasargil MG, Carter LP: Saccular aneurysms of the distal anterior cerebral. J Neurosurg 39:218, 1974

297. Yoshimoto T, Uchida K, Suzuki J: Surgical treatment of distal anterior cerebral artery aneurysms. J Neurosurg 50:40, 1979

Basilar Apex Aneurysms

298. Adamson T, Batjer H: Aneurysm recurrence associated with induced hypertension and hypervolemia. Surg Neurol 29:57, 1988
299. Allcock JM, Drake CG: Postoperative angiography in cases of ruptured intracranial aneurysms. J Neurosurg 20:752, 1963
300. Batjer H, Samson D: Use of extracranial-intracranial bypass in the management of symptomatic vasospasm. Neurosurgery 19:235, 1986
301. Batjer HH, Frankfurt AI, Purdy PD et al: Use of etomidate, temporary arterial occlusion, and intraoperative angiography in large and giant cerebral aneurysm surgery. J Neurosurg 68:234, 1988
302. Batjer HH, Mickey BM, Samson DS: Enlargement and rupture of distal basilar aneurysm following iatrogenic carotid occlusion. Neurosurgery 60:624, 1987
303. Batjer HH, Samson DS: Intraoperative aneurysmal rupture: incidence, outcome, and suggestions for surgical management. Neurosurgery 18:701, 1986
304. Batjer HH, Samson DS: Causes of morbidity and mortality from surgery of aneurysms of the distal basilar artery. Neurosurgery 25:904, 1989
305. Buckland M, Batjer HH, Gieseke AH: Anesthesia for cerebral aneurysm surgery: use of induced hypertension in patients with symptomatic vasospasm. Anesthesiology 69:116, 1988
306. Chou SN, Ortiz-Suarez HJ: Surgical treatment of arterial aneurysms of the vertebrobasilar circulation. J Neurosurg 41:671, 1974
307. Chui M, Battista AF, Kricheff H: Vasospasm of the vertebrobasilar system in cases of ruptured intracranial aneurysm. Neurosurgery 12:542, 1983
308. Drake CG: Bleeding aneurysms of the basilar artery: direct surgical management in four cases. J Neurosurg 18:230, 1961
309. Drake CG: Surgical treatment of ruptured aneurysms of the basilar artery. Experience with 14 cases. J Neurosurg 23:457, 1965
310. Drake CG: Further experience with surgical treatment of aneurysms of the basilar artery. J Neurosurg 29:372, 1968
311. Drake CG: Giant intracranial aneurysms: experience with surgical treatment in 174 patients. Clin Neurosurg 26:12, 1979
312. Drake CG: The treatment of aneurysms of the posterior circulation. Clin Neurosurg 26:96, 1979
313. Drake CG, Friedman AH, Peerless SJ: Failed aneurysm surgery: reoperative in 115 cases. J Neurosurg 61:848, 1984
314. Drake CG, Vanderlinden RG: The late consequences of incomplete surgical treatment of cerebral aneurysms. J Neurosurg 27:226, 1967
315. Feuerberg I, Lindquist C, Lindqvist M et al: Natural history of postoperative aneurysm rests. J Neurosurg 66:30, 1987
316. Finn SS, Stephenson SA, Miller CA et al: Observations on the perioperative management of aneurysmal subarachnoid hemorrhage. J Neurosurg 65:48, 1986
317. Fisher CM, Kistler JP, Davis JM: Relation of cerebral vasospasm to subarachnoid hemorrhage visualized by computerized tomographic scanning. Neurosurgery 6:1, 1980
318. Fox JL: Intracranial Aneurysms. Vol. 1. Springer-Verlag, New York, 1983
319. Gallagher JP: Pilojection for intracranial aneurysms, report of progress. J Neurosurg 21:129, 1964
320. Gentleman D, Johnston R: Postoperative extradural hematoma associated with induced hypertension. Neurosurgery 17:105, 1985
321. Gillingham FJ: Management of aneurysms of posterior circulation. p. 1715. In Youmans JR (ed): Neurological Surgery: A Comprehensive Reference Guide to the Diagnosis and Management of Neurosurgical Problems. Vol. 3. WB Saunders, Philadelphia, 1982
322. Grand W, Hopkins LN: The microsurgical anatomy of the basilar artery bifurcation. Neurosurgery 1:128, 1977
323. Jamieson KG: Aneurysms of the vertebrobasilar system: surgical intervention in 19 cases. J Neurosurg 21:781, 1964
324. Jamieson KG: Aneurysms of the vertebrobasilar system. Further experience with nine cases. J Neurosurg 28:544, 1968
325. Kassell NF, Peerless SJ, Durward QJ et al: Treatment of ischemic deficits from vasospasm with intravascular volume expansion and induced arterial hypertension. Neurosurgery 11:337, 1982
326. Kassell NF, Sasaki T, Colohan ART et al: Cerebral vasospasm following subarachnoid hemorrhage. Stroke 16:562, 1985
327. Kassell NF, Torner JC: Aneurysmal rebleeding: a preliminary report from the Cooperative Aneurysm Study. Neurosurgery 13:479, 1983
328. Kassell NF, Torner JC: The International Cooperative Study on Timing of Aneurysm Surgery: an update. Stroke 15:566, 1984
329. Kodama N, Kamiyama K, Mineura K et al: Surgical treatment of vertebrobasilar aneurysms. Neurol Surg 7:321, 1979
330. Kosnik EJ, Hunt WE: Postoperative hypertension in the management of patients with intracranial aneurysms. J Neurosurg 45:148, 1976
331. Krayenbuhl HA, Yasargil MG: Cerebral Angiography. JB Lippincott, Philadelphia, 1968
332. Kwak R, Niizuma H, Takatsugu D et al: Angiographic study of cerebral vasospasm following rupture of intracranial aneurysms, part 1: time of the appearance. Surg Neurol 11:257, 1979
333. Liliequist B: The subarachnoid cisterns. An anatomic and roentgenologic study. Acta Radiol (Stockh) 185(Suppl):1, 1959
334. Logue V: The surgical treatment of aneurysms in the

posterior fossa. J Neurol Neurosurg Psychiatry 21:66, 1958

335. Mount LA, Taveras JM: Ligation of basilar artery in treatment of an aneurysm at the basilar artery bifurcation. J Neurosurg 19:167, 1962

336. Mullan S, Reyes C, Dawley J et al: Stereotactic copper electric thrombosis of intracranial aneurysms. p. 212. In Krayenbuhl H, Maspes P, Sweet W (eds): Progress in Neurological Surgery. Vol. 3. Karger, Basel, 1969

337. Paine JT, Batjer HH, Samson DS: Intraoperative ventricular puncture. Neurosurgery 22:1107, 1988

338. Peerless SJ, Drake CG: Management of aneurysms of the posterior circulation. p. 1715. In Youmans JR (ed): Neurological Surgery. Vol. 3. WB Saunders, Philadelphia, 1982

339. Peerless SJ, Drake CG: Posterior circulation aneurysms. p. 1422. In Wilkins RH, Rengachary SS (eds): Neurosurgery. McGraw-Hill, New York, 1985

340. Pelz DM, Vineula F, Fox AJ et al: Vertebrobasilar occlusion therapy of giant aneurysms. Significance of angiographic morphology of the posterior communicating arteries. J Neurosurg 60:560, 1984

341. Richardson AE: Surgery of basilar aneurysms. Psychiatr Neurol Neurochir 75:441, 1972

342. Roski PA, Spetzler RF: Carotid ligation. p. 1414. In Wilkins RH, Rengachary SS (eds): Neurosurgery. McGraw-Hill, New York, 1985

343. Sachs M, Hirsch JF, David M: Ruptured saccular aneurysms of the vertebrobasilar system: review of 19 personal and 88 published cases. Acta Neurochir 20:105, 1969

344. Saito I, Sano K: Vasospasm after aneurysm rupture: incidence, onset, and course. p. 294. In Wilkins RH (ed): Cerebral Arterial Spasm. Williams & Wilkins, Baltimore, 1980

345. Samson DS, Batjer HH: Aneurysms of the distal basilar artery—the pterional approach. p. 121. In Samson DS, Batjer HH: Intracranial Aneurysm Surgery—Techniques. Futura, Mount Kisco, NY, 1990

346. Samson DS, Batjer HH: Aneurysms of the distal basilar artery—the subtemporal approach. p. 143. In Samson DS, Batjer HH: Intracranial Aneurysm Surgery—Techniques. Futura, Mount Kisco, NY, 1990

347. Samson DS, Hodosh RM, Clark WK: Microsurgical evaluation of the pterional approach to aneurysms of the distal basilar circulation. Neurosurgery 3:135, 1978

348. Sano K, Saito I: Timing and indication of surgery for ruptured intracranial aneurysms with regard to cerebral vasospasm. Acta Neurochir (Wien) 41:49, 1978

349. Sugita K, Kobayashi S, Shintani A et al: Microneurosurgery for aneurysms of the basilar artery. J Neurosurg 51:615, 1979

350. Terada T, Komai N, Hayashi S et al: Hemorrhagic infarction after vasospasm due to ruptured cerebral aneurysm. Neurosurgery 18:415, 1986

351. Troupp H: The natural history of aneurysms of the basilar bifurcation. Acta Scand 47:350, 1971

352. Uihlein A, Hughes RA: The surgical treatment of intracranial vestigial aneurysms. Surg Clin North Am 35:1071, 1955

353. Weir B: Surgery-specific sites and results of series. p. 475. In Weir B: Aneurysms Affecting the Nervous System. Williams & Wilkins, Baltimore, 1987

354. Weir B, Grace M, Hansen J et al: Time course of vasospasm in man. J Neurosurg 48:173, 1978

355. Wollschlaeger G, Wollschlaeger PB, Lucas FV: Experience and result with post-mortem cerebral angiography performed as routine procedure of autopsy. Am J Roentgenol 101:68, 1967

356. Yamaura A, Ise H, Makino H: Treatment of aneurysms arising from the terminal portion of the basilar artery—with special reference to the radiometric study and accessibility of transsylvian approach. Neurol Med Chir 22:521, 1982

357. Yasargil MG: Operative anatomy. p. 5. In Yasargil MG (ed): Microneurosurgery. Vol. 1. George Thieme Verlag, Stuttgart, 1984

358. Yasargil MG: Pathological considerations. p. 279. In Yasargil MG (ed): Microneurosurgery. Vol. 1. George Thieme Verlag, Stuttgart, 1984

359. Yasargil MG: Vertebrobasilar aneurysms. p. 232. In Yasargil MG (ed): Microneurosurgery. Vol. 2. George Thieme Verlag, Stuttgart, 1984

360. Yasargil MG, Antic J, Laciga R et al: Microsurgical pterional approach to aneurysms of the basilar bifurcation. Surg Neurol 6:83, 1976

361. Yasargil MG, Fox JL, Ray MW: The operative approach to aneurysms of the anterior communicating artery. p. 113. In Krayenbuhl H (ed): Advances and Technical Standards in Neurosurgery. Vol. 2. Springer-Verlag, New York, 1975

Posterior Cerebral and Superior Cerebellar Artery Aneurysms

362. Amacher A, Drake D, Ferguson G: Posterior circulation aneurysms in young people. Neurosurgery 8:315, 1981

363. Chang H, Fukushima T, Miyasaki S et al: Fusiform posterior cerebral artery aneurysm treated with excision and end-to-end anastomosis. J Neurosurg 64:501, 1986

364. Chang H, Fukushima T, Takakura K et al: Aneurysms of the posterior cerebral artery: report of ten cases. Neurosurgery 19:1006, 1986

365. Dandy W: Intracranial Arterial Aneurysms. Comstock, Ithaca, NY, 1944

366. Drake C: Giant intracranial aneurysms: experience with surgical treatment in 174 patients. Clin Neurosurg 26:12, 1979

367. Drake C: The treatment of aneurysms of the posterior circulation. Clin Neurosurg 26:96, 1979

368. Drake C: RMP Donaghy Lecture—Cerebrovascular Surgery, Current Status and Future Prospects. AANS annual meeting, Toronto, 1988

369. Drake C, Amacher A: Aneurysms of the posterior cerebral artery. J Neurosurg 30:468, 1969

370. Hanafee W, Jannetta P: Aneurysm as a cause of stroke. Am J Roentgenol 98:647, 1966

371. Hoffman H, Margolis M, Newton T: The superior cerebellar artery. Normal gross and radiographic anatomy. p. 1809. In Newton T, Potts D (eds): Radiology of the Skull and Brain. Vol. II, book 2. CV Mosby, St. Louis, 1974

372. Hoyt W, Newton T, Margolis T: The posterior cerebral artery. Embryology and developmental anomalies. p. 1540. In Newton T, Potts D (eds): Radiology of the Skull and Brain. Vol. II, book 2. CV Mosby, St. Louis, 1974

373. Hunt W, Hess R: Aneurysm of the posterior cerebral artery with unexpected postoperative neurological deficit. Case report. J Neurosurg 26:633, 1967

374. Krayenbuhl H, Yasargil M: Cerebral Angiography. 2nd Ed. JB Lippincott, Philadelphia, 1968

375. Margolis M, Newton T, Hoyt W: The posterior cerebral artery. Gross and roentgenographic anatomy. p. 1551. In Newton T, Potts D (eds): Radiology of the Skull and Brain. Vol. II, book 2. CV Mosby, St. Louis, 1974

376. Meyer F, Sundt T, Fode N et al: Cerebral aneurysms in childhood and adolescence. J Neurosurg 70:420, 1989

377. Newton T, Hoyt W, Margolis M: The posterior cerebral artery. Pathology. p. 1580. In Newton T, Potts D (eds): Radiology of the Skull and Brain. Vol. II, book 2. CV Mosby, St. Louis, 1974

378. Pedroza A, Dujovny M, Ausman J et al: Microvascular anatomy of the interpeduncular fossa. J Neurosurg 64:484, 1986

379. Peerless S, Drake C: Management of aneurysms of the posterior circulation. p. 1764. In Youmans J (ed): Neurological Surgery. 3rd Ed. WB Saunders, Philadelphia, 1990

380. Peerless S, Nemoto S, Drake C: Acute surgery for ruptured posterior circulation aneurysms. Adv Technical Standards Neurosurg 15:115, 1987

381. Pia H, Fontana H: Aneurysms of the posterior cerebral artery. Locations and clinical pictures. Acta Neurochir 38:13, 1977

382. Rhoton A, Saeki N, Perlmutter D et al: Microsurgical anatomy of common aneurysm sites. Clin Neurosurg 26:248, 1979

383. Sugita K, Kobayashi S: Microneurosurgical Atlas. Berlin, Springer-Verlag, 1985

384. Sundt T: Posterior cerebral artery and superior cerebellar artery. p. 331. In Sundt T (ed): Surgical Techniques for Saccular and Giant Intracranial Aneurysms. Williams & Wilkins, Baltimore, 1990

385. Verlooy J, Piepgras D, Sundt T: Surgical management of posterior cerebral artery aneurysms. An analysis of 32 cases. In preparation.

386. Yasargil M: Microsurgical anatomy of the basal cisterns and vessels of the brain, diagnostic studies, general operative techniques and pathological considerations of the intracranial aneurysms. p. 134. In Microsurgery. Vol. I. Thieme-Stratton, Stuttgart, 1984.

387. Yasargil M: Clinical considerations, surgery of the intracranial aneurysms and results. p. 260. In Microneurosurgery. Vol. II. Thieme-Stratton, Stuttgart, 1984

388. Zeal A, Rhoton A: Microsurgical anatomy of the posterior cerebral artery. J Neurosurg 48:534, 1978

Index

Surgical instruments *(Continued)*
  monopolar coagulation and cutting,
      78
    bayonet forceps, 78, 78f
  nerve hooks, 87
  nerve stimulators in acoustic neuroma
      surgery, 87
  scalp clips, 72
  scalp reflection, 72
  suction tubes, 87–89, 88f
  superiosteal dissection, 72–73, 73f
  tumor-grasping forceps, 81
  turning the bone flap, 73–74
  ultrasonic aspiration, 87
Surgical planning
  infratentorial procedures, 1567–1707.
      See also Infratentorial proce-
      dures, overview.
  supratentorial procedures
    complication prevention, 4–9
    execution of operation, 6–8
    postoperative care, 8–9
Surgical positioning. *See* Positioning.
Surgical side: double-checking identity of,
      8
Surgical table. *See* Operating table.
Surgical team communication, 6
Surgical treatment phases, 5
Surgical wound
  classification, 129, 130–131
  infection. *See also* Infections; Wound
      infection.
    prevention guidelines, 127–128
Surgicel. *See also* Hemorrhage;
      Hemostasis.
  misuse in epidural bleeding, 74, 74f
Suture: for posterior fossa surgery, 1648f,
      1657, 1659, 1659f, 1659t
  microsurgery diameters, 1659t
  size in relation to vessel size, 1659t
Swallowing
  brainstem and control of, 1583–1584
  head injuries and disorders of, 1366
Swallowing reflex, 1572
Sylvian aqueduct, syndrome of, 1584
Sylvian cistern: in middle cerebral artery
      aneurysm surgery, 983
Sylvian fissure
  cleavage plane identification, 79
  craniopharyngiomas migrating to, 321
  frontotemporal approach to, 60
  in lateral microorbitotomy, 665t
  locating lesion in relation to, 54
  in pterional approach to posterior fossa,
      1628t
  retractor blade use, 79
  splitting
    in ACoA aneurysm surgery, 1022,
        1024f
    in carotid bifurcation aneurysm
        surgery, 970, 977f, 978
    in carotid ophthalmic aneurysm
        surgery, 946, 947f

in cavernous sinus surgery, 608–610,
    609f, 614
for cerebral revascularization, 912,
    914f
in intracavernous carotid artery
    aneurysm surgery, 930–931
for lobar AVMs, 1153
in MCA aneurysm surgery, 983, 985,
    989, 999f, 1005f
in parasellar meningioma surgery,
    220–221
in pterional approach, 37
Sylvian vein
  in carotid sinus surgery, 609f
  medial: in carotid bifurcation aneurysm
      surgery, 978
Sympathetic nerves
  in cavernous sinus surgery, 2198
  in subtemporal-infratemporal approach,
      2228
Sympathetic nervous system: brainstem
      and, 1575
Syncope
  glossopharyngeal neuralgia and, 2155
  and vertebrobasilar insufficiency, 1864
Syndrome of inappropriate antidiuretic
      hormone secretion. *See*
      SIADH.
Syndrome of Sylvian aqueduct. *See*
      Parinaud's syndrome.
Syndrome of the trephined, 1385, 1386
Syphilitic gummas, 1415
Syringohydromyelia: and basilar invagina-
      tion, 2030
Syringomyelia, 1985–2001. *See also*
      Chiari malformation.
  and basilar invagination, 2030
  complications, 1986t
  diagnosis, 187f, 1987–1988, 1988f
  surgical technique, 1988–2000
    cyst drainage, 1995
    postoperative care, 2000
Syringoperitoneal shunt: CSF drainage:
      Chiari malformation, 1989
Syringopleural shunt: for CSF drainage in
      Chiari malformation, 1989
Systemic blood pressure. *See also* Blood
      pressure.
  decreasing. *See also* Hypotension,
      induced.
    for intraoperative hemorrhage man-
        agement, 94
Systemic vascular resistance: and SAH-
      induced cerebral vasospasm, 861

T

T₃. *See* Triiodothyronine.
T₄. *See* Thyroxine.
Tachyarrhythmias, supraventricular: as
      perioperative complication,
      170–171

Tachycardia
  and anesthesia, 25–26
  and closed head injuries, 1357
  and malignant hyperthermia, 96
  perioperative: valvular heart disease and,
      168
  and transfusion complications, 95
  ventricular: and head trauma, 1358
Tachypnea: in closed head injury, 1361
Tacking sutures: in craniotomy closure, 66,
      66f
Tactile transfer deficits: from transcallosal
      approach to anterior third ventri-
      cle, 544t, 545
Taenia solium
  brain abscess, 1414
  epidemiology, 1419–1420
  infection with, 1419–1429. *See also*
      Cysticercosis.
  life cycle, 1419–1420
Tantalum cranioplasty, 1388–1389
  inlay method, 1389
  onlay method, 1389
Tantalum mesh
  for congenital cranial malformations,
      1443
  in craniosynostosis repair, 1457, 1458f
Tanycytes, 320
Tardive dyskinesia: differential diagnosis,
      2115, 2118
Tarsorrhaphy, 2173
  after cavernous sinus surgery, 2209
  for cranial nerve palsies, 1679, 2312
  in craniofacial resection, 2309
Taylor-Haughton lines: and cerebral neo-
      plasm localization, 381, 382f
TCD. *See* Transcranial Doppler ultra-
      sonography.
T-cell function: in closed head injury,
      1359–1360
Tearing reflex, 1590
Technical complications: in neurosurgery,
      4t
TEE. *See* Transesophageal echocardiogra-
      phy.
Teflon tube graft: in vertebral artery-to-
      CCA transposition, 1875, 1876f,
      1877
Tegmen tympani, 2335
  and epidural abscess, 1402
Tegretol. *See* Carbamazepine.
Tela choroidea: temporal lobectomy and,
      453
Telangiectasia, 1443
Telecanthus, 1439
Telencephalic arteries, 764
Telencephalon
  embryonic, 722f
  reptilian, 779
Telfa: use and misuse, 76
Temperature
  monitoring
    in anesthesia, 14